# Nursing Skills
# for a Concept-Based Approach to Learning

## North Carolina Custom Edition

Taken from:

*Skills in Clinical Nursing,* Sixth Edition
by Audrey Berman, Shirlee Snyder, and Christina Jackson

*Clinical Nursing Skills: Basic to Advanced Skills,* Seventh Edition
by Sandra F. Smith, Donna J. Duell, and Barbara C. Martin

*Clinical Skills Manual for Maternal and Child Nursing Care,* Second Edition
by Ruth C. Bindler, Jane W. Ball, Marcia L. London, and Patricia W. Ladewig

*Kozier and Erb's Fundamentals of Nursing: Concepts, Process, and Practice,* Eighth Edition
by Audrey Berman, Shirlee J. Snyder, Barbara Kozier, and Glenora Erb

**Learning Solutions**

New York   Boston   San Francisco
London   Toronto   Sydney   Tokyo   Singapore   Madrid
Mexico City   Munich   Paris   Cape Town   Hong Kong   Montreal

Cover Image: Courtesy of Maria Guglielmo

Taken from:

*Skills in Clinical Nursing,* Sixth Edition
by Audrey Berman, Shirlee Snyder, and Christina Jackson
Copyright © 2009 by Pearson Education, Inc.
Published by Prentice Hall
Upper Saddle River, New Jersey 07458

*Clinical Nursing Skills: Basic to Advanced Skills,* Seventh Edition
by Sandra F. Smith, Donna J. Duell, and Barbara C. Martin
Copyright © 2008 by Pearson Education, Inc.
Published by Prentice Hall

*Clinical Skills Manual for Maternal and Child Nursing Care,* Second Edition
by Ruth C. Bindler, Jane W. Ball, Marcia L. London, and Patricia W. Ladewig
Copyright © 2007 by Pearson Education, Inc.
Published by Prentice Hall

*Kozier and Erb's Fundamentals of Nursing: Concepts, Process, and Practice, Eighth Edition*
by Audrey Berman, Shirlee J. Snyder, Barbara Kozier, and Glenora Erb
Copyright © 2008 by Pearson Education, Inc.
Published by Prentice Hall

This special edition published in cooperation with Pearson Learning Solutions.

Pearson Learning Solutions, 501 Boylston Street, Suite 900, Boston, MA 02116
A Pearson Education Company
www.pearsoned.com

Printed in the United States of America

4 5 6 7 8 9 10 V 3 57 14 13 12 11 10

2009380016

DC

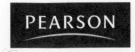

ISBN 10: 0-558-35687-7
ISBN 13: 978-0-558-35687-3

# CONTENTS

## CHAPTER 1
## Comfort

**Skill 1.1** Teaching Controlled Breathing 2
**Skill 1.2** Teaching Progressive Muscle Relaxation 4
**Skill 1.3** Assisting with Guided Imagery 6
**Skill 1.4** Managing a TENS Unit 8
**Skill 1.5** Applying Dry Heat Measures: Hot Water Bottle, Electric Heating Pad, Aquathermia Pad, Disposable Hot Pack 13
**Skill 1.6** Applying Compresses and Moist Packs 15
**Skill 1.7** Assisting with a Sitz Bath 17
**Skill 1.8** Providing Tepid Sponges 17
**Skill 1.9** Monitoring an Infant Radiant Warmer 18
**Skill 1.10** Applying Dry Cold Measures: Ice Bag, Ice Collar, Ice Glove, Disposable Cold Pack 20
**Skill 1.11** Using a Cooling Blanket 21
**Skill 1.12** Meeting the Physiologic Needs of the Dying Client 25
**Skill 1.13** Performing Postmortem Care 28

## CHAPTER 2
## Elimination

**Skill 2.1** Assisting with a Bedpan 33
**Skill 2.2** Assisting with a Urinal 34
**Skill 2.3** Assisting Client to the Commode 36
**Skill 2.4** Applying an External Urinary Device 37
**Skill 2.5** Collecting a Routine Urine Specimen 39
**Skill 2.6** Collecting a Specimen from an Infant 41
**Skill 2.7** Collecting 24-Hour Urine Specimen 41
**Skill 2.8** Collecting a Urine Specimen for Culture and Sensitivity by the Clean-Catch Method 42
**Skill 2.9** Performing Urine Tests 45
**Skill 2.10** Performing Urinary Catheterization 46
**Skill 2.11** Performing Catheter Care and Removal 53
**Skill 2.12** Performing Bladder Irrigation 55
**Skill 2.13** Maintaining Continuous Bladder Irrigation 57
**Skill 2.14** Providing Suprapubic Catheter Care 58
**Skill 2.15** Performing Urinary Ostomy Care 60
**Skill 2.16** Applying a Urinary Diversion Pouch 62
**Skill 2.17** Obtaining Urine Specimen from an Ileal Conduit 64
**Skill 2.18** Removing Fecal Impaction 65
**Skill 2.19** Developing a Regular Bowel Routine 66
**Skill 2.20** Inserting a Rectal Tube 67
**Skill 2.21** Obtaining and Testing Stool Specimen 69

**Skill 2.22** Collecting Infant Stool Specimen 72
**Skill 2.23** Collecting Stool for Bacterial Culture 72
**Skill 2.24** Teaching Parents to Test for Pinworms 73
**Skill 2.25** Collecting Stool for Ova and Parasites 73
**Skill 2.26** Implementing the Zassi Bowel Management System™ 74
**Skill 2.27** Administering an Enema 78
**Skill 2.28** Administering a Retention Enema 80
**Skill 2.29** Applying a Fecal Ostomy Pouch 82
**Skill 2.30** Changing a Bowel Diversion Ostomy Appliance 89
**Skill 2.31** Assisting with Peritoneal Dialysis Catheter Insertion 94
**Skill 2.32** Conducting Peritoneal Dialysis Procedures 96
**Skill 2.33** Providing Hemodialysis 98
**Skill 2.34** Providing Ongoing Care of Hemodialysis Client 100
**Skill 2.35** Terminating Hemodialysis 101
**Skill 2.36** Maintaining Central Venous Dual-Lumen Dialysis Catheter (DLC) 102
**Skill 2.37** Home Setting: Using Clean Technique for Intermittent Self-Catheterization 104
**Skill 2.38** Home Setting: Providing Suprapubic Catheter Care 105
**Skill 2.39** Home Setting: Administering Continuous Ambulatory Peritoneal Dialysis (CAPD) 105
**Skill 2.40** Home Setting: Changing Dressing for a CAPD Client 107
**Skill 2.41** Home Setting: Instructing Client in Colostomy Irrigation 107
**Skill 2.42** Performing the Allen Test 108
**Skill 2.43** Assisting with Arterial Line Insertion 108
**Skill 2.44** Monitoring Arterial Blood Pressure 109
**Skill 2.45** Withdrawing Arterial Blood Samples 111
**Skill 2.46** Removing Arterial Catheter 112

## CHAPTER 3
## Fluids and Electrolytes

**Skill 3.1** Monitoring Intake and Output 116
**Skill 3.2** Establishing Intravenous Infusions 122
**Skill 3.3** Performing Venipuncture with All Variations 126
VARIATION: Inserting a Butterfly (Winged-Tip) Needle 132
**Skill 3.4** Regulating Infusion Flow Rate 134
**Skill 3.5** Using an Infusion Pump or Controller 138
**Skill 3.6** Using a "Smart" Pump 140

**Skill 3.7** Using a Syringe Pump  142

**Skill 3.8** Maintaining Infusions  144

**Skill 3.9** Maintaining Intermittent Infusion Devices  147

**Skill 3.10** Changing Gown for Client with IV  150

**Skill 3.11** Discontinuing Infusion Devices  150

**Skill 3.12** Infusing IV Fluids through a Central Line  153

## CHAPTER 4
# Infection

**Skill 4.1** Hand Hygiene (Medical Asepsis)  157
VARIATION: Using Waterless Antiseptic Agents (Foam or Gels)  159

**Skill 4.2** Latex Precautions  161

**Skill 4.3** Donning and Removing Clean Gloves  161

**Skill 4.4** Donning and Removing Isolation Attire  163

**Skill 4.5** Using a Mask  165

**Skill 4.6** Assessing Vital Signs  166

**Skill 4.7** Removing Items from Isolation Room  166

**Skill 4.8** Utilizing Double-Bagging for Isolation  167

**Skill 4.9** Removing Specimen from Isolation Room  168

**Skill 4.10** Transporting Isolation Client Outside Room  169

**Skill 4.11** Removing Soiled Large Equipment from Isolation Room  169

**Skill 4.12** Performing Surgical Hand Antisepsis/Scrubs  170
VARIATION: Surgical Hand Antisepsis/Hand Scrub Using Alcohol-Based Surgical Hand Rub  172

**Skill 4.13** Donning Sterile Gown and Gloves (Closed Method)  173

**Skill 4.14** Preparing the Surgical Site  174

**Skill 4.15** Preparing the Client for Surgery  175

**Skill 4.16** Pouring from a Sterile Container  178

**Skill 4.17** Preparing a Sterile Field Using Pre-Packaged Supplies  179

**Skill 4.18** Preparing for Dressing Change Using Individual Supplies  179

**Skill 4.19** Changing a Sterile Dressing  180

**Skill 4.20** Removing Sutures  181

**Skill 4.21** Removing Staples  182

**Skill 4.22** Preparing for Client Care  183

**Skill 4.23** Home Setting: Disposing of Waste Material  184

**Skill 4.24** Home Setting: Caring for an AIDS or HIV Client  185

**Skill 4.25** Home Setting: Teaching Preventative Measures  185

**Skill 4.26** Teaching Safer Practices to IV Drug Users  186

## CHAPTER 5
# Metabolism

**Skill 5.1** Serving a Food Tray (see Caring Interventions)  190

**Skill 5.2** Assisting an Adult to Eat  190

**Skill 5.3** Inserting a Nasogastric Tube  192

**Skill 5.4** Flushing/Maintaining Nasogastric (NG) Tube  195

**Skill 5.5** Performing Gastric Lavage  196

**Skill 5.6** Administering Poison Control Agents  197

**Skill 5.7** Removing a Nasogastric Tube  197

**Skill 5.8** Administering a Tube Feeding  198
VARIATION: Feeding Bag (Open System)  199
VARIATION: Syringe (Open System)  199
VARIATION: Prefilled Bottle with Drip Chamber (Closed System)  200
VARIATION: Continuous-Drip Feeding  200

**Skill 5.9** Administering a Gastrostomy or Jejunostomy Feeding  202

**Skill 5.10** Providing Continuous Feeding via Small-Bore Nasointestinal/Jejunostomy Tube  204

**Skill 5.11** Providing Total Parenteral Nutrition  208

**Skill 5.12** Infusing IV Lipids  209

**Skill 5.13** Obtaining a Capillary Blood Specimen and Measuring Blood Glucose  212

**Skill 5.14** Administering Total Nutrient Admixture (TNA) in the Home  215

**Skill 5.15** Monitoring Client on TNA  216

**Skill 5.16** Discontinuing TNA Infusion  216

## CHAPTER 6
# Mobility

**Skill 6.1** Applying Body Mechanics  219

**Skill 6.2** Supporting the Client's Position in Bed  221
VARIATION: Supporting a Client in Fowler's Position  221
VARIATION: Supporting a Client in the Dorsal Recumbent Position  223
VARIATION: Supporting a Client in the Prone Position  223
VARIATION: Supporting a Client in the Lateral Position  224
VARIATION: Supporting a Client in the Sims' Position  224

**Skill 6.3** Positioning a Child for Injections or Intravenous Access  225
VARIATION: Supine Position  225
VARIATION: Sitting Position  225

**Skill 6.4** Positioning a Child for Lumbar Puncture  225

**Skill 6.5** Positioning a Child for an Otoscopic Examination 226
VARIATION: Supine Position 226
VARIATION: Sitting Position 227

**Skill 6.6** Moving a Client Up in Bed 227
VARIATION: A Client with Limited Strength of the Upper Extremities 228
VARIATION: Two Nurses Using a Turn Sheet 228

**Skill 6.7** Turning a Client to the Lateral or Prone Position in Bed 229
VARIATION: Turning the Client to a Prone Position 230

**Skill 6.8** Logrolling a Client 231
VARIATION: Using a Turn or Lift Sheet 232

**Skill 6.9** Assisting the Client to Sit on Side of Bed (Dangle) 232
VARIATION: Teaching a Client How to Sit on the Side of the Bed Independently 233

**Skill 6.10** Transferring between Bed and Chair 234
VARIATION: Angling the Wheelchair 236
VARIATION: Transferring without a Belt 236
VARIATION: Transferring with a Belt and Two Nurses 236
VARIATION: Transferring a Client with an Injured Lower Extremity 236
VARIATION: Using a Sliding Board 237

**Skill 6.11** Transferring between Bed and Stretcher 237
VARIATION: Using a Transfer Board 238

**Skill 6.12** Using a Hydraulic Lift 238

**Skill 6.13** Performing Passive Range of Motion Exercises 240

**Skill 6.14** Using Continuous Passive Motion Device 247

**Skill 6.15** Assisting the Client to Ambulate 249
VARIATION: Two Nurses 250

**Skill 6.16** Assisting the Client to Use a Cane 251

**Skill 6.17** Assisting the Client to Use Crutches 253
VARIATION: Four-Point Alternate Gait 253
VARIATION: Three-Point Gait 254
VARIATION: Two-Point Alternate Gait 254
VARIATION: Swing-to Gait 254
VARIATION: Swing-Through Gait 255
VARIATION: Getting into a Chair 255
VARIATION: Getting Out of a Chair 255
VARIATION: Going Up Stairs 255
VARIATION: Going Down Stairs 256

**Skill 6.18** Assisting the Client to Use a Walker 257

**Skill 6.19** Transporting the Infant 258

**Skill 6.20** Transport of the Toddler 259

**Skill 6.21** Performing Initial Cast Care 260

**Skill 6.22** Performing Ongoing Cast Care 263
VARIATION: Plaster Cast 264
VARIATION: Synthetic Cast 264

**Skill 6.23** Performing Care for a Child with a Cast 265

**Skill 6.24** Caring for Clients in Traction 266
VARIATION: Caring for Client in Skin Traction 266
VARIATION: Skeletal Traction 267

**Skill 6.25** Applying and Monitoring Skin Traction for a Child 270

**Skill 6.26** Positioning Nonhospital Bed for Client Care 271

## CHAPTER 7
# Oxygenation

**Skill 7.1** Deep Breathing and Coughing 275
VARIATION: Pursed-Lip Breathing 276

**Skill 7.2** Collecting a Sputum Specimen 276

**Skill 7.3** Obtaining Nose and Throat Specimens 277
VARIATION: For a Throat Specimen 278
VARIATION: For a Nasal Specimen 278
VARIATION: Obtaining a Nasopharyngeal Culture 279

**Skill 7.4** Oxygen Saturation (Using a Pulse Oximeter) 279

**Skill 7.5** Using an Incentive Spirometer 280
VARIATION: For a Flow-Oriented SMI 280
VARIATION: For All Devices 281

**Skill 7.6** Administering Oxygen by Cannula, Face Mask, or Face Tent 282
VARIATION: Using a Cannula 282
VARIATION: Using a Face Mask 283
VARIATION: Face Tent 283
VARIATION: Nasal Cannula 284
VARIATION: Face Mask or Tent 284

**Skill 7.7** Using an Oxygen Cylinder 284

**Skill 7.8** Providing Oxygen via a Pediatric Tent 285

**Skill 7.9** Measuring Peak Expiratory Flow 286

**Skill 7.10** Preparing Client for Chest Physiotherapy (CPT) 287

**Skill 7.11** Performing Chest Percussion 288

**Skill 7.12** Performing Chest Vibration 288

**Skill 7.13** Inserting an Oropharyngeal Airway 289

**Skill 7.14** Inserting a Nasopharyngeal Airway (Nasal Trumpet) 290

**Skill 7.15** Assisting with Endotracheal Intubation 291

**Skill 7.16** Inflating a Tracheal Tube Cuff 293

**Skill 7.17** Providing Care for Client with Endotracheal Tube 294

**Skill 7.18** Extubating an Endotracheal Tube 294

**Skill 7.19** Oropharyngeal, Nasopharyngeal and Nasotracheal Suctioning 295

**Skill 7.20** Suctioning a Tracheostomy or Endrotracheal Tube 298
VARIATION: Using a Ventilator to Provide Hyperventilation 300
VARIATION: Closed Suction System (In-Line Catheter) 301

**Skill 7.21** Providing Tracheostomy Care 302
VARIATION: Using a Disposal Inner Cannula 305

**Skill 7.22** Capping a Tracheostomy Tube with Speaking Valve 306

**Skill 7.23** Caring for the Client on a Mechanical Ventilator 307

**Skill 7.24** Weaning a Client from a Ventilator 311

**Skill 7.25** Assisting with Chest Tube Insertion 312

**Skill 7.26** Maintaining Chest Tube Drainage 315

**Skill 7.27** Chest Tube Removal 319

**Skill 7.28** Clearing an Obstructed Airway 320
VARIATION: Chest Thrusts 321

**Skill 7.29** Performing Rescue Breathing 324

**Skill 7.30** Administering External Cardiac Compressions 328
VARIATION: CPR Performed by One Rescuer 330
VARIATION: CPR Performed by Two Rescuers 330

**Skill 7.31** Administering Automated External Defibrillation 332

**CHAPTER 8**
## Perfusion

**Skill 8.1** Using Digital Pressure 335

**Skill 8.2** Using Pressure Dressing 336

**Skill 8.3** Applying Antiemboli Stockings (Graduated Compression Stockings and Elastic Stockings) 337

**Skill 8.4** Applying Pneumatic Compression Devices 339

**Skill 8.5** Applying Sequential Compression Devices (SCDs) 340

**Skill 8.6** Monitoring Clients on Telemetry 343

**Skill 8.7** Interpreting an ECG Strip 345

**Skill 8.8** Recording a 12-Lead ECG 350

**Skill 8.9** Monitoring Temporary Cardiac Pacing (Transvenous, Epicardial) 352

**Skill 8.10** Assisting with Pacemaker Insertion 353

**Skill 8.11** Maintaining Temporary Pacemaker Function 355

**Skill 8.12** Providing Permanent Pacemaker Client Teaching 356

**CHAPTER 9**
## Reproduction

**Skill 9.1** Maternal and Newborn Assessments 359

**Skill 9.2** Assisting with a Pelvic Examination 372

**Skill 9.3** Assessing Deep Tendon Reflexes and Clonus 373

**Skill 9.4** Administration of Rh Immune Globulin (RhoGAM, HypRho-D) 374

**Skill 9.5** Assisting during Amniocentesis 375

**Skill 9.6** Assessment of Fetal Well-Being: Nonstress Test (NST) 376

**Skill 9.7** Assessment of Fetal Well-Being: Contraction Stress Test (CST) 377

**Skill 9.8** Assessment of Fetal Well-Being: Biophysical Profile (BPP) 378

**Skill 9.9** Performing an Intrapartal Vaginal Examination 379

**Skill 9.10** Assisting with Amniotomy (AROM: Artificial Rupture of Membranes) 381

**Skill 9.11** Auscultating Fetal Heart Rate 381

**Skill 9.12** External Electronic Fetal Monitoring 382

**Skill 9.13** Internal Electronic Fetal Monitoring: Application of Fetal Scalp Electrode 384

**Skill 9.14** Assisting with and Monitoring of Woman Undergoing Induction of Labor with Pitocin and Cervical Ripening Agents 385

**Skill 9.15** Assisting with and Caring for the Woman with an Epidural during Labor 386

**Skill 9.16** Care of the Woman with Prolapsed Cord 388

**Skill 9.17** Assessing the Uterine Fundus Following Vaginal Birth 388

**Skill 9.18** Evaluating the Lochia 389

**Skill 9.19** Assessing Postpartum Perineal 391

**Skill 9.20** Assisting with Breastfeeding after Childbirth 392

**Skill 9.21** Performing Nasal Pharyngeal Suctioning 394

**Skill 9.22** Suctioning an Infant with a Bulb Syringe 395

**Skill 9.23** Assessing Newborn APGAR Scores 396

**Skill 9.24** Thermoregulation of the Newborn 397

**Skill 9.25** Umbilical Cord Clamp: Application, Care, and Removal 398

**Skill 9.26** Assisting with Circumcision and Providing Circumcision Care 399

**Skill 9.27** Initial Newborn Bath 400

**Skill 9.28** The Infant Receiving Phototherapy 400

**CHAPTER 10**
## Tissue Integrity

**Skill 10.1** Performing a Dry Dressing Change 405

**Skill 10.2** Cleaning a Sutured Wound and Changing a Dressing on a Wound with a Drain 408

**Skill 10.3** Applying Wet-to-Moist Dressings 410

**Skill 10.4** Irrigating a Wound 412

**Skill 10.5** Applying an Abdominal Binder 413

**Skill 10.6** Using Alginates on Wounds 414

**Skill 10.7** Applying Bandages and Binders (Elastic Bandages) 416

**Skill 10.8** Maintaining Closed Wound Drainage 419

**Skill 10.9** Obtaining a Wound Drainage Specimen 420
VARIATION: Obtaining a Specimen for Anaerobic Culture Using a Sterile Syringe and Needle 422

**Skill 10.10** Assessing Ankle-Brachial Index (ABI) 422

**Skill 10.11** Changing a Dressing—Venous Ulcer 422

**Skill 10.12** Preventing Pressure Ulcers 426

**Skill 10.13** Providing Care for Clients with Pressure Ulcers 428

**Skill 10.14** Applying Transparent Film Dressing 429

**Skill 10.15** Using Hydrocolloid Dressing 431

**Skill 10.16** Using Electrical Stimulation 434

**Skill 10.17** Using Noncontact Normothermic Wound Therapy 435

**Skill 10.18** Using Negative Pressure Wound Therapy 437

**Skill 10.19** Applying a Transparent Wound Barrier 440

**Skill 10.20** Positioning and Exercising the Stump 442

**Skill 10.21** Shrinking/Molding the Stump 443

## CHAPTER 11

# Assessments

Skill 11.1 Assessing Appearance and Mental Status 448
Skill 11.2 Assessing the Skin 451
Skill 11.3 Assessing the Hair 456
Skill 11.4 Assessing the Nails 457
Skill 11.5 Assessing the Skull and Face 459
Skill 11.6 Assessing the Eyes and Vision 460
Skill 11.7 Assessing the Ears and Hearing 466
Skill 11.8 Assessing the Nose and Sinuses 469
Skill 11.9 Assessing the Mouth and Oropharynx 471
Skill 11.10 Assessing the Neck 475
Skill 11.11 Assessing the Thorax and Lungs 477
Skill 11.12 Assessing the Heart and Central Vessels 484
Skill 11.13 Assessing the Peripheral Vascular System 487
Skill 11.14 Assessing the Breasts and Axillae 489
Skill 11.15 Assessing the Abdomen 494
Skill 11.16 Assessing the Musculoskeletal System 498
Skill 11.17 Assessing the Neurologic System 501
Skill 11.18 Assessing the Female Genitals and Inguinal Area 510
Skill 11.19 Assessing the Male Genitalia and Inguinal Area 512
Skill 11.20 Assessing the Anus 515
Skill 11.21 Assessing the Client in Pain 516
   VARIATION: Daily Pain Diary 519
   VARIATION: Child Pain Assessment 519
Skill 11.22 Assessing Body Temperature 522
   VARIATION: Measuring an Infant or Child's
   Temperature 523
Skill 11.23 Assessing an Apical-Radial Pulse 529
Skill 11.24 Assessing an Apical Pulse 531
Skill 11.25 Assessing Peripheral Pulses 533
Skill 11.26 Assessing Respirations 535
Skill 11.27 Assessing Blood Pressure 537
Skill 11.28 Assessing Pulse Oximeter 543
Skill 11.29 Measuring Length 544
Skill 11.30 Measuring Height 545
Skill 11.31 Measuring Weight 546
Skill 11.32 Measuring Body Mass Index 546
Skill 11.33 Measuring Head Circumference 547
Skill 11.34 Measuring Chest Circumference 547
Skill 11.35 Measuring Abdominal Girth 548
Skill 11.36 Assessing the Heart Rate 548
Skill 11.37 Assessing the Respiratory Rate 549
Skill 11.38 Assessing Blood Pressure 549
Skill 11.39 Assessing a Child's Body Temperature 551
Skill 11.40 Glasgow Coma Scale 553
Skill 11.41 Neurovascular Assessment 554
Skill 11.42 Intracranial Pressure Monitoring and Daily Care 554
Skill 11.43 Assessing Visual Acuity 555
Skill 11.44 Assessing Hearing Acuity 557

## CHAPTER 12

# Caring Interventions

Skill 12.1 Changing an Unoccupied Bed 562
Skill 12.2 Changing an Occupied Bed 567
Skill 12.3 Providing Morning Care 570
Skill 12.4 Bathing an Adult or Pediatric Client 571
Skill 12.5 Providing Evening Care 581
Skill 12.6 Providing a Back Massage 581
Skill 12.7 Brushing and Flossing the Teeth 583
Skill 12.8 Providing Special Oral Care for the Unconscious
   or Debilitated Client 587
Skill 12.9 Shaving a Male Client 589
Skill 12.10 Providing Hair Care 590
Skill 12.11 Shampooing Hair 591
Skill 12.12 Identifying the Presence of Lice and Nits
   (Lice Eggs) 592
Skill 12.13 Removing Lice and Nits 593
Skill 12.14 Providing Nail Care 595
Skill 12.15 Providing Foot Care 595
Skill 12.16 Providing Routine Eye Care 598
Skill 12.17 Providing Eye Care for Comatose Client 598
Skill 12.18 Providing Postoperative Socket Care 599
Skill 12.19 Removing and Cleaning an Artificial Eye
   (Ocular Prosthesis) 599
Skill 12.20 Removing and Cleaning Contact Lenses 600
Skill 12.21 Removing, Cleaning, and Inserting a Hearing Aid 601
Skill 12.22 Providing Perineal-Genital Care 603
Skill 12.23 Assisting an Adult to Eat 605
Skill 12.24 Serving a Food Tray 607
Skill 12.25 Assisting the Dysphagic Client to Eat 607
Skill 12.26 Preparing for Medication Administration 609
Skill 12.27 Converting Dosage Systems 610
Skill 12.28 Calculating Dosages 611
Skill 12.29 Using the Narcotic Control System 611
Skill 12.30 Using an Automated Dispensing System 613
Skill 12.31 Administering Medication Protocol 614
Skill 12.32 Administering Oral Medications 616
Skill 12.33 Administering Medications by Enteral Tube 619
Skill 12.34 Administering Sublingual Medications 621
Skill 12.35 Administering Ophthalmic Medications 622
Skill 12.36 Administering Otic Medications 624
Skill 12.37 Administering Nasal Medications 625
Skill 12.38 Administering Metered-Dose Inhaler Medications 626
Skill 12.39 Administering Dry Powder Inhaled (DPI)
   Medications 628

**Skill 12.40** Administering Medication by Nonpressurized (Nebulized) Aerosol (NPA) 629

**Skill 12.41** Administering Vaginal Medications 630

**Skill 12.42** Administering Rectal Medications 631

**Skill 12.43** Preparing Injections 633

**Skill 12.44** Administering Intradermal Injections 637

**Skill 12.45** Administering Subcutaneous Injections 638

**Skill 12.46** Preparing Insulin Injections 640

**Skill 12.47** Teaching Client to Use Insulin Delivery System—Insulin Pen 643

**Skill 12.48** Teaching Use of Insulin Pump 644

**Skill 12.49** Administering Suncutaneous Anticoagulates (Heparin, LMWH, Arixtra) 646

**Skill 12.50** Administering Intramuscular (IM) Injections 647

**Skill 12.51** Using Z-Track Method 651

**Skill 12.52** Adding Medications to Intravenous Fluid Containers 654

**Skill 12.53** Administering Intermittent Intravenous Medication Using a Secondary Set 656

**Skill 12.54** Administering Intravenous Medications Using IV Push 658

**Skill 12.55** Managing Pain with a PCA Pump 660

**Skill 12.56** Administering Blood Transfusions 661

**Skill 12.57** Administering Blood Components 663

**Skill 12.58** Managing Central Lines 663

**Skill 12.59** Changing a Central Line Dressing 665

**Skill 12.60** Working with Implanted Vascular Access Devices 667

**Skill 12.61** Home Setting: Bathing Client in the Home 670

**Skill 12.62** Home Setting: Transferring Client to Tub or Shower 670

**Skill 12.63** Home Setting: Adapting Bedmaking to the Home 671

**Skill 12.64** Home Setting: Providing Wound Care 671

**Skill 12.65** Home Setting: Removing Lice 671

**Skill 12.66** Home Setting: Administering Medications 672

**Skill 12.67** Home Setting: Sterilizing Nondisposable Medication Equipment 673

## CHAPTER 13
# Safety

**Skill 13.1** Providing Safety for Clients during a Fire 675

**Skill 13.2** Preventing Thermal/Electrical Injuries 676

**Skill 13.3** Managing Clients in Restraints 677
VARIATION: Applying Torso/Belt Restraints 678

**Skill 13.4** Using a Bed or Chair Exit Safety Monitoring Device 678

**Skill 13.5** Applying Wrist or Ankle Restraint 680

**Skill 13.6** Applying a Papoose Board Immobilizer 681

**Skill 13.7** Applying a Mummy Immobilizer 682

**Skill 13.8** Implementing Seizure Precautions 683

**Skill 13.9** Identifying Eligibility for Medicare Reimbursement 685

**Skill 13.10** Completing Admission Documentation 687

**Skill 13.11** Maintaining Nurses' Safety 687

**Skill 13.12** Assessing Home for Safe Environment 688

**Skill 13.13** Evaluating Client's Safety 689

**Skill 13.14** Assessing Caregiver's Safety 690

**Skill 13.15** Assessing for Elder Abuse 690

## CHAPTER 14
# Assisting with Medical Procedures

**Skill 14.1** Assisting with Invasive Procedures 692

**Skill 14.2** Assisting with Thoracentesis 693

**Skill 14.3** Assisting with Paracentesis 694

**Skill 14.4** Assisting with Lumbar Puncture 695

**Skill 14.5** Assisting with Bone Marrow Aspiration 697

**Skill 14.6** Assisting with Chest Tube Insertion 700

**Skill 14.7** Assisting with Chest Tube Removal 703

**Skill 14.8** Assisting with Percutaneous Central Vascular Catheterization 706

# 1

# Comfort

Skill 1.1    Teaching Controlled Breathing          2

Skill 1.2    Teaching Progressive Muscle
Relaxation                                4

Skill 1.3    Assisting with Guided Imagery          6

Skill 1.4    Managing a TENS Unit                   8

Skill 1.5    Applying Dry Heat Measures: Hot
Water Bottle, Electric Heating Pad,
Aquathermia Pad, Disposable Hot Pack   13

Skill 1.6    Applying Compresses and Moist
Packs                                     15

Skill 1.7    Assisting with a Sitz Bath              17

Skill 1.8    Providing Tepid Sponges                17

Skill 1.9    Monitoring an Infant Radiant
Warmer                                    18

Skill 1.10   Applying Dry Cold Measures:
Ice Bag, Ice Collar, Ice Glove,
Disposable Cold Pack                      20

Skill 1.11   Using a Cooling Blanket                21

Skill 1.12   Meeting the Physiological Needs
of the Dying Client                       25

Skill 1.13   Performing Postmortem Care             28

Experts have studied the effects of deep relaxation on the mind and body. They found that individuals who regularly practice relaxation exercises experience less stress than people who don't.

Guided imagery can help individuals learn how to stop troublesome thoughts and focus on images that help them relax and decrease the negative impact of stressors.

### EXPECTED OUTCOMES

- Client is able to reduce environmental stressors.
- Client is able to identify and alleviate stress caused by mental concerns.

## CULTURAL CONSIDERATIONS

Heathcare personnel working in a variety of settings maintain that pain is a culturally influenced phenomenon. How pain is experienced and expressed varies by cultural group. For example, some cultures (such as the Italians and Jewish people) encourage open expression of feelings like pain, while others (the stoic English, Irish, and Chinese) believe that pain is something to be ignored or endured in silence. This was demonstrated by Zborowski's study done as early as the 1950s. While these general conclusions may lead to stereotyping, it is important to consider the impact of the individual's culture in the assessment of pain level.

*Source:* Spector, R. (2001). *Cultural diversity in health and illness* (5th ed). Upper Saddle River, NJ: Prentice Hall Health.

## Skill 1.1  Teaching Controlled Breathing

### Procedure

1. Instruct client to sit so that his or her back is well supported, with spine straight but not rigid.
2. Have client place feet flat on floor and place hands on legs.
3. If client is lying down, have him or her place hands at side.
4. Suggest client find a comfortable position, close eyes, and take a deep, slow breath through nostrils.
5. Continue giving the client the following instructions.
   a. Extend your abdominal muscles.
   b. Hold your breath for the count of four. Then very slowly release the air through slightly parted lips, making a whoosh sound.
   c. When you think that all the air is out, hold your stomach in to push out even more air.
   d. Repeat this breathing pattern several times so that your body relaxes.
   e. Breathe in through your nostrils to the count of four—1-2-3-4. Hold it—1-2-3-4—and expel the breath all the way out slowly, slowly releasing the air through your mouth.
   f. As the air goes out, feel all of the tension drain out with it.
   g. Now double the count, and breathe in slowly, filling your lungs all the way to the top to the count of eight. 1-2-3-4-5-6-7-8. Hold it—1-2-3-4—and now slowly release the breath—5-6-7-8.

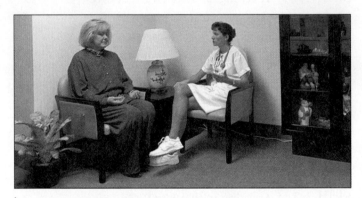

Find a quiet room to teach relaxation process.

   h. Again breathe in slowly to the count of 10 and count for the client—1-2-3-4-5-6-7-8-9-10. Hold it to the count of eight—1-2-3-4-5-6-7-8—and slowly release the air through your mouth to the count of 10—1-2-3-4-5-6-7-8-9-10. Pause.
   i. Continue with your regular breathing pattern, letting the air breathe for you.
6. Stop the process by having the client open his or her eyes.

### CLINICAL TIP

If you are motivated to learn CAM techniques, there are numerous classes available. In fact, to implement certain CAM therapies such as Reiki, therapeutic touch, acupressure, or acupuncture, you will need specialized classes/training.

## TABLE 1–1 NONPHARMACOLOGICAL APPROACHES TO PAIN

| Physical Methods | Advantages |
| --- | --- |
| TENS—stimulating skin with mild electric current—provides pain relief by blocking pain impulses to the brain | Noninvasive method<br>Higher level of activity<br>Studies show more effective for postoperative pain<br>Gives staff confidence they can assist client with pain<br>Choice for chronic pain |
| Acupuncture—ancient Chinese form of treating diseases and pain through insertion and manipulation of needles at specific points on the body | Insertion of thin needles is not painful to the client<br>Pain relieving capacity extends beyond actual procedure<br>Method may provide relief when no other method works |
| Biofeedback—electric monitoring device that feeds back effect of behavior so client can control internal processes (e.g., heartbeat) | Noninvasive method<br>Completely controlled by client<br>Promotes stress reduction as well as pain relief<br>After mastery, instruments are not needed to achieve result |
| Vibration or massage—hands-on manipulation of muscles or electrical form of massage (vibration) | Noninvasive method—electrically alleviates pain by numbness or paresthesia or through touch<br>Increases circulation and endorphins to area<br>Relaxes muscles and reduces tension on nerves and promotes relaxation<br>Useful only for light to moderate pain |
| Cold therapy—cold wraps, gel packs, cold therapy, ice massage; do not use on irradiated tissue or when clients have peripheral vascular disease | Relieves pain faster than heat therapy<br>Numbs nerves and decreases inflammation and spasms<br>Effective for nerve, abdominal, and lower back pain<br>Alters pain threshold<br>Decreases tissue injury response |
| Heat therapy—hot wraps, dry heat, moist heat; do not use on irradiated tissue or tumors | Noninvasive method<br>Decreases pain by reducing inflammation<br>Promotes relaxation of muscles<br>Increases vasodilation and blood flow to area<br>Facilitates clearance of tissue toxins and fluids |
| Counterirritants—mentholated ointments or lotions (Ben-Gay or Icy Hot) | May contain salicylates (reduces inflammation) but dangerous if client has potential bleeding problems<br>May be irritating to the skin—potential skin breakdown |
| Acupressure application—based on the ancient Chinese method of acupuncture, this method involves using specific points located on meridians at various places on the body | Noninvasive method<br>Redirection of energy flow through pressure on meridian points<br>Reduces pain and increases endorphins |
| Chiropractic adjustment | Manipulation of muscles and realignment of spinal column<br>Nerve function is restored<br>Structural integrity and balance are restored |
| **Cognitive–Behavioral Methods** | **Advantages** |
| Relaxation—body relaxation of muscles used with imagery, therapist instruction | Relaxes tense muscles and reduces stress<br>Effective in reducing pain<br>Easy to learn and implement techniques for self-mastery<br>Reduces fear and anxiety connected to pain |
| Imagery—visualization technique of forming sensory images, or seeing in the "mind's eye" an image that distracts from the sensation of pain | Effective in reducing pain<br>Client can control use and timing of technique<br>Reduces high-level anxiety connected to pain |
| Deep breathing—techniques using breath to control pain | Effective in reinforcing body relaxation and visualization<br>Reduces pain through breath control; increases oxygen utilization |
| Hypnosis—creating a state of altered consciousness so that client is susceptible to instruction | Effective with a client who is suggestive and who experiences tension and anxiety accompanying pain |

## CLIENTS IN PAIN

When working with diverse clients in pain, remember:

- Pain is expressed differently across and within cultures.
- Pain has different meanings across and within cultures.
- Use various types of assessment to get at an accurate understanding of a client's pain.
- Use family-centered approaches to care.
- Ensure that language barriers have been overcome with interpreters and written materials in the language of choice of the client and family members/ caregivers.
- Assess the client's explanation for the pain, and what the pain means to the client.
- Show respect for client beliefs, and incorporate folk health care practices that seem safe into care whenever possible.

### CLINICAL ALERT

Perception is reality. The client's self-report of pain is what must be used to determine pain intensity. The nurse is obligated to record the pain intensity as reported by the client. By challenging the believability of the client's report, the nurse is undermining the therapeutic relationship and preventing the fulfillment of advocacy and helping people with pain, which is called for in the ANA's 2005 publication *Scope and Standards of Practice: Pain Management Nursing.*

Expressions of pain vary from culture to culture and may vary from person to person within a culture.

*African Americans*

- Some believe pain and suffering is a part of life and is to be endured.

- Some may deny or avoid dealing with the pain until it becomes unbearable.
- Some believe that prayer and laying on of hands will free a person from suffering and pain.

*Mexican Americans*

- May tend to view pain as a part of life and as an indicator of the seriousness of an illness.
- Some believe that enduring pain is a sign of strength.

*Puerto Ricans*

- Many tend to be loud and outspoken in their expressions of pain. This is a socially learned way to cope and it is important for the nurse to not judge or disapprove.

*Asian Americans*

- Chinese culture values silence. As a result, some clients may be quiet when in pain because they do not want to cause dishonor to themselves and their family.
- Japanese may have a stoic (minimal verbal and nonverbal expressions) response to pain. They may even refuse pain medication.
- Filipino clients may believe that pain is "God's will." Some elderly Filipino clients may refuse pain medication.

*Native Americans*

- In general, Native Americans are quiet, less expressive verbally and nonverbally, and may tolerate a high level of pain. They tend to not request pain medication and may tolerate pain until it physically disables them.

*Arab Americans*

- Pain responses are considered private and reserved for immediate family, not for health professionals. As a result, this may lead to conflicting perceptions between the family members and the nurse regarding the effectiveness of the client's pain relief.

*Note:* From *Transcultural Communication in Nursing,* 2nd ed., by C. Munoz and J. Luckmann, 2005, Clifton Park, NY: Delmar Learning, and *Transcultural Concepts in Nursing Care,* 4th ed., by M. M. Andrews and J. S. Boyle, 2003, Philadelphia: Lippincott Williams & Wilkins.

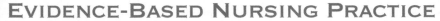

## Skill 1.2  Teaching Progressive Muscle Relaxation

### EVIDENCE-BASED NURSING PRACTICE

**The Opposite of a Stress Response**

In many studies, Herbert Benson, MD, author of *The Relaxation Response,* found that the opposite of a stress response (physiological response) can be achieved by completing only two steps: repeating a prayer, word, sound, phrase, or movement, and disregarding all other thoughts (as in meditation, yoga, etc.).

*Source:* Benson, J. (1984). *The relaxation response.* New York: Times Books.

**Managing Stress**

The results of 153 studies on stress management were analyzed to determine whether there was consensus in definitions and therapy protocols. Most studies endorsed either a cognitive–behavioral approach to stress-coping skills (77%) (examples are problem-focused skills, self-monitoring of stress intensity, record keeping, time management, assertiveness training) or, a less structured approach, breathing, relaxation, imagery, meditation, yoga, and massage therapy (85%).

*Source:* Ong, L., Linden, W., & Young, S. (2004). Stress management, what is it? *Journal of Psychosomatic Research, 56*(1), 133–137.

## EXPECTED OUTCOMES

- Client is able to reduce environmental stressors.
- Client is able to identify and alleviate stress caused by mental concerns.

## Delegation

Noninvasive pain management techniques can be delegated to UAP if they have experience using the technique and are comfortable doing so. The nurse is responsible for assessing the client's willingness to participate in the relaxation or imagery exercise. The nurse instructs UAP to report the client's response to the nurse.

## Equipment

- A printed relaxation script that an individual can read until the client learns the technique. Many are available online and through stress management resource books and tapes.
- Tape recorder and tape (optional). The tape recorder could be used to provide the script for the exercise or for the playing of background music.

## Preparation

Allow 10 to 15 minutes of uninterrupted time for the session. Ensure that the environment is private, quiet, and at a temperature that suits the client. The client should have an empty bladder. ➤*Rationale: Interruptions or distractions interfere with the client's ability to achieve full relaxation. Once clients learn how to use this technique, they will be able to do it in less than 5 minutes as part of self-care and ongoing stress management.*

## Procedure

1. Prior to performing the procedure, introduce self and verify the client's identify using agency protocol. Explain to the client what you are going to do, why it is necessary, and how he or she can participate.
2. Perform hand hygiene and observe other appropriate infection control procedures.
3. Provide for client privacy.
4. Prepare the client:
   - Tell the client how progressive muscle relaxation works.
   - Provide a rationale for the procedure. ➤*Rationale: It has been noted that muscular tension accompanies most stress states. By aiming to reduce muscle tension, the negative effects of stress on the mind–body can be lessened.*
   - Ask the client to identify the stressors operating in the client's life and the reactions to these stressors. ➤*Rationale: Awareness is important as the client learns how to cope effectively.*
   - Demonstrate the method of tensing and relaxing groups of muscles and have client do it with you. It is easy to start with making fists—tensing the muscles with 100% effort the first time, and then with only 50% effort the second time. ➤*Rationale: Demonstration and initial practice*

*enables the client to understand the progression of muscle relaxation more clearly.*
   - Assist the client to a comfortable position.
5. If music is to be used, select music that is instrumental, calming, neutral, and unfamiliar to the client. ➤*Rationale: Music should not be recognizable and should not intentionally elicit memories or emotion. In this way, the music will enhance relaxation. Classical music can sometimes be too "busy" and may evoke memories and emotion that could be distracting for the client.*
   - Ensure that all body parts are supported and the joints slightly flexed with no strain or pull on the muscles (e.g., arms and legs should not be crossed). ➤*Rationale: Assuming a position of comfort facilitates relaxation.*
6. Encourage the client to begin slow, deep diaphragmatic or abdominal breathing to rest the mind and begin relaxing the body. Inhaling through the nose and exhaling through the mouth (pursed lips are best) slows down the breath and enhances relaxation.
7. Instruct the client to tense and then relax each group of muscles starting from the head and moving down the body. Use a tone of voice throughout the exercise that invites participation rather than directs.
   - The following script suggestions are just one way of doing the technique:
     a. Take in a deep breath, and close eyes tightly shut, furrowing your brows and wrinkling your forehead. Hold this contraction with the most effort you can, and then release as you exhale slowly. Again, take a breath and contract these same muscles with half the effort you used last time. Hold, hold, and now release with your breath, feeling the tension leave your body as a soothing wave of relaxation flows over your head and face. . . . You could keep your eyes softly closed throughout this exercise. . . .
     b. You might want to clench your jaw as you breathe in, feeling the muscles in your cheeks and throat and base of your tongue tightening as you hold, hold, and then release. You could repeat this contraction as you inhale, and hold with less tension this time, and then release as you exhale, allowing all of these muscles to soften, allowing your teeth to rest just slightly apart.
     c. Next, pull your shoulders up toward your ears as you take a full and gentle breath in and hold as tightly as you can. Now relax and release your shoulders with your breath, allowing a soothing wave of relaxation to flow into your neck and shoulder area. This time hunch your shoulders up with only half the effort you used last time . . . hold it . . . and release, allowing any tension to run down your arms and through your hands and out the tips of your fingers. . . .
     d. Next, you could inhale and make tight fists of both hands and hold these fists as strongly as you can.

Release your fists and your breath. Take another breath in and make fists again, this time with less effort . . . hold . . . and release, allowing tension to leave your hands, being replaced with softness.

e. Now we can focus on the arms. As you breathe in, think about contracting the muscles of the arms, perhaps making fists again, and feeling the entire length of your arms tightening and flexing. Hold, hold, and release, feeling the tension leaving your arms and flowing out through your hands and fingertips. This time breathe in and tighten your arms with less effort, and then release with your breath, feeling a sense of comfort and peace as the tension leaves you now.

f. You could focus on your abdominal muscles, and pull them in tightly as if to button your navel onto the front of your spine. You may even notice tension in your back muscles, and hold this as tightly as you can. Exhale and release all of these muscles, feeling as if a band of tightness around your midsection is being released. Breathe in and tense this abdominal and low back band of muscles again. Hold more gently this time and then release, exhaling slowly. Enjoy the feelings as your muscles become relaxed and loose.

g. You could inhale deeply and flex your hip and buttock muscles, feeling yourself lift as the muscles contract. Hold, and then release as you exhale. This time, flex these muscles a bit more gently, aware of the peace that is flowing throughout your body as you continue to relax.

h. You could inhale and flex your heels away from your body as you pull your toes hard, hard toward your face. Hold this, feeling your calf and thigh muscles flexing as well, and then release as you exhale. Inhale again and this time press your toes away from your

face and feel the tension throughout the entire length of your leg once again. You can repeat this with less effort, and feel the whole body relax and release.

• Encourage the client to breathe slowly and deeply during the entire procedure. ➤*Rationale: Quiet, full, slow breathing with an emphasis on prolonged exhalation elicits a parasympathetic response that is the opposite of the fight-or-flight response.*

• Speak in a calm voice that encourages relaxation and coach the client to mentally focus on each muscle group being addressed. ➤*Rationale: By suggesting rather than directing throughout the process, you avoid triggering any underlying control issues in the client.*

8. Ask the client to state whether any tension remains after all muscle groups have been tensed and relaxed.
   • Repeat the procedure for muscle groups that are not relaxed.

9. Terminate the relaxation exercise slowly by counting from 1 to 3, suggesting that the client will feel calm and alert.
   • Ask the client to move the body slowly: first the hands and feet, then arms and legs, and finally the head and neck.

10. Remind the client that this technique can be used any time the client needs to release tension or wants to feel more relaxed.

11. Document the client's response to the exercise.

### Documentation

Sample: 7/20/09 2300 Reports "mild" headache, 1–2/10 on pain scale. Also expressing anxiety about recent diagnosis, having difficulty falling asleep. Progressive muscle relaxation taught using relaxation music as a background. Participated fully, stated "headache is gone." Asleep when nurse returned with sleep med. Sleep med held.
——————————————— B. Montgomery, RN

## Skill 1.3   Assisting with Guided Imagery

### Preparation

Allow 10 to 15 minutes for this process. Provide a private, comfortable, quiet environment free of distractions. Ensure thermal comfort and make sure the client has an empty bladder. ➤*Rationale: Comfort and freedom from distractions are necessary for the client to relax and focus on the exercise.*

### Procedure

1. Prior to performing the procedure, introduce self to the client and verify the client's identity using

agency protocol. Explain the rationale and benefits of imagery. Ask the client about the goals for the session. Imagery can provide relaxation and feelings of empowerment, lead to creative problem solving, and facilitate healing. The content used will vary depending on the client's goals. Many books and tapes are available for those who want to learn more about this powerful technique. ➤*Rationale: The client is an active participant in an imagery exercise and can offer direction for the session.*

2. Perform hand hygiene and observe other appropriate infection control procedures.
3. Provide for client privacy.
4. Assist the client to a comfortable position.
   - Assist the client to a reclining position and ask the client to close the eyes. ➤*Rationale: A position of comfort can enhance the client's focus during the imagery exercise.*
5. Implement actions to induce relaxation.
   - Speak clearly in a calming and neutral tone of voice. ➤*Rationale: Positive voice coaching can enhance the effect of imagery. A shrill or loud voice can distract the client from the image.*
   - Ask the client to take slow, full diaphragmatic/ abdominal breaths and to relax all muscles. Use progressive muscle relaxation exercises as needed to assist the client to achieve total relaxation.
   - Guide the client through relaxation breathing and then through muscle relaxation. Then begin to guide the client toward a most beautiful or peaceful place. The client may have been to this place before or may be imagining this place. Do *not* impose your own suggestions as to where they might be. Clients know where they want and need to go! Slowly guide them to approach and then finally enter the place. Prompt them to use all of their senses as they look around the place, listen to the sounds of the place, feel the air, feel what's underfoot, and smell the fragrances of the place. Have them find and move toward a safe spot where they can rest for awhile.
   - While clients are in their safe spot, you can assist them to do some work. For example, if they need stress management or pain relief, they can picture themselves (from the safety of this, their very safe spot) in a potentially tense situation. Then have them inhale and exhale slowly three times, saying to themselves "relax, relax, relax" with each exhalation. For internal healing work, encourage the client to focus on a meaningful image of power and to use it to control the specific problem. Or, the client can be educated beforehand to use anatomical and physiologic imagery for their own healing. These kinds of goals are facilitated with some prior preparation on the part of the nurse and client, and many resources exist to prepare people for this work. Ask the client to use all the senses when practicing imagery. ➤*Rationale: Using all the senses enhances the client's benefit from imagery. Clients may be asked to assign a color to their pain, and then identify a color signifying "no pain." Then they can use imagery to change the color of their pain to the "no-pain color."*

6. Take the client out of the image by suggesting that it is time for the client to leave this most beautiful and safe place. Suggest that the client can return at any time desired and that their breathing will lead the way.
   - Slowly count from 1 to 3, suggesting that it is time for the client to leave this most beautiful and safe place. Suggest that the client come back into the here and now. Tell the client that they will feel rested and refreshed when they open their eyes on 3.
   - Remain until the client is alert. If the client remains in a trancelike state, simply repeat that they will wake up on the number 3 and count to three again. No harm will occur if the client stays "asleep." You can allow them to remain so, or gently touch them to facilitate awakening.
7. Following the experience, ask the client to describe the physical and emotional feelings elicited by the imagery session. The meanings images have for the individual client can be very helpful in the therapeutic process. Direct the client to explore the response to images because this enables the client to modify the imagery for future sessions.
8. Encourage the client to practice the imagery technique.
   - Imagery is a technique that can be done independently by the client once the client knows how.
9. Document the client's response to the exercise, noting signs of increased relaxation and reduced anxiety.

---

## UNEXPECTED OUTCOMES

Client moves into the stage of exhaustion, and stress becomes dangerous to health.

Client refuses to acknowledge that stress is affecting his or her life.

## CRITICAL THINKING OPTIONS

- Immediately take measures to remove stressors through medication, complete rest, and so forth.
- Implement specific stress-reducing measures, such as relaxation processes, visualization, and biofeedback.
- Attempt to elicit feelings of client before giving information about the role of stress and effect on one's body.
- Refer client to resources, articles, and knowledgeable persons who can discuss the effect of stress and the importance of eliminating stressors.

# Skill 1.4  Managing a TENS Unit

## EXPECTED OUTCOMES

- Pain is controlled through nonpharmacological methods such as massage, relaxation techniques, or TENS.
- Client is satisfied with level of pain control.
- Client receives adequate pain medications; pain level does not interfere with ambulation, getting out of bed, etc.
- Client's anxiety level is lowered in relation to pain.

## Delegation

The assessment for and application of a TENS unit requires specialized knowledge and problem solving. It is important that the nurse understand how this method of pain management works. In an acute care health setting, the nurse would not delegate the skill of managing a TENS unit to UAP. A TENS unit is often ordered for home use and the nurse is responsible for teaching the client or caregiver how to safely and effectively use the device.

## Equipment

- TENS unit
- Bath basin with warm water
- Soap
- Washcloth
- Towel
- Conduction cream, gel, or water (see manufacturer's instructions)
- Hypoallergenic tape

## Procedure

1. Prior to performing the procedure, introduce self and verify the client's identity using agency protocol. Explain to the client what you are going to do, why it is necessary, and how he or she can participate. The TENS unit may not completely eliminate pain but should reduce pain to a level that allows the client to rest more comfortably and/or carry out everyday activities.
2. Perform hand hygiene and observe other appropriate infection control procedures.
3. Provide for client privacy.
4. Prepare the equipment.
   - Insert the battery into the TENS unit to test its functioning.
   - With the TENS unit off, plug the lead wires into the battery-operated unit at one end, leaving the electrodes at the other end.
5. Clean the application area.
   - Wash, rinse, and dry the designated area with soap and water. ➤*Rationale: This reduces skin irritation and facilitates adhesion of the electrodes to the skin for a longer period of time.*

6. Apply the electrodes to the client.
   - If the electrodes are not pre-gelled, moisten them with a small amount of water or apply conducting gel. (Consult the manufacturer's instructions.) ➤*Rationale: This facilitates electrical conduction.*
   - Place the electrodes on a clean, unbroken skin area. Choose the area according to the location, nature, and origin of the pain.
   - Ensure that the electrodes make full surface contact with the skin. Tape all sides evenly with hypoallergenic tape. ➤*Rationale: This prevents an inadvertent burn.*
7. Turn the unit on.
   - Ascertain that the amplitude control is set at level 0.
   - Slowly increase the intensity of the stimulus (amplitude) until the client notes a slight increase in discomfort.
   - When the client notes discomfort, slowly decrease the amplitude until the client notes a pleasant sensation. Once this has been achieved, keep the TENS unit set at this level to maintain blockage of the pain sensation. Most clients select frequencies between 60 and 100 Hz.
8. Monitor the client.
   - If the client complains of itching, pricking, or burning, explore the following options:
     a. Turn the pulse-width dial down.
     b. Check that the entire electrode surface is in contact with the skin.
     c. Increase the distance between the electrodes.
     d. Select another type of electrode suitable for the model of TENS unit in use.
     e. Discontinue the TENS and consider the possibility of another brand of TENS.
   - If the sensation of the stimulus is unpleasant, too intense, or distracting, turn down both the amplitude and pulse-width dial.
   - If the client complains of headache or nausea during application or use, turn down both the amplitude and the pulse-width dial. Repositioning of the electrodes may also be helpful.
   - If further troubleshooting is not effective, discontinue the use of the TENS unit and notify the primary care provider.
9. After the treatment:
   - Turn off the controls and unplug the lead wires from the control box.
   - Clean the electrodes according to the manufacturer's instructions. Clean the client's skin with soap and water.
   - Replace the used battery pack with a charged battery. Begin recharging the used battery.
   - If continuous therapy is used, remove the electrode patches and inspect the skin at least once daily.

10. Provide client teaching.
    - Review instructions for use with the client and verify that the client understands.
    - Have the client demonstrate the use of the TENS unit and verbalize ways to troubleshoot if headache, nausea, or unpleasant sensations occur.
    - Instruct the client not to submerge the unit in water but instead to remove and reapply it after bathing.
11. Document all relevant information.
    - Record the date and time TENS therapy was initiated, the location of electrode placement and status of skin in that area, the character and quality of the pain, settings of TENS unit used, and side effects experienced and the client's response.

**Documentation**

Sample: 7/30/09 1100 C/o sharp pain in right hip that radiates down back of right leg. Rates pain at 3/10, and achieves some relief with positional changes that take weight off of hip. TENS applied over lateral aspect of right hip at 70 Hertz. _____ M. Johnstone, RN

7/30/09 1110 c/o nausea. Frequency reduced to 60 Hertz; nausea resolved. _____ M. Johnstone, RN

7/30/09 1140 TENS discontinued. Rates pain at 0–1/10. No c/o nausea. Skin intact. _____ M. Johnstone, RN

## SETTING OF CARE

TENS units are frequently ordered for home use to relieve chronic pain. Instruct the client or caregiver on:

- How to use and care for the TENS equipment.
- How to troubleshoot if side effects or problems occur and who to call if the equipment malfunctions.
- Where and how to obtain supplies needed for the TENS unit.
- How to remove the electrodes daily and check for skin breakdown at the electrode sites.
- Teach client to keep a pain diary to monitor pain onset, activity before pain, pain intensity, use of analgesics or other relief measures, and so on.

- Instruct client to contact a health care professional if planned pain control measures are ineffective.
- Teach the use of preferred and selected nonpharmacologic techniques such as relaxation, guided imagery, distraction, music therapy, massage, and so on.
- Instruct the client to use pain control measures before the pain becomes severe.
- Inform the client of the effects of untreated pain.
- Provide appropriate information about how to access community resources, home care agencies, and associations that offer self-help groups and educational materials.

## DEVELOPMENTAL CONSIDERATIONS

### Infant

- Giving an infant, particularly a very-low-birth-weight infant, a water and sucrose solution administered through a pacifier is effective in reducing pain during procedures that may be painful, but should not replace anesthetic or analgesic medications when indicated.

### Child

- Distract the child with toys, books, or pictures.
- Hold the child to console and promote comfort.
- Explore misconceptions about pain and correct in concrete, developmentally appropriate terms (e.g.,

avoid language such as "put to sleep" to describe anesthesia during surgery—this might remind of family pet who was euthanized and be very frightening).
- Children can use their imagination during guided imagery. To use the "pain switch," ask the child to imagine a pain switch (even give it a color) and tell them to visualize turning the switch off in the area where there is pain. A "magic glove" or "magic blanket" is an imaginary object that the child applies on areas of the body (e.g., hand, thigh, back, hip) to lessen discomfort.
- Offer PCA whenever appropriate.

*(continued)*

---

**DEVELOPMENTAL CONSIDERATIONS** (CONTINUED)

**Elders**

- Focus on the client's control in dealing with the pain (drug and nondrug measures that have worked in the past should be encouraged).
- Spend time with the client and listen carefully.

- Clarify misconceptions. Encourage independence whenever possible.
- Carefully review the treatment plan to avoid drug–drug, food–drug, or disease–drug interactions.

---

| **UNEXPECTED OUTCOMES** | **CRITICAL THINKING OPTIONS** |
|---|---|
| Client achieves no relief from massage. | • Try combining method with use of medications (i.e., while waiting for the medication to take effect). |
| | • Client has to trust the technique before it can be effective. Have client talk to another person who has found technique helpful. |
| Client cannot focus on relaxation technique. | • Start with very simple breathing techniques and progress slowly to relaxation and visualization. |

---

## APPLYING HEAT AND COLD MEASURES

Heat and cold are applied to the body to promote the repair and healing of tissues. The form of thermal application generally depends on its purpose. Cold applied to a body part draws heat from the area; heat, of course, warms the area. The application of heat or cold produces physiologic changes in the temperature of the tissues, size of the blood vessels, capillary blood pressure, capillary surface area for exchange of fluids and electrolytes, and tissue metabolism. The duration of the application also affects the response. See Table 1–2 for a summary of the physiologic effects of heat and cold.

### EXPECTED OUTCOMES

- Inflammatory response is controlled.
- Bleeding and edema are reduced/controlled.
- Local anesthetic response is achieved.
- Local cryotherapy causes no undesired effects.
- Core body temperature is reduced.

**TABLE 1–2 PHYSIOLOGIC EFFECTS OF HEAT AND COLD**

| Heat | Cold |
|---|---|
| Vasodilation | Vasoconstriction |
| Increases capillary permeability | Decreases capillary permeability |
| Increases cellular metabolism | Decreases cellular metabolism |
| Increases inflammation | Slows bacterial growth, decreases inflammation |
| Sedative effect | Local anesthetic effect |

## TABLE 1-3 SELECTED INDICATIONS FOR THE USE OF HEAT AND COLD

| Indication | Effect of Heat | Effect of Cold |
|---|---|---|
| Muscle spasm | Relaxes muscles and increases their contractility. | Relaxes muscles and decreases muscle contractility. |
| Inflammation | Increases blood flow, softens exudates. | Vasoconstriction decreases capillary permeability, decreases blood flow, slows cellular metabolism. |
| Pain | Relieves pain, possibly by promoting muscle relaxation, increasing circulation, and promoting psychological relaxation and a feeling of comfort; acts as a counterirritant. | Decreases pain by slowing nerve conduction rate and blocking nerve impulses; produces numbness, acts as a counterirritant, increases pain threshold. |
| Joint contracture | Reduces contracture and increases joint range of motion by allowing greater distention of muscles and connective tissue. | |
| Joint stiffness | Reduces joint stiffness by decreasing viscosity of synovial fluid and increasing tissue distensibility. | |
| Traumatic injury | | Decreases bleeding by constricting blood vessels; decreases edema by reducing capillary permeability. |

## TABLE 1-4 TEMPERATURES FOR HOT AND COLD APPLICATIONS

| Description | Temperature | Application |
|---|---|---|
| Very cold | Below 15°C (59°F) | Ice bags |
| Cold | 15–18°C (59–65°F) | Cold pack |
| Cool | 18–27°C (65–80°F) | Cold compresses |
| Tepid | 27–37°C (80–98°F) | Alcohol sponge bath |
| Warm | 37–40°C (98–104°F) | Warm bath, aquathermia pads |
| Hot | 40–46°C (104–115°F) | Hot soak, irrigations, hot compresses |
| Very hot | Above 46°C (above 115°F) | Hot water bags for adults |

## VARIABLES AFFECTING PHYSIOLOGIC TOLERANCE TO HEAT AND COLD

- *Body part.* The back of the hand and foot are not very temperature sensitive. In contrast, the inner aspect of the wrist and forearm, the neck, and the perineal area are temperature sensitive.
- *Size of the exposed body part.* The larger the area exposed to heat and cold, the lower the tolerance.
- *Individual tolerance.* The very young and the very old generally have the lowest tolerance. Persons who have neurosensory impairments may have a high tolerance, but the risk of injury is greater.
- *Length of exposure.* People feel hot and cold applications most while the temperature is changing. After a period of time, tolerance increases.
- *Intactness of skin.* Injured skin areas are more sensitive to temperature variations.

## CONTRAINDICATIONS TO THE USE OF HEAT AND COLD THERAPIES

Determine the presence of any conditions contraindicating the use of heat:

- *The first 24 hours after traumatic injury.* Heat increases bleeding and swelling.
- *Active hemorrhage.* Heat causes vasodilation and increases bleeding.
- *Noninflammatory edema.* Heat increases capillary permeability and edema.
- *Localized malignant tumor.* Because heat accelerates cell metabolism and cell growth and increases circulation, it may accelerate metastases (secondary tumors).
- *Skin disorder that causes redness or blisters.* Heat can burn or cause further damage to the skin.

Determine the presence of any conditions contraindicating the use of cold:

- *Open wounds.* Cold can increase tissue damage by decreasing blood flow to an open wound.
- *Impaired circulation.* Cold can further impair nourishment of the tissues and cause tissue damage. In clients with Raynaud's disease, cold increases arterial spasm.
- *Allergy or hypersensitivity to cold.* Some clients have an allergy to cold that may be manifested by an inflammatory response, for example, erythema, hives, swelling, joint pain, and occasional muscle spasm. Some react with a sudden increase in blood pressure, which can be hazardous if the person is hypertensive.

Determine the presence of any conditions indicating the need for special precautions during heat and cold therapy:

- *Neurosensory impairment.* Persons with sensory impairments are unable to perceive that heat is damaging the tissues and are at risk for burns, or they are unable to perceive discomfort from cold and are unable to prevent tissue injury.
- *Impaired mental status.* Persons who are confused or have an altered level of consciousness need monitoring and supervision during applications to ensure safe therapy.
- *Impaired circulation.* Persons with peripheral vascular disease, diabetes, or congestive heart failure lack the normal ability to dissipate heat via the blood circulation, which puts them at risk for tissue damage with heat applications. Cold applications are contraindicated for these people.
- *Open wounds.* Tissues around an open wound are more sensitive to heat and cold.

## DEVELOPMENTAL CONSIDERATIONS

ELDERLY CLIENTS ARE MORE SUSCEPTIBLE TO INJURY FROM HEAT AND COLD THERAPY AS A RESULT OF PHYSIOLOGIC CHANGES OR MEDICAL CONDITIONS.

- The epidermal cells are replaced more slowly in the elderly.
- Skin in the elderly is thin and contains less moisture.
- The elderly have a reduced sensitivity to pain, and therefore may not feel untoward effects of heat and cold treatment.
- Temperature should be reduced when using heat therapy because the elderly client's skin burns more easily.

VITAL SIGNS AND FREQUENT ASSESSMENT MAY BE NECESSARY DURING HEAT AND COLD THERAPY, AS VASODILATION FROM HEAT OR VASOCONSTRICTION FROM COLD CAN CAUSE CHANGES IN CARDIAC FUNCTION AND BLOOD PRESSURE

- Peripheral circulation may be compromised due to atherosclerosis or microvascular disease.
- Sensation in distal extremities may be impaired in elderly clients with neuropathy due to diabetes.
- The elderly may take medications that decrease sweating (anticholinergics for Parkinson's) or increase heat production (CNS stimulants or lithium).
- Temperature threshold for sweating is higher in the elder client and ability to mount a metabolic response to temperature loss is limited.
- Living conditions and financial limitations may not afford adequate environmental control.
- Hemodynamic responses to heat/cold therapies may be more unpredictable.

# Skill 1.5   Applying Dry Heat Measures: Hot Water Bottle, Electric Heating Pad, Aquathermia Pad, Disposable Hot Pack

## EXPECTED OUTCOMES

- Circulation is increased to area.
- Client reports decrease in pain.
- Inflammation is enhanced.
- Tissue fluid is mobilized/edema reduced.
- Normal body temperature is achieved.

## Delegation

Application of certain heat measures (e.g., baths) may be delegated to unlicensed assistive personnel (UAP) if they meet the general criteria for delegation. Sometimes, heat is applied as a component of wound care. However, in all cases, assessment of the client and the determination that the measure is safe to employ are the responsibility of the nurse. UAP may observe the area being treated during usual care and must report abnormal findings to the nurse. Abnormal findings must be validated and interpreted by the nurse.

## Equipment

- Hot water bottle (bag)
  - Hot water bottle with a stopper
  - Cover
  - Hot water and a thermometer
- Electric heating pad
  - Electric pad and control
  - Cover (waterproof if there will be moisture under the pad when it is applied)
  - Gauze ties (optional)
- Aquathermia pad
  - Pad
  - Distilled water
  - Control unit
  - Cover
  - Gauze ties or tape (optional)
- Disposable hot pack
  - One or two commercially prepared disposable hot packs

## CLINICAL ALERT

Do not allow the client to lie on a "constant heat source" such as a heating pad or aquathermic pad.

## Preparation

- Test all equipment for proper functioning and integrity (lack of leaks) before taking it to the client if possible.

## Procedure

1. Prior to performing the procedure, introduce self and verify the client's identity using agency protocol. Explain to the client what you are going to do, why it is necessary, and how he or she can participate. Discuss how the results will be used in planning further care or treatments.
2. Perform hand hygiene and observe other appropriate infection control procedures.
3. Provide for client privacy.
   - Expose only the area to be treated.
4. Apply the heat.

## VARIATION: Hot Water Bottle

- Measure the temperature of the water. Follow agency practice for the appropriate temperature. The following temperatures are commonly used:
  a. 46° to 52°C (115° to 125°F) for a normal adult
  b. 40.5° to 46°C (105° to 115°F) for a debilitated or unconscious adult
- Fill the hot water bottle about two-thirds full.
- Expel the air from the bottle. ➤*Rationale: Air remaining in the bottle prevents it from molding to the body part being treated.*
- Secure the stopper tightly.
- Hold the bottle upside down, and check for leaks.
- Dry the bottle.
- Wrap the bottle in a towel or hot water bottle cover.
- Apply the bottle to the body part using pillows to support it if necessary.

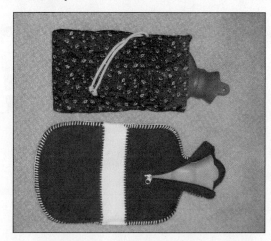

● Hot water bottle and cloth covers.

**VARIATION: Electric Heating Pad**

- Ensure that the body area is dry. ➤*Rationale: Electricity in the presence of moisture can conduct a shock.*
- Check that the electric pad is functioning and in good repair. The cord should be free from cracks, wires should be intact, heating components should not be exposed, and temperature distribution over the pad should be even.
- Place the cover on the pad. Some models have waterproof covers to be used when the pad is placed over a moist dressing. ➤*Rationale: Moisture could cause the pad to short circuit and burn or shock the client.*
- Plug the pad into the electric socket.
- Set the control dial for the correct temperature.
- After the pad has heated, place the pad over the body part to which heat is being applied.
- Use gauze ties instead of safety pins to hold the pad in place, if needed. ➤*Rationale: A pin might strike a wire, damaging the pad and giving an electric shock to the client.*

**VARIATION: Aquathermia Pad (Also Called a K-Pad)**

- Fill the unit with distilled water until it is two-thirds full. The unit will warm the water, which circulates through the pad.
- Secure the lid.
- Regulate the temperature with the key if it has not been preset. Normal temperature is 40.5°C (105°F). Check the manufacturer's instructions.
- Cover the pad with a towel or pillowcase.
- Plug in the unit.
- Check for any leak or malfunctions of the pad before use.
- Use tape or gauze ties to hold the pad in place. Never use safety pins. They can cause leakage.
- If unusual redness or pain occurs, discontinue the treatment, and report the client's reaction.

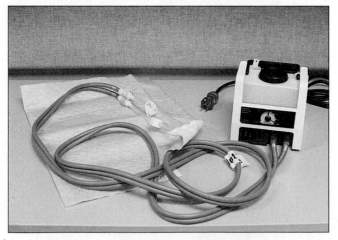

● An aquathermia heating unit.

**VARIATION: Disposable Hot Pack**

- Microwave, strike, squeeze, or knead the pack according to the manufacturer's directions.
- Note the manufacturer's instructions about the length of time that heat is produced.
- Depending on the type of pack, wrap in a towel or enclose in a cover prior to application.

5. Give the client the following instructions:
   - Do not insert any sharp, pointed object (e.g., a pin) into the bottle, pack, or pad.
   - Do not lie directly on the bottle or pad. ➤*Rationale: The surface below the object promotes heat absorption instead of normal heat dissipation.*
   - To prevent injury, avoid adjusting the heat higher than specified. ➤*Rationale: The degree of heat felt shortly after application will decrease, because the body's temperature receptors quickly adapt to the temperature. This adaptive mechanism can lead to tissue injury if the temperature is adjusted higher.*
   - Call the nurse if any discomfort is felt.

6. Leave the heat in place for only the designated period of time to avoid the rebound phenomenon, usually 30 minutes. Check the application and skin area after 5 to 10 minutes to be sure the area is not becoming burned.

7. Document the application of the heat and the client's response in the client record, using forms or checklists supplemented by narrative notes when appropriate.

---

**DEVELOPMENTAL CONSIDERATIONS**

**Infant/Child**

- The temperature of water in a hot water bottle should be 40.5° to 46°C (105° to 115°F) for a child under 2 years of age.

**Elders**

- Use special care in assessing the area to be treated and in evaluating the effects of the treatment because elders have many of the conditions predisposing to injury with heat measures.

---

**CLINICAL ALERT**

Contraindications to heat therapies include acute injury or inflammation, recent or potential hemorrhage, deep-vein thrombophlebitis, impaired circulation, impaired sensation, and impaired mentation.

> ## CLINICAL ALERT
>
> When treating an area where skin is not intact, cover lesion with sterile gauze and insulating barrier before applying heat.

> ## CLINICAL ALERT
>
> Do not apply heat to an edematous area until the reason for edema has been determined.

| UNEXPECTED OUTCOMES | CRITICAL THINKING OPTIONS |
|---|---|
| Client experiences pain, asks about alternative measures for relief. | • Cold therapy may be an option, or heat/cold alternating therapy as counterirritants; these therapies alter nerve transmission.<br>• Assess if application is too hot.<br>• Ensure that temperature is not over 110 degrees F (43.3 degrees C) if heating pad is used. |
| Swelling is not reduced with heat therapy. | • Ensure that acute inflammation is not present, as heat therapy is contraindicated during this phase, but is beneficial for subacute and chronic inflammation.<br>• Reassess to determine that area being treated has sufficient circulation.<br>• Support venous return by elevating the part.<br>• Reinforce importance of resting area until swelling is reduced.<br>• Consult physician regarding discontinuation of therapy after a 2-day trial and possible need for anti-inflammatory medication or reevaluation. |
| Aquathermic pump signals "Over Temp." | Check reservoir water level it may be low or empty.<br>Be sure to use room temperature (not hot) distilled water in reservoir.<br>Check that hoses are not kinked or hose clamps closed. |
| Pump continues to signal "Over Temp" after previous actions. | Disconnect, label, and send to BioMed department.<br>Obtain a different pump. |

# Skill 1.6   Applying Compresses and Moist Packs

## Delegation

Application of unsterile compresses or packs may be delegated to UAP if they meet the general criteria for delegation. However, in all cases, assessment of the client and the determination that the measure is safe to employ are the responsibility of the nurse. UAP may observe the area being treated during usual care and must report abnormal findings to the nurse. Abnormal findings must be validated and interpreted by the nurse.

## Equipment

Use sterile equipment and supplies for an open wound.

### Compress

- Disposable gloves or sterile gloves (for an open wound)
- Container for the solution
- Solution at the strength and temperature specified by the primary care provider or the agency
- Thermometer
- Gauze squares
- Sterile gloves, forceps, and cotton applicator sticks (if compress must be sterile)
- Petroleum jelly
- Insulating towel
- Plastic wrap
- Ties (e.g., roller gauze or masking tape)
- Hot water bottle or aquathermia pad (optional)

  *or*

- Ice bag (optional)
- Sterile dressing, if required

### *Moist Pack*

- Clean gloves
- Flannel pieces or towel packs
- Hot-pack machine for heating the packs

  *or*

- Basin of water with some ice chips
- Thermometer if a specific temperature is ordered for the pack
- Sterile gloves, forceps, and cotton applicator sticks (if sterility must be maintained)
- Petroleum jelly
- Insulating material (e.g., flannel or towels)
- Plastic wrap
- Hot water bottle (optional)

  *or*

- Ice bag (optional)
- Sterile dressing, if required

### Preparation

- If possible, perform care so that the application of the compress or pack will not need to be interrupted for other activities such as toileting.

### Procedure

1. Prior to performing the procedure, introduce self and verify the client's identity using agency protocol. Explain to the client what you are going to do, why it is necessary, and how he or she can participate. Discuss how the results will be used in planning further care or treatments.
2. Perform hand hygiene and observe other appropriate infection control procedures.
3. Provide for client privacy.
   - Expose only the area to be treated.
4. Prepare the client.
   - Assist the client to a comfortable position, and support the body part requiring the application.
   - Expose the area for the compress or pack.
   - Provide support for the body part requiring the compress or pack.
   - Apply clean gloves, and remove the wound dressing, if present. A dry, sterile dressing is often placed over open wounds between applications of moist heat or cold. Remove and discard gloves. Perform hand hygiene.
5. Moisten the compress or the pack.
   - Place the gauze in the solution.

     *or*

   - Heat the flannel or towel in a steamer, or chill it in the basin of water and ice chips.
6. Protect the surrounding skin as indicated.
   - With a cotton swab or an applicator stick, apply petroleum jelly to the skin surrounding the wound, not on the wound or open areas of the skin. ▸*Rationale: Jelly protects the skin from possible burns, maceration, and the irritating effects of some solutions.*
7. Apply the moist compress or pack.
   - Wring out the gauze compress so that the solution does not drip from it. For a sterile compress, use sterile forceps or sterile gloves to wring out the gauze.
   - Apply the gauze lightly and gradually to the designated area and, if tolerated by the client, mold the compress close to the body. Pack the gauze snugly against all wound surfaces. ▸*Rationale: Air is a poor conductor of cold or heat, and molding excludes air.*

     *or*

   - Wring out the flannel (for a sterile pack, use sterile gloves).
   - Apply the flannel to the body area, molding it closely to the body part.
8. Immediately insulate and secure the application.
   - Cover the gauze or flannel quickly with a dry towel and a piece of plastic wrap. ▸*Rationale: This step helps maintain the temperature of the application and thus its effectiveness.*
   - Secure the compress or pack in place with gauze ties or tape.
   - *Optional:* Apply a hot water bottle, aquathermia pad, or ice bag over the plastic wrap to maintain the heat or cold.
9. Monitor the client.
   - Assess the client for discomfort at 5- to 10-minute intervals. If the client feels any discomfort, assess the area for erythema, numbness, maceration, or blistering.
   - For applications to large areas of the body, note any change in the pulse, respirations, and blood pressure.
   - In the event of unexpected reactions, terminate the treatment and report to the nurse in charge.
10. Remove the compress or pack at the specified time.
    - Compresses and packs with an external heat or cold source on top may remain in place 1 to 2 hours. Without external heat or cold, they need to be changed every few minutes.
    - Apply a sterile dressing if one is required.
11. Document the application of the compress or pack and the client's response in the client record using forms or checklists supplemented by narrative notes when appropriate.

# Skill 1.7 Assisting with a Sitz Bath

## Equipment

Disposable sitz bath with tubing and bag
Warm water (40°–43°C) *Note:* Cold temperature may be indicated for client's situation.
Towels for drying
 Thermometer
 Clean gloves

## Preparation

1. Verify physician's order for sitz bath, duration and frequency of treatments.
2. Raise toilet seat and place sitz bath basin with "FRONT" facing the front of the toilet bowl.
3. Fill basin with warm water (40°–43°C ) 1/2 to 2/3 full.
4. Close flow tubing clamp.
5. Open top of plastic bag and fill with hot water (40°–43°C).
6. Hang bag at a level higher than the sitz basin so that fluid will flow by gravity.
7. Insert tubing through front or rear entry hole in sitz bath, then snap or secure tubing into channel or "eye" in bottom of basin.
8. Perform hand hygiene.

## Procedure

1. Identify client by checking identaband and asking client to state name.
2. Explain procedure and rationale for sitz bath.
3. Assist client to treatment area with accessible call bell.
4. Provide privacy by placing sign on door.
5. Check to ensure that temperature of thermotherapy water is 40.5°–43.3°C. *Note:* Most hospitals control water temperature so that it will not exceed 110°F or 43.3°C.

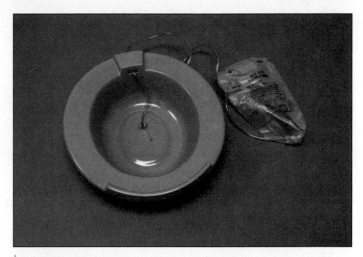

● Individual disposable sitz bath units are used for infection control purposes.

6. Assist client to sit in sitz bath for 15–20 minutes.
7. Maintain water temperature by continually adding water of appropriate temperature to bag. ➤*Rationale:* Overflow will drain into toilet through openings in back of basin.
8. Upon completion, assist client to dry area and allow client to sit briefly to allow normalization of blood pressure and to prevent hypotension upon standing. ➤*Rationale:* Orthostatic hypotension may occur with rapid position change following warm sitz bath due to vasodilation.
9. Don clean gloves, empty and rinse client's sitz basin, and store in convenient location for future use.
10. Discard soiled linen.
11. Perform hand hygiene.

# Skill 1.8 Providing Tepid Sponges

## EVIDENCE-BASED NURSING PRACTICE

**Effective Ways to Reduce Fever**
There is no statistical difference in fever reduction between use of cooling blanket vs. tepid water sponge bathing; however, cooling blankets are associated with significantly *more* shivering. Cooling blankets do appear to reduce fever effectively in heavily sedated or paralyzed critically ill clients.

*Source:* Manthous (1995). *American Journal of Respiratory Critical Care Medicine,* 151, 10–14.

## Equipment

Water or other coolant at prescribed temperature
Basin or tub
Washcloth and towels
Bath blanket
Electric fan
Tympanic or temporal artery thermometer
Cardiac monitor
Automated blood pressure unit

## Preparation

1. Review order for cooling method.
2. Gather equipment and bring to client's room. Check two forms of client ID and introduce yourself.
3. Provide privacy and explain procedure.
4. Perform hand hygiene.
5. Obtain baseline vital signs.
6. Apply ongoing blood pressure and cardiac monitoring equipment.

## Procedure

1. Remove client's clothing to allow for cooling and observation. Use bath blanket for privacy.
2. Monitor skin color and vital signs every 15–30 minutes during cooling. Immerse washcloths or material for sponging in ordered solution, generally 21°–27°C. ➤*Rationale:* Cool application reduces heat by conduction.
3. Wring out excess solution and place cloths on neck, axillae, groin. ➤*Rationale:* The vascularity of these areas promotes cooling.
4. Depending on type of bath, change cloths every 5 minutes. ➤*Rationale:* This prevents cloths from warming and losing effectiveness.

5. Cool the ambient temperature to 68°–72°F. ➤*Rationale:* This enhances therapy by convection and evaporation.
6. Direct a warm fan onto client to promote evaporation. ➤*Rationale:* This enhances cooling by evaporation.
7. Observe client for early signs of shivering (ECG tremor artifact, facial muscle twitching).
8. Stop treatment if client begins to shiver and notify physician. ➤*Rationale:* Shivering raises core temperature, defeating purpose of cooling intervention. The physician may order IV medication such as chlorpromazine.
9. Monitor client's temperature frequently. When temperature has decreased to desired level, dry skin and replace light covering over client and reposition for comfort. ➤*Rationale:* A thin client will cool faster than one with more subcutaneous fat.
10. Continue to monitor vital signs, cardiac rhythm, I&O, and blood pressure.
11. Provide fluids and a high-calorie diet. ➤*Rationale:* Increased temperatures cause an increased metabolic rate. Carbohydrates, proteins, and 2500–3000 mL fluid intake is essential for maintaining homeostasis.
12. Place cloths in linen hamper and return equipment to utility or storage area.
13. Perform hand hygiene.

### CLINICAL ALERT

Do not immerse the client in cold or ice slush. Resulting peripheral vasoconstriction will impair body cooling and induce shivering which produces heat.

# Skill 1.9   Monitoring an Infant Radiant Warmer

## Equipment

Radiant warmer with skin or rectal probe
Bedding appropriate for warmer

## Preparation

1. Several different radiant warmers, or infant care centers, are available. Follow the manufacturer's operating instructions for safety and to determine if a manual or proportional controller is used. (General operating instructions and protocols are presented here.)
2. Check caster locks to make certain that each caster is in locked position.
3. Adjust procedure table to desired position.
4. Plug line cord into a three-wire receptacle.

5. Turn power switch ON; the red pilot light and the alarm indicator should glow. Turn alarm switch ON to test alarm system.
6. Turn manual knob to automatic.
7. Install skin or rectal probe in controller and set switch to either rectal or skin, depending on which probe is being used.
8. Warm unit for 7 minutes.
9. Adjust temperature to degree ordered; temperature is dialed on digital temperature set switch.
10. Perform hand hygiene.

## Procedure

1. Check two forms of infant ID.
2. Place infant in warmer.

3. Attach skin probe.
   a. Place 1-cm skin probe with polished surface touching skin to left of the umbilicus.
   b. Use a rectal probe is hospital protocol permits.
4. Monitor placement of skin probe.
   a. Inspect infant's skin under probe at regular intervals. ➤*Rationale:* Infant's skin is delicate and irritates easily.
   b. Change the probe location is irritation begins to appear.
   c. Do not use adhesive tape or pads. ➤*Rationale:* These may cause skin irritation or allergic reactions. Infant's skin is very thin and fragile.
5. Allow 3–5 minutes for probe to reach infant's temperature.
6. Activate audible alarm by setting switch to ON. ➤*Rationale:* If the infant's temperature exceeds 102 degrees F (38.8 degrees C), the audible alarm sounds and the visible alarm light flashes.
7. Perform hand hygiene.

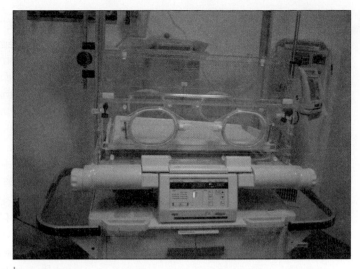

● Type 2: Infant radiant warmer used to maintain body temperature—used without clothes on infant.

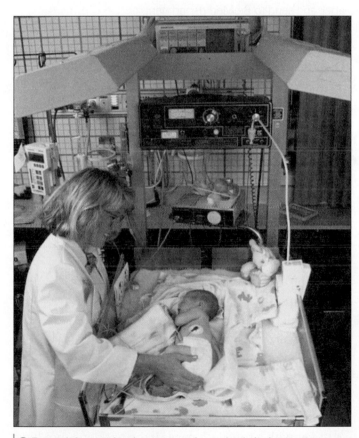

● Type 1: Infant overhead warmer used to maintain body temperature.

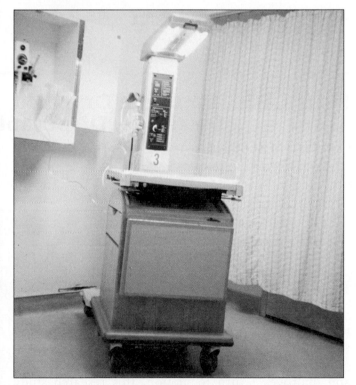

● Type 3: Infant warmer most often used in birthing room to maintain body heat while examining newborn.

## ▌ LEGAL ALERT

*Salter v. Deaconess Family Medicine Center* (1999). The nurse and hospital were found liable for injuries to an infant's foot following a nurse's application of a wet washcloth which had been heated for one full minute in a microwave oven then applied to the infant's heel to facilitate drawing blood. Application of the hot cloth was the proximate cause of second-degree burns to the infant's heel.

*Source:* Westlaw.com

| UNEXPECTED OUTCOMES | CRITICAL THINKING OPTIONS |
|---|---|
| Client experiences pain, asks about alternative measures for relief. | • Cold therapy may be an option, or heat/cold alternating therapy as counterirritants; these therapies alter nerve transmission.<br>• Assess if application is too hot.<br>• Ensure that temperature is not over 110 degrees F (43.3 degrees C) if heating pad is used. |
| Swelling is not reduced with heat therapy. | • Ensure that acute inflammation is not present, as heat therapy is contraindicated during this phase, but is beneficial for subacute and chronic inflammation.<br>• Reassess to determine that area being treated has sufficient circulation.<br>• Reinforce importance of resting area until swelling is reduced.<br>• Consult physician regarding discontinuation of therapy after a 2-day trial and possible need for anti-inflammatory medication or reevaluation. |
| Aquathermic pump signals "Over Temp." | • Check reservoir water level; it may be low or empty.<br>• Be sure to use room temperature (not hot) distilled water in reservoir. Check that hoses are not kinked or hose clamps closed. |
| Pump continues to signal "Over Temp" after previous actions. | • Disconnect, label, and send to BioMed department.<br>• Obtain a different pump. |

# Skill 1.10   Applying Dry Cold Measures: Ice Bag, Ice Collar, Ice Glove, Disposable Cold Pack

## EXPECTED OUTCOMES

• Inflammatory response is controlled.
• Bleeding and edema are reduced/controlled.
• Local anesthestic response is achieved.
• Local cryotherapy causes no undesired effects.
• Core body temperature is reduced.

## EVIDENCE-BASED NURSING PRACTICE

**Postoperative Cold Therapy**

While several studies have demonstrated that the use of cold over compression reduces bleeding and swelling and improves return to motion, this research study concludes that compression is just as effective as cold post total knee surgery, and is more cost effective.

*Source:* Smith, J., et al. (2002). A randomized, controlled trial comparing compression bandaging and cold therapy in postoperative total knee replacement surgery. *Orthopaedic Nursing,* 21(2), 61–66.

## Delegation

Application of certain cold measures (e.g., cooling baths) may be delegated to UAP if they meet the general criteria for delegation. However, in all cases, assessment of the client and the determination that the measure is safe to employ are the responsibility of the nurse. UAP may observe the area being treated during usual care and must report abnormal findings to the nurse. Abnormal findings must be validated and interpreted by the nurse.

## Equipment

• Ice bag, collar, glove, or cold pack
• Ice chips
• Protective covering
• Roller gauze, a binder or a towel, and tape

## VARIATION: Disposable Cold Pack

• Strike, squeeze, or knead the cold pack according to the manufacturer's instructions. ▶*Rationale: The action activates the chemical reaction that produces the cold.*
• Cover with a soft cloth cover if the pack does not have a cover. Most commercially prepared cold packs have soft outer coverings to permit application directly to the body part.
1. Instruct the client as follows:
   • Remain in position for the duration of the treatment.
   • Call the nurse if discomfort is felt.
2. Monitor the client during the application.
   • Assess the client in terms of comfort and skin reaction (e.g., pallor, mottled appearance) as frequently as necessary for the client's safety (e.g., every 5 to 10 minutes).

## CLINICAL ALERT

Never apply a fully cooled reusable cold pack directly to the skin; also do not over insulate the area.

Bony areas (knee, ankle, elbow) usually require half the treatment time as fatty areas. Superficial nerves at these joint sites are especially vulnerable to cold-induced neuropathy, especially if cold is combined with compression.

Check more often if client has had previous negative responses to applications and or client has difficulty reporting problems.

- Report untoward reactions and remove the application. Disposable ice bag.

### Procedure

1. Prior to performing the procedure, introduce self and verify the client's identity using agency protocol. Explain to the client what you are going to do, why it is necessary, and how he or she can participate. Discuss how the results will be used in planning further care or treatments.
2. Perform hand hygiene and observe other appropriate infection control procedures.
3. Provide for client privacy.
   - Expose only the area to be treated, and provide warmth to avoid chilling.
4. Prepare the client.
   - Assist the client to a comfortable position, and support the body part requiring the application.
5. Apply the cold measure.

### VARIATION: Ice Bag, Collar, or Glove

- Fill the device one-half to two-thirds full of crushed ice. ➤*Rationale:Partial filling makes the device more pliable so that it can be molded to a body part.*
- Remove excess air by bending or twisting the device. ➤*Rationale: Air inflates the device so that it cannot be molded to the body part.*
- Insert the stopper securely into an ice bag or collar, or tie a knot at the open end of a glove. ➤*Rationale: This prevents leakage of fluid when the ice melts.*

## CLINICAL ALERT

Do not apply an instant chemical pack to the face and never use pins to secure pack. Leakage of chemical contents can cause serious injury. In contents are exposed to skin, immediately flush with copious amount of water and notify physician.

- Hold the device upside down, and check it for leaks.
- Cover the device with a soft cloth cover, if it is not already equipped with one. ➤*Rationale: The cover absorbs moisture that condenses on the outside of the device. It is also more comfortable for the client.*
- Hold the device in place with roller gauze, ties, a binder, or a towel. Secure with tape as necessary.
1. Leave the cold in place for only the designated period of time. ➤*Rationale: Avoid the rebound phenomenon and the harmful effects of prolonged cold.*
2. Document the application of the cold and the client's response in the client record using forms or checklists supplemented by narrative notes when appropriate.

### Documentation

Sample: 3/30/09 2245 Rt foot and ankle swollen toes to lower calf. Reports pain is 7/10. Moves toes and ankle, pedal pulses present. Skin warm, no bruising or wounds noted. Padded ice pack applied ×10 minutes. Reports pain 5/10.
_____ P. Wilder, RN

## CLINICAL ALERT

- Gel packs provide more aggressive cooling than ice bags, so deserve greater caution.
- During cold therapy, erythema will occur.
- The client will experience four stages of cold progression: cold/stinging/burning/numbness.
- Discontinue therapy upon numbness.

# Skill 1.11 Using a Cooling Blanket

## EVIDENCE-BASED NURSING PRACTICE

**Hypothermia Improves Stroke Outcome**

A study of stroke patients indicates that induced hypothermia to 32°C for a 3-hour period with cooling blankets and ice water/alcohol bath improved outcomes. Hypothermia reduces ischemic damage and reperfusion injury following thrombolysis, and reduces bleeding risk associated with administration of tPA. It may also help prevent hyperthermia associated with shift of the third ventricle during an intracerebral hemorrhage.

*Source:* Mitka, M. (2001). Playing it cool in stroke research. *Journal of the American Medical Association, 285*(10), 1282.

## Equipment

Thermal (heating/cooling) unit
Distilled water
Rectal thermometer probe and lubricant, tympanic,
  or temporal artery thermometer
Clean gloves
Disposable thermal (cooling) blanket
1 sheet or thin blanket
Covering for client
4 towels
Tape
Lower extremity (or foot) compression wraps
Sphygmomanometer
Stethoscope
Continuous ECG monitoring (if indicated)
Supplemental oxygen therapy equipment

## Preparation

1. Check physician's orders for desired client temperature.
2. Identify medications client has received (narcotic, sedative).
3. Gather equipment and take to client's room.
4. Connect power cord to grounded outlet.
5. Ensure that reservoir (distilled water) level is adequate.
6. Perform hand hygiene.
7. Identify client using two forms of ID and explain procedure.
8. Provide privacy.
9. Obtain baseline vital signs.

## Procedure

1. Place the cooling blanket on bed, and connect it to the machine. ➤*Rationale:* The cooling blanket increases heat transfer from client and reduces body temperature by conduction.
   a. Push the tubing tab to insert male tubing connector of the cooling pad into inlet opening. Release the tab.
   b. Repeat connection using the outlet opening.
   c. Turn the unit ON by pushing power switch.
2. Place a sheet or a thin bath blanket over the cooling blanket.
3. Place client on the cooling blanket. Wrap client's legs and feet in compression wraps. ➤*Rationale:* This helps to prevent thrombus formation and reduces edema.
4. Wrap client's lower arms and hands and lower legs and feet (and scrotum if indicated) in towels and tape to secure. ➤*Rationale:* This provides insulation to prevent tissue injury and prevents stimulation of skin thermoreceptors that initiate shivering.
5. Set the master temperature control to either automatic or manual operation. ➤*Rationale:* There are two separate temperature controls, one for automatic and one for manual operation.

*For Automatic Control*

   a. Don clean gloves.
   b. Insert lubricated temperature probe into client's rectum 2 inches.
   c. Set temperature control at the desired temperature (fluid temperature set point).
   d. Turn automatic mode light on and press "START."
      ➤*Rationale:* The pad fluid temperature will adjust automatically to bring client's temperature to a selected set point.
   e. Check that the pad temperature limits are set as ordered.
   f. Remove and clean rectal probe every 4 hours.

*For Manual Control*

   a. Don clean gloves.
   b. Insert lubricated temperature probe into client's rectum 2 inches.
   c. Observe that the manual mode light is on.
   d. Monitor the fluid set point, which indicates temperature of pad. ➤*Rationale:* This ensures pad temperature is maintained at desired level.

6. Set the temperature control to 37°C, and begin lowering temperature 1°C every 15 minutes until 33° or 34°C is reached (or set temperature as ordered). ➤*Rationale:* Thermal blanket will cool client at this temperature independent of client's temperature.
7. Monitor client's temperature every 15 minutes. ➤*Rationale:* To prevent excessive cooling. Tympanic measurement reflects core temperature since the hypothalamus and tympanic membrane share a common blood supply.
8. Observe client for signs predicting onset of shivering: ECG muscle tremor artifact, visible facial muscle twitchings, hyperventilation, and verbalized sensations. Palpate jaw line for a "hum" sensation.
9. If manifestations of shivering occur discontinue therapy and notify physician. ➤*Rationale:* Shivering causes an increase in core temperature, thus defeating the purpose of treatment. Shivering imposes a heavy metabolic burden. Oxygen consumption doubles.

| CLASSIFICATION OF HYPOTHERMIA | | |
|---|---|---|
| Mild | 32°–37°C | 89.6°–98.6°F |
| Moderate | 28°–32°C | 82.4°–89.6°F |
| Severe | 20°–28°C | 68.0°–82.4°F |

10. While client undergoes hypothermia, monitor vital signs every 15–30 minutes during reduction of temperature control and then every 2 hours. ➤*Rationale:* Monitoring allows for continual evaluation of client response.
11. Monitor ECG if the client has cardiac disease (possible arrhythmias) or hypokalemia. ➤*Rationale:* Serum potassium levels fluctuate with induced hypothermia.
12. Observe obese clients for fluid balance alterations.
13. Monitor client's serum glucose. ➤*Rationale:* Insulin levels are decreased with induced hypothermia. Glucose levels may rise with shivering.
14. Remove and clean rectal temperature probe every 4 hours.
15. Check physician's order for compression wraps. ➤*Rationale:* To prevent venous stasis.
16. Turn and deep-breathe client every 30 minutes.
17. Monitor client's skin condition and bony prominences every 2 hours. ➤*Rationale:* Client is at risk for pressure ulcers when skin temperature is lowered.
18. Turn off unit when client's temperature is 1°–3°C above desired temperature. ➤*Rationale:* Cooling will continue upon discontinuation of therapy.

> ## CLINICAL ALERT
> Effectiveness and safety of cooling blankets for treatment of fever are poorly demonstrated. They may be dangerous in some instances. Use of cooling blanket is discouraged except for environmental hyperthermia.

19. Monitor vital signs every 15 minutes during warming.
20. Observe for edema. ➤*Rationale:* This is caused by increased cell permeability, acidosis due to shivering, fluid imbalance, and hypothermia.
21. Clean and return equipment to central supply following use. Dispose of blanket.
22. Monitor client's vital signs frequently after discontinuation of treatment. Overshoot hypothermia may occur.
23. Make client comfortable.
24. Perform hand hygiene.

| UNEXPECTED OUTCOMES | CRITICAL THINKING OPTIONS |
|---|---|
| Local edema is not reduced. | • Elevate extremity above level of heart.<br>• Ensure that body surface is sufficiently covered with cold application to cause vasoconstriction. Check that area is not overinsulated. |
| Bleeding continues even with cold applications. | • Reassess area for possible "bleeders," which may require cautery or ligation by the physician.<br>• Apply pressure to site to stop bleeding.<br>• Assess pulse distal to bleed. |
| Area to be treated is near superficial nerve. | • Use caution: reduce time and duration of cold application.<br>• Ask client to report any itching or tingling and discontinue therapy if these occur. |
| Hand develops waxy white sheen, mottling, and blisters during local ice therapy. | • Immerse part in moving water at 40°–42°C until area flushes (about 30 minutes).<br>• Do not apply dry heat, keep area uncovered at room temperature.<br>• Do not rub part; keep part elevated. |
| Cold cycling pad is not cooling properly. | • Examine if pad or hose is folded or kinked.<br>• Determine if securing straps are too tight and restricting flow of cold water.<br>• Make sure pump inside cooler is completely covered with ice water.<br>• Check all connections between hose and treatment pad.<br>• If still not cooling properly, disconnect, label and send to BioMed.<br>• Obtain different machine. |
| Client's core temperature decreases rapidly to desired level. | • Turn off cooling blanket or discontinue tepid sponging. |

*(continued)*

| UNEXPECTED OUTCOMES (cont.) | CRITICAL THINKING OPTIONS (cont.) |
|---|---|
| Client begins to shiver. | • Stop the procedure or warm the solution a few degrees (or both).<br>• Monitor temperature because shivering causes an increase in the metabolic rate leading to an increase in heat production.<br>• Monitor temperature every 15 minutes to detect additional temperature decrease.<br>• Contact physician for medication order (narcotic or sedative agent).<br>• Provide supplemental oxygen therapy. |
| Client's core temperature is not reduced. | • Discuss need for cold water spray and warm air fan to reduce client's temperature.<br>• Consider that cutaneous vasoconstriction due to external cooling may be conserving core body heat.<br>• Discuss need for more aggressive internal cooling measures (e.g., cold peritoneal lavage). |
| Cooling blanket does not function properly. | • Check that plug is connected to the outlet.<br>• Check that the fluid level is sufficient and that unit freezing has not occurred.<br>• Check that the thermistor probe is properly connected.<br>• Check that the cool limit on the pad is not set too high.<br>• Check that there is no constriction through pads or tubing. |

# THE PHYSIOLOGIC NEEDS OF THE DYING CLIENT

Nurses may interact with dying clients and their families or caregivers in a variety of settings, from fetal demise (death of an unborn child), to the adolescent victim of an accident, to the elderly client who finally succumbs to a chronic illness. Death can be viewed as a person's final opportunity to experience life in ways that bring significance and fulfillment. It is the nurse's role to provide or facilitate physical, emotional, and spiritual care of the dying client and the client's family.

Caring for the dying and the bereaved (those persons mourning the dead) is one of the nurse's most complex and challenging responsibilities, bringing into play all skills needed for holistic physiologic and psychosocial care. This skills chapter emphasizes physical care. It is beyond the scope of the chapter to address in detail, theoretical concepts such as grief and grieving or legal aspects such as the process of organ donation and living wills. The reader is referred to a fundamentals or concepts book for additional material.

**EXPECTED OUTCOMES**
• Client is able to progress through stages of grief with support of family and nursing staff.
• Client is accepting of loss and eventual outcome of grief process.
• Client is as pain free as possible.
• Client's cultural beliefs are considered throughout the dying process.
• Client found internal sources to support acceptance of death.
• Family members are supported throughout the dying process.

## CLINICAL ALERT

The goal of care for the dying client changes from curative to palliative care. Helping the client achieve a measure of comfort and knowing that family members are significant others are being supported during this process is a comfort for the client.

# Skill 1.12   Meeting the Physiological Needs of the Dying Client

## Delegation

Comfort measures and supportive care strategies for care of clients at the end of life are often delegated to unlicensed assistive personnel (UAP). The nurse reviews with the UAP those measures and strategies needed for a specific client. UAPs must inform the nurse if the client appears in unanticipated or unrelieved distress.

## Equipment

* Needed equipment depends on the specific comfort measures being provided. Items may include medications, linens, and hygiene supplies.

## Preparation

* The physiologic needs of people who are dying are related to a slowing of body processes and to homeostatic imbalances. Interventions include providing personal hygiene measures; controlling pain; relieving respiratory difficulties; assisting with movement, nutrition, hydration, and elimination; and providing measures related to sensory changes.

## Procedure

1. Introduce self and verify the client's identity using agency protocol. Explain to the client what you are going to do, why it is necessary, and how he or she can participate. Discuss how the results will be used in planning further care or treatments.
2. Perform hand hygiene and observe other appropriate infection control procedures.
3. Provide for client privacy depending on the specific interventions.
4. Perform bathing/hygiene.
   * Provide frequent baths and linen changes if diaphoretic, incontinent, or need for odor control. ➤*Rationale: Dying persons may have wounds, fever, or loss of sphincter control that are both uncomfortable when substances are left on the skin and cause distressing smells.*
   * Give mouth care as needed for dry mouth.
   * Apply moisturizing creams and lotions for dry skin, and moisture-barrier skin preparations for incontinent clients.
   * Cleanse skin areas around wounds or that collect wound drainage.

5. Provide pain control.
   * Pain control is essential to enable clients to maintain some quality in their life and their daily activities, including eating, moving, and sleeping. Many drugs have been used to control the pain associated with terminal illness: morphine, heroin, methadone, and alcohol.
   * Usually the primary care provider determines the dosage, but the client's opinion should be considered; the client is the one ultimately aware of personal pain tolerance and fluctuations of internal states. Because primary care providers usually prescribe a range for the dosage of pain medication, nurses use their own judgment as to the specific amount and frequency of pain medication needed to provide client relief.
   * Because of decreased blood circulation, if analgesics cannot be administered orally, they are given by intravenous infusion, sublingually, or rectally, rather than subcutaneously or intramuscularly. ➤*Rationale: Subcutaneous or intramuscular injections given to clients with impaired circulation will not reach the desired receptors and, thus, will be ineffective.*
   * Clients on narcotic pain medications also require implementation of a protocol to treat opioid-induced constipation.
   * Under periods of stress, the brain releases endorphins, morphine-like substances that modulate pain perception. Although studied primarily in animal models and in near-death experiences, some scientists believe that large amounts of endorphins may be released at the time of death. This could explain the seemingly peaceful sense of dissociation from the reality of pain, floating outside the body, seeing a tunnel, or moving toward the light that is expressed by some persons.
6. Provide respiratory support.
   * For clients with difficulty clearing their own airway, place in Fowler's position if conscious, lateral position if unconscious. ➤*Rationale: Fowler's position makes breathing easier. The lateral position allows secretions to drain out rather than entering the client's airway.*
   * Perform oral throat suctioning as needed, especially for conscious clients who express discomfort.
   * Apply nasal oxygen for hypoxic clients. ➤*Rationale: Supplemental oxygen may relieve the signs and symptoms of oxygen deprivation such as confusion.*

- Anticholinergic medications (e.g., atropine, hyoscine hydrobromide) may be indicated to help dry secretions. Note that noisy respirations, sometimes referred to as the *death rattle* are believed to be more distressing to those who have to listen to the sounds than the condition is for the dying client.
- For clients who have air hunger (the sensation of needing to breathe), open windows or use a fan to circulate air. Morphine may be indicated in an acute episode.

7. Assist with movement.
   - Assist client out of bed periodically, if able.
   - Regularly change client's position.
   - Support client's position with pillows, blanket rolls, or towels as needed.
   - Elevate client's legs when sitting up.
   - Implement pressure ulcer prevention program and use pressure-relieving surfaces as indicated.

8. Provide nutrition and hydration.
   - Administer antiemetics or a small amount of an alcoholic beverage to stimulate appetite.
   - Encourage favorite foods as tolerated.
   - Support family members who may be very concerned that their loved one is not eating or drinking and that failure to push nutrition signifies giving up and failure. In some states, a feeding tube cannot be removed from a person in a PVS without a prior directive from the client, but in other states the removal is allowed at the family's request or a physician's order.
   - Teach family that clients with dehydration and alterations in electrolytes at the end of life may not be experiencing discomfort. In addition, dehydration actually reduces secretions and the need for elimination.

9. Assist with elimination.
   - For constipation, provide dietary fiber as tolerated, stool softeners or laxatives as needed.
   - Perform meticulous skin care in response to incontinence of urine or feces.
   - Keep the bedpan, urinal, or commode chair within easy reach and the call light within reach for assistance onto bedpan or commode.
   - Use absorbent pads under incontinent clients; change linen as often as needed.
   - Urinary catheterization may be performed, if necessary.
   - Keep the room as clean and odor-free as possible.

10. Be aware of sensory changes.
    - Check the client's preference for a light or dark room. Position to be able to view the television, favorite items or photos, or a window as desired.
    - Hearing is not diminished; speak clearly and do not whisper. Use music as desired.
    - Touch sensation is diminished, but client will feel pressure of touch.
    - Provide gown, clothing, and bedding that feels and looks as the client prefers.
    - Facilitate client interaction with others as desired. This may require flexing agency rules regarding visiting hours or presence of pets. Advocate for the client as much as possible about these.
    - Implement a pain management protocol if indicated; medicate for other sensory alterations such as itching.

11. Family members should be encouraged to participate in the physical care of the dying person as much as they wish to and are able. The nurse can suggest they assist with bathing, speak or read to the client, and hold hands. The nurse must not, however, have specific expectations for family members' participation. Those who feel unable to care for or be with the dying person also require support from the nurse and from other family members. They should be shown an appropriate waiting area if they wish to remain nearby.

12. Sometimes, it seems as if the client is "holding on," possibly out of concern for the family not being ready. It may be therapeutic for both the client and the family for the family to verbally give permission to the client to "let go," to die when he or she is ready. This is a painful process, and the nurse must be prepared to encourage and support the family through saying their last good-byes.

13. Consider how routine care should be modified based on the dying client. Often vital signs are measured less frequently, blood and other laboratory tests no longer performed, and active, invasive, or expensive treatment measures (such as antibiotics for infection) suspended. Caring for dying clients who have agreed to organ donation can also be complex in terms of determining which medications, treatments, or equipment must be continued until the time for harvesting the organs has arrived.

14. Document all client care, especially the effectiveness of symptom management activities.

## Documentation

Sample: 12/20/09 23:30

S  "I am so tired. Please don't make me turn right now. Could you give me some ice chips?"

O  Lotion and massage to reachable back and extremities. Repositioned slightly to shift weight off bony prominences. Ice chips given and placed within reach.

A  Care modified to support dying client autonomy.

P  Turn q 3 h instead of q 2 if the client prefers. Reinforce need to assess and treat dependent skin areas. Assess need for analgesics before each turn. Request pressure-reducing mattress.

_____ S. Amber, RN

## CLINICAL MANIFESTATIONS

### Impending Clinical Death

#### Loss of Muscle Tone

- Relaxation of the facial muscles (e.g., the jaw may sag)
- Difficulty speaking
- Difficulty swallowing and gradual loss of the gag reflex
- Decreased activity of the gastrointestinal tract, with subsequent nausea, accumulation of flatus, abdominal distention, and retention of feces, especially if narcotics or tranquilizers are being administered
- Possible urinary and rectal incontinence due to decreased sphincter control
- Diminished body movement

#### Slowing of the Circulation

- Diminished sensation
- Mottling and cyanosis of the extremities

- Cold skin, first in the feet and later in the hands, ears, and nose (the client, however, may feel warm if there is a fever)
- Slower and weaker pulse
- Decreased blood pressure

#### Changes in Respirations

- Rapid, shallow, irregular, or abnormally slow respirations
- Noisy breathing, referred to as the death rattle, due to collecting of mucus in the throat
- Mouth breathing, dry oral mucous membranes

#### Sensory Impairment

- Blurred vision
- Impaired senses of taste and smell
- Various consciousness levels may exist just before death. Some clients are alert, whereas others are drowsy, stuporous, or comatose. Hearing is thought to be the last sense lost.

---

### CLIENT TEACHING CONSIDERATIONS

Caregivers of a dying person need ongoing support and ongoing teaching as the client's condition changes. Some of these teaching needs include:

- Ways to feed the client when swallowing becomes difficult.
- Ways to transfer and reposition the client safely.
- Ways to communicate if verbalization becomes more difficult.
- Nonpharmacological methods of pain control.
- Comfort measures, such as frequent oral care and frequent repositioning.

### SETTING OF CARE

People facing death may need help accepting that they have to depend on others. Some dying clients require only minimal care; others need continuous attention and services. People need help, well in advance of death, in planning for the period of dependence. They need to consider what will happen and how and where they would like to die.

A major factor in determining whether a person will die in a health care facility or at home is the availability of willing and able caregivers. If the dying person wishes to be at home, and family or others can provide care to maintain symptom control, the nurse should facilitate a referral to outpatient hospice services. Hospice staff and nurses will then conduct a full assessment of the home and care providers' skills.

---

 ## CULTURAL CONSIDERATIONS

Singer and Blackhall, in the article, "Negotiating Cross-Cultural Issues at the End of Life," state that culture is an important part of how everyone understands their world and how this impacts their decisions, especially on health care issues. This includes health care professionals as well. Cultural influences the way people make meaning out of illness and dying; therefore, it also influences how they utilize the medical community at the end of life. Each individual has a perspective that is also influenced by factors such as personal psychology, gender, and life experiences. There is a wide variation of beliefs and behaviors within any ethnic population. This leads us to realize that each client needs to be treated individually. Health care

professional must not influence clients with their own beliefs or cultures. Failure to take the client's cultural background seriously means we fail to understand the values held by the client

Lack of cultural sensitivity and skills can lead to inappropriate clinical outcomes and poor interaction with clients and families at a very crucial point in their end-of-life process. Addressing and respecting cultural differences will increase trust, leading to a more satisfactory end-of-life process for both the client and the family.

*Source:* Kagawa-Singer, M. & Blackhall, I. J. (2001), December 19). Negotiating cross-cultural issues at the end of life. *Journal of the American Medical Association.* 286 (23), 2992–3001.

## CULTURAL DIVERSITY AT THE END OF LIFE

The 2000 census revealed that whites make up about 65% of the U.S. population; 13% are black; 13% are Hispanic; 4.5% are Asian-Pacific Islander; and 1.5% are American-Indian/Alaskan native. The remaining 2.5% list themselves as bi-ethnic. With the makeup of the United States changing, health care workers must become more aware of how cultural factors influence clients' reactions to serious illness and how they make decisions and cope with end-of-life issues. There are three basic dimensions in end-of-life treatment that vary culturally; communications of "bad news"; locus of decision-making; and attitudes toward advance directives and end-of-life care. Many ethnic health care workers conceal adverse diagnoses from clients, believing that it is disrespectful, impolite, or even harmful to the client. Decisions on end-of-life care are most often made by the family or the family in consultation with the physician, not the client. Advance Directives are usually not completed by specific ethnic minority clients because they have a distrust of the U.S. health care system.

*Source:* Searight, R., & Galford, J. (2005, February 1). Cultural diversity at the end of life: Issues and guidelines for family physicians. *American Family Physician,* 71(3).

## Skill 1.13  Performing Postmortem Care

### EXPECTED OUTCOMES
- Postmortem care is completed maintaining client's dignity.
- Client's relatives are supported by staff during grief process.
- Appropriate procedures are carried out for organ donations.

### Delegation

Postmortem care can be delegated to UAPs after the activities described above have been completed so that the UAP knows what tubes or other medical devices can be removed or other special care provided.

### Equipment

- Shroud or other linens used by the agency to wrap the body
- Washcloths, towels
- Absorbent pads
- Clean gloves
- Patient gown (if the family will be viewing the body)
- Bags for personal belongings and the medical record document used to record transfer of the belongings and valuables

### Preparation

- Consider whether more than one person is needed to perform the postmortem care since turning the body is involved. For caregivers who are performing postmortem care for the first time, it is especially advised that at least two caregivers work together to provide the care.
- Postmortem care can be time consuming. Arrange for someone to cover the caregiver's other clients during this time.

## EVIDENCE-BASED NURSING PRACTICE

**Critical Care Family Needs Inventory**
A meta-analysis of several studies using the Critical Care Family Needs Inventory led to a summary of the ten most important needs of families of critically ill dying clients:

1. To be with the person.
2. To be helpful to the dying person.
3. To be informed of the dying person's changing condition.
4. To understand what is being done to the client and why.
5. To be assured of the client's comfort.
6. To be comforted.
7. To ventilate emotions.
8. To be assured that their decisions were right.
9. To find meaning in the dying of their loved one.
10. To be fed, hydrated, and rested.

Aspects of major recommendations based upon the review include preparation of the client, family and clinical team; ensuring the comfort of the client; withdrawal of life-sustaining treatments; terminal extubation versus terminal wean; special issues in communicating with families near the time of death; special ethical issues.

*Source:* Truog, R.D., Cist, A.F., Brackett, S. E., Burns, J. P., Curley, M. A., Danis, M., et al. (2001, December). Recommendations for end-of-life care in the intensive care unit: The Ethics Committee of the Society of Critical Care Medicine. *Critical Care Medical,* 2332–2348.

## Procedure

1. Observe appropriate infection control procedures. Apply clean gloves.
2. Because the deceased person's family often wants to view the body immediately after death, and because it is important that the deceased appear natural and comfortable, nurses need to position the body, place dentures in the mouth, and close the eyes and mouth before rigor mortis sets in.
   - Normally the body is placed in a supine position with the arms either at the sides, palms down, or across the abdomen.
   - After blood circulation has ceased, the red blood cells break down, releasing hemoglobin, which discolors the surrounding tissues. This discoloration, referred to as livor mortis, appears in the lowermost or dependent areas of the body. One pillow is placed under the head and shoulders to prevent blood from discoloring the face by settling in it.
   - The eyelids are closed and held in place for a few seconds so they remain closed.
   - Dentures are usually inserted to help give the face a natural appearance. The mouth is then closed.

   *If the body will be viewed in the hospital:*
   - Place a clean gown on the client, and brush and comb the hair.
   - Adjust the top bed linens neatly to cover the client to the shoulders.
   - Provide tissues, soft lighting, and chairs for the family.
3. If the deceased's family or friends wish to view the body immediately after death, it is important to make the environment as clean and pleasant as possible and to make the body appear natural and comfortable. All equipment, soiled linen, and supplies should be removed from the bedside.
4. Some agencies require that all tubes in the body remain in place; in other agencies, tubes may be cut to within 2.5 cm (1 in.) of the skin and taped in place; in others, all tubes may be removed. In some cases, if a central IV line is in place, it may be left to assist with the process of preserving the body (embalming) (Marthaler, 2005). Use the same careful handling you would use with a living body. ▶*Rationale: As the body cools, the skin loses its elasticity and can easily be broken when removing dressings and adhesive tape.*
5. Soiled areas of the body are washed; however, a complete bath is not necessary, because the body will be washed by the mortician (also referred to as an undertaker), a person trained in care of the dead.
6. Absorbent pads are placed under the buttocks to take up any feces and urine released because of relaxation of the sphincter muscles.
7. Remove all jewelry, except a wedding band in some instances, which is taped to the finger.
8. The deceased's wrist identification tag is left on. After the body has been viewed by the family, additional identification tags are applied. ▶*Rationale: Mislabeling can create legal problems if the body is inappropriately identified and prepared incorrectly for burial or a funeral.*
9. Wrap the body in a shroud, a large piece of plastic or cotton material used to enclose a body after death. Apply identification to the outside of the shroud.
   - If the dentures were placed in the mouth for the viewing, secure the jaw with a strap or remove them so they do not fall out as the mouth muscles relax (Beattie, 2006).
   - Remove and discard gloves. Perform hand hygiene.

### CLINICAL ALERT

Inform the funeral home if the client has tuberculosis or any other infectious disease so appropriate care can be taken to prevent contamination of the environment.

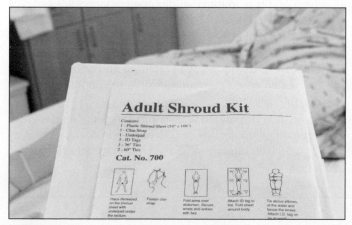

● Shroud contents.

● A body wrapped in a shroud.

10. Take the body to the morgue if arrangements have not been made to have a mortician pick it up from the client's room. Nurses have a duty to handle the deceased with dignity and to label the body appropriately. ➤*Rationale: Mishandling can cause emotional distress to survivors.*

11. Document the postmortem care in the client record and on forms designed for this purpose. Include what items were removed from the body, whether the body was viewed by the family, and whether the body was taken to the morgue or picked up from the room.

**UNEXPECTED OUTCOMES**

Client is not identified properly when sent to the morgue

Donated organs are needed

**CRITICAL THINKING OPTIONS**

- Check identaband and shroud label before releasing client to mortician
- Request another nurse to check labels
- Provide support to family and give an opportunity for questions.
- Obtain signatures for consent form (Kidneys should be removed within 1 hour after death. Eyes should be removed within 6–24 hours after death.)
- Examine reverse side of driver's license, or remind the charge nurse to call mortician if burial plans have been made previously, to check on permission for organ donation through a living will.

## DEVELOPMENTAL CONSIDERATIONS

### Children

- Children's response to death or loss depends on the messages they get from adults and others around them as well as their understanding of death. When adults are able to cope effectively with a death, they are more likely to be able to support children through the process.
- Comprehension of death evolves as the person develops.
- From infancy to 5 years: the child does not understand concept of death. An infant's sense of separation forms basis for later understanding of loss and death. They believe death is reversible, a temporary departure, or sleep.
- 5 to 9 years: Understands that death is final. Believes own death can be avoided. Associates death with aggression or violence. Believes wishes or unrelated actions can be responsible for death.
- 9 to 12 years: Understands death as the inevitable end of life. Begins to understand own mortality, expressed as interest in afterlife or as fear of death.
- 12 to 18 years: Fears a lingering death. May fantasize that death can be defied, acting out defiance through reckless behaviors (e.g., dangerous driving, substance abuse). Seldom thinks about death, but views it in religious and philosophic terms. May seem to reach "adult" perception of death but be emotionally unable to accept it. May still hold concepts from previous developmental stages.

- One of the saddest situations is that of parents who experience the death of a child. They will likely feel shock, disbelief, and many other emotions. The nurse supports the parents by giving concrete and specific information about the child's condition, arranging for the parents to be close to the child for extended time as they desire, and facilitating parent participation in the child's care (Ball, & Bindler, 2008). The challenges of providing "competent, compassionate, and consistent care that meets their physical, emotional, and spiritual needs" to dying children and their families has been well described in a report by the Institute of Medicine (Field & Behrman, 2003), available to read free online.

### Elders

- Elders who are dying often have a need to know that their lives had meaning. An excellent way to assure them of this is to make audiotapes or videotapes of them telling stories of their lives. This gives the client a sense of value and worth and also lets him or her know that family members and friends will also benefit from it. Doing this with children and grandchildren often eases communication and support during this difficult time.
- Elders fear prolonged illness and see death as having multiple meanings (e.g., freedom from pain, or reunion with already deceased family members).

**Three Out of Four Elderly People Die of Heart Disease, Cancer, or Stroke**

- Heart disease is leading cause of death, although it has declined since 1968.
- Death rates from cancer have decreased, but lung cancer has increased in women.
- Death statistics for people in the 65–74 age group: heart disease accounted for 38%; cancer, 30% of deaths.
- Two thirds of hospice clients are over 65 years of age.

**Death in the Life Cycle**

- In American culture, the obsession with youth often results in denial of death as a natural phase of the life cycle, and death is not considered a positive process.
- Elderly may see death as an end of suffering and loneliness.
- Death is usually not feared if the person has lived a long and fulfilled life, having completed all developmental tasks.
- Spiritual beliefs or philosophy of life are important.

 # CULTURAL CONSIDERATIONS

**Death Rituals Vary from One Culture to Another**

Arab-Americans do not openly anticipate death or grieve for a dying person. Most of the Arab-American clients prefer to die in the hospital. There are special rituals after the death, such as washing the body and all orifices. The designated head of the family determines how family members will be notified of the death. Organ donation is usually not allowed out of respect for burying the body whole. They will probably not choose a DNR order; in fact, the family may lose trust in the health care system if this option is offered them.

Black Americans vary with respect to dying at home or in the hospital. Many families care for the clients at home until death is imminent, then bring them to the hospital. Some believe it is bad luck to die at home. There are no rituals associated with care of the body. Cremation is usually not done. Organ donation is usually not done except for an immediate family need.

Chinese-Americans may be fatalistic when faced with a terminal illness and death. They usually do not talk about it. Chinese believe that dying at home brings bad luck, but others believe the spirit will get lost if death occurs in the hospital. Each client and family should be supported in their belief. Organ donation and autopsy should be kept intact.

Native Americans embrace the present. Some tribes avoid contact with the dying, while others will want to be present 24 hours a day. Eating, playing games, and making jokes in the hospital are seen as appropriate for some tribes. Many of the tribes will bring healers to attend to the spiritual health of the dying client. Some family members will wrap the body for burial and not allow a mortuary to prepare the body, while others may avoid all contact with the body. Organ donation is generally not accepted.

# 2

# Elimination

Skill 2.1    Assisting with a Bedpan    33

Skill 2.2    Assisting with a Urinal    34

Skill 2.3    Assisting Client to the Commode    36

Skill 2.4    Applying an External Urinary Device    37

Skill 2.5    Collecting a Routine Urine Specimen    39

Skill 2.6    Collecting a Specimen from an Infant    41

Skill 2.7    Collecting 24-Hour Urine Specimen    41

Skill 2.8    Collecting a Urine Specimen for Culture and Sensitivity by the Clean-Catch Method    42

Skill 2.9    Performing Urine Tests    45

Skill 2.10    Performing Urinary Catheterization    46

Skill 2.11    Performing Catheter Care and Removal    53

Skill 2.12    Performing Bladder Irrigation    55

Skill 2.13    Maintaining Continuous Bladder Irrigation    57

Skill 2.14    Providing Suprapubic Catheter Care    58

Skill 2.15    Performing Urinary Ostomy Care    60

Skill 2.16    Applying a Urinary Diversion Pouch    62

Skill 2.17    Obtaining Urine Specimen from an Ileal Conduit    64

Skill 2.18    Removing a Fecal Impaction    65

Skill 2.19    Developing a Regular Bowel Routine    66

Skill 2.20    Inserting a Rectal Tube    67

Skill 2.21    Obtaining and Testing Stool Specimen    69

Skill 2.22    Collecting Infant Stool Specimen    72

Skill 2.23    Collecting Stool for Bacterial Culture    72

Skill 2.24    Teaching Parents to Test for Pinworms    73

Skill 2.25    Collecting Stool for Ova and Parasites    73

Skill 2.26    Implementing the Zassi Bowel Management System™    74

Skill 2.27    Administering an Enema    78

Skill 2.28    Administering a Retention Enema    80

Skill 2.29    Applying a Fecal Ostomy Pouch    82

Skill 2.30    Changing a Bowel Diversion Ostomy Appliance    89

Skill 2.31    Assisting with Peritoneal Dialysis Catheter Insertion    94

Skill 2.32    Conducting Peritoneal Dialysis Procedures    96

Skill 2.33    Providing Hemodialysis    98

Skill 2.34    Providing Ongoing Care of Hemodialysis Client    100

Skill 2.35    Terminating Hemodialysis    101

Skill 2.36    Maintaining Central Venous Dual-Lumen Dialysis Catheter (DLC)    102

Skill 2.37    Home Setting: Using Clean Technique for Intermittent Self-Catheterization    104

Skill 2.38    Home Setting: Providing Suprapubic Catheter Care    105

**Skill 2.39** Home Setting: Administering Continuous Ambulatory Peritoneal Dialysis (CAPD)    105

**Skill 2.40** Home Setting: Changing Dressing for a CAPD Client    107

**Skill 2.41** Home Setting: Instructing Client in Colostomy Irrigation    107

**Skill 2.42** Performing the Allen Test    108

**Skill 2.43** Assisting with Arterial Line Insertion    108

**Skill 2.44** Monitoring Arterial Blood Pressure    109

**Skill 2.45** Withdrawing Arterial Blood Samples    111

**Skill 2.46** Removing Arterial Catheter    112

Elimination from the urinary tract is usually taken for granted. Only when a problem arises do most people become aware of their urinary habits and any associated symptoms. The nurse's role in urinary elimination may be to (1) assist the client with urinary control, (2) obtain a urine specimen (voided or catheterized), or (3) establish bladder emptiness through catheterization.

# Skill 2.1   Assisting with a Bedpan

## EXPECTED OUTCOMES
- Client understands purpose of test.
- Client is able to follow procedure of collection when appropriate.
- Dietary restrictions (if appropriate to test) were adhered to by client prior to test.
- Specimen collected is adequate for test.

## Delegation

Unlicensed assistive personnel (UAP) commonly assist clients with bedpans. The nurse must determine if the specific client has unique needs that would require special training of the UAP in the use of the bedpan. Ensure that personnel are aware of any specimens that need to be collected. Abnormal findings must be validated and interpreted by the nurse.

## Equipment
- Clean bedpan and cover
- Toilet tissue
- Basin of water, soap, washcloth, and towel
- Equipment for a specimen if required (see Skill 2.3)
- Clean gloves
- Disposable absorbent pad

## Preparation
- Adjust the bed to a height appropriate to prevent back strain.
- Elevate the rail on the opposite side of the bed. ➤*Rationale: This prevents the client from falling and provides a hand grasp for the client if needed.*

## Procedure
1. Prior to performing the procedure, introduce self to the client and verify the client's identity using agency protocol. Explain to the client what you are going to do, why it is necessary, and how he or she can participate.
2. Perform hand hygiene and observe other appropriate infection control procedures (e.g., clean gloves).
3. Apply clean gloves.
4. Provide for client privacy.
5. Prepare the client.
   - For clients who can assist by raising their buttocks, fold down the top bed linen on the near side to expose the hip, and adjust the gown so that it will not fall into the bedpan. ➤*Rationale: A pie fold of the top bed linens exposes the client minimally and facilitates placement of the bedpan.*
   - For clients who cannot raise their buttocks onto and off a bedpan, fold the top bed linens down to the hips.
6. Place client on the bedpan.
   - For clients who can lift their buttocks:
     a. Ask the client to flex the knees, rest their weight on the back and the heels, and then raise the buttocks. The client can use a trapeze, if present, or grasp the side rail for support. Assist the client to lift the buttocks by placing the hand nearest the person's head palm up under the lower back, resting the elbow on the mattress, and using the forearm as a lever. ➤*Rationale: Use of appropriate body mechanics by both client and nurse prevents unnecessary muscle strain and exertion.*
     b. Place the absorbent pad on the bed where the bedpan will be located. Position a regular bedpan under the buttocks with the narrow end toward the foot of the bed and the buttocks resting on the smooth, rounded rim. Place a slipper (fracture) pan with the flat end under the client's buttocks. ➤*Rationale: Improper placement of the bedpan can cause skin abrasion to the sacral area and spillage of the bedpan's contents.*
   - For clients who cannot lift their buttocks:
     a. Assist the client to a side-lying position.
     b. Place the bedpan against the buttocks with the open rim toward the foot of the bed.

c. Smoothly roll the client onto the bedpan while holding the bedpan against the buttocks.

7. Elevate the head of the bed to a semi-Fowler's position. ➤*Rationale: This position relieves strain on the client's back and permits a more normal position for elimination.* Recheck the position of the bedpan because it may have been repositioned while the head of the bed was being raised.
   - If the person is unable to assume a semi-Fowler's position, place a small pillow under the back, or help the client to another comfortable position.

8. Replace the top bed linen.

9. Provide the client with toilet tissue, raise the side rail, lower the bed height, and ensure that the call light is readily accessible. Ask the client to signal when finished. Leave only when, in your judgment, it is safe to do so. ➤*Rationale: Having necessary items within reach prevents falls.*

### Removing a Bedpan

10. Return the bed to the position used when giving the bedpan.
    - Hold the bedpan steady to prevent spillage of its contents.
    - Cover the bedpan, and place it on an adjacent chair with a pad or towel under it. ➤*Rationale: Covering the bedpan reduces offensive odors and reduces the client's embarrassment.*

11. Assist the client with any needed hygienic measures.
    - Wrap toilet tissue several times around the gloved hand, and wipe the person from the pubic area to the anal area, using one stroke for each piece of tissue. ➤*Rationale: Cleaning in this direction—from the less soiled area to the more soiled area—helps prevent the spread of microorganisms.*
    - Place the soiled tissue in the bedpan.

- Wash the anal area with soap and water as indicated, and thoroughly dry the area. ➤*Rationale: Adequate washing and drying prevents skin abrasion and excessive accumulation of microorganisms.*
- Remove the disposable absorbent pad or replace the drawsheet if it is soiled.
- Offer the client materials to wash and dry the hands. ➤*Rationale: Handwashing following elimination is a practice that helps prevent the spread of microorganisms.*

12. Attend to any unpleasant odors in the environment.
    - Spray the air with an air freshener as needed unless contraindicated because of respiratory problems, allergies, or because it is offensive. ➤*Rationale: Elimination odor can be embarrassing to clients and visitors alike. However, sprays may be harmful to people with respiratory problems, and some perfume sprays are offensive to some people.*

13. Attend to the used bedpan.
    - Acquire a specimen if required. Place it in the appropriately labeled container.
    - Empty and clean the bedpan. Provide a clean bedpan cover, if necessary, before returning it to the client's unit.
    - Remove and discard gloves. Perform hand hygiene.

14. Document findings (e.g., color, odor, amount, and consistency of feces) in the client record using forms or checklists supplemented by narrative notes when appropriate.

---

### CLINICAL ALERT

Individuals, especially children, may use very different terms for a bowel movement. The nurse may need to try several different common words before finding one the client understands.

---

# Skill 2.2   Assisting with a Urinal

### EXPECTED OUTCOMES
- Client voids 200–500 mL of urine without discomfort or difficulty.
- Bladder does not become distended.
- Genitourinary system is free of infection.

In preparing to assist the client with the use of a urinal, determine if there are any restrictions in positioning the client. Inquire whether the client has used a urinal previously. If so, determine if the client has any unique needs related to the use of the urinal.

### Delegation

Assisting the client with a urinal is often delegated to unlicensed assistive personnel (UAP). Ensure that UAP are aware of any specimens that need to be collected. The nurse must validate and interpret abnormal findings.

### Equipment
- Clean urinal
- Toilet tissue
- Equipment for specimen if required
- Clean gloves

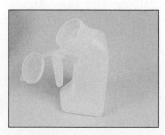

● Male urinal.

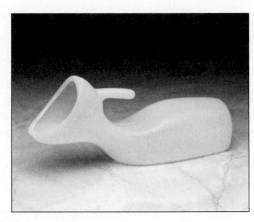

● Female urinal.

## Preparation

- Assist the client to an appropriate position.
- Both males and females confined to bed may prefer a semi-Fowler's position, or the male may prefer a standing position at the side of the bed if health permits.

## Procedure

1. Prior to performing the procedure, introduce self and verify the client's identity using agency protocol. Explain to the client what you are going to do, why it is necessary, and how he or she can participate. Discuss how the results will be used in planning further care or treatments.
2. Perform hand hygiene and observe other appropriate infection control procedures.
3. Provide for client privacy.
4. Assist the client with using the urinal:
   - Offer the urinal so that the client can position it independently.
   *or*

- Place the urinal between the client's legs with the handle uppermost so that urine will flow into it.
- Leave the signal cord within reach of the person.
  ➤*Rationale: The client can then call for assistance if required.*
- Leave for 2 to 3 minutes or until the client signals.
  *or*
- Remain if the client needs support to stand at the bedside or other assistance.
5. Assist the client with removing the urinal as needed.
   - Apply clan gloves. Remove the urinal.
   - If wet, wipe the area around the urethral orifice with a tissue. Dry the perineum.
   - Change the linens or pad under the client if wet.
   - Provide the client with handwipes, a dampened washcloth, or water, soap, and a towel to wash and dry hands.
6. Attend to the urine as required.
   - Measure the urine if the client is on monitored intake and output, and transfer a specimen to the appropriate container if required.
   - Empty and rinse out the urinal, and return it to the bedside unit. If the male client prefers, the urinal may be hung on the side rail by its handle for easy access.
   - Remove and discard gloves. Perform hand hygiene.
7. Document findings in the client record using forms or checklists supplemented by narrative notes when appropriate. Record the amount of urine, if it was measured, and all assessment data (e.g., cloudy urine, reddened perineum).

## Documentation

Sample: 4/22/09 13:20 Assisted with use of urinal due to arm in cast. Voided 450 mL dark yellow, clear, odorless urine. Specimen to lab for UA. Encouraged to drink more fluids; ice water and juice placed at bedside. Client verbalizes agreement to increase intake.

_____ K. Clark, R.N.

## DEVELOPMENTAL CONSIDERATIONS

### Infant

- Babies have no conscious control, and the urine is released after a small amount accumulates in the bladder.

### Children

- In children, 50 to 200 mL stimulates stretch receptors in the bladder.
- Urinary control normally takes place between 2 and 4 1/2 years of age. Boys are usually slower than girls in developing this control.
- Teaching proper perineal hygiene can reduce infection. Girls should learn to wipe from front to back and wear cotton underwear. ➤*Rationale: Wiping from*

*front to back prevents stool or vaginal secretions from contaminating the urethral meatus.* Wearing cotton underwear is recommended over nylon because it "breathes" and is less likely to support bacterial growth.

- Teach children and parents that they should go to the bathroom as soon as the sensation to void is felt and not try to hold the urine in.

### Elders

- Bladder capacity decreases, as does ability to completely empty the bladder.
- Decreased muscle tone may lead to nocturia, frequency, and increased residual.

*(continued)*

## DEVELOPMENTAL CONSIDERATIONS (CONTINUED)

- Altered cognition may lead to incontinence since it prevents the person from understanding the need to urinate and the actions needed to perform the activity.
- Many older men have enlarged prostate glands, which can inhibit complete emptying of the bladder, resulting in urinary retention and urgency, which sometimes causes incontinence.
- Women past menopause have decreased estrogen, which results in a decrease in perineal tone and

support of bladder, vagina, and pelvic tissues. This often results in urgency and stress incontinence and can even increase the incidence of urinary tract infections.
- Increased stiffness and pain in joints, previous joint surgery, and neuromuscular problems can impair mobility and often make it difficult to get to the bathroom.

# Skill 2.3   Assisting Client to the Commode

### EXPECTED OUTCOMES

- Client voids 200–500 mL of urine without discomfort or difficulty.
- Bladder does not become distended.
- Genitourinary system is free of infection.
- Client transferred to commode for voiding.

### Equipment

Commode with locking wheels or rubber-tipped legs
Toilet tissue
Nurse's call bell
Slippers
Bath blanket

### Procedure

1. Place commode at foot of bed. Be sure to lock wheels on commode if needed.
2. Place slippers on client.
3. Raise head of bed to facilitate moving client to edge of bed.
4. Move client to edge of bed and assist to a sitting position at edge of bed. Instruct client to place feet flat on floor.
5. Stand directly in front of client, blocking client's toes with your feet and client's knees with your knees.
   ▸*Rationale: Prevents client from buckling knees.*
6. Flex your knees.
7. Place your arms securely around client's waist.
   ▸*Rationale: Stabilizes client for transfer.*
8. When starting to transfer, avoid bending at the waist. ▸*Rationale: Prevents back strain.*
9. Instruct client to push self off bed and support his/her own weight.
10. Straighten your knees and hips as you raise client to standing position.
11. Pivot client in front of commode. Instruct client to grasp arm rest on farthest side.

12. Lower client onto commode, using correct body mechanics (flexing your hip and knees but not your back) to ensure client is securely positioned on commode.
13. Place toilet tissue within easy reach.
14. Cover client with bath blanket for warmth and privacy.
15. Place call bell within easy access of client.
16. Provide privacy by closing curtains and shutting door.
17. Perform hand hygiene.

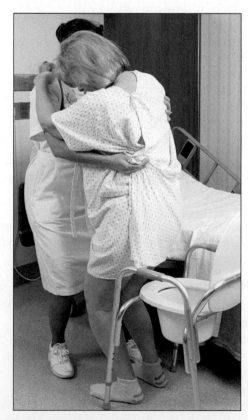

● Pivot with client and bend knees when seating client.

### Documentation

- Amount, color, appearance, and odor of urine
- Techniques effective in stimulating voiding

- Equipment used (e.g., commode, bedpan)
- Type of support needed for transfer to commode

| UNEXPECTED OUTCOMES | CRITICAL THINKING OPTIONS |
|---|---|
| Unable to turn and has difficulty raising hips. | • Use a fracture pan rather than a bedpan. Powder the fracture pan.<br>• Insert the fracture pan with the flat side toward the head, under the client's thighs.<br>• Assess reason.<br>• Maintain complete privacy. |
| Unable to void on bedpan. | • Run water in sink.<br>• Massage the lower abdomen.<br>• Place a hot washcloth on the abdomen.<br>• Pour warm water over the perineum with client positioned on toilet or bedpan.<br>• Give client a sitz bath after obtaining an order. |

# CULTURAL CONSIDERATIONS

Some cultures incorporate the participation of family members to provide personal care, particularly assistance with using a bedpan or bedside commode, to maintain modesty. Puerto Ricans, African-Americans, and clients of Arab descent should be questioned as to their preferences for assistance with personal care.

# Skill 2.4   Applying an External Urinary Device

### EXPECTED OUTCOMES

- Client remains dry with condom catheter for urine collection.
- Skin irritation does not occur with condom catheter use.

Discuss the use of external urinary devices with the client and/or family. Research has shown that condom catheters may be more comfortable and cause fewer urinary tract infections than indwelling catheters (Saint et al., 2006). Determine if the client has had an external catheter previously and any difficulties with it. Perform any procedures that are best completed without the catheter in place; for example, weighing the client would be easier without the tubing and bag.

### Delegation

Applying a condom catheter may be delegated to UAP. However, the nurse must determine if the specific client has unique needs such adhering condoms, or those with Velcro, tape, or other external securing device.

### Equipment

- Condom sheath of appropriate size: small, medium, large, extra-large. Use the manufacturer's size guide

as indicated. Use latex-free silicone for clients with latex allergies. Use self-adhering condoms, or those with Velcro, tape, or other external securing device.

- Leg drainage bag if ambulatory or urinary drainage bag with tubing
- Clean gloves
- Basin of warm water and soap
- Washcloth and towel

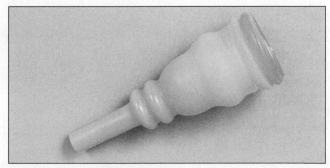

● An external or condom catheter.

## Preparation

- Assemble the leg drainage bag or urinary drainage bag for attachment to the condom sheath.
- If the condom supplied is not rolled onto itself, roll the condom outward onto itself to facilliatee easier application. On some models, an inner flap will be exposed. This flap is applied around the urinary meatus to prevent the reflux of urine.

## Procedure

1. Prior to performing the procedure, introduce self and verify the client's identity using agency protocol. Explain to the client what you are going to do, why it is necessary, and how he can participate.
2. Perform hand hygiene and observe other appropriate infection control procedures.
3. Apply clean gloves.
4. Position the client in either a supine or a sitting position. Provide for client privacy.
   - Drape the client appropriately with the bath blanket, exposing only the penis.
5. Inspect and clean the penis.
   - Clean the genital area and dry it thoroughly. ➤*Rationale: This minimizes skin irritation and excoriation after the condom is applied.*
6. Apply and secure the condom.
   - Roll the condom smoothly over the penis, leaving 2.5 cm (1 in.) between the end of the penis and the rubber or plastic connecting tube. ➤*Rationale: This space prevents irritation of the tip of the penis and provides for full drainage of urine.*
   - Secure the condom firmly, but not too tightly, to the penis. Avoid catching pubic hair if possible. Some condoms have an adhesive inside the proximal end that adheres to the skin of the base of the penis. Many condoms are packaged with special tape. If neither is present, use a strip of elastic tape or Velcro around the base of the penis over the condom. Ordinary tape is contraindicated because it is not flexible and can stop blood flow.

7. Securely attach the urinary drainage system.
   - Make sure that the tip of the penis is not touching the condom and that the condom is not twisted. ➤*Rationale: A twisted condom could obstruct the flow of urine.*
   - Attach the urinary drainage system to the condom.
   - Remove and discard gloves. Perform hand hygiene.
   - If the client is to remain in bed, attach the urinary drainage bag to the bed frame.
   - If the client is ambulatory, attach the bag to the client's leg. ➤*Rationale: Attaching the drainage bag to the leg helps control the movement of the tubing and prevents twisting of the thin material of the condom appliance at the tip of the penis.*
8. Teach the client about the drainage system.
   - Instruct the client to keep the drainage bag below the level of the condom and to avoid loops or kinks in the tubing.
9. Inspect the penis 30 minutes following the condom application and at least every 4 hours. Check for urine flow. Document these findings.
   - Assess the penis for swelling and discoloration. ➤*Rationale: This indicates that the condom is too tight.*
   - Assess urine flow if the client has voided. Normally, some urine is present in the tube if the flow is not obstructed.
10. Change the condom as indicated and provide skin care. In most settings, the condom is changed daily.
    - Remove the elastic or Velcro strip, apply clean gloves, and roll off the condom.
      - Wash the penis with soapy water, rinse, and dry it thoroughly.
      - Assess the foreskin for signs of irritation, swelling, and discoloration.
      - Apply a new condom.
      - Remove and discard gloves. Perform hand hygiene.
11. Document in the client record using forms or checklists supplemented by narrative notes when appropriate. Record the application of the condom, the time, and pertinent observations, such as irritated areas on the penis.

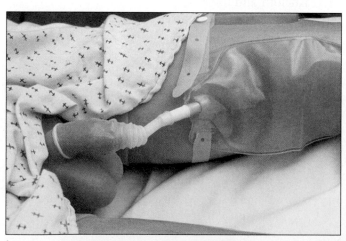

The condom rolled over the penis.

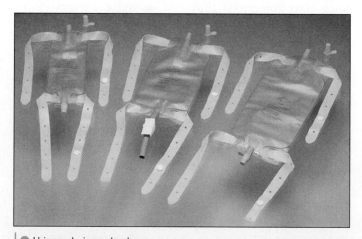

Urinary drainage leg bags.
(Courtesy of Bard Medical Division)

## Documentation

Sample: 4/22/09 22:45 Condom cath applied per client request for the night. Glans clean, skin intact. Cath attached to bedside collection bag.
_____ L. Chan, R.N.

> Use of an external urine collection system is recommended for incontinent men without urine retention. These devices are comfortable, and there is less bacteriuria than with indwelling catheters.

| UNEXPECTED OUTCOMES | CRITICAL THINKING OPTIONS |
|---|---|
| Condom catheter leaks. | • Use smaller size condom to provide wrinkle-free fit.<br>• Replace adhesive strips for better condom adherence.<br>• Make sure penis is thoroughly dry before applying condom system.<br>• Ensure that drainage collection system is dependent of condom tubing to promote gravity flow. |
| Penis becomes reddened with condom catheter use. | • Remove condom.<br>• Notify wound care specialist/physician for topical medication order.<br>• Apply adult brief and change frequently until problem resolves.<br>• Make sure penis is clean and dry and protective coating is applied before condom application.<br>• Clip rolled portion of condom to prevent constriction at base of penis. |

# Skill 2.5   Collecting a Routine Urine Specimen

## Delegation

UAP may be assigned to collect a routine urine specimen. Provide the UAP with clear directions on how to instruct the client to collect his or her own urine specimen or how to correctly collect the specimen for the client who may need to use a bedpan or urinal.

## Equipment

• Clean gloves as needed
• Clean bedpan, urinal, or commode for clients who are unable to void directly into the specimen container
• Wide-mouthed specimen container
• Completed laboratory requisition
• Completed specimen identification label

## Preparation

Obtain needed equipment. Determine if the client requires supervision or assistance in the bathroom. Clients who are seriously ill, physically incapacitated, or disoriented may need to use a bedpan or urinal in bed. A fracture bedpan may be needed for a client with a hip fracture.

## Procedure

1. Prior to performing the procedure, introduce self and verify the client's identity using agency protocol. Explain to the client what you are going to do, why it is necessary, and how he or she can participate. Discuss how the results will be used in planning further care or treatments. Give ambulatory clients the following information and instructions:
   • Explain the purpose of the urine specimen and how the client can assist.
   • Explain that all specimens must be free of fecal contamination, so voiding needs to occur at a different time from defecation.
   • Instruct clients to discard the toilet tissue in the toilet or in a waste bag rather than in the bedpan. ➤*Rationale: Tissue in the specimen makes laboratory analysis more difficult.*
   • Give the client the specimen container, and direct the client to the bathroom to void into it.
2. Perform hand hygiene and observe other appropriate infection control procedures such as gloves to handle specimen containers.
3. Provide for client privacy.
4. Assist clients who are seriously ill, physically incapacitated, or disoriented. Provide required assistance in the bathroom or help the client to use a bedpan or urinal in bed.
5. Ensure that the specimen is sealed and the container clean.
   • Put the lid tightly on the container. ➤*Rationale: This prevents spillage of the urine and contamination of other objects.*
   • If the outside of the container has been contaminated by urine, apply clean gloves and clean it with soap and water. ➤*Rationale: This prevents the spread of microorganisms.*
   • Remove and discard gloves. Perform hand hygiene.

6. Label and transport the specimen to the laboratory, using appropriate biohazard specimen bags or containers.
   - Ensure that the specimen label and the laboratory requisition have the correct information on them. Attach them securely to the specimen container. ➤*Rationale: Inappropriate identification of the specimen can lead to errors of diagnosis or therapy for the client.*
   - Arrange for the specimen to be taken immediately to the laboratory or placed in a refrigerator. ➤*Rationale: Urine deteriorates relatively rapidly from bacterial contamination when left at room temperature; specimens should be analyzed immediately after collection. If the urine specimen is delayed from reaching the lab by more than 1 hour, a new specimen may be needed.*

7. Document the collection of the specimen on the client's chart. Include the date and time of collection and the appearance and odor of the urine.

## DEVELOPMENTAL CONSIDERATIONS

### Infant

- The process for cleaning the perineal area and the urethral opening is similar to the process for an adult. A specimen bag, however, is used to collect the urine specimen. The specimen bag has an adhesive backing that attaches to the skin. After the infant has voided a desired amount, gently remove the bag from the skin.
- If you are having trouble obtaining a bagged urine specimen from an infant, try cutting a hole in the diaper (front for a boy and middle for a girl) and pulling part of the bag through. You can see when urine is collected without having to untape the diaper.

### Child

- When collecting a routine urine specimen, explain the procedure in simple, nonmedical terms to the child and ask the child to void using a potty chair or a bedpan placed inside the toilet.
- Give the child a clean specimen container to play with.
- Allow a parent to assist the child, if possible. The child may feel more comfortable with a parent.

### Elders

- For a clean-catch urine specimen, an older adult may have difficulty controlling the stream of urine.
- An older female adult with arthritis may have difficulty holding the labia apart during the collection of a clean-catch urine specimen.

## CLINICAL ALERT

When applying the urine bag on girls, begin by placing the bag below the vaginal opening and then allow it to adhere to the labia. For boys, be sure the bag is adhered on the scrotum and the scrotum is not inside the bag's opening. Cutting a hole in the diaper so the end of the bag can pass through makes it easier to visualize when the infant has urinated.

## SETTING OF CARE

- Assess the client's ability and willingness to collect a timed urine specimen. If poor eyesight or hand tremors are a problem, suggest using a clean funnel to pour the urine into the container.
- Always wash hands well with warm, soapy water before and after collecting urine samples.
- Always wear gloves if handling another person's urine.
- The home should have a refrigerator or other method for cooling the urine samples. Tell the client to keep the specimen container in a plastic or paper bag in the refrigerator, separate from other refrigerator contents. The client may also use a cooler with ice.

# Skill 2.6   Collecting a Specimen from an Infant

## Equipment

Cleansing solution
Towel
Pediatric urine collector
Diapers
Appropriate specimen containers
Clean gloves (2 pair)
Clean specimen container
Label for specimen

## Procedure

1. Gather equipment.
2. Perform hand hygiene. Don clean gloves.
3. Identify correct child by checking two forms of infant ID.
4. Cleanse and dry child's perineum.
5. Remove paper backing from the adhesive on the urine collector.
6. Apply urine collector to child's perineum, avoiding extension over anus to prevent contamination.
   - Male: Place child's penis through the opening of the collector.
   - Female: Place the opening of the collection bag over the child's urinary meatus.
7. Remove gloves.
8. Place a diaper on the child to help hold the collector in place.
9. Perform hand hygiene.
10. Check the collector every 15 minutes until a specimen is obtained.

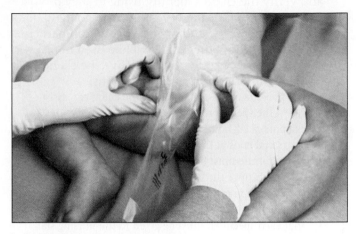

● Remove adhesive backing from urine collection bag and place securely over penis.

11. Don clean gloves.
12. Remove the collector and place in a urine specimen container.
13. Place clean diaper on child.
14. Remove gloves and perform hand hygiene.
15. Send the urine specimen to the lab by either placing the urine collection bag in a urine container or pouring urine from collection bag into the urine container.
16. Label the container with the child's name, date and time of collection, and the initials of the nurse doing the collection.

# Skill 2.7   Collecting 24-Hour Urine Specimen

Determine the client's ability to understand instructions and to provide urine samples independently. Are there any fluid or dietary requirements associated with the test? Are there any medication restrictions or requirements for the test?

## Delegation

UAP may be assigned to assist in the collection of a timed urine specimen. Provide clear directions about the collection procedure, proper storage of the specimen container, and the importance of saving all of the client's urine to avoid the need to restart the collection process.

## Equipment

- Appropriate specimen containers with or without preservative in accordance with the specific test
- Completed specimen identification labels

- Completed laboratory requisition
- Bedpan or urinal
- Sign on or near the bed indicating the specific times for urine collection
- Clean gloves, as needed
- Ice-filled container if a refrigerator is not available

## Preparation

Obtain a specimen container with preservative (if indicated) from the laboratory. Label the container with identifying information for the client, the test to be performed, time started, and time of completion. Provide a clean receptacle to collect urine (bedpan, commode, or toilet collection device). Post signs in the client's chart, Kardex, room, and bathroom alerting personnel to save all urine during the specified time.

**Procedure**

1. Prior to performing the procedure, introduce self and verify the client's identity using agency protocol. Explain to the client what you are going to do, why it is necessary, and how he or she can participate. Discuss how the results will be used in planning further care or treatments. Give the client the following information and instructions:
   - The purpose of the test and how the client can assist.
   - When the specimen collection will begin and end. (For example, a 24-hour urine test commonly begins at 0700 hours and ends at the same hour the next day.)
   - That all urine must be saved and placed in the specimen containers once the test starts.
   - That the urine must be free of fecal contamination and toilet tissue.
   - That each specimen must be given to the nursing staff immediately so that it can be placed in the appropriate specimen bottle.
2. Perform hand hygiene and observe other appropriate infection control procedures.
3. Provide for client privacy.
4. Start the collection period.
   - Ask the client to void in the toilet or bedpan or urinal. *Discard* this urine (check agency procedure), and document the time the test starts with this discarded specimen. Collect all subsequent urine specimens, including the one specimen collected at the end of the period.
   - Ask the client to ingest the required amount of liquid for certain tests or to restrict fluid intake. Follow the test directions.
   - Intake and output should be implemented and documented.
   - Instruct the client to void all subsequent urine into the bedpan or urinal and to notify the nursing staff when each specimen is provided. Some tests require voiding at specified times.

- Number the specimen containers sequentially (e.g., 1st specimen, 2nd specimen, 3rd specimen) if separate specimens are required.
5. Collect all of the required specimens.
   - Place each specimen into the appropriately labeled container. For some tests, each specimen is not kept separately but is poured into a large bottle.
   *Note:* All urine specimens must be collected for timed collections. If one voiding is missed, the timed urine collection may need to be restarted.
   - If the outside of the specimen container is contaminated with urine, put on gloves and clean it with soap and water. ►*Rationale: Cleaning prevents the transfer of microorganisms to others.*
   - Ensure that each specimen is refrigerated throughout the timed collection period. If not refrigerated, specimens are often kept on ice. ►*Rationale: Refrigeration or other form of cooling prevents bacterial decomposition of the urine.*
   - Measure the amount of each urine specimen if required.
   - Ask the client to provide the last specimen 5 to 10 minutes before the end of the collection period.
   - Inform the client that the test is completed.
   - Remove the signs and the specimen equipment from the client's unit and bathroom.
   - Remove and discard gloves. Perform hand hygiene.
6. Document all relevant information.
   - Record the starting time of the test, the name of the test, and completion of the specimen collection on the client's chart. Include the date and specific time. In addition, if indicated for the specific test, note the time each urine specimen was collected, the volume of each specimen, the appearance of the urine, and other relevant data such as fluid intake or restrictions.

> ## CLINICAL ALERT
>
> Note an dietary restriction or medication precautions in preparation for 24-hour urine collection.

---

# Skill 2.8    Collecting a Urine Specimen for Culture and Sensitivity by the Clean-Catch Method

**Delegation**

UAP may perform the collection of a clean-catch or midstream urine specimen. It is important, however, that the nurse inform the UAP how to instruct the client in the correct process for obtaining the specimen. Proper cleansing of the urethra should be emphasized to avoid contaminating the urine specimen.

**Equipment**

Equipment used varies from agency to agency. Some agencies use commercially prepared disposable clean-catch kits. Others use agency-prepared sterile trays. Both prepared trays and kits generally contain the following items:

- Clean gloves
- Antiseptic towelettes

- Sterile specimen container
- Specimen identification label

In addition, the nurse needs to obtain the following:
- Completed laboratory requisition form
- Urine receptacle, if the client is not ambulatory
- Basin of warm water, soap, washcloth, and towel for the nonambulatory client

## Preparation

Collect the necessary equipment needed for the collection of the specimen. Use visual aids, if available, to assist the client to understand the midstream collection technique.

## Procedure

1. Prior to performing the procedure, introduce self and verify the client's identity using agency protocol. Explain to the client that a urine specimen is required, give the reason, and explain the method to be used to collect it. Discuss how the results will be used in planning further care or treatments.
2. Perform hand hygiene and observe other appropriate infection control procedures.
3. Provide for client privacy.
4. For an ambulatory client who is able to follow directions, instruct the client on how to collect the specimen.
   - Direct or assist the client to the bathroom.
   - Ask the client to wash and dry the genitals and perineal area with soap and water. ➤*Rationale: Washing the perineal area reduces the number of skin and transient bacteria, decreasing the risk of contaminating the urine specimen.*
   - Ask the client if they are sensitive to any antiseptic or cleansing agents. ➤*Rationale: This will avoid unnecessary irritation of the genitals or perineum.*
   - Instruct the client on how to clean the urinary meatus with antiseptic towelettes. ➤*Rationale: The antiseptic further reduces bacterial contamination of the urinary meatus and the risk of contaminating the specimen.*

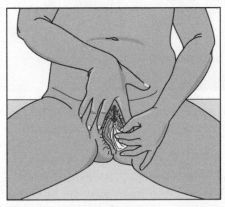

🔵 Cleansing the female urinary meatus. Spread the labia minora with one hand and with the other hand, cleanse perineal area from front to back.

### For Female Clients
- Use each towelette only once. Clean the perineal area from front to back and discard the towelette.
- Use all towelettes provided (usually two or three). ➤*Rationale: Cleaning from front to back cleans the area of least contamination to the area of greatest contamination.*

### For Male Clients
- If uncircumcised, retract the foreskin slightly to expose the urinary meatus.
- Using a circular motion, clean the urinary meatus and the distal portion of the penis.
- Use each towelette only once, then discard. Clean several inches down the shaft of the penis. ➤*Rationale: This cleans from the area of least contamination to the area of greatest contamination.*

5. For a client who requires assistance, prepare the client and equipment.
   - Apply clean gloves.
   - Wash the perineal area with soap and water, rinse, and dry.
   - Assist the client onto a clean commode or bedpan. If using a bedpan or urinal, position the client as upright as allowed or tolerated. ➤*Rationale: Assuming a normal anatomic position for voiding facilitates urination.*
   - Remove and discard gloves. Perform hand hygiene.
   - Open the clean-catch kit, taking care not to contaminate the inside of the specimen container or lid. Place the lid in the upright position. ➤*Rationale: It is important to maintain sterility of the specimen container to prevent contamination of the specimen.*
   - Apply clean gloves.
   - Clean the urinary meatus and perineal area as described in step 4.
6. Collect the specimen from a nonambulatory client or instruct an ambulatory client on how to collect it.
   - Instruct the client to start voiding. ➤*Rationale: Bacteria in the distal urethra and at the urinary meatus are cleared by the first few milliliters of urine expelled.*

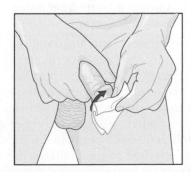

🔵 Cleansing the male urinary meatus. Restract the foreskin if needed. Using a towelette, cleanse the urinary meatus by moving in a circular motion from center of urethral opening around the glans and down the distal portion of the shaft of the penis.

- Place the specimen container into the midstream of urine and collect the specimen, taking care not to touch the container to the perineum or penis. ➤*Rationale: It is important to avoid contaminating the interior of the specimen container and the specimen itself.*
- Collect urine in the container.
- Cap the container tightly, touching only the outside of the container and the cap. ➤*Rationale: This prevents contamination or spilling of the specimen.*
- If necessary, clean the outside of the specimen container with disinfectant. ➤*Rationale: This prevents transfer of microorganisms to others.*
- Remove and discard gloves. Perform hand hygiene.

7. Label the specimen and transport it to the laboratory.
   - Ensure that the specimen label is attached to the specimen cup, not the lid, and the laboratory requisition provides the correct information. Place the specimen in a plastic bag that has a biohazard label on it. Attach the requisition securely to the bag. ➤*Rationale: Inaccurate identification or information on the specimen container can result in errors of diagnosis or therapy.*
   - Arrange for the specimen to be sent to the laboratory immediately. ➤*Rationale: Bacterial cultures must be started immediately before any contaminating organisms can grow, multiply, and produce false results.*

8. Document pertinent data.
   - Record collection of the specimen, any pertinent observations of the urine such as color, odor, or consistency, and any difficulty in voiding that the client experienced.
   - Indicate on the lab slip if the client is taking any current antibiotic therapy or if the client is menstruating.

### Documentation

Sample: 6/15/2009 0800 Informed of MD order for clean-catch urine for C&S. Instructed how to perform. Stated she understood. Urine specimen cloudy. States she continues to have burning on urination. Urine specimen sent to lab. Antibiotic started per MD orders.

_____ T. Sanchez, RN

### VARIATION: Obtaining a Urine Specimen from a Closed Drainage System

Sterile urine specimens can be obtained from closed drainage systems by inserting a sterile needle attached to a syringe through a drainage port in the tubing. Aspiration of urine from catheters can be done only with self-sealing rubber catheters—not plastic, silicone, or Silastic catheters. When self-sealing rubber catheters are used, the needle is inserted just above the location where the catheter is attached to the drainage tubing. The area from which to obtain urine may be marked by a patch on the catheter.

Newer closed drainage urinary systems now have needleless ports, meaning that a needle is no longer

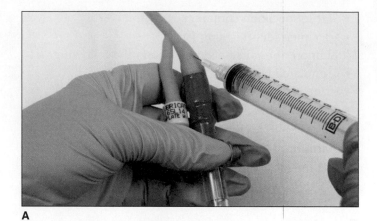

A

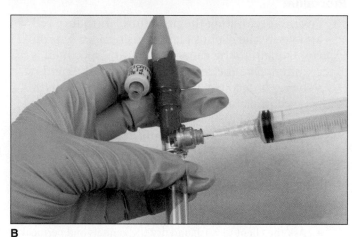

B

● Obtaining a urine specimen from a retention catheter: **A,** from a specific area near the end of the catheter; **B,** from an access port in the tubing.

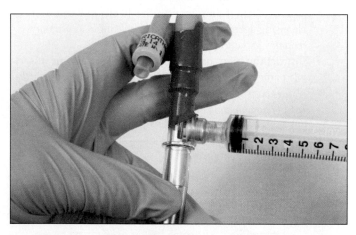

● Obtaining a urine specimen from a retention catheter using a needleless port.

needed to obtain a sample. This protects the nurse from a needlestick injury and maintains the integrity and sterility of the catheter system by eliminating the need to puncture the tubing (Davis, 2004). The needleless port accepts a Luerlock syringe.

Position the syringe perpendicular to the center of the port and insert, twist, and lock into the port. When the specimen is obtained and the syringe removed, the port seals itself.

To collect a specimen from a Foley (retention) catheter or a drainage tube, follow these steps:

- Apply clean gloves.
- If there is no urine in the catheter, clamp the drainage tubing at least 8 cm (3 in.) below the sampling port for about 30 minutes. ➤*Rationale: This allows fresh urine to collect in the catheter.*
- Wipe the area where the needle or Luer lock syringe will be inserted with a disinfectant swab. The site should be distal to the tube leading to the balloon to avoid puncturing this tube. ➤*Rationale: Disinfecting the needle insertion site removes any microorganisms on the surface of the catheter thereby avoiding contamination of the needle and the entrance of microorganisms into the catheter.*
- Insert the needle at a 30- to 45-degree angle. This angle of entrance facilitates self-sealing of the rubber.

Insert the Luer lock syringe at a 90-degree angle for the needleless port.

- Withdraw the required amount of urine, for example, 3 mL for a urine culture or 10 mL for a routine urinalysis.
- Unclamp the catheter.
- Transfer the urine to the specimen container. If a sterile culture tube is used, make sure the needle or syringe (depending on the system) does not touch the outside of the container.
- Discard the syringe and needle or syringe (depending on the system) in an appropriate sharps container.
- Cap the container.
- Remove and discard gloves. Perform hand hygiene.
- Label the container, and send the urine to the laboratory immediately for analysis or refrigeration.
- Record collection of the specimen and any pertinent observations of the urine on the appropriate records.

# Skill 2.9   Performing Urine Tests

### Delegation

Urine testing may be performed by UAP. It is important for the UAP to understand the specific specimen collection procedure and report the results of the test to the nurse. Inform the UAP to save the urine sample to allow the nurse to repeat the test if necessary.

### Equipment

*For All Tests*

- Clean gloves

*For Specific Gravity*

- Multiple-test dipstick that has a separate reagent area for specific gravity

*For Urine pH*

- Dipstick or litmus paper (red or blue)

*For Glucose*

- Reagent tablet or reagent test strip
- Appropriate color chart
- Clean test tube and a dropper, if a tablet is used

*For Ketone Bodies*

- Reagent tablet or dipstick

*For Occult Blood*

- Reagent strip

### Preparation

- Use a fresh urine sample.
- Determine the appropriate equipment and testing product for the client.
- Follow the manufacturer's instructions.

### Procedure

1. Prior to performing the procedure, introduce self and verify the client's identity using agency protocol. Explain to the client what you are going to do, why it is necessary, and how he or she can participate. Discuss how the results will be used in planning further care or treatments.
2. Perform hand hygiene and observe other appropriate infection control procedures.
3. Provide for client privacy.
4. To measure specific gravity:
   - Put on clean gloves and place dipstick into the urine specimen.
   - Observe the color and compare it to a standardized color chart on the bottle.
5. To measure pH:
   - Put on a glove and dip a strip of either red or blue litmus paper into the urine specimen.
   - Observe the color of the litmus paper and compare it to a standardized color chart on the bottle. The blue litmus paper, more commonly used, remains blue if the urine is alkaline and turns red if it is acidic. The red litmus paper

remains red in the presence of acidic urine and turns blue if the urine is alkaline. Whichever litmus strip is used, red always indicates acidic urine and blue always indicates alkaline urine.

6. To test for glucose:
   - Obtain a freshly voided specimen. Most agencies require a second-voided specimen: Ask the client to void, and in 30 minutes to void again, providing a specimen for the test this time. ➤*Rationale: A second-voided specimen more accurately reflects the present condition of the body. Urine that has accumulated in the bladder (e.g., overnight) reflects the condition of the body at the time the urine was produced (e.g., 0300 hours).*
   - To carry out the test, put on gloves and follow the directions specified by the manufacturer. If Clinitest tablets are used, be careful not to touch the bottom of the test tube because it becomes extremely hot when the tablet boils in the presence of urine and water.

7. To test for ketone bodies:
   - Put on a glove and place one or two drops of urine on a reagent tablet (e.g., an Acetest tablet) or dip a reagent test strip (e.g., Ketostix) into the urine.
   - Observe and compare the results with the appropriate color chart to determine the quantity of ketones present.

8. To test for occult blood:
   - Put on a glove, and dip the reagent strip (e.g., Hemastix) into a sample of urine.
   - Compare the color change with a color chart in the same manner as with other reagent strips.

9. For all tests:
   - Discard the urine following the tests. Clean the equipment with soap and water.
   - Remove and discard gloves. Perform hand hygiene.

10. Document the results in accordance with the product used and agency practice.

---

# Skill 2.10   Performing Urinary Catheterization

## EVIDENCE-BASED NURSING PRACTICE

### Regaining Voiding Ability

In hip surgery patients, those receiving intermittent catheterization regained satisfactory voiding quicker than those with an indwelling catheter.

*Source:* Cravens, D., & Sweig, S. (2000). Urinary catheter management. *American Family Physician, 61*(2), 369–375.

### Risks for Urinary Retention

In this study, risks for urinary retention were greated in elderly patients receiving over 4000 mL of IV fluids perioperatively in a 24-hour period, and on prolonged bedrest (over 24 hours). Length of anesthesia time, history of urinary problems, and type of analgesic did not correlate with incidence of urinary retention.

*Source:* Wynd, C., et al. (1996). Factors influencing postoperative urinary retention following orthopaedic surgical procedures. *Orthopaedic Nursing, 15*(1), 43–49.

### Foley Catheter Cautions

Some studies have shown that the standard Foley catheter with a solitary drainage hole at its tip (1.5 cm above the base of the balloon) allows residual urine to accumulate, may lead to inaccurate measurement of urine output and may increase risk for urinary tract infections.

*Source:* Fallis, Wendy. (2005, April). Indwelling Foley catheters: Is the current design a source of erroneous measurement of urine output? *Critical Care Nurse, 25*(2).

Allow adequate time to perform the catheterization. Although the entire procedure can require as little as 15 minutes, several sources of difficulty could result in a much longer time period.

If possible, it should not be performed just prior to or after the client eats. Some clients may feel uncomfortable being catheterized by nurses of the opposite gender. If this is the case, obtain the client's permission. Also consider whether agency policy requires or encourages having a person of the client's same gender present for the procedure.

### EXPECTED OUTCOMES

- Catheterization is avoided with use of bladder scanner.
- Sterile technique is maintained throughout catheterization procedure.
- Catheter enters bladder as evidenced by urine outflow.
- Client remains free of urine leakage around retention catheter.
- Urinary tract infection does not occur secondary to catherization.

### Delegation

Due to the need for sterile technique and detailed knowledge of anatomy, insertion of a urinary catheter is not delegated to UAP.

### Equipment

- Sterile catheter of appropriate size (An extra catheter should also be at hand.)
- Catheterization kit or individual sterile items:
  - Sterile gloves

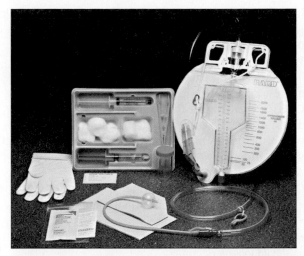

A

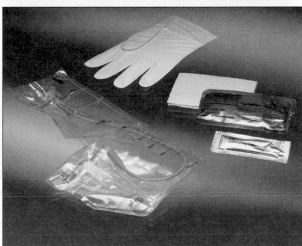

B

| Catheter insertion kits: **A,** indwelling; **B,** straight.
(Courtesy of Bard Medical Division)

- Waterproof drape(s)
- Antiseptic solution
- Cleansing balls
- Forceps
- Water-soluble lubricant
- Urine receptacle
- Specimen container
- For an indwelling catheter:
  - Syringe prefilled with sterile water in amount specified by catheter manufacturer
  - Collection bag and tubing
- 5–10 mL 2% Xylocaine gel or water-soluble lubricant for urethral injection (if agency permits)
- Clean gloves
- Supplies for performing perineal cleansing
- Bath blanket or sheet for draping the client
- Adequate lighting (Obtain a flashlight or lamp if necessary.)

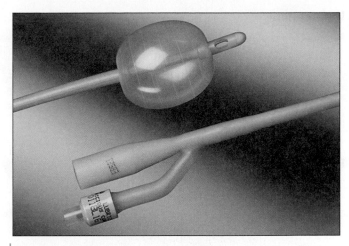

| A retention (Foley) catheter with the balloon inflated.
(Courtesy of Bard Medical Division)

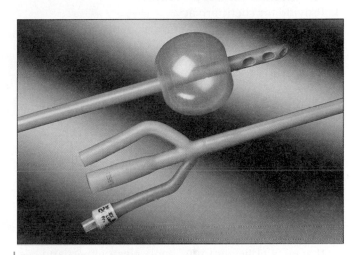

| Three-way Foley catheter.
(Courtesy of Bard Medical Division)

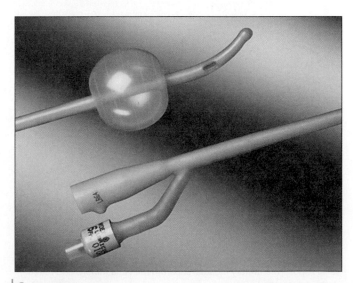

| Coude catheter tip.
(Courtesy of Bard Medical Division)

## Preparation

- If using a catheterization kit, read the label carefully to ensure that all necessary items are included.
- Apply clean gloves and perform routine perineal care to cleanse the meatus from gross contamination. For women, use this time to locate the urinary meatus relative to surrounding structures.
- Remove and discard gloves. Perform hand hygiene.

## Procedure

1. Prior to performing the procedure, introduce self and verify the client's identity using agency protocol. Explain to the client what you are going to do, why it is necessary, and how he or she can participate.
2. Perform hand hygiene and observe other appropriate infection control procedures.
3. Provide for client privacy.
4. Place the client in the appropriate position and drape all areas except the perineum.
   - *Female:* supine with knees flexed, feet about 2 feet apart, and hips slightly externally rotated, if possible
   - *Male:* supine, thighs slightly abducted or apart
5. Establish adequate lighting. Stand on the client's right if you are right-handed, on the client's left if you are left-handed.
6. If using a collecting bag and it is not contained within the catheterization kit, open the drainage package and place the end of the tubing within reach. ►*Rationale: Since one hand is needed to hold the catheter once it is in place open the package while two hands are still available.*
7. If agency policy permits, apply clean gloves and inject 10 to 15 mL Xylocaine gel or water-soluble

lubricant into the urethra of both males and females (Head, 2006). In males, wipe the underside of the penile shaft to distribute the gel up the urethra. Wait at least 5 minutes for the gel to take effect before inserting the catheter. Remove and discard gloves. Perform hand hygiene.

8. Open the catheterization kit. Place a waterproof drape under the buttocks (female) or penis (male) without contaminating the center of the drape with your hands.
9. Apply sterile gloves.
10. Organize the remaining supplies:
    - Saturate the cleansing balls with the antiseptic solution.
    - Open the lubricant package.
    - Remove the specimen container and place it nearby with the lid loosely on top.
11. Attach the prefilled syringe to the indwelling catheter inflation hub and test the balloon.
    ►*Rationale: If the balloon malfunctions, it is important to replace it prior to use.*
12. Lubricate the catheter 2.5 to 5 cm (1 to 2 in.) for females, 15–17.5 cm (6 to 7 in.) for males and place it with the drainage end inside the collection container.
13. If desired, place the fenestrated drape over the perineum, exposing the urinary meatus.
14. Cleanse the meatus. *Note:* The nondominant hand is considered contaminated once it touches the client's skin.
    - *Women:* Use your nondominant hand to spread the labia so the meatus is visible. Establish a firm but gentle position. The antiseptic may make the tissues slippery but the labia must not be allowed to return over the cleaned mea-

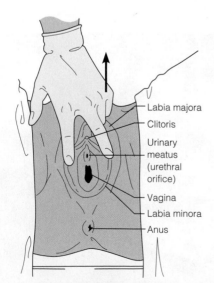

● To expose the urinary meatus, separate the labia minora and retract the tissue upward.

Labia majora
Clitoris
Urinary meatus (urethral orifice)
Vagina
Labia minora
Anus

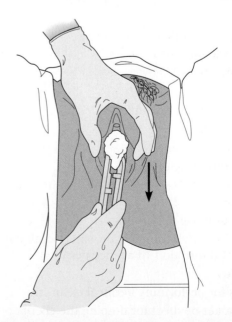

● When cleaning the labia minora, move the swab downward.

tus. *Note:* Location of the urethral meatus is best identified during the cleansing process. Pick up a cleansing ball with the forceps in your dominant hand and wipe one side of the labia majora in an anteroposterior direction.

- Use great care that wiping the client does not contaminate this sterile hand. Use a new ball for the opposite side. Repeat for the labia minora. Use the last ball to cleanse directly over the meatus.

- *Men:* Use your nondominant hand to grasp the penis just below the glans. If necessary, retract the foreskin. Hold the penis firmly upright, with slight tension. ➤*Rationale: Lifting the penis in this manner helps straighten the urethra.* Pick up a cleansing ball with the forceps in your dominant hand and wipe from the center of the meatus in a circular motion around the glans to the base. Use great care that wiping the client does not contaminate this sterile hand. Use a new ball and repeat three more times. The antiseptic may make the tissues slippery but the foreskin must not be allowed to return over the cleaned meatus nor the penis be dropped.

15. Insert the catheter.
    - Grasp the catheter firmly 5 to 7.5 cm (2 to 3 in.) from the tip. Ask the client to take a slow deep breath and insert the catheter as the client exhales. Slight resistance is expected as the catheter passes through the sphincters. If necessary, twist the catheter or hold pressure on the catheter until the sphincter relaxes.
    - Advance the catheter 5 cm (2 in.) farther after the urine begins to flow through it. ➤*Rationale: This is to be sure it is fully in the bladder, will not easily fall out, and the balloon is into the bladder completely.* For male clients, some experts recommend advancing the catheter to the "Y" bifurcation of the catheter (Senese, Hendricks, Morrison, & Harris, 2006b). Check your agency's policy.
    - If the catheter accidentally contacts the labia or slips into the vagina, it is considered contaminated and a new, sterile catheter must be used. The contaminated catheter may be left in the vagina until the new catheter is inserted to help avoid mistaking the vaginal opening for the urinary meatus.

16. Hold the catheter with the nondominant hand.

17. For an indwelling catheter, inflate the retention balloon with the designated volume.
    - Without releasing the catheter (and, for females, without releasing the labia), hold the inflation valve between two fingers of your nondominant hand while you attach the syringe (if not left attached earlier when testing the balloon) and inflate with your dominant hand. If the client complains of discomfort, immediately withdraw the instilled fluid, advance the catheter further, and attempt to inflate the balloon again.
    - Pull *gently* on the catheter until resistance is felt to ensure that the balloon has inflated and to place it in the trigone of the bladder.

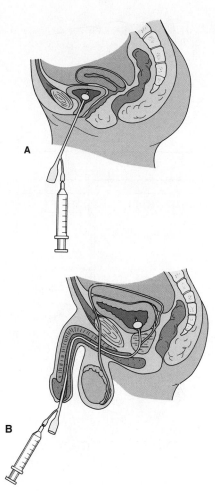

● Placement of catheter and inflated balloon: **A,** female client; **B,** male client.

## CLINICAL ALERT

Chronic irritation and inflammation of bladder mucosa due to long-term (over 8 months) presence of an indwelling catheter (urethral or suprapubic) is associated with an increased risk for bladder cancer.

18. Collect a urine specimen if needed. For a straight catheter, allow 20 to 30 mL to flow into the bottle without touching the catheter to the bottle. For an indwelling catheter preattached to a drainage bag, a specimen may be taken from the bag this initial time only.

19. Allow the straight catheter to continue draining into the urine receptacle. If necessary, attach the drainage end of an indwelling catheter to the collecting tubing and bag.

20. Examine and measure the urine. In some cases, only 750 to 1,000 mL of urine are to be drained

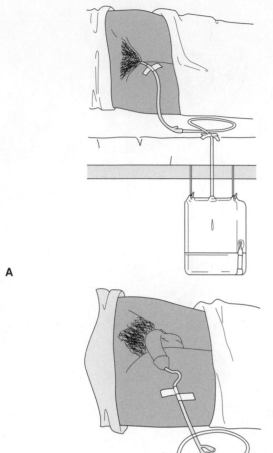

**A**

**B**

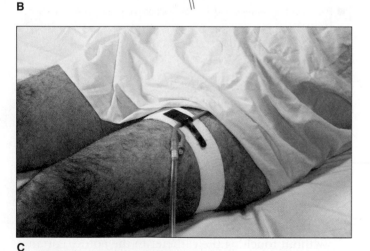

**C**

● Tape the catheter to the **A,** inside of a female's thigh; **B,** thigh or abdomen of a male client; **C,** or use a catheter securement device.
(Courtesy of Dale Medical Products, Inc.)

from the bladder at one time. Check agency policy for further instructions if this should occur.
21. Remove the straight catheter when urine flow stops. For an indwelling catheter, secure the catheter tubing to the inner thigh for female clients or the upper

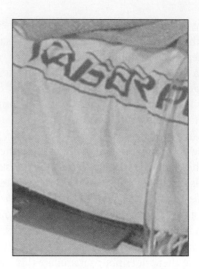

● Correct position for urine drainage bag and tubing.

thigh or abdomen for male clients with enough slack to allow usual movement. Tape or a manufactured catheter-securing device should be used to secure the catheter tubing to the client. This prevents unnecessary trauma to the urethra. Research comparing the effectiveness of a device specifically designed to prevent movement of the catheter versus tape, Velcro, or other method has shown that a securing device can reduce symptomatic urinary tract infection (Darouiche et al, 2006). Next secure the collecting tubing to the bed linens and hang the bag below the level of the bladder. No tubing should fall below the top of the bag.
22. Wipe the perineal area of any remaining antiseptic or lubricant. Replace the foreskin if retracted earlier. Return the client to a comfortable position. Instruct the client on positioning and moving with the catheter in place.
23. Discard all used supplies in appropriate receptacles.
24. Remove and discard gloves. Perform hand hygiene.
25. Document the catheterization procedure including catheter size and results in the client record using forms or checklists supplemented by narrative notes when appropriate.

## CLINICAL ALERT

Recommended urinary catheter sizes:
Infant—4–5 French
Toddler and Preschooler—6 French
School-Age Child—6–10 French
Adolescent—8–12 French

## CLINICAL ALERT

The use of urinary catheters is one of the most common causes of hospital-acquired infections.

### Documentation

Sample: 2/24/09 0530 Client agreed to insertion of cath for pre-op as per orders. #16 Ch 3-way Foley c̄ 10-mL balloon inserted s̄ difficulty, secured to inner thigh, connected to straight drainage. Immediate return of 100 mL pale, clear yellow urine.

_____ G. Hampton, R.N.

## DEVELOPMENTAL CONSIDERATIONS

### Infants/Children

*   Adapt the size of the catheter for pediatric clients.
*   Ask a family member to assist in holding the child during catheterization, if appropriate.

### Elders

*   Obtaining consent and cooperation may take longer than with younger clients.
*   When catheterizing elders, be very attentive to problems of limited movement, especially in the hips. Arthritis, or previous hip or knee surgery, may limit elders movement and cause discomfort. Modify the position (e.g., side-lying) as needed to perform the procedure safely and comfortably. For women, obtain the assistance of another nurse to flex and hold the client's knees and hips as necessary or place her in a modified Sims' position.
*   If the female meatus cannot be visualized, insert a gloved finger into the vagina and press gently upward. ➤*Rationale: This action may straighten the urethra and make the meatus visible.* (Senese, Hendricks, Morrison, & Harris, 2006a).

## CLINICAL ALERT

Recommended urinary catheter sizes:
Infant—4–5 French
Toddler and Preschooler—6 French
School-Age Child—6–10 French
Adolescent—8–12 French

## CLINICAL ALERT

For indwelling catheters, instruct the client to:

*   Never pull on the catheter.
*   Keep the catheter tubing attached to your leg using a catheter securing device.
*   Ensure that there are no kinks or twists in the tubing.
*   Keep the urine drainage bag below the level of the bladder.
*   Report signs and symptoms of urinary tract infection including burning, urgency, abdominal pain, cloudy urine; in older adults, confusion may be an early sign.
*   Maintain adequate oral intake of fluids.

Clients who have indwelling catheters for lengthy periods of time need to have the catheter and bag changed at regular intervals. Changing equipment once a month is often the standard, although agency policy may differ. Inform the client of this routine. Also, issues of sexuality must be discussed with clients who have indwelling catheters at home. Nurses who are not familiar or comfortable with providing the client this information must request another health care provider to assume this responsibility.

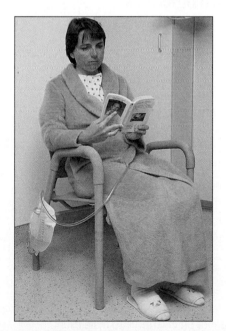

● Positioning the collecting bag and tubing when sitting in a chair.

## SETTING OF CARE

- Clients with spinal cord injuries who are unable to stimulate voiding may use intermittent straight catheterization every few hours. The client or another caregiver can perform this procedure once taught by a nurse. Often, the client will use clean rather than sterile technique and reuse equipment since the microorganisms to which the client is exposed are his or her own.

- For intermittent self-catheterization, instruct the client to:
  - Follow instructions for clean technique.
  - Wash hands well with warm water and soap prior to handling equipment or performing catheterization.
  - Monitor for signs and symptoms of urinary tract infection including burning, urgency, abdominal pain, and cloudy urine; in elders, confusion may be an early sign.
  - Ensure adequate oral intake of fluids.
  - After each catheterization, assess the urine for color, odor, clarity, and the presence of blood.

- Wash reusable catheters thoroughly with soap and water after use, dry, and store in a clean place.

- For ambulatory clients, those in the home, or those in wheelchairs who have indwelling catheters, modifications are needed in securing the catheter and maintaining the collection bag below bladder level. A leg bag may substitute for a hanging bag for those who are upright.

- Discuss with the client and family ways to minimize urinary tract infections in those requiring frequent catheterization. Increased fluid intake and urine acidification through drinking cranberry juice are two examples. Also discuss modifications in hygiene and sexual intercourse that may be indicated for persons with indwelling catheters.

- Teach the client and family when and how to empty the collection bag and to assess the urine for signs of infection, bleeding, or other complications.

- Clients with an indwelling catheter should take a shower rather than a tub bath. ➤*Rationale: Sitting in a tub allows bacteria easier access into the urinary tract.*

| UNEXPECTED OUTCOMES | CRITICAL THINKING OPTIONS |
|---|---|
| Bladder scan gives no reading. | • Make certain adequate conducting gel has been used.<br>• Have obese client bend knees so that feet are flat on the bed.<br>• Have thin client partially sit up to compress abdomen.<br>• Apply more pressure with scanhead, depressing 1–2 inches into client's abdomen. |
| Catheter is contaminated during procedure. | • Obtain new kit (or sterile catheter) and repeat procedure.<br>• Keep catheter tip in lubricant packet until ready to catheterize.<br>• If catheter has tear-away sleeve, leave catheter within it while catheterizing client. |
| Catheter is inserted into female client's vagina. | • Leave the catheter in place and follow these actions:<br>    Have someone obtain a new sterile catheter and gloves<br>    Reposition fingers to better visualize urethral meatus<br>    Obtain an assistant to provide direct lighting<br>    Insert new catheter pointing upward (toward client's umbilicus) as downward angle insertion tends to follow vaginal inlet<br>• Place obese client in side-lying position and flex upper leg for catheterization. |
| Catheter cannot be inserted into male client. | • Obtain new catheter kit and follow these actions:<br>    Hold penis vertical to client's body<br>    Insert catheter while applying slight traction by gently pulling upward on the shaft of the penis<br>    If resistance encountered, rotate catheter, increase traction, and lower angle of penis<br>    Ask client to cough<br>    Try using a condé or 12 Fr catheter |

*(continued)*

| **UNEXPECTED OUTCOMES** *(cont.)* | **CRITICAL THINKING OPTIONS** *(cont.)* |
|---|---|
| Urine flow upon catheterization immediately exceeds 700 mL. | • Inflate catheter balloon, but clamp catheter for 10 minutes, then resume urine drainage.<br>• Monitor client's vital signs; watch for hypotension, pallor, diaphoresis with rapid bladder decompression. |
| Urine leaks around retention catheter. | • Inflate catheter balloon with full amount of sterile water in syringe (10 mL) to fill balloon and catheter inflation lumen as well.<br>• Do not increase catheter size as this increases bladder irritation, spasm, and leakage.<br>• Obtain urine culture and sensitivity as leakage may be sign of urinary tract infection.<br>• Obtain order for anticholinergic medication to relieve bladder spasms. |
| Client develops urinary tract infection while catheterized. | • Remind physician that client has a catheter; reevaluate need for continued use.<br>• Obtain order for antimicrobial prophylaxis if client has history of UTIs.<br>• Keep urine collection system below level of client's bladder—avoid any chance of urinary reflux.<br>• Encourage fluid intake of 3 L/day unless contraindicated.<br>• Maintain client and system positioning so that continuous urine drainage is unobstructed.<br>• Make certain that catheter is secured properly (thigh of female, abdomen of male).<br>• Maintain/coil drainage tubing to allow straight drainage into urine collection bag.<br>• Provide daily perineal care with soap and water only.<br>• Don clean gloves to empty urine collection bag; avoid contamination of drain port.<br>• Suggest suprapubic catheter placement for long-term use.<br>• Suggest external collection system (condom catheter) for male client. |

# Skill 2.11   Performing Catheter Care and Removal

If the catheter requires changing, an entire new system with collecting bag must be used.

### Delegation

Routine care of the client with an indwelling catheter may be delegated to UAP. Abnormal findings must be validated and interpreted by the nurse. Removal of an indwelling catheter may be performed by UAP according to agency policy, provided they have been thoroughly trained in the procedure and are aware of conditions that could arise that require the assistance of a nurse.

### Equipment

• Clean gloves (3 pairs)
• Washcloth, soap, and towels

For catheter removal:

• Paper towel or waste receptacle
• Luer lock or slip tip syringe at least as large as the size of the retention balloon (printed on the inflation port)

### Preparation

Determine an appropriate time for catheter care or removal, and client's knowledge and need for teaching.

### Procedure

1. Prior to performing the procedure, introduce self and verify the client's identity using agency protocol. Explain to the client what you are going to do, why it is necessary, and how he or she can participate. Discuss how the results will be used in planning further care or treatments.
2. Perform hand hygiene and observe other appropriate infection control procedures.

> ### CLINICAL ALERT
> Do not aspirate balloon vigorously. Doing so may collapse inflation lumen and prevent balloon deflation.

# EVIDENCE-BASED NURSING PRACTICE

### Cranberry for Urinary Tract Infection Prophylaxis

There is growing accumulation of evidence-based information in support of use of cranberry in UTI prevention. Its beneficial effect is not by acidifying urine, but by inhibiting adherence of E. coli and other gram-negative uropathogens to urinary tract epithelial cells. A recent randomized controlled trial demonstrated that one table of concentrated cranberry extract (300–400 mg) twice daily or 8 oz. of pure unsweetened cranberry juice three times daily is safe and effective for up to 12 months. Cranberry may increase urinary oxalate levels and so may increase risk of kidney stone formation in patients with a history of oxalate calculi.

Cranberry also seems to inhibit the aggregation of dental plaque bacteria.

*Source:* Lynch, Darren. (2004). Cranberry for prevention of urinary tract infections. *American Family Physician,* 70 (11), 2175.

### Reminder Reduces Urinary Catheterization Use

This study demonstrated that catheter use could be decreased if physicians received automatic computerized (or written) reminders that their clients had catheters and how long they had been in place. Because urinary catheters are a major source of nosocomial infection, their use should be as brief as possible.

*Source:* Saint, S., et al. (2005). A reminder reduces urinary catheterization in hospitalized patients. *Journal on Quality and Patient Safety,* August.

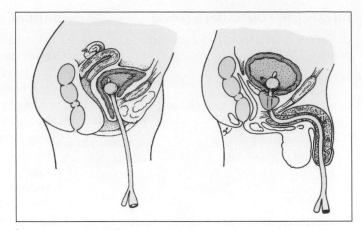

● Balloon must be deflated before removing to prevent damage to urethra.

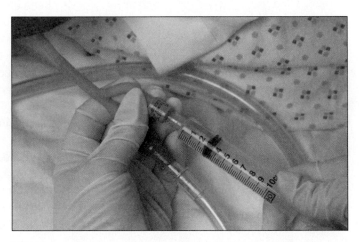

● Insert syringe hub into balloon port and withdraw fluid from retention catheter balloon.

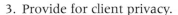

3. Provide for client privacy.
4. Prepare the client.
   - Ask the client to assume a back-lying position.
   - Obtain a sterile urine specimen if ordered or recommended by agency protocol.
5. Perform catheter care.
   - Apply clean gloves.
   - Wash the urinary meatus and the proximal catheter with soap and water. Dry gently.
   - Remove and discard gloves. Perform hand hygiene.
6. Empty the collection bag at least every 8 hours and whenever close to half full.
   - Apply clean gloves.
   - Obtain the graduated container used for measuring urine for that client.
   - Place a paper towel on the floor below the bag.
   - Remove the end of the drainage tube from its protective housing on the collection bag without touching the end.
   - Point the tube into the container and release the clamp.
   - After the bag is completely emptied, cleanse the end of the tube according to agency policy (e.g., with an alcohol swab), clamp the tube, and replace it into the protective housing.
   - Note the volume and characteristics of the urine. Empty the container into the toilet if the urine does not need to be saved.
   - Rinse the container and return it to its storage location.
   - Remove and discard gloves. Perform hand hygiene.
7. To remove the catheter:
   - Place a towel or receptacle between the client's legs.
   - Detach the catheter from where it has been secured to the client's skin.
   - Apply clean gloves.
   - Insert the hub of the syringe into the inflation tube of the catheter.
   - Withdraw all the fluid from the balloon. ➤*Rationale: This will permit the balloon to deflate.* If not all fluid can be removed, report this fact to the nurse in charge before proceeding. *Do not pull* the catheter while the balloon is inflated. ➤*Rationale: The urethra may be injured if the inflated balloon is pulled through it.*

- Gently withdraw the catheter, observe for intactness, and place in the towel or waste receptacle. ➤*Rationale: If the catheter is not intact, parts may remain in the bladder. Report this immediately to the nurse in charge or primary care provider.*
  - Wash and dry the perineal area.
8. Measure the urine in the drainage bag (see step 6 above).
9. Discard all used supplies in appropriate receptacles,
  - Remove and discard gloves. Perform hand hygiene.
10. Document the procedure and assessment data.
  - Record the time the catheter was removed; the intactness of the catheter; and the amount, color, and clarity of the urine.
11. Determine time of first voiding and the amount voided over the first 8 hours. Compare this with the fluid intake. ➤*Rationale: When the fluid output is considerably less than the fluid intake, the bladder may be retaining urine.* If urine retention is suspected, scan or palpate the bladder for fullness. Use noninvasive methods to encourage voiding such as allowing the client to hear running water or placing the client's hand in water. Notify the primary care provider if the client has not voided in 8 hours (or another interval specified by policy) because the client may need to be recatheterized. Record the voiding or other action taken.

### Documentation

Sample: 7/3/09 1015 Foley removed intact after aspirating balloon for 9.5 mL fluid s̄ difficulty. Moderate amount white sediment noted around catheter tip. Peri care provided. Skin intact and s̄ lesions. Taught to continue goal intake of fluids of 150 mL/hour. Verbalized agreement.

_____ S. Brown, RN

7/3/09 1645 Up to BR. Voided 600 mL amber urine. c/o slight burning at start of urination. Will continue fluid intake as much as can.

_____ S. Brown, RN

# Skill 2.12   Performing Bladder Irrigation

Before irrigating a catheter or bladder, check (1) the reason for the irrigation; (2) the order authorizing the continuous or intermittent irrigation (in most agencies, a primary care provider's order is required); (3) the type of sterile solution, the amount, and strength to be used, and the rate (if continuous); and (4) the type of catheter in place. If these are not specified on the client's charge, check agency protocol.

### Delegation

Due to the need for sterile technique, urinary irrigation is generally not delegated to UAP. If the client has continuous irrigation, the must be validated and interpreted by the nurse.

### Equipment

- Clean gloves (2 pairs)
- Retention catheter in place
- Drainage tubing and bag (if not in place)
- Drainage tubing clamp
- Antiseptic swabs
- Sterile receptacle
- Sterile irrigating solution warmed or at room temperature (Label the irrigant clearly with the words *Bladder Irrigation*, including the information about any medications that have been added to the original solution, and the date, time, and nurse's initials.)
- Infusion tubing
- IV pole

### Procedure

1. Prior to performing the procedure, introduce self and verify the client's identity using agency protocol. Explain to the client what you are going to do, why it is necessary, and how he or she can participate. The irrigation should not be painful or uncomfortable. Discuss how the results will be used in planning further care or treatments.
2. Perform hand hygiene and observe other appropriate infection control procedures.
3. Provide for client privacy.
4. Apply clean gloves.
5. Empty, measure, and record the amount and appearance of urine present in the drainage bag. Discard urine and gloves. ➤*Rationale: Emptying the drainage bag allows more accurate measurement of urinary output after the irrigation is in place or completed. Assessing the character of the urine provides baseline data for later comparison.*
6. Prepare the equipment.
  - Perform hand hygiene.
  - Connect the irrigation infusion tubing to the irrigating solution and flush the tubing with solution, keeping the tip sterile. ➤*Rationale: Flushing the tubing removes air and prevents it from being instilled into the bladder.*
  - Apply clean gloves and cleanse the port with antiseptic swabs.
  - Connect the irrigation tubing to the input port of the three-way catheter.

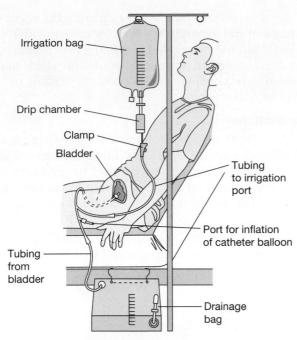

Irrigation bag

Drip chamber

Clamp

Bladder

Tubing to irrigation port

Port for inflation of catheter balloon

Tubing from bladder

Drainage bag

● A continuous bladder irrigation (CBI) setup.

- Connect the drainage bag and tubing to the urinary drainage port if not already in place.
- Remove and discard gloves. Perform hand hygiene.

7. Irrigate the bladder.
- For closed continuous bladder irrigation using a three-way catheter, open the clamp on the urinary drainage tubing (if present). ➤*Rationale: This allows the irrigating solution to flow out of the bladder continuously.*
  a. Apply clean gloves.
  b. Open the regulating clamp on the irrigating fluid infusion tubing and adjust the flow rate as prescribed by the primary care provider or to 40 to 60 drops per minute if not specified.
  c. Assess the drainage for amount, color, and clarity. The amount of drainage should equal the amount of irrigant entering the bladder plus expected urine output. Empty the bag frequently so that it does not exceed half full.
- For closed intermittent irrigation, determine whether the solution is to remain in the bladder for a specified time.
  a. If the solution is to remain in the bladder (a bladder irrigation or instillation), apply the clamp to the urinary drainage tubing. ➤*Rationale: Closing the flow clamp allows the solution to be retained in the bladder and in contact with bladder walls.*
  b. If the solution is being instilled to irrigate the catheter, no flow clamp on the urinary drainage tubing is used. ➤*Rationale: Irrigating solution will flow through the urinary drainage port and tubing, removing mucous shreds or clots.*

  c. If a three-way catheter is used, open the flow clamp to the irrigating fluid infusion, allowing the specified amount of solution to infuse. Then close the clamp on the infusion tubing.
  *or*
  a. If a two-way catheter is used, connect an irrigating syringe with a needleless adapter to the injection port on the drainage tubing and instill the solution.
  b. After the specified period the solution is to be retained has passed, open the drainage tubing flow clamp and allow the bladder to empty.
  c. Assess the drainage for amount, color, and clarity. The amount of drainage should equal the amount of irrigant entering the bladder plus expected urine output.
- Remove and discard gloves. Perform hand hygiene.

8. Assess the client and the urinary output.
- Assess the client's comfort.
- Empty the drainage bag and measure the contents. Subtract the amount of irrigant instilled from the total volume of drainage to obtain the volume of urine output.
- Remove and discard gloves. Perform hand hygiene.

9. Document findings in the client record using forms or checklists supplemented by narrative notes when appropriate.
- Note any abnormal constituents such as blood clots, pus, or mucous shreds.

**VARIATION: Open Irrigation Using a Two-Way Indwelling Catheter**

1. Assemble the equipment. Use an irrigation set or assemble individual items, including:

**Equipment**

- Clean gloves
- Disposable water-resistant towel
- Sterile irrigating solution
- Sterile basin
- Sterile 30- to 50-mL irrigating syringe
- Antiseptic swabs
- Sterile protective cap for drainage tubing

2. Prepare the client (see steps 1 through 5 of main procedure for catheter irrigation).

---

CLINICAL ALERT

Opening a closed urinary drainage system is indicated as a last resort to reestablish catheter patency. Manual irrigation should NOT be performed with transurethral resection of a bladder tumor due to risk of bladder rupture.

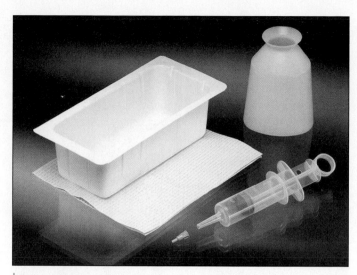

● An irrigation set.
(Courtesy of Bard Medical Division)

3. Prepare the equipment.
   - Perform hand hygiene.
   - Using aseptic technique, open supplies and pour the irrigating solution into the sterile basin or receptacle. ➤*Rationale: Aseptic technique is vital to reduce the risk of instilling microorganisms into the urinary tract during the irrigation.*
   - Place the disposable water-resistant towel under the catheter.
   - Apply clean gloves.

- Disconnect catheter from drainage tubing and place the catheter end in the sterile basin. Place the sterile protective cap over end of drainage tubing. *Rationale: The end of the drainage tubing will be considered contaminated if it touches bed linens or skin surfaces.*
- Draw the prescribed amount of irrigating solution into the syringe, maintaining the sterility of the syringe and solution.

4. Irrigate the bladder.
   - Insert the tip of the syringe into the catheter opening.
   - Gently and slowly inject the solution into the catheter at approximately 3 mL per second. In adults, about 30 to 40 mL generally is instilled for catheter irrigations; 100 to 200 mL may be instilled for bladder irrigation or instillation. ➤*Rationale: Gentle instillation reduces the risks of injury to bladder mucosa and of bladder spasms.*
   - Remove the syringe and allow the solution to drain back into the basin.
   - Continue to irrigate client's bladder until the total amount to be instilled has been injected or when fluid returns are clear and/or clots are removed.
   - Remove protective cap from drainage tube and wipe with antiseptic swab.
   - Reconnect catheter to drainage tubing.
   - Remove and discard gloves. Perform hand hygiene.
   - Assess the drainage for amount, color, and clarity. The amount of drainage should equal at least the amount of irrigant entering the bladder plus any urine that may have been dwelling in the bladder.

5. Assess the client and the urinary output and document the procedure as in steps 8 and 9 above.

## Skill 2.13   Maintaining Continuous Bladder Irrigation

### Equipment

Irrigating solution (2000 mL sterile normal saline) as
   prescribed
IV tubing with roller clamp
IV pole
Antiseptic swabs
Clean gloves

### Procedure

1. Check physician's orders and client care plan.
2. Note if client has triple lumen indwelling catheter and drainage bag.
3. Identify client.
4. Explain procedure to client and provide privacy.
5. Perform hand hygiene and don clean gloves.
6. Remove protective covering from spike on tubing, and insert spike into insertion port of solution container. Use aseptic technique.

7. Hang irrigating solution container on IV pole and prime tubing. Height of pole is usually 24–36 inches above bladder.
   a. Remove protective cover from end of tubing using aseptic technique.
   b. Open roller clamp, and allow irrigating solution to run through tubing until all air is expelled. ➤*Rationale: This prevents air from entering bladder and causing discomfort.*
   c. Close roller clamp.
8. Connect tubing to catheter irrigating (indwelling) lumen using aseptic technique.
9. Remove gloves.
10. Adjust drip rate of irrigating solution by adjusting the clamp on the tubing to increase or decrease based on urine outflow color.
    a. Infuse continuously to keep urine drainage pink to clear.

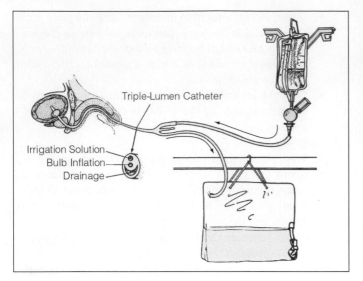

● Maintain continuous bladder irrigation by using a triple-lumen catheter for procedure.

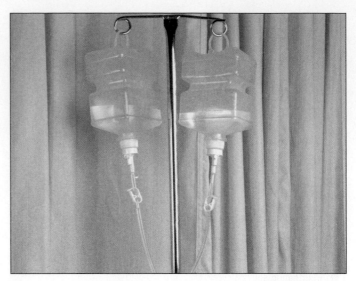

● Hang irrigating solution on IV pole at height of 24–36 inches above bladder.

b. When drainage is dark red or contains tissue or blood clots, increase drip rate. ►*Rationale: Increased drip rate will clear the drainage and flush out debris and clots.*

c. Change irrigation solution bottle using aseptic technique.

11. Check for bladder distention or abdominal pain; note urine color.

12. Monitor urine output at least every hour to observe patency of system.

13. Empty drainage bag as needed. Subtract amount of irrigant infused from total output to obtain urine output and record.

14. Maintain catheter traction if taped to thigh. ►*Rationale: This promotes venous hemostasis.*

15. Remove gloves and perform hand hygiene.

*Note:* Procedure is done to flush clots and debris from bladder following prostatic surgery, and to prevent catheter obstruction and promote patency. Immediately report bright red urine outflow as this indicates an arterial bleed.

# Skill 2.14   Providing Suprapubic Catheter Care

**EXPECTED OUTCOMES**

• Suprapubic catheter remains intact.
• Client remains free of urinary tract infection.
• Client is able to void naturally.

**Equipment**

Closed drainage system, including Foley catheter tubing and bag
Catheter clamp and plug
Dry sterile dressing and tape if ordered
Cleansing solution
Clean gloves
Sterile gloves

**Preparation**

1. Check physician's orders and client care plan.
2. Identify client and explain purpose of catheter.
3. Describe procedure for continuous or intermittent urinary drainage.
4. Perform hand hygiene.
5. Provide privacy.

**Procedure**

1. Observe catheter for patency. ►*Rationale: The most common problem with suprapubic catheters is occlusion with sediment or clots.*
   a. First 24 hours: check the catheter every hour to detect possible obstruction. Urine output should be in excess of 30 mL/hour.
   b. Second day: check the catheter every 8 hours.
   c. Third day: check the catheter when the catheter is unclamped.
2. Maintain a closed drainage system. Do not open system to irrigate or obtain urine sample.
3. Observe for signs of urinary tract infection (color, odor, presence of sediment).

4. Keep the dressing dry around site of insertion. Apply a new dressing, maintaining sterile technique, every morning and as necessary.
   a. Perform hand hygiene and don clean gloves.
   b. Remove old dressing, discard gloves, and dispose in appropriate container.
   c. Perform hand hygiene and open sterile supplies.
   d. Open cleansing solution and pour over sterile gauze.
   e. Don sterile gloves.
   f. Assess skin surrounding suprapubic catheter.
   g. Cleanse area with cleansing solution. Allow to dry.
   h. Apply sterile dressing and secure with tape.
   i. Remove gloves and supplies and discard in appropriate container.
   j. Perform hand hygiene.
5. Perform clamping protocol according to physician orders for intermittent urinary drainage.
   a. Explain the clamping procedure and ask client to help monitor the clamping.
   b. Instruct client to report if he or she feels fullness in the bladder during clamping.
   c. Don clean gloves.
   d. Clamp the catheter.
6. Empty the drainage bag or remove drainage tubing from catheter, maintaining aseptic technique.
   a. Place drainage tubing in sterile package to maintain sterility.
   b. Place catheter plug in catheter end.
   c. Remove gloves and perform hand hygiene.
   d. Record urine output on I&O record.
   e. Leave the catheter clamped or plugged for 3–4 hours depending on client's level of comfort and physician's orders.
7. At 3- to 4-hour intervals, or when client feels bladder fullness, ask client to void normally. Don clean gloves to measure the urine and record output on I&O bedside record.
8. Immediately after client voids, unclamp catheter and leave unclamped for 5 minutes, collecting the residual urine.
   a. Don clean gloves to measure the residual urine following unclamping of the catheter.
   b. Reclamp catheter.
   c. Send a urine specimen to laboratory after the first clamping. ▶*Rationale: This checks for the presence of microorganisms.*
9. Repeat clamping protocol every 3–4 hours according to physician orders. The catheter may be open to drainage from bedtime until 6 in the morning.

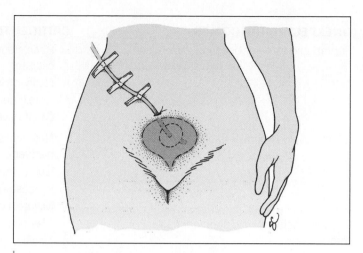

● Tape catheter and connect to a closed system.

10. When the client is voiding normally, clamp the catheter throughout the night in preparation for its removal.
11. When the client's residual urine output is less than 100 mL or retains less than 20% of residual urine on two successive checks, notify the physician for removal of the catheter.
12. Apply a 2 × 2 sterile dressing over the insertion site.
13. Dispose of the catheter in biohazard bag.
14. If the client is discharged from the hospital with the catheter, provide the following teaching for home care:
    a. Instruct the client to drink one glass of fluid every hour while awake.
    b. Instruct client to follow clamping procedure when awake or as instructed by physician.
    c. Instruct the client to leave the catheter open to the drainage system at night. (Drainage system may be urinary tubing and bag or leg bag.)
    d. Tell client to notify physician if dysuria occurs when voiding or if urine becomes cloudy, odorous, or has sediment.

### Documentation

- Time catheter clamped
- Length of time clamped
- Client's ability to void spontaneously
- Client's feelings of fullness
- Time specimen sent to laboratory
- Color, amount, and odor of urine obtained
- Color, amount, and odor of residual urine

| UNEXPECTED OUTCOMES | CRITICAL THINKING OPTIONS |
|---|---|
| Suprapubic catheter becomes dislodged. | • Place sterile dressing over catheter insertion site; do not attempt to replace catheter.<br>• Notify physician.<br>• Obtain new catheter to prepare for insertion by physician.<br>Client develops urinary tract infection. |
| Client develops urinary tract infection. | • Note signs and symptoms of UTI: cloudy malodorous urine with sediment, bladder discomfort/spasms, elevated temperature.<br>• Notify physician to obtain order for urinalysis and antimicrobial therapy.<br>• Increase fluid intake to at least 2 L/day (unless cantraindicated).<br>• Maintain continuous urine drainage per suprapubic catheter. |
| Client is unable to void spontaneously through urethra. | • Maintain suprapubic urine drainage. through urethra.<br>• Notify physician. |

# Skill 2.15  Performing Urinary Ostomy Care

## EXPECTED OUTCOMES
• Pouching system does not leak.
• Client demonstrates self-care skills.
• Urine specimen is readily obtained from urinary diversion system.
• Peristomal skin remains intact and healthy.

Review the client's record to determine the type of urinary diversion. Determine when the device was last changed and any pertinent findings at that time. Generally, a urinary diversion appliance adheres to the client's skin for 3 to 5 days.

## Delegation

Due to the complexity of the procedure, the need for assessment skills, and use of aseptic technique, changing a urostomy device is not delegated to UAP. However, aspects of ostomy function are observed during usual care and may be recorded by persons other than the nurse. Abnormal findings must be validated and interpreted by the nurse.

## Equipment

- One- or two-piece urinary pouch
- Tail closure clamp
- Clean gloves
- Cleaning materials, including tissues, warm water, mild soap (optional), cotton balls, washcloth or gauze pads, towel
- Skin barrier/prep (gel, liquid, powder, or film)
- Stoma measuring guide
- Pen or pencil and scissors
- Deodorant liquid drops (optional)
- Bedpan or graduated cylinder

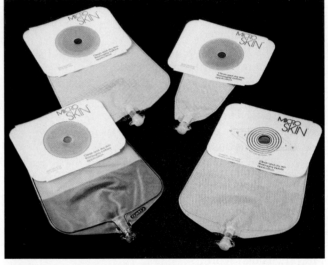

A

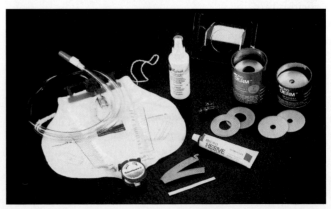

B

 **A,** one piece urostomy system; **B,** urostomy supplies.
(Courtesy of Cymed Ostomy Company)

## Preparation

- Determine the need for an appliance change.
- Assess the used appliance for leakage of urine. ➤*Rationale: Urine irritates the peristomal skin.*
- Ask the client about any discomfort at or around the stoma. ➤*Rationale: A burning sensation may indicate breakdown beneath the faceplate of the pouch.*
- Assess the fullness of the pouch. ➤*Rationale: The weight of an overly full bag may loosen the faceplate and separate it form the skin, causing the urine to leak and irritate the peristomal skin.*
- If there is pouch leakage or discomfort at or around the stoma, change the appliance.
- Select an appropriate time to change the appliance.
- Avoid times close to meals or visiting hours. ➤*Rationale: Ostomy odor may reduce appetite or embarrass the client.*

## Procedure

1. Prior to performing the procedure, introduce self and verify the client's identity using agency protocol. Explain to the client what you are going to do, why it is necessary, and how he or she can participate. Discuss how the results will be used in planning further care or treatments. Changing an ostomy appliance should not cause discomfort, but it may be distasteful to the client. Communicate acceptance and support to the client. It is important to change the appliance competently and quickly. Include support persons as appropriate.
2. Perform hand hygiene and observe other appropriate infection control procedures.
3. Provide for client privacy.
4. Assist the client to a comfortable sitting or lying position in bed or a sitting or standing position in the bathroom. ➤*Rationale: Lying or standing positions may facilitate smoother pouch application.*
5. Empty and remove the ostomy appliance. *Note:* Because urine flows continuously, if the stoma can be measured for the new appliance with the appliance in place, perform step 8 first. This can usually be accomplished if the pouch is thin or transparent enough to fit the measuring guide snugly over the stoma while it is in place.
   - Apply clean gloves.
   - Empty the pouch through the bottom opening into a bedpan or graduated cylinder. ➤*Rationale: Emptying before removing the pouch prevents spillage of urine onto the client's skin.*
   - Peel the bag off slowly while holding the client's skin taut. ➤*Rationale: Holding the skin taut minimizes client discomfort and prevents abrasion of the skin.*
   - Place tissue or gauze pad over the stoma, and change as needed. ➤*Rationale: This absorbs urine seepage from the stoma.*

6. Clean and dry the peristomal skin and stoma.
   - Use warm water, mild soap (optional), and damp cotton balls, gauze, or a washcloth and towel to clean the skin and stoma. Check agency practice on the use of soap. ➤*Rationale: Soap is sometimes not advised because it can be irritating to the skin.*
   - Dry the area thoroughly by patting with a towel or cotton balls. ➤*Rationale: Excess rubbing can abrade the skin.*
7. Assess the stoma and peristomal skin.
   - Inspect the stoma for color, size, shape, and bleeding.
   - Inspect the peristomal skin for any redness, ulceration, or irritation. Transient redness after removal of adhesive is normal.
8. Prepare and apply the new pouch.
   - Use the guide to measure the size of the stoma.
   - On the backing of the skin barrier, trace a circle the same size as the stomal opening.
   - Cut out the traced stoma pattern to make an opening in the skin barrier. Make the opening no more than 0.3 cm (1/8 in.) larger than the stoma. ➤*Rationale: This allows space for the stoma to expand slightly when functioning and minimizes the risk of urine contacting peristomal skin.*
   - Remove the backing to expose the sticky adhesive side of the barrier. The backing can be saved and used as a pattern when making an opening for future skin barriers.
   - Apply the peristomal skin barrier to the faceplate of the ostomy appliance or around the stoma depending on the manufacturer's recommendations. Skin barrier powder may be used on irritated skin, but Skin-Prep liquid may not be applied to irritated skin.
   - Center the faceplate over the stoma, and gently press it onto the client's skin, smoothing out any wrinkles or bubbles. Hold in place for about 30 seconds. ➤*Rationale: The heat and pressure help activate the adhesives in the skin barrier.*
   - Remove the air from the pouch. ➤*Rationale: Removing the air helps the pouch lie flat against the abdomen.*
   - *Optional:* Place approximately 10 drops of deodorant in the pouch.
   - Close the pouch by turning up the bottom a few times, fanfolding its end lengthwise, and securing it with a tail closure clamp or replacing the drainage outlet cap.
   - Discard all used supplies in appropriate receptacles.
   - Remove and discard gloves, and perform hand hygiene.
9. Document findings in the client record using forms or checklists supplemented by narrative notes when appropriate.

## Documentation

Sample: 8/31/09 0900 Urostomy bag changed due to slight leakage. Had been in place for 6 days. No redness or irritation around stoma. Stoma pink, bled a few drops when washed. Client states home care RN changes the appliance when home.

_____ M. Earl, RN

| UNEXPECTED OUTCOMES | CRITICAL THINKING OPTIONS |
|---|---|
| Pouching system leaks. | • Check area for crease or dip in skin, which allows urine to pool and leak out.<br>• Fill in dip area with skin barrier to prevent pooling.<br>• Apply belt to improve fit.<br>• Apply another type of pouch (e.g., convex).<br>• Change more frequently if leak is due to dissolving of skin barrier—or use different barrier.<br>• Advise client to avoid using soaps or wipes to clean area because they interfere with pouch adhesion. |
| Client is unable to manage own urinary diversion. | • Simplify pouch procedure if possible.<br>• Provide detailed instruction in more simplified manner.<br>• Include caregiver in teaching to assist and support client.<br>• Refer client to home health agency for follow-up care. |
| Client is offended by odor in urine collection system. | • Recommend urine acidifying agent (e.g., vitamin C, 500 mg b.i.d. to t.i.d.); collection system. avoid alkaline ash citrus juices.<br>• Wash reusable equipment with mild soap and water and rinse in vinegar weekly, or use commercial deodorant.<br>• Inform client that certain foods and drugs (asparagus, vitamin B complex) give odor to urine. Empty pouch frequently if these are ingested.<br>• Inform client that cloudy urine and strong odor may indicate urinary tract infection. Advise physician and collect sterile urine specimen. |
| No urine is obtained from conduit. | • Rotate catheter, or position client on side to allow urine to flow into catheter. As little as 1 mL is needed for urine culture and sensitivity testing.<br>• Have client drink water. |
| Erythematous vesicular rash appears on peristomal skin. | • Suspect possible allergic reaction; obtain patch test for allergy.<br>• Avoid use of chemical wipes and perfumed soaps.<br>• Suspect yeast infection; report to physician. |

# Skill 2.16   Applying a Urinary Diversion Pouch

## Equipment

One- or two-piece urinary pouch with skin barrier, flange, and spigot at bottom of pouch to empty urine
Items to clean stoma (e.g., soft cloth or gauze sponges) and warm water
Plastic bag for disposal of used equipment
Gauze for drying skin and for wicking stoma
Underpad to protect bedding
Scissors if indicated
Protective barriers such as skin prep, skin gel, or protective barrier film if necessary
Stoma measuring guide
Clean gloves

## Preparation

1. Check physician's order and client care plan. Pouch should be changed every 3–7 days.
2. Gather equipment.
3. Perform hand hygiene.

4. Identify client and explain procedure.
5. Provide privacy.
6. Place client in a position that promotes visualization and self-care.
7. Place protective pad under client.
8. Place bath blanket over client's chest and position top covers over lower abdomen without impeding client's visualization of procedure.

## Procedure

1. Don clean gloves.
2. Empty, then remove old pouch, and discard in plastic bag.
3. Wash skin with warm water and dry thoroughly. ▸*Rationale: Chemical or perfumed wipes can irritate skin or may interfere with pouch seal. Note:* Stoma may bleed slightly when wiped.
4. Prepare new urinary pouch. First measure stoma site with measuring guide, unless pouch has precut opening.

5. Trace size of stoma on wafer and cut ¹⁄₁₆–¹⁄₈ inch larger than size. ➤*Rationale: This small opening prevents leakage of effluent onto skin; however, the size is large enough to prevent pressure on the stoma from the wafer rubbing on skin.*

6. Snap pouch onto flange.

7. Check stoma for healing; it should be bright but not dark red and moist, and raised ½–1 inch above skin surface (or may be flush). Check for mucocutaneous separation. *Note:* This may be an appropriate time to teach client to check status of stoma and skin around stoma.

8. Wick stoma with gauze. ➤*Rationale: To keep urine from contact with skin during pouch change.*

9. Check skin surrounding stoma to ensure urine hasn't been draining under wafer causing skin irritation.

10. Apply protective barrier (only if indicated) to skin surrounding stoma or to wafer. ➤*Rationale: Protective barriers contain alcohol and cause burning, and may interfere with seal.* In addition, barrier must be removed with adhesive remover.

11. Let dry thoroughly.

12. Remove paper from adhesive on wafer of one- or two-piece appliance.

13. Remove wick and center wafer over stoma; apply to dry skin, starting at bottom, and working up around stoma. If two-piece pouch, attach pouch to wafer flange.

14. Attach pouch to gravity drainage bag only while client is in bed. Pouch has a spout at end to drain urine. Empty pouch when one-third full.

15. Discard equipment in appropriate receptacle.

16. Remove gloves and perform hand hygiene.

---

## CLINICAL ALERT

Thin plastic tubes (stents) may be placed in each ureter during surgery. These exit stoma and remain in place for up to 10 days. They serve to maintain patency until swelling has subsided at ureteroileal anastamosis site (6–10 days). Their presence and length of exposure should be documented. The surgeon should be notified when they wash out into collection pouch.

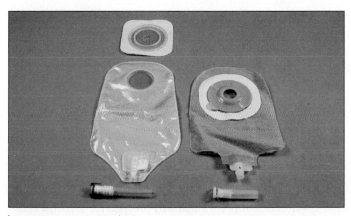

● One-piece and two-piece urinary diversion pouches.

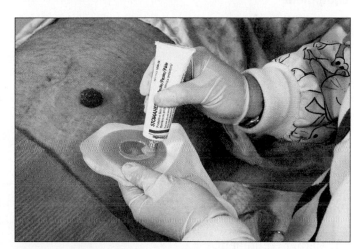

● Apply protective barrier paste to wafer, only if indicated.

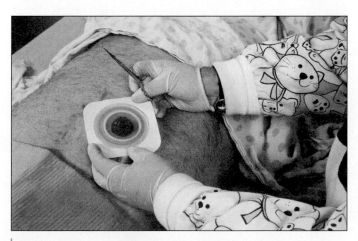

● Cut wafer opening slightly larger than stoma.

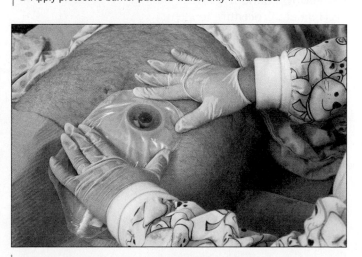

● Apply pouch and press firmly to facilitate seal.

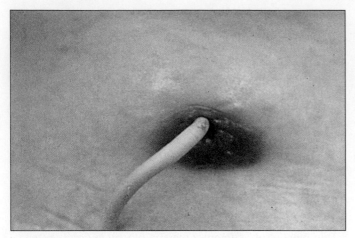

● Catheter is used to obtain specimen from ileal conduit.

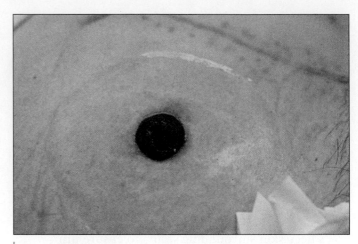

● Ileal conduit stoma.

# Skill 2.17   Obtaining Urine Specimen from an Ileal Conduit

## Equipment

Sterile catheter kit
Prep solution
Sterile saline or water
Underpad
New urinary pouch
Supplies to apply new pouch
Bath blanket, towels
Clean gloves
Soap and water
Pitcher of water and glass
Biohazard bag

## Preparation

1. Check physician's orders and client care plan.
2. Gather equipment.
3. Perform hand hygiene.
4. Explain procedure to client.
5. Provide privacy.
6. Place bath blanket over client's chest and position top covers over lower abdomen.
7. Place towels around stoma. ➤*Rationale: Urine will leak around catheter.*
8. Don gloves.

## Procedure

1. Open sterile packages.
2. Remove pouch or snap pouch off wafer flange. *Note:* Do not use pouch contents to obtain urine specimen. Remove gloves.
3. Put on sterile gloves.

4. Place sterile drape over stoma.
5. Remove lid from specimen container, and place end of catheter into container.
6. Apply lubricant to catheter.
7. Use forceps to pick up cotton ball and prep stoma with solution and rinse with sterile saline or water.
8. Insert tip of catheter into stoma approximately 1½ inches.
9. When urine specimen is obtained (usually not more than 5–25 mL), remove catheter. If no urine obtained, have client drink water.
10. Return lid to specimen container and apply label.
11. If wafer removed, wash and dry peristomal area.
12. Replace pouch, or apply new pouch.
13. Remove gloves and perform hand hygiene.
14. Place specimen container in biohazard bag and send specimen to lab immediately or refrigerate.

## Elimination—Waste Products

Elimination of the waste products of digestion from the body is essential to health. The excreted waste products are referred to as feces or stool. Defecation is the expulsion of feces from the anus and rectum. It is also called a bowel movement. The frequency is highly individual, varying from several times per day to two or three times per week. The amount defecated also varies from person to person. When peristaltic waves move the feces into the sigmoid colon and the rectum, the sensory nerves in the rectum are stimulated and the individual becomes aware of the need to defecate.

# Skill 2.18 Removing a Fecal Impaction

### Delegation

Due to the potential results of stimulation of the vagus nerve during the procedure, digital removal of an impaction is generally not delegated to UAP.

### Equipment

- Bath blanket
- Disposable absorbent pad
- Bedpan and cover
- Toilet tissue
- Clean gloves
- Lubricant
- Soap, water, and towel
- Topical lidocaine (if agency permits)

### Preparation

- Check agency policy to determine if a primary care provider's order is required. ➤*Rationale: Rectal manipulation can cause stimulation of the vagus nerve, resulting in a slowing of the heart rate.*
- If the agency permits the use of the topical anesthetic lidocaine, 1 to 2 mL should be inserted into the anal canal 5 minutes prior to the procedure. ➤*Rationale: This will numb the anal and rectal areas, reducing the pain of the procedure.*

### Procedure

1. Prior to performing the procedure, introduce self and verify the client's identity using agency protocol. Explain to the client what you are going to do, why it is necessary, and how he or she can participate. Discuss how the results will be used in planning further care or treatments. This procedure is distressing, tiring, and uncomfortable, so the person may desire the presence of another nurse or support person.
2. Perform hand hygiene and observe other appropriate infection control procedures.
3. Apply clean gloves.
4. Provide for client privacy.
5. Assist the client to a right or left lateral or Sims' position with the back toward you. ➤*Rationale: When the person lies on the right side, the sigmoid colon is uppermost; thus, gravity can aid removal of the feces. Positioning on the left side allows easier access to the sigmoid colon.*
6. Place the disposable absorbent pad under the client's hips, and arrange the top bedclothes so that they fall obliquely over the hips, exposing only the buttocks.

7. Place the bedpan and toilet tissue nearby on the bed or a bedside chair.
8. Lubricate the gloved index finger. ➤*Rationale: Lubricant reduces resistance by the anal sphincter as the finger is inserted.*
9. Remove the impaction. Have the client take slow, deep breaths during the procedure.
   - Gently insert the index finger into the rectum, moving toward the umbilicus.
   - Gently massage around the stool. ➤*Rationale: Gentle action prevents damage to the rectal mucosa. A circular motion around the rectum dislodges the stool, stimulates peristalsis, and relaxes the anal sphincter.*
   - Work the finger into the hardened mass of stool to break it up.
   - If you cannot break up the impaction with one finger, insert two fingers and try to break up the impaction scissor style.
   - Work the stool down to the anus, remove it in small pieces, and place them in the bedpan.
   - Carefully continue to remove as much fecal material as possible; at the same time, assess for bleeding or signs of pallor, feelings of faintness, shortness of breath, perspiration, or changes in pulse rate. Terminate the procedure if these occur. ➤*Rationale: Manual stimulation could result in mucosal damage, excessive vagal nerve stimulation, and subsequent cardiac arrhythmia.*
   - Assist the client to a position on a clean bedpan, commode, or toilet. ➤*Rationale: Digital stimulation of the rectum may induce the urge to defecate.*
10. Assist the client with hygienic measures as needed.
    - Wash the rectal area with soap and water and dry gently.
    - Remove and discard gloves. Perform hand hygiene.
11. Document the results of the procedure in the client record using forms or checklists supplemented by narrative notes when appropriate.

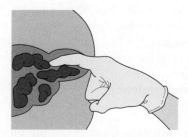

● Digital removal of fecal impaction.

# Skill 2.19   Developing a Regular Bowel Routine

## EVIDENCE-BASED NURSING PRACTICE

### Management of Constipation in Older Adults

Studies conducted in Britain and the United States indicate that between 10% and 18% of otherwise healthy adults have frequent straining on defecation. Constipation appears to be more common in women than men, and about 20% of the elderly identify the problem. Constipation is not a physiological consequence of the aging process; however, decreased GI motility is a contributing factor to the prevalence in older adults. Constipation may occur secondary to other conditions such as colorectal cancer or strictures. It is also associated with contributing factors such as inadequate fluid intake, absence of dietary fiber, caloric intake, and lack of exercise. In a recent study of clients who considered themselves constipated, 40% were using over-the-counter medications known to cause constipation. In addition to these factors, clients in the hospital may have a lack of privacy and inconvenience or lack of toilet facilities, which can lead to constipation.

A variety of products have been studied to determine if any of them prevent constipation. Some studies support the effectiveness of supplementing the diet with bran but its effectiveness has not been supported by randomized controlled trials.

Other studies suggest that fiber may be effective in improving bowel movement frequency in the ambulatory client, while stimulant and osmotic laxatives may be more effective than bulk-forming agents for the immobilized client. A current study supports establishing a bowel-training program to establish regularity. Additional studies support incorporating regular exercise to reduce the risk of constipation.

*Source:* (a) Management of constipation in older adults, Best Practice, 3(1), 1999. (b) Hsieh, C. Treatment of constipation in older adults. *American Family Physician* (2005, Dec).

### Equipment

Clean gloves, 1 or 2 pair
Lubricant
Bedpan or commode
Absorbent pad
Specific enema if ordered
Washcloth and towel

### Preparation

1. Check physician's orders and client care plan.
2. Identify the correct client, and explain procedure.
3. Identify time of day client usually evacuates bowels.
4. Evaluate diet, exercise, former use of medications for bowel evacuation.
5. Administer the following drugs as ordered:
   a. Stool softener (Colace, Dialose, DCS, coloxyl) daily.
   b. Bulk former (Metamucil or FiberCon)—daily to t.i.d.
   c. Mild laxative (Senokot, Doxidan, Dulcolax) 8 hours before program.
   d. Suppository (glycerin or Dulcolax) just before digital stimulation.
6. Perform hand hygiene.

### Procedure

1. Don gloves. You may want to double-glove to prevent contamination if glove tears.

2. Perform digital stimulation ½ hour after dinner or breakfast or according to client's time schedule for evacuation (see previous intervention). ➤*Rationale: Food stimulates bowel activity.*
3. Place client on toilet or commode. (Use bedpan if client is on bed rest.) ➤*Rationale: Assuming normal posture for bowel movement facilitates evacuation.*
4. Encourage client to contract abdominal muscles or bend forward while bearing down. ➤*Rationale: Increases abdominal pressure and helps evacuate the bowel.*
5. Remove gloves.
6. Perform hand hygiene.
7. Provide privacy and sufficient time for evacuation.
8. Don gloves.
9. Wash and dry perineal area if client is unable to do so.
10. Remove gloves.
11. Place client in wheelchair or bed and position for comfort.
12. Perform hand hygiene.
13. Wean client away from suppositories and laxatives when spontaneous bowel movements occur with digital stimulation.

## BOWEL TRAINING

Good bowel training programs include

- Initiation of defecation on demand with digital stimulation and abdominal massage
- Evacuation at same time each day; best time 20–40 minutes after a meal
- Proper diet, increased fiber and fluids
- Daily physical exercise regimen
- Client and family education

## DEVELOPMENTAL CONSIDERATIONS

**Recommendations for Preventing Constipation in the Older Adult Population**

- Identify bowel patterns using a bowel diary.
- Increase fluids to 1500–2000 mL/day; minimize caffeine and alcohol intake.
- Promote regular consistent toileting.
- Tailor physical activity to client's physical abilities.
- Assess constipation by obtaining the client's history; including information regarding the amount of fluid intake, food ingested, and dietary fiber.
- Review medications associated with an increased risk of developing constipation; screen for polypharmacy.

*Source:* www.guidelines.gov, "Prevention of Constipation in the Older Adult Population." RNAO Registered Nurses Association of Ontario, National Clearing House, March 2005.

# Skill 2.20   Inserting a Rectal Tube

### Equipment

Rectal tube: size 22–24 straight (French) for adults and size 12–18 French for children
Small plastic bag or stool specimen container
Hypoallergenic paper tape
Water-soluble lubricant
Bed protector
Clean gloves

### Procedure

1. Check physician's orders and client care plan.
2. Perform hand hygiene.
3. Gather equipment.
4. Identify the correct client with two forms of identification and explain the procedure.
5. Provide privacy. Place client on left side in a recumbent position and drape. ➤*Rationale: This position facilitates insertion of tube following the normal curve of rectum and sigmoid colon.*
6. Place bed protector under client.
7. Tape the plastic bag around the distal end of the rectal tube or insert the tube into the stool specimen container.
8. Vent the upper side of the plastic bag to prevent inflation.
9. Don gloves.
10. Lubricate the proximal end of the rectal tube with water-soluble lubricant.
11. Gently separate buttocks, and ask client to take in a deep breath. Gently insert the tube into the client's rectum, past the external and internal anal sphincters (2–4 inches in adults, 1–3 inches in children). ➤*Rationale: Taking a deep breath relaxes the anal sphincter and prevents tissue trauma during tube insertion.*
12. With adults, gently tape the tube in place, using hypoallergenic paper tape. With children, hold the tube in place manually.
13. Take client's pulse. ➤*Rationale: Alterations in pulse rate can indicate a vagal stimulation and the rectal tube may need to be removed.* This can occur particularly in a client with a cardiac condition.
14. Leave the tube in place no longer than 20 minutes. ➤*Rationale: Prolonged stimulation of the anal sphincter may result in a loss of the neuromusclar response.* The prolonged presence of a catheter may cause pressure necrosis of the mucosal surface.
15. Remove the tube, and provide perianal care as needed.
16. Help the client assume a comfortable position.
17. Clean the tubing, and replace in bathroom if to be reused. Remove and discard the plastic bag.

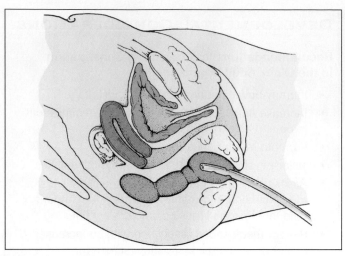

18. Instruct client that chewing gum, sucking on candy, drinking liquids through a straw, carbonated beverages, and smoking tend to promote the swallowing of air and increase abdominal distention.
19. Remove gloves, and perform hand hygiene.

● Insert rectal tube past the external and internal anal sphincters.

| UNEXPECTED OUTCOMES | CRITICAL THINKING OPTIONS |
|---|---|
| When digital stimulation is performed, client exhibits reflex spasm that prevents stool expulsion. | • Apply local anesthetic around rectum and anus, if ordered.<br>• Wait for spasm to relax, and then proceed with stimulation. |
| Client develops diarrhea. | • Identify possible cause of diarrhea.<br>• Observe dietary intake for possible cause. Provide for bulk.<br>• Hold the laxatives and stool softeners temporarily.<br>• Instruct client to eat yogurt and drink milk if not contraindicated by condition.<br>• Inform physician of diarrhea and obtain orders for Kaopectate. Administer 2 teaspoons after each loose stool for 24 hours.<br>• Check with physician if medications should be readjusted for bowel training as needed. |
| Client exhibits signs and symptoms of vagal response during removal of fecal impaction. | • Immediately discontinue procedure.<br>• Place client in shock position.<br>• Monitor vital signs every 5–15 minutes until condition is stable.<br>• Notify physician of findings and request medication order for antispasmodic such as atropine.<br>• Be prepared for "Code" situation, even though it is not likely to occur. |
| Effective bowel evacuation program is not established. | • Ask dietitian for altered diet (including more fruits and vegetables).<br>• Check if contraindication exists for increasing fluids to 3000 mL daily.<br>• Obtain order from the physician to administer a different stool softener and bulk former or increase dosage.<br>• Have client increase physical activity, especially exercise of the abdominal muscles if not contraindicated by condition.<br>• Ensure that client begins bowel training program 1/2 hour after a meal. |
| No relief of abdominal distention. | • Reposition client at an angle that raises the lower part of the body (e.g., in a prone position with the foot of the bed raised).<br>• Instruct client to circle, raise, and lower his or her legs.<br>• Reinsert the tube after 2–3 hours.<br>• Remove the tube and check for feces that may be clogging the outlet. Clean tube, and reinsert. |

*(continued)*

**UNEXPECTED OUTCOMES** *(cont.)*

Fecal impaction lower in rectum prevents insertion of rectal tube.

Client is impacted with stool even after stool modification program is instituted.

Stool becomes liquid when using the BMS.

Irrigant will not infuse or infuses slowly through BMS.

BMS catheter is expelled.

**CRITICAL THINKING OPTIONS** *(cont.)*

• Perform digital examination with gloved finger and water-soluble lubricant. Break up impaction if present.
• Position client on left side in Fowler's position.
• Reinsert the rectal tube.
• Irrigate aggressively to loosen stool.
• Irrigate q 8–12 hours if necessary to maintain loose stool.
• Administer enema and/or laxatives.
• Obtain physician's order for antidiarrheal agent.
• Use large-bore syringe to clear occlusion.
• Place 100–200 mL of irrigant into catheter through flush/sampling port, milk across anal canal and douche to clear occlusion.
• Ensure that no external traction is applied to catheter, i.e., catheter is caught in bed linen.
• Clean catheter and reinsert but increase retention cuff pressure.

# Skill 2.21  Obtaining and Testing Stool Specimen

## EXPECTED OUTCOMES

• Client understands purpose of test.
• Client is able to follow procedure of collection when appropriate.
• Dietary restrictions (if appropriate to test) were adhered to by client prior to test.
• Specimen collected is adequate for test.

## Delegation

UAP may obtain and collect stool specimen(s). The nurse, however, needs to consider the collection process before delegating this task. For example, a random stool specimen collected in a specimen container may be delegated, but a stool culture requiring a sterile swab in a test tube should be done by the nurse. Use of an incorrect collection technique can cause inaccurate test results.

The task of obtaining and testing a stool specimen for occult blood may be performed by UAP. It is important that the nurse instruct the UAP to tell the nurse if blood is detected and/or if the test is positive. In addition, the stool specimen should be saved to allow the nurse to repeat the test.

## Equipment

*Collecting a Stool Specimen*

• Clean bedpan or bedside commode
• Clean gloves
• Cardboard or plastic specimen container (labeled) with a lid or, for stool culture, a sterile swab in a test tube, as policy dictates

• Two tongue blades
• Paper towel
• Completed laboratory requisition

*Testing the Stool for Occult Blood*

• Clean bedpan or bedside commode
• Clean gloves
• Two tongue blades
• Paper towel
• Test product

## Preparation

Assemble the needed equipment. Post a sign in the client's bathroom if a timed specimen is required (e.g., "Save All Stools").

## Procedure

1. Prior to performing the procedure, introduce self and verify the client's identity using agency protocol. Explain to the client what you are going to do, why it is necessary, and how he or she can participate. Discuss how the results will be used in planning further care or treatments. Give ambulatory clients the following information and instructions:
   • The purpose of the stool specimen and how the client can assist in collecting it.
   • Defecate in a clean bedpan or bedside commode.
   • Do not contaminate the specimen, if possible, with urine or menstrual discharge. Void before the specimen collection.

- Do not place toilet tissue in the bedpan after defecation, because contents of the paper can affect the laboratory analysis.
- Notify the nurse as soon as possible after defecation, particularly for specimens that need to be sent to the laboratory immediately after collection.

2. Perform hand hygiene and observe other appropriate infection control procedures.
   - When obtaining stool samples, that is, when handling the client's bedpan, when transferring the stool sample to a specimen container, and when disposing of the bedpan contents, the nurse follows medical aseptic technique meticulously.

3. Provide for client privacy.

4. Assist clients who need help.
   - Assist the client to a bedside commode or a bedpan placed on a bedside chair or under the toilet seat in the bathroom.
   - Apply gloves to prevent hand contamination, and clean the client as required. Inspect the skin around the anus for any irritation, especially if the client defecates frequently and has liquid stools.

5. Transfer the required amount of stool to the stool specimen container.
   - Use one or two tongue blades to transfer some or all of the stool to the specimen container, taking care not to contaminate the outside of the container. The amount of stool to be sent depends on the purpose for which the specimen is collected. Usually, 2.5 cm (1 in.) of formed stool or 15 to 30 mL of liquid stool is adequate. For some timed specimens, however, the entire stool passed may need to be sent. Visible pus, mucus, or blood should be included in the sample.
   - For a culture, dip a sterile swab into the specimen, preferably where purulent fecal matter is present in the feces. Place the swab in a sterile test tube using sterile technique.
   - For an occult blood test, see step 7.
   - Wrap the used tongue blades in a paper towel before disposing of them in a waste container. ➤*Rationale: These measures help prevent the spread of microorganisms by contact with other articles.*
   - Place the lid on the container as soon as the specimen is in the container. ➤*Rationale: Putting the lid on immediately prevents the spread of microorganisms.*

6. Ensure client comfort.
   - Empty and clean the bedpan or commode, and return it to its place.
   - Remove and discard the gloves. Perform hand hygiene.

7. Label and send the specimen to the laboratory.
   - Ensure that the specimen label and the laboratory requisition have the correct information on them and are securely attached on the specimen container. ➤*Rationale: Inappropriate identification of the specimen can lead to errors of diagnosis or therapy for the client.*

- Ensure that specimens are placed in appropriate biohazard containers or specimen bags.
- Arrange for the specimen to be taken to the laboratory. Specimens to be cultured or tested for parasites need to be sent immediately. If this is not possible, follow the directions on the specimen container. In some instances, refrigeration is indicated because bacteriologic changes take place in stool specimens left at room temperature. Never place a stool specimen in a refrigerator that contains food or medication. ➤*Rationale: This prevents contamination of "clean" items with "dirty" items. It also follows OSHA standards for biohazard materials.*

*To Test the Stool for Occult Blood:*

- Select a test product.
- Apply clean gloves.

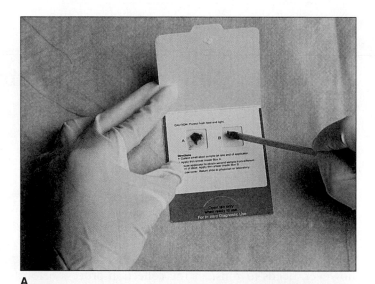

**A**

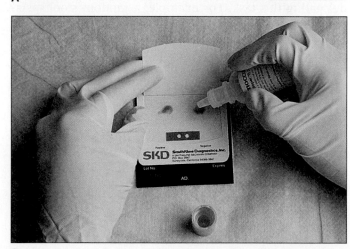

**B**

● **A,** Opening the front cover of a Hemoccult slide and applying a thin smear of feces on the slide. **B,** Opening the flap on the back of the slide and applying two drops of developing fluid over each smear.
(Photographer: Elena Dorfman)

- Follow the manufacturer's directions. For example:
  a. For a guaiac test, smear a thin layer of feces on a paper towel or filter paper with a tongue blade, and drop reagents onto the smear as directed.
  b. For a Hematest, smear a thin layer of feces on filter paper, place a tablet in the middle of the specimen, and add two drops of water as directed.
  c. For a Hemoccult slide, smear a thin layer of feces over the circle inside the envelope, and drop reagent solution onto the smear.
- Note the reaction. For all tests, a blue color indicates a positive result—that is, the presence of occult blood.
- Remove and discard gloves. Perform hand hygiene.
8. Document all relevant information.
- Record the collection of the specimen on the client's chart. Include the date and time of the collection and all nursing assessments (e.g., color, odor, consistency, and amount of feces); presence of abnormal constituents, such as blood or mucus; results of test for occult blood if obtained; discomfort during or after defecation; status of perianal skin; any bleeding from the anus after defecation.
- For an occult blood test, record the type of test product used and the reaction.

---

## DEVELOPMENTAL CONSIDERATIONS

### Infants

- To collect a stool specimen for an infant, the stool is scraped from the diaper, being careful not to contaminate the stool with urine.

### Children

- A child who is toilet trained should be able to provide a fecal specimen, but may prefer being assisted by a parent.
- When explaining the procedure to the child, use words appropriate for the child's age rather than medical terms. Ask the parent what words the family normally uses to describe a bowel movement.
- A specimen for pinworms is collected by the parent early in the morning, after sleep and before the child has a bowel movement. Scotch tape is attached to a tongue blade and the sticky side is laid flat against the perineum and anus to pick up any eggs or small worms. The tongue blade is then examined under a microscope.

### Elders

- Elders may need assistance if serial stool specimens are required.

---

| UNEXPECTED OUTCOMES | CRITICAL THINKING OPTIONS |
|---|---|
| Client is embarrassed by having to give stool specimen. | • Place a bedpan or other collection device under the toilet seat in bathroom to obtain specimen.<br>• If client is confined to bed, pull sheets over client's legs and draw curtains around the bed until procedure is completed.<br>• If odor occurs from passage of stool, spray room with air freshener. |
| Client is unable to pass adequate stool for specimen collection. | • Notify physician to obtain order to give a normal saline or tap water enema. |
| Client passes liquid stools. | • Determine if part of entire specimen is required for test.<br>• Obtain a plastic container with a cover and several large cotton swabs. Dip cotton swabs into the liquid stool. Place swabs in plastic container. After procedure, pay close attention to skin care. A protective ointment may be necessary to protect skin from liquid stools. |

---

## CARE SETTING

- Ask the client or caregiver to call when the stool specimen is obtained. If a laboratory test is needed, the home health nurse can pick up the specimen or a family member may take it to the laboratory.

- Place the stool specimen inside a plastic biohazard bag. Carry the bag in a sealed container marked "Biohazard" and take it to the laboratory promptly. Do not expose the specimen to extreme temperatures in the car.

# Skill 2.22 Collecting Infant Stool Specimen

## Equipment

Diaper
Plastic diaper liner
Waxed cardboard or plastic container with cover
Cotton swabs
Label for container
Clean gloves

## Procedure

1. Perform hand hygiene and identify infant using two forms of ID.
2. Place a clean, disposable diaper on the child or infant.
3. Check diaper frequently so that you obtain a specimen that is not contaminated with urine.
4. If child is passing liquid stools, place a plastic liner inside the diaper.
5. Don clean gloves before taking diaper off child and collecting specimen.
6. Use cotton swabs to procure the specimen.
7. Place specimen in stool container.
8. Remove gloves, perform hand hygiene, label, and send to lab immediately with client's name and medical record number.

# Skill 2.23 Collecting Stool for Bacterial Culture

## Equipment

Waxed cardboard container with cover
Tongue blade
Label for container
Clean bedpan or bedside commode
Clean gloves

## Procedure

1. Follow steps for Collecting Adult Stool Specimen (in bulleted list below). Don clean gloves before collecting stool specimen.
   - Check 2 forms of client ID, and explain the procedure to the client.
   - Determine if dietary restrictions are required prior to specimen collection.
   - Before collecting stool specimen, ask the client to void.
   - Tell client not to void on the specimen. ➤*Rationale: This prevents contamination of specimen with urine, which could result in inaccurate test results.*
   - Don gloves.
   - Clean out all urine from the bedpan or bedside commode.
   - Raise the head of the bed so that client can assume a squatting position on the bedpan, or help client sit on the bedside commode.
   - Provide privacy until client has passed a stool.
   - Remove the bedpan or bedside commode. If necessary, help the client clean perineum.
   - Use tongue blade to obtain and place a small portion (2 teaspoons) of the formed stool in a waxed cardboard or plastic container. (For some tests you may need to collect the entire specimen.) Do not contaminate inside of container.
   - Discard remaining stool, and clean bedpan or bedside commode.
   - Remove gloves, and perform hand hygiene.
   - Label container with client's name.
   - Fill out laboratory request for appropriate test.
   - Take specimen to laboratory immediately. *Rationale: Specimen may need to be refrigerated or examined immediately after collection.*
2. Collect exudate, mucus, and blood with all specimens.
3. Place a small amount of feces in a waxed cardboard container (if entire specimen is not needed).
4. Remove gloves, perform hand hygiene, and send entire specimen to the laboratory immediately after collection. If there is any delay, the specimen must be iced.
5. Report and calculate on the basis of daily output any stool specimens that are to undergo chemical analysis.

# Skill 2.24   Teaching Parents to Test for Pinworms

### Equipment
Specimen container with paddle
Clean gloves

### Procedure

1. Explain procedure to child and parent. *Note:* This test is rarely done or seen in hospital settings, so if pinworms are suspected, the parents can be taught how to obtain specimen at home.
2. Parents may choose to wear clean gloves.
3. Instruct parents to make collection upon arising in the morning before bathing, cleansing, or passing a bowel movement. *Note:* For very active children, specimens may be collected a few hours after going to bed, while the child is sleepy and more cooperative. ➤*Rationale: Pinworms, when present, migrate out of the anus to lay eggs during sleep.*
4. Remove cap in which is inserted a plastic paddle with one side coated with a nontoxic, adhesive material. This side is marked "sticky side." Do not touch this side with fingers.
5. Separate buttocks and press the sticky side against several areas around anus using moderate pressure.
6. Replace the paddle in tube. Be sure there is no stool on paddle.
7. Label container with your full name, medical record number, and date.
8. Keep specimen at room temperature until all specimens are collected (on consecutive days). Return all tubes to the doctor.

### CLINICAL **ALERT**

After treatment (drug of choice is mebendazole) and to prevent reinfection, use meticulous cleaning practices and teach parents of child to do the same.

# Skill 2.25   Collecting Stool for Ova and Parasites

### Equipment
Waxed cardboard or plastic container with cover
Tongue blade
Label for container
Clean bedpan or bedside commode
Clean gloves

### Procedure

1. Follow the steps for Collecting Adult Stool Specimen. Don clean gloves to collect stool specimen.
2. Collect exudate, mucus, and blood with all specimens.
   a. Place stool into container (with a preservative fluid).
   b. Mash the specimen in the container until mixed well with preservative. ➤*Rationale: Parasites thrive in this type of medium.*
3. Replace and tighten cup. Shake the contents until mixed well.
4. Keep specimens at body temperature to be examined within 30 minutes. ➤*Rationale: Organisms must be seen in their active stages, as loose, fluid stools are likely to contain trophozoites or intestinal amoebas and flagellates.*
5. There is usually no need to maintain well-formed or semiformed stool specimens at body temperature or to examine them quickly even though they may contain ova or cystic form of parasites.
6. Collect complete stools after purgative medications are administered.
7. When the presence of tapeworms is suspected, all stools must be examined in their entirety in order to find the head of the parasite.
8. Do not give barium, oil, and laxatives containing heavy metals that interfere with the extraction process for 7 days prior to stool examination. ➤*Rationale: Ova or cysts are not revealed.*
9. Use only normal saline solution or tap water if an enema must be administered to collect specimens. Do not use soap suds or other substances.
10. Do not contaminate the specimen with urine as it kills amoeba.
11. Collect three random, normally passed stool specimens to ensure accurate test results.
12. Provide air freshener, if needed.

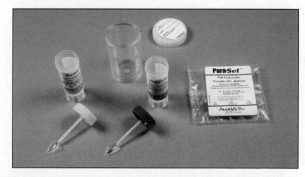

● Equipment necessary for collecting ova and/or parasite specimen.

# Skill 2.26   Implementing the Zassi Bowel Management System™

## EXPECTED OUTCOMES

- Client establishes regular bowel evacuation program.
- Constipation is prevented.
- Fecal impaction is removed.
- Client is able to evacuate bowel at a convenient and consistent time.
- Client is free of pain, flatus, and discomfort.
- Digital stimulation is performed without cardiac complications.
- Rectal tube insertion relieves flatus.
- BMS is effective to prevent skin excoriation for clients with diarrhea.

## Equipment

1 hydrocolloid dressing, cut in half
2 pieces of tape, 2 cm width
1 irrigation set
20-mL syringe
Bowel Management System Catheter; 4 cm or 6 cm
Retention cuff
Large-capacity collection bag
Gloves, 2 pair
Water-soluble lubricant
Container with 100 mL water
500 mL lukewarm irrigant (water or saline)

## Preparation

1. Identify the client using two forms of identification.
2. Review client history to determine if a contraindication to catheter placement has occurred.
   a. Severe strictures of distal rectum or anal canal.
   b. Presence of impacted or formed stool. ➤*Rationale: Client must have loose stool flow prior to insertion of BMS.*
   c. Recent history of rectal anastomosis (less than 6 weeks)
   d. History of recent anal or sphincter reconstruction.
   e. Compromised rectal wall integrity.
3. Explain procedure to client. RNs or MDs may insert catheter.
4. Determine need for analgesia. If analgesia is necessary, notify MD or check orders to determine appropriate medication.

## Procedure

1. Perform hand hygiene and don clean gloves.
2. Position client in left lateral, knee-chest position. ➤*Rationale: Provides maximal sphincter relaxation.*
3. Perform digital rectal exam.
   a. Assess rectum and anal canal for pathology, size, stool, fecal impaction.
   b. Rectum must be cleared of stool.
   c. Determine length of anal canal. If 2.5 cm or less, a 4-cm BMS is used. If greater than 2.5 cm, a 6-cm BMS is used. Follow directions on package.
4. Remove gloves and discard. Don new clean gloves.
5. Open package containing catheter and bag.
6. Check catheter for appropriate functioning of system:
   a. Draw up 20 mL air in syringe.
   b. Inflate intralumenal balloon (red connector) with 20 mL air. Disconnect syringe. Status of connector pilot balloon indicates inflated state of intralumenal balloon.
   c. Fill syringe with 35–40 mL water. Fill retention cuff (blue connector) with 35–40 mL water. Disconnect syringe. Verify that pilot balloon indicates inflated state of retention cuff.
   d. Inspect cuff and balloon for leaks and check pilot balloons to indicate the inflated state of the intralumenal balloon or retention cuff.
   e. After verifying proper function, insert syringe and slowly and completely aspirate ALL fluid from cuff and balloon. Disconnect syringe. Connector pilot balloons indicate deflated state of intralumenal balloon and retention cuff.
   f. Inject water through the irrigation lumen (clear connector) to confirm lumen patency. Close white tethered cap and continue with preparations for insertion.
   g. Ensure the system does not come into contact with sharp edges such as lubricating packet. This could damage the system.
7. Connect end of catheter drain tube to collection bag by inserting catheter connector into bag connector and twisting clockwise to lock in place, after closing off collection bag drain tube with red clamp.
8. Draw up 25 mL air into syringe, attach syringe to intralumenal balloon, and inflate balloon via red connector. Disconnect syringe. *Note:* An additional 5 mL of air is infused for added rigidity to perform the introducer function. Normal inflation is 20 mL air.
9. Apply water-soluble lubricant generously over inflated intralumenal balloon, fully collapse retention cuff around anus and anal canal.
10. Grasp the lubricated catheter directly behind the retention cuff with triple lumen connector tubing oriented anteriorly. At the time of maximum sphincter relaxation, insert the balloon end of the catheter into the distal rectum.
11. Maintain anterior orientation of the triple lumen connector tubing throughout insertion.
12. Fill the syringe with 35–40 mL lukewarm water and insert into retention cuff via blue connector.

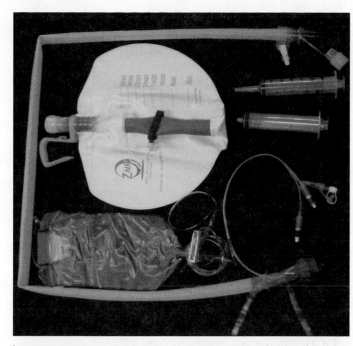

● Equipment needed for inserting and managing Bowel Management System.

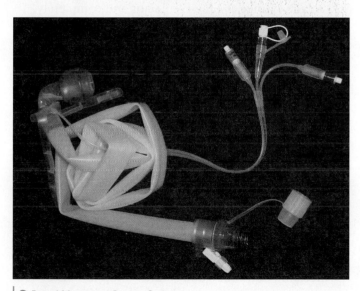

● Bowel Movement System Catheter.

### ZASSI BOWEL MANAGEMENT SYSTEM

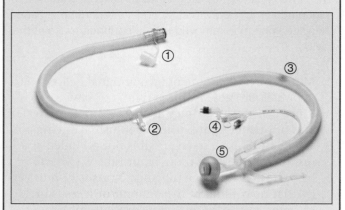

1. Drain tube connector and cup used to prevent leakage when bag disconnected.
2. Adjustable sheet clamp used to maintain the position of the drain tube.
3. Flush/Sampling port provides access for specimen collection and catheter cleaning.
4. Connectors are color coded and accept leur tip syringes. Pilot balloons on the intralumenal balloon and retention cuff indicate inflation status of catheter.
5. Transphincteric catheter zone allows normal sphincter function during use and after removal.

(*Note:* Courtesy of Zassi BMS/Zassi Medical.)

Disconnect syringe. Connect catheter to collection bag.

13. Following catheter placement insert syringe into red connector and aspirate 25 mL of air from intralumenal balloon. Disconnect syringe.
14. Confirm pilot balloon is fully collapsed.
15. Confirm catheter fit is tension free with gentle tug and recoil to "seal" retention cuff (fit of 1 cm or greater gap between anchor strap faceplate and anus).

16. Secure catheter with anchor straps to "seat" retention cuff on rectal floor.
    a. Apply hydrocolloid dressing to each buttock.
    b. Check that catheter is not twisted, anchor straps are lateral, triple lumen connector is anterior.
    c. Tape anchor straps to hydrocolloid dressing.
    d. Ensure straps do not apply tension on catheter.
17. Hang collection bag and position catheter to facilitate gravity drainage. ►*Rationale: This allows for unobstructed flow of fecal matter from catheter to collection bag.*
18. Secure catheter drain tube to sheet using sheet clip.
19. Maintain system by verifying system patency with open flow configuration (intralumenal balloon deflated) and irrigate with 50 mL water.
20. Ensure client is in comfortable position.
21. Remove gloves and discard.
22. Perform hand hygiene.

*For Maintaining Bowel Management System*

1. Maintain system throughout catheter insertion. Catheters can remain in place up to 29 days.
2. Follow strict Stool Modification Plan and irrigation protocol.

> ## Clinical Alert
>
> The BMS is contraindicated for use in clients with impacted stool. The BMS catheter must be removed and then the impaction removed before continuing use of the BMS.

3. Monitor deflated state of intralumenal balloon (via pilot balloon) at least three times per day.
4. Rinse catheter two times per day with 60 mL water at room temperature, using the flush/sampling port.
5. Check BMS q 2 h to ensure it is not occluded as a result of client lying on tube, or tube is twisted.
6. Inspect BMS drainage tube near anus q 12 h to verify that no column of irrigant and/or feces is in catheter. If irrigant or feces is present, milk into collection bag.
7. Assess perianal region q 12 h to observe for mucous or feces leakage in region. Cleanse area and place absorbent pad over area.
8. Check retention cuff volume weekly or according to physician orders by: aspirating all fluid from retention cuff and disconnect syringe; observe that cuff is deflated by checking pilot balloon; refill retention cuff with 35–40 mL room temperature water.
9. Provide the following interventions to maintain a stool modification plan. ➤*Rationale: To maintain a functioning BMS system.*
   a. Add fiber either in a tube feeding or through use of bulk laxatives.
      1. Citrucel (methyl cellulose), psyllium, prune juice, 6 oz every 8 hours.
      2. Add water to the diet when administering fiber.
   b. Add stool softeners such as Ducosate (Colace) 100–200 milligrams q 12 h.
   c. Administer osmotic laxatives such as Lactulose 30 mL q 12 h or Mira Lax, 17 grams daily for 14 days.

*Note:* Increasing the frequency and/or dose of stool modifying agents may improve results.

### For Irrigating Bowel Management System

#### Equipment

60 mL Luer tip syringe
Irrigation bag with connector
Lukewarm irrigant 300 to 1000 mL per order

#### Procedure

1. Perform hand hygiene and don clean gloves.
2. Empty collection bag unless it can accommodate additional 2 liters of irrigant.
3. Fill irrigation bag with 300–1000 mL lukewarm tap water or saline and hang from IV pole 50–100 cm above client's anus.

4. Position client in Sims' or left side position with head down.
5. Connect irrigation bag administration set to clear connector. Ensure the irrigation bag is connected to correct catheter connector.
6. Draw up 20 mL air into syringe, inflate intralumenal balloon via red connector. Inflate with 20 mL air only.
7. Infuse 500 mL of water in approximately 10 minutes. If flow rate is less than optimal, attempt to squeeze gravity bag to clear occlusion.
8. Following irrigant infusion, allow solution to dwell for 5 to 10 minutes.
9. Connect syringe to red connector. Aspirate the 20 mL of air from the intralumenal balloon. Disconnect syringe and confirm pilot balloon is fully collapsed. ➤*Rationale: This allows drainage of fluid and feces out of rectum and colon.*
10. Position client with head slightly raised and feet in downward position to facilitate gravity drainage, if necessary.
11. Disconnect administration set from clear connector upon completion of irrigation procedure.
12. Attach syringe to blue connector and completely aspirate all water from retention cuff and then refill to 35 to 45 mL water if additional water was added to prevent leakage.
13. Milk all remaining feces and irrigant in catheter, from anchor straps to collection bag. Empty contents of bag.
14. Remove and dispose of gloves and perform hand hygiene.

### For Emptying Collection Bag

1. Perform hand hygiene and don clean gloves.
2. Remove drain tube plug.
3. Remove drain tube clamp from holster by sliding upward.
4. Open drain tube clamp and empty bag into secondary container.
5. Reclamp drain tube and return clamp to holster after emptying completed.
6. Replace drain tube plug.
7. Dispose of contents according to facility policy, maintaining standard precautions.
8. Dispose of gloves and perform hand hygiene.

### For Removing Catheter

1. Perform hand hygiene and don clean gloves.
2. Insert 20 mL syringe into intralumenal balloon via red connector and inflate with 20 mL air. Disconnect syringe.
3. Insert 60 mL syringe into blue connector of catheter retention cuff and deflate by slowly aspirating all water from the retention cuff. Disconnect syringe.

## CLINICAL ALERT

If client experiences cramping or leakage, the irrigation solution may be too hot or too cold, or the infusion rate is too fast. Check the solution temperature and monitor the rate of infusion carefully. You may need to stop the infusion until the cramping is alleviated. If leakage occurs, infuse additional water into retention cuff (blue connector) to prevent leakage.

4. Verify state of retention cuff by confirming blue connector pilot balloon is collapsed.
5. Grasp catheter at external retention faceplate, ask client to bear down and apply steady traction to slide catheter out the anal orifice.
6. If catheter does not come out easily, add water-soluble lubricant to anal canal and attempt to slide catheter again.
7. Discard catheter in biohazard container maintaining standard precautions.
8. Remove and discard gloves and perform hand hygiene.

### Documentation

- Type and number of suppositories used
- Digital stimulation used
- Approximate time used for digital stimulation
- Amount, consistency, characteristics of stool
- Protocol for bowel evacuation for client
- Untoward complications of bowel training program
- Nursing interventions needed to correct complications
- Time rectal tube inserted, size of tube
- Amount, color, and consistency of feces collected
- Time rectal tube removed
- Presence, absence, or change in abdominal distention
- Client's reaction to procedure
- Any unexpected outcomes and measures taken to treat these outcomes
- Pulse rate before and during procedure
- BMS insertion and maintenance
- Interventions related to stool modification plan
- Irrigation solution; type and amount

---

| UNEXPECTED OUTCOMES | CRITICAL THINKING OPTIONS |
|---|---|
| When digital stimulation is performed, client exhibits reflex spasm that prevents stool expulsion. | • Administer 2 teaspoons after each loose stool for 24 hours.<br>• Apply local anesthetic around rectum and anus, if ordered.<br>• Wait for spasm to relax, and then proceed with stimulation. |
| Client develops diarrhea. | • Identify possible cause of diarrhea.<br>• Observe dietary intake for possible cause. Provide for bulk.<br>• Hold the laxatives and stool softeners temporarily.<br>• Instruct client to eat yogurt and drink milk if not contraindicated by condition.<br>• Inform physician of diarrhea and obtain orders for Kaopectate. Administer 2 teaspoons after each loose stool for 24 hours.<br>• Check with physician if medications should be readjusted for bowel training as needed. |
| Client exhibits signs and symptoms of vagal response during removal of fecal impaction. | • Immediately discontinue procedure.<br>• Place client in shock position.<br>• Monitor vital signs every 5–15 minutes until condition is stable.<br>• Notify physician of findings and request medication order for antispasmodic such as atropine.<br>• Be prepared for "Code" situation, even though it is not likely to occur. |
| Effective bowel evacuation program is not established. | • Ask dietitian for altered diet (including more fruits and vegetables).<br>• Check if contraindication exists for increasing fluids to 3000 mL daily.<br>• Obtain order from the physician to administer a different stool softener and bulk former or increase dosage.<br>• Have client increase physical activity, especially exercise of the abdominal muscles if not contraindicated by condition.<br>• Ensure that client begins bowel training program ½ hour after a meal. |

*(continued)*

| UNEXPECTED OUTCOMES *(cont.)* | CRITICAL THINKING OPTIONS *(cont.)* |
|---|---|
| No relief of abdominal distention. | • Reposition client at an angle that raises the lower part of the body (e.g., in a prone position with the foot of the bed raised).<br>• Instruct client to circle, raise, and lower his or her legs.<br>• Reinsert the tube after 2–3 hours.<br>• Remove the tube and check for feces that may be clogging the outlet. Clean tube, and reinsert. |
| Fecal impaction lower in rectum prevents insertion of rectal tube. | • Perform digital examination with gloved finger and water-soluble lubricant.<br>• Break up impaction if present.<br>• Position client on left side in Fowler's position.<br>• Reinsert the rectal tube. |
| Client is impacted with stool even after stool modification program is instituted. | • Irrigate aggressively to loosen stool.<br>• Irrigate q 8–12 hours if necessary to maintain loose stool.<br>• Administer enema and/or laxatives. |
| Stool becomes liquid when using the BMS. | • Obtain physician's order for antidiarrheal agent. |
| Irrigant will not infuse or infuses slowly through BMS. | • Use large-bore syringe to clear occlusion.<br>• Place 100–200 mL of irrigant into catheter through flush/sampling port, milk across anal canal and douche to clear occlusion. |
| BMS catheter is expelled. | • Ensure that no external traction is applied to catheter, i.e., catheter is caught in bed linen.<br>• Clean catheter and reinsert but increase retention cuff pressure. |

# Skill 2.27   Administering an Enema

## EXPECTED OUTCOMES
• Clients experience increased comfort and relief from abdominal distention.
• Enema administered without difficulty.
• Returns are clear if preparing client for diagnostic examination or surgery.
• Relief obtained from fecal impaction or constipation.
• Return of solution plus formed, soft feces is complete.

## Planning

Before administering an enema, determine that there is a primary care provider's order. At some agencies, a primary care provider must order the kind of enema and the time to give it, for example, the morning of an examination. At other agencies, enemas are given at the nurses' discretion (i.e., as necessary on a prn order). In addition, determine the presence of kidney or cardiac disease that contraindicates the use of a hypotonic solution.

## Delegation

Administration of some enemas may be delegated to UAP. However, the nurse must ensure the personnel are competent in the use of standard precautions. Abnormal findings such as inability to insert the rectal tip, client inability to retain the solution, or unusual return from the enema must be validated and interpreted by the nurse.

## Equipment
• Disposable linen-saver pad
• Bath blanket
• Bedpan or commode
• Clean gloves
• Water-soluble lubricant if tubing not prelubricated
• Paper towel

*Large-Volume Enema*
• Solution container with tubing of correct size and tubing clamp
• Correct solution, amount, and temperature

*Small-Volume Enema*
• Prepackaged container of enema solution with lubricated tip
• Assuming a left lateral position for an enema. Note the commercially prepared enema.

## Preparation

- Lubricate about 5 cm (2 in.) of the rectal tube (some commercially prepared enema sets already have lubricated nozzles). ➤*Rationale: Lubrication facilitates insertion through the sphincter and minimizes trauma.*
- Run some solution through the connecting tubing of a large-volume enema set and the rectal tube to expel any air in the tubing, then close the clamp. ➤*Rationale: Air instilled into the rectum, although not harmful, causes unnecessary distention.*

## Procedure

1. Prior to performing the procedure, introduce self and verify the client's identity using agency protocol. Explain to the client what you are going to do, why it is necessary, and how he or she can participate. Discuss how the results will be used in planning further care or treatments. Indicate that the client may experience a feeling of fullness while the solution is being administered. Explain the need to hold the solution as long as possible.
2. Perform hand hygiene and observe other appropriate infection control procedures.
3. Apply clean gloves.
4. Provide for client privacy.
5. Assist the adult client to a left lateral position, with the right leg as acutely flexed as possible and the linen-saver pad under the buttocks. ➤*Rationale: This position facilitates the flow of solution by gravity into the sigmoid and descending colon, which are on the left side. Having the right leg acutely flexed provides for adequate exposure of the anus.*
6. Insert the enema tube.
   - For clients in the left lateral position, lift the upper buttock. ➤*Rationale: This ensures good visualization of the anus.*
   - Insert the tube smoothly and slowly into the rectum, directing it toward the umbilicus. ➤*Rationale: The angle follows the normal contour of the rectum. Slow insertion prevents spasm of the sphincter.*
   - Insert the tube 7 to 10 cm (3 to 4 in.). ➤*Rationale: Because the anal canal is about 2.5 to 5 cm (1 to 2 in.) long in the adult,*

*insertion to this point places the tip of the tube beyond the anal sphincter into the rectum.*
   - If resistance is encountered at the internal sphincter, ask the client to take a deep breath, then run a small amount of solution through the tube. ➤*Rationale: This relaxes the internal anal sphincter.*
   - Never force tube or solution entry. If instilling a small amount of solution does not permit the tube to be advanced or the solution to freely flow, withdraw the tube. Check for any stool that may have blocked the tube during insertion. If present, flush it and retry the procedure. You may also perform a digital rectal examination to determine if there is an impaction or other mechanical blockage. If resistance persists, end the procedure and report the resistance to the primary care provider and nurse in charge.
7. Slowly administer the enema solution.
   - Raise the solution container, and open the clamp to allow fluid flow
   *or*
   - Compress a pliable container by hand.
   - During most low enemas, hold or hang the solution container no higher than 30 cm (12 in.) above the rectum. ➤*Rationale: The higher the solution container is held above the rectum, the faster the flow and the greater the force (pressure) in the rectum.* During a high enema, hang the solution container about 45 cm (18 in.). ➤*Rationale: The fluid must be instilled farther to clean the entire bowel.* See agency protocol.
   - Administer the fluid slowly. If the client complains of fullness or pain, lower the container or use the clamp to stop the flow for 30 seconds, and then restart the flow at a slower rate. ➤*Rationale: Administering the enema slowly and stopping the flow momentarily decreases the likelihood of intestinal spasm and premature ejection of the solution.*
   - If you are using a plastic commercial container, roll it up as the fluid is instilled. This prevents subsequent suctioning of the solution.
   - After all the solution has been instilled or when the client cannot hold any more and feels the desire to defecate (the urge to defecate usually indicates that sufficient fluid has

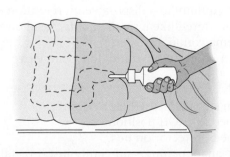

● Assuming a left lateral position for an enema. Note the commercially prepared enema.

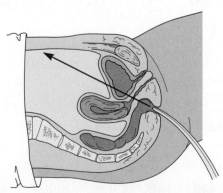

● Inserting the enema tube following the direction of the rectum.

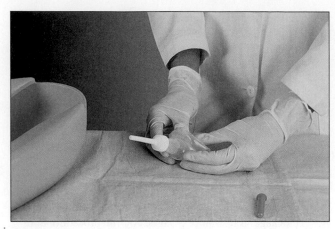

● Rolling up a commercial enema container.

been administered), close the clamp and remove the enema tube from the anus.

- Place the enema tube in a disposable towel as you withdraw it.

8. Encourage the client to retain the enema.

- Ask the client to remain lying down. ➤*Rationale: It is easier for the client to retain the enema when lying down than when sitting or standing, because gravity promotes drainage and peristalsis.*
- Request that the client retain the solution for the appropriate amount of time, for example, 5 to 10 minutes for a cleansing enema or at least 30 minutes for a retention enema.

9. Assist the client to defecate.

- Assist the client to a sitting position on the bedpan, commode, or toilet. A sitting position facilitates the act of defecation.
- Ask the client who is using the toilet not to flush it. The nurse needs to observe the feces.

- If a specimen of feces is required, ask the client to use a bedpan or commode.
- Remove and discard gloves. Perform hand hygiene.

10. Document the type and volume, if appropriate, of enema given. Describe the results.

### Documentation

Sample: 8/2/2009 1000. States last BM five days ago. Abdomen distended and firm. Bowel sounds hypoactive. Fleet's enema given per order resulting in large amount of firm brown stool. States he "feels better"

———————————— M. Lopez, RN

### VARIATION: Administering an Enema to an Incontinent Client

Occasionally a nurse needs to administer an enema to a client who is unable to control the external sphincter muscle and thus cannot retain the enema solution for even a few minutes. In that case, after the rectal tube is inserted, the client assumes a supine position on a bedpan. The head of the bed can be elevated slightly, to 30 degrees if necessary for easier breathing, and pillows support the client's head and back.

### VARIATION: Administering a Return-Flow Enema

For a return-flow enema, the solution (100 to 200 mL for an adult) is instilled into the client's rectum and sigmoid colon. Then the solution container is lowered so that the fluid flows back out through the rectal tube into the container, pulling the flatus with it. The inflow–outflow process is repeated five or six times (to stimulate peristalsis and the expulsion of flatus), and the solution is replaced several times during the procedure if it becomes thick with feces.

Document type of solution; length of time solution was retained; the amount, color, and consistency of the returns; and the relief of flatus and abdominal distention in the client record using forms or checklists supplemented by narrative notes when appropriate.

## Skill 2.28   Administering a Retention Enema

### Equipment

Commercially prepared disposable oil retention enema
Oil: Adult 150–200 mL, child 75–100 mL, 91° F
Water-soluble lubricant
Bedpan or commode
Bed protector
Skin care items (e.g., soap, water, towels)
Clean gloves

### Preparation

1. Identify and prepare client as for any enema.
2. Provide privacy.

3. Gather equipment—disposable oil retention enema is administered like a small enema. Read directions on enema container.
4. Perform hand hygiene and don clean gloves.

### Procedure

1. Explain steps of procedure to client.
2. Raise bed to HIGH position.
3. Place bed protector on bed.
4. Expose anal opening, and gently insert rectal tube tip of container 3–4 inches. Commercially prepared enemas are prelubricated.

5. Squeeze contents slowly, and empty entire amount into rectum.
6. Keep container compressed and remove rectal tube gently. ➤*Rationale: To prevent solution from being drawn back into container.*
7. Lower bed.
8. Discard equipment and gloves, following standard precautions. Perform hand hygiene.
9. Explain to client that oil should be retained for 30–60 minutes before it is expelled. ➤*Rationale: Purpose of enema is to soften stool.*
10. A cleansing enema may need to be given to remove oil and stimulate defecation.

---

### SETTING OF CARE

Teach the caregiver or client the following:

- To make saline solution, mix 1 teaspoon of table salt with 500 mL of tap water.
- Use enemas only as directed. Do not rely on them for regular bowel evacuation.
- Prior to administration, make sure a bedpan, commode, or toilet is nearby.

---

| UNEXPECTED OUTCOMES | CRITICAL THINKING OPTIONS |
|---|---|
| Client expels solution prematurely. | • Calm and ease client's distress by reassuring him or her as you clean the equipment.<br>• Place bedpan under client. Place client in semi-Fowler's position with knees flexed.<br>• Hold the rectal tube in client's rectum between thighs. Slow the water flow, and continue with the enema. |
| Client complains of severe and sudden abdominal pain, nausea, and distention. | • Remove tubing, and notify physician immediately of possible perforation. (This is an uncommon complication.)<br>• Assess vital signs. If you suspect cardiac dysrhythmias, remove bedpan and notify physician immediately.<br>• Be prepared to administer emergency drugs, such as atropine.<br>• If an IV is not in place, start an IV of 5% dextrose in water ($D_5W$) using a large-bore needle for emergency use. |
| The flow of water is impeded or an obstruction is felt. | • Open clamp on tubing. Allow a small amount of solution to flow. (The warm solution may help relax the internal sphincter.)<br>• Withdraw tube slightly, and reinsert.<br>• Gently perform a digital examination for the possibility of fecal impaction. Break up impaction if present. Ask physician for order to give a retention enema, followed by a cleansing enema 2–3 hours later. |
| Client cannot return enema solution. | • Gently massage client's abdomen if not contraindicated.<br>• Replace rectal tube. Lower the enema bag below the level of the bed.<br>• If client is not uncomfortable, do nothing. If client complains of discomfort or pain, notify physician. |
| Enema returns are not clear prior to surgery or diagnostic testing. | • Repeat enema. If, after three enemas, returns are still not clear, notify physician of findings.<br>• May need to give an enema with a stronger solution.<br>• Physician may need to order magnesium citrate or electrolyte solution (i.e., GoLYTELY). |
| Fecal impaction is not relieved. | • Check orders for oil retention enema.<br>• Check catheter size needed.<br>• Obtain order for and use digital stimulation and manual extraction of feces if not contraindicated by diagnosis of cardiac or neurologic involvement. |

## DEVELOPMENTAL CONSIDERATIONS

### Infants/Children

- Provide a careful explanation to the parents and child before the procedure.
- The enema solution should be isotonic (usually normal saline). Some hypertonic commercial solutions (e.g., Fleet phosphate enema) can lead to hypovolemia and electrolyte imbalances. In addition, the osmotic effect of the enema may produce diarrhea and subsequent metabolic acidosis.
- Infants and small children do not exhibit sphincter control and need to be assisted in retaining the enema. The nurse administers the enema while the infant or child is lying with the buttocks over the bedpan, and the nurse firmly presses the buttocks together to prevent the immediate expulsion of the solution. Older children can usually hold the solution if they understand what to do and are not required to hold it for too long a period. It may be necessary to ensure that the bathroom is available for an ambulatory child before starting the procedure or to have a bedpan ready.
- Enema temperature should be 37.7°C (100°F) unless otherwise ordered.
- Large-volume enemas consist of 50 to 200 mL in children less than 18 months old; 200 to 300 mL in children 18 months to 5 years; and 300 to 500 mL in children 5 to 12 years old.
- Careful explanation is especially important for the preschool child. An enema is an intrusive procedure and therefore threatening.

- For infants and small children, the dorsal recumbent position is frequently used. Position them on a small padded bedpan with support for the back and head. Secure the legs by placing a diaper under the bedpan and then over and around the thighs. Place the underpad under the client's buttocks to protect the bed linen, and drape the client with the bath blanket.
- Insert the tube 5 to 7.5 cm (2 to 3 in.) in the child and only 2.5 to 3.75 cm (1 to 1.5 in.) in the infant.
- For children, lower the height of the solution container appropriately for the age of the child. See agency protocol.
- To assist a small child in retaining the solution, apply firm pressure over the anus with tissue wipes, or firmly press the buttocks together.

### Elders

- Elders may fatigue easily.
- Elders may be more susceptible to fluid and electrolyte imbalances. Use tap water enemas with great caution.
- Monitor the client's tolerance during the procedure, watching for vagal episodes (e.g., slow pulse) and dysrhythmias.
- Protect older adults' skin from prolonged exposure to moisture.
- Assist older clients with perineal care as indicated.

# Skill 2.29    Applying a Fecal Ostomy Pouch

## EXPECTED OUTCOMES

- Pouch remains intact without leakage for 3–5 days.
- Pouching system provides maximal skin protection.
- Pouching system remains odorproof for 3–5 days.
- Client gradually assumes an active role in applying the pouch.
- Client's skin remains free of erythema, excoriation, and infection.

## Equipment

1 or 2 piece transparent ostomy pouch with adhesive
  wafer
Warm water
Soft cloths
Bath blanket

Plastic bag for pouch disposal
Tail closure or night adaptor for pouch
Clean gloves
Measuring guide
Tissues
Ostomyscissors

## Preparation

1. Check client care plan and identify client using two forms of identification.
2. Determine exact supplies client uses.
3. Gather equipment.
4. Explain procedure to client.
5. Provide privacy.
6. Raise bed to high position.
7. Perform hand hygiene and don gloves.

## Procedure

1. Place bath blanket over client. Place absorbent pad or towels under client. ➤*Rationale: To protect bed from spillage.*
2. Observe placement of stoma. ➤*Rationale: To determine normal amount of output and consistency.* (Immediately after surgery, all stomas will have very liquid stool and high flatus output.)
3. Empty old pouch into graduate, bedpan, or toilet.
4. Remove old pouch by pushing against skin as you pull backing from skin and discard in plastic bag. Save tail closure on bottom of pouch.
5. Measure output, if ordered.
6. Clean skin and stoma gently with warm water and soft cloth. ➤*Rationale: Oily substances can interfere with pouch adhesive.*
7. Dry skin well with soft cloth. Keep tissues available if stoma functions while pouch is off.
8. Observe skin and stoma for changes in size, ulceration, and color (stoma should be a beefy red).
9. Measure stoma at the base with measuring guide.
10. Trace measured pattern on pouch.
11. Cut pouch to pattern, making sure opening is large enough (at least ¼ inch) to encircle stoma without pushing on edges. ➤*Rationale: No skin should appear between the pouch edge and the stoma.*
12. If using a two-piece pouch, snap the wafer and pouch together: (See photo sequence for alternate method of using two-piece pouch.)
13. Remove paper from skin barrier on pouch and save it. ➤*Rationale: This may be used as a pattern for next pouch change.*
14. Apply a ring of skin barrier paste to opening on pouch.
15. Apply Stomadhesive powder to denuded skin only.
16. Remove paper from outer ring.

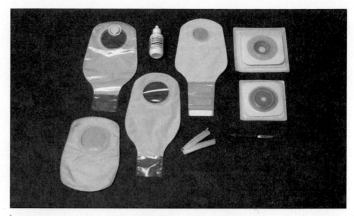

● Fabric pouches, convexity faceplates, pouch with filter.

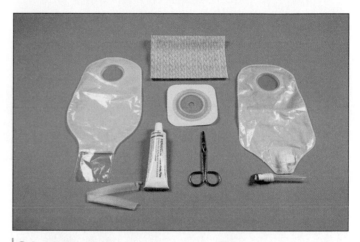

● Supplies needed to change two-piece pouches.

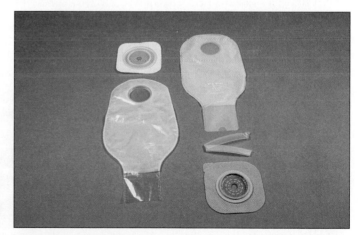

● Two-piece fecal pouches.

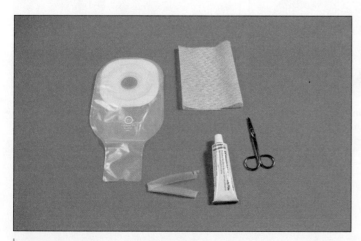

● Supplies needed to change one-piece pouches.

## CLINICAL ALERT

To promote the client's self-esteem and body image, be aware of your own body language. Even subtle changes in the way you look at the stoma could indicate disgust or disapproval and an altered self-esteem could result.

17. Center and apply pouch to clean and dry skin. Smooth edges of adhesive to skin. ➤*Rationale: If adhesive is wrinkled, it may result in leakage from pouch.*

18. Pouches can be applied over an incision. ➤*Rationale: Incisions are sealed within 24 hours of surgery.*

19. Close and secure end of pouch with tail closure.
    a. Ensure bowed end is next to body. ➤*Rationale: This provides a better fit to body, and prevents outpouching of clamp through clothing.*
    b. Lay hook on top of bag and fold bag 1 inch over end of pouch.
    c. Squeeze clamp together to close.

20. Remove soiled pouch and tissues from bedside.

21. Remove gloves and perform hand hygiene.

22. Position client for comfort. Return bed to low position.

23. Put away supplies and reorder as necessary.

> ## CLINICAL ALERT
>
> Clients with ostomies will need a nutritional consult and a written dietary guide. They need to limit the amount of hard-to-digest foods for at least the first 2–3 weeks post op. Also, limiting gas-producing foods will prevent gas-forming odors.

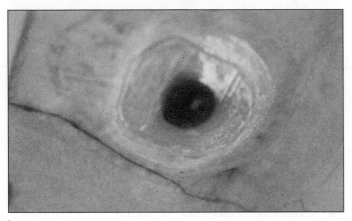

● Viable stoma.

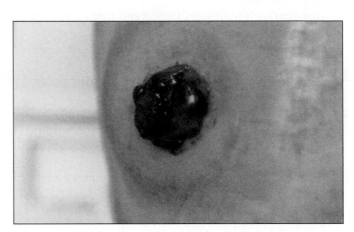

● Nonviable parastomal hernia.

### Changing One-Piece Fecal Ostomy Pouch

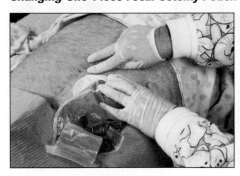

❶ Starting at upper corner, remove old pouch.

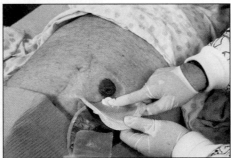

❷ As you remove old pouch, push against skin while pulling on pouch.

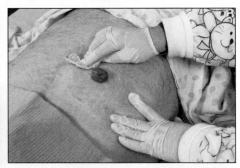

❸ Clean skin with warm water; dry well.

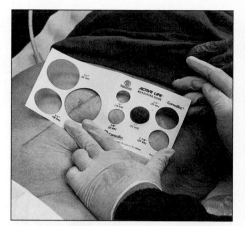

④ Measure stoma size.

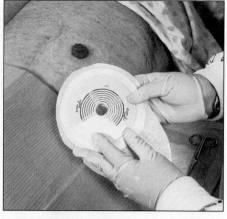

⑤ Remove plastic covering from one-piece pouch.

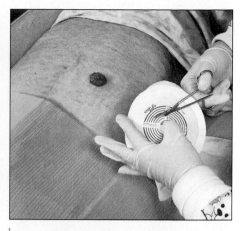

⑥ Cut pouch opening to exact size of stoma.

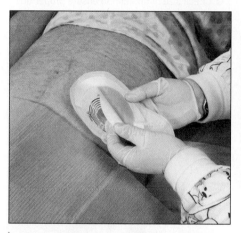

⑦ Remove paper from inner wafer. Save pattern for future pouch changes.

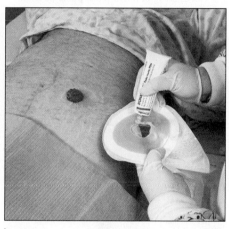

⑧ Apply ring of paste to opening on pouch.

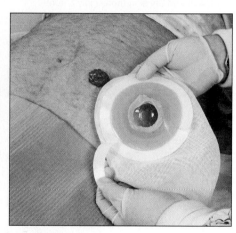

⑨ Remove paper from outer adhesive ring of pouch.

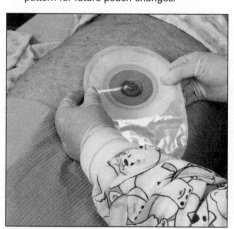

⑩ Center and apply pouch to clean, dry skin.

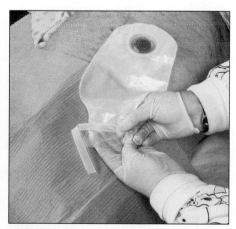

⑪ After applying one-piece pouch, clamp bottom of pouch.

## Applying Two-Piece Fecal Ostomy Pouch

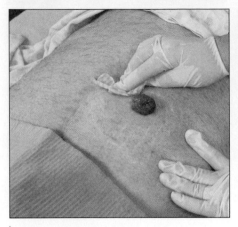

❶ Clean and dry skin thoroughly before applying two-piece pouch.

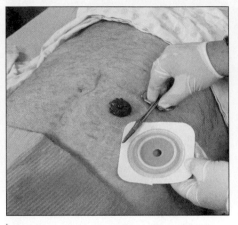

❷ Cut opening of a two-piece pouch to exact size of stoma.

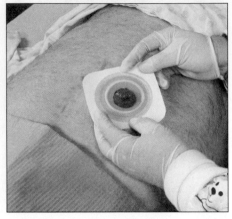

❸ Check size of opening to ensure proper fit.

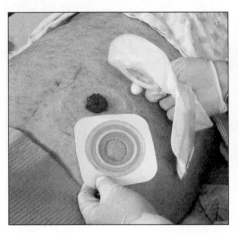

❹ Snap pouch onto wafer when using a two-piece pouch.

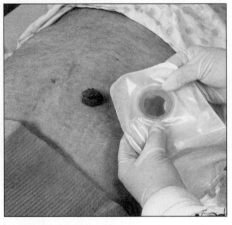

❺ Check for secure fit by tugging at bottom of pouch.

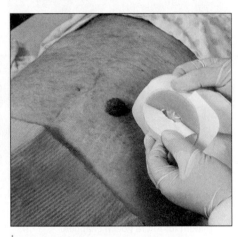

❻ Remove paper from inner barrier.

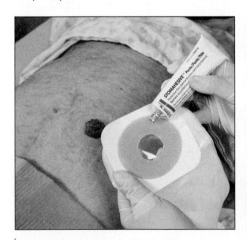

❼ Apply paste to inner circle of wafer.

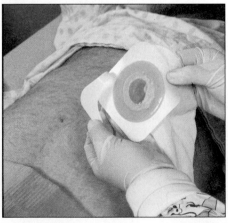

❽ Remove paper from outer adhesive ring.

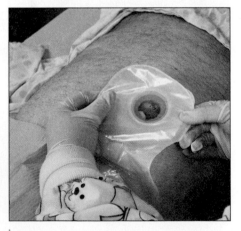

❾ Center pouch over stoma and press onto skin.

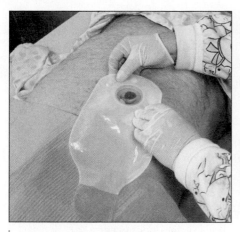

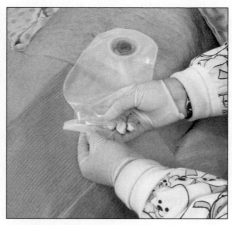

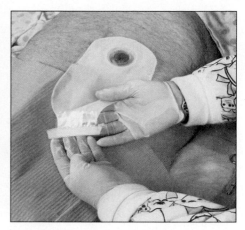

⑩ Secure adhesive to skin.

⑪ Clamp bottom of pouch.

⑫ Check that pouch clamp is secure.

## CLIENT TEACHING

- Empty pouch when one-third full of stool or flatus.
  a. Empty into toilet.
  b. Pouch should last for 3–4 days.
- Rinse pouch using room temperature water and a rubber ear syringe (squirt into pouch).
- Use pouch deodorant if desired.
- Empty each morning and last thing at night even if not one-third full.

- Check seal on daily basis for tight fit, change if needed.
- Instruct client to always carry a supply of ostomy equipment for emergency use.
- Instruct client on emptying and cleaning pouch, opening and closing clamp, observing and cleaning periostomal area, and changing pouch.
- Have client return demonstration until able to perform activities correctly.

## LOOP COLOSTOMY WITH ROD

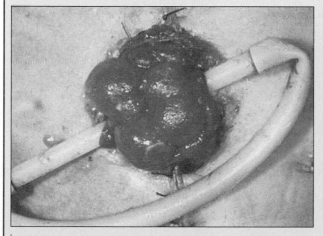

● A loop of bowel is brought onto abdomen and is supported by a plastic rod.

## LOOP COLOSTOMY WITH ROD REMOVED

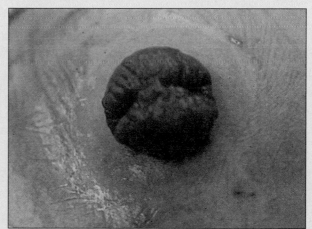

● Two openings are made in colostomy.
Proximal loop is functional and discharges fecal material.
Distal end is nonfunctional and discharges only mucus.

| UNEXPECTED OUTCOMES | CRITICAL THINKING OPTIONS |
|---|---|
| Stoma appears dark, dusky-colored, or black. | • Notify physician of findings, and document in chart. (Usually indicates stoma is ischemic.) |
| Stoma becomes ulcerated or cut. | • Examine pouching system to see if opening of pouch may be cutting into stoma.<br>• Recut opening to exact size of stoma. |
| Bleeding occurs when stoma is touched. | • Observe and note—usual occurrence postoperatively. |
| Erythematous rash at site of pouch. | • Assess for allergic reaction to product being used.<br>• May need to change to different type of adhesive on pouch or change to a pouch with no adhesive. |
| Papular rash appears on peristomal skin. | • Assess for possible yeast sensitivity.<br>• Be sure skin is clean and dry before applying pouch.<br>• Do not rinse pouch with water because this traps water under wafer.<br>• May need to use antifungal powder on skin with each pouch change until skin clears. |
| Peristomal skin complications occur. | • Evaluate cause of leakage.<br>• Be sure pouch is cut to correct size.<br>• Measure stoma at each pouch change for 4–6 weeks. Size will change as edema subsides.<br>• Measure stoma at base.<br>• May need to fill any creases around stoma with skin barrier paste.<br>• Apply thin layer of ostomy powder over area and seal with an alcohol-free coating.<br>• May need to use secondary skin barrier like Eakin seal.<br>• May need to attach belt to minimize lateral leakage.<br>• Change to a product like Durahesive that swells around stoma preventing leakage and holds up well to liquid output.<br>• Be sure pouch is emptied before it is over ⅓ full of stool or flatus, since an overfull pouch can break seal of pouch.<br>• Pouches should not be changed more than once daily. |
| Ostomy is flush or below the surface. | • Apply convex pouch system to assist ostomy to protrude.<br>• Apply ostomy belt. |
| Ostomy is in skin fold or crease. | • Apply a one-piece pouch for more flexibility.<br>• Fill deep crevices with caulking material. |
| Client experiences itching or burning under appliance | • May be a sign that stool is undermining seal of pouch. |
| Client not coping with altered body image. | • Refer to United Ostomy Associations of America, Inc., the Crohn's and Colitis Foundation of America, American Cancer Society or the local Enterostomal Therapy nurse. |

## DEVELOPMENTAL CONSIDERATIONS

• Elderly clients frequently have concomitant cardiac problems, which can be affected by vagal stimulation during fecal removal or enema administration. Check with the physician before these skills are performed on elderly clients. Monitor the pulse carefully during the procedure.

• Fecal impaction is not uncommon with elderly clients due to decreased mobility and exercise, dietary habits, and tendency to overuse enemas and laxatives.

• Encourage clients to decrease use of laxatives and enemas, increase fluid intake and fiber in diet, and increase exercise. Dehydration resulting from inadequate fluid intake leads to constipation and fecal impaction.

• To select the proper ostomy appliance for an elderly client, the nurse must determine if the client has any physical limitations that could influence the type of appliance needed. These limitations include poor vision, use of only one hand, arthritis, and inability to perform cleaning and pouching procedure.

# Skill 2.30  Changing a Bowel Diversion Ostomy Appliance

## EXPECTED OUTCOMES
- Pouch remains intact without leakage for 3–5 days.
- Pouching system provides maximal skin protection.
- Pouching system remains odorproof for 3–5 days.
- Client gradually assumes an active role in applying the pouch.
- Client's skin remains free of erythema, excoriation, and infection.

Review features of the appliance to ensure that all parts are present and functioning correctly.

## Delegation

Care of a *new* ostomy is not delegated to UAP. However, aspects of ostomy function are observed during usual care and may be recorded by persons other than the nurse. Abnormal findings must be validated and interpreted by the nurse. In some agencies, UAP may remove and replace well-established ostomy appliances.

## Equipment

- Clean gloves
- Bedpan
- Moisture-proof bag (for disposable pouches)
- Cleaning materials, including warm water, mild soap (optional), washcloth, towel
- Tissue or gauze pad
- Skin barrier (optional)
- Stoma measuring guide
- Pen or pencil and scissors
- New ostomy pouch with optional belt

- Tail closure clamp
- Deodorant for pouch (optional)

## Preparation

- Determine the need for an appliance change.
- Assess the used appliance for leakage of stool. ▶Rationale: *Stool can irritate the peristomal skin.*
- Ask the client about any discomfort at or around the stoma. ▶Rationale: *A burning sensation may indicate breakdown beneath the faceplate of the pouch.*

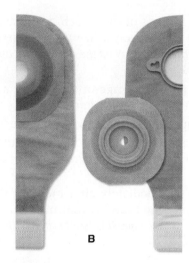

**A,** One-piece ostomy appliance of pouching system; **B,** two-piece ostomy or pouching system.
(Courtesy of Hollister, Inc.)

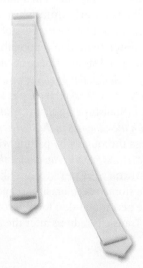

● Adjustable ostomy belt.
(Courtesy of Hollister, Inc.)

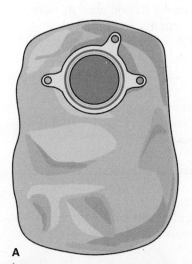
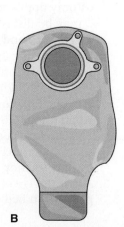

● **A,** Closed pouch; **B,** drainable pouch.
(Courtesy of Convatec, a Bristol-Meyers Squibb Company)

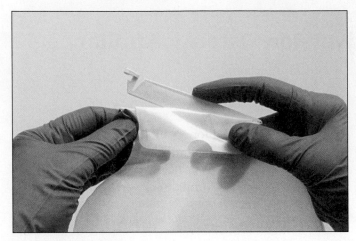

● Applying a pouch clamp.

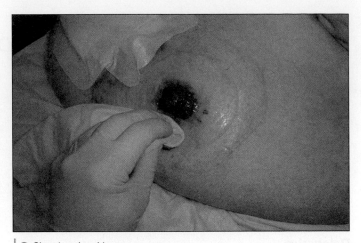

● Cleaning the skin.
(Courtesy of Cory Partrick Hartley, San Ramon Regional Medical Center, San Ramon, CA. Reprinted with permission.)

- Assess the fullness of the pouch. ➤*Rationale: The weight of an overly full bag may loosen the skin barrier and separate it from the skin, causing the stool to leak and irritate the peristomal skin.*
- If there is pouch leakage or discomfort at or around the stoma, change the appliance.
- Select an appropriate time to change the appliance.
- Avoid times close to meal or visiting hours. ➤*Rationale: Ostomy odor and stool may reduce appetite or embarrass the client.*
- Avoid times immediately after meals or the administration of any medications that may stimulate bowel evacuation. ➤*Rationale: It is best to change the pouch when drainage is least likely to occur.*

## Procedure

1. Prior to performing the procedure, introduce self and verify the client's identity using agency protocol. Explain to the client what you are going to do, why it is necessary, and how he or she can participate. Discuss how the results will be used in planning further care or treatments. Changing an ostomy appliance should not cause discomfort, but it may be distasteful to the client. Communicate acceptance and support to the client. It is important to change the appliance competently and quickly. Include support persons as appropriate.
2. Perform hand hygiene and observe other appropriate infection control procedures.
3. Apply clean gloves.
4. Provide for client privacy preferably in the bathroom, where clients can learn to deal with the ostomy as they would at home.
5. Assist the client to a comfortable sitting or lying position in bed or preferably a sitting or standing position in the bathroom. ➤*Rationale: Lying or standing positions may facilitate smoother pouch application that is, avoid wrinkles.*
6. Unfasten the belt if the client is wearing one.
7. Empty the pouch and remove the ostomy skin barrier.
   - Empty the contents of a drainable pouch through the bottom opening into a bedpan or toilet. ➤*Rationale: Emptying before removing the pouch prevents spillage of stool onto the client's skin.*
   - If the pouch uses a clamp, do not throw it away because it can be reused.
   - Assess the consistency, color, and amount of stool.
   - Peel the skin barrier off slowly, beginning at the top and working downward, while holding the client's skin taut. ➤*Rationale: Holding the skin taut minimizes client discomfort and prevents abrasion of the skin.*
   - Discard the disposable pouch in a moisture-proof bag.
8. Clean and dry the peristomal skin and stoma.
   - Use toilet tissue to remove excess stool.
   - Use warm water, mild soap (optional), and a washcloth to clean the skin and stoma. Check agency practice on the use of soap. ➤*Rationale: Soap is sometimes not advised because it can be irritating to the skin.* If soap is allowed, do not use deodorant or moisturizing soaps. ➤*Rationale: They may interfere with the adhesives in the skin barrier.*
   - Dry the area thoroughly by patting with a towel. ➤*Rationale: Excess rubbing can abrade the skin.*
9. Assess the stoma and peristomal skin.
   - Inspect the stoma for color, size, shape, and bleeding.
   - Inspect the peristomal skin for any redness, ulceration, or irritation. Transient redness after the removal of adhesive is normal.

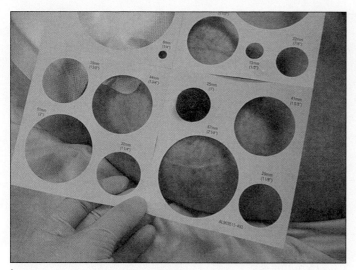

● A guide for measuring the stoma.

(Courtesy of Cory Partrick Hartley, San Ramon Regional Medical Center, San Ramon, CA. Reprinted with permission.)

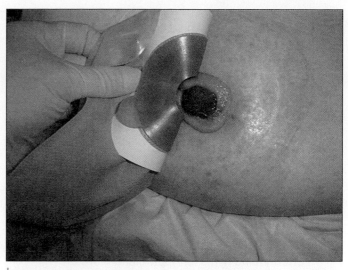

● Centering the skin barrier over the stoma.

(Courtesy of Cory Partrick Hartley, San Ramon Regional Medical Center, San Ramon, CA. Reprinted with permission.)

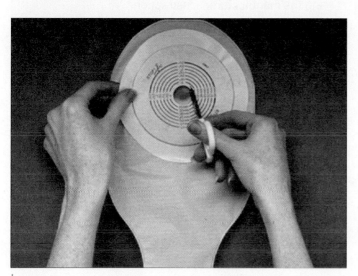

● The nurse is making a stoma opening on a disposable one-piece pouch.

(Courtesy of Convatec, a Bristol-Meyers Squibb Company)

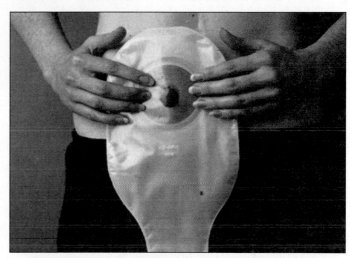

● Pressing the skin barrier of a disposable one-piece pouch for 30 seconds to activate the adhesives in the skin barrier.

(Courtesy of Convatec, a Bristol-Meyers Squibb Company)

10. Place a piece of tissue or gauze over the stoma, and change it as needed. ➤*Rationale: This absorbs any seepage from the stoma while the ostomy appliance is being changed.*

11. Prepare and apply the skin barrier (peristomal seal).
    - Use the guide to measure the size of the stoma.
    - On the backing of the skin barrier, trace a circle the same size as the stomal opening.
    - Cut out the traced stoma pattern to make an opening in the skin barrier. Make the opening no more than ⅛ to ¼ inch larger than the stoma (Erwin-Toth, 2003).
      ➤*Rationale: This allows space for the stoma to expand slightly*

*when functioning and minimizes the risk of stool contacting peristomal skin.*
    - Remove the backing to expose the sticky adhesive side. The backing can be saved and used as a pattern when making an opening for future skin barriers.

### For a One-Piece Pouching System

- Center the one-piece skin barrier and pouch over the stoma, and gently press it onto the client's skin for 30 seconds. ➤*Rationale: The heat and pressure help activate the adhesives in the skin barrier.*

## PRACTICE GUIDELINES

### Irrigating a Colostomy

- Fill the solution bag with 500 mL of warm (body temperature) tap water or other solution as ordered.
- Hang the solution bag on an IV pole so that the bottom of the container is at the level of the client's shoulder or 30 to 45 cm (12 to 18 in.) above the stoma.
- Attach the colon catheter securely to the tubing.
- Open the regulator clamp, and run fluid through the tubing to expel air from it. Close the clamp until ready for the irrigation.
- Provide privacy.
- Perform hand hygiene. Apply clean gloves.
- Assist the client who must remain in bed to a side-lying position. Place a disposable pad on the bed in front of the client, and place the bedpan on top of the disposable pad, beneath the stoma, or assist an ambulatory client to sit on the toilet or on a commode in the bathroom.
- Remove the colostomy bag and dispose of used pouch in a plastic bag.
- Center the irrigation drainage sleeve over the stoma and attach it snugly. Direct the lower, open end of the drainage sleeve into the bedpan or between the client's legs into the toilet.

- Lubricate the tip of the stoma cone or colon catheter.
- Using a rotating motion, insert the catheter or stoma cone through the opening in the top of the irrigation drainage sleeve and gently through the stoma. Insert a catheter only 7 cm (3 in.); insert a stoma cone just until it fits snugly. Use of a stoma cone avoids the risk of perforating the bowel.
- Open the tubing clamp, and allow the fluid to flow into the bowel. If cramping occurs, stop the flow until the cramps subside and then resume the flow.
- After all the fluid is instilled, remove the catheter or cone and allow the colon to empty, usually 10 to 15 minutes.
- Cleanse the base of the irrigation drainage sleeve, and seal the bottom with a drainage clamp, following the manufacturer's instructions.
- Encourage an ambulatory client to move around for about 30 minutes to completely empty the colon.
- Empty and remove the irrigation sleeve.
- Clean the area around the stoma, and dry it thoroughly.
- Apply skin barrier and colostomy appliance as needed.

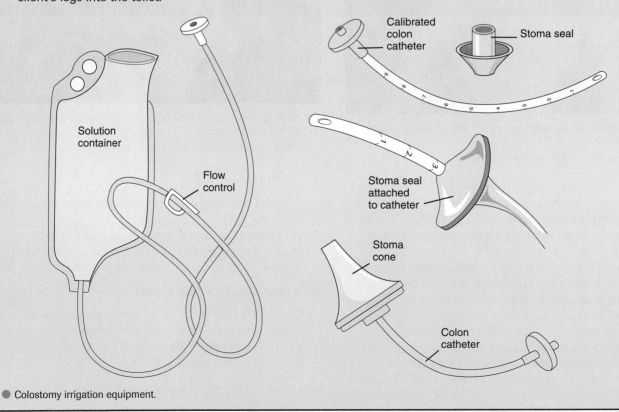

Colostomy irrigation equipment.

### For a Two-Piece Pouching System

- Center the skin barrier over the stoma and gently press it onto the client's skin for 30 seconds.
- Remove the tissue over the stoma before applying the pouch.
- Snap the pouch onto the flange or skin barrier wafer.
- For drainable pouches, close the pouch according to the manufacturer's directions.
- Remove and discard gloves. Perform hand hygiene.
12. Document the procedure in the client record using forms or checklists supplemented by narrative notes when appropriate. Report and record pertinent assessments and interventions. Report any increase in stoma size, change in color indicative of circulatory impairment, and presence of skin irritation or erosion. Record on the client's chart discoloration of the stoma, the appearance of the peristomal skin, the amount and type of drainage, the client's reaction to the procedure, the client's experience with the ostomy, and skills learned by the client.

### Documentation

Sample: 8/3/2009 0900 Colostomy bag changed. Moderate to large amount of semi-formed brown stool.

Stoma reddish color. No redness or irritation around stoma. Client looked at stoma today and started asking questions about how she will be able to change the pouch when she is home. Asked if she would like to do the next changing of the pouch. Stated "yes."

_____ G. Hsu, RN

### VARIATION: Emptying a Drainable Pouch

- Empty the pouch when it is one-third to one-half full of stool or gas. ➤*Rationale: Emptying before it is overfull helps avoid breaking the seal with the skin and stool then coming in contact with the skin.*
- While wearing gloves, hold the pouch outlet over a bedpan or toilet. Lift the lower edge up.
- Unclamp or unseal the pouch.
- Drain the pouch. Loosen feces from sides by moving fingers down the pouch.
- Clean the inside of the tail of the pouch with a tissue or a premoistened towelette.
- Apply the clamp or seal the pouch.
- Dispose of used supplies.
- Remove and discard gloves. Perform hand hygiene.
- Document the amount, consistency, and color of stool.

| UNEXPECTED OUTCOMES | CRITICAL THINKING OPTIONS |
|---|---|
| Stoma appears dark, dusky-colored, or black. | • Notify physician of findings, and document in chart. (Usually indicates stoma is ischemic.) |
| Stoma becomes ulcerated or cut. | • Examine pouching system to see if opening of pouch may be cutting into stoma.<br>• Recut opening to exact size of stoma. |
| Stoma remains a persistent pale pink. | • Request physician to order Hgb, Hct (usually the result of low Hgb).<br>• Instruct client to monitor effluent for constipation if iron preparation ordered. |
| Bleeding occurs when stoma is touched. | • Observe and note—usual occurrence postoperatively. |
| Erythematous rash at site of pouch. | • Assess for allergic reaction to product being used.<br>• May need to change to different type of adhesive on pouch or change to a pouch with no adhesive. |
| Papular rash appears on peristomal skin. | • Assess for possible yeast sensitivity.<br>• Be sure skin is clean and dry before applying pouch.<br>• Do not rinse pouch with water because this traps water under wafer.<br>• May need to use antifungal powder on skin with each pouch change until skin clears. |
| Peristomal skin complications occur. | • Evaluate cause of leakage.<br>• Be sure pouch is cut to correct size.<br>• Measure stoma at each pouch change for 4–6 weeks. Size will change as edema subsides.<br>• Measure stoma at base.<br>• May need to fill any creases around stoma with skin barrier paste. |

*(continued)*

**UNEXPECTED OUTCOMES** *(cont.)*

**CRITICAL THINKING OPTIONS** *(cont.)*

- Apply thin layer of ostomy powder over area and seal with an alcohol-free coating.
- May need to use secondary skin barrier like Eakin seal.
- May need to attach belt to minimize lateral leakage.
- Change to a product like Durahesive that swells around stoma preventing leakage and holds up well to liquid output.
- Be sure pouch is emptied before it is over ⅓ full of stool or flatus, since an overfull pouch can break seal of pouch.
- Pouches should not be changed more than once daily.

Ostomy is flush or below the surface.

- Apply convex pouch system to assist ostomy to protrude.
- Apply ostomy belt.

Ostomy is in skin fold or crease.

- Apply a one-piece pouch for more flexibility.
- Fill deep crevices with caulking material.

Client experiences itching or burning under appliance.

- May be a sign that stool is undermining seal of pouch.

Client not coping with altered body image.

- Refer to United Ostomy Associations of America, Inc., the Crohn's and Colitis Foundation of America, American Cancer Society, or the local Enterostomal Therapy nurse.

---

## SETTING OF CARE

- Provide the client with the names and phone numbers of a WOCN, supply vendor, and other resource people to contact when needed. Provide pertinent Internet resources for information and support.
- Inform the client of signs to report to a health care provider (e.g., peristomal redness, skin breakdown, and changes in stomal color).
- Provide client and family education regarding care of the ostomy and appliance when traveling.

- Educate the client and family regarding infection control precautions, including proper disposal of used pouches since these cannot be flushed down a toilet.
- Younger clients may have special concerns about odor and appearance. Provide information about ostomy care and community support groups. A visit from someone who has had an ostomy under similar circumstances may be helpful.

---

# Skill 2.31   Assisting with Peritoneal Dialysis Catheter Insertion

Anuria (lack of urine production), oliguria (inadequate urine production), and both acute and chronic renal failure can occur as a result of kidney disease, severe heart failure, burns, and shock. These conditions can be fatal if some other means is not used to remove the body waters. Dialysis is the technique by which blood is filtered for the removal of these wastes and of excess fluid. When hemodialysis is used, intravascular needles or catheters are inserted directly into blood vessels so that the blood can be removed from the body, cycled through machines that filter the blood, and then returned to the body. This chapter describes another type of dialysis: peritoneal dialysis.

### Delegation

Assisting with peritoneal catheter insertion is a sterile procedure and not delegated to unlicensed assistive personnel (UAP).

### Equipment

- Sterile gloves, masks, caps, goggles, and gowns for primary care provider, nurse, and anyone assisting; mask for client
- Peritoneal catheter
- Local anesthetic (e.g., lidocaine), 25-gauge ⅝-inch needle, and 3-mL syringe
- Alcohol sponges

- Scalpel with a blade
- Precut gauze to place around the catheter
- Drape
- Tubing and clamp
- Dialysate filter (if specified by agency policy)
- Sutures, needles, and needle driver
- Trocar (the sharp, needle-like instrument used to make a hole in body tissues)
- Connector
- 4 × 4 gauze square
- Specimen container
- Antiseptic ointment (e.g., povidone-iodine)
- Protective catheter cap
- 10-mL syringe and 1.5-inch needle
- Scissors
- Skin preparation/dressing set containing:
- Chlorhexidine gluconate 2%, povidone-iodine, or other disinfecting solution
- Razor and blade or scissors
- Gauze sponges
- Nonallergenic tape

### Preparation

Although the primary care provider will have already done initial client and family teaching, the nurse reinforces key elements. Review the technique of peritoneal dialysis and its purpose with the client and family.

- Explain that since the kidneys are not functioning properly, this procedure will rid the blood and body of excess waste and fluid that are normally excreted by the kidneys.
- Explain that inserting the trocar (which is the primary care provider's responsibility) may be uncomfortable. The discomfort can be reduced by the client tensing the abdominal muscles as if for a bowel movement.
- Explain that the purpose of the masks, gowns, gloves, and caps is to reduce the possibility of contaminating the site during insertion. Then explain that the client will also need to wear a mask for the same reason.

### Procedure

1. Prior to performing the procedure, introduce self and verify the client's identity using agency protocol. Explain to the client what your role will be, why it is necessary, and how he or she can participate. Remind the client that additional teaching will be done at the time of the actual peritoneal dialysis treatment.

2. Perform hand hygiene and observe other appropriate infection control procedures throughout the various phases of the procedure. Assist the client with use of the mask.
3. Provide for client privacy.
4. Prepare the client.
   - Ask the client to urinate before the procedure. In some cases, bowel cleansing is also done prior to catheter insertion. ➤*Rationale: Emptying the bladder and bowels lessens the danger that they will be punctured by the trocar.*
   - Assist the client to a supine position, and arrange the bedding to expose the area around the umbilicus. ➤*Rationale: The insertion site is usually in the midline just below the umbilicus.*
5. Prepare the solution and the tubing.
6. Implement surgical aseptic practices and body fluid precautions according to agency protocol.
   - Apply masks. ➤*Rationale: Applying masks prior to breaking the seals on the packages reduces the chance of contamination.*
   - Apply cap, gown, and goggles.
   - Open the dialysis set and any sterile supplies not part of the set.
   - Apply sterile gloves.
7. Assist the primary care provider as needed during and after the catheter insertion.
   - Connect the end of the tubing from the solution to the catheter.
   - Connect the drainage receptacle to the outflow tubing. Close the outflow tubing clamp.
   - Cover the catheter site with the precut sterile gauze, and tape the occlusive dressing in place.
   - Remove and discard gloves. Perform hand hygiene.
8. Administer prophylactic antibiotics as ordered. The medication can be administered prior to or following the catheter insertion. ➤*Rationale: A single dose of a first- or second-generation cephalosporin is recommended to reduce wound and exit site infections (Flanigan & Gokal, 2005).*
9. Document findings in the client record using forms or checklists supplemented by narrative notes when appropriate. Record the date and time of the procedure, client's response, appearance of exit site and dressing.

### Documentation

Sample: 5/19/09 1430 Double-cuff coiled Tenckhoff peritoneal catheter inserted in right lower quadrant by Dr. Novar under local anesthesia using sterile technique throughout. VS stable during and after procedure. Catheter taped to abdominal skin. Dry, sterile, occlusive dressing applied to exit site.

_____ U. Schmidt, RN

# Skill 2.32 Conducting Peritoneal Dialysis Procedures

## Delegation

Conducting peritoneal dialysis procedures is not delegated to UAP. However, the client's status is observed during usual care and may be recorded by persons other than the nurse. Abnormal findings must be validated and interpreted by the nurse.

## Equipment

### For Infusing the Dialysate

- Container of peritoneal solution at body temperature, of the amount and kind ordered by the primary care provider. Bags range in size from 1 to 3 liters.
- IV pole
- Sterile peritoneal dialysis administration set (separate or combined pieces):
- Y connector
- IV-type tubing for dialysate
- Drainage bag with tubing
- Dialysis log or flow sheet
- Clean gloves
- Mask and goggles
- Povidone-iodine swabs (or other antiseptic per agency protocol). Some agencies recommend a sterile bowl and antiseptic for soaking the transfer set tubing.

### For Changing the Catheter Site Dressing

- Sterile gloves and masks (gowns and goggles as needed)
- Sterile cotton-tipped applicators
- Chlorhexidine gluconate, povidone-iodine solution, or soap and water as specified by agency protocol
- Povidone-iodine ointment
- Precut sterile 2 × 2 gauze or slit transparent occlusive dressing
- Nonallergenic tape

## Preparation

- Determine when the last dressing change was performed. The dressing should be changed when wet, soiled, loose, or at intervals specified by agency policy.

## Procedure

1. Prior to performing the procedure, introduce self and verify the client's identity using agency protocol. Explain to the client what you are going to do, why it is necessary, and how he or she can participate. Discuss how the results will be used in planning further care or treatments.
2. Perform hand hygiene and observe other appropriate infection control procedures.
3. Provide for client privacy.
4. Prepare the solution and the tubing.
   - Examine the label on the container and the dialysate itself. The dialysate solution should be clear and the seals unbroken. Check the expiration date.
   - Warm the dialysate using an approved warmer (not a microwave oven) to at least body temperature. *Rationale: Warmed solution enhances exchange and is more comfortable for the client.*
   - Add any prescribed medication to the dialysate solution. Heparin is sometimes added. ➤*Rationale: This prevents the accumulation of fibrin in the catheter.* Potassium is often added. ➤*Rationale: This prevents excessive loss of potassium.*
   - Spike the solution container, close the clamp, and hang the container on the IV pole.
   - Prime the tubing: Remove the protective cap and hold the tubing over a cup or basin. Maintain the sterility of the end of the tubing and the cap. Open the clamp and let the fluid run through the tubing, removing all bubbles. Close the tubing clamp. ➤*Rationale: This rids the tubing of air that could enter the peritoneal cavity, causing discomfort and preventing free drainage outflow.*
5. Connect the solution to the catheter.
   - Apply clean gloves, mask, and goggles.
   - Free the catheter end from the dressing if necessary.
   - Cleanse or soak the transfer set connections with povidone-iodine or other specified disinfectant for the time listed in the agency protocol (usually 5 minutes). Remove the cap from the transfer set and attach the Y connector and end of the tubing from the solution to the catheter.
   - Connect the drainage receptacle to the outflow tubing. Close the outflow tubing clamp.
   - If necessary, cover the catheter site with the precut sterile gauze, and tape the dressing in place.
   - Remove and discard gloves. Perform hand hygiene.

6. Infuse the peritoneal dialysate.
   - Open the clamp on the inflow tubing so that the dialysate can flow into the peritoneal cavity for the time specified by the order. If no rate is specified, the client can usually tolerate a steady open flow.
   - After the fluid has infused, clamp the inflow tubing. ➤*Rationale: With the tubing clamped air will not enter the peritoneal cavity.*
   - Leave the fluid in the cavity for the designated time.
7. Ensure client comfort and safety.
   - Assist the client into a comfortable position.
   - Monitor the client's vital signs.
   - Periodically assess the client's comfort during the dwell time.
8. Remove the fluid.
   - Unclamp the outflow tubing, and permit the fluid to drain into the drainage bag by gravity for about 30 minutes.
   - If the fluid does not drain freely, assist the client to change position, or raise the head of the bed. If specified, drain only the amount ordered.
9. Assess the outflow fluid.
   - Observe the appearance of the outflow fluid. ➤*Rationale: A cloudy pink-tinged or blood-tinged return may indicate peritonitis (infection/inflammation of the peritoneal cavity).* During the first two to four exchanges, the return may be blood tinged but should quickly progress to a straw-color return.
   - Apply clean gloves.
   - Measure the amount of outflow fluid, and discard the fluid and used supplies in an appropriate area.
10. Calculate the fluid balance for each exchange.
    - Compare the amount of outflow fluid with the amount of solution infused for each exchange.
    - If more fluid was infused than removed, the client's fluid balance is positive (+); if more fluid was removed than infused, the fluid balance is negative (–). *Example:*

      + 2,000 mL dialysate solution infused
      <u>– 1,500 mL fluid returned in drainage bag</u>
      =   500 mL balance for this exchange
    - Repeat steps for each exchange.
11. Calculate the cumulative fluid balance. The cumulative fluid balance should be negative.
    - Add the balance from each exchange (from step 10) to the total exchange balance:

*Example:*

| | |
|---|---|
| Previous cumulative exchange balance | +100 mL |
| Present exchange balance | –500 mL |
| Cumulative exchange balance | –400 mL |

12. Check the dressing at the catheter site if present.
    - Assess the dryness or wetness of the dressing. ➤*Rationale: The dressing should remain dry during dialysis.*
    - To change the catheter site dressing, use the supplies listed above. Do not forcibly remove crusts or scabs. ➤*Rationale: This may irritate skin and increase the risk of exit site infection.* Dressings may not be necessary for well-healed insertion sites.
13. Disconnect the catheter from the tubing, and cover the end of the catheter with a new sterile cap. ➤*Rationale: This allows the catheter to remain in place between each of the exchanges without contamination of the catheter.*
14. Remove and discard gloves. Perform hand hygiene.
15. Document findings in the client record using forms or checklists supplemented by narrative notes when appropriate. Include the time during which the fluid infused; exchange number; dialysate and additives used; details of the exchange balance; color of outflow dialysate return from client; client's response; appearance of exit site and dressing; and client's weight before and after the set of exchanges (daily). These may be written in the nurse's notes or on a flowchart.

**Documentation**

Sample: 5/20/09 0830 First 1L dialysate infused over 20 minutes thru PD catheter. VS unchanged, no complaints of discomfort. Insertion site dressing clean & dry. Up in chair for breakfast

_____ S. Everley, RN

5/20/09 1230 VS stable, drsg dry & intact. 950mL pink-tinged fluid returned from PD catheter by gravity flow over 20 minutes. PD bag #2, 1L, infused in 15 minutes. Amb in hall independently.

_____ S. Everley, RN

## SETTING OF CARE

Most clients undergoing peritoneal dialysis perform these procedures themselves at home. The nurse performs initial teaching and documents that the client and family are knowledgeable and able to demonstrate the techniques involved. In addition, the nurse assists with arrangements for all equipment and supplies that the client requires for home care.

For clients using CAPD, the empty dialysate solution bag can be left attached to the catheter during dwelling and is then used as the drainage bag. A special belt that stabilizes the catheter and holds the administration set between uses is available. Many clients begin with CAPD and then transition to CCPD over time.

Teach the client and family:

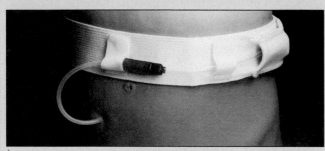

● Peritoneal dialysis belt with tubing pouch stored in place.

- Store supplies in a clean, cool, dry place.
- Examine the solution for any signs of contamination before using it.
- Warm the dialysate using a heating pad for about 1 hour.
- Hang dialysate bag at approximately shoulder height for infusion. Assist the client with obtaining an IV pole or other hanging device.
- Perform thorough hand cleansing and wear a surgical mask when changing tubing.
- Record weight and dialysis fluid balance daily or as ordered.
- Report any signs of peritonitis:
  - Fever.
  - Nausea or vomiting.
  - Redness or pain around the exit site.

# Skill 2.33   Providing Hemodialysis

## EXPECTED OUTCOMES

- Dialysis proceeds without complication (excess fluids and wastes removed from blood.)
- Vascular access site remain patent.
- Client demonstrates self-care after teaching.

## Equipment

Dialyzer (types are hollow fiber or cellulose acetate)
1000-mL bag of 0.9% normal saline IV solution
Machine blood lines
Fistula needles, ¹⁵⁄₁₆ gauge, 1–1½ inches in length
Sterile gauze pads, alcohol swabs, and povidone–iodine or Chloroprep swabs
Two 3-mL syringes
Two 20-mL syringes
Drape
Client mask
Hemostats, cannula clamps
Tape
Sterile gloves and clean gloves
Gown
Protective goggles and face mask or visor shield
12-mL syringe
Heparin solution 1000 U/mL
Hemastix

## Preparation

1. Obtain dialysate bath composition as ordered.
2. Set up 1000-mL IV of normal saline using IV tubing in blood line set.
3. Load heparin pump (e.g., 8 mL heparin) per manufacturer's instructions. ➤*Rationale: Heparin is added to system just before blood enters dialyzer to prevent clotting. The clotting mechanism is activated when blood moves outside body and is in contact with foreign substances.*
4. Check location of nearest emergency power outlet. ➤*Rationale: To maintain electric current if routine power fails.*
5. Test dialysis machine for presence of bleach with Hemastix. ➤*Rationale: This detects presence of caustic agents that could result in client complications.*
6. Prime dialyzer and arterial and venous blood lines with saline.
7. Hang additional IV solution of saline. ➤*Rationale: Saline infusions must be available immediately for rapid reversal of hypotension or discontinuation of dialysis.*
8. Connect pressure monitor lines to both arterial and venous drip chambers. ➤*Rationale: This monitors the amount of hydrostatic pressure exerted on blood in the*

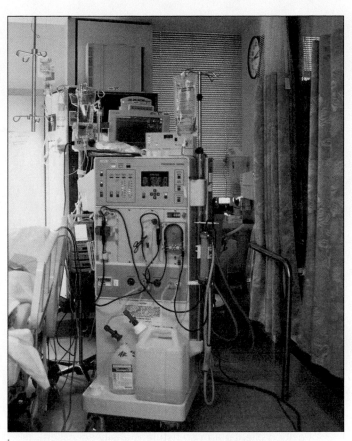

● Hemodialysis unit used to treat renal failure clients.

## THE HEMODIALYSIS PROCESS

Hemodialysis works by removing blood from the client's arterial access site (graft, fistula, or catheter) circulating it through a tubing system to a dialyzer. In the dialyzer, which acts like a semipermeable membrane, fluid, electrolytes, and toxins are removed from the blood through a process of convection, osmosis, and diffusion. The blood then flows from the dialyzer through a tubing system to the client's venous access site. Fluid is removed through the use of hydrostatic pressure applied to the blood and a negative hydrostatic pressure applied to the dialysate bath. The difference between these two pressures is termed transmembrane pressure and this results in the process of ultrafiltration.

## CLINICAL ALERT

When a hemodialysis client is hospitalized:
1. Place an identifying bracelet on access arm.
2. Post safety precautions at head of bed (e.g., "Do not use access arm for blood pressure or venipuncture," and "Fluid restriction specified").
3. Notify dialysis specialty nurse of client's admission to hospital.

*ultrafiltration process used to extract fluid throughout dialysis treatment.*

9. Set the alarm pressures—high and low.
10. Connect air leak detector to venous drip chamber.
11. Test all machine alarms—venous and arterial pressure, air detector, and blood leak detector.
12. Connect arterial and venous lines for recirculation with adapter, and turn blood pump to 200 mL/min.
13. Document alarm checks in dialysis log.

**Procedure**

*For AV Fistula or Graft*

1. Place blood line at the same level as the bed.
2. Don mask and gown. Put on goggles, and perform hand hygiene.
3. Don clean gloves, and remove dressing, if used. Remove and discard gloves and perform hand hygiene.
4. Don sterile gloves.
5. Clean access site using Chloroprep or alcohol swab, then povidone–iodine swab. Using a circular motion, cleanse from needle insertion site outward. Allow to dry. ►*Rationale: Cleansing occurs from cleanest to dirtiest area preventing contamination of the site.*

6. Insert needles into fistula or graft. Tape securely to extremity.
7. Obtain blood for predialysis blood samples as ordered by the physician. (Usually electrolytes, hematocrit, clotting time, etc.)
8. After blood is drawn for lab work, heparin bolus should be given to client according to physician's order—start heparin pump at ordered rate.
9. Prime the extracorporeal circuit with blood.
   a. Connect arterial tubing of the blood line to client's arterial site.
   b. Connect venous tubing.
   c. Unclamp venous blood line.
   d. Unclamp arterial blood line.
   e. Clamp saline infusion line.
10. Note time of dialysis initiation.
11. Tape all connections securely; secure blood tubing to client's extremity.
12. Set alarm pressures—high and low.
13. Establish blood flow rate (usually 300–450 mL/min).
14. Ensure that access connections are visible.
15. Check client's blood pressure and pulse once dialysis has been initiated, then every 30 minutes unless otherwise indicated.

## BLOOD FLOW FOR DIALYSIS

An adequate vascular access should permit blood flow to the dialyzer of 200–450 mL/min. Optimal blood access and blood flow to the dialyzer influences dialysis efficiency.

## SAFETY PRECAUTIONS FOR FISTULA OR GRAFT

- Feel for vibration (thrill) over access site regularly.
- Do not measure blood pressure on extremity.
- Do not perform venipuncture in extremity.
- Counsel client not to wear constrictive clothing on extremity.
- Counsel client to avoid lying on extremity.
- Avoid carrying heavy loads with access extremity.
- Immediately report swelling, discoloration, drainage, or coldness, numbness, or weakness of hand.

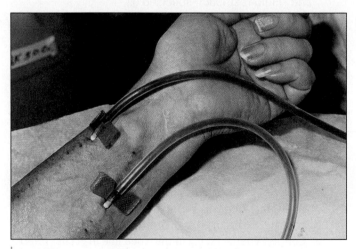

● Arterial and venous needles placed in graft for hemodialysis.

16. Assess client at least every 30 minutes for vital signs and potential complications.
17. Administer any ordered medication through the venous line. ▶*Rationale: Medication infuses into client, not machine.*
18. Turn heparin infusion off last 30–60 minutes or as ordered.

## ■ CULTURAL COMPETENCE

- African-Americans have a more rapid decline in glomerular filtration rate than do Caucasians.
- Hypertensive African-Americans have decreased renal excretion of sodium, making sodium restriction an important factor in treatment.
- Hypertension, diabetes, and end stage renal disease (ESRD) are 3–4 times more common in African-Americans and American Indians than in Caucasians.

## ASSESSING ARTERIOVENOUS FISTULA

- Perform hand hygiene.
- Position client's arm so fistula is easily accessed.
- Palpate the area to feel for thrill (vibration). This indicates arterial to venous blood flow and fistula patency.
- Auscultate with a stethoscope to detect a bruit (swishing noise). This indicates a patent fistula.
- Palpate pulses distal to fistula to check circulation.
- Observe capillary refill in extremity digits.
- Assess for numbness, tingling, coldness, pallor, or alternation in sensation in digits of fistula extremity.
- Assess for signs and symptoms of infection: redness, edema, soreness, warmth, or increased temperature.

# Skill 2.34  Providing Ongoing Care of Hemodialysis Client

### Procedure

1. Limit fluid intake to prescribed amount (e.g., 1500 mL/day).
2. Maintain individualized diet as prescribed: high-quality protein 1.1 g/kg ideal body wt/day; sodium 70 mEq/day; potassium, average 70 mEq/day.
3. Check BP for hypertension/hypotension; check temperature for possible infection.
4. Auscultate heart and lung sounds for signs of fluid overload (pulmonary edema and pericarditis).
5. Provide access site care.
6. Observe mental status—indicative of fluid and electrolyte imbalance.
7. Administer Epogen, if ordered, to improve hemoglobin level (given at time of dialysis).
8. Encourage regular rest periods.

9. Weigh daily to assess fluid accumulation.
10. Use antibacterial soap and lotion to bathe. ➤*Rationale: This decreases risk of staphylococcal infections.*
11. Determine that client understands when and how to take medications (e.g., Tums with meals).
12. Provide continued emotional support.
    a. Allow for expression of feelings about change in body image and role performance.
    b. Encourage expression of fears.
    c. Encourage caregiver support.
    d. Give support for required change in lifestyle.

*Note:* Dialysis adequacy is improved with increased prescription, conversion of catheters to grafts or fistulas, and by not shortening treatments.

# Skill 2.35   Terminating Hemodialysis

## Equipment

Clean gloves
Gown
Goggles
Mask
Nonsterile pads
Tubing clamps

## Procedure

1. Don gloves, gown, goggles, and protective mask.
2. Remove tape and dressing to visualize needle insertion site.
3. Place pads under connectors.
4. Open IV of normal saline to return blood on the arterial side of tubing.
5. Start blood pump at 200 mL/min.
6. Return venous blood.
7. Clamp lines.
8. Remove needles according to unit protocol and apply pressure to sites.
9. Remove protective gear, discard, and perform hand hygiene.
10. Measure and record postdialysis vital signs and weight.

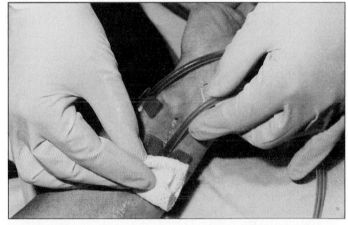

● Remove arterial and venous needles, using needle safety shields.

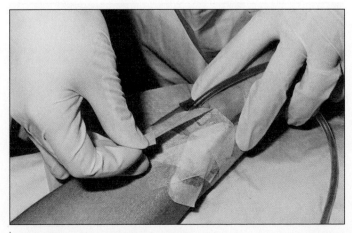

● Carefully remove tape from needle sites.

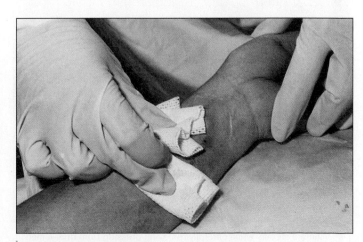

● Apply pressure over needle site for 5 to 10 minutes.

# EVIDENCE-BASED NURSING PRACTICE

**Survival Rate in Hemodialysis Clients**

This study revealed that elderly ESRD clients receiving hemodialysis during morning hours have a higher survival rate than those undergoing dialysis in the afternoon.

Previously identified risk factors for this study did not account for these differences.

*Source:* Bliwise, D., et al. (2001). Survival by time of day of hemodialysis in an elderly cohort. JAMA, 286(21), 2690–2694.

# Skill 2.36 Maintaining Central Venous Dual-Lumen Dialysis Catheter (DLC)

## Equipment

Heparin 1000 U/mL
Sterile normal saline for injection
Betadine spray
Sterile 4 × 4 gauze pads
Sterile transparent occlusive dressings if indicated
Tape
Luer-Lok catheter caps
Nonsterile drape
Two 3-mL syringes
Two 20-mL syringes
Clean gloves
Two masks
Sterile gloves

## Preparation

1. Perform hand hygiene.
2. Fill two 20-mL syringes with 20 mL each of normal saline, and two 3-mL syringes with 3 mL of 1000 µ/mL heparin.
3. Mask client and self, and don clean gloves.
4. Place drape under catheter lumens.
5. Remove gauze wrap from lumens, if present, and discard in appropriate receptacle.
6. Remove gloves and perform hand hygiene.

## Procedure

1. Open sterile supplies.
2. Holding corner of 4 × 4, place under catheter lumens.
3. Spray lumens with Betadine and allow to dry.
4. Don sterile gloves.
5. Remove old lumen caps.
6. Use 4 × 4 gauze to pick up new caps and place on lumens.
7. Unclamp and inject 20 mL saline solution into each lumen using positive pressure technique.
8. Inject 3 mL heparin into each catheter using positive pressure technique.
9. Reclamp lumens.

## CLINICAL ALERT

Central venous dual-lumen dialysis catheter (DLC) maintenance (heparin "pack" and site dressing) is performed only by the nephrology nurse following a dialysis treatment. These catheters are not maintained the way CVADs are. Instead, they are "packed" with undiluted heparin following dialysis, then "unpacked" (3 mL blood withdrawn from catheter) prior to the next dialysis treatment.

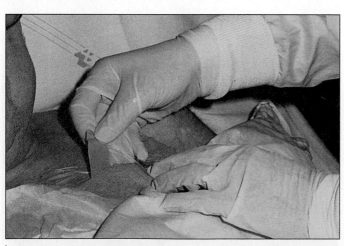

● Maintain sterility while carefully removing dressing from dual-lumen catheter.

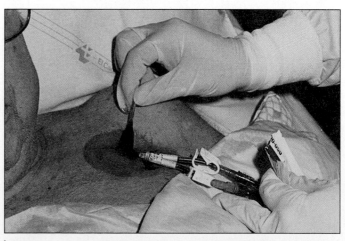

● Cleanse catheter insertion site with antimicrobial swabs.

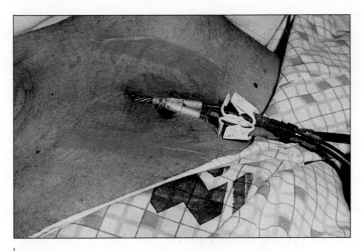
● Monitor frequently for signs of infection, bleeding, or catheter displacement.

10. Remove old dressing, and discard in biohazard receptacle.
11. Cleanse area surrounding catheter with antimicrobial swabs.
12. Place sterile transparent dressing over catheter insertion site.

*Note:* Provide catheter site care after each dialysis treatment. Dressing is not required after permanent catheter site epithelializes around catheter (about 2 weeks).

13. If desired, wrap lumens in gauze and tape.
    ➤*Rationale: To prevent skin irritation from lumen clamps.*
14. Dispose of equipment in biohazard receptacle.
15. Remove gloves and mask, and discard.
16. Perform hand hygiene.
17. Monitor daily for signs of infection, bleeding, or displacement of catheters.

---

## SETTING OF CARE

### Urinary Elimination

Home care clients who require assistance with emptying their bladders are usually placed on intermittent clean catheterization protocols rather than having an indwelling catheter. This procedure assists in preventing penoscrotal abscess formation, overwhelming infection, and altered body image. Fluid intake needs to be monitored and restricted to 1500 mL per day to avoid bladder distention. If spontaneous voiding returns, frequency of catheterizations can be extended to every 12 hours and discontinued when the residual urine is consistently less than 100 mL in 24 hours.

When an indwelling catheter is used, it is important to be aware that it may lead to urinary tract infection. The nurse must teach the client and family to observe for signs and symptoms of urinary tract infections and sepsis. They should note odor, color, and consistency of the urine. Catheter changes are the responsibility of the nurse and are usually performed once a month. Encouraging fluids becomes a major role assumed by family members and monitored by the nurse. Urinary antiseptics are adjunctive measures when catheterizations are required.

Home care dialysis is common in many areas of the country. The principles and procedures are similar to those in a hospital or free-standing dialysis unit. The major change is the advent of portable dialysis methods such as continuous ambulatory peritoneal dialysis (CAPD) and continuous cycling peritoneal dialysis (CCPD). These procedures allow individuals to participate in a normal lifestyle. However, use of these methods requires monitoring by the nurse and specific teaching of the essential components to prevent complications and promote health. Peritoneal dialysis (PD) reflects more normal kidney function than hemodialysis. Fluid and electrolytes are removed gradually and, therefore, clients have fewer complications with blood pressure alterations and disequilibrium syndrome. There are fewer dietary and fluid restrictions, allowing clients to lead a more normal life. PD provides the client with a more flexible schedule, allowing him or her to work, travel, and participate in activities. One major restriction, besides ensuring the ordered number of exchanges each day, is the monthly appointment at the dialysis center for lab work and consultation with the physician or nurse.

The catheter is placed in a dependent position in the peritoneal cavity to minimize the chance of catheter obstruction or erosion into other abdominal organs. The catheter is placed outside of the abdomen to decrease infections. There are several devices that are placed around the catheter that prevent fluid leak from the peritoneal cavity. These devices impede the migration of bacteria.

There are three types of PD: continuous ambulatory peritoneal dialysis (CAPD), continuous cycling peritoneal dialysis (CCPD), and intermittent peritoneal dialysis (IPD). The two most common types for home care clients are CAPD and CCPD.

*(continued)*

---

**SETTING OF CARE** (CONTINUED)

**Bowel Elimination**

Most skills involving care of the bowel are the same as those performed in the hospital setting. Colostomy irrigations are usually not taught or initiated in the hospital, as there is little supporting evidence for the need to irrigate a colostomy. It was thought that irrigating the colostomy would help regulate the bowel and there would not be bowel eruptions at various times of the day. It has been found that the bowel will return to presurgical habits of elimination. If bowel movements occurred erratically before surgery, this pattern will continue after surgery. To irrigate or not to irrigate is basically a preference by the client.

---

# Skill 2.37    Home Setting: Using Clean Technique for Intermittent Self-Catheterization

## Equipment

Straight catheters in clean container, plastic bag, or wrapped in aluminum foil
Washcloth, soap, water
Water-soluble lubricant (K–Y; Surgilube)
Plastic bags
Basin or container
Mirror

## Procedure

*For Female Client*

1. Attempt to urinate. If unable to do so, continue to follow these steps.
2. Perform hand hygiene and gather equipment. (Keep equipment in one large container.)
3. Assume sitting position on bed or commode. (Place plastic under towel if bed is used.)
4. Separate labia with one hand while cleaning with soap and water front to back with other hand.
5. Position mirror to visualize urinary meatus.
6. Remove catheter from container (plastic bag or aluminum foil).
7. Lubricate end of catheter with water-soluble lubricant and place other end in container to catch urine.
8. While holding labia apart with one hand, insert catheter about 3 inches or until urine flows.
9. Press down with abdominal muscles to promote bladder's emptying.
10. Pinch off catheter after all urine has drained and withdraw gently, holding tip of catheter upright.
11. Wash and dry perineal area.
12. Wash catheter in warm, soapy water.
13. Rinse with clear water and dry outside with paper towel.
14. Place in plastic bag for storage.
15. Use catheters for 2–4 weeks and then discard.
16. Perform hand hygiene.

*For Male Client*

1. Attempt to urinate. If unable to do so, continue to follow these steps.
2. Perform hand hygiene and gather equipment. (Keep equipment in one large container.)
3. Assume sitting position on the bed or commode. (Place plastic under towel if bed is used.)
4. Retract the foreskin, if present, and wash tip of penis with soap and water.
5. Remove catheter from container (plastic bag or aluminum foil).
6. Lubricate the first 7–10 inches of catheter with water-soluble lubricant. Place other end in container to catch urine.
7. Hold penis at right angle to body, keeping foreskin retracted. Insert catheter 7–10 inches into penis or until urine begins to flow. Then insert catheter 1 inch farther.
8. Press down with abdominal muscles to promote bladder's emptying.
9. Pinch off catheter after all urine has drained and gently withdraw, holding tip of catheter upright.
10. Wash and dry area. Replace foreskin, if present.
11. Wash catheter in warm, soapy water.
12. Rinse with clear water and dry outside with paper towel.
13. Place in plastic bag for storage.
14. Use catheters for 2–4 weeks and then discard.
15. Perform hand hygiene.

# Skill 2.38  Home Setting: Providing Suprapubic Catheter Care

**Equipment**

Catheter plug and clamp
Closed drainage system
Sterile dressings if necessary
Clean gloves
Receptacle to drain urine from drainage bag
Normal saline solution or mild soap and water
White vinegar
Applicator sticks
4 × 4 gauze pads
Paper tape

**Procedure**

1. Instruct client to gather equipment for specific skill to be done.
2. Perform hand hygiene and don gloves.
3. Clean around catheter site with normal saline solution or mild soap and water. Use applicator sticks to remove material from around catheter opening.
4. Ensure catheter is not pulling on exit site. Tape catheter to skin so a gentle curve is present to prevent tugging on catheter.
5. Empty catheter bag. Some clients use leg bags. Empty into container and then dispose of contents in toilet or, if removing bag, empty directly into toilet.
6. Clean drainage bags with warm water and soap every day or two. Place one teaspoon of vinegar in rinse water to reduce odor.
7. Replace catheter bag on catheter.
8. Remove gloves and perform hand hygiene.
9. Instruct client in bladder testing:
   a. Wash hands and catheter connections with soap and water.
   b. Clamp the suprapubic tube so it does not drain. Use catheter plug or clamp.
   c. Have client attempt to void when client feels urge to urinate. Measure amount of urine.
   d. Unclamp the suprapubic tube immediately after voiding; empty urine into container and measure residual urine amount.
   e. Instruct client to keep a log of each voiding and residual amount.
   f. Call physician with findings when residual amount is less than 20% voided amount. Usually, this amount is about 60 mL. Usually, the suprapubic tube is removed when client is able to urinate without complications.
10. Instruct client to monitor carefully for signs of urinary tract infection and notify physician immediately. Check for bladder pain, bleeding, temperature over 100° F, chills, cloudy urine, drainage or edema around the suprapubic tube.

# Skill 2.39  Home Setting: Administering Continuous Ambulatory Peritoneal Dialysis (CAPD)

**Equipment**

Sterile dialysate solution, warmed
Transfer set, either Y tubing or straight, and cap
Hook on wall of room used for dialysis
Clamp
Paper towels
Low stool or table
Intake and output record
Clean gloves
Mask
Antibacterial soap

**Preparation**

1. Perform hand hygiene thoroughly, dry using paper towel.
2. Obtain container of sterile dialysate.
3. Check that strength and amount of solution are accurate as ordered.
4. Take equipment to clean area for assembly.

**Procedure**

*for Draining Fluid*

1. Perform hand hygiene and don clean gloves.
   ➤*Rationale: Infection control precaution for caregiver when there is potential contact with blood or body fluids.*
2. Don mask.
3. Uncap catheter maintaining aseptic technique.
4. Attach sterile bag and transfer set to catheter for draining dialysate.
5. Place bag on low stool or table below level of client's abdomen. ➤*Rationale: This position allows fluid to drain by gravity from client's peritoneal cavity.*
6. Unclamp tubing.
7. Allow fluid to drain into bag from abdomen until flow ceases, approximately, 10–20 minutes.
8. Reclamp tubing.

9. Examine drainage for discoloration or cloudiness. ➤Rationale: Change in color may indicate presence of infection.

10. Disconnect tubing from drainage bag while maintaining aseptic technique. Unscrew catheter from tubing and attach Mini Cap, according to clinic's instruction. ➤Rationale: The glucose in the dialysate solution predisposes the client to infections.

11. Weigh drainage bag on scale. Effluent should weigh at least 4 and ½ pounds. This is equal to 2 liters of fluid. ➤Rationale: To ensure all fluid is drained from abdomen.

12. Dispose of effluent into toilet.

13. Double bag tubing and drainage bag. Place biohazardous label on bag. Discard by placing in biohazardous container. Tubing is usually disposed of following each exchange.

14. Remove and discard gloves and mask.

15. Perform hand hygiene.

16. Check blood pressure and pulse. ➤Rationale: Rapid fluid shift may cause hypotension.

Note: Mini Cap disinfects dialysis tubing between exchanges.

### For Infusing Dialysate

1. Warm dialysate. The bag can be encased in a heating pad for 1 hour. DO NOT PLACE IN MICROWAVE. ➤Rationale: Microwave heating will produce uneven heating and can cause burning in the client.

2. Perform hand hygiene for 3 minutes with antibacterial soap. ➤Rationale: To prevent contamination.

3. Gather equipment, don gloves.

4. Open plastic wrap on dialysate solution and inspect solution bag for expiration date and color and consistency of dialysate, and assess bag for possible leaks.

5. Add medications as ordered. Maintain sterile technique in this step. ➤Rationale: Some clients add routine drugs to dialysate, such as insulin.

6. Connect tubing to dialysate bag by removing protective cover from port and spiking into dialysate bag. Maintain sterility throughout this step. Each manufacturer has a slightly different mechanism for connecting the tubing and bag. Follow manufacturer's directions. See box: Transfer Sets.

7. Hang new dialysate bag on hook, which is positioned above client at shoulder height.

8. Open clamp and adjust height to ensure inflow of solution by gravity over a 10- to 20-minute period.

9. Clamp tubing.

10. Discard empty dialysate bag or place in a holding pouch at client's waist, according to type of transfer set being used.

11. Allow fluid to remain in peritoneal cavity approximately 4 hours.

12. Remove gloves.

13. Perform hand hygiene.

14. Repeat procedure four times daily, the last time at bedtime, allowing fluid to remain in peritoneal cavity overnight.

15. Ensure that client and caregiver are knowledgeable in strict aseptic technique.

16. Instruct client to notify physician if there is evidence of infection.

17. Document findings and bring to physician at each visit.

---

## TRANSFER SETS

Transfer sets are tubing that connects bag of dialysate solution to catheter. There are two types being used for CAPD.

### Straight Tubing

Straight tubing stays connected to the catheter. For each exchange, the "free" end is connected to the solution. With this type of transfer set, the empty bag from solution is rolled up and worn under clothing. That bag is then unrolled, placed on the floor, and used to drain dialysate from the abdomen. After draining is completed, tubing is disconnected from the straight transfer set and a new solution bag and tubing are connected to the catheter.

### Y-Set Tubing

This type of tubing is disconnected between exchanges. The base of the Y is connected to the catheter. One branch of the Y is connected to a new bag of solution and the other to an empty bag. The base of the Y is closed and a small amount of solution is drained from the full bag into the empty bag. This is done to rid the transfer set of any bacteria that might be in the tubing. The branch that leads to the empty bag is then closed and the solution flows into the abdomen. Once the solution bag is empty, the Y-set is disconnected from the catheter. This removes the need to wear the bag around the waist while solution is in abdomen. The catheter is then reconnected to the Y-set and solution is drained into an empty bag to discard. A new bag of solution is hung and the process continues. The Y-set is filled with disinfectant when not in use. The disinfectant is flushed out with the used dialysate. The Y-set can be reused for several months.

---

## CLINICAL ALERT

Observe draining dialysate for indications of fibrin, a white gelatin-like material. This indicates a shedding of the peritoneal lining's old skin; an increase in this fibrin indicates potential peritonitis.

# Skill 2.40  Home Setting: Changing Dressing for a CAPD Client

## Equipment

Dressing according to facility policy
Antimicrobial swabs
Sterile saline
Sterile gloves (two pair)
Forceps (optional)

## Procedure

1. Perform hand hygiene.
2. Don gloves.
3. Remove old dressing with sterile gloves.
4. Inspect site for infection (erythema, edema, warmth, exudate).
5. Remove any dried blood or drainage with warm, soapy water.
6. Rinse area with normal saline.
7. Dry area thoroughly.
8. Change gloves.
9. Cleanse area surrounding catheter with antimicrobial swab.
10. Apply dressing according to facility policy.
11. Remove gloves and perform hand hygiene.

# Skill 2.41  Home Setting: Instructing Client in Colostomy Irrigation

## Equipment

Solution container with 1000 mL warm water
Irrigating tubing with cone
Three pair of clean gloves
Irrigating sleeve cut long enough to reach water level in toilet
Items to clean skin and stoma (e.g., washcloths or gauze sponges)
Plastic bag for disposal of used pouch
Clean pouch and closure device
Skin barriers
Water-soluble lubricant
Hook near toilet

## Procedure

1. Instruct client in benefits of relaxing and taking periodic deep breaths.
2. Perform hand hygiene and don clean gloves.
3. Remove and dispose of used pouch in plastic bag.
4. Clean stoma and skin with warm water and soft cloth. Assess skin for signs of irrigation or breakdown.
5. Apply irrigation sleeve to peristomal skin, and place belt around waist.
6. Fill container with 1000 mL lukewarm water (500 mL for first irrigation). ➤*Rationale: Lukewarm water temperature is 105°–110°F. This temperature prevents injury from hot solutions and cramping from cold solutions.*
7. Suspend container on bathroom hook at level of client's shoulders (no higher than 18 inches above stoma).
8. Open roller clamp and allow solution to run through tubing; close clamp. ➤*Rationale: This removes air from tubing and prevents discomfort for client.*
9. Assist client to sit on toilet or on chair in front of toilet.
10. Place sleeve between client's thighs and direct end into toilet.
11. Lubricate cone tip with water-soluble lubricant.
12. Position cone in sleeve by placing through top opening. If cone cannot be inserted easily do not force it.
13. Hold cone snugly against stoma. ➤*Rationale: This prevents back flow of solution.*
14. Open roller clamp on tubing and allow water to run through cone while inserting cone into stoma.
15. Instill solution (750–1000 mL) over 5–10 minutes. ➤*Rationale: The container height and rate of water flow affects results obtained.* If client complains of feeling light-headed or has vertigo, take pulse and stop instillation. ➤*Rationale: These are symptoms of a vagal response.*
16. Clamp tubing for a few minutes if cramping occurs. Instruct client to take a deep breath when solution is instilled. ➤*Rationale: Deep breathing relaxes abdominal muscles.*
17. Remove cone, and close off or fold over top of sleeve after solution is instilled.
18. Allow client to remain seated while the majority of stool and solution return, usually 10–15 minutes.
19. Remove gloves and discard.
20. Instruct client to rinse sleeve with water. Dry bottom of sleeve and close end of sleeve.
21. Ask client to wear sleeve in this manner for 30–60 minutes. Client may sit in chair, walk around, or proceed with other activities during this time. ➤*Rationale: This provides additional time for expelling solution or feces and thus prevents accidental evacuation.*
22. Instruct client to remove sleeve, clean, and store in designated area of bathroom.

> ### CLINICAL ALERT
>
> A distended colon can cause a vagal response resulting in hypotension, bradycardia, and even loss of consciousness.

> ### CLINICAL ALERT
>
> The danger of perforation of the colon is much greater when irrigating a colostomy with a catheter. The use of an irrigation cone results in safer administration and better water flow.

23. Instruct client to cleanse skin and stoma with warm water and dry thoroughly.
24. Instruct client on how to apply skin barriers and clean pouch.
25. Instruct client to reorder supplies as needed.
26. Place discarded supplies in client's trash.
27. Remove gloves and perform hand hygiene.

Direct blood pressure monitoring allows continuous measurement of the client's systolic, diastolic, and mean arterial pressures (MAP) to facilitate evaluation of perfrusion to vital organs. A short single lumen catheter is placed in the client's radial artery (brachial artery may be used), then attached to a pressure transducer and high-pressure infusion system and a display monitor. Direct pressure readings are typically 20–30 mm Hg higher than simultaneously measured indirect (cuff) readings.

### EXPECTED OUTCOMES

- Blood supply to hand to adequate before and following arterial catheter placement.
- Arterial cannulation is accomplished without complication.
- Arterial blood pressure monitoring system functions reliably and accurately.
- Arterial blood samples are obtained.

## Skill 2.42   Performing the Allen Test

### Procedure

1. Perform the Allen test to determine distal peripheral perfusion. ►*Rationale: This procedure assesses blood supply to client's hand to determine that radial and ulnar artery are functioning before an arterial line is inserted.*
2. Compress both arteries at client's wrist for about 1 minute.
3. Instruct client to clench and unclench fist several times. ►*Rationale: This causes blanching in the hand and palm.*
4. With client's hand in open, relaxed position, release pressure on ulnar artery.
5. Observe how quickly (≤7 seconds) the palm color flushes. ►*Rationale: If color returns quickly, good collateral blood supply to the hand exists. If normal color does not return, there is insufficient collateral circulation to the hand should radial artery occlusion occur.*
6. Repeat procedure with release of the radial artery.
7. Report to physician if collateral blood flow is insufficient. ►*Rationale: A Doppler flow study may be used to help determine collateral blood flow.*

## Skill 2.43   Assisting with Arterial Line Insertion

### Equipment

20-gauge Teflon catheter with introducer and flexible guidewire
500 mL normal saline for flush
Heparin 1,000 units/mL
One mL unit dose syringe
Pressure bag for flush infusion
IV tubing
Short wide-bore, high-pressure tubing
Three-way stopcocks with nonvented caps
Established pressure monitor system
Clean gloves, sterile gloves
Razor
Personal protection equipment (PPE)
Sterile towels and drape
Skin prep solution (2% chlorhexidine)
Sterile 4 × 4 gauze sponges
Sterile 2 × 2 gauze sponges
Lidocaine 1% (without epinephrine)
3-mL syringe with 18- and 25-gauge needles for topical anesthetic
Alcohol wipes

000 silk suture (if used)
Transparent dressing
Atropine for reversal of bradycardia

## Preparation

1. Validate that informed consent has been obtained.
2. Determine if client has received anticoagulant therapy. ➤*Rationale: Coagulation studies may be indicated.*
3. Identify client, check identaband and ask client to state name and birthdate.
4. Explain rationale for procedure and verbally reassure client.
5. Gather equipment.
6. Perform hand hygiene.
7. Add heparin to NS solution, and label bag with additive and date (commonly 2 units heparin/mL fluid). Follow hospital protocols.
8. Connect IV tubing to solution bag.
9. Remove all air from flush solution bag.
10. Insert flush infusion bag into pressure bag, and hang bag on IV pole.
11. Prepare and assemble pressurized monitoring system (transducer, continuous flush device, and stopcocks) following manufacturer's instructions.
12. Level stopcock above transducer to client's phlebostatic axis.
13. Shave or prepare site as needed.
14. Inflate pressure bag to 300 mm Hg, using hand pump on bag.

## Procedure

1. Don gloves and PPE, and prepare to assist the physician as needed.
   a. Skin is prepped briskly with 2% chlorhexidine for 3 seconds.
   b. Lidocaine vial is cleansed with alcohol wipe.
   c. Physician dons sterile gloves.
   d. Sterile drape is placed over arterial insertion site.
   e. Physician aspirates lidocaine with 18-gauge needle, changes needle, and injects client's skin with 25-gauge needle. ➤*Rationale: For local anesthesia.*
   f. Percutaneous insertion is made at arterial insertion site, and arterial catheter is inserted.
   g. Physician advances catheter in artery.
   h. Arterial catheter is sutured in place with 000 silk suture or taped with tape or transparent membrane dressing (Tegaderm).
2. Observe for pulsating bright-red blood spurting retrograde into catheter. ➤*Rationale: This evidence ensures arterial catheter position.*
3. Attach catheter to primed pressure-monitoring system tubing—make certain all connections are secure.
4. Press fast flush valve to clear system.
5. Observe oscilloscope for arterial waveform.
6. Apply sterile occlusive dressing to site after catheter is sutured into place.
7. Remove gloves and perform hand hygiene.
8. Set monitor alarms for both HIGH and LOW parameters.

---

### CLINICAL ALERT

Arterial catheter alarms should always be enabled to detect disconnection, alterations in blood pressure, or pulseless electrical activity.

---

# Skill 2.44  Monitoring Arterial Blood Pressure

## Equipment

Disposable pressure transducer, dome, and amplifier
Flush valve with flush system
Display monitor (oscilloscope)
Sterile stopcock cap
2 × 2 gauze sponges
Tape
Gloves
Carpenter's level
Marker

## Procedure

1. Leveling and zeroing (calibrating) the system.
   a. Calibrate system at beginning of each shift. ➤*Rationale: Monitor readings are altered by changes in atmospheric pressure.*
   b. Position client with HOB flat or up to 45° elevation.
   c. Using carpenter's level, align stopcock above transducer level with client's left atrium (phlebostatic axis) and mark client's chest for future readings. ➤*Rationale: Readings will be inaccurately high or low if stopcock above transducer is not level with client's phlebostatic axis.*

d. To zero ("calibrate") the system, turn stopcock near transducer off to client. Remove cap from stopcock, opening it to air.

e. Depress "zero" button on monitor, release button, and note monitor reading is zero. ➤*Rationale: Zero reading indicates monitor is calibrated to atmospheric pressure.*

f. Replace cap or place new sterile cap on stopcock.

g. Turn stopcock so transducer is open to client.

2. Observe waveform at eye level for the sharp systolic upstroke, peak, dicrotic notch, and end diastole.

3. Compare direct and indirect blood pressure measurements at least every 4 hours. ➤*Rationale: In normovolemic clients, the direct blood pressure measure is typically 5–10 mm Hg higher than indirect readings. If there is greater disparity, equipment malfunction or errors in leveling and zeroing are likely.* Cuff (indirect) measure of blood pressure in the hypovolemic client is unreliable.

4. Fast flush line with valve device. ➤*Rationale: To keep system airfree.*

5. Ensure pressure bag is maintained at 300 mm Hg.

6. Leave cannulated extremity uncovered for easy observation. Assess site for signs of infection every shift.

7. Assess circulation, motion, and sensation of extremity distal to cannulation site every 2 hours initially, then every 8 hours.

8. Immobilize extremity if necessary.

9. Change flush solution and tubing every 96 hours (according to agency policy).

10. Change dressing weekly or if it becomes wet or soiled. ➤*Rationale: Wet dressings increase risk of infection at site.*

a. Put on gloves.

b. Remove dressing, and discard in biohazard container.

c. Cover with occlusive dressing.

d. Tape securely.

11. Remove gloves and PPE and perform hand hygiene.

12. Monitor site to ensure hemostasis occurs.

13. Monitor extremity distally for adequacy of perfusion.

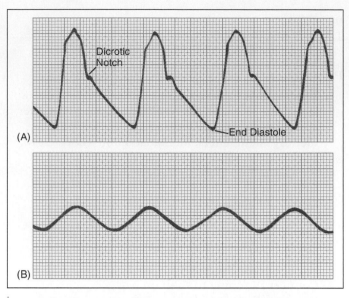

● **A,** Arterial line–normal waveform. **B,** Arterial line–flattened waveform. Flattened arterial waveform indicates damping. Damping results from obstruction in arterial line or imbalance of transducer.

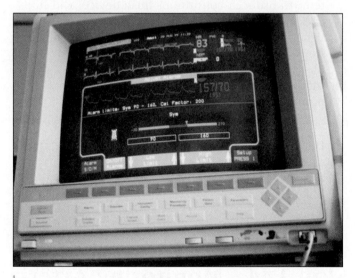

● Arterial line allows direct measurement of blood pressure–monitor displays digital and wave form.

# EVIDENCE-BASED NURSING PRACTICE

**Monitoring Arterial Blood Pressure**

There is no absolute correlation between direct arterial blood pressure monitoring and indirect blood pressure measurement methods. Good correlation between the two methods does not mean the arterial pressure monitoring system is functioning properly.

*Source:* McGhee, B., & Bridges, E. (2002). Monitoring arterial blood pressure: What you may not know. *Critical Care Nurse, 22*(2), 60–79.

| TABLE 2–1 CAUSES OF ACID–BASE IMBALANCE | |
|---|---|
| **Acidemia** | **Alkalemia** |
| Hypovolemia | Hyperventilation |
| Hypoventilation | Hypokalemia |
| COPD | Pulmonary embolus |
| Cardiac arrest | Diuretics/steroids |
| Diabetic ketoacidosis | Prolonged vomiting |
| Severe diarrhea | NG suction |
| Renal failure | |

# Skill 2.45   Withdrawing Arterial Blood Samples

## Equipment

One 6-mL sterile syringe

ABG kit with one 3-mL syringe with dry lithium heparin; air filter device Or: Vacutainer with Luer-Lok adapter cannula; blood specimen tubes

Gloves

Face shield

Container with ice (paper cup, emesis basin)

Two specimen labels

Bubble packaging

Biohazard specimen bag

Gauze sponges/pads

## Preparation

1. Identify client, check identaband, and ask client to state name and birthdate.
2. Gather equipment and explain procedure to client.
3. Attach label to specimen syringe with client's name, hospital number, room number, time, and date. Also add client's current temperature and FIO2.
4. For blood gas specimen, maintain client's current oxygen delivery setting for 20 minutes prior to obtained specimen.
5. Fill paper cup or emesis basin with ice.
6. Perform hand hygiene and don gloves.

## Procedure

1. Momentarily disengage arterial alarms.
2. Turn stopcock off to client.
3. Remove protective cap from open blood sampling port on three-way stopcock closest to arterial line insertion site.
4. Attach syringe or Vacutainer with Luer-Lok adapter cannula to open port of three-way stopcock.
5. Turn stopcock off to flush solution.
6. Attach syringe or blood specimen tube into Vacutainer to establish blood draw.
7. Discard obtained sample. ►*Rationale: This discard ensures a specimen that is free of heparin or flush solution. Note: For an ABG blood sample, discard volume should be twice the dead space volume of the catheter and tubing up to the sampling site. For coagulation studies, discard volume should be six times the dead space volume.*
8. Engage ABG specimen tube into Vacutainer.
9. Obtain arterial blood gas specimen.
10. Turn stopcock off to open port. ►*Rationale: This reestablishes flow between flush solution and client.*
11. Remove Vacutainers for Blood Conservatory Process.

### For Blood Conservatory Process

a. Don clean gloves.
b. Aspirate blood into reservoir tubing.
c. Close stopcock to reservoir tubing.
d. Access sampling port (closest to client) using blunt cannula with tube holder (Vacutainer).
e. Engage blood collection tubes into tube holder and allow to fill. ►*Rationale: Obtaining specimens using a blood conservatory system helps to prevent nosocomial anemia.*
f. When sampling is complete, remove blunt cannula and tube holder.
g. Open stopcock to reservoir tubing and return contents to client.

12. Place arterial blood gas specimen tubes in container filled with ice.
13. Fast flush remaining blood onto gauze pad.
14. Reattach protective cap on open port.
15. Validate good arterial waveform on monitor.
16. Reactivate monitor alarms.

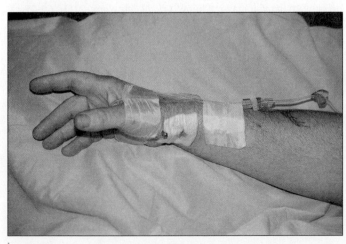

● Radial artery catheter provides continuous blood pressure monitoring and easy access for blood sampling.

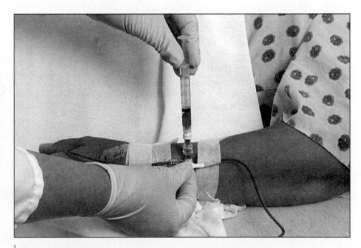

● Engage syringe or vacutainer to sample port to obtain arterial blood.

17. Wrap syringe/specimen in bubble packaging and place in biohazard bag with ice.
18. Remove gloves and perform hand hygiene.
19. Send specimens to laboratory immediately and notify lab that tubes are being sent.

## CLINICAL ALERT

"In-line" blood sampling systems eliminate the need for discarding blood, thus reducing blood loss and associated risks.

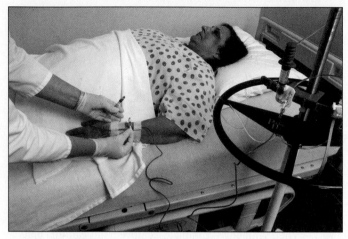

● When sampling is complete, open stopcock to reservoir tubing and return contents to client-blood conservatory system.

### TABLE 2-2 ARTERIAL BLOOD GAS VALUES IN ACID–BASE IMBALANCES

| Respiratory Acidosis | | Compensation |
|---|---|---|
| pH: decreased | <7.35 | 7.35 |
| $PCO_2$: increased | >45 mm Hg | |
| $HCO_3-$: normal | 24 | >26 mEq |
| **Respiratory Alkalosis** | | **Compensation** |
| pH: increased | >7.45 | 7.45 |
| $PCO_2$: decreased | <35 mm Hg | |
| $HCO_3-$: normal | 24 | <22 mEq |
| **Metabolic Acidosis** | | **Compensation** |
| pH: decreased | <7.35 | 7.35 |
| $HCO_3-$: decreased | <22 mEq | |
| $PCO_2$: normal | 40 | <35 mm Hg |
| **Metabolic Alkalosis** | | **Compensation** |
| pH: increased | >7.45 | 7.45 |
| $HCO_3-$: increased | ≥26 mEq | |
| $PCO_2$: normal | 40 | >45 mm Hg |
| **Normal ABG Values** | | |
| pH | 7.35–7.45 | |
| $PCO_2$ | 35–45 mm Hg | |
| $HCO_3$ | 22–26 mEq | |

## ▮ EVIDENCE-BASED NURSING PRACTICE

**Mean Arterial Blood Pressure**

In general, the MAP (mean arterial pressure) provides a more accurate interpretation of a patient's hemodynamic status. It provides the best estimate of central aortic pressure and is less sensitive to over-and under-damping distortions.

*Source:* McGhee, B., & Bridges, E. (2002). Monitoring arterial blood pressure: What you may not know. *Critical Care Nurse,* 22(2), 60–79.

## Skill 2.46   Removing Arterial Catheter

### Equipment

Gloves
Personal protective equipment
Two 4 × 4 gauze pads
Suture removal set
Tape

### Preparation

1. Check physician's orders.
2. Check client's coagulation lab results (values).
3. Gather equipment.
4. Perform hand hygiene.

5. Identify client; check identaband, have client state name and birthdate, and explain procedure to client.
6. Disarm monitor alarms.

**Procedure**

1. Don gloves and PPE.
2. Remove tape from site.
3. Remove dressing, and discard in appropriate container.
4. Clip retaining sutures if present.
5. Apply finger pressure approximately 2 cm above skin puncture site. ➤*Rationale: The artery puncture site is proximal to the skin puncture site.*
6. Place folded 4 × 4 gauze pad over cannula site with nondominant hand, and apply gentle pressure.
7. Pull arterial cannula straight out of artery with quick, even pressure.
8. Apply firm pressure over and just above cannula site for at least 5–10 minutes. ➤*Rationale: This action*

> ### CLINICAL ALERT
> Apply pressure to puncture site for at least 10 minutes if client is on anticoagulation or antithrombotic therapy.

*achieves hemostasis and prevents formation of a hematoma.*
9. Place folded 4 × 4 gauze pad over puncture site, and tape tightly. ➤*Rationale: This provides additional pressure to site to prevent bleeding.*
10. Discard supplies, remove gloves, PPE, and perform hand hygiene.
11. Check cannulation site frequently. ➤*Rationale: To observe for bleeding or thrombosis.*
12. Check distal extremity for temperature, circulation, motion, and sensation intermittently for several hours, then routinely after catheter removal. ➤*Rationale: Delayed complications (thrombosis) may occur.*

| UNEXPECTED OUTCOMES | CRITICAL THINKING OPTIONS |
|---|---|
| Absence of collateral circulation noted when performing the Allen test (negative Allen test). | • Assess contralateral extremity.<br>• Avoid radial artery.<br>• Notify physician. (An alternate artery may be selected—femoral.) |
| Cannulated extremity develops diminished distal perfusion. | • Check periphery for changes in color, temperature, motion and sensation resulting from possible thrombus occlusion or circulatory "steal."<br>• Notify physician immediately.<br>• Prepare for catheter removal. |
| Hypotension and bradycardia occur during arterial puncture or catheter removal. | • Reverse response with atropine administration. |
| Hematoma or bleeding occurs at arterial insertion site. | • Apply direct pressure over artery while you check for leaks in the system. Check all stopcocks: check if catheter is inserted in artery as it should be.<br>• Keep cannulated extremity exposed for observation.<br>• Remove catheter if oozing continues. |
| Signs of infection or inflammation appear at insertion site. | • Always use aseptic technique with dressing changes; change dressing weekly.<br>• Cap open port on stopcock to maintain asepsis.<br>• Do not apply ointment to insertion site.<br>• Change tubing every 24–48 hours using sterile technique.<br>• Flush open port after obtaining blood specimens.<br>• Prepare for catheter removal if infection suspected. |
| Arterial waveform loses definition and digital pressures drop. | • Reverse response with atropine administration.<br>• Use low compliance (rigid) short (3–4 ft) monitor tubing.<br>• Check for thrombus formation by aspirating blood through stopcock and then flushing system.<br>• Be sure to fast-flush arterial line thoroughly after arterial blood samples are obtained or system is zeroed. |

*(continued)*

## UNEXPECTED OUTCOMES *(cont.)*

## CRITICAL THINKING OPTIONS *(cont.)*

- Make sure all stopcocks are closed to air.
- Keep 300 mm Hg pressure in pressure bag.
- Ensure secure fit of all stopcocks and connections. Avoid adding stopcocks and line extensions.
- Change position of extremity in which catheter is placed.

Direct blood pressure readings vary significantly.

- Flick tubing system to remove tiny air bubbles escaping the flush solution.
- Recheck transducer and client position to ensure accurate data.
- Recalibrate transducer.
- Flush system after sampling and zeroing.
- Keep flush bag adequately filled and cleared of air.
- Maintain bag external pressure at 300 mm Hg.
- Check that connections are tightly secured.

Arterial blood sample is unobtainable.

- Suspect arterial spasm; allow spasm of artery to stop, then attempt to aspirate blood with gentle pressure using a 6-mL syringe rather than Vacutainer.
- Reposition client's arm, making sure there is no pressure at catheter insertion site.
- Check that catheter is in artery (note waveform on oscilloscope), flush catheter, then attempt to obtain sample.

# Fluids and Electrolytes

**Skill 3.1**  Monitoring Intake and Output  116

**Skill 3.2**  Establishing Intravenous Infusions  122

**Skill 3.3**  Performing Venipuncture
with All Variations  126

VARIATION: Inserting a Butterfly
(Winged-Tip) Needle  132

**Skill 3.4**  Regulating Infusion Flow Rate  134

**Skill 3.5**  Using an Infusion Pump or Controller  138

**Skill 3.6**  Using a "Smart" Pump  140

**Skill 3.7**  Using a Syringe Pump  142

**Skill 3.8**  Maintaining Infusions  144

**Skill 3.9**  Maintaining Intermittent Infusion
Devices  147

**Skill 3.10**  Changing Gown for Client with IV  150

**Skill 3.11**  Discontinuing Infusion Devices  150

**Skill 3.12**  Infusing IV Fluids through
a Central Line  153

In good health, a delicate balance of fluids, electrolytes, and acids and bases is maintained in the body, This balance, or physiologic **homeostasis,** depends on multiple physiologic processes that regulate fluid intake and outcome the movement of water and the substances dissolved in it between body compartments.

The measurement and recording of all fluid intake and output (I&O) during a 24-hour period provides important data about the client's fluid and electrolyte balance.

Input in children is measured as for adults, recording the fluids delivered to the child through parenteral or oral routes in milliliters (mL).

Output is a measurement of what is expelled, drained, secreted, or suctioned from the body. Output sources include urine, stool, vomitus, sweat, drainage from wounds, and nasogastric suction. Output for older children can be measured as for adults with a graduated cylinder, and is recorded in milliliters (mL).

Accurate measurement of I and O is documented for adults and children, such as those receiving IV fluids or certain medications, after major surgery, and those with serious infections, renal disease or kidney damage, congestive heart failure, diabetes mellitus, dehydration or hypovolemia, or severe thermal burns.

### TABLE 3–1   AVERAGE DAILY FLUID INTAKE FOR AN ADULT

| Source | Amount (mL) |
| --- | --- |
| Oral fluids | 1,200 to 1,500 |
| Water in foods | 1,000 |
| Water as by-product of food metabolism | 200 |
| Total | 2,400 to 2,700 |

### TABLE 3–2   AVERAGE DAILY FLUID OUTPUT FOR AN ADULT

| Source | Amount (mL) |
| --- | --- |
| Urine | 1,400 to 1,500 |
| Insensible losses | |
| Lungs | 350 to 400 |
| Skin | 350 to 400 |
| Sweat | 100 |
| Feces | 100 to 200 |
| Total | 2,300 to 2,600 |

# Skill 3.1   Monitoring Intake and Output

## EXPECTED OUTCOMES

- Client's intake and output are maintained within expected parameters of 200–300 mL of each other.
- Fluid intake is at least 2500 mL unless contraindicated by diagnosis.
- Client's fluid status, vital signs, and mental status are within normal range.
- Output is maintained at more than 30 mL/hour.
- IV flow rate is maintained at prescribed rate.
- All sources of fluid intake and output are recorded.
- Client's intake and output balance.

## Delegation

Measurement and recording of normal oral fluid intake or urinary and gastrointestinal output may be delegated to UAP. Measurement of parenteral fluid intake and output from wounds and tubes is generally not delegated to UAP.

## Equipment

- Graduated measuring containers
- I & O records
- Signs to post in room if client is on I & O recording
- A sample 24-hour fluid intake and output record.

## Preparation

Three clinical measurements of fluid balance that the nurse can initiate independently are daily weights, vital signs, and fluid intake and output.

Assessing fluid intake and output is an ongoing process that requires the nurse to have measuring devices and methods of recording easily accessible. Most agencies have a form for recording incremental I & O, usually a bedside record on which the nurse lists all items measured and the quantities per shift. These values will then be transferred onto the permanent chart record in the appropriate place (often on the vital signs record).

## CLINICAL ALERT

Hourly urine output less than 30mL/hr for two consecutive hours or 24-hour urine output less than 500 mL can indicate dehydration or internal bleeding and can result in acute renal failure.

### Procedure

1. Prior to performing the procedure, introduce self and verify the client's identity using agency protocol. Explain to the client what you are going to do, why it is necessary, and how he or she can participate. Discuss how the results will be used in planning further care or treatments.
2. Perform hand hygiene and observe appropriate infection control procedures.
3. If necessary, record on the Kardex or nursing care plan that the client's I & O are to be measured, including when if more often than every shift.
4. *Recording intake:* Clients who wish to be involved in recording fluid intake measurements need to be taught how to compute the values and what to measure.
   - Record each fluid item taken, specifying the time and type of fluid. All of the following fluids need to be recorded:
   - *Oral fluids.* Water, milk, juice, soft drinks, coffee, tea, cream, soup, and any other beverages. Include water taken with medications. To assess the amount of water taken from a water pitcher, measure what remains and subtract this amount from the volume of the full pitcher. Then refill the pitcher.
   - *Ice chips.* Record the fluid as approximately one-half the volume of the ice chips. For example, if the ice chips fill a cup holding 200 mL and the client consumed all of the ice chips, the volume consumed would be recorded as 100 mL.
   - *Foods that are or tend to become liquid at room temperature.* These include ice cream, sherbet, custard, and gelatin. Do not measure foods that are pureed, because purees are simply solid foods prepared in a different form.
   - *Tube feedings.* Remember to include the 30- to 60-mL water flush at the end of intermittent feedings or during continuous feedings.

## CLINICAL ALERT

Use client's own graduated receptacle when measuring output. Change gloves and perform hand hygiene between each client. The CDC calls for decontamination of hands after removing gloves. Gloves should also be changed and hands decontaminated when moving from a contaminated body site to a clean one on the same client.

- *Parenteral fluids.* The exact amount of intravenous fluid administered is to be recorded, since some fluid containers may be overfilled. Blood transfusions are included.
- *Intravenous medications.* Intravenous medications that are prepared with solutions such as normal saline (NS) and are administered as an intermittent or continuous infusion must also be included (e.g., ceftazidime 1 g in 50 mL of sterile water). Most intravenous medications are mixed in 50 to 100 mL of solution.
- *Catheter or tube irrigants.* Fluid used to irrigate urinary catheters, nasogastric tubes, and intestinal tubes or remaining after peritoneal dialysis must be measured and recorded if not immediately withdrawn.

5. *Recording output:* Inform clients, family members, and all caregivers that accurate measurements of the client's fluid intake and output are required, explaining why and emphasizing the need to use a bedpan, urinal, commode, or in-toilet collection device (unless a urinary drainage system is in place). Instruct the client not to put toilet tissue into the container with urine. Clients who wish to be involved in recording fluid output measurements need to be taught how to handle the fluids and to compute the values.
   - To measure fluid output, measure the following fluids (remember to observe appropriate infection control precautions):
     - *Urinary output.* Following each voiding, pour the urine into a measuring container, observe the amount, and record it and the time of voiding on the I & O form. For clients with retention catheters, empty the drainage bag into a measuring container at the end of the shift (or at prescribed times if output is to be measured more often). Sometimes, urine output is measured hourly. If the client is incontinent of urine, estimate and record these outputs. For example, for an incontinent client the nurse might record "Incontinent × 3" or "Drawsheet soaked in 12-in. diameter." A more accurate estimate of the urine output of infants and incontinent clients may be obtained by first weighing diapers or incontinent pads that are dry, and then subtracting this weight from the weight of the soiled items. Each gram of weight left after subtracting is equal to 1 mL of urine. If urine is frequently soiled with feces, the number of voidings may be recorded rather than the volume of urine.
     - *Vomitus and liquid feces.* The amount, appearance, and type of fluid and the time need to be specified.
     - *Tube drainage, such as gastric or intestinal drainage.* The amount, appearance, and type of fluid and the time need to be specified.
     - *Wound drainage and draining fistulas.* Wound drainage may be recorded by documenting the type and number of dressings or linen saturated with drainage or by measuring the exact amount of drainage collected in a vacuum drainage (e.g., Hemovac) or gravity drainage system.

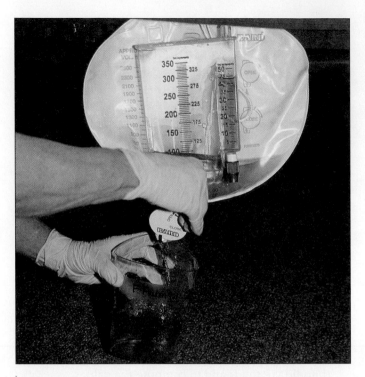

● Empty urinal, bedpan, or Foley drainage bag into client's individual (labeled) graduate and note amount of urine.

6. Document in the client record using forms or checklists supplemented by narrative notes when appropriate. Fluid intake and output measurements are totaled at the end of the shift (every 8 to 12 hours), and the totals are recorded in the client's permanent record. Usually the staff on night shift totals the amounts of I & O recorded for each shift and records the 24-hour total.
   - Consume six to eight glasses of water daily.
   - Avoid excess amount of fluids high in salt, sugar, and caffeine.
   - Limit alcohol intake because it has a diuretic effect.
   - Increase fluid intake before, during, and after strenuous exercise, particularly when the environmental temperature is high, and replace lost electrolytes from excessive perspiration as needed with commercial electrolyte solutions.
   - Learn about and monitor side effects of medications that affect fluid balance (e.g., diuretics) and ways to handle side effects.
   - Recognize possible risk factors for fluid imbalance such as prolonged or repeated vomiting, frequent watery stools, or inability to consume fluids because of illness.
   - Seek prompt professional health care for notable signs of fluid imbalance such as sudden weight gain or loss, decreased urine volume, swollen ankles, shortness of breath, dizziness, or confusion.

## Monitoring Fluid Intake and Output

- Teach and provide the rationale for monitoring fluid intake and output to the client and family as appropriate. Include how to use a commode or collection device ("hat") in the toilet, how to empty and measure urinary catheter drainage, and how to count or weigh diapers.
- Instruct and provide the rationale for regular weight monitoring to the client and family. Weigh at the same time of day, using the same scale and with the client wearing the same amount of clothing.
- Educate and provide the rationale to the client and family on when to contact a health care professional, such as in the cases of a significant change in urine output; any change of 5 pounds or more in a 1- to 2-week period; prolonged episodes of vomiting, diarrhea, or inability to eat or drink; dry, sticky mucous membranes; extreme thirst; swollen fingers, feet, ankles, or legs; difficulty breathing, shortness of breath, or rapid heartbeat; and changes in behavior or mental status.

## Maintaining Fluid Intake

- Establish a 24-hour plan for ingesting the fluids. Generally, half of the desired total volume is given during the day, and the other half is divided between the evening and night, with most of that ingested during the evening. For example, if 2,500 mL is to be ingested in 24 hours, the plan may specify 7–3 (1,500 mL); 3–11 (700 mL); and 11–7 (300 mL). Try to avoid the ingestion of large amounts of fluid immediately before bedtime to prevent the need to urinate during sleeping hours.
- Set short-term outcomes that the client can realistically meet. Examples include ingesting a glass of fluid every hour while awake or a pitcher of water by 12 noon.
- If the client is on enteral or intravenous fluids and feeding at home, teach and provide the underlying rationale to caregivers about proper administration and care. Contact a home health or home intravenous service to provide services and teaching.
- Explain to the client the reason for the required intake and the specific amount needed.
- Identify fluids the client likes and make available a variety of those items, including fruit juices, soft drinks, and milk (if allowed). Remember that beverages such as coffee and tea have a diuretic effect, so their consumption should be limited.
- Help clients to select foods that tend to become liquid at room temperature (e.g., gelatin, ice cream, sherbet, custard), if these are allowed.

- Encourage clients when possible to participate in maintaining the fluid intake record. This assists them to evaluate the achievement of desired outcomes.
- Be alert to any cultural implications of food and fluids. Some cultures may restrict certain foods and fluids and view others as having healing properties.

### Helping Clients Increase Fluid Intake

- Teach family members the rationale for the importance of offering fluids regularly to clients who are unable to meet their own needs because of age, impaired mobility or cognition, or other conditions such as impaired swallowing due to a stroke.
- For clients who are confined to bed, supply appropriate cups, glasses, and straws to facilitate appropriate fluid intake and keep the fluids within easy reach.
- Make sure fluids are served at the appropriate temperature: hot fluids hot and cold fluids very cold.

### Helping Clients Restrict Fluid Intake

- Explain the reason for the restricted intake and how much and what types of fluids are permitted orally. Many clients need to be informed that ice chips, gelatin, and ice cream, for example, are considered fluid.
- Help the client decide the amount of fluid to be taken with each meal, between meals, before bedtime, and with medications.
- Identify fluids or fluid-like substances the client likes and make sure that these are provided, unless contraindicated. A client who is allowed only 200 mL of fluid for breakfast, for example, should receive the type of fluid the client favors.
- Set short-term goals that make the fluid restriction more tolerable. For example, schedule a specified amount of fluid at one or two hourly intervals between meals. Some clients may prefer fluids only

## DEVELOPMENTAL CONSIDERATIONS

### Infants and Children

Infants are at high risk for fluid and electrolyte imbalance because

- Their immature kidneys cannot concentrate urine.
- They have a rapid respiratory rate and proportionately larger body surface area than adults, leading to greater insensate loss through the skin and respirations.
- They cannot express thirst, nor actively seek fluids.

Vomiting and/or diarrhea in infants and young children can lead quickly to electrolyte imbalance. Oral rehydration therapy (ORT) (e.g., electrolyte solutions such as Pedialyte) should be used to retore fluid and electrolyte balance in mild to moderate dehydration (American Medical Association et al., 2004). Prompt treatment with ORT can prevent the need for intravenous therapy and hospitalization (Spandorfer, Alessandrine, Joffe, Localio & Shaw, 2005). Even if the child is nauseated and vomiting small sips of ORT can be helpful.

### Elders

Certain changes related to aging place the elder at risk for serious problems with fluid and electrolyte imbalance, if homeostatic mechanisms are compromised. Some of the changes are

- Decrease in thirst sensation.
- A decrease in ability of the kidneys to concentrate urine.
- A decrease in intracellular fluid and in total body water.
- A decrease in response to body hormones that help regulate fluid and electrolytes.

Other factors that may influence fluid and electrolyte balance in elders are

- Increased use of diuretics for hypertension and heart disease.
- Decreased intake of food and water, especially in elders with dementia or who are dependent on others to feed them and offer them fluids.
- Preparations for certain diagnostic tests that have the client NPO for a long period of time or cause diarrhea from laxative preps.
- Clients with impaired renal function, such as elders with diabetes.
- Those having certain diagnostic procedures. (Dyes used for some procedures, such as arteriograms and cardiac catheterizations, may cause further renal problems. Always see that the client is well hydrated before, during, and after the procedure to help in diluting and excreting the dye. If the client is NPO for the procedure, the nurse should check with the primary care provider to see if IV fluids are needed.)
- Any condition that may tax the normal compensatory mechanism, such as a fever, influenza, surgery, or heat exposure.

All of these conditions increase elders' risk for fluid and electrolyte imbalance. The change can happen quickly and become serious in a short time. Astute observations and quick actions by the nurse can help prevent serious consequences. A change in mental status may be the first symptom of impairment and must be further evaluated to determine the cause.

between meals if the food provided at mealtime helps relieve thirst.

- Place allowed fluids in small containers such as a 4-ounce juice glass to allow the perception of a full container.

- Periodically offer the client ice chips as an alternative to water, because ice chips when melted are approximately half of the frozen volume.

- Provide frequent mouth care and rinses to reduce the thirst sensation.

- Instruct the client to avoid ingesting or chewing salty or sweet foods (hard candy or gum), because these foods tend to produce thirst. Sugarless gum may be an alternative for some clients.

### Referrals

- Make appropriate referrals to home health or community social services for assistance with resources such as intravenous infusions and access, enteral feedings, and homemaker or home health aide services to help with ADLs.

- Provide a list of sources for supplies such as commodes, catheters and drainage bags, measuring devices, tube feeding formulas, and electrolyte replacement drinks.

## CLINICAL ALERT

Check all drainage receptacles such as Foley bag and NG canister at the beginning of each shift to ensure they were emptied from the previous shift and that there has not been excessive drainage.

## CARE SETTING

Assess for the following:

### Client

- Risk factors for imbalance: the client's age, medications required such as diuretic therapy or corticosteroids, and presence of chronic diseases such as diabetes mellitus, heart disease, lung disease, or dementia

- Self-care abilities for maintaining fluid intake: mobility; ability to swallow, to access fluids and respond to thirst

- Current level of knowledge (as appropriate) about any fluid restrictions, actions and side effects of prescribed medications, regular weight monitoring, gastric tube care and enteral feedings, central line or PICC catheter care, and parenteral fluids and nutrition

### Family

- Caregiver availability, skills, and responses: availability and willingness to assume responsibility for care, knowledge and ability to provide assistance with maintaining adequate intake of fluids, knowledge of risk factors and early warning signs of problems

- Family role changes and coping: effect on financial status, parenting and spousal roles, social roles

## EVIDENCE-BASED NURSING PRACTICE

**How Prevalent Is Chronic Dehydration in Elders?**

Previous research has documented that dehydration is a problem in hospitalized elders, and low fluid intake has been documented to be a problem in nursing home residents. The authors questioned whether chronic dehydration is also a problem in elders living in the community. The researchers conducted a descriptive, retrospective study of 185 elders ranging from 75 to 100 years old. This group of elders visited a hospital emergency department during a 1-month period of time. Dehydration was defined as a ratio of blood urea nitrogen to creatine (BUN:Cr) greater than 20:1. Forty-eight percent of the group were dehydrated on admission to the emergency department. The elders from a residential facility were most likely to be dehydrated (65%); however, 44% of the elders living in the community were dehydrated.

### Implications

The results demonstrated that dehydration is a problem with both elders living in the community as well as elders living in residential facilities. Prevention of dehydration is an important intervention for nurses working with elders. Nursing interventions need to include talking with elders and their families about the dangers of dehydration and suggesting strategies to prevent dehydration.

*Note:* From "Unrecognized Chronic Dehydration in Older Adults, Examining Prevalence Rate and Risk Factors," by J.A. Bennett, V. Thomas, and B. Riegel, 2004, *Journal of Gerontological Nursing*, 30(1), pp. 22–28. Copyright © 2004 SLACK, Inc. Reprinted with permission.

| UNEXPECTED OUTCOMES | CRITICAL THINKING OPTIONS |
|---|---|
| Recorded I&O do not balance. | • Correlate I&O imbalance with weight changes.<br>• Emphasize importance of accurate measures to client and family.<br>• Check that entries into computer are accurate (i.e., entering 100 mL instead of 1,000 mL).<br>• Identify possible nonmeasurable sources of I or O.<br>• Report to charge nurse so she can assure that all nurses are keeping accurate records.<br>• Check if client or family can help with keeping the I&O record.<br>• Check the addition on the I&O record to see if an error was made. |
| Client unable to maintain an intake of at least 1500 mL/day. | • Ensure that fluid restriction is not ordered.<br>• Offer fluids in small amounts more frequently.<br>• Determine client's fluid preferences.<br>• Determine client preference for fluid to be hot, cold, or room temperature.<br>• Consider "other" fluids such as Jell-O, Popsicles.<br>• Assess client's ability to use a straw (hemiplegic client is often unable to suck through a straw).<br>• Check if client is able to drink fluids independently or if assistance is needed.<br>• Ensure that adequate fluids are accessible at the bedside for the client.<br>• Do not administer fluids with a bulb syringe.<br>• Address client's toileting needs q 2 hours—some clients restrict their fluid intake for fear of incontinence.<br>• Use a thickening additive to liquids to facilitate swallowing for the client with aspiration precautions. |
| IV flow not maintained at appropriate rate. | • Monitor IV fluid intake hourly.<br>• Observe IV site for complications.<br>• Restart IV immediately when infiltrated to ensure continuous IV fluid intake.<br>• Document IV fluid intake every shift.<br>• Account for interruption of primary infusion and the delivery of intermittent infusions of medications.<br>• Check accuracy of IV administration equipment: electronic device, dial-a-flow, etc.<br>• Inform physician of alterations in fluid received from what was ordered. |
| Client voids in toilet. | • Document "voided in toilet" on I&O record.<br>• Review instructions for accurate I&O monitoring with client.<br>• Post sign above toilet: "All urine must be measured and recorded."<br>• Place "hat" receptacle in toilet. |
| Family members obtain fluids for client without notifying staff. | • Post sign indicating need to record all fluid intake.<br>• Remind family of importance of I&O monitoring; provide cups with measured increments and paper for them to record fluids given (unless fluids are restricted). |
| Fluid intake and output do not balance (intake greater than output). | • Initiate daily weight measurement (weigh before breakfast, after voiding, same scale, same clothing).<br>• Compare losses or gains with client's daily weight measurement.<br>• Determine whether treatment goal is to rehydrate or diurese the client.<br>• Use graduated container to accurately measure output in "hat."<br>• Search for sources of unmeasured output (fever, wound drainage, diarrhea). |
| Fluid output is greater than intake. | • Analyze whether treatment goal (rehydration, diuresis) has been achieved.<br>• Reposition client cautiously, monitoring for possible orthostatic hypotension.<br>• Identify when "dry weight" has been achieved (intake balances output following therapy received).<br>• Search for sources of unrecorded intake (family offerings, flush solutions, ice chips, full-liquid foods). |

# Skill 3.2   Establishing Intravenous Infusions

Many clients require administration of fluids or medications directly into the vascular system through **intravenous** (within or into the vein) devices. Nurses provide a significant amount of this type of therapy both in the hospital and in ambulatory settings and must have substantial knowledge and skill to do so with safety. New intravenous (IV) devices and strategies are always in development such that continuing education regarding IV therapy is an ongoing nursing responsibility.

## EXPECTED OUTCOMES

- Fluid and electrolyte needs are met.
- Appropriate IV site is selected and IV inserted without difficulty.
- IV fluids infuse at prescribed rate without complications.
- Appropriate IV equipment for client.
- IV site is maintained using sterile technique.
- Fluids are administered without adverse effects.
- IV site remains clean, without signs of infection or infiltration.
- IV is converted to a saline lock and is functioning properly.
- Client's gown is changed while maintaining IV placement.
- IV is discontinued intact and site remains free of infection or bleeding.
- Central vascular line is properly placed without complication.
- Central vascular line remains patent and free of infection.
- CVP monitoring guides fluid management.
- Central vascular catheter dressing is changed without complications.
- BIOPATCH is applied and potential infection prevented.
- Access cap replaced maintaining sterile technique.
- StatLock prevents catheter displacement.
- IV catheter maintains patency with use of CLC2000 device.
- Catheter site remains free of infection.
- Blood samples are obtained without difficulty.
- Infusions of medications or fluids are accomplished without difficulty.

## Delegation

Due to the use of sterile technique, intravenous infusion therapy is not delegated to UAP. UAP may care for clients receiving IV therapy, and the nurse must ensure that the UAP knows how to perform routine tasks such as bathing and positioning without disturbing the IV. The UAP should also know what complications or adverse signs, such as leakage, should be reported to the nurse.

In many states, a licensed practical nurse or licensed vocational nurse with special IV therapy training may start intravenous infusions. Check the state's nurse practice act.

## Equipment

- Clean gloves
- Infusion set and adapters if needed
- Container of sterile parenteral solution
- Labels for IV tubing and container
- IV pole
- Nonallergenic tape
- Electronic infusion device or pump, as determined by the nurse

## Preparation

- If possible, select a time to establish the infusion that is convenient for the client. Unless initiating IV therapy is urgent, provide any scheduled care before initiation to minimize excessive movement of the affected limb.
- Make sure that the client's clothing or gown can be removed over the IV apparatus if necessary. Some agencies provide special gowns that open over the shoulder and down the sleeve for easy removal.

## Procedure

1. Prior to performing the procedure, introduce self and verify the client's identity using agency protocol. Explain to the client what you are going to do, why it is necessary, and how he or she can participate. If possible, explain how long the infusion will need to remain in place.
2. Perform hand hygiene and observe other appropriate infection control procedures.
3. Position the client appropriately.
   - Assist the client to a comfortable position, either sitting or lying. Expose the limb to be used but provide for client privacy.
4. Apply a medication label to the solution container if a medication was added.
   - In many agencies, medications and labels are applied to IV bags in the pharmacy; if they are not, apply the label upside down on the container. ➤*Rationale: The label is applied upside down so it can be read easily when the container is hanging up.*
5. Apply a timing strip to the solution container.
   - Mark the strip to indicate the anticipated fluid level at hourly intervals.
   - The timing strip may be applied at the time the infusion is started. Follow agency practice. See discussion of regulating infusion flow rates.

6. Open and prepare the infusion set.
   - Remove tubing from the container, and straighten it out.
   - Slide the tubing clamp along the tubing until it is just below the drip chamber to facilitate its access.
   - Close the clamp.
   - Leave the ends of the tubing covered with the plastic caps until the infusion is started. ➤*Rationale: This will maintain the sterility of the ends of the tubing.*

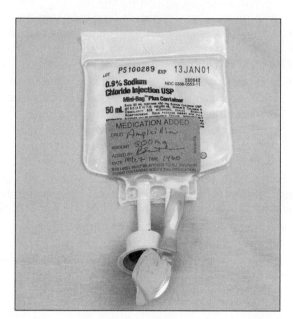

● Medication in a labeled infusion bag.

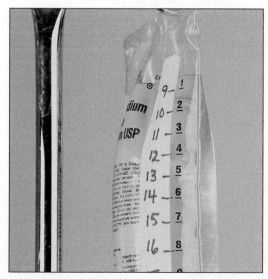

● Timing label on an IV container. The first time marked (0900 hours) would be correct for a bag hung at 0800 hours with a rate of 100 mL per hour.
Photographer: Elena Dorfman

7. Spike the solution container.
   - Expose the insertion site of the bag or bottle.
   - Remove the cap from the spike, and insert the spike into the insertion site.
8. Hang the solution container on the pole.
   - Adjust the pole so that the container is suspended about 1 m (3 ft) above the client's head. ➤*Rationale: This height is needed to enable gravity to overcome venous pressure and facilitate flow of the solution into the vein.*
9. Partially fill the drip chamber with solution. (*Note:* Steps 4 through 10 may be performed outside of the client's room and then the system transported to the client's bedside.)
   - Squeeze the chamber gently until it is half full of solution. ➤*Rationale: The drip chamber is partly filled with solution to prevent air from moving down the tubing.*

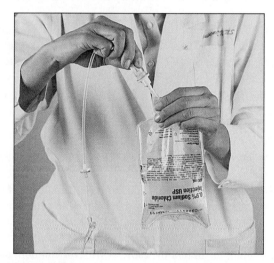

● Inserting the spike.
Photographer: Elena Dorfman

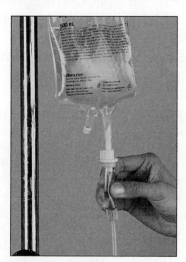

● Squeezing the drip chamber.
Photographer: Elena Dorfman

10. Prime the tubing as described below. The term "prime" means "to make ready" but in common use refers to flushing the tubing to remove air.
    - Remove the protective cap, and hold the tubing over a container. Maintain the sterility of the end of the tubing and the cap.
    - Release the clamp, and let the fluid run through the tubing until all bubbles are removed. Tap the tubing if necessary with your fingers to help the bubbles move. *➤Rationale: The tubing is primed to prevent the introduction of air into the client. Air bubbles smaller than 0.5 mL usually do not cause problems in peripheral lines.*
    - Reclamp the tubing, and replace the tubing cap, maintaining sterile technique.
    - For caps with air vents, do not remove the cap when priming this tubing. *➤Rationale: The flow of solution through the tubing will cease when the cap is moist with one drop of solution.*
    - If an infusion control pump, electronic device, or controller is being used, follow the manufacturer's directions for inserting the tubing and setting the infusion rate (see Skill 3.3).
11. Disconnect the used tubing or remove the cap on an intermittent device.
    - Apply clean gloves.
    - Place a sterile swab under the hub of the catheter. *➤Rationale: This absorbs any leakage that might occur when the tubing is disconnected.*
    - Clamp the tubing. With the fourth or fifth finger of the nondominant hand, apply pressure to the vein above the end of the catheter. *➤Rationale: This helps prevent blood from coming out of the needle during the change of tubing.*
    - Holding the hub of the catheter with the nondominant hand, remove the tubing or cap with the dominant hand, using a twisting and pulling motion. *➤Rationale: Holding the catheter firmly but gently maintains its position in the vein.*
    - Place the end of the used tubing or cap in a basin or other receptacle.

**VARIATION: Starting an Infusion on a Central Line**

**(See also Skills 3.8 and 3.9)**

- Apply clean gloves and mask.
- Clean the junction of the catheter and tubing or cap with antiseptic, as required by agency protocol. *➤Rationale: This prevents the transfer of microorganisms from the client's skin to the open catheter hub when it is detached; it also decreases the number of microorganisms at the catheter-tubing junction.*
- Clamp the catheter, disconnect the tubing or cap, using a twisting, pulling motion. If the catheter does not have a clamp, ask the client to perform Valsalva's maneuver (that is, to take a deep breath and bear down) and to turn the head away while you detach the tubing or cap. *➤Rationale: Performance of Valsalva's maneuver increases intrathoracic pressure, which reduces*

*the risk of air entering the catheter. Turning the head to the side reduces the chances of contaminating the equipment.*

12. Connect the new tubing, and establish the infusion.
    - Continue to hold the catheter and grasp the new tubing with the dominant hand.
    - Remove the protective tubing cap and, maintaining sterility, insert the tubing end securely into the needle hub.
    - Open the clamp to start the solution flowing.
13. Ensure appropriate infusion flow.
    - Remove and discard gloves. Perform hand hygiene.
    - Apply a padded arm board to splint the joint, as needed.
    - Adjust the infusion rate of flow according to the order.
14. Label the IV tubing.
    - Label the tubing with the date and time of attachment and your initials. This labeling may also be done when the container is set up. *➤Rationale: The tubing is labeled to ensure that it is changed at regular intervals (i.e., every 24 to 96 hours according to agency policy).*
15. Loop the tubing and secure it with tape to the client's skin. *➤Rationale: Looping and securing the tubing prevent the weight of the tubing or any movement from pulling on the needle or catheter.*
16. Document all assessments and interventions.
    - Record the infusion in the client's chart. Some agencies provide a special form for this purpose. Include the date and time of beginning the infusion; amount and type of solution used, including any additives (e.g., kind and amount of medications); container number; flow rate; and the client's general response.

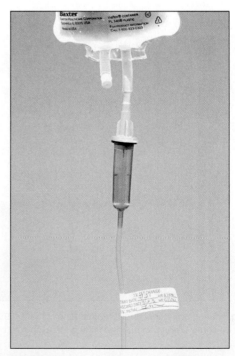

● Tubing labeled with date, time, and nurse's initials.

Division of Nursing
Oakland, California 94609

## VENIPUNCTURE

| DATE | TIME | SITE CODE | TYPE / GAUGE NEEDLE | INIT. | DC DATE | INIT. |
|------|------|-----------|---------------------|-------|---------|-------|
|      |      |           |                     |       |         |       |
|      |      |           |                     |       |         |       |
|      |      |           |                     |       |         |       |
|      |      |           |                     |       |         |       |
|      |      |           |                     |       |         |       |
|      |      |           |                     |       |         |       |

## CODES

**SITE LOCATION:**

| | | | |
|---|---|---|---|
| RH | HAND | LH | HAND |
| RF | FOREARM | LF | FOREARM |
| RA | ANTECUBITAL | LA | ANTECUBITAL |
| RU | UPPER ARM | LU | UPPER ARM |
| RS | SUBCLAVIAN | LS | SUBCLAVIAN |
| RJ | JUGULAR | LJ | JUGULAR |
| RL | LEG | LL | LEG |
| VA | VASCULAR ACCESS | | |

**SITE CONDITION:**
A. PATENT WITHOUT REDNESS OR SWELLING
   OCCLUSIVE DRESSING INTACT
B. PATENT WITH MILD REDNESS AND/OR SWELLING
   OCCLUSIVE DRESSING INTACT
C. DRAINAGE (SEE NOTE)
D. DISLODGED / OCCLUDED
E. INFILTRATED
F. OCCLUSIVE DRESSING CHANGED

## I.V. ORDERS

| DATE ORDERED | INITIALS TRANS. | INITIALS CHECK | SOLUTION / ADDITIVE(S) | INFUSION RATE | DURATION |
|--------------|-------|-------|------------------------|---------------|----------|
|              |       |       |                        |               |          |
|              |       |       |                        |               |          |
|              |       |       |                        |               |          |
|              |       |       |                        |               |          |
|              |       |       |                        |               |          |
|              |       |       |                        |               |          |

## I.V.'s ADMINISTERED

| DATE | TIME | INIT. | SITE LOC. | BOTTLE NUMBER | SOLUTION / ADDITIVE(S) | SHIFT | AMOUNT ABSORBED | AMOUNT REMAINING | TIME TUBING CHANGE | SITE COND. | TOTAL INFUSED |
|------|------|-------|-----------|---------------|------------------------|-------|-----------------|------------------|--------------------|------------|---------------|
|      |      |       |           |               |                        | 0600  |                 |                  |                    |            |               |
|      |      |       |           |               |                        | 1400  |                 |                  |                    |            |               |
|      |      |       |           |               |                        | 2200  |                 |                  |                    |            |               |
|      |      |       |           |               |                        | 0600  |                 |                  |                    |            |               |
|      |      |       |           |               |                        | 1400  |                 |                  |                    |            |               |
|      |      |       |           |               |                        | 2200  |                 |                  |                    |            |               |
|      |      |       |           |               |                        | 0600  |                 |                  |                    |            |               |
|      |      |       |           |               |                        | 1400  |                 |                  |                    |            |               |
|      |      |       |           |               |                        | 2200  |                 |                  |                    |            |               |
|      |      |       |           |               |                        | 0600  |                 |                  |                    |            |               |
|      |      |       |           |               |                        | 1400  |                 |                  |                    |            |               |
|      |      |       |           |               |                        | 2200  |                 |                  |                    |            |               |
|      |      |       |           |               |                        | 0600  |                 |                  |                    |            |               |
|      |      |       |           |               |                        | 1400  |                 |                  |                    |            |               |
|      |      |       |           |               |                        | 2200  |                 |                  |                    |            |               |
|      |      |       |           |               |                        | 0600  |                 |                  |                    |            |               |
|      |      |       |           |               |                        | 1400  |                 |                  |                    |            |               |
|      |      |       |           |               |                        | 2200  |                 |                  |                    |            |               |

## SIGN.

| INIT. | SIGNATURE / TITLE | INIT. | SIGNATURE / TITLE | INIT. | SIGNATURE / TITLE |
|-------|-------------------|-------|-------------------|-------|-------------------|
|       |                   |       |                   |       |                   |
|       |                   |       |                   |       |                   |

SUMMIT
MEDICAL CENTER

# Intravenous Therapy Record

AFFIX PATIENT
I.D. LABEL HERE

MPN-105 86-6105-0

IV flow record.

# Skill 3.3 Performing Venipuncture with All Variations

Review the client record regarding previous venipuncture. Note any difficulties encountered and how they were resolved.

## Description

Kozier and Erb p. 1361 "Before preparing the infusion, the nurse first verifies the primary care provider's order including the type of solution, the amount to be administered, the rate of flow of the infusion, and client allergies (e.g., to tape or povidine-iodine)."

## Delegation

Due to the need for knowledge of anatomy and use of sterile technique, venipuncture is not delegated to unlicensed assistive personnel (UAP). UAP may care for clients with intravenous needles inserted, and the nurse must ensure that the UAP knows how to perform routine tasks such as bathing and positioning without disturbing the IV. The UAP should also know what complications or adverse signs, such as leakage, should be reported to the nurse. In many states, this procedure may be delegated to the Licensed Practical nurse.

## Equipment

Substitute appropriate supplies if the client has tape, antiseptic, or latex allergies.

- Clean gloves
- Tourniquet or blood pressure cuff
- Antiseptic swabs such as 10% povidone-iodine or 2% chlorhexidine gluconate. Chlorhexidine is the preferred agent (Hadaway, 2006).
- Antiseptic ointment, such as povidone-iodine (depending on dressing and agency policy)

---

### PRACTICE GUIDELINES

#### Vein Selection

- Use distal veins of the arm first. ▸*Rationale: If an IV site develops complications such as leakage, a site more proximal to that vein may still be used (depending on the specific complication).*
- Use the client's nondominant arm whenever possible. ▸*Rationale: This minimizes the client's restricted mobility and function.*
- Select a vein that is:
  a. Easily palpated and feels soft and full.
  b. Naturally splinted by bone.
  c. Large enough to allow adequate circulation around the catheter.
- Avoid using veins that are:
  a. In areas of flexion (e.g., the antecubital fossa).
  b. Highly raised/visible. ▸*Rationale: These veins tend to roll away from the needle.*
  c. Damaged by previous use, phlebitis, infiltration, or sclerosis.
  d. Continually distended with blood, knotted, or tortuous.
  e. In a surgically compromised or injured extremity (e.g., following a mastectomy). ▸*Rationale: These sites may have impaired circulation and cause discomfort for the client.*
  f. In the foot or legs unless arm veins are inaccessible, and with a primary care provider's order. ▸*Rationale: Lower extremity sites are more prone to thrombus formation and subsequent emboli.*

---

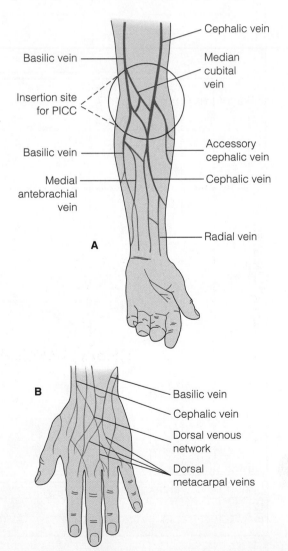

● Commonly used venipuncture sites of the **A,** arm; **B,** hand. **A** also shows the site used for a peripherally inserted central catheter (PICC).

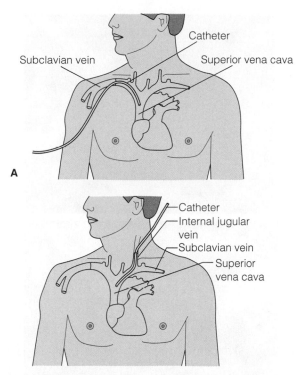

A

B

● Central venous lines with **A,** subclavian insertion; **B,** left jugular vein insertion.

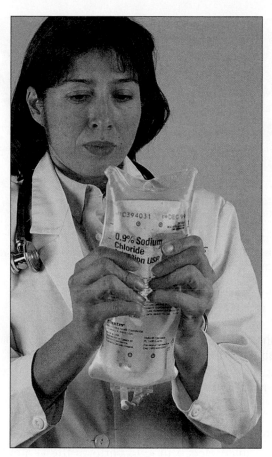

● A plastic intravenous fluid container.

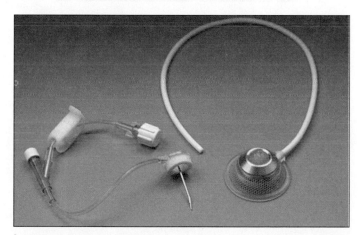

● An implantable venous access device (right) and a Huber needle with extension tubing.

- Intravenous catheter/needle (Choose an IV needle of the appropriate type and size based on the size of the vein and the purpose of the needle. A 20- to 22-gauge needle is indicated for most adults. Always have an extra needle and ones of different sizes available.)
- Sterile gauze dressing or transparent occlusive dressing
- Splint, if required
- Towel or bed protector
- Local anesthetic (optional and per agency policy)

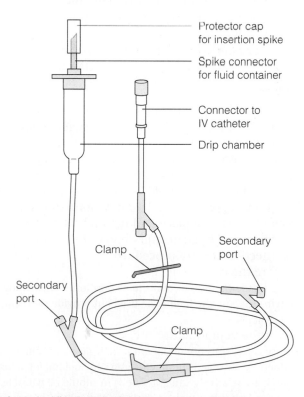

● A standard IV administration set.

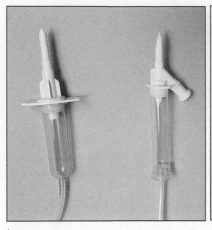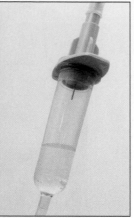

● Infusion set spikes and drip chambers: nonvented macrodrip, vented macrodrip, nonvented microdrip.

## CLINICAL ALERT

Peripheral IVs should be started using aseptic technique. IVs started without proper asepis, for example, in an emergency or outside the hospital, should be replaced at the earliest opportunity, and within 24 hours.

### Preparation

- If possible, select a time to perform the venipuncture that is convenient for the client. Unless initiating IV therapy is urgent, provide any scheduled care before insertion to minimize excessive movement of the affected limb.
- Visitors or family members may be asked to leave the room if desired by the nurse or the client.

### Procedure

1. Prior to performing the procedure, introduce self and verify the client's identity using agency protocol. Explain to the client what you are going to do, why it is necessary, and how he or she can participate. Venipuncture can cause discomfort for a few seconds, but there should be no ongoing pain after insertion. If possible, explain how long the IV will need to remain in place and how it will be used.
2. Perform hand hygiene and observe other appropriate infection control procedures.
3. Prepare the client.
   - Assist the client to a comfortable position, either sitting or lying. Expose the limb to be used but provide for client privacy.
4. Select the venipuncture site.
   - Use the client's nondominant arm, unless contraindicated. Identify possible venipuncture sites by looking for veins that are relatively straight. The vein should be palpable, but may not be visible, especially in clients with dark skin.

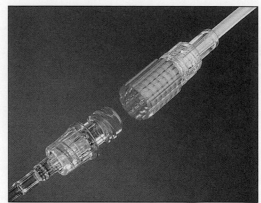

A

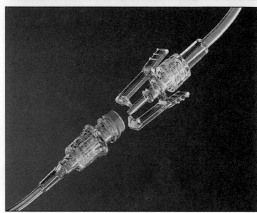

B

● Needleless cannulae used to connect the tubing of secondary sets to primary tubing: **A,** threaded cannula; **B,** lever-lock cannula.

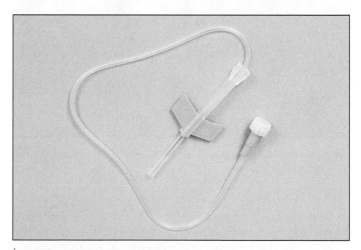

● A butterfly IV needle.

Consider the catheter length; look for a site sufficiently distal to the wrist or elbow where the tip of the catheter will not be at a point of flexion. ►*Rationale: Sclerotic veins may make initiating and maintaining the IV difficult. Joint flexion increases the risk of irritation of vein walls by the catheter.*

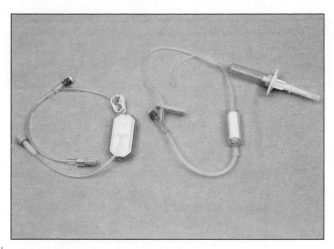

● Two types of IV filters.

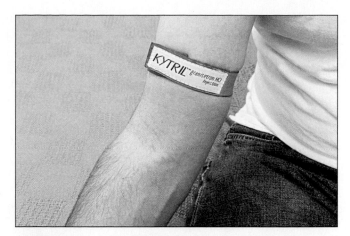

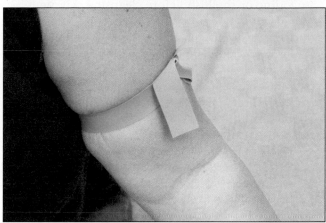

● Two types of tourniquets.

- Check agency protocol about shaving if the site is very hairy. ➤*Rationale: Shaving can cause microabrasions, which increase the risk of infection.*
- Place a towel or bed protector under the extremity to protect linens (or furniture if in the home).

5. Dilate the vein.
- Place the extremity in a dependent position (lower than the client's heart). ➤*Rationale: Gravity slows venous return and distends the veins. Distending the veins makes it easier to insert the needle properly.*
- Apply a tourniquet firmly 15 to 20 cm (6 to 8 in.) above the venipuncture site. Explain that the tourniquet will feel tight. ➤*Rationale: The tourniquet must be tight enough to obstruct venous flow but not so tight that it occludes arterial flow. Obstructing arterial flow inhibits venous filling. If a radial pulse can be palpated, the arterial flow is not obstructed. Use the tourniquet on only one client. This avoids cross-contamination to other clients.*
- For elders with fragile skin, instead of applying a tourniquet, place the arm in a dependent position to allow the veins to engorge. ➤*Rationale: The tourniquet can cause tissue damage and may not be needed to allow the vein to dilate.*
- If the vein is not sufficiently dilated:
  a. Massage or stroke the vein distal to the site and in the direction of venous flow toward the heart. ➤*Rationale: This action helps fill the vein.*
  b. Encourage the client to clench and unclench the fist. ➤*Rationale: Contracting the muscles compresses the distal veins, forcing blood along the veins and distending them.*

## CLINICAL ALERT

Do not shave the venipuncture site. Shaving can facilitate the development of infection through the multiplication of organisms in resulting microabrasions. Hairy sites can be clipped with scissors.

c. Lightly tap the vein with your fingertips. ➤*Rationale: Tapping may distend the vein.*
- If the preceding steps fail to distend the vein so that it is palpable, remove the tourniquet and wrap the extremity in a warm, moist towel for 10 to 15 minutes. ➤*Rationale: Heat dilates superficial blood vessels, causing them to fill.* Then repeat step 5.

6. Minimize insertion pain as much as possible.
- Although the pain of insertion should be brief, prevention can and should be offered. Simple refrigeration of the skin by placing ice topically for 3 minutes provides enough analgesia to carry out the insertion with minimal pain (Movahedi, Rostami, Salsali, Keikhaee, & Moradi, 2007). Transdermal analgesic creams (e.g., EMLA, Synera) may also be used, depending on policy. Allow 20 minutes for the topical analgesic to take effect (Pain patch, 2006).
- If desired and permitted by policy, inject 0.05 mL of 1% lidocaine or normal saline intradermally over the site where you plan to insert the IV needle (be sure to first apply gloves and clean the skin site as described in step 7 below). Allow 5 to 10 seconds for the anesthetic to take effect.

## CLINICAL ALERT

If using needleless angiocath system, once the "flash" is noted and the catheter is advanced, the retract button is pushed and the needle automatically shielded.

7. Apply clean gloves and clean the venipuncture site. ➤*Rationale: Gloves protect the nurse from contamination by the client's blood.* Clean the skin at the site of entry with a topical antiseptic swab (e.g., 2% chlorhexidine gluconate, or alcohol). Some institutions may use an anti-infective solution such as povidone-iodine (check agency protocol). Check for allergies to iodine or shellfish before cleansing skin with povidone-iodine or iodine products.
   - Use a circular motion, moving from the center outward for several inches. ➤*Rationale: This motion carries microorganisms away from the site of entry.*
   - Permit the solution to dry on the skin. Povidone-iodine should be in contact with the skin for 1 minute to be effective.
8. Insert the catheter and initiate the infusion.
   - Remove the catheter assembly from its sterile packaging. Review instructions for using the catheter—especially since a variety of needle-safety devices are manufactured. Remove the cover of the needle.
   - Use the nondominant hand to pull the skin taut below the entry site. ➤*Rationale: This stabilizes the vein and makes the skin taut for needle entry. It can also make initial tissue penetration less painful.*
   - Holding the over-the-needle catheter at a 15- to 30-degree angle with the needle (stylet) bevel up, insert the catheter through the skin and into the vein. Sudden lack of resistance is felt as the needle enters the vein. Jabbing, stabbing, or quick thrusting should be avoided because it may cause rupture of delicate veins (Phillips, 2005).

## CLINICAL ALERT

Some agencies allow only certified IV therapists to perform venipuncture.

- Once blood appears in the lumen or clear "flashback" chamber of the needle, lower the angle of the catheter until it is almost parallel with the skin, and advance the needle and catheter approximately 0.5 to 1 cm (about 1/4 in.) farther. Holding the needle assembly steady, advance the catheter until the hub is at the venipuncture site. The exact technique depends on the type of device used. ➤*Rationale: The catheter is advanced to ensure that it, and not just the stylet, is in the vein.*
- If there is no blood return, try redirecting the catheter assembly again toward the vein. If the stylet has been withdrawn from the catheter even a small distance, or the catheter tip has been pulled out of the skin, the catheter must be discarded and a new one used. ➤*Rationale: Reinserting the stylet into the catheter can result in slicing the catheter apart. A catheter that has been removed from the skin is considered contaminated and cannot be reused.*

## CLINICAL ALERT

If no blood is observed and you did not feel the catheter enter the vein, pull back on entire catheter apparatus without exiting skin. Reassess vein position, then reattempt venipuncture. If you are not successful, remove catheter and look for a different site. Remember the catheter is now contaminated and cannot be used again. Most facilities allow the nurse to attempt two venipunctures; if unsuccessful, they must notify another professional to attempt venipuncture.

● Blood is noted in the flashback chamber once the stylet has entered the vein.

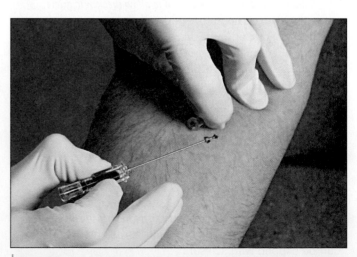

● Occlude the vein with one finger while removing the stylet.

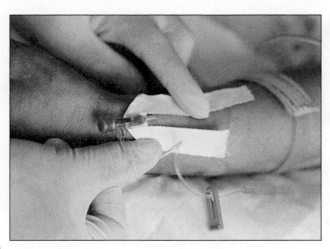

● Taping an IV catheter using the U method.

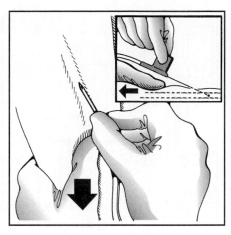

● Inserting a butterfly needle.

- If blood begins to flow out of the vein into the tissues as the needle is inserted, creating a hematoma, the insertion is unsuccessful. This is sometimes referred to as a blown vein. Immediately release the tourniquet and remove the needle, applying pressure over the insertion site with dry gauze. Attempt the venipuncture in another site, in the opposite arm if possible. ➤*Rationale: Placing the tourniquet back on the same arm above the unsuccessful site may cause it to bleed. Placing the IV below the unsuccessful site could result in infusing fluid into the already punctured vein, causing it to leak.*
- Release the tourniquet.
- Put pressure on the vein proximal to the catheter to eliminate or reduce blood oozing out of the catheter. Stabilize the hub with thumb and index finger of the nondominant hand.
- Remove the protective cap from the distal end of the tubing and hold it ready to attach to the catheter, maintaining the sterility of the end.
- Stabilize the catheter hub and apply pressure distal to the catheter with your finger. ➤*Rationale: This prevents excessive blood flow through the catheter.*
- Carefully remove the stylet, engage the needle-safety device, and attach the end of the infusion tubing to the catheter hub. Place the stylet directly into a sharps container. If this is not within reach, place the stylet into its original package and dispose in a sharps container as soon as possible.
- Initiate the infusion or flush the catheter with sterile normal saline. ➤*Rationale: Blood must be removed from the catheter lumen and tubing immediately. Otherwise, the blood*

*will clot inside the lumen.* Watch closely for any signs that the catheter is infiltrated. **Infiltration** occurs when the tip of the IV is outside the vein and the fluid is entering the tissues instead. It is manifested by localized swelling, coolness, pallor, and discomfort at the IV site. ➤*Rationale: Inflammation or infiltration necessitates removal of the IV needle or catheter to avoid further trauma to the tissues.*

9. Tape the catheter. In some cases, the hub is secured with tape while in other settings only a transparent dressing (step 10) is used. Use paper tape if the skin is fragile.
   - Tape the catheter by the U method or according to the manufacturer's instructions. If using an already opened roll of tape, discard the first rotation of tape around the roll. ➤*Rationale: The first rotation has been shown to be highly colonized with infectious organisms* (Redelmeier & Livesley, 1999). Using three strips of adhesive tape, each about 7.5 cm (3 in.) long:
     a. Place one strip, sticky side up, under the catheter's hub.
     b. Fold each end over so that the sticky sides are against the skin.
     c. Place the second strip, sticky side down, over the catheter hub.
     d. Place the third strip, sticky side down, over the tubing hub. Do not tape directly over the insertion site. ➤*Rationale: The tape is not sterile and may contaminate the site.*

## CLINICAL ALERT

Meticulous care must be used to insert the winged-tipped needle because these needles lead to many reported needle stick injuries.

## CLINICAL ALERT

All tape placed under transparent dressings should be sterile. Check facility policy before securing IV site. Some hospitals do not allow tape under the transparent dressing.

*Source:* Intravenous Nurses Society, Standard 49, 2006.

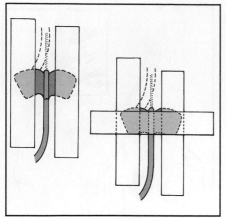

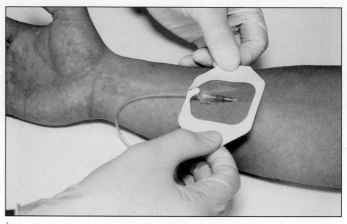

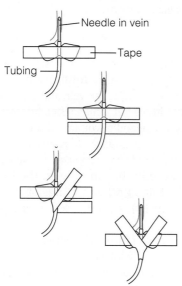

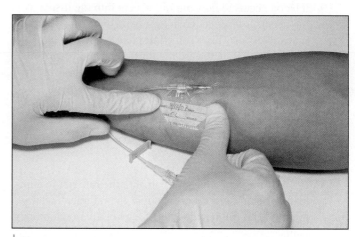

● Cover insertion site with a transparent dressing.

Needle in vein
Tape
Tubing

● Taping the butterfly needle by the H and chevron methods.

● Label IV site with date, time, size of needle, and initials.

### VARIATION: Inserting a Butterfly (Winged-Tip) Needle

- Hold the needle, pointed in the direction of the blood flow, at a 30-degree angle, with the bevel up, and pierce the skin beside the vein about 1 cm (1/2 in.) below the site planned for piercing the vein.
- Once the needle is through the skin, lower the needle so that it is almost parallel with the skin. ➤*Rationale: Lowering the needle reduces the chances of puncturing both sides of the vein.* Follow the course of the vein, and pierce one side of the vein. Sudden lack of resistance can be felt as blood enters the needle.
- When blood flows back into the needle tubing, gently advance the needle to its hub. If the butterfly is a plastic catheter with a stylet, remove the stylet and activate the safety mechanism. Place the stylet directly into a sharps container. If this is not within reach, place the stylet into its original package and dispose in a sharps container as soon as possible.
- Release the tourniquet, attach the injection cap, or begin the infusion.

### Securing a Butterfly Needle

- Tape the butterfly needle securely by the crisscross (chevron) or H method. Place a small gauze square under the hub, if required. ➤*Rationale: The gauze keeps the needle in position in the vein.* Do not tape directly over the insertion site. ➤*Rationale: The tape is not sterile and may contaminate the site.*

## DEVELOPMENTAL CONSIDERATIONS

### Infant/Child

- For infants, veins in the scalp are used for venipuncture.

- Because infants do not have large veins in the antecubital fossa, blood specimens for examination are usually taken from the external jugular and femoral veins.

- Use a doll to demonstrate venipuncture for children and explain the procedure to the parents.

- Explain the procedure to the young client, encourage questions, and be alert for nonverbal cues. Children may not understand things that seem obvious to adults. For example, a child may think the IV therapy is a punishment.

- Venipuncture can be extremely frightening for children. Simply numbing the skin with ice prior to insertion will reduce the discomfort. When prior planning is an option, EMLA cream (lidocaine and prilocaine) topical anesthetic can be applied ahead of time with an occlusive dressing to cover. Remove all of the cream and clean the site prior to insertion.

- Even with analgesia, many children will resist, cry, and even become combative. Parents, in turn, may become upset. Offering distractions and rewards may help. Helping the child to take deep, slow breaths can also trigger some degree of relaxation. Sometimes it is necessary to restrain the child.

Most pediatric professionals believe that it is best if a person other than the child's parent holds the child, so the child doesn't associate the parent with the fear and pain. It is important for the parent to remain with the child, soothing the child with voice, closeness, and touch. Some parents are not able to do this, and they need support and understanding from nursing staff. A calm demeanor on the nurse's part (and relaxation breathing) will help ease this potentially upsetting situation for all concerned.

- A 24-gauge needle is commonly indicated for use with children.

- Apply age-appropriate restraints, arm boards, or other devices to protect the IV site.

### Elders

- Skin is often fragile and bruises easily. Select an IV site with adequate healthy tissue to support the needle.

- To distend the vein, tap only lightly to prevent trauma.

- Consider not using a tourniquet. Elders' superficial veins are often large enough to insert the needle without further distention. Using a tourniquet can cause the vein to burst when the needle enters.

- Minimize the use of alcohol and tape to avoid irritating sensitive skin.

---

10. Dress and label the venipuncture site and tubing according to agency policy.
    - Unless there is an allergy, a sterile transparent occlusive dressing is applied. This permits assessment of the site without disturbing the dressing. This type of dressing can be left on for 72 hours, then changed.
    - Loop any tubing and secure it with tape. ➤*Rationale: Looping and securing the tubing prevent the weight of the tubing or any movement from pulling on the needle or catheter.*
    - Label the dressing with the date and time of insertion, type, gauge of catheter used, and your initials.
    - Discard the tourniquet. Remove and discard gloves. Perform hand hygiene.

## CLINICAL ALERT

The CDC has not established a recommendation for hang time of IV fluids. Follow hospital policy and change fluids accordingly.

11. Apply a padded arm board to splint the joint, as needed.
12. Discard all used disposable supplies in appropriate receptacles. Cleanse any blood spills according to agency policy. Clean any reusable supplies.
13. Document all assessments and interventions.
    - Record the venipuncture on the client's chart. Some agencies provide a special form for this purpose. Include the date and time of the venipuncture; type and gauge of the needle or catheter; venipuncture site; and the client's general response.

### Documentation

Sample: 4/7/2009 0815 Inserted 20-gauge angiocath saline lock in (L) forearm on first attempt. Explained reason for IV. Stated understanding.

_____ A. Luis, RN

# Skill 3.4   Regulating Infusion Flow Rate

### Equipment

Electronic infusion device (pump)
Device-compatible IV administration set
Needleless cannula
Gloves

### Procedure

1. Spike IV solution bag.
2. Close regulating clamp on the set tubing before hanging bag.
3. Fill drip chamber to minimum 1/3 full. ➤*Rationale: This amount allows sufficient air space in drip chamber.*
4. Prime tubing by opening regulating clamp slowly and allowing tubing to fill with IV solution. If using a cassette-type tubing, follow package instructions to correctly prime the cassette portion of the tubing that engages into the control device.

*Note:* Check if tubing has anti-free-flow device that must be opened prior to primary tubing.

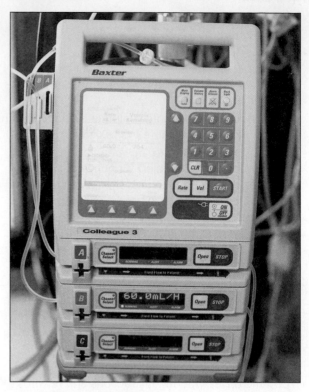

Baxter: Multiple Channel Pump.

---

## IF ALARM SOUNDS, CHECK THE FOLLOWING

Most devices have a message system that specifies the exact problem. You should be prepared to troubleshoot various components of the system.

- *Infusion Complete:* When the exact volume to be delivered is set and the volume limit has been reached, an alarm sounds and the machine goes to a KVO "keep-open" mode. Establish if the total volume of the container has been delivered; change the solution contained if needed, and reset the volume to be infused.

- *Occlusion:* All devices sound an alarm when they cannot maintain delivery in the face of increasing resistance. In this instance, check the insertion site for infiltration, and look for position problems, pinched tubing, closed clamp, turned stopcock, or clogged filter.

- *Other Problems:* Other messages may indicate "air in the line," "low battery," "cassette (improperly loaded), or "free flow."

- *Nursing Action:* Check trouble spot carefully, readjust, and restart the infusion.

## CLINICAL ALERT

Observe IV site frequently when pumps are used. IV pumps do not normally detect infiltration at the IV site. Infiltration does not produce enough pressure to trigger an alarm. Check for edema, cool skin, discomfort, and tenderness at the IV site.

5. Follow manufacturer's instructions to load administration set into device, taking care to fit tubing and cassette into appropriate receptor sites. (One type of pump is a multiple channel pump that can infuse four different IV solutions at one time.)
6. Close device door and latch.
7. Perform hand hygiene and don gloves.
8. Check that client's venipuncture site is free from signs of vein irritation or infiltration.
9. Connect administration set tubing to establish infusion site protective cap using a needleless cannula.
10. Open regulating clamp on administration set.
11. Turn device ON.

## IV CALORIE CALCULATION

- 1000 mL $D_5W$ provides 50 g of dextrose.
- 50 g of dextrose provides 4 Cal/g (actually 3.4 Cal); therefore, multiply 50 g $\times$ 4 Cal.
- 1000 mL $D_5W$ provides 200 Cal.
- Usual IV fluid maintenance is 2000–3000 mL/day (400–600 Cal/day).

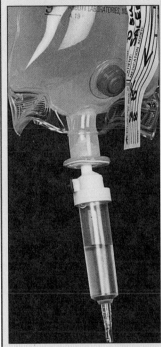 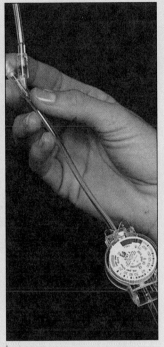

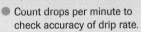 Count drops per minute to check accuracy of drip rate.

● Set dial-a-flow to prescribed mL drip rate per hour.

## FACTORS THAT INFLUENCE IV FLOW RATES WHEN USING GRAVITY FOR INFUSION

- Warm fluids drip faster than cold fluids.
- The higher the bag is above insertion site, the faster the infusion.
- The more IV administration is tilted, the larger each drop from drip chamber.
- The larger the catheter diameter, the faster the flow rate.
- The longer the catheter, the slower the flow rate because of resistance.
- Increased blood pressure or coughing will slow the flow rate (this is a temporary situation usually).

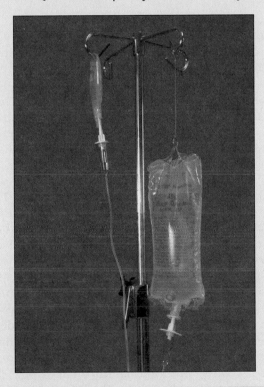

*Note:* Because of these variables, manual control of IVs is not recommended. IV pumps are the most predictable method of infusing fluids.

12. Set device parameters for operation, again following manufacturer's instructions or machine's setup prompts. Parameters may include:
    a. Infusion (e.g., primary).
    b. Volume to be infused.
    c. Rate (mL/hr).
    d. Pressure (measure can vary; e.g., mm Hg, cm $H_2O$, or psi).
13. START device when parameters are set.
14. Observe that infusion is running properly.
15. Remove gloves and perform hand hygiene.
16. Check client's infusion site frequently.

Nurses need to check infusions at least every hour to ensure that the indicated milliliters per hour have infused and to assess the IV site. A strip of adhesive marking the exact time and/or amount to be infused should be taped to the solution container. Some agencies make pre-marked labels available. Do not write directly on the IV bag. Writing directly on the IV bag with a ballpoint pen could damage the bag and contaminate the solution. A felt-tip pen should not be used directly on the bag or on the label because the ink could penetrate the label or bag

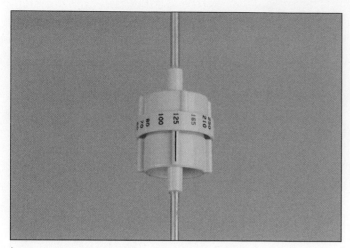

● The Dial-A-Flo in-line IV rate control device.

Photographer: Elena Dorfman

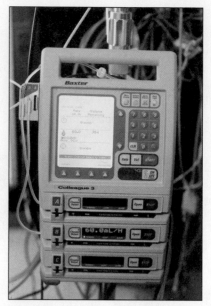

● Programmable infusion pump.

surface, causing contamination of the solution. Additionally, the writing from felt-tip pens may become illegible with time.

The *Dial-A-Flo* in-line device is a manual regulator that controls the amount of fluid to be administered. The Dial-A-Flo may be used in situations where a pump is not available or required, but prevention of fluid overload is important. The nurse presets the volume to be infused by rotating the dial to the desired rate. Another variation is a *volume-control set,* or *Volutrol,* which is used if the volume of fluid administered is to be carefully controlled. The set, which holds a maximum of 100 mL of solution, is attached below the solution container, and the drip chamber is placed below the set. Volume control sets are frequently used in pediatric settings, where the volume administered is critical.

Devices such as battery-operated controllers and infusion pumps with alarm systems facilitate a regulated flow. Newer systems are programmable and include drug libraries with dose rate calculators, automatic flushing between medications, dual or triple simultaneous line control, memory, multiple alarm settings (air in line, pressure/resistance, battery), schedule reminders, volume settings down to 0.1 mL, panel locks, and digital. Pumps can exert pressure on the tubing or on the fluid if restrictions develop (increased venous resistance) to maintain the fluid flow.

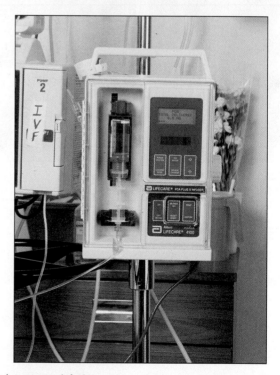

● An intravenous infusion pump.

Photographer: Jenny Thomas

| UNEXPECTED OUTCOMES | CRITICAL THINKING OPTIONS |
|---|---|
| Client develops unexplained fever with chills and rising pulse rate. | • Unexplained fever may be associated with catheter-related sepsis. Report to physician.<br>• Assess IV site for signs of infection.<br>• Ensure that IV solutions hang for no more than 24 hours.<br>• Check client's vital signs: temperature usually above 100°F when caused by IV-related sepsis.<br>• Check for other symptoms of pyrogenic reactions (e.g., backache, headache, malaise, nausea, and vomiting).<br>• Stop the infusion.<br>• Obtain blood specimens, if ordered. |
| IV solution does not flow properly. | • Ensure that the control clamp is open.<br>• Check that blood pressure readings are not taken on arm in which IV is running, as flow is impeded and a clot can form on the end of the needle.<br>• Ensure that IV administration set is properly loaded. Check pump for flow problem indicator (e.g., cassette seating, air in line).<br>• Check IV tubing from insertion site to IV solution for kinks/obstructions.<br>• Check for extremity causing positional obstruction to flow (e.g., elbow bent, arm rotated). |
| IV solution appears to be infiltrating resulting in tissue swelling. | • Decrease the flow rate. (Remove from pump for "keep open" rate.)<br>• Lower bag of IV solution; if blood returns, cannula may be in the vein but fluid may be leaking into surrounding tissue via existing puncture in vein wall.<br>• Discontinue infusion and establish a new site. |
| Phlebitis is suspected at infusion site (tenderness, warmth, erythema, and pain). | • Check infusion solution and medications being administered. (Potassium chloride and hypertonic solutions are particularly irritating to veins.)<br>• Discontinue IV.<br>• Apply warm compress per hospital policy. |
| Postinfusion phlebitis may also occur after the IV has been discontinued in response to either chemical or mechanical factors of the preexisting IV. | • Check IV solution; hypertonic solution causes irritation necessitating use of large veins and changing IV sites more frequently.<br>• Follow hospital policy for treatment. Warm compresses to the site are generally recommended.<br>• Elevate extremity. |
| Venipuncture is unsuccessful for needle insertion. | • Remove needle, apply pressure at insertion site until bleeding stops. (This prevents ecchymosis at site.) Apply Band-Aid.<br>• Apply small pressure dressing if client on anticoagulant therapy.<br>• Select another site more proximal in vein, or use another extremity.<br>• Avoid the one-step entry method since this frequently results in a through-and-through vein puncture.<br>• After two failed attempts, seek a more experienced person to perform venipuncture.<br>• Place extremity in dependent position prior to placing tourniquet. Allows vein to fill.<br>• Place warm compress on extremity to increase vasodilation, prior to placing tourniquet. |
| Vein rolls and is difficult to enter. | • Apply traction with thumb and index finger to stabilize skin and vein; maintain traction until venipuncture complete.<br>• Select a smaller gauge catheter.<br>• Advance catheter slowly. |
| Vein is fragile and "balloons" around needle on vein entry. | • Release tourniquet as soon as vein entry is evident.<br>• Avoid use of tourniquet if veins are very fragile or client is taking an anticoagulant.<br>• Enter vein with needle bevel down. |
| Infiltration occurs. | • Place warm moist pack, using warm towel, enclose area from fingertips to elbow. Place extremity in plastic bag with open end at elbow. Leave in place no more than 10 minutes. |
| Vesicant drug infuses into tissue. | • Clamp IV tubing.<br>• Infuse antidote for specific medication, according to physician orders. |

# Skill 3.5 Using an Infusion Pump or Controller

## Delegation

Due to the need for sterile technique and technical complexity, use of infusion devices is not delegated to UAP. UAP may care for clients with such devices, and the nurse must ensure that the UAP knows how to perform routine tasks such as positioning and changing gowns when a device is in place. The UAP should also know what complications or adverse signs, such as alarms, should be reported to the nurse.

In many states, a licensed practical nurse or licensed vocational nurse with special IV therapy training may manage infusions. Check the state's nurse practice act.

## Equipment

- Infusion pump or controller
- IV solution or medication
- IV pole
- IV administration set with compatible IV tubing
- Alcohol swabs and tape
- Label for tubing
- Time strip for container

## Preparation

- Review the use of the pump outside of the client's room. Read all appropriate materials and confirm how to set the device.
- Ensure that the tubing is the correct one for the device. Each manufacturer and model may require different tubing.

## Procedure

1. Prior to performing the procedure, introduce self and verify the client's identity using agency protocol. Explain to the client what you are going to do, why it is necessary, and how he or she can participate. Explain what the device sounds like during normal use, the various alarms, and to notify the nurse if an alarm sounds.
2. Perform hand hygiene and observe other appropriate infection control procedures.
3. Prepare the client.
   - Check the client's identification band against the IV fluid container. ➤*Rationale: This ensures that the correct client receives the infusion.*
   - Assist the client to a comfortable position, either sitting or lying. Expose the limb as needed but provide for client privacy. Make sure that the clothing or gown can be removed over the IV apparatus if necessary. Some agencies provide special gowns that open over the shoulder and down the sleeve for easy removal.

### Infusion Controller

1. Attach the controller to the IV pole.
   - Attach the controller to the IV pole so that it will be below and in-line with the IV container.
   - Plug the machine into the electric outlet, unless battery power is used.
2. Set up the IV infusion.
   - Open the IV container, maintaining the sterility of the port, and spike the container with the administration set.
   - Place the IV container on the IV pole, and position the drip chamber 76 cm (30 in.) above the venipuncture site. ➤*Rationale: This provides sufficient gravitational pressure for the fluid to flow into the client.*
   - Fill the drip chamber of the IV tubing one-third full. ➤*Rationale: If the drip chamber is filled more than halfway, the drops may be miscounted.*
   - Prime the tubing according to the manufacturer's directions, and close the clamp.
3. Attach the IV drop sensor, and insert the IV tubing into the controller.
   - Attach the IV drop sensor (electronic eye) to the drip chamber so that it is below the drip orifice and above the fluid level in the drip chamber. ➤*Rationale: This placement ensures an accurate drop count. If the sensor is placed too high, it can miss drops; if placed too low it may mistake splashes for drops.*

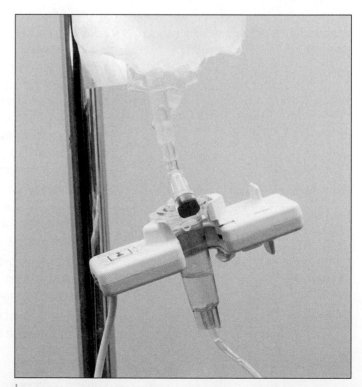

The IV controller drop sensor.

- Make sure the sensor is plugged into the controller.
- Insert the tubing into the controller according to the manufacturer's instructions.

4. Initiate the infusion.
   - Perform a venipuncture or connect the tubing to the existing IV catheter.

5. Set volume control for the appropriate volume per hour.
   - Press the power button.
   - Close the door to the controller, and ensure that all tubing clamps are wide open. ➤*Rationale: This enables the controller to regulate the fluid flow.*
   - Set the controls on the front of the controller to the appropriate infusion rate and volume.
   - Press the start button.
   - Count the drops for 15 seconds, and multiply the result by 4. ➤*Rationale: This verifies that the rate has been correctly set and the controller is operating accurately.*

*Note:* In some cases the drops may fall at an uneven rate. If so, count the drops for 30 to 60 seconds to verify that the per-minute rate is correct. Continue with step 6 below.

### Infusion Pump

1. Attach the pump to the IV pole.
   - Attach the pump at eye level on the IV pole. ➤*Rationale: Because the pump does not depend on gravity pressure, it can be placed at any level. Eye level is convenient for checking its functioning.*
   - Plug the machine into an electric outlet, unless battery power is used.

2. Set up the infusion.
   - Check the manufacturer's directions before using an IV filter or before infusing blood. ➤*Rationale: Infusion pump pressures may damage filters or cause rate inaccuracies. Certain models may also cause hemolysis of red blood cells.*
   - Open the IV container, maintaining the sterility of the port, and spike the container with the administration set.
   - Place the IV container on the IV pole above the pump.
   - Fill the drip chamber.
   - Prime the tubing, and close the clamp. Some pumps have a cassette that must also be primed. Manufacturers give instructions for doing this. Often, the cassette must be tilted to be filled with fluid. Some pumps must have the power on and the tubing and cassette in place in order to perform priming.

3. Insert the IV tubing into the pump.
   - Press the power button to the on position.
   - Load the machine according to the manufacturer's instructions.

## CLINICAL ALERT

Observe IV site frequently when pumps are used. IV pumps do not normally detect infiltration at the IV site. Infiltration does not produce enough pressure to trigger an alarm. Check for edema, cool skin, discomfort, and tenderness at the IV site.

4. Initiate the infusion.
   - Perform venipuncture or connect the tubing to the IV catheter.

5. Set the controls for the required drops per minute or milliliters per hour.
   - Press the start button.
   - Check the drip chamber to ensure that fluid is flowing from the container.

6. Set the alarms. ➤*Rationale: The alarms notify the nurse when a set volume of fluid has been infused or indicates malfunctioning of the equipment.*

7. Monitor the infusion.
   - Check the volume of fluid infused at least every hour, and compare it with the time tape on the IV container. This confirms the actual volume of fluid infused.
   - If the volume infused does not coincide with the time tape or the alarm sounds, begin at the client level and check that:
     a. The IV has not infiltrated or clotted at the insertion site.
     b. The tubing is not pinched, kinked, or disconnected.
     c. The appropriate tubing clamps are fully open.
     d. The sensors are correctly placed.
     e. The rate/volume settings are accurate.
     f. The drip chamber is correctly filled.
     g. The container still has solution.
     h. The time tape is accurate.
     i. The IV container is correctly placed.

8. Document relevant information.
   - Record the date and time of starting the infusion, the type and amount of fluid being infused, the rate at which it is being infused, the infusion device used, the status of the IV insertion site, and any adverse responses of the client.

## DEVELOPMENTAL CONSIDERATIONS

### Infant/Children

- Emphasize to children that the IV controller or pump is not a toy and should not be touched unless an adult is present. Children are naturally curious and will want to examine the equipment.
- Use a volume control infusion set (Volutrol, Buretrol, or Coluset) with the pump/controller for pediatric clients.
- Explain the procedure to the young client, encourage questions, and be alert for nonverbal cues. Children may not understand things that seem obvious to adults. For example, a child may think the IV therapy is a punishment.

### Elders

- Check the IV flow rate frequently for older adults. Elders are at increased risk to develop fluid overload if IV fluid is infused too rapidly.
- For older clients, check the IV site often for signs of infiltration. Veins become more fragile with aging.

# Skill 3.6  Using a "Smart" Pump

### Equipment

Point-of-care computer specific to nursing unit
IV tubing
IV fluids and/or IV medications

### Procedure

1. Identify client and explain pump's function.
2. Assemble equipment and bring to client's bedside.
3. Perform hand hygiene.
4. Verify IV site is patent and absent signs of infiltration.
5. Plug pump into electrical outlet.
6. Insert the pump module into the point-of-care computer ("brain").
7. Spike IV fluid bag.
8. Prime IV tubing with appropriate solution.
9. Insert the IV tubing into the pump module and close the door to the pump. (Follow photos for inserting tubing into cassette.)
10. View screen will ask which client care area is being used. ➤*Rationale: The pump automatically configures itself to provide the infusion parameters for that area.*
11. Choose the intended drug and concentration from

---

### USING A BAR CODE MEDICATION ADMINISTRATION SYSTEM

- If the facility uses a bar code medication administration (BCMA) system, a computerized prescriber order entry (CPOE), automatic medication dispensing, and electronic medication records, smart pumps can provide a very high level of client safety. The system will tell you which IV medications were ordered via a CPOE for your client and when the medication is due.

- When the nurse enters the client's room with the scanning device, she/he scans the bar-code labels on the medication, the client's ID band, and the nurse's ID badge. The information from the bar-code label attached to the medication IV bag will be transmitted wirelessly to and programmed into the infusion pump.

- The pump will begin infusing only when scanning of all pieces of information is completed.

- The pump automatically communicates with a computer in the pharmacy, providing the status of the infusion.

---

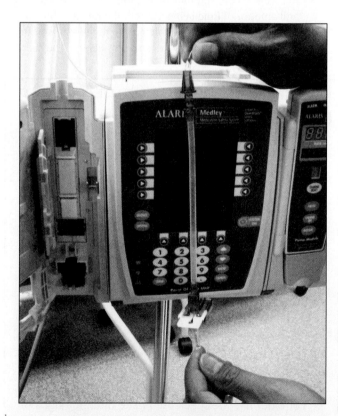

❶ Hang IV bag on pole. Prime tubing and insert into pump module cassette.

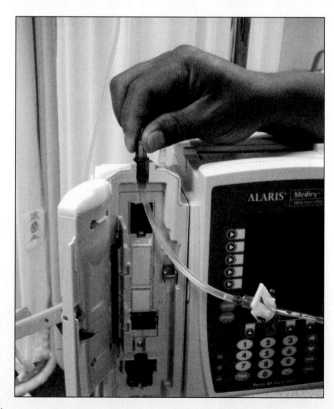

❷ Place top of IV tubing into top of cassette, listen for click indicating it is seated.

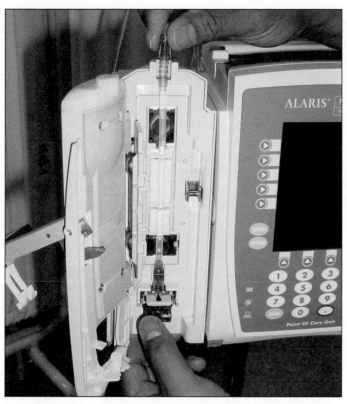

③ Insert white slide clamp into cassette, listen for click.

## CLINICAL ALERT

Check the facility's policies and procedures to determine whether the pump can be run with the override or whether a verbal verification of the order with a physician or pharmacist must be obtained before proceeding.

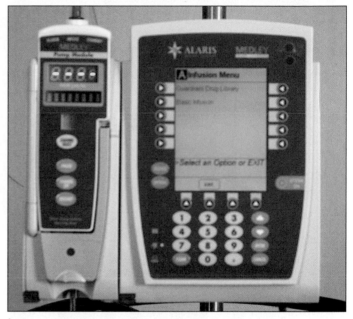

⑤ Select medication to be infused.

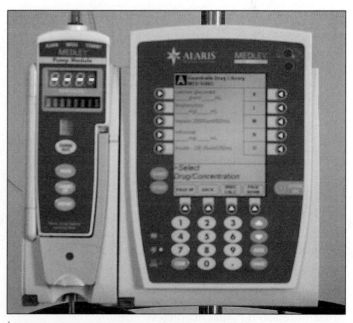

④ Close pump module door and lower locking level.

⑥ Check screen for drug name and infusion rate.

## LEGAL ALERT

By 2006, the FDA has mandated that all drug manufacturers must label most prescription medications and certain over-the-counter drugs with machine-readable bar codes, using the National Drug Code number that uniquely identifies each drug, its dosage form and strength. The FDA predicts that using bar codes will prevent up to 500,000 adverse drug events and transfusion errors over the next 20 years.

*Source:* U.S. Food and Drug Administration. (2005, September). FDA Issues Bar Code Regulation, 2004. www.fda.gov/oc/initiatives/barcode.

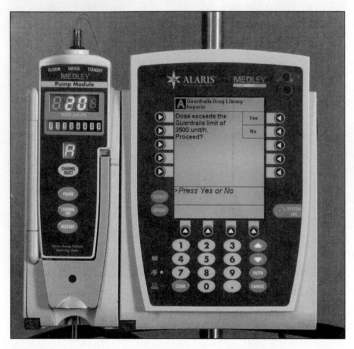

**⑦** Check screen when "soft alert" sounds to determine problem.

the list outlined on the screen.

12. Enter the ordered dose and infusion rate; the pump checks this information against the drug library. If what was programmed matches the pump's drug library, the pump allows the infusion to begin.

13. If an audible and visual alert occurs, the pro-

## EVIDENCE-BASED NURSING PRACTICE

### Smart Pump Technology Reduces Errors

There has been little IV error-prevention data published that documents the actual frequency of IV medication errors with infusion devices.

In a study conducted in the intensive care unit and operating room areas at Massachusetts General Hospital where use of an electronic drug library was implemented, a 50% reduction in the number of drug administration errors involving syringe pumps occurred over a 3-month period using the smart pump. The study indicated that logs from the 135 smart pumps showed:

- 40,644 infusion starts (potential for error)
- 693 alert messages (1.7% of start-ups)
- 158 programming changes (0.4% of start-ups, 22.8% of alert messages).

*Source:* Reves, Jerry. (2003). "Smart pump" technology reduces errors. www.apsf.org/resource_center, 2003. Information was based on a study by Ellen Kinnealey, BSN, Infusion pumps with "drug libraries" at the point of care: A solution for safer drug delivery.

grammed data is outside the specified limits. The alert informs you about which parameter is out of the recommended range.

14. Depending on the medication or client care area, the pump will sound a "soft" alarm or a "hard" alarm. Some facilities allow a "soft" alarm to be overridden. If you override the alarm, the infusion will begin. This alarm is considered a minor error.

15. When "hard" alarm occurs, the pump shuts down. It cannot be overridden. Reprogram the pump with settings that are within your facility's specified limits to begin infusing when a "hard" alarm sounds.

*Note:* The smart pump's software logs and tracks all alerts, recording the time, date, drug, concentration, and infusion rate, as well as any action taken, whether the pump is overridden or not.

16. Observe the screen to ensure medication is infusing at prescribed rate.

## Skill 3.7  Using a Syringe Pump

### Equipment

Battery or electronic operated syringe infusion pump
Pharmacy-prepared and labeled syringe with prescribed medication
Microbore tubing with needleless cannula
2% chlorhexidine antimicrobial wipe

### Procedure

1. Check syringe label with physician's order for drug, dosage, and amount of drug to be delivered over specified time.

2. Assure that medication is compatible with primary infusing solution.

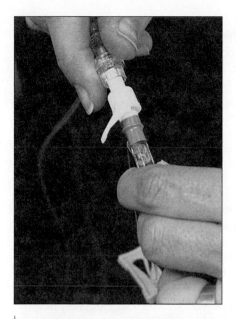

❶ Attach luer access pin to microbore tubing.

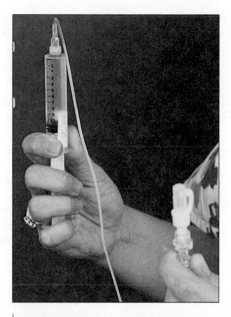

❷ Expel air from syringe before priming tubing.

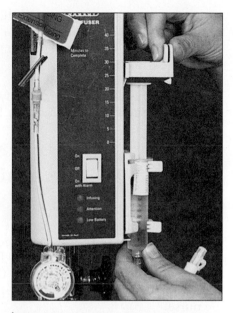

❸ Insert syringe into cradle of pump.

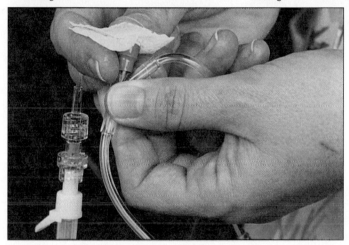

❹ Prep port closest to client before "piggybacking" syringe pump.

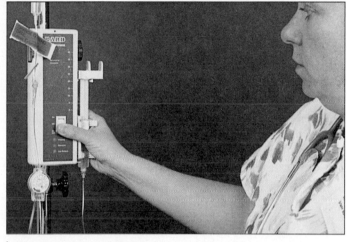

❺ Set infusion rate for drug delivery as prescribed. (Dial-a-flow).

3. Calculate amount of medication to be delivered per minute.
4. Attach microbore tubing to syringe, and holding syringe upright, expel air from medication syringe before priming tubing.
5. Holding syringe downward, carefully prime microbore tubing with medication (about 0.5 mL).
6. Insert syringe into cradle of pump, squeezing clamp around designated parts of syringe; attach pusher to plunger.
7. Verify that IV site is free from infiltration or vein irrigation.
8. Swab primary IV tubing port closest to client.
9. Insert microbore cannula into port.

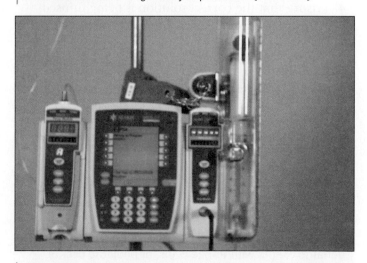

❻ Smart Pumps have syringe modules available to be attached to the point of care computers. To attach module, follow manufacturer's directions.

10. Set rate for drug delivery according to pharmacy specifications on syringe label, or as prescribed. Drug will be infused independent of the primary infusion rate.
11. Start syringe pump.
12. Check infusion indicator to verify pump is infusing.
13. Monitor site and pump function frequently.

14. For subsequent doses, pharmacy dispenses a new syringe but microbore tubing may be reused for 48–72 hours (according to agency policy). A sterile cap is used each time client's primary tubing is accessed.

*Note:* For other brands of syringe pumps, follow directions for setup and delivery of meds with their product.

# Skill 3.8  Maintaining Infusions

## Delegation

Due to the need for sterile technique and technical complexity, inspection of IV sites and regulation of IV rates is not delegated to UAP. UAP may care for clients with such devices, and the nurse must ensure that the UAP knows what complications or adverse signs should be reported to the nurse.

In many states, a licensed practical nurse or licensed vocational nurse with special IV therapy training may manage infusions. Check the state's nurse practice act.

## Equipment

None

## Performance

1. Prior to performing the procedure, introduce self and verify the client's identity using agency protocol. Explain to the client what you are going to do, why it is necessary, and how he or she can participate.
2. Perform hand hygiene and observe other appropriate infection control procedures.
3. Position the client appropriately.
   - Assist the client to a comfortable position, either sitting or lying.
   - Expose the IV site but provide for client privacy.
4. Ensure that the correct solution is being infused.
   - Compare the label on the container (including added medications) to the order. If the solution is incorrect, slow the rate of flow to a minimum to maintain the patency of the catheter. If the infusing solution is contraindicated for the client, stop the infusion and saline-lock the catheter. ►*Rationale: Just stopping the infusion may allow a thrombus to form in the IV catheter. If this occurs, the catheter must be removed and another venipuncture performed before the infusion can be resumed. Because IV tubing contains approximately 12 to 15 mL,*

*it may be desirable to prevent even this much additional incorrect solution to infuse when the correct IV solution container is hung on existing tubing. In this case, all tubing should be removed until new tubing, primed with the correct solution, can be started.*
   - Change the solution to the correct one, using new tubing if indicated.
   - Document and report the error according to agency protocol.
5. Observe the rate of flow every hour.
   - Compare the rate of flow at least hourly against the infusion schedule. ►*Rationale: Infusions that are off schedule can be harmful to a client.* To read the volume in an IV bag, pull the edges of the bag apart at the level of the fluid and read the volume remaining. ►*Rationale: Stretching the bag allows the fluid meniscus to fall to the proper level.*
   - Observe the position of the solution container. If it is less than 1 m (3 ft) above the IV site, readjust it to the correct height of the pole. ►*Rationale: If the container is too low, the solution may not flow into the vein because there is insufficient gravitational pressure to overcome the pressure of the blood within the vein.*
   - If too much fluid has infused in the time interval, check agency policy. The primary care provider may need to be notified.
   - In some agencies, you will slow the infusion to less than the ordered rate so that it will be completed at the planned time. ►*Rationale: Solution administered too quickly may cause fluid overload.* If the client has received significantly more fluid than planned, assess for manifestations of hypervolemia: dyspnea; rapid, labored breathing; cough; crackles (rales); tachycardia; and bounding pulses.
   - In other agencies, if the order is for a specified amount of fluid per hour, the IV may be adjusted to the correct rate

**CLINICAL ALERT**

Clients receiving hypertonic, acidic, or irritating agents, geriatric clients with fragile veins, or pediatric clients who are active are at particular risk for IV site problems.

**CLINICAL ALERT**

To check for extravasation, place constrictive band proximal to infusion site tight enough to restrict blood flow through the vein. Set tubing roller clamp to a "keep open" (or slow) rate, and remove tubing from infusion pump. If the infusion continues to drip, fluid is extravasating into the surrounding tissue.

**Division of Nursing**
Oakland, California 94609

## VENIPUNCTURE

| DATE | TIME | SITE CODE | TYPE / GAUGE NEEDLE | INIT. | DC DATE | INIT. |
|------|------|-----------|---------------------|-------|---------|-------|
|      |      |           |                     |       |         |       |
|      |      |           |                     |       |         |       |
|      |      |           |                     |       |         |       |
|      |      |           |                     |       |         |       |
|      |      |           |                     |       |         |       |
|      |      |           |                     |       |         |       |
|      |      |           |                     |       |         |       |

## CODES

**SITE LOCATION:**

| | | | |
|---|---|---|---|
| RH | HAND | LH | HAND |
| RF | FOREARM | LF | FOREARM |
| RA | ANTECUBITAL | LA | ANTECUBITAL |
| RU | UPPER ARM | LU | UPPER ARM |
| RS | SUBCLAVIAN | LS | SUBCLAVIAN |
| RJ | JUGULAR | LJ | JUGULAR |
| RL | LEG | LL | LEG |
| VA | VASCULAR ACCESS | | |

**SITE CONDITION:**
A. PATENT WITHOUT REDNESS OR SWELLING OCCLUSIVE DRESSING INTACT
B. PATENT WITH MILD REDNESS AND/OR SWELLING OCCLUSIVE DRESSING INTACT
C. DRAINAGE (SEE NOTE)
D. DISLODGED / OCCLUDED
E. INFILTRATED
F. OCCLUSIVE DRESSING CHANGED

## I.V. ORDERS

| DATE ORDERED | INITIALS TRANS. | INITIALS CHECK | SOLUTION / ADDITIVE(S) | INFUSION RATE | DURATION |
|--------------|--------|--------|------------------------|---------------|----------|
|              |        |        |                        |               |          |
|              |        |        |                        |               |          |
|              |        |        |                        |               |          |
|              |        |        |                        |               |          |
|              |        |        |                        |               |          |
|              |        |        |                        |               |          |
|              |        |        |                        |               |          |
|              |        |        |                        |               |          |

## I.V.'s ADMINISTERED

| DATE | TIME | INIT. | SITE LOC. | BOTTLE NUMBER | SOLUTION / ADDITIVE(S) | SHIFT | AMOUNT ABSORBED | AMOUNT REMAINING | TIME TUBING CHANGE | SITE COND. | TOTAL INFUSED |
|------|------|-------|-----------|---------------|------------------------|-------|-----------------|------------------|--------------------|------------|---------------|
|      |      |       |           |               |                        | 0600  |                 |                  |                    |            |               |
|      |      |       |           |               |                        | 1400  |                 |                  |                    |            |               |
|      |      |       |           |               |                        | 2200  |                 |                  |                    |            |               |
|      |      |       |           |               |                        | 0600  |                 |                  |                    |            |               |
|      |      |       |           |               |                        | 1400  |                 |                  |                    |            |               |
|      |      |       |           |               |                        | 2200  |                 |                  |                    |            |               |
|      |      |       |           |               |                        | 0600  |                 |                  |                    |            |               |
|      |      |       |           |               |                        | 1400  |                 |                  |                    |            |               |
|      |      |       |           |               |                        | 2200  |                 |                  |                    |            |               |
|      |      |       |           |               |                        | 0600  |                 |                  |                    |            |               |
|      |      |       |           |               |                        | 1400  |                 |                  |                    |            |               |
|      |      |       |           |               |                        | 2200  |                 |                  |                    |            |               |
|      |      |       |           |               |                        | 0600  |                 |                  |                    |            |               |
|      |      |       |           |               |                        | 1400  |                 |                  |                    |            |               |
|      |      |       |           |               |                        | 2200  |                 |                  |                    |            |               |
|      |      |       |           |               |                        | 0600  |                 |                  |                    |            |               |
|      |      |       |           |               |                        | 1400  |                 |                  |                    |            |               |
|      |      |       |           |               |                        | 2200  |                 |                  |                    |            |               |

## SIGN.

| INIT. | SIGNATURE / TITLE | INIT. | SIGNATURE / TITLE | INIT. | SIGNATURE / TITLE |
|-------|-------------------|-------|-------------------|-------|-------------------|
|       |                   |       |                   |       |                   |
|       |                   |       |                   |       |                   |

**SUMMIT** MEDICAL CENTER

# Intravenous Therapy Record

AFFIX PATIENT
I.D. LABEL HERE

MPN-105 86-6105-0

IV flow record.

and the client monitored for signs of fluid overload. In this case, make the appropriate revisions on the container time strip.

- If the rate is too slow, adjust the IV to the prescribed rate. Also, check agency policy. Some agencies permit nursing personnel to adjust an IV that is behind time by a specified percent. Adjustments above this amount may require a primary care provider's order. ➤*Rationale: Solution that is administered too slowly can supply insufficient fluid, electrolytes, or medication for a client's needs.*
- If the prescribed rate of flow is 150 mL/h or more, check the rate of flow more frequently, for example, every 30 minutes.

6. Inspect the patency of the IV tubing and needle.
   - Observe the drip chamber. If it is less than half full, squeeze the chamber to allow the correct amount of fluid to flow in.
   - Open the drip regulator and observe for a rapid flow of fluid from the solution container into the drip chamber. Then close the drip regulator to reestablish the prescribed rate of flow. ➤*Rationale: Rapid flow of fluid into the drip chamber indicates patency of the IV line. Close the drip overload.*

- Inspect the tubing for pinches, kinks, or obstructions to flow. Arrange the tubing so that it is lightly coiled and under no pressure. Sometimes the tubing becomes caught under the client's arm and the weight of the arm blocks the flow.
- Observe the position of the tubing. If it is dangling below the venipuncture site, coil it carefully on the surface of the bed. ➤*Rationale: The solution may not flow upward into the vein against the force of gravity.*
- If the infusion is dripping at less than the prescribed rate even when adjusted, lower the solution container below the level of the infusion site, and observe for a return flow of blood from the vein. ➤*Rationale: A return flow of blood indicates that the needle is patent and in the vein. Blood returns because venous pressure is greater than the fluid pressure in the IV tubing (siphoning). Absence of blood return may indicate that the needle is no longer in the vein or that the tip of the catheter is partially obstructed by a thrombus, the vein wall, or a valve in the vein. (Note: With some catheters, no blood may appear even with patency because the soft catheter walls collapse during siphoning.)*
- If the infusion is dripping at less than the prescribed rate even when adjusted, determine whether the bevel of the

## CLINICAL ALERT

Some facilities use a single secondary tubing for all agents. The tubing is back-flushed with the primary solution prior to administering a new agent providing the agents are compatible.

## CLINICAL ALERT

Regarding IV systems as closed sterile systems and maintain as such. All entries into the tubing should be made through injection ports that are disinfected just before entry.

catheter is against the wall of the vein. Carefully raise or lower the hub of the needle. If the flow rate improves, tape a sterile gauze pad under or over the hub to secure the modified position of the catheter bevel.

- If there is leakage, locate the source. If the leak is at the catheter connection, tighten the tubing into the catheter. If the leak is elsewhere in the tubing, slow the infusion and replace the tubing. Estimate the amount of solution lost, if it was substantial. If fluid is leaking at the insertion site, the needle may be blocked. Check agency policy regarding irrigating potentially clotted needles.

7. Inspect the insertion site for fluid infiltration.
   - If infiltration is present, stop the infusion and remove the catheter. Restart the infusion at another site.
   - Apply a warm compress to the site of the infiltration. ➤*Rationale: Warmth promotes comfort and vasodilation, facilitating absorption of the fluid from interstitial tissues.*
   - If the infiltration involves a **vesicant** drug (one that causes blistering when in the tissues but not in the vascular system), it is called **extravasation** and other measures may be indicated. Extravasated vesicant drugs can cause severe tissue injury or destruction. The extravasation of a vesicant drug should be considered an emergency. Usually, vesicants are administered only through central venous infusions and by specially certified nurses. An example of a vesicant is the chemotherapy medication paclitaxel.
     a. Stop the infusion immediately. Disconnect the tubing as close to the catheter hub as possible and attempt to aspirate any drug remaining in the hub. If an injectable antidote is available, the catheter should remain in place.

   b. The nursing supervisor and primary care provider should be notified and, if ordered, the antidote administered.
   c. Depending on the drug, heat or cold therapy should be implemented. Inspect the insertion site for **phlebitis** (inflammation of a vein).
- Inspect the site. Phlebitis can occur as a result of mechanical trauma or chemical irritation (such as from intravenous electrolytes, especially potassium and magnesium, and certain medications). Signs of phlebitis are redness, warmth, and swelling at the intravenous site and burning pain along the course of the vein.
- If phlebitis is detected, discontinue the infusion, and apply warm compresses to the venipuncture site. Do not use this injured vein for further infusions.

8. Inspect the intravenous site for bleeding.
   - Oozing or bleeding into the surrounding tissues can occur while the infusion is freely flowing but is more likely to occur after the needle has been removed from the vein.
   - Observation of the venipuncture site is extremely important for clients who bleed readily, such as those receiving anticoagulants.

9. Document relevant information.
   - Record the status of the IV insertion site and any adverse responses of the client.
   - Document the client's IV fluid intake at least every 8 hours according to agency policy. Include the date and time; amount and type of solution used; container number; flow rate; and the client's general response. In most agencies, the amount remaining in each IV container is also recorded at the end of the shift.

# Skill 3.9   Maintaining Intermittent Infusion Devices

## Delegation

Due to the need for sterile technique and technical complexity, use of IV devices is not delegated to UAP. UAP may care for clients with such devices, and the nurse must ensure that the UAP knows what complications or adverse signs should be reported to the nurse.

In many states, a licensed practical nurse or licensed vocational nurse with special IV therapy training may manage intermittent infusion devices. Check the state's nurse practice act.

## Equipment

- Intermittent infusion cap or device
- Clean gloves
- Sterile 2 × 2 or 4 × 4 gauze
- Sterile saline for injection (without preservative) or heparin flush solution (10 units/mL or 100 units/mL)

in a prefilled syringe, a 3-mL syringe with a 25-gauge needle, or a needleless infusion device
- Isopropyl alcohol wipes
- Tape

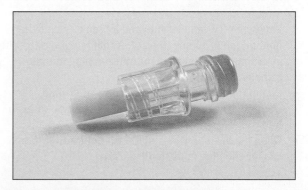

● Intermittent infusion device with injection port.

## EVIDENCE-BASED NURSING PRACTICE

### Flushing with Low-Dose Heparin

There are many conflicting studies indicating outcomes that are both pro and con for using low-dose heparin with peripheral venous catheters. In one study, low-dose heparin infused continuously through peripheral venous catheters required further study to determine effectiveness in prolonging catheter life. Studies have proven that using heparin in arterial catheters is of benefit. Using intermittent heparin flushes for peripheral IV catheters also requires further validation, as it seems to be no more effective than using NS flushes.

*Source:* Randolph, A., et al. (1998, March 28). Benefit of heparin in peripheral venous and arterial catheters: Systematic review and meta-analysis of randomized controlled trials. *British Medical Journal, 316,* 969–975.

### Flushing Using Saline or Heparin

In a second study completed at the Mayo Clinic, Rochester, MN, a prospective, randomized, and double-blind study was completed on 73 hospitalized pregnant women between 24 and 42 weeks gestation. The clients were randomly assigned to receive a peripheral intermittent IV lock flush of either saline or heparin after each medication administration, or at least every 24 hours. The IV sites were assessed every 12 hours for signs of phlebitis. The results of the study indicated there were no statistically significant differences in IV lock patency or in phlebitis between heparin or normal saline flushes. The conclusion was that the study provides support for both normal saline and heparin in the doses studied as being equally effective in the maintenance of peripheral IV locks. With the small number of participants, the authors suggest additional studies are needed to determine optimal therapy over time.

*Source:* Niesen, K. M., Harris, D. Y., Parkin, I. S., et al. (2003). The effects of heparin versus normal saline for maintenance of peripheral intravenous locks in pregnant women. *Journal of Obstetric, Gynecologic, Neonatal Nursing, 32*(4), 503–508.

### Procedure

1. Prior to performing the procedure, introduce self and verify the client's identity using agency protocol. Explain to the client what you are going to do, why it is necessary, and how he or she can participate. Explain the reason for the intermittent device and that changing an IV to a heparin or saline lock should cause no discomfort other than that associated with removing tape from the IV tubing.
2. Perform hand hygiene and observe other appropriate infection control procedures.
3. Assist the client to a comfortable position, either sitting or lying. Expose the IV site but provide for client privacy.
4. Assess the IV site and determine the patency of the catheter (see Skill 3.4). If the catheter is not fully patent or there is evidence of phlebitis or infiltration, discontinue the catheter and establish a new IV site.
   - Expose the IV catheter hub and loosen any tape that is holding the IV tubing in place or that will interfere with insertion of the intermittent infusion plug into the catheter.
   - Clamp the IV tubing to stop the flow of IV fluid.
   - Open the gauze pad and place it under the IV catheter hub.
   - Open the alcohol wipe and intermittent infusion cap, leaving the plug in its sterile package.

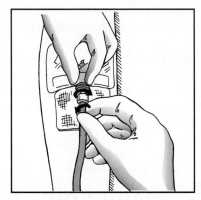

● Separating the IV catheter from the infusion tubing.

5. Remove the IV tubing and insert the intermittent infusion plug into the IV catheter.
   - Apply clean gloves.
   - Stabilize the IV catheter with your nondominant hand and use the little finger to place slight pressure on the vein above the end of the catheter. Twist the IV tubing adapter to loosen it from the IV catheter and remove it.
   - Pick up the intermittent infusion plug from its package and remove the protective sleeve from the male adapter, maintaining its sterility. Insert the plug into the IV catheter, twisting it to seat it firmly or engage the Luer-Lok.

## CLIENT TEACHING CONSIDERATIONS

Teach the client how to maintain the lock.

- Avoid manipulating the catheter or infusion plug and protect it from catching on clothing or bedding. A gauze bandage such as Kerlix or Kling may be wrapped over the plug to protect it when it is not in use.
- Cover the site with an occlusive dressing when showering; avoid immersing the site.
- Flush the catheter with saline or heparin solution as directed.
- Notify the care provider if the plug or catheter comes out: if the site becomes red, inflamed or painful; or if any drainage or bleeding occurs at the site.

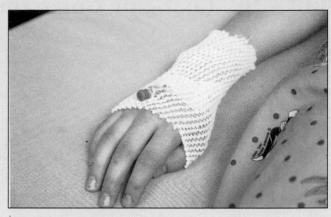

● Intermittent infusion device in place.

6. Instill saline or heparin solution per agency policy. ➤*Rationale: Saline or heparin is used to maintain patency of the IV catheter when fluids are not infusing through the catheter.*

7. Tape the intermittent infusion plug in place using a chevron or U method. ➤*Rationale: Tape provides added security to prevent the infusion plug from coming out of the intravenous catheter. It also promotes comfort, preventing the plug from catching on clothing or bedding.*

## CLINICAL ALERT

If the gauge of the catheter is small, i.e., 22 gauge or smaller, it is possible that you may not get a blood return. This can be due to the collapse of the tip of the catheter as negative pressure is applied when attempting to aspirate blood. This does not always mean that the catheter is occluded. You may attempt to gently inject the saline while feeling for resistance. If any resistance is felt, it is possible that the catheter is occluded and needs to be removed and a new catheter inserted.

## CLINICAL ALERT

Studies indicate that there is no significant difference in the use of saline or heparin to maintain catheter patency, maintain dwell time, and avoid phlebitis. Some hospitals still use a small amount of dilute heparin for flushing peripheral locks; it is usually prepared with 1 mL heparin (1000 units/mL) added to 9 mL normal saline to produce 100 units/mL solution. Prepared heparin for infusion comes in 10 units/mL. Caution should be exercised because heparin-induced thrombocytopenia can occur with as little as 500 units of heparin/day.

8. Access the device to infuse fluids or medication:
   - Cleanse the cap with povidone-iodine or alcohol according to agency policy.
   - Use a threaded lock needleless connector for infusions.
9. Flush the device with prescribed solution after each use or every 8 to 12 hours if not in use, according to agency policy.
10. Remove and discard gloves. Perform hand hygiene.
11. Document relevant information.
    - Record the date and time of converting the infusion device, the status of the IV insertion site, and any adverse responses of the client.

# Skill 3.10 Changing Gown for Client with IV

## Equipment

Clean gown
Bath blanket
Bathing supplies, if needed

## Procedure

1. Check client care plan for infusion drip rate, type of solution, and any special considerations.
2. Perform hand hygiene.
3. Identify client using two descriptors.
4. Take equipment to client's room and explain procedure to client.
5. Untie back of gown, and remove gown from unaffected arm. If available, select gown with snap sleeve closure.
6. Support arm with IV and slip gown down arm to IV tubing.
7. Place clean gown over client's chest and abdomen.
8. Use tubing clamp to slow infusion to "keep open" rate and remove tubing from infusion pump if in use.
9. Remove IV bag from hook and slip sleeve over bag, keeping bag above client's arm. ➤*Rationale: This prevents backflow of blood into tubing. Do not jar or pull tub-ing.* ➤*Rationale: IV tubing may become dislodged and infiltrate into surrounding tissue.*
10. Place your hand up through distal end of clean gown sleeve and grasp IV bag. Pull bag and tubing out through clean gown sleeve.
11. Rehang bag on hook, and check to see that infusion is running according to ordered drip rate.
12. Replace tubing into infusion pump, unclamp and reestablish prescribed infusion flow rate.
13. Guide sleeve of gown up client's arm to shoulder.
14. Assist client to put other arm through remaining sleeve.
15. Tie gown at the back.
16. Check IV infusion rate and IV tubing to determine that solution is flowing unimpeded into client's vein. ➤*Rationale: Kinks in tubing impede solution flow.*
17. Return bed to comfortable position for client.
18. Remove dirty linen from room.
19. Perform hand hygiene.

*Note:* Most facilities provide "IV gowns" that snap from the shoulder down the sleeve of the gown for ease in removal without disturbing the IV.

# Skill 3.11 Discontinuing Infusion Devices

## Delegation

In some states and agencies, removal of a peripheral IV catheter may be delegated to UAP. In others removal of IV infusions or devices is not delegated to UAP. In any case, the nurse must ensure that the UAP knows what complications or adverse signs following removal should be reported to the nurse.

In many states, a licensed practical nurse or licensed vocational nurse with special IV therapy training may discontinue infusions. Check the state's nurse practice act.

## Equipment

- Clean gloves
- Dry or antiseptic-soaked swabs, according to agency practice
- Small sterile dressing and tape

## Procedure

1. Prior to performing the procedure, introduce self and verify the client's identity using agency protocol. Explain to the client what you are going to do, why it is necessary, and how he or she can participate. Explain the reason for discontinuing the IV and that the procedure should cause no discomfort other than that associated with removing the tape.
2. Perform hand hygiene and observe other appropriate infection control procedures.
3. Assist the client to a comfortable position, either sitting or lying. Expose the IV site but provide for client privacy.
4. Prepare the equipment.
   - Clamp the infusion tubing. ➤*Rationale: Clamping the tubing prevents the fluid from flowing out of the needle onto the client or bed.*

- Loosen the tape at the venipuncture site while holding the needle firmly and applying countertraction to the skin. ➤*Rationale: Movement of the needle can injure the vein and cause discomfort to the client. Countertraction prevents pulling the skin and causing discomfort.*
- Apply clean gloves, and hold a sterile gauze above the venipuncture site.

5. Withdraw the needle or catheter from the vein.
   - Withdraw the needle or catheter by pulling it out along the line of the vein. ➤*Rationale: Pulling it out in line with the vein avoids pain and injury to the vein.*

- Immediately apply firm pressure to the site, using sterile gauze, for 2 to 3 minutes. ➤*Rationale: Pressure helps stop the bleeding and prevents hematoma formation.*
- Hold the client's arm or leg above heart level if any bleeding persists. ➤*Rationale: Raising the limb decreases blood flow to the area.*
- Teach the client to inform the nurse if the site begins to bleed at any time or the client notes any other abnormalities in the area.

---

## DEVELOPMENTAL CONSIDERATIONS

### ELDERLY CLIENTS' VEINS ARE FRAGILE AND ROLL EASILY, AND FREQUENTLY THE NEEDLE PUNCTURES THE WALL OF THE VESSEL

- Insert small-gauge winged catheter in distal vein first to preserve proximal vessel.
- Tourniquet (constricting band) may not be necessary for venipuncture. If used, it should be applied loosely.
- If used, release tourniquet as soon as venipuncture yields blood return to prevent excessive pressure in vein.
- Maintain close assessment of IV sites to promote long-term use of vessel.

### ELDERLY CLIENTS ARE PRONE TO FLUID AND ELECTROLYTE DISORDERS AS A RESULT OF THE NORMAL AGING PROCESS

- Thirst mechanism is decreased.
- Renal threshold is altered.
- Total body fluid is less due to decreased lean muscle mass.
- Fluid replacement therapy requires close monitoring to prevent fluid overload, leading to pulmonary edema and electrolyte imbalance.
- Dehydration is a common reason for IV therapy.
- When infusing IV fluids, monitor closely for signs of fluid volume overload.
- Monitor BUN and electrolytes regularly for signs of overload.

- Use IV pump whenever infusing fluids into elderly clients. If dextrose solution is being infused, IV pumps *must* be used. Dextrose overload can lead to cerebrain edema if infused too rapidly.

### STABILIZING IV CATHETER AND DRESSING IS PROBLEMATIC DUE TO CLIENT'S FRAGILE SKIN

- Avoid excessive use of tape.
- Apply skin protector solution before dressing site.
- Use stretch mesh gauze to cover site and tubing to prevent catching on bed (avoid roll-type gauze).

### PROTECT FRAGILE SKIN THAT IS MORE SUSCEPTIBLE TO INJURY, INFILTRATION, AND DISCOMFORT FROM IRRITATING DRUGS

- Observe IV site carefully for signs of infiltration. Because of skin's loose folds and decreased tactile sensation, a large amount of fluid can sequester in subcutaneous tissue and go unnoticed before client complains of pain.
- Check IV site frequently when client receives drugs that can cause irritation and even necrosis if they infiltrate.
- At first sign of phlebitis or infiltration, remove IV and restart in a new site.
- If client complains of discomfort during IV therapy, apply a moist and warm pack to site, decrease rate of fluid infusion.

6. Examine the catheter removed from the client.
   - Check the catheter to make sure it is intact. ➤*Rationale: If a piece of tubing remains in the client's vein, it could move centrally (toward the heart or lungs) and cause serious problems.*
   - Report a broken catheter to the nurse in charge or primary care provider immediately.
   - If the broken piece can be palpated, apply a tourniquet above the insertion site. ➤*Rationale: Application of a tourniquet decreases the possibility of the piece moving until a primary care provider is notified.*

7. Cover the venipuncture site.
   - Apply the sterile dressing. ➤*Rationale: The dressing continues the pressure and covers the open area in the skin, preventing infection.*
   - Remove and discard gloves. Perform hand hygiene.

8. Read the amount remaining in the IV solution container, if infusions are being discontinued, and discard the used supplies appropriately.

9. Document all relevant information.
   - Record the amount of fluid infused on the intake and output record and in the record, according to agency practice. Include the container number, type of solution used, time of discontinuing the infusion, and the client's response.

| UNEXPECTED OUTCOMES | CRITICAL THINKING OPTIONS |
| --- | --- |
| Client develops unexplained fever with chills and rising pulse rate. | • Unexplained fever may be associated with catheter-related sepsis. Report to physician.<br>• Assess IV site for signs of infection.<br>• Ensure that IV solutions hang for no more than 24 hours.<br>• Check client's vital signs: temperature usually above 100°F when caused by IV-related sepsis.<br>• Check for other symptoms of pyrogenic reactions (e.g., backache, headache, malaise, nausea, and vomiting).<br>• Stop the infusion.<br>• Obtain blood specimens, if ordered. |
| IV solution does not flow properly. | • Ensure that the control clamp is open.<br>• Check that blood pressure readings are not taken on arm in which IV is running, as flow is impeded and a clot can form on the end of the needle.<br>• Ensure that IV administration set is properly loaded. Check pump for flow problem indicator (e.g., cassette seating, air in line).<br>• Check IV tubing from insertion site to IV solution for kinks/obstructions.<br>• Check for extremity causing positional obstruction to flow (e.g., elbow bent, arm rotated). |
| IV solution appears to be infiltrating resulting in tissue swelling. | • Decrease the flow rate. (Remove from pump for "keep open" rate.)<br>• Lower bag of IV solution; if blood returns, cannula may be in the vein but fluid may be leaking into surrounding tissue via existing puncture in vein wall.<br>• Discontinue infusion and establish a new site. |
| Phlebitis is suspected at infusion site (tenderness, warmth, erythema, and pain). | • Check infusion solution and medications being administered. (Potassium chloride and hypertonic solutions are particularly irritating to veins.)<br>• Discontinue IV.<br>• Apply warm compress per hospital policy. |
| Postinfusion phlebitis may also occur after the IV has been discontinued in response to either chemical or mechanical factors of the preexisting IV. | • Check IV solution; hypertonic solution causes irritation necessitating use of large veins and changing IV sites more frequently.<br>• Follow hospital policy for treatment. Warm compresses to the site are generally recommended.<br>• Elevate extremity. |

# Skill 3.12 Infusing IV Fluids through a Central Line

## Equipment

Primed IV fluid administration set with needleless Luer-Lok connector
Infusion delivery pump
Antimicrobial swabs
10-mL needleless syringe with 5 mL normal saline solution
CLC 2000 Positive Pressure Cap
Clean gloves

## Preparation

1. Check physician's order sheet and client's Medication Record for IV order.
2. Check IV order with IV solution bag.
3. Take equipment to client's room.
4. Identify client using two descriptors.
5. Explain procedure to client and provide privacy.

> **CLINICAL ALERT**
>
> To minimize pressure on the catheter during injection NEVER use less than a 10-mL syringe for central lines. Smaller syringes increase pressure within the catheter.

## Procedure

1. Perform hand hygiene and don gloves.
2. Hang IV solution on IV stand.
3. Wipe access port with antimicrobial swab and allow to dry.
4. Insert needleless cannula from saline flush syringe and unclamp lumen. (Clamp is not found on PICC lines or Groshong valve catheter).
5. Aspirate for blood return, using very little force, to check for lumen patency and placement.
6. Instill saline solution slowly. The CVD and tubing has a volume of 1–3 mL; therefore, about 5 mL

> **CLINICAL ALERT**
>
> Nontunneled central vascular access devices have the highest infection rate of all types of CVADs; therefore, it is crucial that aseptic techniques be used in all aspects of catheter care.

should be used to thoroughly flush the catheter. ➤*Rationale: To clear lumen of inline dilute heparin.*

7. Maintain positive pressure when withdrawing syringe by clamping catheter before removing syringe or by maintaining pressure on syringe plunger before you clamp or use the CLC 2000 Positive Pressure Cap. ➤*Rationale: This prevents aspiration of blood into lumen and decreases risk of catheter occlusion.*
8. Swab access port again with antimicrobial swabs.
9. Insert IV tubing with Luer-Lok connector into access port. Unclamp lumen.
10. Set electronic device to prescribed rate and begin infusing IV fluids.
11. Ensure central line dressing is clean and intact.
12. Remove gloves and perform hand hygiene.

Positive fluid displacement and positive end-pressure prevent blood reflux into catheter lumen. The device automatically provides the saline flush to prevent clotting of catheter.

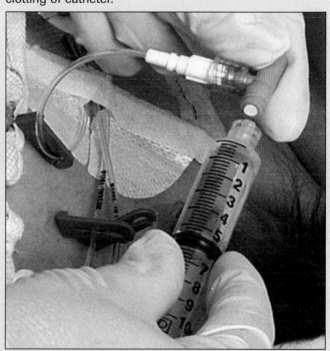

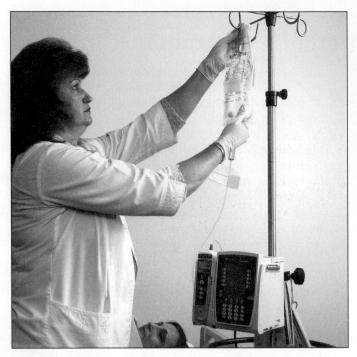

① Hang IV solution on IV stand.

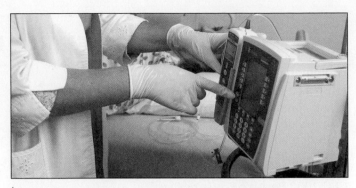

② Attach point-of-care module and program.

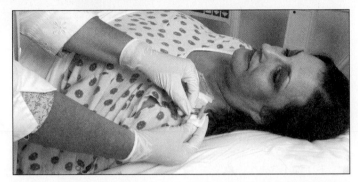

③ Wipe access cap or positive pressure clamp with antimicrobial swab and allow to dry.

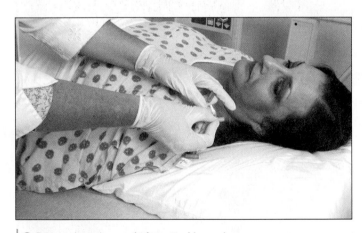

④ Ensure clamp is open before attaching syringe.

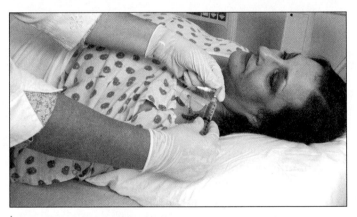

⑤ Attach 10 mL needleless syringe with saline to pressure valve.

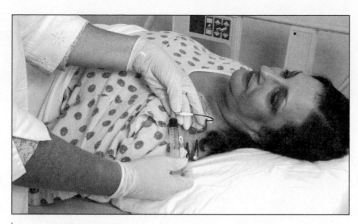

⑥ Aspirate and check for blood return before infusing saline solution.

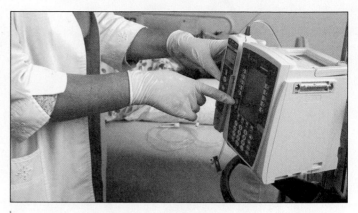

⑦ After connecting IV tubing to catheter, turn on electric device to prescribed use.

# 4

# Infection

Skill 4.1    Hand Hygiene (Medical Asepsis)    157

VARIATION: Using Waterless Antiseptic
Agents (Foam or Gels)    159

Skill 4.2    Latex Precautions    161

Skill 4.3    Donning and Removing Clean Gloves    161

Skill 4.4    Donning and Removing Isolation
Attire    163

Skill 4.5    Using a Mask    165

Skill 4.6    Assessing Vital Signs    166

Skill 4.7    Removing Items from Isolation Room    166

Skill 4.8    Utilizing Double-Bagging for Isolation    167

Skill 4.9    Removing Specimen from Isolation
Room    168

Skill 4.10    Transporting Isolation Client Outside
Room    169

Skill 4.11    Removing Soiled Large Equipment
from Isolation Room    169

Skill 4.12    Performing Surgical Hand
Antisepsis/Scrubs    170

VARIATION: Surgical Hand Antisepsis/
Hand Scrub Using Alcohol-Based
Surgical Hand Rub    172

Skill 4.13    Donning Sterile Gown and Gloves
(Closed Method)    173

Skill 4.14    Preparing the Surgical Site    174

Skill 4.15    Preparing the Client for Surgery    175

Skill 4.16    Pouring from a Sterile Container    178

Skill 4.17    Preparing a Sterile Field Using
Pre-Packaged Supplies    179

Skill 4.18    Preparing for Dressing Change Using
Individual Supplies    179

Skill 4.19    Changing a Sterile Dressing    180

Skill 4.20    Removing Sutures    181

Skill 4.21    Removing Staples    182

Skill 4.22    Preparing for Client Care    183

Skill 4.23    Home Setting: Disposing
of Waste Material    184

Skill 4.24    Home Setting: Caring for
an AIDS or HIV Client    185

Skill 4.25    Home Setting: Teaching
Preventative Measures    185

Skill 4.26    Teaching Safer Practices
to IV Drug Users    186

Planned nursing strategies to reduce the risk of transmission of organisms from one person to another include the use of meticulous asepsis. Asepsis is the freedom from infection or infectious material. There are two basic types of asepsis: medical and surgical. Medical asepsis includes all practices intended to confine a specific microorganism to a specific area, limiting the number, growth, and spread of microorganisms. Surgical asepsis, or sterile technique, refers to those practices that keep an area or objects free of all microorganisms; it includes practices that destroy all microorganisms and spores (microscopic dormant structures formed by some pathogens that are very hardy and often survive common cleaning techniques).

## BASIC MEDICAL ASEPSIS

### EXPECTED OUTCOMES

- Decreased number of bacteria on hands from client to client.
- Delivered care with pathogen-free hands to clients.
- Prevented spread of microorganisms from health care workers or environment to clients.
- Prevented cross-contamination between clients.
- Prevented client-to-client spread of endogenous and exogenous flora.
- Protected hospital personnel from becoming infected.
- Prevented immunosuppressed clients from acquiring nosocomial infections.
- Reduced transference of organisms from hospital environment to clients.

## EVIDENCE-BASED NURSING PRACTICE

**Intervention Improves Handwashing Practice**

After implementing an educational hand hygiene program, researchers found that before the program 51% of all health care workers complied with handwashing guidelines and after the intervention 83% did. For nurses, compliance went up from 56% to 89% after the intervention. The program included a handout that specified how important handwashing is and described the proper technique as well as the CDC's hand hygiene guidelines. Five posters were placed around the nurses' station.

*Source:* Creedon, S. A. (2006). Health care workers' hand decontamination practices: An Irish study. *Clinical Nursing Research*, 15(1), 6.

## Skill 4.1 Hand Hygiene (Medical Asepsis)

### EVIDENCE-BASED NURSING PRACTICE

**Improving Hand Hygiene**

The leading cause of heath care-acquired infections and spread of multiorganisms is inappropriate or inadequate hand hygiene. Nine studies (between 1977 and 2000) demonstrated the impact of hand hygiene on the risk of acquiring infections. One of these studies showed that endemic MRSA was eliminated in 7 months in a neonatal ICU following the introduction of a new hand antiseptic.

*Source:* Webster, J., Faoagil, J., Cartwright, D. (1994). Elimination of MRSA from a neonatal ICU after hand washing with Triclosan. *Journal of Pediatric Child Health*, 30, 59–64.

### Equipment

Nonantimicrobial soap (according to 1997 HICPAC recommendations) for routine handwashing
Orangewood stick for cleaning nails, if available
Running warm water
Paper towels
Trash basket

### Procedure

1. Stand in front of but away from sink. ➤*Rationale: Uniform should not touch sink to avoid contamination.*
2. Ensure that paper towel is hanging down from dispenser.
3. Turn on water using foot pedal or faucet so that flow is adequate, but not splashing.
4. Adjust temperature to warm. ➤*Rationale: Cold does not facilitate sudsing and cleaning; hot is damaging to skin.*

## COMPLIANCE STUDIES FOR HAND HYGIENE

- A study of 2,800 opportunities for handwashing showed only a 48% compliance.
- Another study showed hands were washed only 8.5–9.5 seconds; a minimum of 10–15 seconds is necessary to prevent spread of infection.
- Compliance with handwashing technique is higher among nurses than physicians and other health care personnel; however, it is estimated to be only 30–50%.

*Source:* Centers for Disease Control and Prevention.

## CLINICAL ALERT

Nurses must wash hands for 10–15 seconds before and after each direct contact with a client or each use of client care items to prevent spread of infection.

5. Wet hands under running water. ➤*Rationale: Wet hands facilitate distribution of soap over entire skin surface.*
6. Place a small amount, one to two teaspoons (3–5 mL) of liquid soap on hands. Soap should come from a dispenser, not bar soap. ➤*Rationale: This prevents spread of microorganisms.*
7. Rub vigorously, using a firm, circular motion, while keeping your fingers pointed down, lower than wrists. Start with each finger, then between fingers, then palm and back of hand. ➤*Rationale: This creates friction on all surfaces.*
8. Wash your hands for least 10–15 seconds. ➤*Rationale: Duration of washing is important to produce mechanical action and to allow antimicrobial products time to achieve desired effect.*
9. Clean under your fingernails with an orangewood stick. (This should be done at least at start of day and if hands are heavily contaminated.)
10. Rinse your hands under running water, keeping fingers pointed downward. ➤*Rationale: This position prevents contamination of arms.*

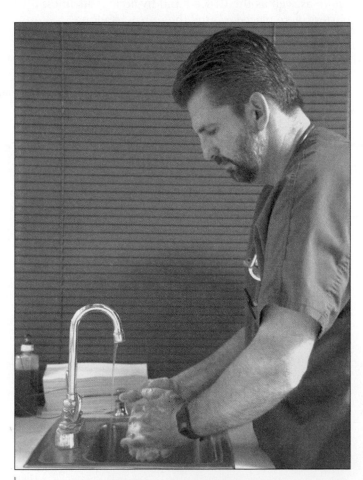

● The single most important nursing action to decrease the incidence of hospital-based infection is washing your hands.

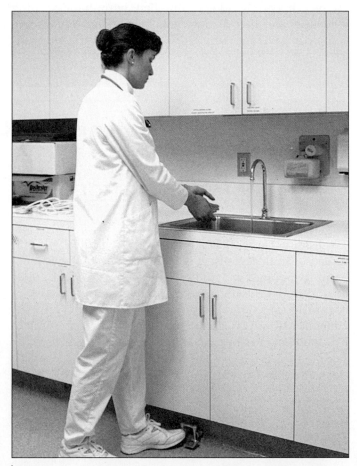

● Use foot pedals when available to prevent contamination of hands.

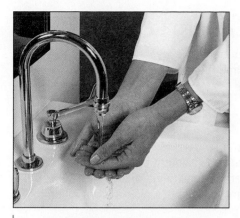

● Wet hands thoroughly before applying soap to facilitate removal of pathogens.

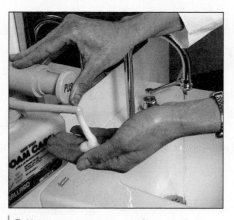

● Use a generous amount of soap and friction during handwashing procedure.

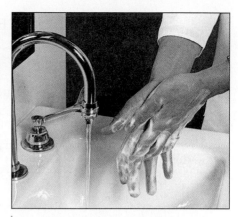

● Keep fingers pointed down during hand-washing to prevent contaminating arms.

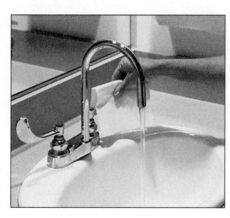

● If foot pedal is not available, turn water faucet off using paper towel.

11. Resoap your hands, rewash, and rerinse if heavily contaminated.
12. Dry hands thoroughly with a paper towel, while keeping hands positioned with fingers pointing up. ➤*Rationale: Moist hands tend to gather more microorganisms from the environment.*
13. Turn off water faucet with dry paper towel, if not using foot pedal. ➤*Rationale: To avoid recontaminating hands.*
14. Restart procedure at step 5 if your hands touch the sink anytime between steps 5 and 13.

## CLINICAL ALERT

CDC Alert: The CDC has stated that health care workers in contact with clients must remove all fake fingernails to maintain infection control principles.

**VARIATION: Using Waterless Antiseptic Agents (Foam or Gels)**

1. Check dirt on hands and use waterless agent only if hands are clean. ➤*Rationale: Hands soiled with dirt or organic matter require soap or detergents that contain antiseptic and water to effectively clean.*
2. Apply small amount of alcohol-based rub, foam, or gel (3–5 mL), on palm or hand.
3. Rub hands together vigorously, covering all surfaces, sides of hands and fingers. ➤*Rationale: Failure to cover all surfaces can leave contaminated areas on the hands.*
4. Rub hands until dry—waterless agent will dry quickly and automatically without using a towel.
5. *Note:* There are now available disposable germicidal wipes that are effective at killing 99.99% of harmful bacteria. These wipes are also effective at removing soil from hands because of natural friction when wiping. The wipes are made from cloth saturated with ethyl alcohol solution, free of fragrance and dye. These products are approved by the EPA for both hepatitis B and viruses.

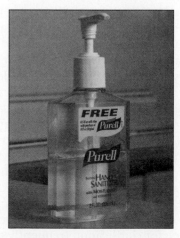

● Waterless hand sanitizer kills 99.9% of the most common germs in 15 seconds.

# EVIDENCE BASED NURSING PRACTICE

## Nail Polish and Microbial Threat

Studies show that chipped nail polish or polish worn more than 4 days is linked to higher microbial load than unpolished or freshly polished nails.

*Source:* Recommended practices for surgical hand antisepsis/hand scrubs. (2004). *AORNJ,* 79(2), 416.

## CLINICAL ALERT

OSHA requires that hands be washed with soap and water every third time the hands are cleansed.

## CLINICAL ALERT

Antimicrobial soap or waterless agent should be used when there is identified resistant bacteria, colonization outbreaks, or hyperendemic infections with the exception of *c. difficile* and *norovirus*, which are not killed by an alcohol-based gel.

| UNEXPECTED OUTCOMES | CRITICAL THINKING OPTIONS |
|---|---|
| Infection occurs in client. | • Assess mode of transmission of microorganism.<br>• Administer antibiotics specific to microorganism as ordered.<br>• Review handwashing technique.<br>• Attend in-service program on infection control procedures.<br>• Notify nurse manager of allergy. |
| Latex allergy identified in health care worker or client. | • Institute latex safety procedures for staff and client (if identified).<br>• Educate staff about latex allergy.<br>• Replace latex-containing objects (particularly gloves) with nonlatex alternatives.<br>• Create a latex-free environment in which those who are allergic can work safely. |

# CULTURAL CONSIDERATIONS

It is imperative that nurses remember the unfamiliar and overwhelming nature of health care settings. Most clients are uncomfortable in a clinical environment, especially when they are undergoing procedures, hearing unfamiliar terminology, and receiving care from people who may be wearing masks and gloves. Imagine if English is not a client's primary language, or if the client is deaf. The challenges to client's psychoemotional and even physical safety increase. When clarity of communication is compromised, therapeutic efficacy and client safety are compromised. It is essential to clarify all aspects of care with clients, and to provide trained interpreters whenever necessary. It is also necessary for members of the health care team to make sure that they themselves understand each other, because English may not be the primary language of every nurse, UAP, physician, or other health care provider. Asking for clarification frequently and not mak-

ing assumptions are two habits that can help prevent clinical care errors. When in doubt ask.

When it comes to cultural diversity, it is especially important to ask the client about nutritional and exercise patterns, health and healing practices, family organization and roles, social support network, spiritual and religious beliefs and practices, communication styles, gender relation patterns, and relationship toward authority. Personal space issues, time orientation, and the client's explanation of his or her health status are also important to explore.

For essential resources regarding cultural considerations in health care environments, search the web for Culturally and Linguistically Appropriate Services (CLAS) for health care settings. *Holistic Nursing: A Handbook for Clinical Practice* (Fossey, Keegan & Guzzetta 2005) also includes resources and cultural assessments for nurses to incorporate into their admissions and clinical care processes.

# Skill 4.2 Latex Precautions

## Equipment

- Latex-free gloves, syringes, and IV ports on IV bags/lines
- Latex-free bellows on ventilator
- Latex-free bags on masks
- Stockinette and latex-free tape
- Medications and equipment for treatment of anaphylactic reaction

## Preparation

1. Reduce and/or eliminate the amount of latex used in agencies by eliminating use of latex gloves where feasible as well as reducing the amount of other latex products used; when latex gloves are used, they should be nonpowdered. ➤*Rationale: Powder in latex gloves contains latex which is spread into the environment when the gloves are donned.*
2. Identify latex-free materials and supplies in the agency.
3. Be aware of signs of latex sensitivity.
4. Assess all patients for a history of latex allergy or significant risk factors.
5. Be prepared for emergency resuscitation if needed.

## Procedure

1. When patients are identified as latex sensitive or allergic, prepare the environment before their entry and continue practices as long as they remain.
2. Remove all latex-containing products (gloves, tourniquets, tape, etc.) from the room. If latex products cannot be removed, the items should be located in a closed storage area, such as cabinets and drawers.
3. After removing latex items, thoroughly clean the room/exam area using latex-free (nitrile or vinyl) gloves to remove contaminated latex-containing dust. Do not wear latex or rubber gloves to clean the room. When an allergic individual has surgery or other procedure, the room should be properly prepared and the case should be the first of the day.
4. Mattresses/exam tables may contain latex and should be covered completely with a nonlatex protective cover.
5. Stock rooms with latex-free material and latex-free gloves.
6. Place a latex precaution sign on the patient's door/exam area.
7. Place all monitoring devices and cord/tubes (oximeter, blood pressure, electrocardiograph wires, ports on intravenous tubing) in stockinette, and tape with nonlatex tape to prevent direct skin contact. Items sterilized in ethylene oxide must be rinsed before use. Residual ethylene oxide can cause an allergic response in a latex-allergic patient.
8. Use stopcocks to inject drugs rather than latex ports.
9. Label the patient's medical record, medication form, and identification bands with allergy alerts.
10. Document measures taken.
11. Report promptly and document any signs of sensitivity or allergy.
12. Teach patients and families about latex allergy and how to avoid latex products.
13. Instruct the family about foods that commonly cause allergies in those with latex allergy, and avoid feeding them to the patient. They include bananas, avocados, kiwis, plums, peaches, cherries, apricots, figs, papayas, tomatoes, potatoes, and chestnuts.

# Skill 4.3 Donning and Removing Clean Gloves

## EVIDENCE-BASED NURSING PRACTICE

### The Effectiveness of Gloves

Numerous studies have proven the effectiveness of gloves in preventing contamination of health care worker's hands. One study found that those who wore gloves during client contact had contaminated hands with an average bacterial count of 3/minute of client care compared to a count of 6/minute for those not wearing gloves.

*Source:* Pitlet, D., et al. (1999). Bacterial contamination of the hands of hospital staff during routine client care. *Archives of Internal Medicine, 159,* 821–826.

### The Importance of Wearing Gloves in Client Care

This study demonstrated that nurses doing "clean" activities such as lifting clients; taking blood pressure, pulse, or oral temperatures; or even touching a client could contaminate their hands with a bacterial count of 100 to 1,000 CFU of *Klebsiella* during such a procedure.

*Source:* Caswell, M., Phillips, I. (1997). Hands as route of transmission for *Klebsiella* species. *British Medical Journal, 2,* 1315–1317.

## Equipment

Clean gloves
Trash receptacle

## Procedure

1. Complete hand hygiene. ➤*Rationale: Donning gloves with unclean hands can transfer microorganisms outside gloves.*
2. Remove glove from glove receptacle.
3. Hold glove at wrist edge and slip fingers into openings. Pull glove up to wrist.
4. Place gloved hand under wrist edge of second glove and slip fingers into opening.
5. Remove glove by pulling off, touching only outside of glove at cuff, so that glove turns inside out.
6. Place rolled-up glove in palm of second hand.
7. Remove second glove by slipping one finger under glove edge and pulling down and off so that glove turns inside out. Both gloves are removed as a unit.
8. Dispose of gloves in proper container, not at bedside.
9. Complete hand hygiene.

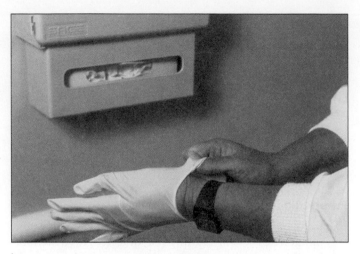

❸ Hold glove at wrist edge and slip fingers into openings. Pull glove up

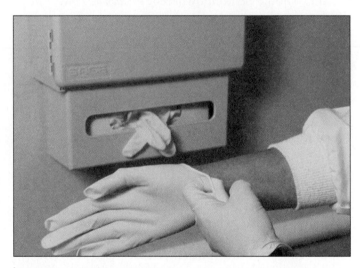

❹ Place gloved hand under wrist edge of second glove and slip fingers into opening.

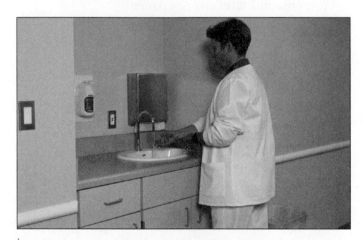

❶ Wash your hands or complete hand hygiene.

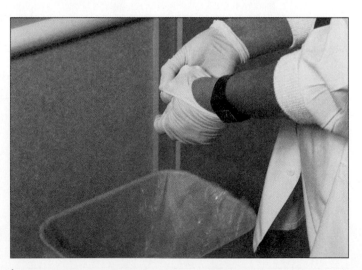

❺ Remove glove by pulling off. Touch only outside of glove at cuff, so that glove turns inside out.

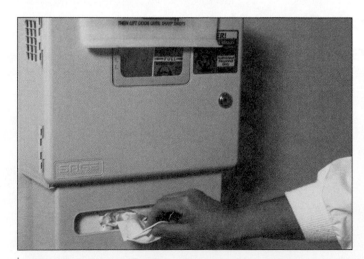

❷ Remove glove from dispenser.

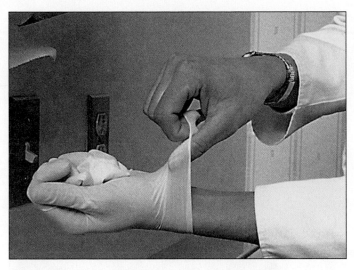

⑥ Place rolled-up glove in palm of second hand. Remove second glove by slipping one finger under glove edge and pulling down and off so that glove turns inside out. Both gloves are removed as a unit.

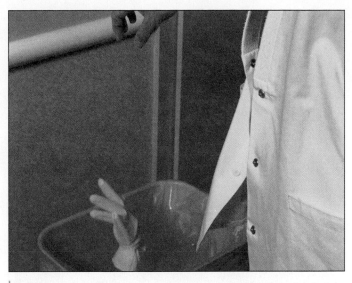

⑦ Dispose of gloves in proper container, not at bedside. Complete hand hygiene.

## CLINICAL ALERT

Ungloved hands should not touch anything that is moist coming from a body surface. The moisture coming from a body surface should be considered potentially contaminated.

# Skill 4.4 Donning and Removing Isolation Attire

## Equipment

Gown
Clean gloves

## Procedure (for Donning Attire)

1. Complete hand hygiene.
2. Take gown from isolation cart or cupboard. Put on a new gown each time you enter an isolation room.
3. Hold gown so that opening is in back when you are wearing the gown.
4. Put gown on by placing one arm at a time through sleeves. Pull gown up and over your shoulders.
5. Wrap gown around your back, tying strings at your neck.
6. Wrap gown around your waist, making sure your back is completely covered. Tie strings around your waist.
7. Don eye shield and/or mask, if indicated. ➤*Rationale: Mask is required if there is a risk of splashing fluids.*
8. Don clean gloves and pull gloves over gown wristlets. ➤*Rationale: Prevents contamination of exposed skin.*

*Note:* Hospital policy in the United States may require staff to use plastic aprons instead of long-sleeved gowns for isolation protocol. This alternative is acceptable for infection control as long as gloves are worn, skin on arms is intact, and rigorous handwashing includes the arms.

## Procedure (for Removing Attire)

1. Untie gown waist strings.
2. Remove gloves and dispose of them in garbage bag.
3. Next, untie neck strings, bringing them around your shoulders so that gown is partially off your shoulders.
4. Using your dominant hand and grasping clean part of wristlet, pull sleeve wristlet over your nondominant hand to pull sleeve wristlet over your dominant hand.
5. Grasp outside of gown through the sleeves at shoulders. Pull gown down over your arms.
6. Hold both gown shoulders in one hand. Carefully draw your other hand out of gown, turning arm of gown inside out. Repeat this procedure with your other arm.

7. Hold gown away from your body. Fold gown up inside out.
8. Discard gown in appropriate place.
9. Remove eye shield and/or mask and place in receptacle.
10. Complete hand hygiene. ➤*Rationale: This prevents cross-infection to other clients.*

## CLINICAL ALERT

Some isolation gowns do not tie at the neck. They skip over the head. When removing these gowns, pull shoulders forward to loosen the Velcro at the neck area. Remove gown in the same manner as you would if tied at the neck.

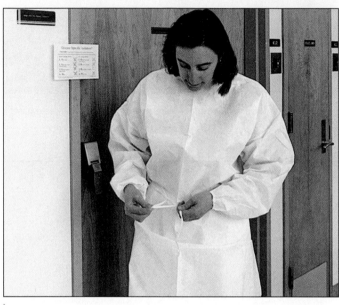

❶ Donning: Isolation gown is put on before mask, eye shield, or gloves.

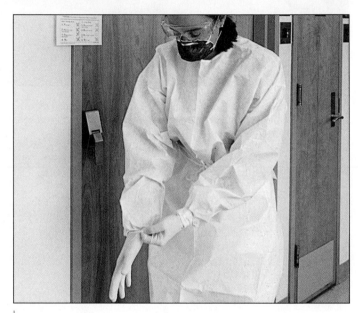

❷ Donning: Cover wristlets completely to prevent contamination of exposed skin.

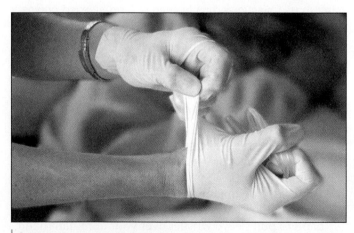

❶ Removing: Remove gloves before gown, mask, or eye shield.

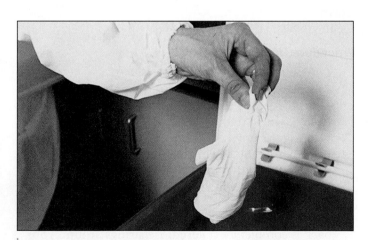

❷ Removing: Dispose of gloves in appropriate receptacle.

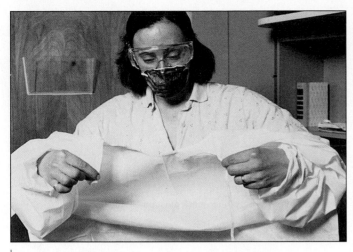

❸ Removing: Pull gown off shoulders, then down over arms.

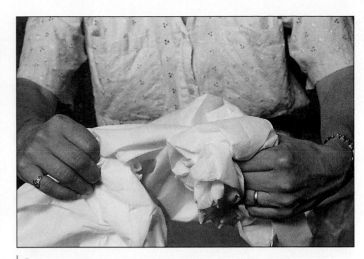

❹ Removing: Hold gown away from body when rolling inside out.

## CARE SETTINGS

- All aspects of standard precautions apply equally in the clinic, home, or long-term care setting.
- Ensure that the supply of gloves, gowns, masks, and eyewear is adequate.
- Ensure that procedures are in place for removal and disposal of used materials.
- Teach the client and family appropriate aspects of standard precautions.

## PEDIATRIC CONSIDERATIONS

Isolation precautions can increase an already stressful situation for a hospitalized child. Younger children have limited cognitive abilities to understand the implications of isolation. Particularly frightening for them is the presence of people in gowns and masks. To help decrease their fears, preparation is important. Letting the children see and play with the equipment lessens some of the anxiety. Health care workers should introduce themselves to the child before donning a mask. Frequent visits to the child can also lessen the fear and loneliness associated with isolation.

# Skill 4.5   Using a Mask

### Equipment

Clean mask

### Procedure

1. Obtain mask from box.
2. Position mask to cover your nose and mouth.
3. Bend nose bar so that it conforms over bridge of your nose.
4. If you are using a mask with string ties, tie top strings on top of your head to prevent slipping. If you are using a cone-shaped mask, tie top strings over your ears.
5. Tie bottom strings around your neck to secure mask over your mouth. There should be no gaps between the mask and your face.

## CLINICAL ALERT

Respiratory N95 or HEPA (high-efficiency particulate air) masks are recommended for suspected or confirmed multidrug-resistant tuberculosis.

- Masks are fitted to worker.
- Wear mask until it becomes difficult to breathe. This indicates mask is clogged.
- When not in use, store mask in zip-lock bag in safe area.
- Masks are expensive and can be used repeatedly until it is difficult to breathe through them.

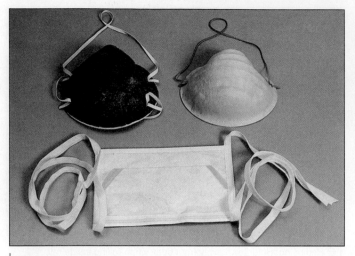

● Sample masks used for isolation protocol.

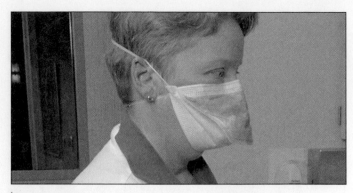

● Particulate filter respirator mask must be airtight.

---

## CLINICAL ALERT

Protective eyewear such as goggles and face shields are worn when there is a risk of splashes or sprays from blood, secretions, excretions, or body fluids. Eyewear is removed before taking off mask.

---

6. *Important:* Change mask every 30 minutes or sooner if it becomes damp. ➤*Rationale: Effectiveness is greatly reduced after 30 minutes or if mask is moist.*
7. Complete hand hygiene before removing mask.
8. To remove mask, untie lower strings first, or slip elastic band off without touching mask. ➤*Rationale: Only strings are considered clean.*
9. Discard mask in a trash container.
10. Complete hand hygiene.

---

# Skill 4.6    Assessing Vital Signs

## Equipment

Thermometer
Stethoscope
Blood pressure cuff and sphygmomanometer
Thermometer stand
Watch with sweep second hand
Isolation clothing

## Procedure

1. Complete hand hygiene and use two forms of client ID.

2. Don isolation clothing as required by type of isolation.
3. Proceed to take vital signs as you would for any client.
4. Place equipment in appropriate area if it is to be left in room. Follow appropriate protocol to remove equipment from isolation room.
5. Remove isolation clothing according to protocol.
6. Complete hand hygiene.
7. Wipe watch if accidentally contaminated. Use appropriate solution.

---

# Skill 4.7    Removing Items from Isolation Room

## Equipment

Large red isolation bags
Specimen container
Plastic bag with biohazard label
Laundry bag
Red plastic container for sharps
Cleaning articles

## Procedure

1. Place laboratory specimen in biohazard plastic bag.
2. Dispose of all sharps in appropriate red plastic container in room.
3. Place all linen in linen bag.
4. Place reusable equipment such as procedure trays in plastic bags. ➤*Rationale: Appropriate separation of*

*equipment from isolation room alerts central supply staff that it is contaminated and special handling needs to be carried out.*

5. Dispose of all garbage in plastic bags.
6. Double bag all material from isolation room. Follow procedure for Utilizing Double-Bagging for Isolation. ➤*Rationale: All material removed from an isolation room is potentially contaminated. This will prevent spread of microorganisms.*

7. Replace all bags, such as linen bag and garbage bag, in appropriate container in room.
8. Clean client's room as necessary, using germicidal solution, according to facility protocol.
9. Prepare to leave the client's room.

# Skill 4.8 Utilizing Double-Bagging for Isolation

**Equipment**

Two isolation bags
Items to be removed from room
Gloves

**Procedure**

1. Follow dress protocol for entering isolation room, or, if you are already in the isolation room, continue with Step 2.
2. Close isolation bag when it is one-half to three-fourths full. Close bag inside the isolation room.
3. Double bag for safety if outside of bag is contaminated, if the bag could be easily penetrated, or if contaminated material in the bag is heavy and could break bag.
4. Set up a new bag for continued use inside room. Bag is usually red with the word "Biohazard" written on outside of bag.
5. Place bag from inside room into a bag held open by a second health care worker outside room if double-bagging is required. Second health care worker makes a cuff with the top of the bag and places hands under cuff. ➤*Rationale: This prevents hands from becoming contaminated.*
6. Place bag into second bag without contaminating outside of the bag. Secure top of bag by tying a knot in top of bag.
7. Take bag to designated area where biohazard material is collected, usually "dirty" utility room.
8. Remove gloves and complete hand hygiene.

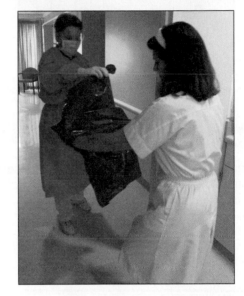

● Place bag from inside room into bag held open from outside room.

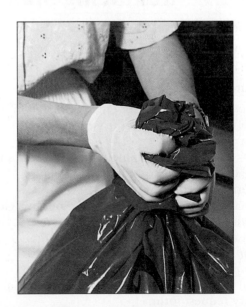

● Close bag securely and label contents, if necessary.

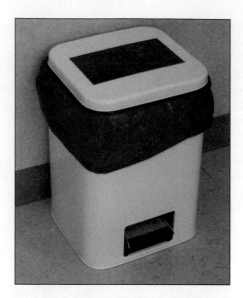

● Set up new biohazard bag for continued use in client's room.

## CLINICAL ALERT

Linen and burnable trash are disposed of in same manner. Ensure that when placing bags in containers in "dirty" utility room you place in correct container according to bag contents.

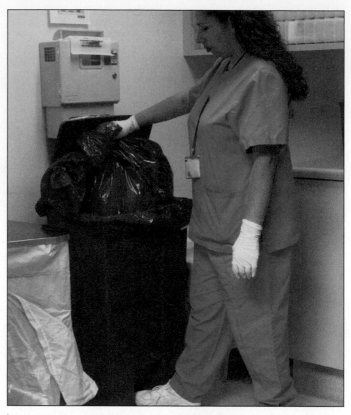

● Place red biohazard bag in specified area for disposal.

# Skill 4.9   Removing Specimen from Isolation Room

## Equipment

Specimen container
Clean biohazard bag

## Procedure

1. Follow dress protocol for entering isolation room, or, if you are already in the isolation room, continue with Step 2.
2. Mark a specimen container with the client's name, type of specimen, and the word "isolation" before entering an isolation room.
3. Collect specimen, and place container in a clean plastic biohazard bag outside the room. ➤*Rationale: Use clear bags so that laboratory personnel can see the specimen easily.*
4. Complete hand hygiene.
5. Send specimen to laboratory with appropriate laboratory request form.

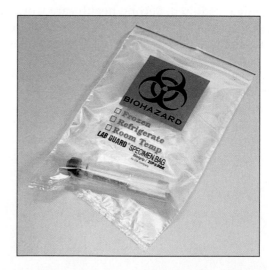

● Biohazard bag for transportation of specimens from isolation room.

# Skill 4.10   Transporting Isolation Client Outside Room

## Equipment

Transport vehicle
Bath blanket
Mask for client if needed

## Procedure

1. Explain procedure to client.
2. If client is being transported from a respiratory isolation room, instruct him or her to wear a mask for the entire time out of isolation. ➤*Rationale: This prevents the spread of airborne microbes.*
3. Cover the transport vehicle with a bath blanket if there is a chance of soiling when transporting a client who has a draining wound or diarrhea.
4. Help client into transport vehicle. Cover client with a bath blanket.
5. Tell receiving department what type of isolation client needs and what precautions hospital personnel should follow.
6. Remove bath blanket, and handle as contaminated linen when client returns to room.

7. Instruct all hospital personnel to complete hand hygiene before they leave the area.
8. Wipe down transportation vehicle with an antimicrobial solution if soiled.

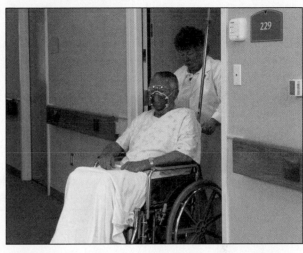

● Place surgical mask on client if he needs to be transported outside room.

# Skill 4.11   Removing Soiled Large Equipment from Isolation Room

## Equipment

Antimicrobial agent and articles needed to wash
  equipment
Plastic bag

## Procedure

1. Don isolation garb as recommended.
2. Wash equipment with an antimicrobial agent.
   ➤*Rationale: Washing is preferred to spraying in order to ensure all surfaces are cleaned.*
3. Cover equipment with a plastic bag.
4. Remove garb, and complete hand hygiene outside the room. Take equipment to the decontamination area of CSR.

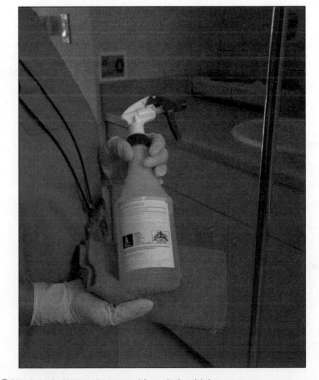

● Wash isolation equipment with antimicrobial agent.

---

### PROTOCOL FOR LEAVING ISOLATION ROOM

Untie gown at waist.

Take off gloves.

Untie gown at neck.

Pull gown off and place in laundry hamper.

Take off goggles or face shield.

Take off mask.

Complete hand hygiene.

## GUIDELINES FOR DISPOSING OF CONTAMINATED EQUIPMENT

- **Disposable glass:** Place in isolation bag separate from burnable trash and direct to appropriate hospital area for disposal.
- **Glass equipment:** Bag separately from metal equipment and return to CSR.
- **Metal equipment:** Bag all equipment together, label, and return to CSR.
- **Rubber and plastic items:** Bag items separately and return to CSR for gas sterilization.
- **Dishes:** Require no special precautions unless contaminated with infected material; then bag, label, and return to kitchen.
- **Plastic or paper dishes:** Dispose of these items in burnable trash.
- **Soiled linens:** Place in laundry bag, and send to separate area of laundry room for special care. If possible, place linens in hot-water–soluble bag. This method is

safer for handling, as bag may be placed directly into washing machine. (Double-bagging is usually required because these bags are easily punctured or torn. They also dissolve when wet.)

- **Food and liquids:** Dispose of these items by putting them in the toilet—flush thoroughly.
- **Needles and syringes:** Do not recap needles; place in puncture-resistant container.
- **Sphygmomanometer and stethoscope:** Require no special precautions unless they are contaminated. If contaminated, disinfect using the appropriate cleaning protocol based on the infective agent.
- **Thermometers:** Dispose of electronic probe cover with burnable trash. If probe or machine is contaminated, clean with appropriate disinfectant for infective agent. If reusable thermometers are used, disinfect with appropriate solution.

# BASIC SURGICAL TECHNIQUE

## Skill 4.12    Performing Surgical Hand Antisepsis/Scrubs

### Delegation

Surgical hand antisepsis/scrub is performed by a perioperative nurse or RNFA. It can be, however, delegated to a UAP or LVN/LPN in some agencies. The AORN believes that individuals who are not licensed to practice professional nursing and who perform in the role of scrub person are performing a delegated technical function under the supervision of a perioperative registered nurse (AORN, 2007, p. 407).

### Equipment

- Deep sink with foot, knee, or elbow controls
- Antimicrobial solution
- Nail-cleaning tool, such as a file or orange stick
- Surgical scrub brush
- Sterile towels for drying the hands

### Preparation

- Ensure that all of the surgical garb is in place (i.e., shoe covers; cap, which should completely cover all the hair; face mask; and protective eyewear).

### Procedure

1. Prepare for the surgical hand antisepsis/scrub.
   - Remove wristwatch, bracelets, and all rings. Ensure that fingernails are trimmed. ➤*Rationale: Jewelry and long finger-*

*nails harbor microorganisms. Removal of jewelry permits full skin contact with the antimicrobial agent.*

   - Turn on the water, using either the foot, knee, or elbow control, and adjust the temperature to lukewarm. ➤*Rationale: Warm water removes less protective oil from the skin than hot water. Soap irritates the skin more when hot water is used.*

2. Wash hands.
   - Wet the hands and forearms under running water, holding the hands above the level of the elbows so that the water runs from the fingertips to the elbows. ➤*Rationale: The hands will become cleaner than the elbows. The water should run from the least contaminated to the most contaminated area.*
   - Apply 2 to 4mL (1tsp) antimicrobial solution to the hands.
   - Use firm, rubbing, and circular movements to wash the palms and backs of the hands, the wrists, and the forearms. Interlace the fingers and thumbs, and move the hands back and forth. Continue washing for 20 to 25 seconds. ➤*Rationale: Circular strokes clean most effectively, and rubbing ensures a thorough and mechanical cleaning action. (Other areas of the hands still need to be cleaned, however.)*
   - Hold the hands and arms under the running water to rinse thoroughly, keeping the hands higher than the elbows. ➤*Rationale: The nurse rinses from the cleanest to the least clean area.*

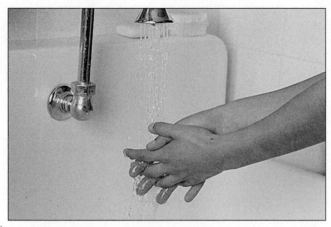

❶ Interlacing the fingers during hand washing.

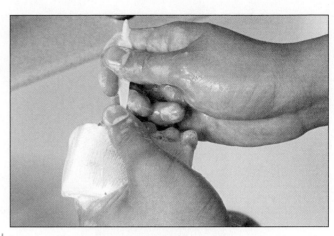

❸ Cleaning the fingernails.

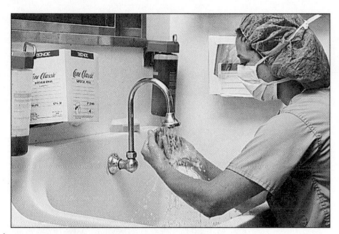

❷ Rinse hands and arms, letting water run from the fingertips to the elbows.

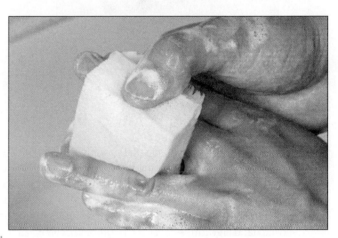

❹ Scrubbing side of finger.

- Check the nails, and clean them with a file or orange stick if necessary. Rinse the nail tool after each nail is cleaned. ➤*Rationale: Sediment under the nails is removed more readily when the hands are moist. Rinsing the nail tool after cleaning each nail prevents the transmission of sediment from one nail to another.*

3. Perform surgical hand antisepsis/scrub (with brush/sponge).
   - Apply antimicrobial agent to wet hands and forearms and lather hands again. Using a scrub brush or sponge, scrub each hand. Visualize each finger and hand as having four sides. Wash all four sides effectively. Repeat this process for opposite fingers and hand (AORN, 2004). ➤*Rationale: Scrubbing loosens bacteria, including those in the creases of the hands.*
   - Using the scrub brush or sponge, scrub from the wrists to 5 cm (2 in.) above each elbow. Visualize each arm as having four sides. Using agency protocol (e.g., scrubbing by number of strokes or length of time), wash all parts of the arms: lower forearm, upper forearm, and antecubital space

to marginal area above elbows. Continue to hold the hands higher than the elbows. ➤*Rationale: Scrubbing thus proceeds from the cleanest area (hands) to the least clean area (upper arm).*
   - Discard the scrub brush or sponge.
   - Rinse hands and arms thoroughly so that the water flows from the hands to the elbows. ➤*Rationale: Rinsing removes resident and transient bacteria and sediment.*
   - Avoid splashing water onto surgical attire. ➤*Rationale: A sterile gown put over wet or damp surgical attire would be considered contaminated.*
   - If a longer scrub is required, use a second brush and scrub each hand and arm with the antimicrobial agent for the recommended time.
   - Discard second brush, and rinse hands and arms thoroughly.
   - Turn off the water with the foot or knee pedal.
   - Keeping hands elevated and away from the body, enter the operating room by backing into the room. ➤*Rationale: This position of the hands maintains the cleanliness of the hands and backing into the room prevents accidental contamination.*

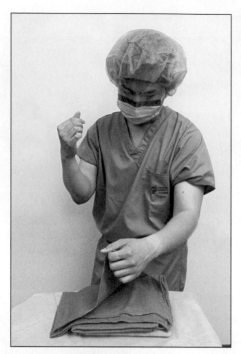

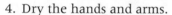 Picking up sterile towel to dry hands and arms.

4. Dry the hands and arms.
  - Use a sterile towel to dry one hand thoroughly from the fingers to the elbow. Use a rotating motion. Use a second sterile towel to dry the second hand in the same manner. In some agencies, towels are of a sufficient size that one half can be used to dry one hand and arm and the second half for the second hand and arm. ➤*Rationale: The nurse dries the hands (the cleanest area) to the least clean area. Using a new towel or the opposite end of a towel prevents the transfer of microorganisms from one elbow (least clean area) to the other hand (cleanest area).*
  - Discard the towel(s).
  - Keep the hands in front and above the waist. ➤*Rationale: This position maintains the cleanliness of the hands and prevents accidental contamination.*

## VARIATION: Surgical Hand Antisepsis/Hand Scrub Using Alcohol-Based Surgical Hand Rub

- Prepare for the surgical hand antisepsis/scrub and wash hands (see steps 1 and 2 above).
- Dry hands and forearms thoroughly with a paper towel.
- Follow the manufacturer's directions for use of the brushless surgical hand antisepsis product. Following is an example of how to use one brushless product. Note, however, that many products are available and it is imperative to use a product according to the manufacturer's guidelines. ➤*Rationale: Following the manufacturer's guidelines helps ensure effective surgical hand antisepsis, which is needed to prevent surgical site infections.*

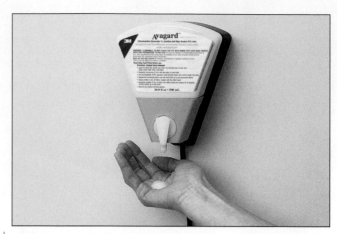

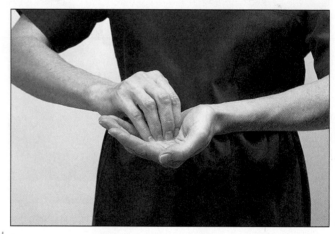 Dispensing hand rub.
Courtesy 3M.

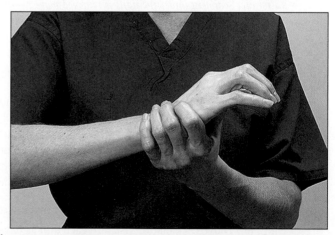 Dip fingers into hand *prep*.
Courtesy 3M.

 Reapply hand rub to both hands up to wrists.
Courtesy 3M.

- Using a foot pump, dispense one pump (2 mL) of the surgical hand rub product into the palm of one hand. ➤*Rationale: A foot pump avoids contamination of the hands.*
- Dip fingertips of the opposite hand into the hand-rub product and work under fingernails. Spread remaining hand-rub product over the hand and up to just above the elbow.

- Dispense another pump (2 mL) of the surgical hand-run product into the palm of the opposite hand and repeat procedure.
- Dispense a final pump (2 mL) of hand-rub product into either hand and reapply to all aspects of both hands up to the wrists.
- Rub thoroughly until dry. Do not use towels.

# Skill 4.13   Donning Sterile Gown and Gloves (Closed Method)

## Delegation

- Applying a sterile gown and sterile gloves is performed by a perioperative nurse or RNFA. It can be, however, delegated to a UAP or LVN/LPN in some agencies. A UAP often assists the RN or RNFA or scrub person by preparing the sterile pack containing the sterile gown and gloves.

## Equipment

- Sterile pack containing a sterile gown and sterile gloves

## Preparation

- Ensure the sterility of the sterile pack.

## Procedure

1. Perform surgical hand antisepsis/scrub.

### Applying a Sterile Gown

1. Apply the sterile gown.
   - Grasp the sterile gown at the crease near the neck, hold it away from you, and permit it to unfold freely without touching anything, including the uniform. ➤*Rationale: The gown will not be sterile if its outer surface touches any unsterile objects.*
   - Put the hands inside the shoulders of the gown without touching the outside of the gown.
   - Work the hands down the sleeves only to the beginning of the cuffs.
   - Have a coworker wearing a hair cover and mask reach inside arm seams and pull gown over shoulders.
   - Coworker grasps the neck ties without touching the outside of the gown and pulls the gown upward to cover the neckline of the scrub person's uniform in front and back.

### Apply Sterile Gloves (Closed Method)

1. Open the sterile glove wrapper while the hands are still covered by the sleeves.
2. Put the glove on the nondominant hand.
   - With the dominant hand, pick up the opposite glove with the thumb and index finger, handling it through the sleeve.

- Position the dominant hand palm upward inside the sleeve. Lay the glove on the opposite gown cuff, thumbside down, with the glove opening pointed toward the fingers.
- Use the nondominant hand to grasp the cuff of the glove through the gown cuff, and firmly anchor it.
- With the dominant hand working through its sleeve, grasp the upper side of the glove's cuff, and stretch it over the cuff of the gown.
- Pull the sleeve up to draw the cuff over the wrist as you extend the fingers of the nondominant hand into the glove's fingers.
3. Put the glove on the dominant hand.
   - Place the fingers of the gloved hand under the cuff of the remaining glove.
   - Place the glove over the cuff of the second sleeve.
   - Extend the fingers into the glove as you pull the glove up over the cuff.

### Completion of Gowning

1. Complete gowning as follows.
   - Have a coworker hold the waist tie of your gown, using sterile gloves or a sterile forceps or drape. ➤*Rationale: This approach keeps the ties sterile.*
   - Make a three-quarter turn, then take the tie and secure it in front of the gown.
     *or*
   - Have a coworker take the two ties at each side of the gown and tie them at the back of the gown, making sure that the scrub person's uniform is completely covered.
   - When worn, sterile gowns should be considered *sterile* in front from the waist to the shoulder. Once the nurse approaches a table, the gown is considered contaminated from the waist or table down, whichever is higher. The sleeves should be considered sterile from the cuff to 5 cm (2 in.) above the elbow, since the arms of a scrubbed person must move across a sterile field. Moisture collection and friction areas such as the neckline, shoulders, underarms, back, and sleeve cuffs should be considered unsterile.

# Skill 4.14  Preparing the Surgical Site

## Equipment

Absorbent pad
Bath blanket or drape
Scissors or electric clippers (optional)
Disposable prep kit (for shaving)
If kit not available:
Disposable razor (number according to area to be shaved)
2 sterile bowls
4 × 4 gauze pads
Emesis basin
Applicator sticks
Cleansing solution
Sterile water
Clean gloves
Depilatory
Antiseptic solution
Tongue blade
4 × 4 gauze pad

## Procedure

1. Refer to physician's orders for specific operative site or area to be prepared. If orders do not state preference for site, refer to procedure manual for appropriate area to be prepared, based on surgical procedure.

> *Note:* Many surgeons do not require hair to be shaved for a surgical site unless it interferes with the surgical procedure or wound closure. Based on clinical research, it has been found that shaving the hair does not prevent surgical site infections, but it does interfere with the client's psychological status. Client's body image can be impaired and he or she senses a loss of control with shaving of the hair, particularly of the head or pubic area.

2. Determine type of preparation to be done: clipping of hair, shaving site, or hair removal using depilatory. Gather equipment.
3. Check two forms of client ID and introduce yourself.
4. Explain procedure to client, and provide privacy.
5. Adjust light to ensure good visualization.
6. Perform hand hygiene.
7. Position client for maximum comfort and site exposure.
8. Drape client for comfort and to prevent undue exposure.
9. Protect bed with absorbent pad.
10. Arrange equipment for your convenience.
11. Put on clean gloves.

## EVIDENCE-BASED NURSING PRACTICE

**Surgical Site Infection (SSI)**

A preoperative antiseptic shower or bath decreases skin microbial colony count. In a study of over 700 clients who received two preoperative antiseptic showers, chlorhexidine reduced bacterial colony counts ninefold. Iodine or triclocarban-medicated soap reduced colony counts 1.3- to 1.9-fold, respectively.

Chlorhexidine gluconate—containing products require several applications to obtain maximum antimicrobial benefit, so repeated antiseptic showers are indicated. Even though these showers reduce the colony count, they have not definitively shown a reduction in SSI rate.

*Source:* Mangram, A. J., et al. (1999). The Hospital Infection Control Practices Advisory Committee. Infection Control and Hospital Epidemiology, 20(4), 247–280.

12. Assess surgical site before skin preparation for moles, warts, rash, and other skin conditions.
    ➤*Rationale: Inadvertent removal of lesions traumatizes skin and may contribute to infection.*

*Note:* CDC standards indicate that clients are to shower or bathe with an antiseptic agent at least the night before surgery. The FDA has also shown that antimicrobial activity of the antiseptic agent prevents skin infections.

13. Prepare site using scissors or clippers according to facility policy/procedures.
    a. Use scissors or electric clippers and cut hair 1 cm above surgical site or according to facility policies.
    b. Clip small amount of hair each time.
    c. Cut in direction hair grows.
    d. Remove all hair from site, and discard.
14. Prepare site using depilatory.
    a. Clip hair before applying cream.
    b. Apply cream to designated area using tongue blade or gloved hand.
    c. Leave on skin for designated time, according to directions on package, usually 10 minutes.
    d. Remove cream by rubbing off with tongue blade or moistened 4 × 4 gauze pads.
    e. Wash skin with antiseptic soap; dry area thoroughly.
    f. Remove all hair with washing. ➤*Rationale: This provides clean, smooth skin, free of abrasions and cuts.*

15. Prepare site using razor.
    a. Lather skin with antiseptic soap and 4 × 4 gauze pads. ➤*Rationale: Wet shave results in fewer microabrasions to the skin. Shaving should be done in direction of hair growth.*
    b. Discard soiled sponges frequently.
    c. Using sharp razor, shave hair moving away from incision site. With free hand, stretch skin taut and shave, following the hair growth pattern and using firm, steady strokes. Shave small area at one time. ➤*Rationale: Shave is closer and nicks are prevented.*
    d. Change razor as often as necessary. Avoid nicking the skin. Report if skin is nicked. ➤*Rationale: Nicks, if severe, can cause infection by bacteria normally found on the skin.*
    e. Wash all hair off site with 4 × 4 gauze pads or use sticky mitt or tape to remove hair.
    f. The shave should be completed close to the time of surgery. The shave prep is completed before the client enters the operating room. ➤*Rationale: Shaving and clipping hair immediately before surgery is associated with a lower risk of infection than if done the night before.*
16. After removing hair, apply antiseptic solution with 4 × 4 pads or use disposable prep kit.
17. Begin at incision site and, with light friction, make ever-widening circles, moving outward from the center to the most distant line of area. ➤*Rationale: Working from most clean to least clean area prevents contamination. Scrub area for 2–3 minutes.*
18. Rinse area with warm water and blot dry with 4 × 4 gauze pads.
19. Remove and dispose of equipment; scissors and razors are disposed of in sharps container.
20. Remove gloves, and discard.
21. Perform hand hygiene.
22. Assist client to put on clean gown.
23. Position the client for comfort.

## EVIDENCE-BASED NURSING PRACTICE

**Skin Preparation and Surgical Site Infections**

Many studies show that hair removal with a razor or clippers can cause skin abrasion, or even nicks in the skin. This can lead to subsequent surgical site infections (SSIs). In a study discussed in the CDC Guideline for Prevention of Surgical Site Infection, it was identified that SSIs occurred in 5.6% of clients who had their hair removed by razor shave, compared to an 0.6% rate among those who had hair removed by depilatory, or had no hair removed at all. The CDC advises that if hair is to be removed, it should be done so immediately before surgery, and preferably with electric hair clippers.

*Source:* Mangram, A. J. (1999). Hospital Infection Control Practices Advisory Committee. *Infection Control and Hospital Epidemiology*, 29(4), 247–280.

### CLINICAL ALERT

If hair must be removed, scissors or clippers should be used and procedure completed before the client reaches the operating room suite. Many hospitals use the minimal shave and scrub preparation approach. The shaved area may be as small as 2 cm surrounding the surgical incision site. Refer to the policy and procedure manual and physician's orders before beginning the surgical prep.

### CLINICAL ALERT

Electric or battery powered clippers are preferred to razors to prevent skin irritation and microscopic cuts to the skin. Clippers must have a disposable head that is changed between clients. Handles should be disinfected.

# Skill 4.15   Preparing the Client for Surgery

**Equipment**

Preoperative checklist
Operative permit
Specific equipment needed to provide physical care as ordered, such as enema equipment, nasogastric tube, Foley catheter
Antiseptic agent for shower

**Procedure**

1. Check two forms of client ID and introduce yourself.
2. Obtain client's signature on surgical consent form and check agency policy. Ensure all preoperative forms are complete, with no blank areas.
3. Assist client to complete anesthesia questionnaire if required.

## CLINICAL ALERT

The Association of PeriOperative Registered Nurses (AORN) recommends preop skin prep should be an antimicrobial agent that has a broad germicidal range and is non-toxic.

The most common antiseptic agents used for preoperative skin preparation and surgical scrubs include alcohol, chlorhexidine, iodine/iodophors, and Triclosan.

**Alcohol** has the most rapid microbial action, which denatures proteins and is effective against both gram-positive and gram-negative bacteria, viruses, and fungi.

**Chlorhexidine** has an intermediate rapidity of action, disrupting the cell membrane. It should not be used on mucous membranes, eyes, or brain tissue (neurotoxic). It works well against gram-positive bacteria, and less well against gram-negative bacteria.

**Iodine/iodophors** has an intermediate action and is acceptable for use against a wide range of bacteria, fungi, and viruses.

**Triclosan** disrupts the cell wall and has an acceptable kill rate against bacteria. Even though alcohol has microbial action, it is not often used as a surgical skin prep because it does not stay on the skin.

## LEGAL ALERT

In 2001 JCAHO reported surgical mistakes were on the rise. After this report a study was completed. The study analyzed 126 cases involving surgical mistakes and found 76% of the cases involved operating on the wrong body part, 13% involved the wrong client, and 11% involved the wrong surgical procedure.

*Source:* http://Medical Malpractice Lawyers.us.

13. Remove earrings, necklaces, medals, watch, rings (ring may be taped to finger or toe in some facilities). If possible, remove body piercing jewelry. Cover with tape if not possible to remove. ➤*Rationale: Protect skin from possible burns from electrical arcing generated by electrical cautery machines.*
14. Remove contact lenses, glasses, hairpieces, and dentures. Some hospitals/anesthesiologists allow full dentures to remain if using a mask.

4. Assess if bowel prep was completed at home. ➤*Rationale: Most clients complete bowel prep before admission to facility. Administer an enema if ordered.*
5. Assist client to shower if not completed at home. Instruct on how to shower and specific time guidelines according to facility guidelines.
6. Complete skin prep, if ordered. Follow facility guidelines for skin prep.
7. Assess for latex allergy. If present, ensure allergy band is applied, physician is notified, and OR staff personnel are notified. ➤*Rationale: All latex products must be removed from OR and client must be scheduled for first case in morning.*
8. Enquire for symptoms and observe for signs of cold or upper respiratory infection.
9. Explain need for client to be NPO for 8–10 hours preoperatively.
10. Remove lipstick and nail polish if required by hospital policy.
11. Insert Foley catheter if ordered.
12. Take and record vital signs.

Surgical preoperative checklist.

● Surgical consent form.

● Preanesthesia evaluation form.

# CLINICAL ALERT

## Universal Protocol for Preventing Wrong Site, Wrong Procedure, and Wrong Person Surgery

- Pre-operative validation of the right client, procedure, and site should occur when the client is awake, aware, and before he/she leaves the preoperative area of enters the surgical suite.

- Person performing the procedure must do the marking.

- Incision site must be marked, using a marker that is not easily removed, at or near the incision site.

- DO NOT MARK any non-operative site(s) unless necessary for some other aspect of care.

- Use initials, word "yes" or a line indicating proposed incision site to prevent ambiguous marks.

- Mark must be visible after client is prepped and draped.

- Final verification of site mark must take place in the location where the procedure will take place. This time is identified as the "Time Out" period. Nothing happens until this has occurred. The entire team must be present during this check.

- Verification must include
  a. Correct client identity.
  b. Correct site and side.
  c. Agreement on procedure to be done.
  d. Correct client position.
  e. Availability of any special equipment or implants needed for procedure.

## Exemptions from Marking Procedure

- Single organ cases: e.g., C-section, cardiac surgery.

- Interventional cases: insertion site of instrument/catheter not pre-determined.

- Premature infants: for whom the mark may cause permanent mark.

*Source:* www.jcaho.org/accredited+organizations/patient 2003.

15. Assist client to void if catheter not inserted, and record time and amount.
16. Check identaband, blood band, and allergy bracelet. During this stage the client must be identified by at least two identifiers (i.e., medical record number, birth date, name, charge number).
17. Put antiembolic stockings on client as ordered.
18. Administer preoperative medications.
19. The operative site needs to be verified and marked, both site and side, by the physician while the client is awake.
20. Place side rails in UP position and bed in low position following administration of medications.
21. Darken room, and provide quiet environment following administration of medications.
22. Check client 15 minutes after medication administered to observe for possible side effects.

# Skill 4.16   Pouring from a Sterile Container

## Equipment

Sterile container
Nonsterile container
Sterile solution

## Procedure

1. Perform hand hygiene.
2. Gather equipment.
3. Open sterile container according to procedure.
4. Place container on firm surface.
5. Take cap off the bottle and invert the cap before laying on firm surface. ▶*Rationale: This keeps the cap sterile.*
6. Hold the bottle with the label facing up.
7. Pour a small amount of liquid into a nonsterile container. ▶*Rationale: This action cleans the lip of the bottle.*
8. Pour the liquid into the sterile container while keeping the label facing up and not touching the container with the bottle. Do not reach over a sterile field if the container has been placed on one.
   ▶*Rationale: Crossing over a sterile field can lead to contamination of the field.*
9. Replace the cap if liquid remains in the bottle. If total contents have been used, dispose of bottle in trash.
10. Date and initial bottle if reusing.
11. Replace partially filled bottle to storage area if it is to be reused.

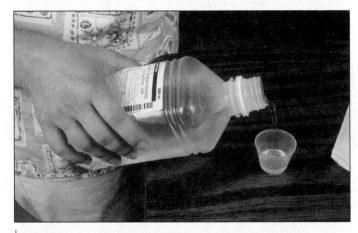

● First pour a small amount of liquid into nonsterile container.

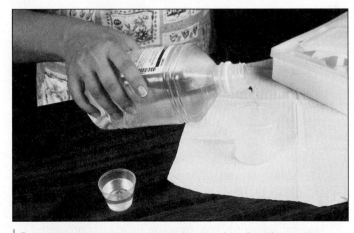

● Pour liquid by placing container close to edge of sterile area.

# Skill 4.17  Preparing a Sterile Field Using Pre-Packaged Supplies

## Equipment

Packaged supplies

## Procedure

1. Perform hand hygiene.
2. Ensure working surface is clean and dry. Client's over-bed table is frequently used as preparation area. ➤*Rationale: This prevents contamination of sterile package.*
3. Remove outer plastic wrap.
4. Place package in center of work area and position so that you first open package flap away from you. ➤*Rationale: This prevents reaching across the sterile field as you continue to open package.*

5. Grasp edge of the first flap of the wrapper, move it away from you, and place it on the working surface.
6. Grasp the first side flap, lift it up; grasp the second side flap and together move both hands out toward the sides. Place the flaps down on the working surface.
7. Grasp the last flap of the wrapper and open it toward you, taking care not to touch the inside of the flap or any of the contents of the package. ➤*Rationale: This prevents contamination of the supplies.*

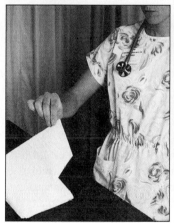

● Grasp edge of top flap of wrapper and lift it away from you.

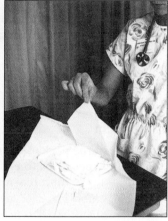

● Open last flap toward you—do not cross over sterile field.

# Skill 4.18  Preparing for Dressing Change Using Individual Supplies

## Equipment

Antiseptic cleaner or cleaning solution
Number and type of dressings needed (i.e., 4 × 4 gauze pads, ABD pads, application sticks, transparent dressings)
Tape
Clean gloves
Sterile gloves
Disposal bag
Mask, if needed

## Procedure

1. Perform hand hygiene.
2. Clean off bedside stand and wash thoroughly with antiseptic solution. Dry thoroughly.
3. Place supply packages on table in configuration that allows you to open packages without reaching over sterile field. ➤*Rationale: Reaching over sterile field will contaminate supplies.*
4. Grasp cover of 4 × 4 pad plastic container and pull flap back and away from sterile area. Place cover in disposal bag.

5. Grasp edge of transparent dressings package, peel back top covering. Place open package on work surface. Do not cross over any open supply packages.
6. Continue to open all supplies using above steps.

7. Pour solution over pads in plastic container, if ordered.
8. Open sterile gloves. Place in position on table where you do not pass over a sterile field.

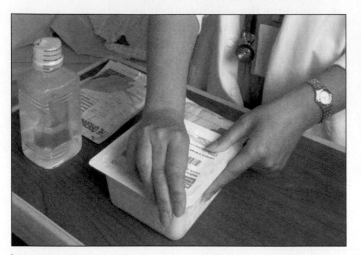

● Open sterile 4 × 4 pads container by pulling back on flap.

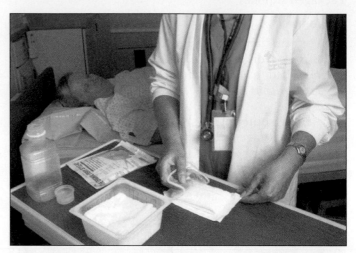

● Open transparent dressing packet.

# Skill 4.19   Changing a Sterile Dressing

## Equipment

Sterile gloves
Clean gloves
Mask
Gown
Disposal bag for used dressings
Dressing supplies, as needed
Micropore tape
Sterile normal saline, optional
Package sterile cotton swabs, or 4 × 4 pads
Bath blanket or sheet

## Preparation

1. Check physician's orders and client care plan.
2. Perform hand hygiene.
3. Gather equipment.
4. Identify the client, and explain procedure.
5. Provide privacy.
6. Clean off over-bed table.
7. Place sterile supplies on over-bed table.
8. Raise bed to HIGH position, and lower side rails, if appropriate.
9. Place bag for soiled dressings near incision site.
10. Fanfold linen to expose incision area.
11. Cover client with bath blanket or sheet, leaving incision area exposed.

12. Open sterile packages, and place on over-bed table. Arrange packages to ensure you don't cross over the sterile field when reaching for dressings. ➤*Rationale: Commercially prepared sterile packages can be opened and used for the sterile field because the inside of the package is sterile.*
13. Cut tape into appropriate length strips.

## Procedure

1. Remove tape slowly by pulling tape toward the wound. ➤*Rationale: Pulling toward the wound decreases the pain of tape removal by not putting pressure on the incision line.*
2. Don clean gloves.
3. Remove soiled dressings, and dispose of in the proper bag. Wet dressing with sterile normal saline if it adheres to the suture line.
4. Assess incision area for erythema, edema, or drainage. ➤*Rationale: Persistent drainage, edema, or temperature above 100.4°F 2 days post-op indicates a complication is occurring.*
5. Assess color of incision. (A healing incision looks pink or red.) ➤*Rationale: Redness that does not fade 48 hours after surgery may indicate impaired healing.*
6. Remove clean gloves, and discard.
7. Move over-bed table next to working area.
8. Don sterile gloves.

9. Cleanse incision area with sterile swabs or 4 × 4 pads soaked in normal saline, according to hospital policy. Cleanse from incision line outward, cleaning from top to bottom, using the swab only once. Discard swabs or 4 × 4 pads in disposal bag. ➤*Rationale: Cleaning outward from incision cleans from least to most contaminated area. Cleaning from top to bottom prevents contamination from secretions that accumulate at the bottom of the wound.*

10. Place 4 × 4 gauze pads over incision area, being careful not to touch incision or client with your gloves. ➤*Rationale: Touching the incision or client contaminates the gloves. You need to reglove if this occurs.*

11. Place abdominal pad over incision, being careful not to contaminate the gloves.

12. Remove gloves and discard.

13. Tape dressing securely.

14. Discard trash in appropriate receptacle.

15. Lower bed and raise side rails. Position client for comfort.

16. Perform hand hygiene.

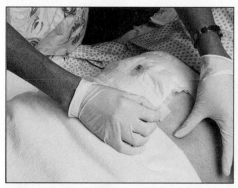
❶ Remove tape by gently lifting toward wound.

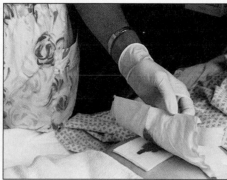
❷ Remove soiled dressing carefully.

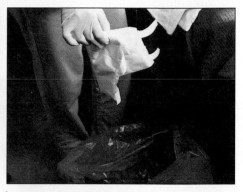
❸ Dispose of dressing in appropriate container.

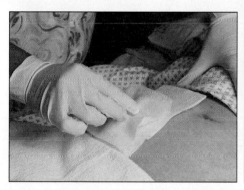
❹ Do not touch incision when applying dressing.

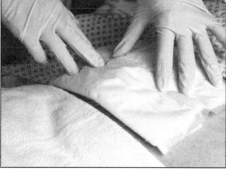
❺ Place abdominal pad over center of incision.

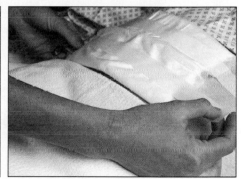
❻ Tape dressing securely to prevent slipping.

# Skill 4.20   Removing Sutures

## Equipment

Sterile suture removal set
Antiseptic solution
Tape
Butterfly tape
Paper bag for disposal of dressings
Two pair clean gloves (1 pair optional)

## Procedure

1. Gather equipment.
2. Perform hand hygiene and don clean gloves.
3. Remove dressing and discard in disposal bag. (Discard gloves only if soiled.)
4. Open suture removal set, and don gloves if second pair needed.
5. Pick up forceps with nondominant hand.
6. Grasp suture at the knot with forceps and lift away from skin.
7. Pick up suture scissors with dominant hand.
8. Place curved tip of suture scissors under suture, next to knot.

9. Cut suture, and with forceps, pull suture through skin with one movement.
10. Discard suture into disposal bag.
11. Check that entire suture is removed.
12. Continue to remove remaining sutures according to hospital policy. Some policies state that every other suture is removed and then remaining sutures are removed at a later time. ➤*Rationale: This prevents wound dehiscence.*
13. Cleanse suture site with antiseptic solution.
14. Remove gloves, and place in disposal bag.
15. Place dressing or butterfly tape over incision area, if ordered.
16. Discard disposal bag into contaminated waste container.
17. Perform hand hygiene.

> ### TOPICAL GLUE FOR WOUND CLOSURE
>
> A new product to replace sutures and staples (estimated at 80–90 million procedures annually) was approved by the FDA after proving itself in clinical trials. This super-glue is called Dermabond. It is a synthetic, noninvasive glue that mitigates trauma and post-procedure inflammation while providing a waterproof seal and protecting underlying tissue without the need for bandages. Dermabond is also painless, fast and simple to apply, and naturally sloughs off in 7–10 days.

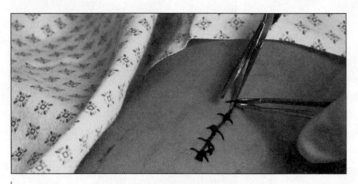

● Grasp suture at the knot with forceps and lift away from skin.

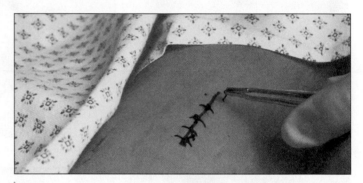

● After cutting suture, grasp suture at knot and pull through skin.

# Skill 4.21 Removing Staples

### Equipment

Sterile staple remover
Disposal bag
Two pair clean gloves (1 pair optional)
Dressings
Tape or butterfly tape
Antiseptic solution

### Procedure

1. Gather equipment, and open sterile staple remover.
2. Perform hand hygiene and don clean gloves.
3. Remove dressing, and discard in disposal bag. (Discard gloves only if soiled.)
4. Don gloves if necessary.
5. Place lower tip of staple remover under staple.
6. Press handles together to depress center of staple.
7. Lift staple remover upward, away from incision site when both ends of staple are visible.
8. Place staple removal device over disposal bag and release handles to release staple.

> ### DISCHARGE CLIENT TEACHING
>
> - Instruct client to eat foods high in protein, carbohydrates, vitamins, and minerals to promote wound healing.
> - Splint wound when coughing or moving from chair or bed to prevent separation of wound edges.
> - Provide list of signs and symptoms of wound infection or delayed healing. Include when to notify physician.
> - Encourage use of daily showers; water may run over wound.
> - Instruct not to use soap, lotions, or vitamin creams on incision.
> - Instruct in dressing change procedure.
> - Instruct to not lift heavy objects (anything over 10 pounds).
> - Instruct in measures to promote elimination.

9. Remove all staples or as directed by hospital policy. Some policies indicate every other staple is removed with remaining staples done at a later time.
   ➤*Rationale: To prevent wound dehiscence.*
10. Cleanse incision area with antiseptic solution if ordered.
11. Remove gloves, and place in disposal bag.
12. Place dressing over incision and secure with tape, or place butterfly tape over incision.
13. Discard disposal bag in contaminated waste container.
14. Perform hand hygiene.

### Home Setting

In the home setting, medical asepsis, or clean technique, is often used instead of sterile technique. The major reasons for this protocol change are the nature of the setting and the personnel providing care.

The greatest infection control problem in hospitals is nosocomial infections due to the large numbers of antibiotic-resistant organisms present in a hospital setting. Although people are able to survive in what may be considered a less-than-desirable environment without acquiring infections, they would not be protected or possess the acquired immunity to the bacteria in a hospital setting.

When clients are in their own environment, however, they tend to develop fewer infections because they are subjected to fewer organisms. In the home setting, focus is on protecting home care staff and family, not other clients. There is minimal data on the incidence of home care acquired infections. Infection preventing strategies in the home should focus on IV therapy, urinary tract, respiratory and wound care.

Nevertheless, sterile technique and equipment, such as prepackaged catheter and irrigation kits, parenteral fluid equipment, and dressings, are often purchased for home care. When sterile technique is required, it is the responsibility of the nurse to provide the instruction and evaluate the family's ability to perform the skill accurately. Hospital techniques may need to be modified for the home setting, and ideal environmental working conditions may not be present. Therefore, adaptations must be made, but the essential infection control measures must be maintained.

Just as in the hospital, effective hand hygiene is the most effective means of infection control in the home setting. There is one major difference between hospital and home. Equipment (soap, running water, and paper towels) that is readily available to the nurse in the hospital may not be available in the home. Even if running water is available, there may not be soap or clean towels. The nurse must carry handwashing supplies with her or him.

According to the *Home Healthcare Nurse Journal* (Feb. 2000, "Improving Infection Control in Home Care: From Ritual to Science-Based Practice"), many of the home care infection control practices have been based on ritual, rather than scientific principles. Many changes in infection control procedures in the home are occurring based on a scientific approach.

If the home care client is suspected of or diagnosed as having an infectious disease or the client is infected or colonized with VRE or MSRA, the nurse should use the same personal protective equipment and protocol used in the hospital setting. The equipment includes gloves, disposable gown or apron, mask, cap, and goggles. Reusable equipment, such as stethoscopes and blood pressure cuffs, should stay in the home and not be used on other home care clients. If possible, these clients should be seen at the end of the day.

# Skill 4.22  Preparing for Client Care

### Equipment

Community health nursing bag
Liquid soap
Antibacterial gel for hand hygiene
Disposable gloves
Disposable apron or gown
Goggles
Masks, air-purifying mask
Thermometers (oral and rectal)
Thermometer sheaths
NexTemp (disposable thermometer)

Vaseline or lubricant
Cotton balls
Alcohol, one small bottle
Antimicrobial wipes
Cotton-tipped applicators
Tongue depressors
Sterile 4 × 4s
Band-Aids
Bandage scissors
Nonallergic tape
Plastic bags with ties

Ketodiastix and chemstrips
Sphygmomanometer
Stethoscope
Paper cups
Bleach, one small bottle

### Procedure

1. Arrange equipment in bag prior to making home visit so that hand hygiene equipment is accessible. Bring only the supplies needed. ➤*Rationale: This procedure decreases the possibility of cross-contamination.*

2. Place bag on flat, dry surface to establish a clean work area during visit. Use of disposable barrier under bag is recommended.

3. Perform hand hygiene.
   a. Use liquid soap and paper towels from bag and client's water supply; or
   b. Use antimicrobial gel as alternative for handwashing when soap and water are not available. Squeeze small amount of germicide onto palm of hand and rub for 30 seconds along all surfaces of hands, fingers, and nails. Germicide evaporates into air, making towels unnecessary.

4. Don disposable gloves when appropriate for infection control, especially when handling blood and body fluids.

5. Take other equipment that will be needed during the visit out of the bag and place on clean work surface.

6. Keep bag closed when not in use to promote cleanliness, safety, and security. Care should be taken not to reenter bag wearing soiled gloves. Washing hands between reentering bag is not necessary unless soiled.

> ### CLINICAL ALERT
>
> If item is soiled and cannot be returned to the bag, place in separate container for transport to agency. Clean item when it is returned to agency. Most items for home care are disposable.

7. Wear disposable apron or gown, goggles, or masks if necessary. ➤*Rationale: This protects the caregiver from blood or body fluid exposure.*

8. Cleanse thoroughly any equipment that left clean area and is to be returned to the bag on completing care.
   a. Rinse equipment (such as bandage scissors, forceps) under cold water, wash with soap and water. Use client's personal equipment or disposable equipment whenever possible.
   b. Return stethoscope and blood pressure cuff to nursing bag. ➤*Rationale: Clean items can be returned to nursing bag if no visible soiling.*

9. Ensure nursing bag is monitored regularly for safety.
   a. Keep bag out of reach of children.
   b. Keep bag in trunk of car or keep in your home overnight. ➤*Rationale: Unattended bags in cars are more often stolen.*
   c. Clean bag monthly and prn.

> By California state mandate, mercury thermometers are confiscated by home health nurses. Clients are given digital thermometers.

# Skill 4.23   Home Setting: Disposing of Waste Material

### Equipment

Plastic bags, heavy duty
Disposable gloves
Receptacle, rigid and puncture-proof
Bleach
Germicide

### Procedure

1. Dispose of wastes contaminated with blood or body fluids.
   a. Place waste products in impenetrable, heavy-duty plastic bag.
   b. Remove plastic gloves by rolling inside out (so contaminated side is on inside) and drop into plastic bag.
   c. Seal plastic bag with tie.
   d. Discard in client's trash.
   e. Perform hand hygiene with soap and water or germicide.

> ### CLINICAL ALERT
>
> All items contaminated with blood, exudates, or other body fluids should be considered to present a risk of transmission of HIV or hepatitis B. These items should be disposed of by incineration if possible. Use mechanisms for disposal of waste into normal trash only when incineration is not available.

2. Dispose of body wastes, such as urine, feces, respiratory secretions, vomitus, and blood, by flushing them down the toilet. (This is true whether the toilet empties into a septic tank or a sewage system.)

3. Dispose of needles and sharp objects.
   a. Do not remove needle from syringe or bend, break, clip, or recap after use.

b. Drop entire disposable safety syringe intact into rigid, puncture-proof receptacle provided by agency.
c. Wash hands.
4. Discard other trash.
   a. Place in plastic bag.
   b. Discard in client's trash.

*Note:* Clothes and bedding do not need to be destroyed. They are laundered separately in hot water with a 10% bleach solution added to the detergent in the washer.

# Skill 4.24  Home Setting: Caring for an AIDS or HIV Client

**Equipment**

Gloves
Disposable mask, gown, or apron
Protective eyewear
Specimen container if needed
Plastic bag for transport of specimen
Chlorine bleach solution (Clorox)

**Procedure**

1. Perform hand hygiene before and after client care and after disposing of soiled materials.
2. Don disposable gloves for any procedure.
   a. Don double gloves if tearing is likely during the procedure.
   b. If staff member has any type of open wound or weeping dermatitis, she or he should not administer care (even with gloves) until condition is resolved.
3. Don disposable gown or apron to protect clothing from soilage.
4. Put on mask and protective eyewear if splattering is anticipated during the procedure (e.g., suctioning, wound irrigations).
5. Collect specimens in appropriate containers. Place in plastic sealable biohazard bags.
6. Use extraordinary care to avoid puncture wounds with needles and other sharp objects.
   a. If puncture occurs, bleed wound and wash with soap and water.
   b. Notify supervisor immediately, and fill out unusual occurrence report.
7. Transport all specimens in an impermeable container, keeping the container separate from nurse's bag and supplies.
8. Clean spills of blood and body fluids with 10% bleach solution (one part liquid chlorine bleach to nine parts water). Make solution fresh each visit.
9. Wash eating utensils (dishes and silverware) in hot soapy water. Water should be hot enough to need gloves to tolerate the temperature. No other special precautions are required. It is best to use a dishwasher, if available. It is not necessary to wash client's dishes separately.
10. Store linens and laundry soiled with body fluids in a plastic bag and then wash separately with very hot water. Use a detergent and a 10% bleach solution. (Nonchlorine bleaches such as Clorox II are acceptable for colored clothing.)
11. Dispose of gown or apron in plastic bag after completing care.
12. Take off gloves by peeling them down and turning them inside out so that contaminated side is on the inside. Place in plastic bag.
13. Perform hand hygiene.
14. Take off mask and goggles.
15. Perform hand hygiene.

# Skill 4.25  Home Setting: Teaching Preventative Measures

**Procedure**

1. Discuss the inadvisability of allowing any person who is ill or who has depressed immune function to come in contact with the client.
2. Teach the client these appropriate hygiene principles:
   a. Wash hands after use of toilet or contact with any body fluids.
   b. Do not share thermometers, razors, razor blades, toothbrushes, douche, or enema equipment.
   c. Do not cough without covering mouth.
   d. Be careful to dispose of nasal secretions in tissue, then in plastic bags.

3. Teach these guidelines for sharing kitchens and bathrooms:
   a. Good household cleaning practices prevent spread of infection.
   b. Don't share eating and drinking utensils. After use, they must be cleaned with hot water (hot enough to necessitate use of gloves) and soap. Use of a dishwasher and soap is appropriate.
   c. Kitchen and bathroom surfaces should be cleaned every day with scouring powder or with chlorine bleach solution (10%, one part bleach to nine parts water). Use disposable bathroom cups. Use covered individual toothbrush holders.
   d. Clean refrigerators regularly with soap and water; remove old food to prevent mold.
   e. Mop floors in bathroom and kitchen weekly. Pour dirty water down the toilet and disinfect with bleach solution.
   f. Clean toilet, tub, and shower weekly or as often as necessary with 10% bleach solution. If urine or diarrhea spills on toilet or floor, wipe immediately with the 10% bleach solution.
   g. Sponges used to clean floors or body fluid spills should be soaked for 5 minutes in a 10% bleach solution.
4. Teach the following principles of food preparation:
   a. Discuss the fact that people infected with HIV may prepare food for others. They should follow usual practices for safe food preparation and be especially diligent about handwashing.
   b. Wash hands thoroughly before any food preparation.
   c. Do not lick fingers or taste from the mixing spoon while cooking.
   d. Avoid unpasteurized milk (danger of contact with Salmonella); do not eat old or moldy food (danger of food poisoning); and carefully wash and thoroughly cook chicken.
   e. Wash all fresh (raw) fruits and vegetables before eating.
5. Teach how to care for linens and laundry.
   a. When clothing or linen is soiled with blood or body fluids, it should be stored separately in a plastic bag. Wash separately with very hot water, detergent, and bleach. Use Clorox II for colored clothing.
   b. Wear disposable gloves when touching soiled clothes or linen.
   c. Do not share used towels or washcloths, and wash separately. (Towels and washcloths are, however, safe to use after washing.)
   d. Change towels and washcloths daily.
6. Inform client and family of measures for disposing of trash.
   a. Flush body wastes down the toilet.
   b. Discard dressings, diapers, Chux, or any materials soiled with secretions in a plastic bag. Discard into the regular trash.
   c. Sharp items (e.g., razors, needles) should be placed in a rigid, puncture-proof container with a solution of 10% bleach. Incinerate when container is full. Pharmacies collect the used containers in some areas.
7. Discuss procedures for caring for pets.
   a. Clean birdcages wearing gloves. Birds can spread psittacosis (*Chlamydia psittaci*) or *Cryptococcus*.
   b. Clean cat litter boxes wearing gloves to prevent spread of toxoplasmosis.
   c. Tropical fish tanks should not be cleaned by the person with AIDS to prevent spread of *Mycobacterium*.
8. Teach general principles of preventing cross-infection.
   a. Wear gloves when handling body fluids, linens, or other objects contaminated with body fluids.
   b. Disposable gowns or aprons protect clothing from becoming soiled.
   c. Caregivers should not provide care when ill themselves. If this is not possible they should wear a mask when in close contact with the person with AIDS. AIDS clients are very susceptible to infections.
   d. Maintain adequate ventilation in the living quarters.
9. Medical supplies should be kept in a clean, dry location. If refrigeration is required, place medications in sealed plastic storage bag.

# Skill 4.26   Teaching Safer Practices to IV Drug Users

**Procedure**

1. Inform persons of risk behaviors and factors associated with IV drug use.
   a. Direct transmission occurs with shared needles and syringes; permits blood-to-blood contact, the most direct method of transmitting the AIDS virus and hepatitis B.
   b. Transmission to sexual partners; permits contact of body fluids.
   c. Transmission to fetus during pregnancy.
   d. Suppression of the immune system caused by alcohol or drug use.
   e. Impaired judgment while under the influence of drugs.
2. Teach IV drug users how to reduce the risk.
   a. Do not share needles or syringes with others.
   b. Clean needles and other equipment vigorously. Wash twice with full-strength bleach or alcohol; rinse twice with water.
   c. Boil needles and other equipment for 15 minutes.

d. Do not borrow or use needles or equipment from others, even if they appear healthy or say that they do not have AIDS.

3. Teach basic health maintenance measures.
   a. Decrease use of all immunosuppressive drugs (marijuana, speed, cocaine, alcohol).
   b. Maintain an adequate, nutritionally sound diet.

c. Reduce stress on self through stress-reduction practices, or removing self from a stressful situation (living with others who routinely use drugs).
d. Obtain regular medical and dental care.
e. Follow lifestyle that provides adequate rest and exercise.
f. Obtain counseling to assist in living life without dependence on drugs.

## LIFESPAN CONSIDERATIONS

### Children

Infections are an expected part of childhood. The majority of these infections are caused by viruses. In some cases, severe, even life-threatening infections occur. Considerations related to children include the following:

- Newborns may not be able to respond to infections due to an underdeveloped immune system. As a result, in the first few months of life, infections may not be associated with typical signs and symptoms (e.g., an infant with an infection may not have a fever).
- Newborns are born with some naturally acquired immunity transferred from the mother across the placenta.
- Breast-fed infants enjoy higher levels of immunity against infections than formula-fed infants.
- Children who are immune compromised (e.g., leukemia, HIV) or have a chronic health condition (e.g., cystic fibrosis, sickle cell disease, congenital heart disease) need extra precautions to prevent exposure to infectious agents.

### Elders

Normal aging may predispose elders to increased risk of infection and delayed healing. Anatomical and physiological agents that are protective when a person is younger often change in structure and function with increasing age and then provide a decrease in their protective ability. Changes take place in the skin, respiratory tract, gastroin-testinal system, kidneys, and immune system. Special considerations for elders include the following:

- Nutrition may be poor in older adults. Certain components, especially adequate protein, are necessary to build up and maintain the immune system.
- Diabetes mellitus, which occurs more frequently in elders, increases the risk of infection and delayed healing by causing an alteration in nutrition and impaired peripheral circulation, which decrease the oxygen transport to the tissues.
- The normal inflammatory response is delayed. This often causes atypical responses to infections with unusual presentations. Instead of displaying the redness, swelling, and fever usually associated with infections, atypical symptoms such as confusion and disorientation, agitation, incontinence, falls, lethargy, and general fatigue are often seen first.

Recognizing these changes in elders is important in the early detection and treatment of the related potential for infections and delayed healing. Nursing interventions to promote prevention include the following:

- Provide and teach ways to improve nutritional status.
- Use strict aseptic technique (especially in health care facilities).
- Encourage elders to have regular immunizations for flu and pneumonia.
- Be alert to subtle atypical signs of infection and act quickly to diagnose and treat.

## CLIENT TEACHING CONSIDERATIONS

### Infection Control

- Describe ways to manipulate the bed, the room, and other household facilities to prevent injury or to contain possible cross-contamination.
- Instruct to clean obviously soiled linen separately from other laundry. Wash in hot water if possible, adding a cup of bleach or phenol-based disinfectant such as Lysol concentrate to the wash, and rinse in cold water.

- Based on assessment of client and family knowledge, teach proper hand hygiene (e.g., before handling foods, before eating, after toileting, before and after any required home care treatment, and after touching any body substances such as wound drainage) and related hygienic measures to all family members.
- Promote nail care. Keep fingernails short, clean, and well manicured to eliminate rough edges or hangnails, which can harbor microorganisms.

*(continued)*

## CLIENT TEACHING CONSIDERATIONS (CONTINUED)

- Instruct not to share personal care items such as toothbrushes, washcloths, and towels. Describe how infections can be transmitted from shared personal items.
- Discuss antimicrobial soaps and effective disinfectants.
- Discuss the relationship between hygiene, rest, activity, and nutrition in the chain of infection.
- Instruct about cleaning reusable equipment and supplies. Use soap and water, and disinfect with a chlorine bleach solution.
- Teach the client and family members the signs and symptoms of infection, and when to contact a health care provider. Determine by verbal questions the level of understanding of the topic after each teaching session.

- Teach the client and family members how to avoid infections.
- Suggest techniques for safe food preservation and preparation (e.g., wash raw fruits and vegetables before eating them, refrigerate all opened and unpackaged foods).
- Remind to avoid coughing, sneezing, or breathing directly on others. Cover the mouth and nose to prevent the transmission of airborne microorganisms.
- Inform of the importance of maintaining sufficient fluid intake to promote urine production and output. This helps flush the bladder and urethra of microorganisms.
- Emphasize the need for proper immunizations of all family members.

## AMBULATORY AND COMMUNITY SETTINGS

### Infection Control

- Assist with injury-proofing the home to prevent the possibility of tissue injury (e.g., use of padding, handrails, removal of hazards).
- Explore ways to control the environmental temperature and airflow (especially if client has an airborne pathogen).

- Determine the advisability of visitors and family members in proximity to an infected client.
- Ensure access to and proper use of hand-cleansing supplies, gloves, and other barriers as indicated by the type of infection or risk.

# 5

# Metabolism

**Skill 5.1**    Serving a Food Tray (see Skill 12.24 in "Caring Interventions")    190

**Skill 5.2**    Assisting an Adult to Eat    190

**Skill 5.3**    Inserting a Nasogastric Tube    192

**Skill 5.4**    Flushing/Maintaining Nasogastric (NG) Tube    195

**Skill 5.5**    Performing Gastric Lavage    196

**Skill 5.6**    Administering Poison Control Agents    197

**Skill 5.7**    Removing a Nasogastric Tube    197

**Skill 5.8**    Administering a Tube Feeding    198

VARIATION: Feeding Bag (Open System)    199

VARIATION: Syringe (Open System)    199

VARIATION: Prefilled Bottle with Drip Chamber (Closed System)    200

VARIATION: Continuous-Drip Feeding    200

**Skill 5.9**    Administering a Gastrostomy or Jejunostomy Feeding    202

**Skill 5.10**    Providing Continuous Feeding via Small-Bore Nasointestinal/ Jejunostomy Tube    204

**Skill 5.11**    Providing Total Parenteral Nutrition    208

**Skill 5.12**    Infusing IV Lipids    209

**Skill 5.13**    Obtaining a Capillary Blood Specimen and Measuring Blood Glucose    212

**Skill 5.14**    Administering Total Nutrient Admixture (TNA) in the Home    215

**Skill 5.15**    Monitoring Client on TNA    216

**Skill 5.16**    Discontinuing TNA Infusion    216

**Nutrition** is the sum of all interactions between an organism and the food it consumes. In other words, nutrition is what a person eats and how the body uses it. **Nutrients** are organic, inorganic, and energy-producing substances found in foods and required for body functioning. People require the essential nutrients in foods for the growth and maintenance of all body tissues and the normal functioning of all body processes.

## ENTERAL NUTRITION

An alternative feeding method to ensure adequate nutrition includes **enteral** (through the gastrointestinal system) methods. **Enteral nutrition (EN),** also referred to as **total enteral nutrition (TEN),** is provided when the client is unable to ingest foods or the upper gastrointestinal tract is impaired and the transport of food to the small intestine is interrupted. Enteral feedings are administered through nasogastric and small-bore feeding tubes, or through gastrostomy or jejunostomy tubes.

## Skill 5.1 Serving a Food Tray (See Skill 12.24 in "Caring Interventions")

## Skill 5.2 Assisting an Adult to Eat

### Delegation

Assisting or feeding a client is often delegated to UAP. It is, however, the responsibility of the nurse to assess the client's ability to eat and to identify actual or potential risk factors that may impact the client's nutritional status. The nurse must instruct the UAP about strategies that promote the client's nutritional health as well as the importance of the UAP reporting any unusual or different client behaviors to the nurse.

### Equipment

• Meal tray with the correct food and fluids
• Extra napkin or small towel
• Straw, special drinking cup, weighted glass, or other adaptive feeding aid as required

### Preparation

Prepare the client and overbed table.

• Assist the client to the bathroom or onto a bedpan or commode if the client needs to urinate.
• Offer the client assistance in washing the hands prior to a meal. If the client has problems with oral hygiene, brushing the teeth or using a mouthwash can improve the taste in the mouth and hence the appetite.
• Clear the overbed table so that there is space for the tray. If the client must remain in a lying position in bed, arrange the overbed table close to the bedside so that the client can see the food.

### Procedure

1. Prior to performing the procedure, introduce self and verify the client's identity using agency protocol. Explain to the client what you are going to do, why it is necessary, and how he or she can participate.
2. Perform hand hygiene and observe other appropriate infection control procedures.
3. Provide for client privacy.
4. Position the client and yourself appropriately.
   • Assist the client to a comfortable position for eating. Most people sit during a meal; if it is permitted, assist the client to sit in bed or in a chair.
   • If the client is unable to sit, assist the client to a lateral position. ➤*Rationale: People will swallow more easily in these positions than in a back-lying position.*
   • If the client requires assistance with feeding, assume a sitting position, if possible, beside the client. ➤*Rationale: This conveys a more relaxed presence and encourages the client to eat an adequate meal.*

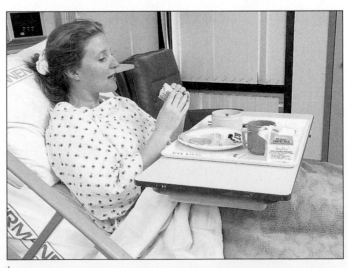

● A supported sitting position contributes to a client's comfort while eating.

5. Assist the client as required.
   - Check tray for the client's name, the type of diet, and completeness. If the diet does not seem to be correct, check it against the client's chart. Do *not* leave an incorrect diet for a client to eat.
   - Encourage the client to eat independently, assisting as needed. Do not take over the feeding process. ➤*Rationale: Participation by the client enhances feelings of independence.*
   - Remove the food covers, butter the bread, pour the drink, and cut the meat, if needed.
   - For a client with a visual impairment, identify the placement of the food as you would describe the time on a clock. For instance, say "The potatoes are at 8 o'clock, the chicken at 12 o'clock, and the green beans at 4 o'clock."
   - If the client needs assistance with feeding:
     a. Ask in which order the client desires to eat the food.
     b. Use normal utensils whenever possible. ➤*Rationale: Using ordinary utensils enhances self-esteem.*
     c. If the client cannot see, tell which food you are giving.
     d. Warn the client if the food is hot or cold.
     e. Allow ample time for the client to chew and swallow the food before offering more.
     f. Provide fluids as requested or, if the client is unable to ask, offer fluids after every three or four mouthfuls of solid food.
     g. Use a straw or special drinking cup for fluids that would spill from normal containers.
     h. Make the time a pleasant one, choosing topics of conversation that are of interest to the client, if the person wants to talk.
6. After the meal, ensure client comfort.
   - Assist the client to clean the mouth and hands.
   - Reposition the client.
   - Replace the food covers and remove the food tray from the bedside.

7. Document all relevant information.
   - Note how much and what the client has eaten and the amount of fluid taken.
   - Record fluid intake and calorie count as required.
   - If the client is on a special diet or is having problems eating, record the amount of food eaten and any pain, fatigue, or nausea experienced.
   - If the client is not eating, notify the nurse in charge so that the diet can be changed or other nursing measures can be taken (e.g., rescheduling the meals, providing small, more frequent meals, or obtaining special self-feeding aids).

---

### DEVELOPMENTAL CONSIDERATIONS

**Elders**

- Offer fluids frequently to prevent dry mouth. Initially avoid dry foods such as crackers and sticky foods such as bananas. ➤*Rationale: Saliva production decreases with age.*
- Allow the older client time to eat and offer to rewarm the food if needed. ➤*Rationale: Hand tremors and arthritic joint changes may slow the eating process for older clients.*
- Observe for dysphagia (difficulty swallowing) and adapt the older client's diet accordingly. ➤*Rationale: Esophageal nerve degeneration, which often occurs with aging, can affect the ability to swallow.*
- Older clients may need extra seasoning on food. ➤*Rationale: Aging decreases the ability to taste, especially sweet and salty foods.*

---

### SETTING OF CARE

- Assess the home for adequate facilities to prepare and store food such as a working refrigerator and stove.
- Assess the client's and caregiver's ability to obtain food and prepare meals.
- Evaluate problems that can interfere with eating such as ill-fitting dentures, sore gums, constipation, diarrhea, or a special diet.
- Instruct the caregiver about the importance of regular, nutritious meals and allowing the client to remain independent when possible.
- Provide written guidelines for the client's diet and any special feeding techniques.

● For a client who is visually impaired, the nurse can use the clock system to describe the location of food on the plate.

# Skill 5.3 Inserting a Nasogastric Tube

## Delegation

Insertion of a nasogastric tube is an invasive procedure requiring application of knowledge (e.g., anatomy and physiology, risk factors) and problem solving. In some agencies, only health care providers with advanced training are permitted to insert nasogastric tubes that require use of a stylet. Delegation of this skill to UAP is not appropriate. The UAP however, can assist with the oral hygiene needs of a client with a nasogastric tube.

## Equipment

- Large- or small-bore tube (nonlatex preferred)
- Non-allergenic adhesive tape, 2.5 cm (1 in.) wide
- Clean gloves
- Water-soluble lubricant
- Facial tissues
- Glass of water and drinking straw
- 20- to 50-mL syringe with an adapter
- Basin
- pH test strip or meter
- Bilirubin dipstick
- Stethoscope
- Disposable pad or towel
- Clamp or plug (optional)
- Anti-reflux valve for air vent if Salem sump tube is used
- Suction apparatus
- Safety pin and elastic band
- $CO_2$ detector (optional)

## Preparation

- Assist the client to a high Fowler's position if client's health condition permits, and support the head on a pillow. ➤*Rationale: It is often easier to swallow in this position, and gravity helps the passage of the tube.*
- Place a towel or disposable pad across the chest.

## Procedure

1. Prior to performing the insertion, introduce self and verify the client's identity using agency protocol. Explain to the client what you are going to do, why it is necessary, and how he or she can participate. The passage of a gastric tube is unpleasant because the gag reflex is activated during insertion. Establish a method for the client to indicate distress and a desire for you to pause the insertion. Raising a finger or hand is often used for this.
2. Perform hand hygiene and observe other appropriate infection control procedures (e.g., clean gloves).
3. Provide for client privacy.
4. Assess the client's nares.
   - Apply clean gloves.
   - Ask the client to hyperextend the head and, using a flashlight, observe the intactness of the tissues of the nostrils, including any irritations or abrasions.
   - Examine the nares for any obstructions or deformities by asking the client to breathe through one nostril while occluding the other.
   - Select the nostril that has the greater airflow.
5. Prepare the tube.
   - If a small-bore tube is being used, ensure stylet or guidewire is secured in position. ➤*Rationale: An improperly positioned stylet or guidewire can traumatize the nasopharynx, esophagus, and stomach.*
   - If a large-bore tube (e.g., Salem sump tube) is being used, place the tube in a basin of warm water while preparing the client. ➤*Rationale: This allows the tubing to become more pliable and flexible.*
6. Determine how far to insert the tube. (Measure the tube.)
   - Use the tube to mark off the distance from the tip of the client's nose to the tip of the earlobe and then from the tip of the earlobe to the tip of the xiphoid. ➤*Rationale: This length approximates the distance from the nares to the stomach. This distance varies among individuals.*
   - Mark this length with adhesive tape if the tube does not have markings.

---

### CLINICAL ALERT

Nurses never insert or withdraw an NG tube for clients recovering from gastric surgery. The suture line could be interrupted, or hemorrhage could occur. The physician should be notified of dislodgement.

Never insert an NG tube in a client after nasal, craniofacial, or hypophysectomy surgery.

### CLINICAL ALERT

Coughing and choking are normal responses for some clients; however, choking and coughing plus cyanosis or inability to speak indicate that the tube may be in the airway.

## GASTRIC (SALEM) SUMP TUBE

This gastric tube is a double-lumen radiopaque plastic tube. One lumen is used for decompression. The blue lumen with a blue pigtail provides an air vent to keep pressure from building in the stomach when the tube is attached to suction. It is NOT used for irrigation, obtaining a specimen, etc. However, if the vent lumen is blocked and requires flushing, following the flush, the pigtail should be cleared with an injection of 20 mL air. The pigtail should be kept above the level of the client's stomach to prevent stomach contents from siphoning into the vent lumen, making it dysfunctional.

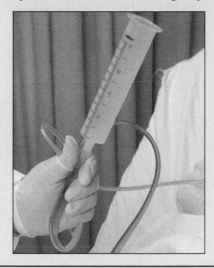

7. Insert the tube.
   - Lubricate the tip of the tube well with water-soluble lubricant or water to ease insertion. ➤*Rationale: A water-soluble lubricant dissolves if the tube accidentally enters the lungs. An oil-based lubricant, such as petroleum jelly, will not dissolve and could cause respiratory complications if it enters the lungs.*

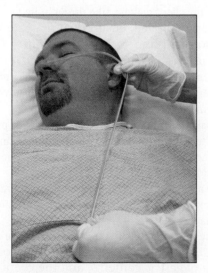

- Insert the tube, with its natural curve toward the client, into the selected nostril. Ask the client to hyperextend the neck, and gently advance the tube toward the nasopharynx. ➤*Rationale: Hyperextension of the neck reduces the curvature of the nasopharyngeal junction.*
- Direct the tube along the floor of the nostril and toward the ear on that side. ➤*Rationale: Directing the tube along the floor avoids the projections(turbinates) along the lateral wall.*
- Slight pressure and a twisting motion are sometimes required to pass the tube into the nasopharynx, and some client's eyes may water at this point. ➤*Rationale: Tears are a natural body response.* Provide the client with tissues as needed.
- If the tube meets resistance, withdraw it, relubricate it, and insert it in the other nostril. ➤*Rationale: The tube should never be forced against resistance because of the danger of injury.*
- Once the tube reaches the oropharynx (throat), the client will feel the tube in the throat and may gag and retch. Ask the client to tilt the head forward, and encourage the client to drink and swallow. ➤*Rationale: Tilting the head forward facilitates passage of the tube into the posterior pharynx and esophagus rather than into the larynx; swallowing moves the epiglottis over the opening to the larynx.*
- If the client gags, stop passing the tube momentarily. Have the client rest, take a few breaths, and take sips of water to calm the gag reflex.
- In cooperation with the client, pass the tube 5 to 10 cm (2 to 4 in.) with each swallow, until the indicated length is inserted.
- If the client continues to gag and the tube does not advance with each swallow, withdraw it slightly, and inspect the throat by looking through the mouth. ➤*Rationale: The tube may be coiled in the throat. If so, withdraw it until it is straight, and try again to insert it.*
- If a $CO_2$ detector is used, after the tube has been advanced approximately 30 cm (12 in.), draw air through the detector. Any change in color of the detector indicates placement of the tube in the respiratory tract. Immediately withdraw the tube and reinsert.

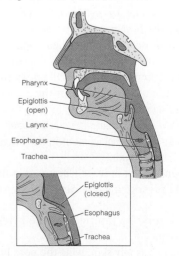

Pharynx
Epiglottis (open)
Larynx
Esophagus
Trachea

Epiglottis (closed)
Esophagus
Trachea

● Measuring the appropriate length to insert a nasogastric tube. Swallowing closes the epiglottis.

## EVIDENCE-BASED NURSING PRACTICE

### Auscultation to Determine Tube Placement

Auscultation of air insufflation as a method for determining tube placement can be dangerously misleading and has no scientific basis. This method does not distinguish whether tube placement is in the lung, esophagus, stomach, or small intestine. Other unreliable methods include:

- Observing for respiratory symptoms (cough, inability to speak)
- Placing tube tip under water to observe for air bubbles

These methods should not be used as the only or primary method for assessing tube placement.

*Source:* Metheny, N., and M. Titler (2001). Assessing placement of feeding tubes. *AJN* Vol. 101(5), 36–46.

8. Ascertain correct placement of the tube.
   - Aspirate stomach contents, and check the pH, which should be acidic. ►*Rationale: Testing pH is a reliable way to determine location of a feeding tube. Gastric contents are commonly pH 1 to 5; pH of 6 or greater would indicate the contents are from lower in the intestinal tract or in the respiratory tract. Some researchers suggest that a pH of greater than 5 should be followed by further confirmation of tube location* (Huffman, Jarczyk, O'Brien, Pieper, & Bayne, 2004).
   - Aspirate can also be tested for bilirubin. Bilirubin levels in the lungs should be almost zero, while levels in the stomach will be approximately 1.5 mg/dL and in the intestine over 10 mg/dL.
   - Almost all nasogastric tubes are radiopaque, and position can be confirmed by x-ray. Check agency policy. If a small-bore tube is used, leave the stylet or guidewire in place until correct position is verified by x-ray. If the stylet has been removed, never reinsert it while the tube is in place. ►*Rationale: The stylet is sharp and could pierce the tube and injure the client or cut off the tube end.*
   - Place a stethoscope over the client's epigastrium and inject 5 to 20 mL of air into the tube while listening for a whooshing sound. Although still one of the methods used, do not use this method as the *primary* method for determining placement of the feeding tube. ►*Rationale: This method does not guarantee tube position.*
   - If the signs indicate placement in the lungs, remove the tube and begin again.
   - If the signs do not indicate placement in the lungs or stomach, advance the tube 5cm (2in.), and repeat the tests.
9. Secure the tube by taping it to the bridge of the client's nose.
   - If the client has oily skin, wipe the nose first with alcohol to defat the skin.
   - Cut 7.5 cm (3 in.) of tape, and split it lengthwise at one end, leaving a 2.5-cm (1-in.) tab at the end.
   - Place the tape over the bridge of the client's nose, and bring the split ends either under and around the tubing, or under the tubing and back up over the nose. Ensure that the tube is centrally located prior to securing with tape to maximize air flow and prevent irritation to the side of the nares. ►*Rationale: Taping in this manner prevents the tube from pressing against and irritating the edge of the nostril.*
10. Once correct position has been determined, attach the tube to a suction source or feeding apparatus as ordered, or clamp the end of the tubing.
11. Secure the tube to the client's gown.
    - Loop an elastic band around the end of the tubing, and attach the elastic band to the gown with a safety pin. *or*
    - Attach a piece of adhesive tape to the tube, and pin the tape to the gown. ►*Rationale: The tube is attached to prevent it from dangling and pulling.* If a Salem sump tube is used, attach the antireflux valve to the vent port (if used) and position the port above the client's waist. ►*Rationale: This prevents gastric contents from flowing into the vent lumen.*
    - Remove and discard gloves. Perform hand hygiene.
12. Document relevant information: the insertion of the tube, the means by which correct placement was determined, and client responses (e.g., discomfort or abdominal distention).
13. Establish a plan for providing daily nasogastric tube care.
    - Inspect the nostril for discharge and irritation.
    - Clean the nostril and tube with moistened, cotton-tipped applicators.
    - Apply water-soluble lubricant to the nostril if it appears dry or encrusted.
    - Change the adhesive tape as required.
    - Give frequent mouth care. Due to the presence of the tube, the client may breathe through the mouth.
14. If suction is applied, ensure that the patency of both the nasogastric and suction tubes is maintained.
    - Irrigations of the tube may be required at regular intervals. In some agencies, irrigations must be ordered by the primary care provider. Prior to irrigation, always recheck placement.
    - If a Salem sump tube is used, follow agency policies for irrigating the vent lumen with air to maintain patency of the suctioning lumen. Often, a sucking sound can be heard from the vent port if it is patent.
    - Keep accurate records of the client's fluid intake and output, and record the amount and characteristics of the drainage.
15. Document the type of tube inserted, date and time of tube insertion, type of suction used, color and amount of gastric contents, and the client's tolerance of the procedure.

## Documentation

Sample: 11/5/09 1030 Feeding tube (#8 Fr) inserted without difficulty through (R) nare with stylet in place. To x-ray to check placement. Radiologist reports tube tip in stomach. Stylet removed. Aspirate pH 4. Tube secured to nose. Verbalizes understanding of need to not pull on tube.

_____ L. Traynor, RN

### DEVELOPMENTAL CONSIDERATIONS

#### Infants and Young Children

- Restraints may be necessary during tube insertion and throughout therapy. ➤Rationale: Restraints will prevent accidental dislodging of the tube.
- Place the infant in an infant seat or position the infant with a rolled towel or pillow under the head and shoulders.
- When assessing the nares, obstruct one of the infant's nares and feel for air passage from the other. If the nasal passageway is very small or is obstructed, an orogastric tube may be more appropriate.

- Measure appropriate nasogastric tube length from the nose to the tip of the earlobe and then to the point midway between the umbilicus and the xiphoid process.
- If an orogastric tube is used, measure from the tip of the earlobe to the corner of the mouth to the xiphoid process.
- Do not hyperextend or hyperflex an infant's neck. ➤Rationale: Hyperextension or hyperflexion of the neck could occlude the airway.
- Tape the tube to the area between the end of the nares and the upper lip as well as to the cheek.

## Skill 5.4   Flushing/Maintaining Nasogastric (NG) Tube

### Equipment

Disposable irrigation set with 50-mL syringe with catheter tip
Emesis basin
Towel
Normal saline irrigation solution
I&O record sheet
Clean gloves

### Preparation

1. Check orders and client care plan.
2. Perform hand hygiene.
3. Check client's identaband and have client state name and birth date.
4. Provide privacy.
5. Explain procedure to client.
6. Place client in semi-Fowler's position.

### Procedure

1. Don clean gloves.
2. Disconnect NG tube from suction source if used.
3. Place towel under NG tube to protect sheets and place emesis basin nearby.
4. Check for NG tube placement by following step 14 in previous skill. ➤Rationale: Solution could be instilled in lungs if NG tube is not in the stomach.

5. Draw up 20–30 mL normal saline into irrigating syringe.
   - Aspirate secretions to check tube placement before instilling saline solution.
   - For irrigating NG tube, draw up 20–30 mL normal saline into irrigating syringe.
   - Gently instill normal saline into NG tube by syringe, or allow solution to flow by gravity.

### CLINICAL ALERT

- If water rather than normal saline is used to flush enteral decompression tubes, the production of gastric secretions will increase and increasing amounts of electrolytes will be washed out. Similarly, if the client is NPO but ingests ice chips ad lib, electrolyte imbalance due to washout can occur, causing metabolic alkalosis.
- Limit the use of ice chips by substituting chips made from an electrolyte solution, and provide oral hygiene to keep the client's mucous membranes moist for comfort.
- If the client is receiving adequate parenteral hydration (IV fluids), excessive thirst should not be experienced.

- Follow Salem tube irrigation with injection of air into blue pigtail to clear, then reinsert blue end of antireflux valve.
6. Gently instill normal saline into NG tube or remove syringe plunger, pour NS into syringe barrel, and allow solution to flow in by gravity.
7. Repeat procedure if necessary.
8. Reconnect NG tube to suction or plug tube.
9. Record instilled amount on I&O record.

10. Remove gloves and perform hand hygiene.
11. Reposition client for comfort.

---

**CLINICAL ALERT**

If secretions siphon into blue vent lumen, clear it by instilling 20 mL of normal saline followed by 20 mL of air. Air vent must be cleared of secretions to restore proper functioning.

---

# Skill 5.5  Performing Gastric Lavage

## Equipment

Large-bore (37–40 Fr) soft Ewald or orogastric tube (client must have cuffed endotracheal tube in place if comatose)
Large irrigating syringe with adapter
Container for aspirate
Lavage fluid, normal saline, or lukewarm water
Activated charcoal for drug/toxin adsorption
Container for specimen
Water-soluble lubricant
Standby suction available
Towel
Pen and tape
Gloves

## Preparation

1. Check physician's orders for gastric lavage and solution to be used.
2. Determine if client is alert or comatose.
3. Gather equipment.
4. Perform hand hygiene and don gloves.

## Procedure

1. Per agency protocol (physician may insert) measure for tube insertion using the following guidelines.
   a. Measure distance from bridge of nose to earlobe to xiphoid process (NEX).
   b. Mark with pen or tape.
2. Place client in head-down, left side-lying position. ➤*Rationale: This reduces risk of aspiration if client vomits.*
3. Lubricate tube with water-soluble lubricant.
4. Insert tube nasogastrically or orogastrically (about 50 cm or 20 inches).
5. Aspirate gastric contents with syringe before instilling solution. Save specimen for analysis.
6. Repeatedly instill 50–100 mL normal saline or water and aspirate contents.

**CLINICAL ALERT**

Gastric lavage assists in arresting hemorrhage and removing liquid from the stomach. It is also used to remove unabsorbed poisons from the stomach. Gastric lavage for poison or drug ingestion is generally ineffective if more than 60 minutes have passed. It is not used for corrosive agents or petroleum distillates due to risk of aspiration. Induced vomiting is no longer considered safe.

7. Carefully monitor volume instilled and character and volume of aspirated contents. ➤*Rationale: This will assist in determining net volume if there is blood loss.*
8. Continue repeating process until gastric return is clear, or as ordered.
9. Stomach will be left empty for decontamination. Activated charcoal maybe instilled (as ordered) or a saline cathartic may be given. ➤*Rationale: Activated charcoal adsorbs drugs in the stomach or intestine.*
10. Pinch tube for removal, wrap in towel, and dispose of equipment.
11. Remove and dispose of gloves and perform hand hygiene.
12. Record vital signs frequently and monitor client's response closely.

**CLINICAL ALERT**

Some authorities recommend water to lavage the stomach of blood since it breaks up clots more easily than saline solution, is less expensive, and is readily available.

# Skill 5.6 Administering Poison Control Agents

## Equipment

Large (37–40 Fr) Soft Ewald tube (physician may insert); comatose client must have endotracheal tube in place.

Lukewarm tap water or saline for lavage

Container for aspirated contents

Large irrigating syringe with catheter tip

50–100 g activated charcoal or prepackaged charcoal/sorbitol product mixed with water to consistency to administer through tube

*or*

Balanced propethylene glycol–electrolyte solution (e.g., GoLYTELY) for bowel irrigation

## Preparation

(See Preparation for Skill 5.3, Inserting a Nasogastric Tube)

## Procedure

1. Place comatose intubated client in a head-down, leftside-lying position or place cooperative alert client on commode.
2. Insert large bore (37–40 Fr) flexible tube nasogastrically or orogastrically.

### CLINICAL ALERT

For a known toxin, one should call a regional poison control center by dialing 800-222-1222.

3. Aspirate gastric contents and save specimen for analysis.
4. Lavage repeatedly with 50–100 mL of fluid until return is clear.
5. Administer activated charcoal slurry and repeat if ordered or, for cooperative client, administer balanced electrolyte solution per NG tube at a rate of 1–2 L/hr until rectal runout is clear.

### ACTIVATED CHARCOAL FOR INGESTED POISONS

Activated charcoal adsorbs significant amounts of certain poisons, especially when a person overdoses. The earlier charcoal is given, the more effective it is. The amount given is 5–10 times that of the suspected poison or, if the poison is unknown, 50–100 g for adults.

# Skill 5.7 Removing a Nasogastric Tube

## Delegation

Due to the need for assessment of client status, the skill of removing a nasogastric tube is not delegated to UAP.

## Equipment

- Disposable pad or towel
- Tissues
- Clean gloves
- 50-mLsyringe (optional)
- Plastic trash bag

## Preparation

- Confirm the primary care provider's order to remove the tube.
- Assist the client to a sitting position if health permits.
- Place the disposable pad or towel across the client's chest to collect any spillage of secretions from the tube.
- Provide tissues to the client to wipe the nose and mouth after tube removal.

## Procedure

1. Prior to performing the removal, introduce self and verify the client's identity using agency protocol. Explain to the client what you are going to do, why it is necessary, and how he or she can participate.
2. Perform hand hygiene and observe other appropriate infection control procedures (e.g., clean gloves).
3. Provide for client privacy.
4. Detach the tube.
   - Apply clean gloves.
   - Disconnect the nasogastric tube from the suction apparatus, if present.
   - Unpin the tube from the client's gown.
   - Remove the adhesive tape securing the tube to the nose.
5. Remove the nasogastric tube.
   - *Optional:* Instill 50 mL of air into the tube. ➤*Rationale: This clears the tube of any contents such as feeding or gastric drainage.*
   - Ask the client to take a deep breath and to hold it. ➤*Rationale: This closes the glottis, thereby preventing accidental aspiration of any gastric contents.*

- Pinch the tube with the gloved hand. ➤*Rationale: Pinching the tube prevents any contents inside the tube from draining into the client's throat.*
- Smoothly withdraw the tube.
- Place the tube in the plastic bag. ➤*Rationale: Placing the tube immediately into the bag prevents the transference of microorganisms from the tube to other articles or people.*
- Observe the intactness of the tube.

6. Ensure client comfort.
   - Provide mouth care if desired.
   - Assist the client as required to blow the nose. ➤*Rationale: Excessive secretions may have accumulated in the nasal passages.*

7. Dispose of the equipment appropriately.
   - Place the pad, bag with tube, and gloves in the receptacle designated by the agency. ➤*Rationale: Correct disposal prevents the transmission of microorganisms.*
   - Remove and discard gloves. Perform hand hygiene.

8. Document all relevant information.
   - Record the removal of the tube, the amount and appearance of any drainage if connected to suction, and any relevant assessments of the client.

## Documentation

Sample: 11/8/09 1500 NG tube removed intact without difficulty. Oral & nasal care given. No bleeding or excoriation noted. States is hungry & thirsty. 60 mL apple juice given. No c/o nausea.

_____ L. Traynor, RN

---

## EVIDENCE-BASED NURSING PRACTICE

**Postoperative GI Motility**

Nurses in this practice project discontinued bowel sound assessment to determine the return of gastrointestinal motility following abdominal surgery, since bowel sounds reflect the normal activity of the small intestine alone but do not represent return of functional GI motility. Primary indicators of the return of GI motility include the return of flatus, bowel movement, client's tolerance of oral intake without nausea or vomiting, return of appetite, and absence of abdominal distension, bloated feeling, and cramps. Recent work on the early feeding and reducing the routine use of nasogastric tubes has also contributed to a growing body of evidence on recovery of postoperative GI motility.

*Source:* Madsen, D., et al. (2005). Listening to bowel sounds: An evidence-based practice project. *AJN*, 105(12), 40.

---

# Skill 5.8   Administering a Tube Feeding

## Delegation

Administering a tube feeding requires application of knowledge and problem solving and it is not usually delegated to UAP. Some agencies, however, may allow a trained UAP to administer a feeding. In this case, it is the responsibility of the nurse to assess tube placement and determine that the tube is patent. The nurse should reinforce major points, such as making sure the client is sitting upright, and instruct the UAP to report any difficulty administering the feeding or any complaints voiced by the client.

## Equipment

- Correct type and amount of feeding solution
- 60-mL catheter-tip syringe
- Emesis basin
- Clean gloves
- pH test strip or meter
- Large syringe or calibrated plastic feeding bag with label and tubing that can be attached to the feeding tube or prefilled bottle with a drip chamber, tubing, and a flow-regulator clamp
- Measuring container from which to pour the feeding (if using open system)
- Water (60 mL unless otherwise specified) at room temperature
- Feeding pump as required

## Preparation

- Assist the client to a Fowler's position (at least 30 degrees elevation) in bed or a sitting position in a chair, the normal position for eating. If a sitting position is contraindicated, a slightly elevated right side-lying position is acceptable. ➤*Rationale: These positions enhance the gravitational flow of the solution and prevent aspiration of fluid into the lungs.*

### Procedure

1. Prior to performing the feeding, introduce self and verify the client's identity using agency protocol. Explain to the client what you are going to do, why it is necessary, and how he or she can participate. Inform the client that the feeding should not cause any discomfort but may cause a feeling of fullness.

2. Perform hand hygiene and observe appropriate infection control procedures (e.g., clean gloves).

3. Provide privacy for this procedure if the client desires it. Tube feedings are embarrassing to some people.

4. Assess tube placement.
   - Apply clean gloves.
   - Attach the syringe to the open end of the tube and aspirate. Check the pH.
   - Allow 1 hour to elapse before testing the pH if the client has received a medication.
   - Use a pH meter rather than pH paper if the client is receiving a continuous feeding. Follow agency policy if the pH is 6 or greater.

5. Assess residual feeding contents.
   - If the tube is placed in the stomach, aspirate all contents and measure the amount before administering the feeding. ➤*Rationale: This is done to evaluate absorption of the last feeding; that is, whether undigested formula from a previous feeding remains. If the tube is in the small intestine, residual contents cannot be aspirated.*
   - If 100 mL(or more than half of the last feeding) is withdrawn, check with the nurse in charge or refer to agency policy before proceeding. The precise amount is usually determined by the primary care provider's order or by agency policy. ➤*Rationale: At some agencies, a feeding is delayed when the specified amount or more of formula remains in the stomach.*
   or
   - Reinstill the gastric contents into the stomach if this is the agency policy or primary care provider's order. ➤*Rationale: Removal of the contents could disturb the client's electrolyte balance.*
   - If the client is on a continuous feeding, check the gastric residual every 4 to 6 hours or according to agency protocol.

6. Administer the feeding.
   - Before administering feeding:
     a. Check the expiration date of the feeding.
     b. Warm the feeding to room temperature. ➤*Rationale: An excessively cold feeding may cause abdominal cramps.*
   c. When an open system is used, clean the top of the feeding container with alcohol before opening it. ➤*Rationale: This minimizes the risk of contaminants entering the feeding syringe or feeding bag.*

### VARIATION: Feeding Bag (Open System)

- Hang the labeled bag from an infusion pole about 30 cm (12 in.) above the tube's point of insertion into the client.
- Clamp the tubing and add the formula to the bag.
  a. Apply a label that indicates the date, time of starting the feeding, and nurse's initials on the feeding bag.
- Open the clamp, run the formula through the tubing, and reclamp the tube. ➤*Rationale: The formula will displace the air in the tubing, thus preventing the instillation of excess air into the client's stomach or intestine.*
- Attach the bag to the feeding tube and regulate the drip by adjusting the clamp to the drop factor on the bag (e.g., 20 drops/mL) if not placed on a pump.

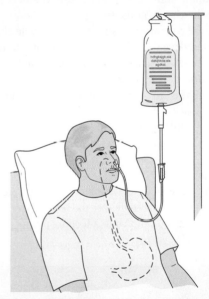

● Using a calibrated plastic bag to administer a tube feeding.

### VARIATION: Syringe (Open System)

- Remove the plunger from the syringe and connect the syringe to a pinched or clamped nasogastric tube. ➤*Rationale: Pinching or clamping the tube prevents excess air from entering the stomach and causing distention.*
- Add the feeding to the syringe barrel.
- Permit the feeding to flow in slowly at the prescribed rate. Raise or lower the syringe to adjust the flow as needed. Pinch or clamp the tubing to stop the flow for a minute if the client experiences discomfort. ➤*Rationale: Quickly administered feedings can cause flatus, cramps, and/or vomiting.*

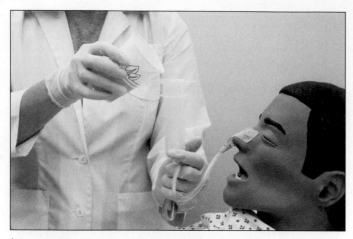

● Using the barrel of a syringe to administer a tube feeding.

## VARIATION: Prefilled Bottle with Drip Chamber (Closed System)

- Remove the screw-on cap from the container and attach the administration set with the drip chamber and tubing.
- Close the clamp on the tubing.
- Hang the container on an intravenous pole about 30 cm (12 in.) above the tube's insertion point into the client. ➤*Rationale: At this height, the formula should run at a safe rate into the stomach or intestine.*
- Squeeze the drip chamber to fill it to one-third to one-half of its capacity.
- Open the tubing clamp, run the formula through the tubing, and reclamp the tube. ➤*Rationale: The formula will displace the air in the tubing, thus preventing the instillation of excess air.*
- Attach the feeding set tubing to the feeding tube and regulate the drip rate to deliver the feeding over the desired length of time or attach to a feeding pump.

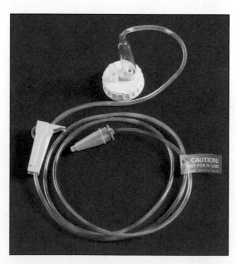

● Feeding set tubing with drip chamber.
(Courtesy of Ross Products, a division of Abbott Laboratories)

7. If another bottle is not to be immediately hung, flush the feeding tube before all of the formula has run through the tubing.
- Instill 50 to 100 mL of water through the feeding tube or medication port. ➤*Rationale: Water flushes the lumen of the tube, preventing future blockage by sticky formula.*
- Be sure to add the water before the feeding solution has drained from the neck of a syringe or from the tubing of an administration set. ➤*Rationale: Adding the water before the syringe or tubing is empty prevents the instillation of air into the stomach or intestine and thus prevents unnecessary distention.*

8. Clamp the feeding tube.
- Clamp the feeding tube before all of the water is instilled. ➤*Rationale: Clamping prevents leakage and air from entering the tube if done before water is instilled.*

9. Ensure client comfort and safety.
- Secure the tubing to the client's gown. ➤*Rationale: This minimizes pulling of the tube, thus preventing discomfort and dislodgment.*
- Ask the client to remain sitting upright in Fowler's position or in a slightly elevated right lateral position for at least 30 minutes. ➤*Rationale: These positions facilitate digestion and movement of the feeding from the stomach along the alimentary tract, and prevent the potential aspiration of the feeding into the lungs.*
- Check the agency's policy on the frequency of changing the nasogastric tube and the use of smaller lumen tubes if a large-bore tube is in place. ➤*Rationale: These measures prevent irritation and erosion of the pharyngeal and esophageal mucous membranes.*
- Remove and discard gloves. Perform hand hygiene.

10. Dispose of equipment appropriately.
- If the equipment is to be reused, wash it thoroughly with soap and water so that it is ready for reuse.
- Change the equipment every 24 hours or according to agency policy.
- Remove and discard gloves. Perform hand hygiene.

11. Document all relevant information.
- Document the feeding, including amount and kind of solution taken, duration of the feeding, and assessments of the client.
- Record the volume of the feeding and water administered on the client's intake and output record.

12. Monitor the client for possible problems.
- Carefully assess client receiving tube feedings for problems.
- To prevent dehydration, give the client supplemental water in addition to the prescribed tube feeding as ordered.

## VARIATION: Continuous-Drip Feeding

- Clamp the tubing at least every 4 to 6 hours, or as indicated by agency protocol or the manufacturer, and aspirate and measure the gastric contents. Then flush the tubing with 30 to 50 mL of water. ➤*Rationale: This determines*

## CLIENT TEACHING

Clients and caregivers need the following instructions to manage these feedings:

- Preparation of the formula. Include name of the formula and how much and how often it is to be given; the need to inspect the formula for expiration date and leaks and cracks in bags or cans; how to mix or prepare the formula, if needed; and aseptic techniques such as swabbing the container's top with alcohol before opening it, and changing the syringe administration set and reservoir every 24 hours.
- Proper storage of the formula. Include the need to refrigerate diluted or reconstituted formula and formula that contains additives.
- Administration of the feeding. Include proper hand washing technique, how to fill and hang the feeding bag, operation of an infusion pump if indicated, the feeding rate, and client positioning during and after the feeding.

- Management of the enteral or parenteral access device. Include site care; aseptic precautions; dressing change, as indicated; how the site should look normally; and flushing protocols (e.g., type of irrigant and schedule).
- Daily monitoring needs. Include temperature, weight, and intake and output.
- Signs and symptoms of complications to report. Include fever, increased respiratory rate, decrease in urine output, increased stool frequency, and altered level of consciousness.
- Whom to contact about questions or problems. Include emergency telephone numbers of home care agency, nursing clinician, and/or primary care provider, or other 24-hour on-call emergency service.

*adequate absorption and verifies correct placement of the tube. If placement of a small-bore tube is questionable, a repeat x-ray should be done.*

- Determine agency protocol regarding withholding a feeding. Many agencies withhold the feeding if more than 75 to 100 mL of feeding is aspirated.
- To prevent spoilage or bacterial contamination, do not allow the feeding solution to hang longer than 4 to 8 hours. Check agency policy or manufacturer's recommendations regarding time limits.

- Follow agency policy regarding how frequently to change the feeding bag and tubing. Changing the feeding bag and tubing every 24 hours reduces the risk of contamination.

### Documentation

Sample: 11/5/09 1330 Aspirated 20 mL pale yellow fluid from NG tube, pH 5. Returned residual. Placed in Fowler's position. 1 liter room-temperature ordered formula begun @ 60 mL/hour on pump. No nausea reported.
————————————————————— L. Traynor, RN

## DEVELOPMENTAL CONSIDERATIONS

### Infants

- Feeding tubes may be reinserted at each feeding to prevent irritation of the mucous membrane, nasal airway obstruction, and stomach perforation that may occur if the tube is left in place continuously. Check agency practice.

### Children

- Position a small child or infant in your lap, provide a pacifier, and hold and cuddle the child during feedings. This promotes comfort, supports the normal sucking instinct of the infant, and facilitates digestion.

### Elders

- Physiologic changes associated with aging may make the elder more vulnerable to complications associated with enteral feedings. Decreased gastric

emptying may necessitate checking frequently for gastric residual. Diarrhea from administering the feeding too fast or at too high a concentration may cause dehydration. If the feeding has a high concentration of glucose, assess for hyperglycemia because with aging, the body has a decreased ability to handle increased glucose levels.
- Conditions such as hiatal hernia and diabetes mellitus may cause the stomach to empty more slowly. This increases the risk of aspiration in a client receiving a tube feeding. Checking for gastric residual more frequently can help document this if it is an ongoing problem. Changing the formula or the rate of administration, repositioning the client, or obtaining a primary care provider's order for a medication to increase stomach emptying may resolve this problem.

**SETTING OF CARE**

- Teach and provide the client or caregiver the rationale for how to assess for tube placement using pH measurement before administering the feeding. Instruct regarding actions to take if the pH is greater than 6.
- Provide instructions and rationale for care of the tube and insertion site.
- Discuss strategies for hanging formula containers if an IV pole is unavailable or inconvenient.

- Plan for optimal timing of feedings to allow for daily activities. Many clients can tolerate having the majority of their feedings run during sleep so they are free from the equipment during the day.
- Teach signs and symptoms to report to the primary care provider or home health nurse.

# Skill 5.9 Administering a Gastrostomy or Jejunostomy Feeding

## Planning

Before commencing a gastrostomy or jejunostomy feeding, determine the type and amount of feeding to be instilled, frequency of feedings, and any pertinent information about previous feedings (e.g., the positioning in which the client best tolerates the feeding).

## Equipment

- Correct amount of feeding solution
- Graduated container and tubing with clamp to hold the feeding
- 60-mL catheter-tip syringe
- Mild soap and water
- Clean gloves
- Petrolatum, zinc oxide ointment, or other skin protectant
- Precut 4 × 4 gauze squares
- Uncut 4 × 4 gauze squares

*For Tube Insertion*

- Clean gloves
- Moisture-proof bag
- Water-soluble lubricant
- Feeding tube (if needed)

## Preparation

- Assist the client to a Fowler's position (at least 30 degrees elevation) in bed or a sitting position in a chair, the normal position for eating. If a sitting position is contraindicated, a slightly elevated right side-lying position is acceptable. ➤*Rationale: These positions enhance the gravitational flow of the solution and prevent aspiration of fluid into the lungs.*

## Procedure

1. Prior to performing the feeding, introduce self and verify the client's identity using agency protocol.

Explain to the client what you are going to do, why it is necessary, and how he or she can participate.
2. Perform hand hygiene and observe other appropriate infection control procedures (e.g., clean gloves).
3. Provide for client privacy.
4. Assess and prepare the client.
   - Apply clean gloves.
5. Insert a feeding tube, if one is not already in place.
   - Wearing gloves, remove the dressing. Then discard the dressing and gloves in the moisture-proof bag.
   - Apply new clean gloves.
   - Lubricate the end of the tube, and insert it into the ostomy opening 10 to 15 cm (4 to 6 in.).
6. Check the location and patency of a tube that is already in place.
   - Determine correct placement of the tube by aspirating secretions and checking the pH.
   - Follow agency policy for amount of residual formula. This may include withholding the feeding, rechecking in 3 to 4 hours, or notifying the primary care provider if a large residual remains.
   - For continuous feedings, check the residual every 4 to 6 hours and hold feedings according to agency policy.
   - Remove the syringe plunger. Pour 15 to 30 mL of water into the syringe, remove the tube clamp, and allow the water to flow into the tube. ➤*Rationale: This determines the patency of the tube. If water flows freely, the tube is patent.*
   - If the water does not flow freely, notify the nurse in charge and/or primary care provider.
7. Administer the feeding.
   - Hold the barrel of the syringe 7 to 15 cm (3 to 6 in.) above the ostomy opening.
   - Slowly pour the solution into the syringe and allow it to flow through the tube by gravity.
   - Just before all of the formula has run through and the syringe is empty, add 30 mL of water. ➤*Rationale: Water flushes the tube and preserves its patency.*

## TABLE 5-1  ADMINISTERING A GASTROSTOMY FEEDING USING AN OPEN SYSTEM

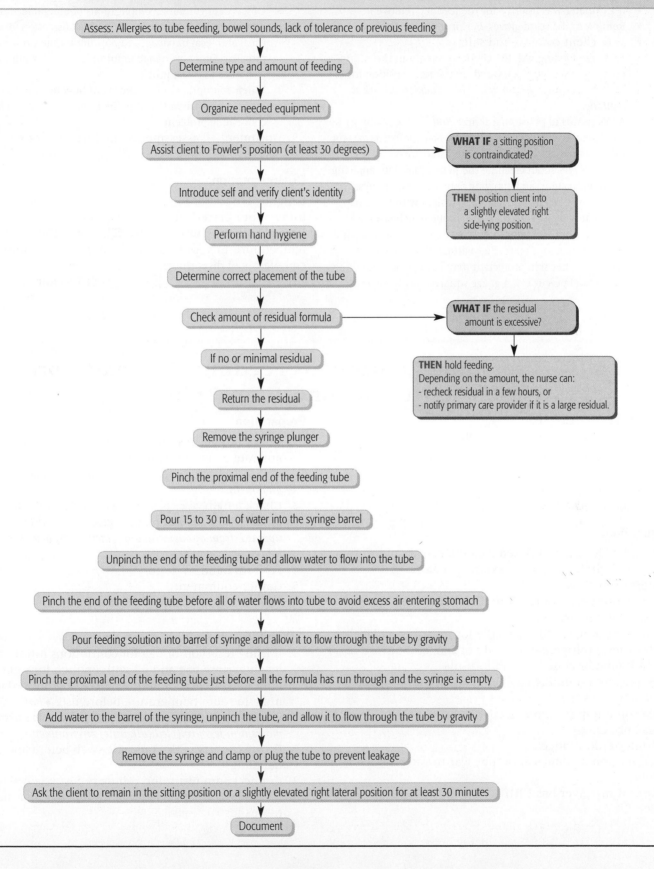

Assess: Allergies to tube feeding, bowel sounds, lack of tolerance of previous feeding

Determine type and amount of feeding

Organize needed equipment

Assist client to Fowler's position (at least 30 degrees)

**WHAT IF** a sitting position is contraindicated?

**THEN** position client into a slightly elevated right side-lying position.

Introduce self and verify client's identity

Perform hand hygiene

Determine correct placement of the tube

Check amount of residual formula

**WHAT IF** the residual amount is excessive?

**THEN** hold feeding.
Depending on the amount, the nurse can:
- recheck residual in a few hours, or
- notify primary care provider if it is a large residual.

If no or minimal residual

Return the residual

Remove the syringe plunger

Pinch the proximal end of the feeding tube

Pour 15 to 30 mL of water into the syringe barrel

Unpinch the end of the feeding tube and allow water to flow into the tube

Pinch the end of the feeding tube before all of water flows into tube to avoid excess air entering stomach

Pour feeding solution into barrel of syringe and allow it to flow through the tube by gravity

Pinch the proximal end of the feeding tube just before all the formula has run through and the syringe is empty

Add water to the barrel of the syringe, unpinch the tube, and allow it to flow through the tube by gravity

Remove the syringe and clamp or plug the tube to prevent leakage

Ask the client to remain in the sitting position or a slightly elevated right lateral position for at least 30 minutes

Document

- If the tube is to remain in place, hold it upright, remove the syringe, and then clamp or plug the tube to prevent leakage.
- If a catheter was inserted for the feeding, remove it.
- Remove and discard gloves. Perform hand hygiene.

8. Ensure client comfort and safety.
   - After the feeding, ask the client to remain in the sitting position or a slightly elevated right lateral position for at least 30 minutes. ➤*Rationale: This minimizes the risk of aspiration.*
   - Assess status of peristomal skin. ➤*Rationale: Gastricor jejunal drainage contains digestive enzymes that can irritate the skin.* Document any redness and broken skin areas.
   - Check orders about cleaning the peristomal skin, applying a skin protectant, and applying appropriate dressings. Generally, the peristomal skin is washed with mild soap and water at least once daily. The tube may be rotated between thumb and forefinger to release any sticking and promote tract formation. Petrolatum, zinc oxide ointment, or other skin protectant may be applied around the stoma, and precut 4 × 4 gauze squares may be placed around the tube. The precut squares are then covered with regular 4 × 4 gauze squares, and the tube is coiled over them.
   - Observe for common complications of enteral feedings: aspiration, hyperglycemia, abdominal distention, diarrhea, and fecal impaction. Report findings to primary care provider. Often, a change in formula or rate of administration can correct problems.
   - When appropriate, teach the client how to administer feedings and when to notify the primary care provider concerning problems.

9. Document all assessments and interventions.

### Documentation

Sample: 1/24/09 2045 No fluid aspirated from gastrostomy tube. Placed in Fowler's position. 30 mL water flowed freely by gravity through tube. 250 mL room-temperature Ensure formula given over 20 minutes. No complaints of discomfort.

_____ L. Traynor, RN

---

## Skill 5.10   Providing Continuous Feeding via Small-Bore Nasointestinal/Jejunostomy Tube

### EXPECTED OUTCOMES
- Clients nutritional needs are met with nasogastric feeding.
- Client's nutritional needs are met with continous enteral feeding.
- Gastrostomy tube site is free of signs of irritation/inflammation.

### Equipment

Prescribed formula in closed container ready to infuse system (preferred). Note expiration date.

Antimicrobial swabs

Formula reservoir or bag if necessary for open system (date and replace daily)

Container of ready to use sterile formula (cover, label for client, refrigerate unused portion, and discard in 48 hours) or closed system formula

Administration tubing compatible with pump (replace daily)

Infusion pump (not to exceed 40 psi)

Label or pen

60-mL sterile syringe

Sterile normal saline solution or warm water

Gloves

Mask (if caregiver has URI)

### Preparation

1. Check physician's order for feeding formula type and rate of administration.
2. Check x-ray report. ➤*Rationale: Validates desired tube placement.*
3. Check length of exposed tubing. ➤*Rationale: An increase in length may indicate tube tip has dislocated upward, from duodenum to stomach, or from stomach into the esophagus.*
4. Perform hand hygiene.
5. Gather equipment.
6. Don clean gloves and mask if indicated.

### Procedure

1. If using reservoir or bag for continuous intestinal feeding, rinse bag and fill with enough formula to limit hang time to 8 hours. *Note:* Bring unused formula to room temperature before use. ➤*Rationale: To reduce risk of infection. Advancement of tube to intestine places it in less protected (alkaline) environment.*
2. Disinfect ports with antiseptic swab before and after handling.
3. Connect administration tubing to formula reservoir (container or bag) and prime tubing per manufacturer's instructions.

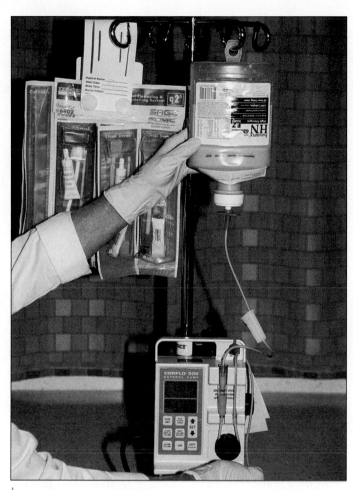

● Limit formula hang to 36 hours for a closed system.

4. Thread tubing through pump per manufacturer's instructions.
5. Note mark on client's feeding tube to determine if migration has occurred.
6. Connect primed formula tubing to client's small-bore nasointestinal tube. Initiate feeding with isotonic (300 mOsml) or slightly hypotonic formula. ➤*Rationale: To prevent dumping syndrome (cramping and diarrhea).*

## CLINICAL ALERT

*Obese clients* cannot efficiently mobilize fat stores, but use protein as a primary source of energy, have marked loss of muscle and lean body mass, and become nutrient depleted when critically ill. Nutrient support, however, can cause *refeeding syndrome* in these as in other protein-deficient clients. This adverse response is characterized by volume overload, heart failure, pulmonary edema, glucose intolerance, excess carbon dioxide production (by product of glucose metabolism), increased respiratory work, and respiratory failure.

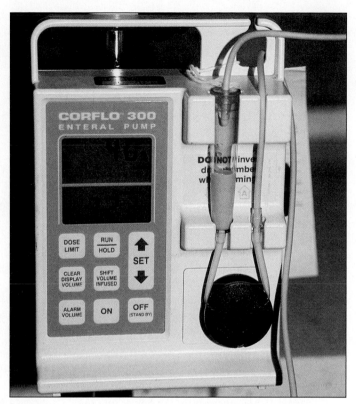

● Thread tubing through pump per manufacturer's instructions. Pump must not exceed 40 psi.

*Note:* Alternate method is to connect formula tubing to client's surgically established jejunostomy feeding tube.

7. Start feeding at slow constant infusion rate (25–50 mL/hr). ➤*Rationale: Slow increase in feeding volume is better tolerated.* (Maximum rate is 100–150 mL/hr).
8. If client tolerates feeding, increase rate in 8–24 hours (increase by 25–50 mL/hr to prescribed rate).
9. Keep client's head of bed elevated at 30–45°, or maintain obese client in reverse Trendelenburg position. ➤*Rationale: To lower intra-abdominal pressure and reduce risk of aspiration.*
10. Prep side port with antimicrobial swab and flush small-bore continuous feeding tube every 4 hours, and before and after medication administration with a minimum of 20 to 30 mL warm tap water, using 60 mL syringe. ➤*Rationale: To prevent tube clogging.*

## CLINICAL ALERT

If possible, administer medications through a prepped side port. Note that some medications precipitate when mixed with formulas. The tube should be flushed pre and post medication administration with 20 to 30 mL warm water.

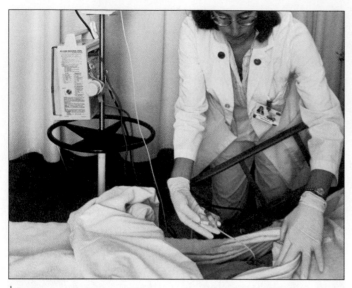

● Connect continuous feeding system to client's surgically placed jejunostomy tube.

11. Check residual volume regularly. ➤*Rationale: Small-bore feeding tube residuals are usually less than 10 mL. Residuals as much as 50 mL may indicate upward displacement from the bowel into the stomach.*

## Documentation for Enteral Tube Feedings

- Date and time of procedure
- Placement of small-bore enteral tube and x-ray validation of proper placement
- External length of exposed tubing
- Methods of validating tube placement
- Quantity and character of aspirated residuals (color, pH, other tests)
- Amount and type of formula administered
- Head of bed elevation during and following feeding
- Frequency of tube irrigation and irrigant used
- Abdominal assessment findings (distention, nausea, vomiting, flatus, bowel movement)
- Bowel elimination pattern and characteristics
- Daily weight
- Intake and output
- Tube exit site assessment
- Application of dressing to exit site
- Oral hygiene provided

### CLINICAL ALERT

The pH method for determining tube placement may not be useful during continuous NG/NI feeding because the infused formula raises gastric pH and lowers intestinal pH. The continuous-feeding aspirate will look like formula; it may be curdled or bile stained. A sudden increase in residual volume may indicate that a nasointestinal tube has become displaced upward into the stomach.

### CLINICAL ALERT

If client is receiving continuous feeding, maintain HOB elevation at 30°–45° at all times. Turn off feeding 1 hour before client must be repositioned at less than 30° for any procedure or transport.

### CLINICAL ALERT

Transition from nutrition support to oral feeding requires careful monitoring. Enteral tubes or parenteral access should not be removed until the client has tolerated oral nutrition for 2–3 days.

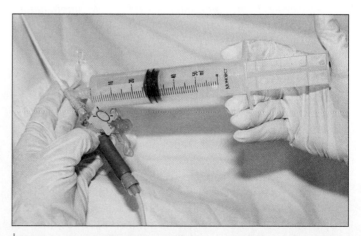

● Maintain head of bed elevation at 30–45° to reduce risk of aspiration in clients receiving continuous enteral feeding.

● Use 60 mL syringe to flush feeding tube with 20-30 mL warm water every 4 hours, and before and after medication administration.

| UNEXPECTED OUTCOMES | CRITICAL THINKING OPTIONS |
|---|---|
| NG tube feedings are delayed/skipped due to large residual volumes. | • Assess for adequate GI function (no abdominal distention; no nausea or vomiting, presence of flatus, bowel movement).<br>• If residual is ≤200 mL, continue feeding but closely monitor client's response. |
| Client develops diarrhea with enteral feeding. | • Use closed system if possible to prevent contamination.<br>• Don clean gloves when setting up or opening system; use sterile technique if client is immunocompromised or critically ill.<br>• Flush bag before refilling with formula.<br>• Use prepackaged, ready-to-use sterile feeding formulas. If using open system, cover, label, and refrigerate unused formula and discard in 24 hours.<br>• Disinfect ports before and after any handling.<br>• Consult dietitian about osmolarity of formula (hyperosmolar or high-fiber formula may cause diarrhea). |
| Small-bore feeding tube fails to advance into duodenum. | • Determine if gastric feeding is acceptable (client does not have gastroparesis, reflux esophagitis, high risk for aspiration, absence of gag or cough reflex).<br>• Administer prokinetic agent before rather than after tube insertion.<br>• Suggest tube be advanced under fluoroscopy. |
| Small-bore feeding tube becomes clogged; occlusion alarm sounds. | • Do not let formula bag run dry.<br>• Use warm water in 50-mL syringe with a gentle push/pull technique for flushing tube. Do not use vigorous pressure.<br>• Do not flush with cola or acidic pH juices such as cranberry juice, as this can precipitate protein and cause tube clogging.<br>• Papain, combinations of activated pancreatic enzymes, and sodium bicarbonate mixed with water may declog the tube.<br>• Flush tube with water every 4–6 hours and before and after any medication administered.<br>• Crush medications fully—do not administer with formula running as this may cause precipitate.<br>• Consider use of papain and sodium bicarbonate with water for flush.<br>• Use declogging system suggested by tube manufacturer—do not reinsert guidewire to unclog tube.<br>• Replace long-term tube every 4 weeks using alternate nostril. |
| Gastrostomy tube site becomes irritated. | • Apply plain antacid (e.g., Mylanta) to area if condition is mild.<br>• Use skin prep barrier followed by antifungal powder followed by skin prep barrier.<br>• Request tube with external bar or disc be replaced with plain tube that is sutured into place (bars and discs may embed into skin). |

# Skill 5.11   Providing Total Parenteral Nutrition

## Planning

Review the client record regarding previous TPN. Note any complications and how they were managed.

## Delegation

Due to the need for sterile technique and technical complexity, administration of TPN is not delegated to UAP. UAP may care for clients receiving TPN, and the nurse must ensure that the UAP knows what complications or adverse signs should be reported to the nurse.

## Equipment

- TPN solution
- Timing tape
- Infusion pump
- Tubing with filter

## Preparation

- Inspect and prepare the solution.
- Remove the ordered TPN solution from the refrigerator 1 hour before use, and check each ingredient and the proposed rate against the order on the chart. ➤*Rationale: Infusion of a cold solution can cause pain, hypothermia, and venous spasm and constriction.*
- Inspect the solution for cloudiness or presence of particles, and ensure that the container is free from cracks. For a lipids, examine the bag for separation of emulsion, fat globules, or froth.
- Before administering any TPN solution:
- Check its expiration date. Most solutions must be used within 24 hours of preparation, unless they are refrigerated.
- Two licensed nurses need to check the nutrients in the bag with the order written by the primary care provider. ➤*Rationale: This is another check that ensures the solution was properly prepared by the pharmacist.*
- Apply a timing tape on the solution container.

## Procedure

1. Prior to performing the procedure, introduce self and verify the client's identity using agency protocol. Explain to the client what you are going to do, why it is necessary, and how he or she can participate.
2. Provide for client privacy and prepare the client.
   - Assist the client to a comfortable position, either sitting or lying. If necessary, expose the central line site but provide for client privacy.
3. Perform hand hygiene and observe appropriate infection control procedures.

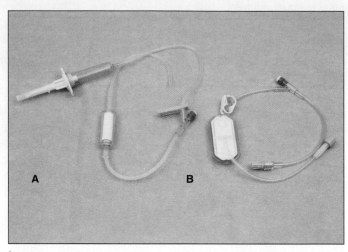

● **A.** A 0.22-micron filter used for TPN; **B.** a 1.22-micron filter for use with TPN containing lipids.

4. Change the solution container to the TPN solution ordered.
   - Ensure that correct placement of the central line catheter has been confirmed by x-ray examination.
   - Ensure that the tubing has an in-line filter connected at the end of the TPN tubing. For plain TPN, use a 0.22-micron filter. A. For TPN with lipids, the filter must be 1.2 microns. B. Plain lipids are infused without a filter. ➤*Rationale: The filter traps bacteria and particles that can form in the TPN solution.*
   - Attach and connect the tubing to an infusion pump, if not present. ➤*Rationale: A pump eliminates the changes in flow rate that occur with alterations in the client's activity and position.*
   - Attach the TPN solution to the IV administration tubing. If a multiple-lumen tube is in place, attach the infusion to the appropriate lumen. If possible, a lumen should be dedicated to TPN use only.
   - If lipids are being infused separately from the TPN, connect the lipid tubing to the injection port closest to the client.
5. Regulate and monitor the flow rate.
   - Establish the prescribed rate of flow and monitor the infusion at least every 30 minutes.
   - Never accelerate an infusion that has fallen behind schedule. ➤*Rationale: Wide fluctuations in blood glucose can occur if the rate of TPN infusion is irregular.*
   - Never interrupt or discontinue the infusion abruptly. If TPN solution is temporarily unavailable, infuse a solution containing at least 5% to 10% dextrose. ➤*Rationale: This prevents rebound hypoglycemia.*

## CLINICAL ALERT

TPN and lipids are frequently infused together in the same bottle to prevent microorganism growth from lipid emulsion.

## CLINICAL ALERT

Do not "catch up" a deficit in infused volume, as doing so could result in complications for the client. To ensure constant flow rate, check rate every two hours.

- During the initial stage of a lipid infusion (i.e., the first hour), closely monitor vital signs and signs of any side effects (e.g., fever, flushing, diaphoresis, dyspnea, cyanosis, headache, nausea, or vomiting).
- Start lipid infusions very slowly according to the primary care provider's orders, the manufacturer's directions, and agency policy. For a 10% emulsion, start at 1 mL/min for the first 5 minutes then up to 4 mL/min for the next 25 minutes. If well tolerated, set ordered rate thereafter.
6. Monitor the client for complications.
- Change the administration set and filter every 24 hours.
- Monitor the vital signs every 4 hours. If fever or abnormal vital signs occur, notify the primary care provider. ➤*Rationale: An elevated temperature is one of the earliest indications of catheter-related sepsis.*
- Collect double-voided urine specimens in accordance with agency policy, and test the urine for specific gravity. If the specific gravity is abnormal, notify the primary care provider, who may alter the constituents of the TPN solution.
- Assess fingerstick blood glucose levels every 6 hours according to agency protocol. ➤*Rationale: Blood glucose is tested to make certain the infusion is not running too rapidly for the body to metabolize glucose or too slowly for caloric needs to be met. Notify the primary care provider of abnormal glucose levels. For hyperglycemia, supplementary insulin may be ordered subcutaneously or added directly to the TPN solution. For hypoglycemia the infusion rate may need to be increased.*

- Measure the daily fluid intake and output and calorie intake. ➤*Rationale: Precise replacement for fluid and electrolyte deficits can then be more readily determined.*
- Monitor the results of laboratory tests (e.g., serum electrolytes and blood urea nitrogen) and report abnormal findings to the primary care provider.
7. Assess weight and anthropometric measurements.
- Weigh the client daily, at the same time and in the same garments. A gain of more than 0.5 kg (1.1 lb) per day indicates fluid excess and should be reported.
- Measure arm circumference and triceps skinfold thickness weekly or in accordance with agency protocol to assess the physical changes.
8. Document all relevant information.
- Record the type and amount of infusion, rate of infusion, vital signs q 4 h, fingerstick blood glucose levels as ordered, client's weight daily, and anthropometric measurements.

## CLINICAL ALERT

- No medication or blood products are to be added or piggy-backed into TPN line.
- No blood specimen should be withdrawn from an IV line infusing TPN.
- TPN is never stopped abruptly. It should be tapered off.

# Skill 5.12   Infusing IV Lipids

**EXPECTED OUTCOMES**
- Lipids infuse within time frame.
- Adequate calories and essential fatty acids are provided to clients unable to ingest orally.
- Parenteral nutrients provided without complications or adverse effects.
- Normal pancreatic function is maintained.

**Equipment**

IV lipid solution in glass container
Nonphthalate vented IV tubing infusion set (to prevent pooling of fat in IV tubing)
Needleless cannula
Antimicrobial swabs
Volume control device

*Note:* Many facilities do not infuse lipids alone but combine with TPN.

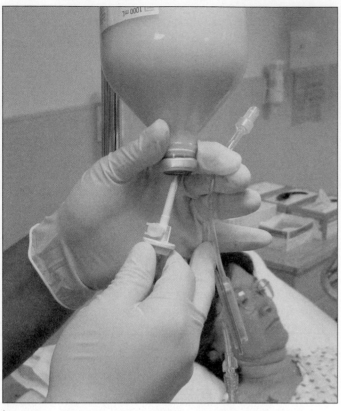

● Lipids are administered from glass container or non-PVC infusion sets.

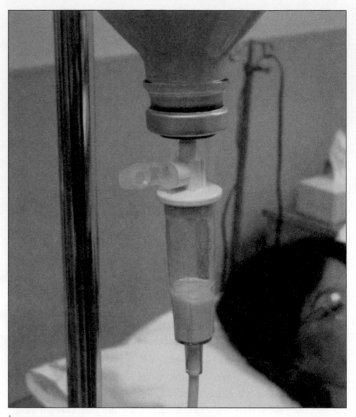

● Vented tubing is required for lipid infusion.

### Preparation

1. Review physician's orders and MAR.
2. Obtain lipid emulsion (refrigerated) from the pharmacy and warm the solution to room temperature.
3. Examine bottle for separation of emulsion into layers or fat globules or for accumulation of froth. Do not use if any of these appear.
4. Label bottle with client name, medical record number, room number, date, time, flow rate, bottle number, and start and stop times.
5. Identify client using two forms of identification.
6. Explain procedure to client.

### Procedure

1. Take vital signs for baseline assessment. ➤*Rationale: Baseline information is needed because an immediate reaction can occur.*
2. Perform hand hygiene, and then swab stopper on IV bottle with antimicrobial swab and allow to dry.
3. Attach vented non-PVC infusion set to bottle, twisting the spike to prevent particles from stopper falling into the emulsion, or spike bag with regular IV tubing.

4. Hang IV bottle at least 30 inches above IV site. ➤*Rationale: Due to solution viscosity, lipid emulsion needs to be at this height to prevent backing up into infusion tubing.*
5. Fill drip chamber two-thirds full, slightly open clamp on the tubing, and prime the tubing slowly. ➤*Rationale: Priming more slowly reduces chance of air bubbles with this solution.*
6. Attach the tubing to the IV site.
7. If piggybacking lipids into hyperalimentation, use port closest to client, below tubing filter.

### CLINICAL ALERT

Administration sets that contain di-(2-ethylhexyl)phthalate (DEHP) plasticizers extract lipids from infusion set. It is recommended to use a separate administration set, glass infusate containers, or special non–polyvinyl chloride (non-PVC) IV bags.

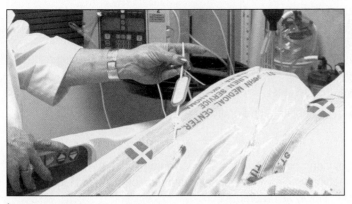

● Check facility policy regarding use of in-line filters for lipid administration. Filters are used with hyperalimentation.

## GUIDELINES FOR IV LIPID INFUSION

- IV lipid solutions are isotonic and provide 1.1 kcal/mL of solution in a 10% solution or 2.0 kcal/mL in a 20% solution.
- Do not put additives into IV lipid bottle.
- Do not use an IV filter because the particles are large and cannot pass through.

### FOR ADULTS

- Lipid 10%: Up to 500 mL 4–6 hours on first day to maximum of 2.5 g/kg body weight per day. Do not exceed 60% of client's total caloric intake per day.
- Liposyn 10%: No more than 500 mL/day in 4–6 hours.

### FOR CHILDREN

- Lipid 10%: Up to 1 g/kg in 4 hours. Do not exceed 60% of total caloric intake.

## CLINICAL ALERT

Lipid emulsions alone promote growth of specific bacteria and yeasts as soon as 6 hours after the infusion. When lipids are combined with TPN (solution of amino acids, lipid emulsion and glucose) in the same bag, it doesn't appear to support any greater microbial growth than non-lipid-containing TPN fluids. Thus TPN solution can hang safely for 24 hours.

## CLINICAL ALERT

In-line filters are not recommended by CDC as a routine infection control measure; however, the Infusion Nurses Society favors the filters. Always check hospital policies and procedures to determine use of filters.

## CLINICAL ALERT

Observe for IV lipid side effects after starting lipid infusion:

| | |
|---|---|
| chills | chest and back pain |
| fever | nausea and vomiting |
| flushing | headache |
| diaphoresis | pressure over the eyes |
| dyspnea | vertigo |
| cyanosis | sleepiness |
| allergic reactions | thrombophlebitis |

8. Infuse lipid solutions initially at 1.0 mL/min for adults and 0.1 mL/min for children for first 15–30 minutes. Then increase rate to 2 mL/min for adults and 0.2 for children.
9. Monitor vital signs according to facility policy and observe for side effects during first 30 minutes of the infusion. If side effects occur, stop the infusion and notify the physician.
10. Adjust flow to prescribed IV rate if no adverse reactions occur.
11. Monitor and maintain the infusion at the ordered rate.
12. Monitor serum lipids 4 hours after discontinuing infusion. ➤Rationale: If you draw blood too soon after infusion is completed, incorrect blood values result.
13. Monitor liver function tests for evidence of impaired liver function. ➤Rationale: These tests indicate the liver's ability to metabolize the lipids.
14. Discard partially used bottles. ➤Rationale: This action prevents contamination.
15. Discard administration set after each unit unless additional units are administered consecutively.
16. Continue to monitor vital signs, and observe client for adverse reactions during the entire process of infusion.
17. Answer any questions the client may have about the procedure, and make client comfortable before leaving room.

**UNEXPECTED OUTCOMES**

Client experiences side effects and cannot continue with lipid infusion.

Client develops dyspnea, cyanosis, or allergic reaction, such as nausea, vomiting, increased temperature, or headache.

Client's serum triglyceride and liver function test results remain elevated.

Client develops hyperlipemia or hypercoagulability.

**CRITICAL THINKING OPTIONS**

- Reassess client's ability to tolerate fat solution.
- Notify physician for order to discontinue fat solution, and administer hyperalimentation solution.
- Monitor liver function test results.
- Stop infusion immediately, and notify physician.

- Hang the solution bottle on an IV stand as you would an IV bottle.
- Begin the feeding with a weaker concentration of formula, and increase the concentration slowly as ordered.
- Monitor laboratory results, particularly liver function tests, and notify physician when any abnormality occurs.

# Skill 5.13 Obtaining a Capillary Blood Specimen and Measuring Blood Glucose

## Equipment

- Blood glucose meter (glucometer)
- Blood glucose reagent strip compatible with the meter
- 2 × 2 gauze
- Antiseptic swab
- Clean gloves
- Sterile lancet (a sharp device to puncture the skin)
- Lancet injector (a spring-loaded mechanism that holds the lancet)

## Preparation

Review the type of meter and the manufacturer's instructions. Assemble the equipment at the bedside.

## Procedure

1. Prior to performing the procedure, introduce self and verify the client's identity using agency protocol. Explain to the client what you are going to do, why it is necessary, and how he or she can participate. Discuss how the results will be used in planning further care or treatments.
2. Perform hand hygiene and observe other appropriate infection control procedures (e.g., gloves).
3. Provide for client privacy.
4. Prepare the equipment.
   - Calibrate the meter and run a control sample according to the manufacturer's instructions.
5. Select and prepare the vascular puncture site.
   - Choose a vascular puncture site (e.g., the side of an adult's finger). Avoid sites beside bone. Hold a finger in a

dependent position. If the earlobe is used, rub it gently with a small piece of gauze. ➤*Rationale: These actions increase the blood flow to the area, ensure an adequate specimen, and reduce the need for a repeat puncture.*
   - Clean the site with the antiseptic swab or soap and water and allow it to dry completely. ➤*Rationale: Alcohol can affect accuracy, and the site burns when punctured if wet with alcohol.*
6. Obtain the blood specimen.
   - Apply clean gloves.
   - Place the injector against the site, and release the needle, thus permitting it to pierce the skin. Make sure the lancet is perpendicular to the site. ➤*Rationale: The lancet is designed to pierce the skin at a specific depth when it is in a perpendicular position relative to the skin.*

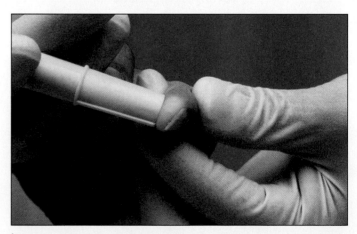

● Place the injector against the site.

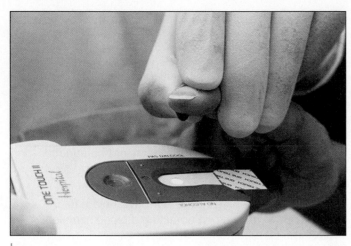

● Gently squeeze a large drop of blood onto the reagent strip.

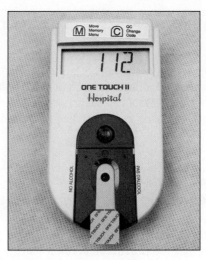

● The glucose meter will display the glucose reading.

- Gently squeeze (but do not touch) the puncture site until a large drop of blood forms. The size of the drop of blood can vary depending on the meter.
- Make sure that the drop of blood is sufficient prior to placing the blood on the strip. Some meters require an amount not much larger than the period at the end of this sentence (Mensing, 2004). ➤*Rationale: An insufficient sample will result in an erroneous reading.*
- Hold the reagent strip under the puncture site until adequate blood covers the indicator square. The pad will absorb the blood and a chemical reaction will occur.

  Do not smear the blood. ➤*Rationale: This will cause an inaccurate reading. Some meters wick the blood by just touching the puncture site with the strip.*
- Ask the client to apply pressure to the skin puncture site with a 2 × 2 or 4 × 4 gauze. ➤*Rationale: Pressure will assist hemostasis (i.e., stop the bleeding). Avoid using an antiseptic swab.* ➤*Rationale: This will cause discomfort or further bleeding at the puncture site.*

7. Expose the blood to the test strip for the period and the manner specified by the manufacturer. As soon as the blood is placed on the test strip:
   - Follow the manufacturer's recommendations on the glucose meter for the amount of time indicated by the manufacturer. ➤*Rationale: The blood must remain in contact with the test pad for a prescribed time to obtain accurate results.*

8. Measure the blood glucose.
   - Place the strip into the meter according to the manufacturer's instructions. (Note that some glucometers have the test strip placed in the machine before the specimen is obtained.) Some devices require that the strip be wiped or blotted after a designated period of time before being inserted in the meter. Other strips do not require blotting or wiping. Refer to the specific manufacturer's recommendations for the specific procedure.
   - After the designated time, most glucose meters will display the glucose reading automatically. Correct timing ensures accurate results.
   - Turn off the meter and discard the test strip and 2 × 2 gauze in a biohazard container. Discard the lancet into a sharps container.
9. Remove and discard gloves. Perform hand hygiene.
10. Document the method of testing and results on appropriate documents in the client's record. If appropriate, record the client's understanding and ability to demonstrate the skill. The client's record may also include a flow sheet on which capillary blood glucose results and the amount, type, route, and time of insulin administration are recorded. Always check if a diabetic flow sheet is being used for the client.
11. Check for orders for sliding scale insulin based on capillary blood glucose results. Administer insulin as prescribed.

## DEVELOPMENTAL CONSIDERATIONS

### Infants

- The outer aspect of the heel is the most common site on neonates and infants for obtaining a capillary blood specimen. Placing a warm cloth on the infant's heel often increases the blood flow to the area.

### Children

- Use the side of a fingertip for a young client older than age 2, unless contraindicated.
- When possible, allow the child to choose the puncture site.
- Praise the young client for cooperating and assure the child that the procedure is not a punishment.

### Elders

- Elders may have arthritic joint changes, poor vision, or hand tremors and may need assistance using the glucose meter or obtaining a meter that accommodates their limitations.
- Elders may have difficulty obtaining diabetic supplies due to financial concerns or homebound status.
- Elders often have poor circulation. Warming the hands by wrapping with a warm washcloth for 3 to 5 minutes may help in obtaining a blood sample.

## CARE SETTINGS

- Assess the client or caregiver's ability and willingness to perform blood glucose monitoring at home.
- Teach the proper use of the lancet and glucose meter, and provide written guidelines. Allow time for a return demonstration. The client may need several visits to completely learn the procedure.
- Ensure the client's ability to obtain supplies and purchase reagent strips. The strips are relatively expensive and may not be covered by the client's insurance.
- Stress the importance of record keeping. Instruct the client on when to do glucose monitoring, how to record the blood glucose levels, and when to notify the primary care provider.
- Diabetic children who need to perform finger-sticks should be taught about safe practices for cleaning blood from surfaces (household bleach is best) and about safe storage of equipment to prevent young children from having access to it. Identify a place in the school where the child can store glucose-monitoring equipment and perform the procedure in private.

### Home Setting

Nutritional support in the home is not significantly different from that in a hospital setting. Gastrostomy and nasogastric tube feedings are frequently performed in the home setting using small feeding tubes and maintained via continuous feeding pumps. The only difference in the procedure at home is that the family is taught how to provide the feeding. The nurse's role is to change the nasogastric tube and to teach and monitor the family's ability to administer the feeding. Intake and output records are maintained by the family and monitored by the nurse when the client's condition warrants it.

Total parenteral nutrition is now being used in the home. The procedure and equipment are similar to that used in the hospital, including the use of sterile technique when preparing and discontinuing the infusion.

Home health agencies have specified policies and procedures for TNA that the nurse must follow to practice within legal parameters. The first infusion of any TNA solution or any IV medication must be given in the hospi-

tal or emergency room (where emergency intervention is available if an adverse reaction occurs).

In the home care setting, the client or family is taught how to administer TNA after the first infusion. TNA is also termed 3-in-1 mixture. It is a combination of amino acids, dextrose, and lipids in one container. Many clients prefer to infuse TNA at night while they sleep, since the procedure takes about 12 hours. The client or family must be taught proper storage, fluid administration, electronic ambulatory infusion pump use, and site care. Most people use pre-prepared TNA solutions that are available at the hospital pharmacy. Clients and families must be given careful instruction on sterile technique used in preparing TNA solutions. Catheter site care is performed the same as in the hospital.

Effective management of clients requiring TNA at home includes:

- A nurse who is an expert in all aspects of TNA administration.

- Knowledge of client monitoring, both fluid infusion and potential complications associated with TNA administration.
- Teaching skills are a must as this procedure is very complicated; family and client (or caregiver) must be versed in all aspects of TNA care to prevent complications and infuse TNA appropriately.

Monitoring for complications includes assessment of clinical and therapeutic response to TNA regimen. Assessment involves monitoring nutritional status and monitoring for potential complications. Weight gain or maintenance, increased strength, and the absence of complications indicate that TNA has a positive effect on client's condition.

# Skill 5.14 Administering Total Nutrient Admixture (TNA) in the Home

## NUTRITIONAL ASSESSMENT

- Height and weight
- Skin integrity
- Elimination
- Behavioral changes
- Mucous membranes
- Nailbeds
- Oral cavity
- State of edema
- Cardiovascular assessment

### Equipment

TNA solution bag
IV tubing with in-line filter
Volutrol
Controller or pump
Padded Kelly forceps, tape
Blood glucose monitoring equipment
Intake and output and TNA record
Clean gloves

### Procedure

1. Remove TNA solution from refrigerator at least 1 hour before using. Parenteral nutrition solutions are stable for 7 days when refrigerated. Without lipids in solution, it is stable for 30–45 days when refrigerated. ➤Rationale: Warming the solution prevents venospasm and hypothermia.
2. Gather equipment.
3. Perform hand hygiene and don gloves.
4. Inspect TNA solution for cloudiness, clarity, and intact bag. If lipids are added, solution will be white. ➤Rationale: Contamination of the solution causes a cloudy or milky precipitate.
5. Prepare to administer TNA solution by spiking bag with tubing, adding filter, and then flushing tubing of all air.

6. Prepare catheter when solution is ready for infusion by clamping catheter with a padded Kelly forceps and removing injection cap.
7. Cleanse end of catheter with antimicrobial swab.
8. Remove protective cap from IV tubing and insert tubing into catheter.
9. Tape connection site. ➤Rationale: Taping prevents accidental dislodging of the tubing from catheter and lessens chance of contamination.
10. Remove gloves, perform hand hygiene.
11. Thread IV tubing through electronic ambulatory infusion machine according to manufacturer's directions and set machine to deliver appropriate rate.
12. Monitor infusion rate, and assess IV site throughout procedure. Procedure takes about 12 hours; therefore, many clients prefer to infuse the solution during their sleeping hours. ➤Rationale: If flow rate is too rapid, excess glucose may cause seizures.
13. Monitor blood glucose daily using Accu-chek or autolet and chemstrips. Report elevated blood glucose levels to physician. ➤Rationale: Insulin may need to be ordered.
14. Instruct client to follow physician's directions for lab work. Blood chemistry profiles and liver function tests are done frequently in the beginning of therapy and progress to every 2–4 weeks.
15. Maintain accurate intake and output and TNA sheet.
16. Instruct client to monitor weight and temperature frequently throughout therapy.

Note: Pumps can deliver single medication as a continuous infusion or as a dual-therapy pump that delivers single medication as a continuous or intermittent infusion.

## CLINICAL ALERT

A 0.2- or 1.2-micron filter is used for parenteral nutrition solutions with amino acids and dextrose. For TNA, a 1.2- or 5-micron filter is used. Filters are changed every 24 hours. If filter becomes occluded, check for precipitation or incompatibility of solutions.

# Skill 5.15 Monitoring Client on TNA

## Equipment

Log book
Scale
Blood glucose monitoring equipment
Thermometer

## Procedure

1. Instruct client or care giver to document assessment data in log book. Bring book to physician during office visit and share with home health nurse during visits.
2. Instruct client to weigh daily at same time and with same clothing, shoes off.
3. Check blood glucose level when first initiating TNA according to the following guidelines:
   a. Before starting TNA. ➤*Rationale: To obtain baseline data.*
   b. Several hours after starting cyclic TNA. ➤*Rationale: To assess peak blood glucose.*
   c. One hour after discontinuing TNA. ➤*Rationale: To observe for rebound hypoglycemia.*
4. Check blood glucose level every 8–12 hours with continuous TNA.

---

### CLINICAL ALERT

A sudden increase in blood glucose in a stable client is an indication of impending sepsis.

---

5. Maintain serum glucose under 200 mg/dL for continuous TNA clients and 240 mg/dL for cyclic TNA clients. Regular insulin on a sliding scale is prescribed for clients on TNA.
6. Measure intake and output daily and record in log book.
7. Instruct client or caregiver on signs of fluid volume deficit (poor skin turgor, dry mucous membranes, etc.) and excess.
8. Explain signs and symptoms associated with electrolyte imbalance (increased fatigue and muscle weakness).
9. Take temperature daily at same time and record in log book.
10. Monitor any drainage for amount, color, consistency, or any changes from usual.
11. Ensure client has routine blood drawn as scheduled.
12. Instruct client to observe for signs of edema and to report these immediately.
13. Instruct client or caregiver to monitor central venous catheter site for signs of infection. Immediately report to home health nurse and do not infuse TNA until nurse observes site. ➤*Rationale: Septicemia is a major cause of morbidity in clients on TNA and accounts for 70% of hospital readmissions.*

*Note:* Developing a worksheet and teaching focus sheet will assist client and caregiver in following client education information and documenting pertinent data. A form will also allow the nurse to quickly assess changes in the client between visits.

---

# Skill 5.16 Discontinuing TNA Infusion

## Equipment

Tape
Sterile injection cap
4 × 4 gauze pad
2 mL normal saline
20-gauge needle
25-gauge needle
2-mL syringe
Alcohol swab
Antimicrobial swab
Padded Kelly clamp
Clean gloves

## Procedure

1. Gather equipment.
2. Perform hand hygiene and don clean gloves.
3. Withdraw 2 mL normal saline into syringe.
4. Turn IV solution off by closing roller clamp and turning off controller or pump.
5. Clamp catheter.

6. Disconnect IV tubing from catheter.
7. Cleanse catheter site with an antimicrobial swab.
8. Place sterile injection cap on catheter.
9. Wipe injection cap with alcohol swab.
10. Inject 2 mL of normal saline solution through cap.
11. Withdraw needle.
12. Coil catheter and place 4 × 4 gauze pad over catheter and tape catheter to chest or abdomen. Site care is performed every 48–72 hours using same sterile technique as in hospital.
13. Discard used equipment.
14. Remove gloves and perform hand hygiene.

*Note:* Refer to Skills 5.7 and 5.9 for NG feeding and G-tube feeding skills.

## COMPLICATIONS ASSOCIATED WITH TNA

### Nutritional Variations

- Fatty acid deficiency if not receiving lipid emulsions
- Vitamin deficiency

### Metabolic Complications

- Fluid and electrolyte imbalances
- Glucose intolerance, hypo- and hyperglycemia
- Liver complications

6

# Mobility

**Skill 6.1** Applying Body Mechanics 219

**Skill 6.2** Supporting the Client's Position in Bed 221

VARIATION: Supporting a Client in Fowler's Position 221

VARIATION: Supporting a Client in the Dorsal Recumbent Position 223

VARIATION: Supporting a Client in the Prone Position 223

VARIATION: Supporting a Client in the Lateral Position 224

VARIATION: Supporting a Client in the Sims' Position 224

**Skill 6.3** Positioning a Child for Injections or Intravenous Access 225

VARIATION: Supine Position 225

VARIATION: Sitting Position 225

**Skill 6.4** Positioning a Child for Lumbar Puncture 225

**Skill 6.5** Positioning a Child for an Otoscopic Examination 226

VARIATION: Supine Position 226

VARIATION: Sitting Position 227

**Skill 6.6** Moving a Client Up in Bed 227

VARIATION: A Client with Limited Strength of the Upper Extremities 228

VARIATION: Two Nurses Using a Turn Sheet 228

**Skill 6.7** Turning a Client to the Lateral or Prone Position in Bed 229

VARIATION: Turning the Client to a Prone Position 230

**Skill 6.8** Logrolling a Client 231

VARIATION: Using a Turn or Lift Sheet 232

**Skill 6.9** Assisting the Client to Sit on Side of Bed (Dangle) 232

VARIATION: Teaching a Client How to Sit on the Side of the Bed Independently 233

**Skill 6.10** Transferring between Bed and Chair 234

VARIATION: Angling the Wheelchair 236

VARIATION: Transferring without a Belt 236

VARIATION: Transferring with a Belt and Two Nurses 236

VARIATION: Transferring a Client with an Injured Lower Extremity 236

VARIATION: Using a Sliding Board 237

**Skill 6.11** Transferring between Bed and Stretcher 237

VARIATION: Using a Transfer Board 238

**Skill 6.12** Using a Hydraulic Lift 238

**Skill 6.13** Performing Passive Range of Motion Exercises 240

| Skill 6.14 | Using Continuous Passive Motion Device | 247 |
| Skill 6.15 | Assisting the Client to Ambulate | 249 |
| | VARIATION: Two Nurses | 250 |
| Skill 6.16 | Assisting the Client to Use a Cane | 251 |
| Skill 6.17 | Assisting the Client to Use Crutches | 253 |
| | VARIATION: Four-Point Alternate Gait | 253 |
| | VARIATION: Three-Point Gait | 254 |
| | VARIATION: Two-Point Alternate Gait | 254 |
| | VARIATION: Swing-to Gait | 254 |
| | VARIATION: Swing-Through Gait | 255 |
| | VARIATION: Getting into a Chair | 255 |
| | VARIATION: Getting Out of a Chair | 255 |
| | VARIATION: Going Up Stairs | 255 |
| | VARIATION: Going Down Stairs | 256 |

| Skill 6.18 | Assisting the Client to Use a Walker | 257 |
| Skill 6.19 | Transporting the Infant | 258 |
| Skill 6.20 | Transport of the Toddler | 259 |
| Skill 6.21 | Performing Initial Cast Care | 260 |
| Skill 6.22 | Performing Ongoing Cast Care | 263 |
| | VARIATION: Plaster Cast | 264 |
| | VARIATION: Synthetic Cast | 264 |
| Skill 6.23 | Performing Care for a Child with a Cast | 265 |
| Skill 6.24 | Caring for Clients in Traction | 266 |
| | VARIATION: Caring for Client in Skin Traction | 266 |
| | VARIATION: Skeletal Traction | 267 |
| Skill 6.25 | Applying and Monitoring Skin Traction for a Child | 270 |
| Skill 6.26 | Positioning Nonhospital Bed for Client Care | 271 |

In this chapter, readers will be given essential guidelines for safe and efficient strategies for assisting clients to move and change positions. The use of assistive equipment, adequate numbers of staff, and proper body alignment of nurse and client are discussed. Skills for assisting clients into various positions, turning clients in bed, and transferring clients from a bed to a chair or stretcher are included. During all positional changes, the comfort and dignity of clients must be protected. Ensure modesty by providing proper coverage throughout the positional change. Protect dignity by giving careful, complete instructions, encouraging patients to help themselves as much as possible, and by using a caring tone of voice and eye contact.

# Skill 6.1   Applying Body Mechanics

**Procedure**

1. Determine need for assistance in moving or turning a client. ➤*Rationale: Half of all back pain is associated with lifting or turning clients. The most common back injury is strain on the lumbar muscle group.*
2. Establish a firm base of support by placing both feet flat on the floor, with one foot slightly in front of the other.
3. Distribute weight evenly on both feet.
4. Slightly bend both knees. ➤*Rationale: Allows strong muscles of legs to do the lifting.*
5. Hold abdomen firm and tuck buttocks in so that spine is in alignment. ➤*Rationale: This position protects the back.*
6. Hold head erect, and secure firm stance.
7. Use this stance as the basis for all actions in moving, turning, and lifting clients.

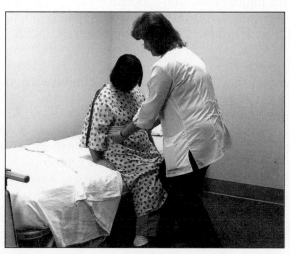

● Gait belts are routinely used to assist in manual transfer in most facilities.

8. Maintain weight to be lifted as close to your body as possible. ➤*Rationale: This position maintains the center of gravity and provides leverage that reduces lower back strain.*

9. Align the three natural curves in your back (cervical, thoracic, and lumbar). ➤*Rationale: Weight of client is evenly distributed throughout spine, lowering risk of back injury.*

10. Prevent twisting your body when moving the client. ➤*Rationale: This prevents injury to the back.*

## EVIDENCE-BASED NURSING PRACTICE

### Use of Back Brace to Prevent Back Injury

Two studies on prevention of low back pain using a back support differed in their conclusions. One study, Linton and van Tulder, researched the literature and found 27 investigations that were consistently negative about the use of back braces to prevent low back pain. There is strong evidence not only that they are ineffective in prevention, but that lumbar supports or back belts are no more beneficial than either no intervention or preventative interventions; in fact, they may be detrimental. The results of the Linton and van Tulder study were consistently negative about the use of lumbar supports. The study indicated that exercises, conversely, showed positive results in the randomized controlled trials, providing consistent evidence of their function in prevention.

The second study, conducted at UCLA by Kraus, McArthur, and Samaniego, found the opposite results. The UCLA study "found compelling evidence that back support can play an important role in helping reduce back injuries among workers who do a lot of lifting." The study, completed in 1994 with 36,000 participants, indicated that low-back injuries are reduced by one-third when workers wear a back support. This study recommends worker training and proper workplace ergonomics design, and that back supports should be part of an overall back injury prevention program.

The National Institute of Occupational Safety and Health reviewed the scientific findings in the UCLA study and issued a report in 1994 that concluded the benefit of back supports remained unproven and did not recommend that they be used. A number of preventive measures have been introduced to prevent work-related back injuries. Training, job screening, and ergonomic modification are recommended by NIOSH, but objective evidence of their effectiveness alone or in combination has been elusive and subject to many issues and problems.

These study results have culminated in a recommendation by the European Guidelines for Prevention in Low

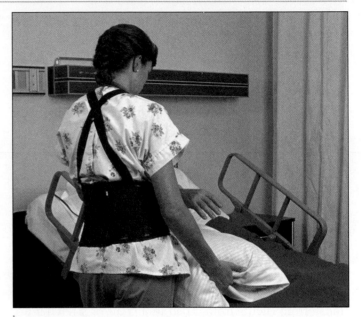

● Use of back brace to support back and keep body in alignment is controversial, and most current studies do not support use of the back brace.

Back Pain (November 2004) to promote prevention of low back pain using activity/exercise, ergonomics, and orthosis. Physical exercise has a positive effect in prevention of back pain.

Various types of activities were reviewed, such as aerobic exercises, physiotherapy, and specific trunk muscle training. The researchers found no specific differences in pain intensity between these interventions. No studies indicated harmful effects of exercise or increased symptoms of pain.

*Source:* Linton and van Tulder. (2001, April 1). Preventive interventions for back and neck problems: What is the evidence?, *Spine*, 26(7), 778–787. Available at: http://www.avenco.com/UCLAStudy/ucla.html, www.backpaineurope.org.

# Skill 6.2 Supporting the Client's Position in Bed

## Delegation

Positioning clients in bed can be delegated to unlicensed assistive personnel (UAP). The nurse must give specific directions to UAP about the appropriate positions for the client and the reporting of any changes in skin integrity. The UAP should be encouraged to have the client participate as much as possible in the position change. The nurse is responsible for evaluating the client's comfort and alignment after the repositioning and for assessing skin integrity, particularly at pressure points.

## Equipment

The following equipment can be used when positioning clients:

- Pillows—one to six depending on client need
- Trochanter rolls
- Footboard
- Hand rolls or wrist splints, if needed
- Folded towel
- Sandbag or rolled towel

## Preparation

- Check the position-change schedule for the next time and type of position change.
- Administer an analgesic, if appropriate, before changing the client's position.
- Obtain required assistance, as needed.

## Procedure

1. Prior to performing the procedure, introduce self and verify the client's identify using agency protocol. Explain to the client what you are going to do, why it is necessary, and how he or she can participate.
2. Perform hand hygiene and observe other appropriate infection control procedures.
3. Provide for client privacy.

## VARIATION: Supporting a Client in Fowler's Position

1. Position the client.
   - Have the client flex the knees slightly before raising the head of the bed. ➤*Rationale: Slight knee flexion prevents the person from sliding toward the foot of the bed as the bed is raised.* Be certain the client's hips are positioned directly over the point where the bed will bend when the head is raised. ➤*Rationale: An appropriate hip position ensures that the client will be sitting upright when the head of the bed is raised.*
   - Raise the head of the bed to 45 degrees or the angle required by or ordered for the client.

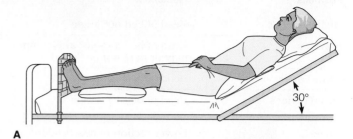

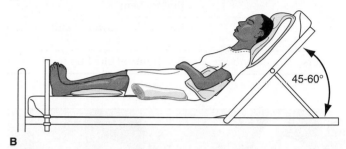

● **A.** Low Fowler's (semi-Fowler's) position (supported); **B.** Fowler's position (supported). The amount of support depends on the needs of the individual client.

2. Provide supportive devices to align the client appropriately.
   - Place a small pillow or roll under the lumbar region of the back if you feel a space in the lumbar curvature. ➤*Rationale: The pillow supports the natural lumbar curvature and prevents flexion of the lumbar spine.*
   - Place a small pillow under the client's head. ➤*Rationale: The pillow supports the cervical curvature of the vertebral column.* Alternatively, have the client rest the head against the mattress. ➤*Rationale: Too many pillows beneath the head can cause neck flexion contracture.*
   - Place one or two pillows under the lower legs from below the knees to the ankles. ➤*Rationale: The pillows provide a broad base of support that is soft and flexible, prevent uncomfortable hyperextension of the knees, and reduce pressure on the heels.* Make sure that no pressure is exerted on the popliteal space and that the knees are flexed. ➤*Rationale: Pressure against the popliteal space can damage nerves and vein walls, predisposing the client to thrombus formation. Keeping the knees slightly flexed also prevents the person from sliding down in the bed.*
   - Avoid using the knee gatch of a hospital bed to flex the client's knees. ➤*Rationale: The position of the knee gatch rarely coincides with the position of the client's knees. Even when the knee gatch does bend at the client's knees, considerable pressure (due to the narrow base of support beneath the knees and the firm, unyielding mattress) can be exerted against the popliteal space and beneath the client's calves.*

### TABLE 6-1 BED POSITIONS FOR CLIENT CARE

| Positions | Placement | Use |
|---|---|---|
| High-Fowler's | Head of bed 60° angle | Thoracic surgery, severe respiratory conditions |
| Fowler's | Head of bed 45°–60° angle; hips may or may not be flexed | Postoperative, gastrointestinal conditions, promotes lung expansion |
| Semi-Fowler's | Head of bed 30° angle | Cardiac, respiratory, neurosurgical conditions |
| Low-Fowler's | Head of bed 15° angle | Necessary degree elevation for ease of breathing, promotes skin integrity, client comfort |
| Knee-Gatch | Lower section of bed (under knees) slightly bent | For client comfort; contraindicated for vascular disorders |
| Trendelenburg | Head of bed lowered and foot raised | Percussion, vibration, and drainage (PVD) procedure; promotes venous return |
| Reverse Trendelenburg | Bed frame is tilted up with foot of bed down | Gastric conditions, prevents esophageal reflux |

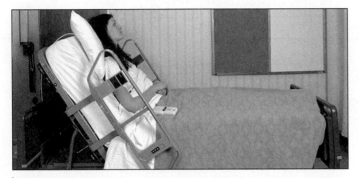

● High-Fowler's position at 60-degree angle.

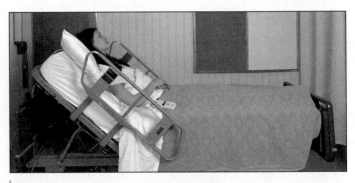

● Fowler's position at 45–60-degree angle.

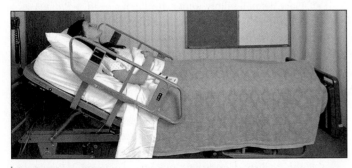

● Semi-Fowler's position at 30-degree angle.

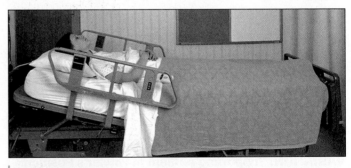

● Low-Fowler's position at 15-degree angle.

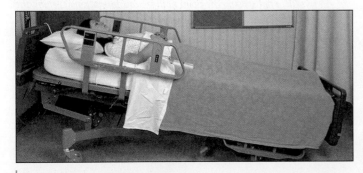

● Reverse Trendelenburg position.

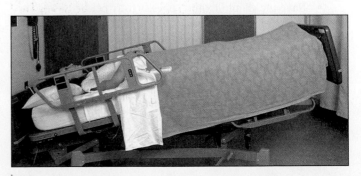

● Trendelenburg position.

- Put a trochanter roll lateral to each femur (optional). ➤*Rationale: This prevents external rotation of the hips.*
- Support the client's feet with a footboard. ➤*Rationale: This prevents plantar flexion.* The footboard should protrude several inches above the toes. ➤*Rationale: This protects the toes from pressure exerted by the top bedding.* The footboard should be placed 1 inch away from the heels. ➤*Rationale: This prevents undue pull on the Achilles tendon and discomfort.*
- Place pillows to support both arms and hands if the client does not have normal use of them. ➤*Rationale: These pillows prevent shoulder and muscle strain from the effects of downward gravitational pull, dislocation of the shoulder in paralyzed persons, edema of the hands and arms, and flexion contracture of the wrist.* Arrange the pillows to support only the forearms and hands, up to the elbow. In this way, the pillows support the shoulder girdle.

## VARIATION: Supporting a Client in the Dorsal Recumbent Position

1. Assist the client to the supine position.
2. Provide supportive devices to align the client appropriately.
   - Place a pillow of suitable thickness under the client's head and shoulders as needed. ➤*Rationale: This prevents hyperextension of the neck. Too many pillows beneath the head may cause or worsen neck flexion contracture.*
   - Place a pillow under the lower legs from below the knees to the ankles. ➤*Rationale: This prevents hyperextension of the knees, keeps the heels off the bed, and reduces lumbar lordosis.*
   - Place trochanter rolls laterally against the femurs (optional). ➤*Rationale: These prevent external rotation of the hips.*
   - Place a rolled towel or small pillow under the lumbar curvature if you feel a space between the lumbar area and the bed. ➤*Rationale: This pillow supports the lumbar curvature and prevents flexion of the lumbar spine.*
   - Put a footboard or rolled pillow on the bed to support the feet. ➤*Rationale: This prevents plantar flexion (footdrop).*
   - If the client is unconscious or has paralysis of the upper extremities, elevate the forearms and hands (*not* the upper arm) on pillows. ➤*Rationale: This position promotes comfort and prevents edema. Pillows are not placed under the upper arms because they can cause shoulder flexion.*
   - If the client has actual or potential finger and wrist flexion deformities, use hand rolls or wrist/hand splints. ➤*Rationale: This prevents flexion contractures of the fingers.* Hand rolls, having a circumference of 13 to 15 cm (5 to

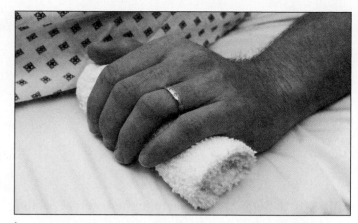

● A hand roll may be made from a folded and rolled washcloth. It is used to maintain functional position of the wrist and fingers and to prevent contractures.

6 in.) exert even pressure over the entire flexor surface of the palm and fingers.

## VARIATION: Supporting a Client in the Prone Position

1. Assist the client to a prone position.
   - See Skill 6.7 later in this chapter.
2. Provide supportive devices to position the client appropriately.
   - Turn the client's head to one side, and either omit the pillow entirely if drainage from the mouth is being encouraged, or place a small pillow under the head to align the head with the trunk. ➤*Rationale: This prevents flexion of the neck laterally.* Avoid placing the pillow under the shoulders. ➤*Rationale: A pillow placed under the shoulders increases lumbar lordosis.*
   - Place a small pillow or roll under the abdomen in the space between the diaphragm (or the breasts of a woman) and the iliac crests. ➤*Rationale: The pillow prevents hyperextension of the lumbar curvature, difficulty breathing, and, for some women, pressure on the breasts. Supports placed too low can increase lumbar lordosis and pressure on bony prominences.*
   - Place a pillow under the lower legs from below the knees to just above the ankles. ➤*Rationale: This raises the toes off the bed surface and reduces plantar flexion. This pillow also flexes the knees slightly for comfort and prevents excessive pressure on the patellae.* Or, position the client on the bed so that the feet are extended in a normal anatomical position over the lower edge of the mattress. ➤*Rationale: There should be no pressure on the toes.*

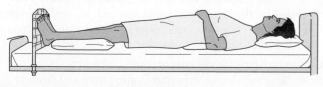

● Dorsal recumbent position (supported).

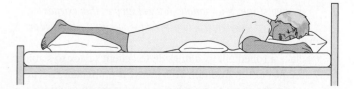

● Prone position (supported).

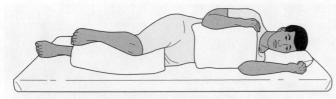

● Lateral position (supported).

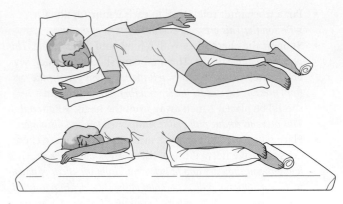

● Sims' position (supported).

## VARIATION: Supporting a Client in the Lateral Position

1. Assist the client to a lateral position.
   - See Skill 6.7 later in this chapter.
2. Provide supportive devices to align the client appropriately.
   - Place a pillow under the client's head so that the head and neck are aligned with the trunk. ➤*Rationale: The pillow prevents lateral flexion and discomfort of the major neck muscles (e.g.,the sternocleidomastoid muscles).*
   - Have the client flex the lower shoulder and position it forward so that the body does not rest on it. Rotate it into any position of comfort. ➤*Rationale: In this way, circulation is not disrupted.*
   - Place a pillow under the upper arm. ➤*Rationale: This prevents internal rotation and adduction of the shoulder and downward pressure on the chest that could interfere with chest expansion during respiration.* If the client has respiratory difficulty, increase the shoulder flexion and position the upper arm in front of the body off the chest.
   - Place two or more pillows under the upper leg and thigh so that the extremity lies in a plane parallel to the surface of the bed. ➤*Rationale: A position parallel to the bed most closely approximates correct standing alignment and prevents internal rotation of the thigh and adduction of the leg. The pillow also prevents pressure caused by the weight of the top leg resting on the lower leg. Such pressure can damage the vein walls in the lower leg and predispose the client to thrombus formation.*
   - Ensure that the two shoulders are aligned in the same plane as the two hips. If they are not, pull one shoulder or hip forward or backward until all four joints are aligned in the same plane. ➤*Rationale: Proper alignment prevents twisting of the spine.*
   - Place a folded towel under the natural hollow at the waistline (optional). ➤*Rationale: This prevents postural scoliosis of the lumbar spine.* Take care to fill in only the space at the waistline. ➤*Rationale: A towel support that extends too high or too low creates undue pressure against the rib cage or iliac crests.*
   - Place a rolled pillow alongside the client's back to stabilize the position (optional). This pillow is not usually needed when the client's upper hip and knee are appropriately flexed.

## VARIATION: Supporting a Client in the Sims' Position
**Procedure**

1. Turn the client as for the prone position.
2. Provide supportive devices to align the client appropriately.
   - Place a small pillow under the client's head, unless drainage from the mouth is being encouraged. ➤*Rationale: The pillow prevents lateral flexion of the neck and cushions the cranial and facial bones and the ear. It is contraindicated if drainage of mucus is required. Too large a pillow produces an uncomfortable lateral flexion of the neck.*
   - Place the lower arm behind and away from the client's body in a position that is comfortable and does not disrupt circulation. ➤*Rationale: This position prevents damage to the nerves and blood vessels in the axillae.*
   - Position the upper shoulder so that it is abducted slightly from the body and the shoulder and elbow are flexed. Place a pillow in the space between the chest and abdomen and the upper arm and bed. ➤*Rationale: This position and support prevent internal shoulder rotation and adduction and maintain alignment of the upper trunk.*
   - Place a pillow in the space between the abdomen and pelvis and the upper thigh and bed. ➤*Rationale: This position prevents internal rotation and adduction of the hip and also reduces lumbar lordosis.*
   - Ensure that the two shoulders are aligned in the same plane as the two hips. If they are not, pull one shoulder or hip forward or backward until all four joints are aligned in the same plane. ➤*Rationale: This prevents twisting of the spine.*
   - Place a support device (e.g., a sandbag or rolled towel) against the lower foot. ➤*Rationale: This device may prevent footdrop.* Efforts to correct plantar flexion in this position, however, are usually unsuccessful.

*Document all position changes carefully, recording:*
   - Time and change of position moved from and position moved to (according to agency protocol).

- Number of personnel required for turning and positioning.
- Safety precautions and the use of any premedications.
- Ways client is able to assist with positioning.
- Any signs of pressure areas or contractures.
- Any difficulty client has with breathing (Fowler's, prone, and Sims' positions).

- Use of support/assistive devices and any special requirements.

### Documentation

Sample: 10/15/09 1030 Turned to (L) side by 2 staff. Pillows under head, upper arm and upper leg. Skin intact without redness over bony prominences.

_____ M. Foti, RN

## Skill 6.3   Positioning a Child for Injections or Intravenous Access

### Preparation

1. Determine if the parent wants to be present during an uncomfortable procedure or to be available after the procedure to comfort the child.
2. When the parent wishes to be present, discuss the parent's role (e.g., holding the child or providing distraction or comfort during the procedure).
3. Make sure the person positioning and holding the child (parent or other assistant) clearly understands what body parts must be held still and how to do this safely.

### Equipment

- Supplies for procedure to be performed
- Infection control supplies as needed.

### Procedure

#### VARIATION: Supine Position

1. Place the child in a supine position on a bed or stretcher. ➤_Rationale: This position allows the child to see what is happening so that some of the child's fear is reduced._
2. Have a parent, a nurse, or an assistant lean over the child to restrain the child's body and extend the

extremity to be used for access or injection.
➤_Rationale: The nurse's body provides a source of human contact as well as securing the child so that the procedure can be done quickly._

#### VARIATION: Sitting Position

Have the child sit on the parent's or assistant's lap with legs held firmly between the assistant's legs. The child's arm closest to the adult can be wrapped around the back of the parent's or assistant's waist.

Have the parent or assistant hold the child firmly against the chest, wrapping arms around the child's upper body. Hold firmly but gently, ensuring that the child has chest expansion, allowing for normal breathing. ➤_Rationale: This hugging position adds comfort as well as security so the procedure can be done quickly._

The child should be restrained by the parent or assistant during intramuscular injections. Alternatively to this technique, the child's arm closest to the adult can be wrapped around the adult waist, leaving just the other arm in front to immobilize. Note that the leg not used for the injection is securely located between the adult's legs. Be certain that the child can breathe freely during restraining procedures.

## Skill 6.4   Positioning a Child for Lumbar Puncture

### Equipment

- Supplies for procedure to be performed.
- Infection control supplies as needed.

### Preparation

1. Determine if the parent wants to be present during an uncomfortable procedure or to be available after the procedure to comfort the child.
2. When the parent wishes to be present, discuss the parent's role (e.g., providing distraction or comfort during the procedure).

3. Make sure the person positioning and holding the child clearly understands what body parts must be held still and how to do this safely.

### Procedure

1. Place the child on his or her side with knees pulled to the abdomen and the neck flexed to the chin. The assistant can hold the child in position by wrapping one arm behind the knees and the other behind the neck, keeping the back curved.
➤_Rationale: This position ensures the best possible access to spinal processes and disk spaces._

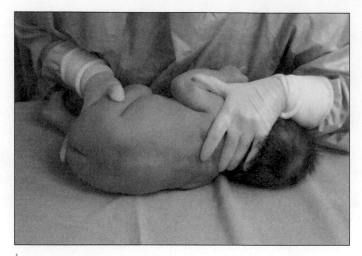

● Infant positioned for a lumbar puncture.

2. The infant can be held in this position easily by holding the neck and thighs in your hands.
3. The older child can be quite strong, and someone with enough strength will be needed to hold him or her in this position. Lean over the child with your entire body, using your forearms against the thighs and around the shoulders and head. Alternatively the older child may be in a seated position, bending forward and supported by the assistant.
4. Be certain that the child has free air exchange. Another assistant may be assigned to monitor respirations and perform other assessments during the procedure.

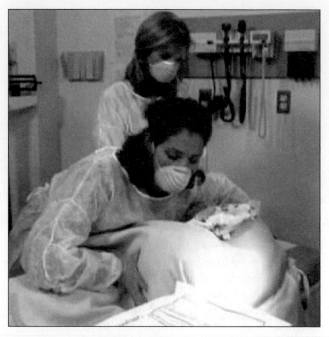

● Child positioned for a lumbar puncture.

## CLINICAL ALERT

Lumbar puncture requires that the child be held still to prevent injury and to ensure success at obtaining fluid. It is advisable to have an experienced staff member hold the child in position for the procedure. Ensure that the child has free air exchange and receives no injuries.

# Skill 6.5   Positioning a Child for an Otoscopic Examination

### Equipment
- Supplies for procedure to be performed.
- Infection control supplies as needed.

### Preparation
1. If the parent will be present, discuss the parent's role (e.g., holding the child or providing distraction or comfort during the procedure).
2. Make sure the person positioning and holding the child (parent or other assistant) clearly understands what body parts must be held and how to do this safely.

### Procedure
### VARIATION: Supine Position
1. Place the child in a supine position on a bed or a stretcher. Have the parent, a nurse, or an assistant lean over the child to position and hold the child's arms and body. The assistant may also assist with stabilizing the child's head.

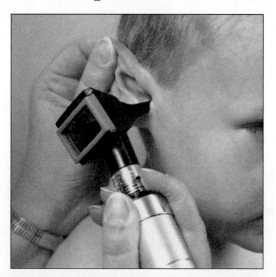

● To straighten the auditory canal: pull the pinna back and up for children over 3 years of age; pull the pinna down and back for children under 3 years of age.

2. Hold the otoscope in the hand closest to the child's face. When the child is cooperative, rest the back of your hand against the child's head. ➤*Rationale: This action provides additional stabilization of the child's head to prevent pain and injury when the otoscope earpiece is inserted into the auditory canal.*

3. Use your other hand to pull the pinna toward the back of the head and either up or down. ➤*Rationale: This action straightens the ear canal so that the tympanic membrane can be visualized.*

### VARIATION: Sitting Position

1. Have the child sit on the parent's or assistant's lap with legs held firmly between the assistant's legs. The child's arms can be wrapped around the parent's or assistant's waist.

2. Have the parent or assistant hold the child's head firmly against the chest with one arm while the other arm holds the arms and upper chest. ➤*Rationale: This position provides comfort to the child while securing the head.*

## Skill 6.6   Moving a Client Up in Bed

### Delegation

The skills of moving and turning clients in bed can be delegated to UAP. The nurse should make sure that any needed equipment and additional personnel are available to reduce risk of injury to the health care personnel. Emphasize the need for the UAP to report changes in the client's condition that require assessment and intervention by the nurse.

### Equipment

Assistive devices such as overhead trapeze, pull and/or turn sheet, sliding board or client moving, and transfer or sliding bar.

### Preparation

*Determine:*

• Assistive devices that will be required.
• Encumbrances to movement such as an IV or a heavy cast on one leg.
• Medications the client is receiving, because certain medications may hamper movement or alertness of the client.
• Assistance required from other health care personnel.

### Procedure

1. Prior to performing the procedure, introduce self and verify the client's identity using agency protocol. Explain to the client what you are going to do, why it is necessary, and how he or she can participate. Listen to any suggestions made by the client or support people.
2. Perform hand hygiene and observe other appropriate infection control procedures.
3. Provide for client privacy.
4. Adjust the bed and the client's position.
   • Adjust the head of the bed to a flat position or as low as the client can tolerate. ➤*Rationale: Moving the client upward against gravity requires more force and can cause back strain.*
   • Raise the bed to the height of your center of gravity.

### EVIDENCE-BASED NURSING

**Use of Draw Sheet for Moving Clients**

Few evidence-based studies disagree that the critical task of repositioning a client in bed places caregivers at an increased risk of back injury due to high spinal loads. Although the two-person draw sheet method of repositioning clients has the lowest low-back disorder risk, spinal loads were still high, thus increasing the risk of a back injury.

Most low back injuries are not the result of a single exposure to a high load but repeated small loads (bending) or a sustained load (sitting). Low back pain is shown to result from repetitive motion and excessive loading.

*Source:* Marras et al. A comprehensive analysis of low-back disorder risk and spinal loading transferring and repositioning of patients using different techniques. *Ergonomics,* 42(7), 904–926, July 1, 1999.

• Lock the wheels on the bed and raise the rail on the side of the bed opposite you.
• Remove all pillows, then place one against the head of the bed. ➤*Rationale: This pillow protects the client's head from inadvertent injury against the top of the bed during the upward move.*
5. Elicit the client's help in lessening your workload.
   • Ask the client to flex the hips and knees and position the feet so that they can be used effectively for pushing. ➤*Rationale: Flexing the hips and knees keeps the entire lower leg off the bed surface preventing friction during movement, and ensures use of the large muscle groups in the client's legs when pushing, thus increasing the force of movement.*
   • Ask the client to:
     a. Grasp the head of the bed with both hands and pull during the move.
        *or*
     b. Raise the upper part of the body on the elbows and push with the hands and forearms during the move.

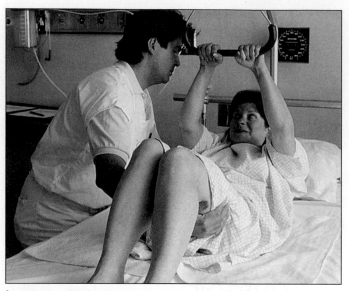

● Moving a client up in bed.

*or*

c. Grasp the overhead trapeze with both hands and lift and pull during the move. ➤*Rationale: Client assistance provides additional power to overcome inertia and friction during the move. These actions also keep the client's arms partially off the bed surface, reducing friction during movement, and make use of the large muscle groups of the client's arms to increase the force during movement.*

6. Position yourself appropriately, and move the client.
   • Face the direction of the movement, and then assume a broad stance with the foot nearest the bed behind the forward foot and weight on the forward foot. Lean your trunk forward from the hips. Flex hips, knees, and ankles.
   • Place your near arm under the client's thighs. ➤*Rationale: This supports the heaviest part of the body (the buttocks).* Push down on the mattress with the far arm. ➤*Rationale: The far arm acts as a lever during the move.*
   • Tighten your gluteal, abdominal, leg, and arm muscles and rock from the back leg to the front leg and back again. Then, shift your weight to the front leg as the client pushes with the heels and pulls with the arms so that the client moves toward the head of the bed.

7. Ensure client comfort.
   • Elevate the head of the bed and provide appropriate support devices for the client's new position.

## VARIATION: A Client with Limited Strength of the Upper Extremities

   • Assist the client to flex the hips and knees as in step 5 previously. Place the client's arms across the chest. ➤*Rationale: This keeps them off the bed surface and minimizes friction during movement.* Ask the client to flex the neck during the move and keep the head off the bed surface.
   • Position yourself as in step 6 previously and place one arm under the client's back and shoulders and the other arm under the client's thighs. ➤*Rationale: This placement of the arms distributes the client's weight and supports the heaviest part of the body (the buttocks).* Shift your weight as in step 6.

## VARIATION: Two Nurses Using a Turn Sheet

Two nurses can use a turn sheet to move a client up in bed. ➤*Rationale: A turn sheet distributes the client's weight more evenly, decreases friction, and exerts a more even force on the client during the move. In addition, it prevents injury of the client's skin, because the friction created between two sheets when one is moved is less than that created by the client's body moving over the sheet.*

   • Place a drawsheet or a full sheet folded in half under the client, extending from the shoulders to the thighs. Each person rolls up or fanfolds the turn sheet close to the client's body on either side.
   • Both individuals grasp the sheet close to the shoulders and buttocks of the client. ➤*Rationale: This draws the weight closer to the nurse's center of gravity and increases the nurse's balance and stability, permitting a smoother movement.* Follow the method of moving clients with limited upper extremity strength as described earlier.

8. Document all relevant information. Record:
   • Time and change of position moved from and position moved to.
   • Any signs of pressure areas.
   • Use of support devices.
   • Ability of client to assist in moving and turning.
   • Response of client to moving and turning (e.g., anxiety, discomfort, dizziness).

## DEVELOPMENTAL CONSIDERATIONS

### Physiologic Age Changes in the Musculoskeletal System that Affect Nursing Care of the Elderly

   • Contractures—muscles atrophy, regenerate slowly; tendons shrink and sclerose.
   • Range of motion of joints decreases—lack of adequate joint motion, ankylosis.
   • Mobility level is limited—muscle strength lessens and gait may be unsteady.

   • Kyphosis occurs—cervical vertebrae may be flexed; intervertebral discs narrow.
   • Bodies of thoracic vertebrae compress slowly with aging leading to the hunchback appearance—loss of overall height results from disk shrinkage and kyphosis.
   • Bone changes—loss of trabecular bones and bones become brittle.

## DEVELOPMENTAL CONSIDERATIONS (CONTINUED)

- Osteoporosis occurs as a result of calcium loss from the bone and insufficient replacement.
- Osteoarthritis increases with age, equally affecting men and women. This condition results in physical stress on joints as a result of long-term mechanical, horizontal, chemical, and genetic factors.

### Psychosocial and Physiological Changes in Elderly Who Are Immobile

- At risk for confusion, depression and disorientation—keep clock and calendar in room to help reorient to time and place.
- More susceptible to hazards of immobility—maintain own ADLs as much as possible and change position every 2 hours.

### Aging and Changes in Ability to Maintain Activity Levels

- As aging occurs, there is a decrease in the rate or speed of activity.

- Loss of muscle mass interferes with activities that require strength such as bending down, dressing, and reaching for objects.
- Dexterity decreases, leading to a change in performing manipulative skills.

### Nursing Care for Positioning Elderly Clients

- Ambulate within limitations of age.
- Alter position every 2 hours; align correctly.
- Prevent osteoporosis of long bones by providing exercises against resistance as ordered.
- Provide active and passive exercises—rest periods necessary and exercise paced throughout the day for the elderly.
- Provide range-of-motion exercises to all joints three times a day.
- Educate family that allowing the client to be sedentary is not helpful.
- Encourage walking, which is best single exercise for the elderly.

## CULTURAL CONSIDERATIONS

Different cultures may have cultural variances regarding distance and space. When clients are being moved, transferred to a bed or gurney, client is brought close to nurse's body. It is important to explain the transfer process to client, particularly Americans, Canadians, and British clients. They may be threatened by invasion of personal space and touch. Japanese, Arabs, and Latin Americans aren't as concerned about personal space.

## Skill 6.7 Turning a Client to the Lateral or Prone Position in Bed

### Preparation

*Determine:*

- Assistive devices that will be required.
- Encumbrances to movement such as an IV or a heavy cast on one leg.
- Medications the client is receiving, because certain medications may hamper movement or alertness of the client.
- Assistance required from other health care personnel.

### Procedure

1. Prior to performing the procedure, introduce self and verify the client's identity using agency protocol. Explain to the client what you are going to do, why it is necessary, and how he or she can participate.
2. Perform hand hygiene and observe other appropriate infection control procedures.

3. Provide for client privacy.
4. Position yourself and the client appropriately before performing the move.
   - Move the client closer to the side of the bed opposite the side the client will face when turned. ➤*Rationale: This ensures that the client will be positioned safely in the center of the bed after turning.* Use a pull sheet beneath the client's trunk and thighs to pull the client to the side of the bed. Roll up the sheet as close as possible to the client's body and pull the client to the side of the bed. Adjust the client's head and reposition the legs appropriately.
   - While standing on the side of the bed nearest the client, place the client's near arm across the chest. Abduct the client's far shoulder slightly from the side of the body and externally rotate the shoulder. ➤*Rationale: Pulling the one arm forward facilitates the turning motion. Pulling the other arm away from the body and externally rotating the shoulder*

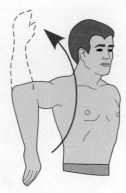

• External rotation of the shoulder prevents the arm from being caught beneath the client's body when the client is turned.

*prevents that arm from being caught beneath the client's body during the roll.*
• Place the client's near ankle and foot across the far ankle and foot. ➤*Rationale: This facilitates the turning motion. Making these preparations on the side of the bed closest to the client helps prevent unnecessary reaching.*
• Raise the side rail next to the client before going to the other side of the bed. ➤*Rationale: This ensures that the client, who is close to the edge of the mattress, will not fall.*
• Position yourself on the side of the bed toward which the client will turn, directly in line with the client's waistline and as close to the bed as possible.

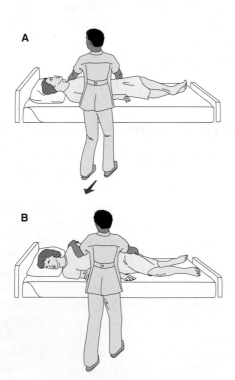

A

B

• Moving a client to a lateral position.

• Lean your trunk forward from the hips. Flex your hips, knees, and ankles. Assume a broad stance with one foot forward and the weight placed on this forward foot.
5. Pull or roll the client toward you to the lateral position.
• Place one hand on the client's far hip and the other hand on the client's far shoulder. ➤*Rationale: This position of the hands supports the client at the two heaviest parts of the body, providing greater control in movement during the roll.*
• Tighten your gluteal, abdominal, leg, and arm muscles; rock backward, shifting your weight from the forward to the backward foot, and roll the client onto the side of the body to face you. ➤*Rationale: Turning the client toward you promotes the client's sense of security.*
• Position the client on his or her side with arms and legs positioned and supported properly.

**VARIATION: Turning the Client to a Prone Position**

To turn a client to the prone position, follow the preceding steps, with two exceptions:
• Instead of abducting the far arm, keep the client's arm alongside the body for the client to roll over. ➤*Rationale: Keeping the arm alongside the body prevents it from being pinned under the client when the client is rolled.*
• Roll the client completely onto the abdomen. ➤*Rationale: It is essential to move the client as close as possible to the edge of the bed before the turn so that the client will be lying on the center of the bed after rolling.* Never pull a client across the bed while the client is in the prone position. ➤*Rationale: Doing so can injure a woman's breasts or a man's genitals.*
6. Document all relevant information. Record:
• Time and change of position moved from and position moved to.
• Any signs of pressure areas.
• Use of support devices.
• Ability of client to assist in moving and turning.
• Response of client to moving and turning (e.g., anxiety, discomfort, dizziness).

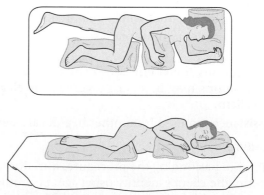

• Lateral position with pillows in place.

# Skill 6.8  Logrolling a Client

**Logrolling** is a technique used to turn a client whose body must at all times be kept in straight alignment (like a log). An example is the client with a spinal injury. Considerable care must be taken to prevent additional injury. This technique requires two nurses or, if the client is large, three nurses. For the client who has a cervical injury, one nurse must maintain the client's head and neck alignment.

## Preparation

*Determine:*

- Assistive devices that will be required.
- Encumbrances to movement such as an IV or a heavy cast on one leg.
- Medications the client is receiving, because certain medications may hamper movement or alertness of the client.
- Assistance required from other health care personnel.

## Procedure

1. Prior to performing the procedure, introduce self and verify the client's identity using agency protocol. Explain to the client what you are going to do, why it is necessary, and how he or she can participate.
2. Perform hand hygiene and observe other appropriate infection control procedures.
3. Provide for client privacy.
4. Position yourselves and the client appropriately before the move.
   - Stand on the same side of the bed, and assume a broad stance with one foot ahead of the other.

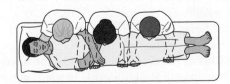

● Correct arm placement for moving a client to the side of the bed: two nurses.

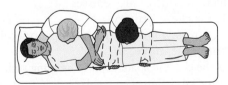

● Correct arm placement for moving a client to the side of the bed: three nurses.

- Place the client's arms across the chest. ➤*Rationale: Doing so ensures that the arms will not be injured or become trapped under the body when the body is turned.*
- Lean your trunk, and flex your hips, knees, and ankles.
- Place your arms under the client as shown below, depending on the client's size. ➤*Rationale: Each staff member then has a major weight area of the client centered between the arms.*
- Tighten your gluteal, abdominal, leg, and arm muscles.

5. Pull the client to the side of the bed.
   - One nurse counts: One, two, three, go. Then, at the same time, all staff members pull the client to the side of the bed by shifting their weight to the back foot. ➤*Rationale: Moving the client in unison maintains the client's body alignment.*
   - Elevate the side rail on this side of the bed. ➤*Rationale: This prevents the client from falling while lying so close to the edge of the bed.*
6. Move to the other side of the bed, and place supportive devices for the client when turned.
   - Place a pillow where it will support the client's head after the turn. ➤*Rationale: The pillow prevents lateral flexion of the neck and ensures alignment of the cervical spine.*
   - Place one or two pillows between the client's legs to support the upper leg when the client is turned. ➤*Rationale: This pillow prevents adduction of the upper leg and keeps the legs parallel and aligned.*
7. Roll and position the client in proper alignment.
   - All nurses flex their hips, knees, and ankles and assume a broad stance with one foot forward.
   - All nurses reach over the client and place hands as shown below. ➤*Rationale: Doing so centers a major weight area of the client between each nurse's arms.*
   - One nurse counts: One, two, three, go. Then, at the same time, all nurses roll the client to a lateral position.
   - Support the client's head, back, and upper and lower extremities with pillows.
   - Raise the side rails and place the call bell within the client's reach.

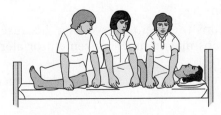

● Correct hand placement for logrolling a client.

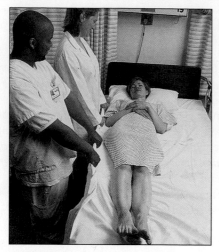

❙● Using a turn sheet, the nurses pull the sheet with the client on it to the edge of the bed.

### VARIATION: Using a Turn or Lift Sheet

- Use a turn sheet to facilitate logrolling. First, stand with another nurse on the same side of the bed. Assume a broad stance with one foot forward, and grasp half of the fanfolded or rolled edge of the turn sheet. On a signal, pull the client toward both of you.
- Before turning the client, place pillow supports for the head and legs, as described in step 6. This helps maintain the client's alignment when turning. Then, go to the other side of the bed (farthest from the client), and assume a stable stance. Reaching over the client, grasp the far edges of the turn sheet, and roll the client toward you.

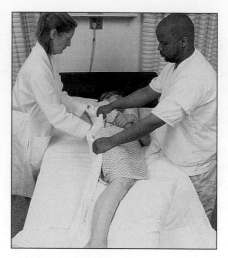

❙● The nurse on the right uses the far edge of the sheet to roll the client toward him; the nurse on the left remains behind the client and assists with turning.

The second nurse (behind the client) helps turn the client and provides pillow supports to ensure good alignment in the lateral position.

8. Document all relevant information. Record:
   - Time and change of position moved from and position moved to.
   - Any signs of pressure areas.
   - Use of support devices.
   - Ability of client to assist in moving and turning.
   - Response of client to moving and turning (e.g., anxiety, discomfort, dizziness).

# Skill 6.9   Assisting the Client to Sit on Side of Bed (Dangle)

The client assumes a sitting position on the edge of the bed to allow neurovascular equilibration before walking, moving to a chair or wheelchair, eating, or performing other activities.

### Preparation

*Determine:*
- Assistive devices that will be required.
- Encumbrances to movement such as an IV or a heavy cast on one leg.
- Medications the client is receiving, because certain medications may hamper movement or alertness of the client.
- Assistance required from other health care personnel.

### Procedure

1. Prior to performing the procedure, introduce self and verify the client's identity using agency protocol. Explain to the client what you are going to do, why it is necessary, and how he or she can participate.

2. Perform hand hygiene and observe other appropriate infection control procedures.
3. Provide for client privacy.
4. Position yourself and the client appropriately before performing the move.
   - Assist the client to a lateral position facing you.
   - Raise the head of the bed slowly to its highest position. ➤*Rationale: This decreases the distance that the client needs to move to sit up on the side of the bed.*
   - Position the client's feet and lower legs at the edge of the bed. ➤*Rationale: This enables the client's feet to move easily off the bed during the movement, and the client is aided by gravity into a sitting position.*
   - Stand beside the client's hips and face the far corner of the bottom of the bed (the angle in which movement will occur). Assume a broad stance, placing the foot nearest the client forward. Lean your trunk forward from the hips. Flex your hips, knees, and ankles.

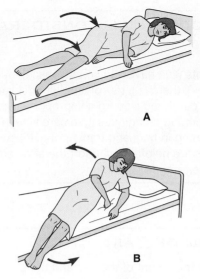

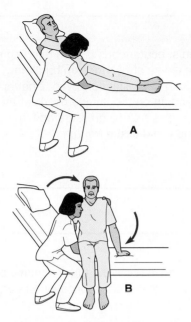

● Moving to a sitting position independently.

● Assisting a client to a sitting position on the edge of the bed.

5. Move the client to a sitting position.
   • Place one arm around the client's shoulders and the other arm beneath both of the client's thighs near the knees. ➤*Rationale: Supporting the client's shoulders prevents the client from falling backward during the movement. Supporting the client's thighs reduces friction of the thighs against the bed surface during the move and increases the force of the movement.*
   • Tighten your gluteal, abdominal, leg, and arm muscles.
   • Lift the client's thighs slightly. ➤*Rationale: This reduces the friction of the client's thighs and the nurse's arm against the bed surface.*
   • Pivot on the balls of your feet in the desired direction facing the foot of the bed while pulling the client's feet and legs off the bed. ➤*Rationale: Pivoting prevents twisting of the nurse's spine. The weight of the client's legs swinging downward increases downward movement of the lower body and helps make the client's upper body vertical. This also gives the client's vascular system a chance to equilibrate after the positional change.*
   • Keep supporting the client until the client is well balanced and comfortable. ➤*Rationale: This movement will help prevent fainting due to orthostatic hypotension.*

   • Assess vital signs (e.g., pulse, respirations, and blood pressure) as indicated by the client's health status.

**VARIATION: Teaching a Client How to Sit on the Side of the Bed Independently**

A client who has had recent abdominal surgery or who is weak may have too much abdominal pain or too little strength to sit straight up in bed. This person can be taught to assume a dangle position without assistance. Instruct the client to:
   • Roll to the side and lift the far leg over the near leg.
   • Grasp the mattress edge with the lower arm and push the fist of the upper arm into the mattress.
   • Push up with the arms as the heels and legs slide over the mattress edge.
   • Maintain the sitting position by pushing both fists into the mattress behind and to the sides of the buttocks.

6. Document all relevant information. Record:
   • Ability of client to assist in moving and turning.
   • Response of client to moving and turning (e.g., anxiety, discomfort, dizziness).

## DEVELOPMENTAL CONSIDERATIONS

### Infants

   • Position infants on their back for sleep, even after feeding. There is little risk of regurgitation and choking, and the rate of sudden infant death syndrome (SIDS) is significantly lower in infants who sleep on their backs.

   • The skin of newborns can be fragile and may be abraded or torn (sheared) if the infant is pulled across a bed.

### Children

   • Carefully inspect the dependent skin surfaces of all infants and children confined to bed at least three times in each 24-hour period. *(continued)*

## DEVELOPMENTAL CONSIDERATIONS (CONTINUED)

### Elders

- In clients who have had cerebrovascular accidents (strokes), there is a risk of shoulder displacement on the paralyzed side from improper moving or repositioning techniques. Use care when moving, positioning in bed, and transferring. Pillows or foam devices are helpful to support the affected arm and shoulder and prevent injury.

- Decreased subcutaneous fat and thinning of the skin place elders at risk for skin breakdown. Repositioning approximately every 2 hours (more or less, depending on the unique needs of the individual client) helps reduce pressure on bony prominences and avoid tissue trauma.

## SETTING OF CARE

- Assess the height of the bed and the person's leg length to ensure that self-movements in and out of the bed are smooth.

- When making a home visit, it is particularly important to inspect the mattress for support. A sagging mattress, a mattress that is too soft, or an under-filled waterbed used over a prolonged period can contribute to the development of hip flexion contractures and low back strain and pain. Bed boards made of plywood and placed beneath a sagging mattress are increasingly recommended for clients who have back problems or are prone to them.

- Assess the caregivers' knowledge and application of body mechanics to prevent injury.

- Demonstrate how to turn and position the client in bed. Observe the caregiver performing a return demonstration. Reevaluate this technique periodically to reinforce correct application of body mechanics.

- Teach caregivers the basic principles of body alignment and how to check for proper alignment after the client has been changed to a new position.

- Warn caregivers of the dangers of lifting and repositioning and encourage the use of assistive devices and a "No Solo Lift" policy.

- Teach the caregiver to check the client's skin for redness and integrity after repositioning the client. Stress the importance of informing the nurse about the length of time skin redness remains over pressure areas after the person has been repositioned. Emphasize that reddened areas should not be massaged because it may lead to tissue trauma.

# Skill 6.10  Transferring between Bed and Chair

### Delegation

The skill of transferring a client can be delegated to UAP who have demonstrated safe transfer technique for the involved client. It is important for the nurse to assess the client's capabilities and communicate specific information about what the UAP should report back to the nurse.

### Equipment

- Robe or appropriate clothing
- Slippers or shoes with nonskid soles
- Transfer (walking) belt
- Chair, commode, wheelchair, or stretcher as appropriate to client need
- Sliding board

### Preparation

- Plan what to do and how to do it.
- Obtain essential equipment before starting (e.g., transfer belt, wheelchair) and check that all equipment is functioning correctly.
- Remove obstacles from the area so clients do not trip, and make sure there are no spills or liquids on the floor on which clients could slip.

## Procedure

1. Prior to performing the procedure, introduce self and verify the client's identity using agency protocol. Explain the transfer process to the client. During the transfer, explain step by step what the client should do, for example, "Move your right foot forward."
2. Perform hand hygiene and observe other appropriate infection control procedures.
3. Provide for client privacy.
4. Position the equipment appropriately.
   - Lower the bed to its lowest position so that the client's feet will rest flat on the floor. Lock the wheels of the bed.
   - Place the wheelchair parallel to the bed as close to the bed as possible. Put the wheelchair on the side of the bed that allows the client to move toward his or her stronger side. Lock the wheels of the wheelchair and raise the footplate.
5. Prepare and assess the client.
   - Assist the client to a sitting position on the side of the bed (see Skill 6.9).
   - Assess the client for orthostatic hypotension before moving the client from the bed.
   - Assist the client in putting on a bathrobe and nonskid slippers or shoes.
   - Place a transfer belt snugly around the client's waist. Check to be certain that the belt is securely fastened.
6. Give explicit instructions to the client. Ask the client to:
   - Move forward and sit on the edge of the bed. ➤*Rationale: This brings the client's center of gravity closer to the nurse's.*
   - Lean forward slightly from the hips. ➤*Rationale: This brings the client's center of gravity more directly over the base of support and positions the head and trunk in the direction of the movement.*
   - Place the foot of the stronger leg beneath the edge of the bed and put the other foot forward. ➤*Rationale: In this way, the client can use the stronger leg muscles to stand and power the movement. A broader base of support makes the client more stable during the transfer.*
   - Place the client's hands on the bed surface so that the client can push while standing. ➤*Rationale: This provides additional force for the movement and reduces the potential for strain on the nurse's back.* The client should **not** grasp your neck for support. ➤*Rationale: Doing so can injure the nurse.*
7. Position yourself correctly.
   - Stand directly in front of the client. Lean the trunk forward from the hips. Flex the hips, knees, and ankles. Assume a broad stance, placing one foot forward and one back. Mirror the placement of the client's feet, if possible. ➤*Rationale: This helps prevent loss of balance during the transfer.*
   - Encircle the client's waist with your arms, and grasp the transfer belt at the client's back with thumbs pointing downward. ➤*Rationale: The belt provides a secure handle for holding on to the client and controlling the movement. Downward placement of the thumbs prevents potential wrist injury as the nurse lifts. By supporting the client in this manner, you keep the client from tilting backward during the transfer.*
   - Tighten your gluteal, abdominal, leg, and arm muscles.

● The wheelchair is placed parallel to the bed as close to the bed as possible. Note that placement of the nurse's feet mirrors that of the client's feet.

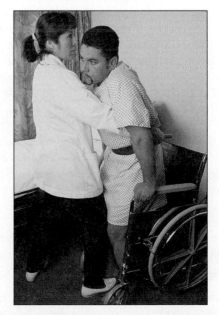

● Using a transfer (walking) belt.

8. Assist the client to stand, and then move together toward the wheelchair.
   - On the count of three, ask the client to push with the back foot, rock to the forward foot, and extend (straighten) the joints of the lower extremities. Push or pull up with the hands, while pushing with the forward foot, rock to the back foot, extend the joints of the lower extremities, and pull the client (directly toward your center of gravity) into a standing position.
   - Support the client in an upright standing position for a few moments. ➤*Rationale: This allows the nurse and the client to extend the joints and provides the nurse with an opportunity to ensure that the client is stable before moving away from the bed.*
   - Together, pivot or take a few steps toward the wheelchair.
9. Assist the client to sit.
   - Ask the client to:
     a. Back up to the wheelchair and place the legs against the seat. ➤*Rationale: Having the client place the legs against the wheelchair seat minimizes the risk of the client falling when sitting down.*
     b. Place the foot of the stronger leg slightly behind the other. ➤*Rationale: This supports body weight during the movement.*
     c. Keep the other foot forward. ➤*Rationale: This provides a broad base of support.*
     d. Place both hands on the wheelchair arms. ➤*Rationale: This increases stability and lessens the strain on the nurse.*
   - Stand directly in front of the client. Place one foot forward and one back.
   - Tighten your grasp on the transfer belt, and tighten your gluteal, abdominal, leg, and arm muscles.
   - On the count of three, have the client shift the body weight by rocking to the back foot. Lower the body onto the edge of the wheelchair seat by flexing the joints of the legs and arms. Place some body weight on the arms, while shifting your body weight by stepping back with the forward foot and pivoting toward the chair while lowering the client onto the wheelchair seat.
10. Ensure client safety.
    - Ask the client to push back into the wheelchair seat. ➤*Rationale: Sitting well back on the seat provides a broader base of support and greater stability and minimizes the risk of falling from the wheelchair. A wheelchair can topple forward when the client sits on the edge of the seat and leans far forward.*
    - Lower the footplates, and place the client's feet on them.
    - Apply a seat belt as required.

**VARIATION: Angling the Wheelchair**

For clients who have difficulty walking, place the wheelchair at a 45-degree angle to the bed. ➤*Rationale: This enables the client to pivot into the chair and lessens the amount of body rotation required.*

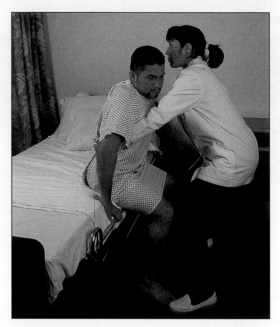

● Transferring without a belt.

**VARIATION: Transferring without a Belt**

- For clients who need minimal assistance, place the hands against the sides of the client's chest (not at the axillae) during the transfer. For clients who require more assistance, reach through the client's axillae and place the hands on the client's scapulae during the transfer. Avoid placing hands or pressure on the axillae, especially for clients who have upper extremity paralysis or paresis.
- Follow the steps described previously.

**VARIATION: Transferring with a Belt and Two Nurses**

- When the client is able to stand, position yourselves on both sides of the client, facing the same direction as the client. Flex your hips, knees, and ankle. Grasp the client's transfer belt with the hand closest to the client, and with the other hand support the client's elbows.
- Coordinating your efforts, all three of you stand simultaneously, pivot, and move to the wheelchair. Reverse the process to lower the client onto the wheelchair seat.

**VARIATION: Transferring a Client with an Injured Lower Extremity**

When the client has an injured lower extremity, movement should always occur toward the client's unaffected (strong) side. For example, if the client's right leg is injured and the client is sitting on the edge of the bed preparing to transfer to a wheelchair, position the wheelchair on the client's left side. ➤*Rationale: In this way, the client can use the unaffected leg most effectively and safely.*

### VARIATION: Using a Sliding Board

• For clients who cannot stand, use a sliding board to help them move without nursing assistance. ➤*Rationale: This method not only promotes the client's sense of independence but also preserves your energy.*

11. Document relevant information:
    • Client's ability to bear weight and pivot.
    • Number of staff needed for transfer and safety measures/precautions used.
    • Length of time up in chair.
    • Client response to transfer and being up in chair or wheelchair.

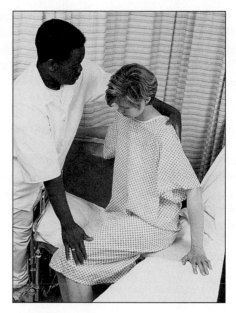

● Using a sliding board.

# Skill 6.11   Transferring between Bed and Stretcher

### Delegation

The skill of transferring a client can be delegated to UAP who have demonstrated safe transfer technique for the involved client. It is important for the nurse to assess the number of staff needed, assistive devices needed, client's ability to assist, and to communicate specific information about what the UAP should report to the nurse.

### Equipment

• Stretcher
• Optional: sliding board or assistive device such as the Slipp® Patient Mover shown in photo

### Preparation

Obtain the necessary equipment and nursing personnel to assist in the transfer.

### Procedure

1. Prior to performing the procedure, introduce self and verify the client's identity using agency protocol. Explain to the client what you are going to do, why it is necessary, and how he or she can participate. Explain the transfer to the nursing personnel who are helping and specify who will give directions (one person needs to be in charge).
2. Perform hand hygiene and observe other appropriate infection control procedures.
3. Provide for client privacy.

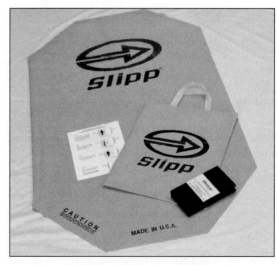

● The Slipp® Patient Mover is a client-moving device that reduces risk of back injuries in staff and maximizes client comfort.
*Note:* Courtesy of Wright Products, hc., Wrightproductsinc.com.

4. Adjust the client's bed in preparation for the transfer.
   • Lower the head of the bed until it is flat or as low as the client can tolerate.
   • Raise the bed so that it is slightly higher than the surface of the stretcher. ➤*Rationale: It is easier to move the client down a slope rather than up.*
   • Ensure that the wheels on the bed are locked.
   • Pull the drawsheet out from both sides of the bed.

5. Move the client to the edge of the bed and position the stretcher.
   - Roll the drawsheet as close to the client's side as possible.
   - Pull the client to the edge of the bed and cover the client with a sheet or bath blanket to maintain comfort.
   - Place the stretcher parallel to the bed next to the client and lock the stretcher wheels.
   - Fill the gap that exists between the bed and the stretcher loosely with the bath blankets (optional).
6. Transfer the client securely to the stretcher.
   - In unison with the other staff members, press your body tightly against the stretcher. ➤*Rationale: This prevents the stretcher from moving.*
   - Roll the pull sheet tightly against the client. ➤*Rationale: This achieves better control over client movement.*
   - Flex your hips and pull the client on the pull sheet in unison directly toward you and onto the stretcher. ➤*Rationale: Pulling downward requires less force than pulling along a flat surface.*
   - Ask the client to flex the neck during the move, if possible, and place the arms across the chest. ➤*Rationale: This prevents injury to these body parts.*
7. Ensure client comfort and safety.
   - Make the client comfortable, unlock the stretcher wheels, and move the stretcher away from the bed.

- Immediately raise the stretcher side rails and/or fasten the safety straps across the client. ➤*Rationale: Because the stretcher is high and narrow, the client is in danger of falling unless these safety precautions are taken.*

### VARIATION: Using a Transfer Board

The transfer board is a lacquered or smooth polyethylene board measuring 45 to 55 cm (18 to 22 in.) by 182 cm (72 in.) with handholds along its edges. Transfer mattresses are also available, as are mechanical assistive devices such as the Slipp® Patient Mover (shown on previous page). It is imperative to have enough people assisting with the transfer to prevent injury to staff as well as clients. Turn the client to a lateral position away from you, position the board close to the client's back, and roll the client onto the board. Pull the client and board across the bed to the stretcher. Safety belts may be placed over the chest, abdomen, and legs.

8. Document relevant information:
   - Equipment used.
   - Number of people needed for transfer and safety measures/precautions used.
   - Destination if reason for transfer is transport from one location to another.

# Skill 6.12   Using a Hydraulic Lift

### Delegation

The skill of using a hydraulic lift can be delegated to UAP who have demonstrated competent use of the equipment for the involved client.

### Equipment

- Hydraulic lift (such as a Hoyer or ceiling-mounted lift) with any necessary accessories.

### Preparation

Obtain the lift and put in the client's room. Arrange for assistance from others at a designated time.

### Procedure

1. Prior to performing the procedure, introduce self and verify the client's identity using agency protocol. Explain to client what you are going to do, why it is necessary, and how he or she can participate. Explain the procedure and demonstrate the lift. ➤*Rationale: Some clients are afraid of being lifted and will be reassured by a demonstration.*
2. Wash hands and observe other appropriate infection control procedures.
3. Provide for client privacy.

4. Prepare the equipment.
   - Lock the wheels of the client's bed and raise the bed to the high position.
   - Put up the side rail on the opposite side of the bed and lower the side rail near you.
   - Position the lift so that it is close to the client.
   - Place the chair that is to receive the client beside the bed. Allow adequate space to maneuver the lift.
   - Lock the wheels, if a chair with wheels is used.
5. Position the client on the sling.
   - Roll the client away from you.
   - Place the canvas seat or sling under the client with the wide lower edge under the client's thighs to the knees and the more narrow upper edge up under the client's shoulders. ➤*Rationale: This places the sling under the client's center of gravity and greatest part of body weight. Correct placement permits the client to be lifted evenly, with minimal shifting.*
   - Raise the bed rail on your side of the bed, and go to the opposite side of the bed. Lower this side rail.
   - Roll the client to the opposite side, and pull the canvas sling through.
   - Roll the client to the supine position and center the client on top of the canvas sling.

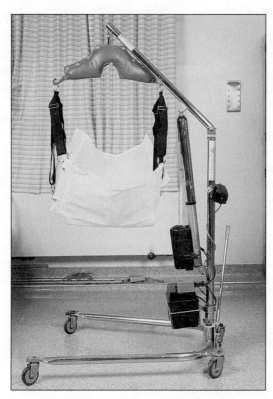

● A one-piece seat hydraulic lift.

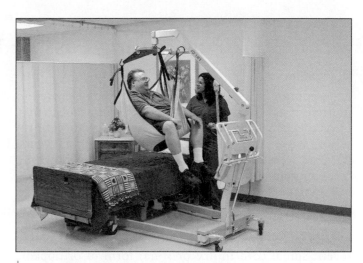

● EZ Lift® is an electric client lift that moves clients from bed, chair, toilet, and floor.

(Courtesy of EZ Way, Inc.)

6. Attach the sling to the swivel bar.
   - Wheel the lift into position, with the footbars under the bed on the side where the chair is positioned. Set the adjustable base at the widest position to ensure stability. Lock the wheels of the lifter.
   - Lower the side rail.
   - Move the lift arms directly over the client and lower the horizontal bar by releasing the hydraulic valve. Lock the valve.
   - Attach the lifter straps or hooks to the corresponding openings in the canvas seat. Check that the hooks are correctly placed and that matching straps or chains are of equal length. Face the hooks away from the client. ➤*Rationale: This prevents the hooks from injuring the client.*

7. Lift the client gradually.
   - Elevate the head of the bed to place the client in a sitting position.
   - Ask the client to remove eyeglasses and put them in a safe place. ➤*Rationale: The swivel bar may come close to the face and cause breakage of eyeglasses.*
   - *Nurse 1:* Close the pressure valve, and gradually pump the jack handle until the client is above the bed surface. ➤*Rationale: Gradual elevation of the lift is less frightening to the client than a rapid rise.*

   - *Nurse 2:* Assume a broad stance, and guide the client with your hands as the client is lifted. ➤*Rationale: This prepares the nurse to hold the client and provide control during the movement.*
   - Check the placement of the sling before moving the client away from the bed.

8. Move the client over the chair.
   - *Nurse 1:* With the pressure valve securely closed, slowly roll the lift until the client is over the chair. Use the steering handle to maneuver the lift.
   - *Nurse 2:* Guide movement by hand until the client is directly over the chair. ➤*Rationale: Slow movement decreases swaying and is less frightening. Guidance also decreases swaying and gives a sense of security.*

9. Lower the client into the chair.
   - *Nurse 1:* Release the pressure valve very gradually. ➤*Rationale: Gradual release is less frightening than a quick descent.*
   - *Nurse 2:* Guide the client into the chair.

10. Ensure client comfort and safety.
    - Remove the hooks from the canvas seat. Leave the seat in place. ➤*Rationale: The seat is left in place in preparation for the lift back to bed.*
    - Align the client appropriately in a sitting position and return the client's eyeglasses, if appropriate.
    - Apply a seat belt or other restraint as needed.
    - Place the call bell within reach.

11. Document the type of equipment, number of assistants needed, safety precautions taken, and the client's physiologic and psychological response.

# Skill 6.13  Performing Passive Range of Motion Exercises

## Delegation

Performing passive ROM exercises can be delegated to unlicensed assistive personnel (UAP). Some agencies may have specially trained nursing assistants who perform restorative activities, such as range of motion, for clients. For UAP who do not have this special training, however, it is important for the nurse to review the general guidelines for performing passive ROM exercises to avoid injury to the UAP or client. Encourage the UAP to perform ROM during the bath. Emphasize the importance of reporting anything unusual to the nurse. If a client has a recent spinal cord injury or some form of orthopedic trauma, the nurse of a physical therapist should do the ROM.

## Equipment

- No special equipment is needed other than a bed.

## Preparation

Prior to initiating the exercises, review any possible restrictions with the primary care provider or physical therapist. Also refer to the agency's protocol.

## Procedure

1. Prior to performing the skill, introduce self and verify the client's identity using agency protocol. Explain to the client what you are going to do, why it is necessary, and how he or she can participate. Listen to any suggestions made by the client or support people. Discuss the importance of ROM exercises in the plan of care. ➤*Rationale: The more a client can assist the better. Whenever possible, progress should be made toward active ROM exercises.*
2. Perform hand hygiene and observe other appropriate infection control procedures.
3. Provide for client privacy, and use client-selected music when possible. ➤*Rationale: The ROM session is an opportunity to use touch with the client in a relaxing and therapeutic manner. Any measures that will enhance relaxation are warranted, such as privacy, scent, and sound.*
4. Assist the client to a supine position near you and expose only the body parts requiring exercise. ➤*Rationale: This ensures thermal comfort and protects modesty.*
5. Place the client's feet together, place the arms at the sides, and leave space around the head and the feet. ➤*Rationale: Positioning the client close to you prevents excessive reaching.*
6. Perform exercises in a head-to-toe format. Follow a repetitive pattern and return to the starting position after each motion. Repeat each motion three to five times on the affected limb. ➤*Rationale: This ensures thoroughness in the movement and reduces chances of forgetting any part of the body.*
7. Support the limb being ranged above and below the joint. ➤*Rationale: This facilitates support and comfort. It also allows the nurse to detect ease/resistance to movement.*
8. Assess for pain by eliciting client self-report before, throughout, and after the session. Observe the client for nonverbal/behavioral cues of discomfort or pain, as well as verbal. Accept the client's self-report or behavioral cues and address pain fully in a timely manner. ➤*Rationale: Pain monitoring is always an essential nursing responsibility. Using verbal self-report and observing behavior will enable the nurse to respond therapeutically to any clients who experience pain, whether or not they are able to verbalize for themselves.*
9. Perform ROM slowly, gently, and smoothly. ➤*Rationale: This will encourage relaxation and lengthening of muscles so they can be ranged further.*
10. Neck (pivot joint)
    - Remove the client's pillow.
    - Flex and extend the neck (ROM: 45 degrees from midline):
      - Place the palm of one hand under the client's head and the palm of the other hand on the client's chin.
      - Move the head from the upright midline position forward until the chin rests on the chest.

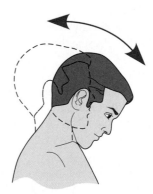

● Flexion/extension of neck.

- Move the head from the flexed position back to the resting supine position without the head pillow.
- Lateral flexion of the neck (ROM: 40 degrees from midline):
  - Place the heels of the hands on each side of the client's cheeks.
  - Move the head laterally toward the right and left shoulders.

- Extension (ROM: 180 degrees from vertical position beside the head):
- Move the arm from a vertical position beside the head forward and down to a resting position at the side of the body.
- Abduction (ROM: 180 degrees):
- Move the arm laterally from the resting position at the side to a side position above the head, palm of the hand away from the head.

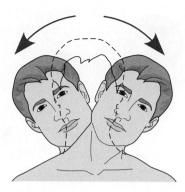

● Lateral flexion of neck.

- Rotation (ROM: 70 degrees from midline):
  - Place the heels of the hands on each side of the client's cheeks.
  - Turn the face as far as possible to the right and left.

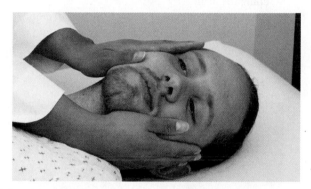

● Rotation of the neck.

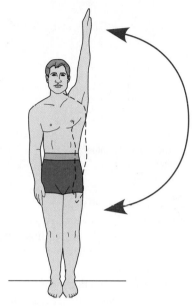

● Abducting the shoulder.

11. Shoulder (ball-and-socket joint)
    - Flexion (ROM: 180 degrees from the side):
      - Begin with the client's arm at the side. Grasp the arm beneath the elbow with one hand and beneath the wrist with the other hand unless otherwise indicated.
      - Raise the arm from a position by the side forward and upward to a position beside the head. The elbow may need to be flexed if the headboard is in the way.

- Adduction (ROM: 230 degrees):
  - Move the arm laterally from the position beside the head downward laterally and across the front of the body as far as possible.

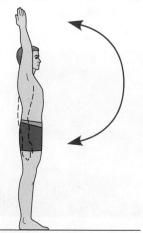

● Flexion/extension of shoulder.

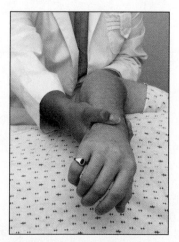

● Adducting the shoulder.

- External rotation (ROM: 90 degrees):
  - With arm held out to the side at shoulder level and the elbow bent to a right angle, fingers pointing down, move the arm upward so that the fingers point up and the back of the hand touches the mattress.

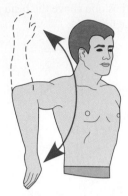

● External/internal rotation of shoulder.

- Internal rotation (ROM: 90 degrees):
  - With the arm held out to the side at shoulder level and the elbow bent to a right angle, fingers pointing up, bring the arm forward and down so that the palm touches the mattress.
- Circumduction (ROM: 360 degrees):
  - Move the arm forward, up, back, and down in a full circle.

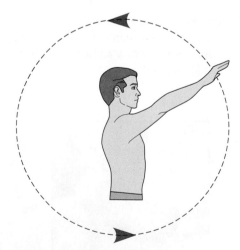

● Circumduction of shoulder.

12. Elbow (hinge joint)
  - Flexion (ROM: 150 degrees):
    - Bring the lower arm forward and upward so that the hand is level with the shoulder.

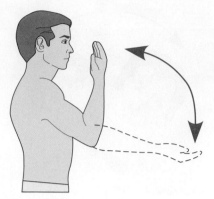

● Flexion/extension of elbow.

- Extension (ROM: 150 degrees):
  - Bring the lower arm forward and downward, straightening the arm.
  - Rotation for supination (ROM: 70 to 90 degrees):
  - Grasp the client's hand as for a handshake and turn the palm upward. Make sure that only the forearm (not the shoulder) moves.

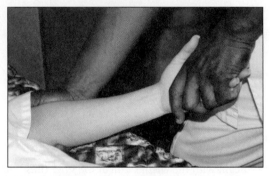

● Supinating the forearm.

- Rotation for pronation (ROM: 70 to 90 degrees):
  - Grasp the client's hand as for a handshake and turn the palm downward. Make sure that only the forearm (not the shoulder) moves.

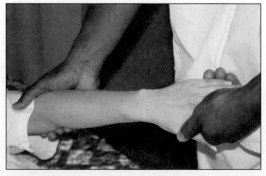

● Pronating the forearm.

13. Wrist (condyloid joint)
    - Flexion (ROM: 80 to 90 degrees):
        - Flex the client's arm at the elbow until the forearm is at a right angle to the mattress. Support the wrist joint with one hand while your other hand manipulates the joint.
        - Bring the fingers of the hand toward the inner aspect of the forearm.

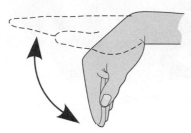

● Flexion/extension of wrist.

- Extension (ROM: 80 to 90 degrees):
    - Straighten the hand to the same place as the arm.
- Hyperextension (ROM 70 to 90 degrees):
    - Bend the fingers of the hand back as far as possible.

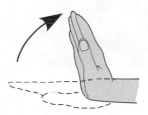

● Hyperextension of wrist.

- Radial flexion (abduction) (ROM: 0 to 20 degrees):
    - Bend the wrist laterally toward the thumb side.

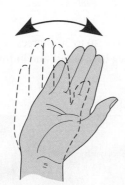

● Radial and ulnar flexion.

- Ulnar flexion (adduction) (ROM: 30 to 50 degrees):
    - Bend the wrist laterally toward the fifth finger.

14. Hand and fingers (metacarpophalangeal joints—condyloid; interphalangeal joints—hinge)
    - Flexion (ROM: 90 degrees):
        - Make a fist.

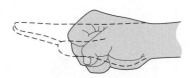

● Flexion/extension of fingers.

- Extension (ROM: 90 degrees):
    - Straighten the fingers.
- Hyperextension (ROM: 30 degrees):
    - Gently bend fingers back.
- Abduction (ROM: 20 degrees):
    - Spread the fingers of the hand apart.

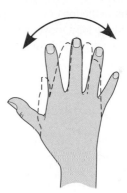

● Abduction/adduction of fingers.

- Adduction (ROM: 20 degrees):
    - Bring fingers together.

15. Thumb (saddle joint)
    - Flexion (ROM: 90 degrees):
        - Move the thumb across the palmar surface of the hand toward the fifth finger.

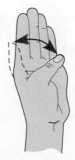

● Flexion/extension of thumb.

- Extension (ROM: 90 degrees):
  - Move the thumb away from the hand.
- Abduction (ROM: 30 degrees):
  - Extend the thumb laterally (can be done when placing fingers in abduction and adduction).

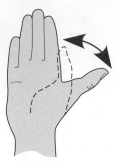

● Abduction/adduction of thumb.

- Adduction (ROM: 30 degrees):
  - Move the thumb back to the hand.
- Opposition:
  - Touch thumb to the top of each finger of the same hand. The thumb joint movements involved are abduction, rotation, and flexion.

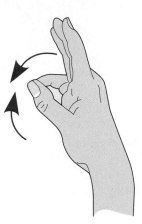

● Opposition.

16. Hip (ball-and-socket joint)
  - To carry out hip and leg exercises, place one hand under the client's knee and the other under the ankle.

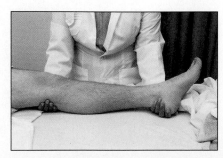

● Position for knee and hip movements.

- Flexion (ROM: knee extended, 90 degrees; knee flexed, 120 degrees):
  - Lift the leg and bend the knee, moving the knee up toward the chest as far as possible.

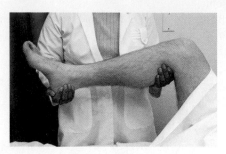

● Flexing the knee and the hop.

- Extension (ROM: 90 to 120 degrees):
  - Bring the leg down, straighten the knee, and lower the leg to the bed.
- Abduction (ROM: 45 to 50 degrees):
  - Move the leg to the side away from the client.

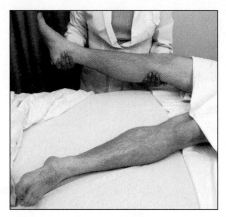

● Abducting the leg.

- Adduction (ROM: 20 to 30 degrees beyond other leg):
  - Move the leg back across and in front of the other leg.

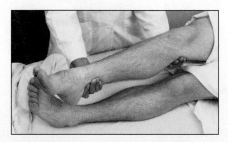

● Adducting the leg.

- Circumduction (ROM: 360 degrees):
  - Move the leg in a circle.

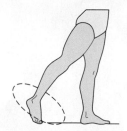

● Circumduction of hip.

- Internal rotation (ROM: 90 degrees):
  - Roll the foot and leg inward.

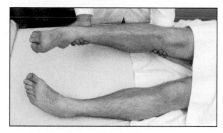

● Internal rotation of hip.

- External rotation (ROM: 90 degrees):
  - Roll the foot and leg outward.

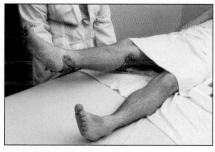

● External rotation of hip.

17. Knee (hinge joint)
    - Flexion (ROM: 120 to 130 degrees):
      - Bend the leg, bringing the heel toward the back of the thigh (done with hip flexion).

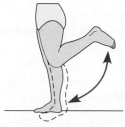

● Flexion/extension of knee.

- Extension (ROM: 120 to 130 degrees):
  - Straighten the leg, returning the foot to the bed.

18. Ankle (hinge joint)
    - Extension (plantar flexion) (ROM: 45 to 50 degrees):
      - Move the foot so the toes are pointed downward.

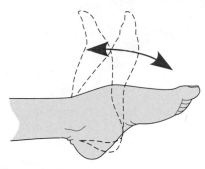

● Extension/flexion of ankle.

- Flexion (dorsiflexion) (ROM: 20 degrees):
  - Move foot so toes are pointed upward.

19. Foot (gliding)
    - Eversion (ROM: 5 degrees):
      - Place one hand under the client's ankle and the other over the arch of the foot.
      - Turn the whole foot outward.

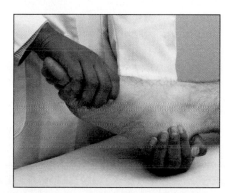

● Everting the foot.

- Inversion (ROM: 5 degrees):
  - Using the same hand placement as above, turn the whole foot inward.

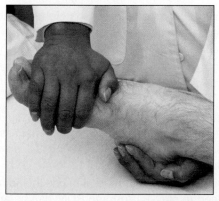

● Inverting the foot.

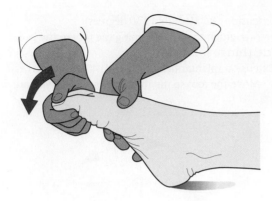

● Flexing the toes.

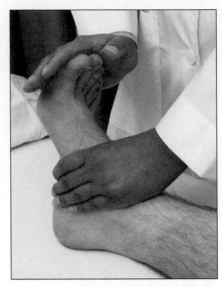

● Extending the toes.

20. Toes (interphalangeal joints—hinge; metatarsophalangeal joints—hinge; intertarsal joints—gliding)
    • Flexion (ROM: 35 to 60 degrees):
        • Place one hand over the arch of the foot.
        • Place the fingers of the other hand over the toes to curl the toes downward.
    • Extension (ROM: 35 to 60 degrees):
        • Place one hand over the arch of the foot.
        • Place the fingers of the other hand under the toes to bend the toes upward.
    • Abduction (ROM: 0 to 15 degrees):
        • Spread the toes apart.
    • Adduction (ROM: 0 to 15 degrees):
        • Bring the toes together.
21. Move to the other side of the bed and repeat exercises for other arm and leg.
22. Document
    • Type of ROM exercise (e.g., active, passive, active-assistive).
    • Joints exercised and their degree of joint motion.
    • Length of exercise.
    • Client's tolerance level to the activity.
    • Any abnormalities.

**Documentation**

Sample: 8/16/09 1000 Passive ROM performed with bath. All joints ranged fully with 4 reps each. Resistance in shoulders resolved when pace slowed. Tolerated well, no c/o pain.

_____ M. Foti, RN

---

## DEVELOPMENTAL CONSIDERATIONS

### Children

• Perform exercises gently and with full range of motion, avoiding hyperextension of joints. ➤Rationale: _Some children may have lax ligaments, and overstretching can cause injury and pain._

• A small roll can be made of soft cloth to place in the palms. ➤Rationale: _The roll is used to prevent contractures of the fingers._

• High-top sneakers or footboards can be used. ➤Rationale: _This helps prevent footdrop (plantar flexion of the foot)._

• In some children with impaired mobility, splinting of the wrist, knees, or ankles may be necessary. ➤Rationale: _Splinting helps prevent severe contractures_ (Hockenberry & Wilson, 2007).

• Children have developmental needs including the need to play. Performing ROM can be an opportunity for fun and for enhancing the child–caregiver relationship.

### Elders

• Avoid hyperextending the joints of elders. ➤Rationale: _Such movements can cause pain or nerve damage because joints become less flexible with age._

• Work slowly and assess for pain when working with elders, especially those who have arthritis. ➤Rationale: _Arthritis changes can cause contractures and enlarged, painful joints._

• Assess for skin breakdown or reddened areas during the range-of-motion procedure. ➤Rationale: _Elders are at risk for skin breakdown due to decreased subcutaneous fat and increased thinning of the skin._

CHAPTER 6  Mobility  **247**

SETTING OF CARE

Teach the client's caregiver:

- The purpose and importance of performing ROM exercises at home.
- To move gently and slowly through each exercise.

- To perform the exercises at least twice daily and to do three to five repetitions of each exercise.
- How to use correct body mechanics to prevent muscle strain while performing the exercises.

# Skill 6.14   Using Continuous Passive Motion Device

### Delegation

The initial application and setting up of the CPM device should not be delegated to UAP because application of scientific and nursing knowledge and potential problem solving are needed. The UAP however, can assist the client with ADLs (e.g., bathing) while the CPM device is being used. The UAP can also assist the nurse in placing the client's limb in the CPM device. The nurse needs to discuss with the UAP what observations to report to the nurse (e.g., client complaint of increased pain, swelling, and/or skin breakdown).

### Equipment

- CPM device
- Padding for the cradle
- Restraining straps
- **Goniometer** (a handheld device used to measure the angle of a joint in degrees)

### Preparation

- Verify the primary care provider's orders and agency protocol.
- Determine the degrees of flexion, extension, and speed initially prescribed.
- Check agency protocol and primary care provider's orders about increases in degrees and speed for subsequent treatments.
- Have another person ready to assist in placing the client's limb in the CPM device.

### Procedure

1. Prior to performing the skill, introduce self and verify the client's identity using agency protocol. Explain to the client what you are going to do, why it is necessary, and how he or she can participate. Listen to any suggestions made by the client or support people. Discuss the importance of CPM in the plan of care.
2. Perform hand hygiene and observe other appropriate infection control procedures.

3. Provide for client privacy.
4. Make sure client has been assisted in toileting prior to beginning.
5. Address client reports of pain prior to beginning, premedicating if necessary.
6. Set up the machine.
   - Place the machine on the bed. Remove an egg-crate mattress, if indicated. ➤*Rationale: This provides a stable surface.*
   - Connect the control box to the CPM machine.
7. Set the prescribed levels of flexion, extension, and speed.
   - Most postoperative clients are started on 10 to 45 degrees of flexion and 0 to 10 degrees of extension.
   - Adjust the speed control to the slow to moderate range for the first postoperative day, and then increase the speed as ordered and tolerated.
   - Place padding on the CPM cradle. ➤*Rationale: This prevents rubbing and pressure.*
   - Run machine through a complete cycle. ➤*Rationale: This ensures that the machine is functioning properly.*
   - Stop the machine in full extension.
8. Position the client and place the leg in the machine.
   - Place the client in a supine position with the head of the bed elevated 15 to 25 degrees.
   - Support the leg and, with the client's help (or another staff member if client is unable to assist), lift the leg and place it in the padded cradle.
   - Adjust the device to the client's extremity. Lengthen or shorten appropriate sections of the frame to fit the machine to the client.
   - Center client's leg on the frame. ➤*Rationale: This avoids the development of pressure areas.*
   - Align the client's knee joint with the hinged joint of the machine.
   - Adjust the foot support so that the foot is supported in either a neutral position or slight dorsiflexion (e.g., 20 degrees). ➤*Rationale: This prevents footdrop.* Check agency protocol.
   - Ensure that the leg is neither internally nor externally rotated. ➤*Rationale: Neutral alignment prevents injury.*

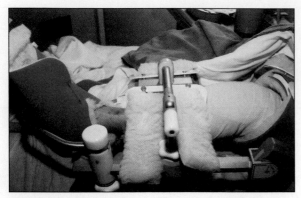

● Extremity secured with straps.

- Secure straps around the thigh and top of the foot and cradle to allow enough space to fit several fingers under the strap.
9. Start the machine.
   - When the machine reaches the fully flexed position, stop the machine, and verify the degree of flexion with a goniometer. ➤*Rationale: This is a double check of the setting and helps prevent possible complications.*
   - Restart the machine, and observe a few cycles of flexion and extension to ensure proper functioning.

10. Ensure continued client safety and comfort.
    - Make sure that the client is comfortable. Observe for non-verbal signs of discomfort.
    - Place within the client's reach the call light, the bedside table, and any items frequently used by the client.
    - Turn off electric bed controls. ➤*Rationale: This prevents client from inadvertently changing alignment of extremity.*
    - Instruct a mentally alert client how to operate the on/off switch.
    - Loosen the straps and check the client's skin at least twice per 8-hour shift.
11. Document the degree of flexion, the degree of extension, the speed, the duration of the therapy, and the client's activity tolerance.

**Documentation**

Sample: 8/17/09 1230 CPM removed. Skin intact, incision without redness or drainage. Reports pain at 3/10. Given Percocet 2.5 mg. per order.

_____ K. Armor, RN

1300 Rates pain at 0/10. Resting comfortably.

_____ K. Armor, RN

1400 CPM resumed @ 30 degrees flexion, 10 degrees extension. Denies pain.

_____ K. Armor, RN

---

## DEVELOPMENTAL CONSIDERATIONS

**Children**

- Explain the use of the CPM device in terms that the child will understand and will not increase the child's anxiety. Use of dolls or stuffed animals may help.
- Arrange for social or creative activities that are developmentally appropriate for the child during the CPM treatment.

**Elders**

- Older clients may have limited joint flexibility.
- Older clients may need to balance period of activity with period of rest.
- If the older client is apprehensive, teach techniques for muscle relaxation and pain control such as guided imagery and progressive relaxation.
- Provide distractions (such as music, TV) and opportunities for socialization.

---

## SETTING OF CARE

The CPM machine can be used at home if the client or caregiver demonstrates competence. Teach the client or caregiver:
- How to set the controls and progressively increase the adjustment as the client's tolerance builds.
- To get assistance from another person and use proper body dynamics to prevent injury to self and client.

- To report excessive pain, swelling, or redness of the affected joints.
- To provide skin care and check for skin breakdown every 4 hours.
- How to clean and care for the equipment.

# Skill 6.15   Assisting the Client to Ambulate

## Delegation

Ambulation of clients is frequently delegated to UAP. However, the nurse should conduct an initial assessment of the client's abilities in order to direct other personnel in providing appropriate assistance. Any unusual events that arise from assisting the client in ambulation must be validated and interpreted by the nurse.

## Equipment

- Transfer belt whether or not the client is known to be unsteady
- Wheelchair for following client, or chairs along the route if the client needs to rest

## Preparation

- Be certain that others are available to assist you if needed. Also, plan the route of ambulation that has the fewest hazards.

## Performance

1. Prior to performing the procedure, introduce self and verify the client's identity using agency protocol. Explain to the client what you are going to do, why ambulation is necessary, and how he or she can participate. Discuss how this activity relates to the overall plan of care.
2. Perform hand hygiene and observe appropriate infection control procedures.
3. Ensure that the client is appropriately dressed to walk and has shoes or slippers with nonskid soles.
4. Prepare the client for ambulation.
   - Apply elastic (antiemboli) stockings as required.
   - Have client sit up in bed for at least 1 minute prior to preparing to dangle legs.
   - Assist the client to sit on the edge of the bed and allow dangling for at least 1 minute (see Skill 6.9).
   - Assess the client carefully for signs and symptoms of orthostatic hypotension (dizziness, light-headedness, or a sudden increase in heart rate) prior to leaving the bedside. ➤*Rationale: Allowing for gradual adjustment can minimize drops in blood pressure (and fainting) that occur with shifts in position from lying to sitting, and sitting to standing.*
   - Assist the client to stand by the side of the bed for at least 1 minute until he or she feels secure.
   - Carefully attend to any IV tubing, catheters, or drainage bags. Keep urinary drainage bags below level of the client's bladder. ➤*Rationale: To prevent backflow of urine into bladder and risk of infection.*
5. Ensure client safety while assisting the client to ambulate.
   - Encourage the client to ambulate independently if he or she is able, but walk beside the client's weak side, if appropriate.

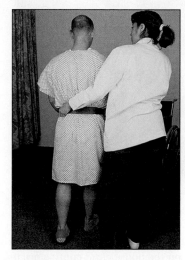

● Using a transfer (walking) belt to support the client.

- Remain physically close to the client in case assistance is needed at any point.
- Use a transfer or walking belt to increase safety. Make sure the belt is pulled snugly around the client's waist and fastened securely. Grasp the belt at the client's back, and walk behind and slightly to one side of the client.
- If it is the client's first time out of bed following surgery, injury, or an extended period of immobility, or if the client is quite weak or unstable, have an assistant follow you and the client with a wheelchair in the event that it is needed quickly.
- If the client is moderately weak and unstable, walk on the client's weaker side and interlock your forearm with the client's closest forearm. Encourage the client to press the forearm against your hip or waist for stability if desired. In addition, have the client wear a transfer or walking belt. ➤*Rationale: You can quickly grab the belt and prevent a fall if the client feels faint.*
- If the client is very weak and unstable, place your near arm around the client's waist, and with your other arm support the client's near arm at the elbow. Walk on the client's stronger side. Again, have the client wear a transfer or walking belt in case of an emergency. Encourage the client to assume a normal walking stance and gait as much as possible.
6. Protect the client who begins to fall while ambulating.
   - If a client begins to experience the signs and symptoms of orthostatic hypotension or extreme weakness, quickly assist the client into a nearby wheelchair or other chair, and help the client to lower the head between the knees.
   - Stay with the client. ➤*Rationale: A client who faints while in this position could fall head first out of the chair.*
   - When the weakness subsides, assist the client back to bed.

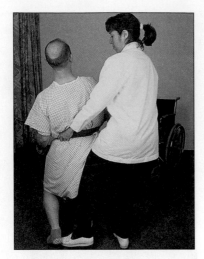

● Lowering a fainting client to the floor.

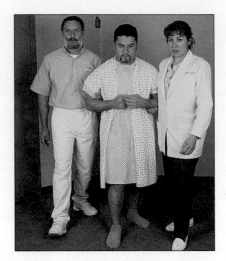

● Two nurses supporting an ambulatory client.

- If a chair is not close by, assist the client to a horizontal position on the floor before fainting occurs.
  a. Assume a broad stance with one foot in front of the other. ➤*Rationale: A broad stance widens your base of support. Placing one foot behind the other allows you to rock backward and use the femoral muscles when supporting the client's weight and lowering the center of gravity (see the next step), thus preventing back strain.*
  b. Bring the client backward so that your body supports the person. ➤*Rationale: Clients who faint or start to fall usually pitch slightly forward because of the momentum of ambulating. Bringing the client's weight backward against your body allows gradual movement to the floor without injury to the client.*
  c. Allow the client to slide down your leg, and lower the person gently to the floor, making sure the client's head does not hit any objects.

## VARIATION: Two Nurses

- After the client stands, assume a position with one nurse at either side. Grasp the inferior aspect of the client's upper arm with your nearest hand and the client's lower arm or hand with your other hand. ➤*Rationale: This provides a secure grip for each nurse.*
- Place a walking belt around the client's waist. Each nurse grasps the side handle with the near hand and the lower aspect of the client's upper arm with the other hand.
- Walk in unison with the client, using a smooth, even gait, at the same speed and with steps the same size as the client's. ➤*Rationale: This gives the client a greater feeling of security.*
- If the client starts to fall and cannot regain strength or balance, slip your arms under the client's axillae, grasp the client's hands, and lower the person gently to the floor or to a nearby chair. ➤*Rationale: Placing the nurse's arms under the client's axillae evenly balances the*

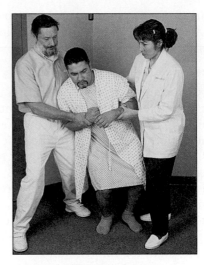

● Two nurses lowering a fainting client to the floor.

*client's weight between the two nurses, preventing injury to both the nurses and the client.*

7. Document distance and duration of ambulation in the client record using forms or checklists supplemented by narrative notes when appropriate. Include description of the client's gait (including body alignment) when walking, pace, activity tolerance when walking (e.g., pulse rate, facial color, any shortness of breath, feelings of dizziness, or weakness), degree of support required, and respiratory rate and blood pressure after initial ambulation to compare with baseline data.

## Documentation

Sample: 8/22/09 1030 Ambulated length of hall and returned with minimal assistance of 2 staff. Steady, aligned gait, tolerated well. VS remain at baseline after walking. _____ B. Snyder, RN

## DEVELOPMENTAL CONSIDERATIONS

### Children

- Children and adolescents who have suffered a sports injury (e.g., sprained ankle) may want to be more active than they should be. A cast, splint, or boot may be put in place to limit activity and assist in healing. Teach children the importance of appropriate activity and the use of assistive devices (e.g., crutches) if necessary. Help them focus on what they can do rather than what they cannot do (e.g., "You can stand at the free-throw line and shoot baskets").

### Elders

- Inquire how the client has ambulated previously and modify assistance accordingly.
- Take into account a decrease in speed, strength, resistance to fatigue, reaction time, and coordination due to a decrease in nerve conduction.
- Be cautious when using a transfer belt with a client with osteoporosis. Too much pressure from the belt can increase the risk of vertebral compression fractures.

- If assistive devices such as a walker or cane are used, make sure clients are supervised in the beginning to learn the proper method of using them. Crutches may be much more difficult for elders due to decreased upper body strength.
- Be alert to signs of activity intolerance, especially in elders with cardiac and lung problems.
- Set small goals and increase slowly to build endurance, strength, and flexibility.
- Be aware of any fall risks the elder may have, such as the following:
  - Effects of medications
  - Neurological disorders
  - Environmental hazards
  - Orthostatic hypotension
  - In elders, the body's responses return to normal more slowly. For instance, an increase in heart rate from exercise may stay elevated for hours before returning to normal.

## SETTING OF CARE

- When making a home visit, assess carefully for safety issues for ambulation. Counsel the client and family about unfastened rugs, slippery floors, and loose objects on the floors.

- Check the surroundings for adequate supports such as railings and grab bars.
- Recommend that nonskid strips be placed on outside steps and inside stairs that are not carpeted.

# Skill 6.16   Assisting the Client to Use a Cane

### Delegation

Due to the extent of knowledge required, teaching the client to use assistive devices is not delegated to UAP. The nurse or the physical therapist does the teaching. However, once the client has demonstrated adequate skill, UAP may assist the client in ambulating with this equipment.

### Equipment

- Appropriately-sized cane with rubber tips

### Preparation

- Ensure that the client's path is free from clutter and hazards.

### Procedure

1. Prior to performing the procedure, introduce self and verify the client's identity using agency protocol. Explain to the client what you are going to do, why it is necessary, and how he or she can participate. Discuss how this activity will be used in planning further care or treatments.
2. Perform hand hygiene and observe appropriate infection control procedures.
3. Ensure that client is appropriately dressed for walking.
4. Prepare the client for walking.
   - Ask the client to hold the cane on the stronger side of the body. ➤*Rationale: This provides support and body alignment when walking. The arm opposite the advancing foot normally swings forward when walking, so the hand holding the cane will come forward and the cane will support the weaker leg.*
   - Position the tip of a standard cane (and the nearest tip of other canes) about 15 cm (6 in.) to the side and 15 cm (6 in.) in front of the near foot, so that the elbow is slightly flexed. ➤*Rationale: This provides the best balance and*

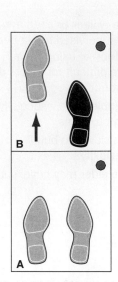
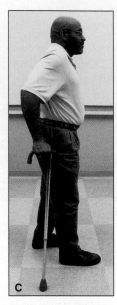

● Steps involved in using a cane to provide maximum support.

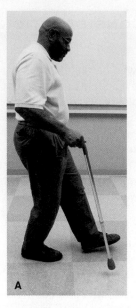
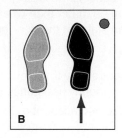

● Steps involved in using a cane when less than maximum support is required.

*prevents the person from leaning on the cane. In this position, the client stands erect, with the center of gravity within the base of support.*

5. When maximum support is required, instruct the client to move as follows:
    • Move the cane forward about 30 cm (1 ft), or a distance that is comfortable while the body weight is borne by both legs.
    • Then, move the affected (weak) leg forward to the cane while the weight is borne by the cane and stronger leg.
    • Next, move the unaffected (stronger) leg forward ahead of the cane and weak leg while the weight is borne by the cane and weak leg.
    • Repeat the above three steps. ➤*Rationale: This pattern of moving provides at least two points of support on the floor at all times.*

6. When the client becomes stronger and requires less support, instruct the client to follow these steps:
    • Move the cane and weak leg forward at the same time, while the weight is borne by the stronger leg.
    • Move the stronger leg forward while the weight is borne by the cane and the weak leg.

7. Ensure client safety.
    • Walk beside the client on the affected side. ➤*Rationale: The client is most likely to fall toward the affected side.*

• Walk the client for the time or distance indicated in the plan of care.
• If the client loses balance or strength and is unable to regain it, slide your hand up to the client's axilla, and take a broad stance to provide a base of support. Have the client rest against your hip until assistance arrives, or gently lower yourself and the client to the floor.
• For stair climbing, the phrase "up with the good, down with the bad" can help clients remember which pattern of movement to use.

8. Document the client's progress in the client record using forms or checklists supplemented by narrative notes when appropriate. Describe the distance ambulated and any difficulties the client experienced.

## CLINICAL ALERT

Instruct clients to use the cane opposite the side of pain or weakness to facilitate balance and decrease weight on painful extremities.

# Skill 6.17   Assisting the Client to Use Crutches

## Preparation

- Ensure that the crutches are the proper length.

## Procedure

1. Assist the client to assume the tripod (triangle) position, the basic crutch stance used before crutch walking.
   - Ask the client to stand and place the tips of the crutches 15 cm (6 in.) in front of the feet and out laterally about 15 cm (6 in.). ➤*Rationale: The tripod position provides a wide base of support and enhances both stability and balance.*
   - Make sure the feet are slightly apart. A tall person requires a wider base than a short person.
   - Ensure that posture is erect; that is, the hips and knees should be extended, the back straight, and the head held straight and high. There should be no hunch to the shoulders and thus no weight borne by the axillae. The elbows should be extended sufficiently to allow weight bearing on the hands.
   - Stand slightly behind and on the client's affected side. ➤*Rationale: By standing behind the client and toward the affected side, the nurse can provide support if the client loses balance.*
   - If the client is unsteady, place a walking belt around the client's waist, and grasp the belt from above, not from below. ➤*Rationale: A fall can be prevented more effectively if the belt is held from above.*

2. Teach the client the appropriate crutch gait.

## VARIATION: Four-Point Alternate Gait

This is the most elementary and safest gait, providing at least three points of support at all times, but it requires coordination. It can be used when walking in crowds because it does not require much space. To use this gait, the client has to be able to bear some weight on both legs. Ask the client to:

- Move the right crutch ahead a suitable distance (e.g., 10 to 15 cm [4 to 6 in.]).

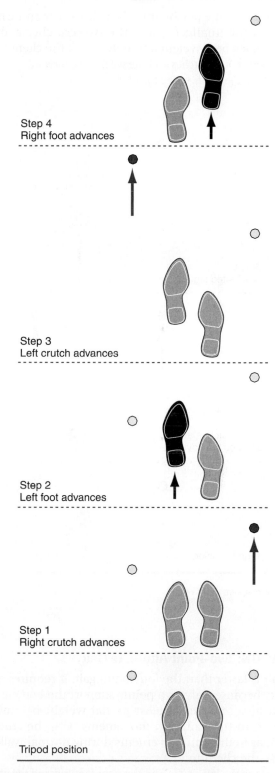

Step 4
Right foot advances

Step 3
Left crutch advances

Step 2
Left foot advances

Step 1
Right crutch advances

Tripod position

● The four-point alternate crutch gait.

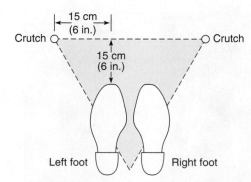

● The tripod position.

- Move the left foot forward, preferably to the level of the crutch.
- Move the left crutch forward.
- Move the right foot forward.

## VARIATION: Three–Point Gait

To use this gait, the person must be able to bear entire body weight on the unaffected leg. The two crutches and the unaffected leg bear weight alternately. Ask the client to:

- Move both crutches and the weaker leg forward.
- Move the stronger leg forward.

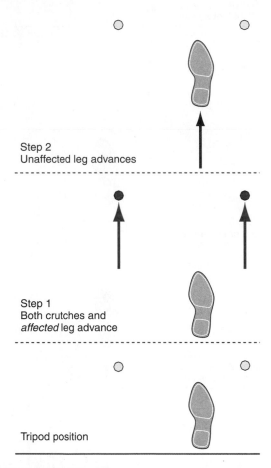

**Step 2**
Unaffected leg advances

**Step 1**
Both crutches and *affected* leg advance

Tripod position

● The three-point crutch gait.

## VARIATION: Two-Point Alternate Gait

This gait is faster than the four-point gait. It requires more balance, because only two points support the body at one time; it also requires at least partial weight bearing on each foot. In this gait, arm movements with the crutches are similar to the arm movements during normal walking. Ask the client to:

- Move the left crutch and the right foot forward together.
- Move the right crutch and the left foot ahead together.

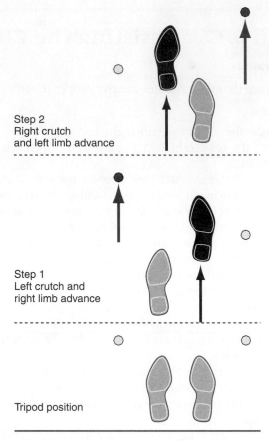

**Step 2**
Right crutch
and left limb advance

**Step 1**
Left crutch and
right limb advance

Tripod position

● The two-point alternate crutch gait.

## VARIATION: Swing-to Gait

People with paralysis of the legs and hips use the swing gaits. Prolonged use of these gaits results in atrophy of the unused muscles. The swing-to gait is the easier of these two gaits.
Ask the client to:

- Move both crutches ahead together.
- Lift body weight by the arms and swing *to* the crutches.

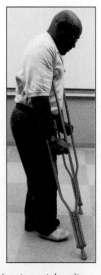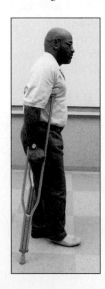

● The swing-to crutch gait.

## VARIATION: Swing-Through Gait

This gait requires considerable client skill, strength, and coordination.

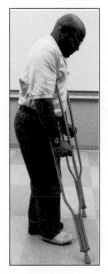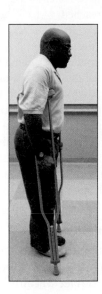

The swing-through crutch gait.

Ask the client to:
- Move both crutches forward together.
- Lift body weight by the arms and swing through and beyond the crutches.

3. Teach the client to get into and out of a chair.

## VARIATION: Getting into a Chair

- Ensure that the chair has armrests and is secure or braced against a wall.
- Instruct the client to:
  a. Stand with the back of the unaffected leg centered against the chair.
  b. Transfer the crutches to the hand on the affected side, hold the crutches by the hand bars, and then grasp the arm of the chair with the hand on the unaffected side. ➤*Rationale: This allows the client to support the body weight on the arms and the unaffected leg.*
  c. Lean forward, flex the knees and hips, and lower into the chair.

## VARIATION: Getting Out of a Chair

- Instruct the client to:
  a. Move forward to the edge of the chair and place the unaffected leg slightly under or at the edge of the chair. ➤*Rationale: This position helps the client stand up from the chair and achieve balance, because the unaffected leg is supported against the edge of the chair.*
  b. Grasp the crutches by the hand bars in the hand on the affected side, and grasp the arm of the chair with the hand on the unaffected side. ➤*Rationale: The body weight is placed on the crutches and the hand on the armrest to support the unaffected leg when the client rises to stand.*

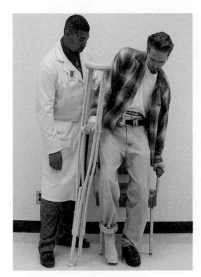

A client using crutches getting into a chair.

  c. Push down on the crutches and the chair armrest while elevating the body out of the chair.
  d. Assume the tripod position before moving.

4. Teach the client to go up and down stairs.

## VARIATION: Going Up Stairs

- Stand behind the client and slightly to the affected side.
- Ask the client to:
  a. Assume the tripod position at the bottom of the stairs.
  b. Transfer the body weight to the crutches and move the unaffected leg onto the step.
  c. Transfer the body weight to the unaffected leg on the step and move the crutches and affected leg up to the step. The crutches always support the affected leg.
- Repeat steps b and c until the top of the stairs is reached.

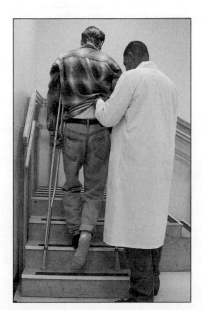

Climbing stairs: Placing weight on the crutches while first moving the unaffected leg onto a step.

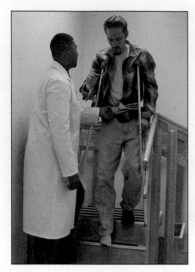

 Descending stairs: Moving the crutches and affected leg to the next step.

## VARIATION: Going Down Stairs

- Stand one step below the person on the affected side.
- Ask the client to:
  a. Assume the tripod position at the top of the stairs.
  b. Shift the body weight to the unaffected leg, and move the crutches and affected leg down onto the next step.

c. Transfer the body weight to the crutches, and move the unaffected leg to that step. The crutches always support the affected leg.
  d. Repeat steps b and c until the bottom of the stairs is reached.
  *or*
- Ask the client to:
  a. Hold both crutches in the outside hand and grasp the handrail with the other hand for support.
  b. Move as in steps b and c, above.

5. Reinforce client teaching.
6. Document the client's progress in the client record using forms or checklists supplemented by narrative notes when appropriate. Describe the distance ambulated and any difficulties the client experienced, including changes in vital signs as compared to baseline.

### Documentation

Sample: 8/22/09 1500 Attempted crutch walking up steps. Unable to lift affected leg to next step, balance remained stable. Became dyspneic and upset. Vital signs (when seated) at baseline after activity. Reassured that this skill takes time. Encouraged to continue seated leg exercises and frequent ambulation. Will re-try tomorrow.
_____ B. Snyder, RN

# CLIENT TEACHING

### Teaching the Client to Use Crutches

- Follow the plan of exercises developed for you to strengthen your arm muscles before beginning crutch walking.
- Have a health care professional establish the correct length for your crutches and the correct placement of the handpieces. Crutches that are too long force your shoulders upward and make it difficult for you to push your body off the ground. Crutches that are too short will make you hunch over and develop an improper body stance.
- The weight of your body should be borne by the arms rather than the axillae (armpits). Continual pressure on the axillae can injure the radial nerve and eventually cause crutch palsy, a weakness of the muscles of the forearm, wrist, and hand.
- Maintain an erect posture as much as possible to prevent strain on muscles and joints and to maintain balance.

- Each step taken with crutches should be a comfortable distance for you. It is wise to start with a small rather than large step.
- Inspect the crutch tips regularly, and replace them if worn.
- Keep the crutch tips dry and clean to maintain their surface friction. If the tips become wet, dry them well before use.
- Wear a shoe with a low heel that grips the floor. Rubber soles decrease the chances of slipping. Adjust shoelaces so they cannot come untied or reach the floor where they might catch on the crutches. Consider shoes with alternative forms of closure (e.g., Velcro), especially if you cannot easily bend to tie laces. Slip-on shoes are acceptable only if they are snug and the heel does not come loose when the foot is bent.

## MEASURING CLIENTS FOR CRUTCHES

When nurses measure clients for axillary crutches, it is most important to obtain the correct length for the crutches and the correct placement of the hand piece. There are two methods for measuring crutch length:

1. The client lies in the supine position, and the nurse measures from the anterior fold of the axilla to a point 2.5 cm (1 in.) lateral from the heel of the foot.
2. The client stands erect and positions the crutch tips 5 cm (2 in.) in front of and 15 cm (6 in.) to the side of the feet. The nurse makes sure the shoulder rest of the crutch is at least three finger widths, that is, 2.5 to 5 cm (1 to 2 in.), below the axilla.

To determine the correct placement of the hand bar:

1. The client stands upright and supports the body weight by the hand grips of the crutches.
2. The nurse measures the angle of elbow flexion. It should be about 30 degrees. A goniometer (a hand-held instrument used to measure joint angles) may be used to verify the correct angle.

### Setting Crutch Height

- While the child is standing, the child's elbows should be slightly and comfortably flexed.
- Place the tip of the crutches about 3 to 6 inches to the upper, outer border of the toes on each foot.
- The upper pad on the crutches should now be lightly placed in the child's axilla.

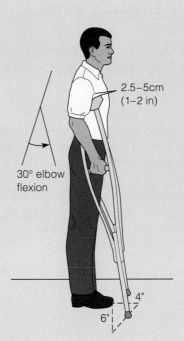

2.5–5cm (1–2 in)

30° elbow flexion

4"

6"

● The standing position for measuring the correct length for crutches.

➤*Rationale: Crutches that are too high can put pressure on the brachial plexus, causing pain and injury.* Crutches that are too low require that the child bend over to walk, and can cause injury or discomfort of the back and neck.

# Skill 6.18   Assisting the Client to Use a Walker

## Preparation

- Ensure client has adequate arm strength to use walker.
- Ensure walker is at correct height
- Ensure client has a clear path free from obstacles.

## Procedure

1. Give the client these instructions when maximum support is required:
   - Move the walker ahead about 15 cm (6 in.) while your body weight is borne by both legs.
   - Then move the right foot up to the walker while your body weight is borne by the left leg and both arms.
   - Next, move the left foot up to the right foot while your body weight is borne by the right leg and both arms.

2. Give the client these instructions if one leg is weaker than the other:
   - Move the walker and the weak leg ahead together about 15 cm (6 in.) while your weight is borne by the stronger leg.
   - Then move the stronger leg ahead while your weight is borne by the affected leg and both arms.

3. Document the client's progress in the client record using forms or checklists supplemented by narrative notes when appropriate. Describe the distance ambulated, any difficulties the client experienced, and changes in vital signs in relation to baseline.

## DEVELOPMENTAL CONSIDERATIONS

### Children

Children learn and adapt quickly to the use of assistive devices. Care should be taken to check regularly that they are using proper technique.

### Elders

- Elders' condition can change rapidly. Check regularly to see that the current assistive device is the most appropriate one and that it fits the client properly.
- Reinforce teaching regarding proper use of mechanical aids. Clients can easily fall into bad habits such as leaning the axillae on the crutches.

## SETTING OF CARE

- When making a home visit, assess carefully for safety issues for ambulation with mechanical devices. Counsel the client and family about unfastened rugs, slippery floors, and loose objects on the floors.
- Recommend nonskid strips be placed on outside steps and inside stairs that are not carpeted.
- Check that appropriate chairs are available.
- Reinforce client teaching about proper gaits with canes, crutches, and walkers.
- Ensure that the equipment is properly maintained and stored out of the way when not in use.
- Tennis balls with a cross cut in them may be applied over walker tips to make sliding easier.

# Skill 6.19   Transporting the Infant

### Equipment

- Transporting vehicle (e.g., stretcher, crib, wheelchair
- Wheeled poles for any necessary equipment
- Necessary supportive equipment such as oxygen tank or ventilation bags/masks
- Blankets

### Preparation

1. Obtain necessary transporting equipment.
2. Securely fasten intravenous lines, feeding lines, ECG leads, and other equipment. ➤*Rationale: Lines that are securely fastened are less likely to be dislodged during transport.*
3. Explain the transport to the family. ➤*Rationale: Adequate explanation helps to decrease anxiety.*

### Procedure

1. Perform an assessment of the child. ➤*Rationale: A baseline assessment provides comparison with later findings.* At times, transport may adversely affect the child's condition. Initial assessment data provide necessary baseline information.
2. The infant is placed in a bassinet or crib for transport. If the bassinet has a bottom shelf, it is used for carrying the IV pump or monitor.
3. Attach intravenous poles and other equipment to the crib. When this is not possible, adequate personnel are needed to push all of the equipment. ➤*Rationale: Lines can be more easily kept intact if they are on one transport vehicle.*
4. Keep the infant covered with blankets. ➤*Rationale: Adequate covers help to prevent hypothermia resulting from a cool environment.*
5. Allow parents to accompany the child on the transport when possible. ➤*Rationale: The parent's presence can provide a sense of security for the young child.*

# Skill 6.20   Transport of the Toddler

### Equipment

- Transporting vehicle (e.g., stretcher, crib, or wheelchair)
- Wheeled poles for any necessary equipment
- Necessary supportive equipment such as oxygen tank or ventilation bags/masks
- Blankets

### Preparation

1. Obtain necessary transporting equipment.
2. Securely fasten intravenous lines, feeding lines, ECG leads, and other equipment. ➤*Rationale: Lines that are securely fastened are less likely to be dislodged during transport.*
3. Explain the transport plan to the family and child. ➤*Rationale: Adequate explanation helps to decrease anxiety.*

### Procedure

1. Transport the toddler in a high-top crib (also used for infants), with the side rails up and the protective top in place. The child may be sitting or lying down. Alternatively, secure the child in a stroller or wheelchair of the proper size for the child's age. ➤*Rationale: Stretchers should not be used because the mobile toddler may roll or fall off.*
2. Be sure to secure the child in the device with the seat safety strap. ➤*Rationale: The child is secured to avoid falls and injury during transport.*

### CLINICAL ALERT

Specialized wheelchairs and other equipment are available to carry enteral feeding solutions, motors necessary for equipment, and other supplies. These transporters are helpful for families when the child has a long-term disability, enabling them to take the child and equipment to school, stores, and other settings.

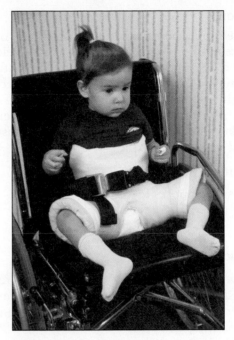

● Toddler in a wheelchair with a safety strap.

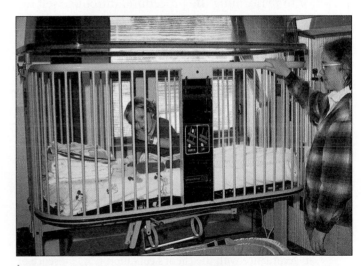

● High-top crib for infant or toddler transport.

# Skill 6.21  Performing Initial Cast Care

## Delegation

The nurse should perform baseline assessment of all new casts. Care of clients with stable casts may be delegated to unlicensed assistive personnel (UAP). The status of the cast is observed during usual care and may be recorded by persons other than the nurse. However, assessment of complications from the cast requires the expertise of a nurse. Abnormal findings detected by UAP must be validated and interpreted by the nurse.

## Equipment

- Pillows to support the casted areas
- Ice packs
- Pen

## Preparation

- Review the client record to determine the reason for the cast and the initial status of the client's extremity. Examine the record regarding pain assessment findings and interventions.

## Procedure

1. Prior to performing the procedure, introduce self to the client and verify the client's identity using agency protocol. Explain to the client what you are going to do, why it is necessary, and how he or she can participate. Discuss how the results will be used in planning further care or treatments.
2. Perform hand hygiene and observe other appropriate infection control procedures.
3. Provide for client privacy as indicated.
4. Assess the neurovascular status of the affected limbs.
   - Assess the toes or fingers for nerve and circulatory impairments every 30 minutes for 4 hours following cast application, and then every 3 hours for the first 24 to 48 hours or until all signs and symptoms of impairment are negative. Increase the frequency of neurovascular assessments in accordance with the client's condition (e.g., presence of circulatory impairment). ➤*Rationale: Rapid swelling under a cast can cause neurovascular problems, necessitating frequent neurovascular assessments by the nurse.*
5. Support and handle the cast appropriately.
   - Immediately after the cast is applied, place it on pillows. Avoid using plastic or rubber pillows. ➤*Rationale: The pillows provide even pressure and support the curves of the cast and promote venous blood return, thereby decreasing the possibility of swelling. Plastic or rubber pillows do not allow the heat of a drying cast to dissipate and so cause discomfort.*
   - Until a cast has set or hardened (10 to 20 minutes), support the cast in the palms of your hands rather than with the fingertips, and extend your fingers so that your fingertips do not touch the plaster. ➤*Rationale: Fingertip pressure can cause dents in unset plaster and subsequent skin pressure areas.*
   - When the cast is set, continue to handle the cast in your palms, but you may then wrap your fingers around the contour of the cast.
6. Implement measures to reduce swelling.
   - Control swelling by elevating arms or legs on pillows or, for a leg fracture, by elevating the foot of the bed. Immediately after injury and surgery, elevate the limb above the level of the client's heart. Generally, three pillows are needed to achieve high elevation of a leg. As circulation improves and healing progresses, the elevation can be gradually reduced to two pillows (moderate elevation) and then to one pillow (low elevation). ➤*Rationale: Swelling can cause neurovascular impairment.*
   - Apply ice packs to control perineal edema associated with a hip spica cast. Although ice packs are a less effective method of control than elevation, elevation of the area is obviously difficult.
   - Report excessive swelling and indications of neurovascular impairment to the primary care provider or nurse in charge. The primary care provider may bivalve a cast if it appears to be too tight. Bivalving a cast is cutting the cast partially or completely and wrapping with bandage material to hold it together. ➤*Rationale: This relieves the pressure of the cast but still provides support.*
7. Use appropriate means to dry the plaster cast thoroughly.
   - Extremity plaster casts usually take 24 to 48 hours to dry completely; spica or body casts require 48 to 72 hours.

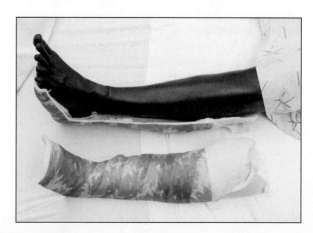

Bivalved cast.

Drying time depends on the temperature, humidity, size of the cast, and method used for drying. The cast is dry when it no longer feels damp. A dry cast feels dry, looks white and shiny, and is odorless, hard, and resonant when tapped. Synthetic casts take only 10 to 15 minutes to harden completely.

- Expose the cast to the circulating air. Place sheets and blankets only over areas that do not have the cast.
- Check agency policy about the recommended turning frequency for clients with different kinds of casts. ➤*Rationale: Frequent turning promotes even drying of the cast.*
- Turn the client with an extremity cast or body spica every 2 to 4 hours.
- Use regular pillows. ➤*Rationale: Plastic or rubber pillows hinder drying and do not allow the heat of a drying cast to dissipate.*
- Avoid the use of artificial means to facilitate drying. These means include fans, hair dryers, infrared lamps, and electric heaters. ➤*Rationale: Artificial methods dry the outer surface of the cast while the inner portion remains soft and spongy. Such a cast cracks readily at points of strain. Natural methods dry the cast evenly.*

8. Monitor bleeding if an open reduction was done or if the injury was a compound fracture.
   - Monitor bloodstains or other drainage on the cast for 24 to 72 hours after surgery or injury or longer if necessary.
   - Outline the stained area with a pen at least every 8 hours if it is changing, and note the time and date, so that any further bleeding can be determined.

9. Assess pain and pressure areas.
   - Never ignore any complaints of pain, burning, swelling or pressure. If a client is unable to communicate, be alert to changes in temperament, restlessness, or fussiness that may indicate a problem. ➤*Rationale:* Compartment syndrome *is a serious complication that can result when swelling and pressure within the closed fascial compartment build to dangerous levels, preventing nourishment from reaching nerve and muscle cells. The skin overlying the area may be red and hard.*

*Apply ice, elevate, and notify primary care provider immediately. An absent or diminished distal pulse necessitates immediate surgical action to allow expansion and blood flow and prevent nerve damage.*

- Determine particularly whether the pain is persistent and if it occurs over a bony prominence or joint.
- Do not disregard a cessation of persistent pain or discomfort complaints from the client. ➤*Rationale: Cessation of complaints can indicate a skin slough. When a skin slough occurs, superficial skin sensation is lost and the client no longer feels pain.*
- When a pressure area under the cast is suspected, the primary care provider may either bivalve the cast so that all of the skin beneath the cast can be inspected or cut a window in the cast over only the area of concern. When a cast is windowed:
  a. Retain the piece (cast and padding) that was cut out. Some primary care providers order that it be taped back if there is no skin problem present but that it be left out if a pressure area is present. ➤*Rationale: Putting back the piece prevents window edema, which occurs when skin pressure at the window is not equal to that from the remainder of the cast.*
  b. Inspect the skin under the window at scheduled time intervals.

10. Document findings in the client record using forms or checklists supplemented by narrative notes when appropriate. Record each assessment (whether or not there are problems).

### Documentation

Sample: 9/18/09 1100 Cast still damp, elevated on one pillow. Fingers warm to touch, color pink, full ROM of fingers, no numbness or tingling. Able to hyperextend R thumb, sensation felt at web space between R thumb and index finger. Arm pain at 2/10. Declined pain med. Will reassess in 30 minutes.

———————————————— E. Mitchell, RN

---

## DEVELOPMENTAL CONSIDERATIONS

### Children

- Teach parents of young children ways to prevent the child from placing small items inside the cast. Parents also need to ensure that the top of a body cast is covered during meals so that food does not fall inside the cast. Serious infections and damage to tissues can occur as a result of sticking anything inside the cast.

- If possible, allow the child to choose the color of the synthetic cast. Wearing a cast can cause distur-

bances in body image and self-concept. Education regarding cast care, how to adapt activities of daily living, efficient ambulation, and what to expect as far as cast removal will help the child cope effectively.

- Reassure the child that the saw used for windowing, bivalving, and removing the cast is not painful. It rapidly vibrates back and forth rather than rotates, so injury from the blade is unlikely. The saw is rather loud and can scare children, so have an adult

*(continued)*

## DEVELOPMENTAL CONSIDERATIONS (CONTINUED)

present to support the child during these procedures. Let the child keep the cast pieces when removed if desired and they are not needed.

**Elders**

- Elders who are immobilized are at increased risk for skin breakdown and pressure ulcers.

- Wound healing may be slower in elders than in younger clients.
- Elders may be less able to manage the additional weight and imbalance caused by the cast.
- Take appropriate steps in planning for use of crutches or other mobility aids to keep elders moving safely.

## SETTING OF CARE

- For itching, suggest that the client use a hair dryer on cool, a vacuum cleaner on reverse, or an ice bag over the outside of the itching area. Emphasize the importance of not putting anything inside the cast, because serious infections and tissue damage can occur (Carmichael & Goucher, 2006). ➤*Rationale: These are safer ways to resolve itching and less irritating to the skin than inserting an object into the cast.*
- Before discharge from the hospital, instruct the client to:
  a. Observe for indications of nerve or circulatory impairment, such as extreme coldness or blueness of toes or fingers; extreme continuous swelling of casted toes or fingers; numbness or tingling ("pins and needles" sensation) in casted toes or fingers; continuous complaints of pain; or inability to move the toes or fingers.
  b. Keep the plaster cast dry.
  c. Avoid strenuous activity and follow medical advice about exercise.

  d. Elevate the arm or leg frequently to prevent dependent edema.
  e. Move the toes or fingers frequently.
  f. Observe the skin around the cast edges frequently, and keep it clean and dry.
  g. Report any increase in pain; unexplained fever; foul odor from within the cast; decreased circulation; numbness; inability to move the fingers or toes; or a weakened, cracked, loose, or tight cast.
- Review modifications that may be necessary in clothing, toileting, sleeping, and other activities of daily living.
- When it is time for cast removal, reassure clients that the saw, though loud, oscillates rather than rotates, and is not dangerous. Skin under the cast will look macerated and pale and hair growth can be increased. Muscle atrophy usually occurs, leading to asymmetry of limbs. Reassure clients and family that the muscles and hair growth will return to normal after 2 weeks of normal activity (Altizer, 2004).

## CLINICAL ALERT

Neurovascular impairment under a cast is an emergency. If assessments indicate impaired circulation or neurologic status, notify the physician immediately. Have a cast cutter at the bedside so the cast can be removed if needed and the pressure relieved.

## CLINICAL ALERT

When casting material inhibits palpation of peripheral pulses, assess capillary refill, assess for edema, comfort level, and other parameters of "CMS" as an indication of neurovascular status.

## CLINICAL ALERT

Do not use abductor bars (incorporated into cast) for moving the client. Move the client as a unit instead.

## CLINICAL ALERT

Casted extremity should be assessed every 1/2 hour for 4 hours and then every 4 hours.

## CLINICAL ALERT

If the client has had open reduction, wound drainage will be absorbed and spread rapidly, or seep down the back of cast. The visible drainage does not necessarily indicate the amount of actual drainage.

Inspect all cast surfaces and mark drainage regularly if it is increasing. Bleeding should not persist after 24 hours.

## CLINICAL ALERT

Diminished or absent pulses, coolness, and pallor are late signs and unreliable indicators of acute compartment syndrome. Always assess active extension, flexion, adduction, and abduction of the fingers, flexion and extension of the toes, and inversion and dorsiflexion of the foot. Pain on passive stretching of the muscle or distal digits in an early indicator of circulatory compromise.

# Skill 6.22    Performing Ongoing Cast Care

### Delegation

Care of clients with stable casts may be delegated to UAP. The status of the cast is observed during usual care and may be recorded by persons other than the nurse. However, assessment of complications from the cast requires the expertise of a nurse. Abnormal findings detected by UAP must be validated and interpreted by the nurse.

### Equipment

Assemble any of the following equipment items necessary to complete client care:

- Pillows to support the casted areas
- Clean gloves
- Damp cloth
- Swab
- Alcohol
- Acetone or nail polish
- Waterproof tape or adhesive strips
- Bib or towels
- Slipper (fracture) bedpan
- Plastic covering
- Soap and water
- Handheld blow dryer
- Mineral, olive, or baby oil

### Preparation

- Review the client record to determine previous status of the cast and the client's extremities. Examine the record regarding pain assessment findings and interventions.

### Procedure

1. Prior to performing the procedure, introduce self to the client and verify the client's identity using agency protocol. Explain to the client what you are going to do, why it is necessary, and how he or she can participate. Discuss how the results will be used in planning further care or treatments.

2. Perform hand hygiene and observe other appropriate infection control procedures.
3. Provide for client privacy as indicated.
4. Continue to assess the client for problems.
   - Apply clean gloves.
   - Assess the neurovascular status of the affected limb at regular intervals in accordance with agency protocol.
   - Inspect the skin near and under the cast edges whenever neurovascular assessments are made and/or whenever the client is turned.
   - Check the cast daily for a foul odor. ➤*Rationale: This kind of odor may indicate skin excoriation from pressure or an infected area beneath the cast.*
5. Implement measures to prevent skin irritation at the edges of the cast.
   - Wash crumbs of plaster from the skin with a damp cloth and feel along the cast edges to check for rough edges or areas that press into the client's skin. ➤*Rationale: As a plaster cast dries, small bits of plaster frequently break off from its rough edges. If they fall inside the cast, they can cause discomfort and irritation.*
   - Remove the resin of synthetic casting materials with a swab moistened with alcohol, acetone, or nail polish remover. Check the manufacturer's directions.
   - When it is dry, cover any rough edges and protect areas of the cast that may come in contact with urine. "Petal" the edges with small strips of waterproof tape as follows:
     a. Cut several strips of 2.5-cm (1-in.) adhesive, 5 to 7.5 cm (2 to 3 in.) long. Then curve all corners of each strip. ➤*Rationale: Square or pointed ends tend to curl.*
     b. Insert one end of each strip as far as possible inside the cast, and bring the other end out over the cast edge.
     c. Press the petals firmly against the plaster.
     d. Overlap successive petals slightly.
6. Provide skin care to all areas vulnerable to pressure.
   - Examine all areas vulnerable to pressure and breakdown at least every 4 hours. For clients with sensitive skin or potential skin problems, provide care every 2 hours during the day and every 3 hours at night.
     a. Reach under the cast edges as far as possible and massage the area.

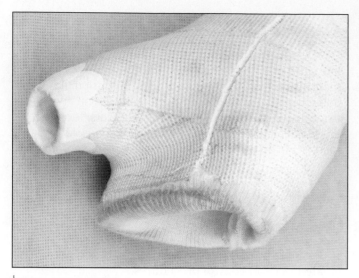

● Completed petalled cast.

b. Also provide skin care over all bony prominences not under the cast (e.g., the sacrum, heels, ankles, wrists, elbows, and feet). ➤*Rationale: These are potential pressure areas if the client is confined to bed.*

7. Keep the cast clean and dry.

**VARIATION: Plaster Cast**

- Place a bib or towel over a body cast to catch spills. If a spill does wet the cast, allow the area to air dry.
- Use a slipper (fracture) bedpan for people with long leg, hip spica, or body casts. ➤*Rationale: The flat end placed correctly under the client's buttocks lessens the chance of spillage and minimizes the amount of lifting required by the client and/or nurse.*
- Before placing the client on the bedpan, tuck plastic or other waterproof material around the top of a long leg cast or around the perineal cutout. For a perineal cutout, funnel one end of the plastic into the bedpan.
- Remove the plastic when elimination is completed. ➤*Rationale: If left in place, waterproof material makes the cast edge airtight and prevents evaporation of perspiration, which is irritating to the skin.*
- For people with long leg casts, keep the cast supported on pillows while the client is on the bedpan. ➤*Rationale: If the cast dangles, urine may run down the cast.*
- For clients with hip spica casts, support both extremities and the back on pillows so that they are as high as the buttocks. ➤*Rationale: This prevents urine from running back into the cast.*
- When removing the bedpan, hold it securely while the client is turning or lifting the buttocks. ➤*Rationale: This prevents dripping and spilling.*
- After removing the bedpan, thoroughly clean and dry the perineal area.

**VARIATION: Synthetic Cast**

- Wash the soiled area with warm water and a mild soap.
- Thoroughly rinse the soap from the cast.
- Dry thoroughly to prevent skin maceration and ulceration under the cast.
- If the cast is immersed in water, dry the cast and underlying padding and stockinette thoroughly. First, blot excess water from the cast with a towel. Then, use a handheld blow dryer on the cool or warm setting, directing the air stream in a sweeping motion over the exterior of the cast for about 1 hour or until the client no longer feels a cold clammy sensation like that produced by a wet bathing suit. ➤*Rationale: This drying procedure is essential to prevent skin maceration and ulceration.*

8. Turn and position the client in correct alignment to prevent the formation of pressure areas.
- Place pillows in such a way that:
  a. Body parts press against the edges of the cast as little as possible.
  b. Toes, heels, elbows, and so on, are protected from pressure against the bed surface.
  c. Body alignment is maintained.
- Plan and implement a turning schedule that will incorporate all of the possible positions. Generally, clients can be placed in lateral, prone, and supine positions unless surgical procedures or any other factors contraindicate them. Attach a trapeze to the overhead frame to enable the client to assist with moving. ➤*Rationale: Repositioning prevents pressure areas.*
- Turn people with large casts or those unable to turn themselves at least once every 4 hours. If the person is at risk for skin breakdown, turn every 1 to 3 hours as needed.
- When turning the client in a long leg cast to the unaffected side, place a pillow between the legs to support the cast.
- Use at least three persons to turn a person in a *damp* hip spica cast. When the cast is dry, the individual can usually turn with the assistance of one nurse. To turn a client from the supine to prone position, follow these steps:
  a. Remove the support pillows only when an assistant is supporting the cast.
  b. Move the client to one side of the bed.
  c. Ask the client to place the arms above the head or along the sides.
  d. Have two assistants go to the other side of the bed while you remain to provide security for the person who is at the edge of the bed.
  e. Place pillows along the bed surface to receive the cast when the client turns.
  f. Roll the client toward the two assistants onto the pillows.
  g. Adjust the pillows as needed so that they provide proper support and comfort, and prevent pressure areas.

9. Encourage range-of-motion (ROM) and isometric exercises.
   - Unless contraindicated, encourage active ROM exercises for all joints on the unaffected extremities, as well as on the joints proximal and distal to the cast. If active exercises are contraindicated, implement active-assistive or passive exercises, depending on the client's abilities and disabilities. ➤*Rationale: Exercise helps prevent joint stiffness, muscle atrophy, and venous stasis.*
   - Encourage the client to move toes and/or fingers of the casted extremity as frequently as possible. ➤*Rationale: Moving these extremities enhances peripheral circulation and decreases swelling and pain.*
   - Teach isometric (muscle-setting) exercises for extremities in a cast. ➤*Rationale: Isometric exercise will minimize muscle atrophy in the affected limb.*
     a. Teach the isometric exercises on the client's unaffected limb before the person applies it to the affected limb.
     b. Demonstrate muscle palpation while the client is carrying out the exercise. ➤*Rationale: Palpation enables the person to feel the changes that occur with muscle contraction and relaxation.*

10. Provide client teaching to promote self-care, comfort, and safety.
    - Teach people immobilized in bed with large body casts ways to turn and to move safely by using a trapeze, the side rails, and other such devices.
    - Instruct clients with leg casts about ways to walk effectively with crutches.
    - Instruct people with arm casts how to apply slings.
    - Teach clients how to resolve itching under the cast safely. Discourage the person from using long sharp objects to scratch under the cast. ➤*Rationale: These objects can break the skin and cause an infection, because bacteria flourish in the warm, dark, moist environment under the cast. Sticking objects under a cast can also cause folding or bunching of padding material and subsequent pressure and discomfort.*
    - When healing is complete and the cast is removed, the underlying skin is usually macerated, pale, flaky, and encrusted, since layers of dead skin have accumulated. Hair growth may be increased, and muscles are usually atrophied (shrunken). Instruct clients to remove this debris gently and gradually. The skin changes, muscle asymmetry and hair growth will return to normal after approximately 2 weeks of regular activity (Altizer, 2004).
      a. Apply oil (e.g., mineral, olive, or baby oil).
      b. Soak the skin in warm water and dry it.
      c. Caution the client not to rub the area too vigorously. ➤*Rationale: Vigorous rubbing can cause bleeding or excoriation of fragile skin.*
      d. Repeat steps a and b for several days. ➤*Rationale: Gradual removal of skin exudates reduces skin irritation.*

11. Remove and discard gloves and soiled materials per agency protocol. Perform hand hygiene.

12. Document findings in the client record using forms or checklists supplemented by narrative notes when appropriate. Record each assessment (whether or not there are problems).

### Documentation

Sample: 9/15/09 1000 Cast intact, leg elevated on 2 pillows. Toes warm to touch, pink, capillary refill 2 seconds. Moves toes readily and fully; states no numbness or tingling. Pain 0/10.

_____ B. Snyder, RN

---

# Skill 6.23   Performing Care for a Child with a Cast

### Equipment
- Cast material (if assisting in application)
- Large basin with water (if assisting in application)
- Pillows with waterproof covering
- Absorbent pads and protectors
- Clean gloves

### Preparation
- Consult the child's chart for description of the injury or surgery.

### Procedure
Following cast application:

1. Elevate a wet cast on pillows covered in plastic. ➤*Rationale: Elevation decreases edema under the cast which can restrict circulation.*
2. Use the palm of the hands when lifting a wet or damp cast. ➤*Rationale: Fingertips can indent plaster and create pressure points.*
3. Circle and note the date and time of any drainage on the cast. ➤*Rationale: Some drainage is common after surgery. Monitoring its presence provides clues to the amount and type of fluid lost.*
4. Assess circulation and neurologic status every 15 minutes after surgery or cast placement and then progress to every 30 minutes, 60 minutes, and 2 hours. Report abnormal findings or changes in condition. Include the following observations on the involved extremities:
   - Distal pulses
   - Color
   - Warmth
   - Sensation

- Capillary refill
- Edema
- Movement
- Pain, tingling
➤*Rationale: Circulation and nerves under the cast can be injured if it is too tight.*

5. Use pain-control measures as needed and reassess pain. Report immediately worsening pain or pain that is not controlled by prescribed medication.
6. Check the edges of the cast for roughness or crumbling. Pull the inner stockinette over the edge of the cast and tape once the cast has dried. ➤*Rationale: These actions can prevent discomfort and skin breakdown.*
7. Keep the cast clean and dry. Cover it with a plastic bag during bathing or toileting.

8. Avoid use of lotions and powders under the cast. ➤*Rationale: These products can cause skin irritation.*
9. Keep shirts or other clothing over the top edges of casts on young children. ➤*Rationale: This action helps to prevent the child from placing objects down into the cast which can result in areas of discomfort or skin damage.*
10. Instruct the family about care of the cast at home and when to return for checks and removal of the cast.
11. Document the cast application, how the child tolerated the procedure, cast care provided, and assessment of vascular and neurologic status.

# Skill 6.24   Caring for Clients in Traction

## Procedure

### VARIATION: Caring for Client in Skin Traction

1. Determine the following: bruises and abrasions in the area where the traction is to be applied; any history of circulatory problems and skin allergies; mental and emotional status and ability to understand activity restrictions.
2. Note the type of traction, and inspect the traction apparatus regularly, that is, whenever you are at the bedside or at prescribed intervals, such as every 2 hours.
3. Maintain the client in the appropriate traction position.
   - Maintain the client in the supine position unless there are other orders. ➤*Rationale: Changing position can change the body alignment and the amount of force supplied by the traction.*
   - Maintain body alignment when turning the client. In some cases, the person can turn to a lateral position if a pillow placed between the legs maintains body alignment. Refer to the client's record for information about permitted movement.
   - Provide a trapeze to assist the client to move and lift the body for back care if he or she is unable to turn.
   - Provide a fracture or slipper bedpan as required to minimize the client's movement during elimination.
4. Assess the neurovascular status of the affected extremity.
   - Conduct a neurovascular assessment 30 minutes following reapplication of the bandage, then every 2 hours for the first 24 hours. If the client's status is "normal," then assess every 4 hours during the traction. If the client's status is not normal, continue assessments hourly.

## ▌EVIDENCE-BASED NURSING PRACTICE

**Traction vs. No Traction for Hip Fracture**

Trials of traction vs. no traction for patients with hip fracture have found no significant differences in pain, operative blood loss, ease of fracture reduction, or length of hospitalization. It seems that providing adequate intravenous analgesia and placing the extremity in a comfortable position are the best measures for reducing preoperative pain.

*Source: Emergency Medicine (2005, July), p. 40.*

5. Provide protective devices and measures to safeguard the skin.
   - Place heel protectors or sheepskins under the heels, sacrum, shoulders, and other pressure areas.
   - Change or clean the sheepskin lining at least weekly.
   - Massage the skin with rubbing alcohol or lotion every 4 hours, or if redness and signs of pressure appear, every 2 hours. ➤*Rationale: Alcohol tends to toughen the skin and leave it less vulnerable to breakdown.* Because alcohol is drying to the skin, however, lotion may be preferred for those who have dry skin (e.g., elderly people).
   - Make sure the spreader bar is wide enough to prevent the traction tape from rubbing on the client's bony prominences.
6. Remove only intermittent nonadhesive skin traction in accordance with agency protocol or orders.
   - To remove a nonadhesive skin traction:
     a. Remove the weights first.

# EVIDENCE-BASED NURSING PRACTICE

### Pin Site Care for Traction

There is no existing standard for traction pin care. Recommended treatments include the use of dressings, cleansing with hydrogen peroxide, alcohol, povidone-iodine, normal saline, soap and water, or sterile water and chlorhexidine gluconate. Almost all of these preparations are associated with pin corrosion, increased infection rates, and delayed healing. Ointments should not be used because they prevent pin site drainage.

Soap and water, sterile water, and normal saline are useful because they soften and allow removal of crusts to promote normal pin site drainage (thereby reducing risk of infection) and are not associated with adverse reactions.

Use of sterile technique and loose application of gauze to the site are advocated by the author. Frequency of pin site care should be based on assessment of crusting and need to promote drainage.

*Source:* McKenzie, L. (1999). In search of a standard for pin site care. *Orthopaedic Nursing,* 18(2), 73–78.

*Note:* There is little research evidence supporting management of skeletal pin sites. Therefore, the applicability of any recommendation for pin site care cannot be assumed.

*Source:* Holmes, Sue & Brown, Sarah. (2005). Pin site care expert panel. Skeletal pin site care (National Association of Orthopaedic Nurses Guidelines for Orthopaedic Nursing. *Orthopaedic Nursing,* 24(2), 99.

### Lifting an Extremity with an External Fixator

A survey of orthopedic surgeons concludes that the best way to lift an extremity with an external fixator is to support the extremity itself, supporting the joint above and below the frame. Repeated lifting and manipulation of the frame itself can lead to pin loosening and fracture malalignment.

*Source:* DeGeorge, P. & Dunwoody, C. (1995). Transfer techniques of the lower extremity with an external fixator. *Orthopaedic Nursing,* 14(6), 17–21.

---

   b. Unwrap the bandage and provide skin care.

   c. Rewrap the limb and slowly reattach the weights.

7. Teach the client ways to prevent problems associated with immobility.

- Teach the client deep-breathing and coughing exercises to prevent hypostatic pneumonia.
- Teach the client appropriate exercises to maintain and develop muscle tone, prevent muscle contracture and atrophy, and promote blood circulation:

   a. Range-of-motion exercises (discussed earlier in this chapter).

   b. Isometric exercises to strengthen the quadriceps include tightening the knees. By pushing the knees down without moving them, the hamstring muscles are also strengthened. Tensing the buttocks and the inner thighs promotes stabilization of the hips. Tensing the inner thighs also helps stabilize the knees.

   c. Circulation to the extremities can be promoted by encouraging the client to flex and extend the feet as well as to perform the isometric exercises.

   d. Specific exercises to strengthen the biceps and triceps in preparation for using crutches can be taught as indicated. For example, raising the buttocks off the bed by pushing down with the arms develops the triceps, and pulling the body up with a trapeze develops the biceps.

8. Document findings in the client record using forms or checklists supplemented by narrative notes when appropriate.

9. Perform a detailed follow-up examination based on findings that deviated from expected or normal for the client. The client should be able to demonstrate

## CLINICAL ALERT

Do not apply Buck's traction over or under a calf compression device. Foot pumps (only around the foot) are acceptable for deep-vein thrombosis prophylaxis.

usual ROM in all unaffected body joints; move all fingers or toes of the affected extremity; feel normal sensation and have normal skin color and temperature in all fingers or toes of the affected extremity; and be free of pressure signs (pallor, redness, increased warmth or tenderness) over pressure areas. Relate findings to previous assessment data if available. Report significant deviations from normal to the primary care provider.

### VARIATION: Skeletal Traction

#### Delegation

Care of clients in traction may be delegated to trained UAP.

#### Equipment

Supplies for providing pin site care according to agency policy (e.g., normal saline, cotton-tipped swabs, gauze dressings, clean or sterile gloves)

#### Preparation

Verify the primary care provider's orders. Determine the degree of movement permitted and any special precautions (e.g., bed positions permitted).

## Procedure

1. Prior to performing the procedure, introduce self to the client and verify the client's identity using agency protocol. Explain to client what you are going to do, why it is necessary, and how he or she can participate. Discuss how the results will be used in planning further care of treatments.
2. Perform hand hygiene and observe other appropriate infection control procedures.
3. Provide for client privacy.
4. Inspect the traction apparatus:
   - Is the appropriate countertraction provided? For example, is the foot of the bed elevated 2.5 cm (1 in.) for every pound of traction or is the knee of the bed flexed 20 to 30 degrees?
   - Are the correct weights applied? For example, Buck's traction should have no more than 5 pounds.
   - Is there free play of the ropes on the pulleys; that is, does the groove of the pulley support the rope? Are the knots positioned no closer than 12 inches to the nearest pulley?
   - Do all weights hang freely and not rest against or on the bed or floor when the bed is in the lowest position?
   - Are the ropes intact, that is, not frayed, knotted, or kinked between their points of attachment?
   - Are the ropes securely attached with slipknots and the short ends of ropes attached with tape?
   - Is the line of the traction straight and in the same plane as the long axis of the bone?
   - Do bedclothes and other objects not impinge on the traction?
   - Is the spreader bar wide enough to prevent the traction tape from rubbing on bony prominences? Skeletal traction can be applied to the skull, the proximal end of the ulna, the distal end of the femur, the proximal and distal ends of the tibia, and the calcaneus (heel bone).

➤Rationale: *Because bone withstands greater stress than skin, heavier weights can be used (e.g.,up to 35 pounds).* Metal pins, wires, or tongs are inserted into the bone to which the traction is applied. Common examples are the Steinmann pin and the Kirschner wire.

- The distal end of a Thomas leg splint and Pearson attachment are attached to a weighted rope for suspension. The Pearson attachment supports the lower leg off the bed and permits the knee to be flexed. The pin or wire drilled through the bone is attached to a spreader, which in turn is attached to ropes, pulleys, and weights. Countertraction is supplied mostly by the body's weight. A weighted rope attached to the proximal end of the Thomas splint, however, counterbalances the suspension weight. To prevent footdrop, a footplate is attached to the Pearson apparatus. To prevent skin breakdown, the ischial ring of the Thomas splint is padded. Sheepskin slings are positioned along the Pearson attachment.
- Skull tongs (e.g., Crutchfield, Burton, Gardner–Wells, or Vinke) are secured to each side of the skull. The center metal bar is attached to ropes, pulleys, and weights and creates a traction pull along the long axis of the spine.

5. Maintain the client in the appropriate traction position. Check that the head, knee, and foot of the bed are properly elevated.
   - For clients with skull tongs or a halo ring, turn the client as a unit. Do not allow the neck to twist. A special bed may be required.
   - If skull tongs or pins become dislodged, support the head, remove the weights, place sandbags or liter fluid bags on either side of the head to maintain alignment, and notify the primary care provider immediately.

6. Assess the neurovascular status of the affected extremity.
   - Conduct a neurovascular assessment every hour for the first 24 hours. If the client's status is "normal," then assess every 4 hours during the traction. If the client's status is not normal, continue assessments hourly.

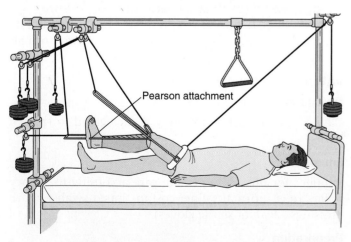

Thomas splint with Pearson attachment for fracture of the femur for balanced suspension skeletal traction.

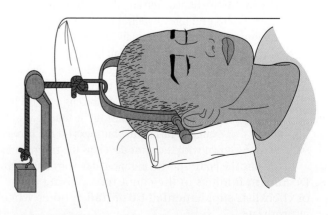

Gardner-Wells skull tongs for skeletal traction immobilizes fractures of cervical and upper thoracic vertebrae.

7. Provide pin site care daily if indicated by the primary care provider's orders and agency protocol.
   - Carefully inspect the site. Regular inspection of the pin site ensures early detection of minor infections, as manifested by signs of serosanguineous drainage, crusting, swelling, and erythema.
   - Use clean or sterile technique as agency protocol dictates. ➤*Rationale: Sterile technique is most often used in the hospital setting, clean technique in the ambulatory setting.*
   - According to agency policy, remove crusts using normal saline or other agent recommended by the agency on cotton-tipped swabs. Use a gentle, rolling technique to reduce irritation to the tissue. ➤*Rationale: Removing crusted secretions permits the pin site to drain freely. Initial crusts around pins do not create a problem and can serve as a barrier to infection, but accumulated crusts around external fixator pins may cause secondary infection.*
   - Apply sterile ointment if ordered. Determine agency practices regarding pin site care; ointment could interfere with proper drainage.
   - Loosely apply gauze dressing around pin site.

   - Adjust frequency of care according to the amount of drainage. If no drainage is present, daily site care is adequate. If drainage is present, perform site care every 8 hours.
   - If purulent (containing pus) drainage is present, notify the primary care provider and obtain specimens for culture and sensitivity.
   - Dispose of soiled equipment according to agency protocol.
   - Remove and discard gloves if used. Perform hand hygiene.

8. Teach the client ways to prevent problems associated with immobility.
9. Document findings in the client record using forms or checklists supplemented by narrative notes when appropriate.

### Documentation

Sample: 9/17/09 1230 Traction maintained at 20 pounds. Skin intact and pink, sensation present, no pain. Pin sites clean and dry without sign of infection.

_____ G. Merritt, RN

## DEVELOPMENTAL CONSIDERATIONS

### Infants/Children

- Bryant's traction is an adaptation of a bilateral Buck's extension. It is used to stabilize fractured femurs or correct congenital hip dislocations in young children under 17.5 kg (35 lb). The skin traction is applied to both the affected and the unaffected leg to maintain the position of the affected leg. A spreader bar attached to the strips or positioning of the pulleys maintains leg alignment. Unless otherwise ordered, the hips are flexed at right angles (90 degrees) to the body with the knees extended, and the buttocks raised about 2.5 cm (1 in.). Pressure areas include skin over the tibia, malleoli, hamstring tendon, soles of feet, and upper back.

### Elders

- Adhesive skin traction should not be used due to the fragility of elders' skin.

- Skin breakdown can occur more easily with any form of traction in the elderly than with younger clients.

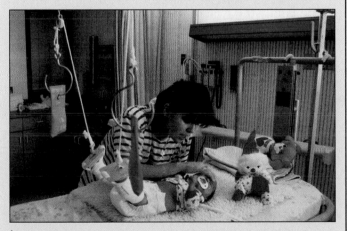

● Bryant's traction. Ensure that the sacrum is elevated sufficiently to allow the nurse to slip a hand between the child's buttocks and the bed.

# Skill 6.25   Applying and Monitoring Skin Traction for a Child

### Equipment

- Poles, pulleys, rope, weight, pads
- Elastic wrap for skin traction

### Preparation

1. Verify the identity of the child. Explain to the child and family the type of traction and what it will involve.
2. Gather equipment needed and review proper setup.
3. Check the weights to be certain they are the same as those ordered by the physician.

### Procedure

1. Set up the prescribed type of traction with proper weights.
2. Apply skin traction as ordered to the particular extremity. Wrap the extremity and apply straps to freely movable prescribed weights.
3. Perform assessments every 30 minutes initially, and then advance to every 1 to 2 hours when stable. Include the following areas:
   - Proper position of traction
   - Proper body alignment
   - Neurovascular status of the extremity
   - Skin condition under and around the traction application
   - Skin on prominences exposed to the surface of the bed
   - Vital signs
   - Pain and psychologic status. ➤*Rationale: Traction can lead to skin breakdown or neurovascular impairment.* Infections can result, especially with internal traction. Regular assess-

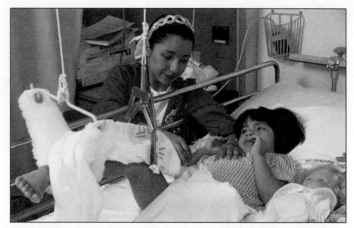

● The child in traction needs close monitoring for alignment and proper traction application. Parents can often provide distraction and activities to help the child pass the time during his or her immobility.

ments help to identify problems early. Children may be pulled out of correct alignment by traction and movement in bed and may require frequent repositioning.
4. Check the child's alignment in bed and reposition as needed.
5. Remove traction according to agency policy, performing assessments and skin care. Reapply as directed in the medical orders.
6. Provide teaching and evaluation of technique if the family will maintain traction at home.

## SETTING OF CARE

Children are increasingly being treated with traction at home. Be certain that the family understands how to set up and maintain the traction. Teach the observations to be made on the extremity involved. Siblings may change the weights or ropes, so close supervision may be needed by parents in some families. A home visit soon after traction begins is often made to evaluate the family's understanding and ability to carry out the regimen.

### Home Setting

Knowledge of body mechanics and how to use these principles when giving care is important to both the health care provider and the client. Correct use of body mechanics decreases the caregiver's potential for injury and provides safety for the client. Recently, there has been an increase in the number of back injury accident claims among home health care providers. One reason for the increase is the improper use of body mechanics while performing skills in the home setting. Also, there may be no one to assist the care provider when lifting and turning clients in the home. The nurse may need to improvise, as the equipment may not be adequate or adjustable. In the home setting, much of the care is given by the family; therefore, it is essential that they also be taught good body mechanics.

# Skill 6.26   Positioning Nonhospital Bed for Client Care

### Procedure

1. Position foam wedges to simulate change in position when head of bed does not move. (High-Fowler's/90 degrees; Fowler's/60 degrees; semi-Fowler's/30 degrees.)
2. Use correct body mechanics to adjust height.
   a. Flex body at knees and keep back straight if bed is only slightly low.
   b. Kneel on pillow by bed or sit in chair alongside bed if bed is extremely low.
3. Lock each wheel or leg of bed in position by securing with bricks or blocks of wood.
4. Make footboard of lumber or item such as a TV tray; position legs of tray under mattress so that tray becomes footboard.

## DEVELOPMENTAL CONSIDERATIONS

### Psychologic Age Changes in the Musculoskeletal System That Affect Nursing Care of the Elderly

- Contractures—muscles atrophy, regenerate slowly; tendons shrink and sclerose.
- Range of motion of joints decreases—lack of adequate joint motion, ankylosis.
- Mobility level is limited—muscle strength lessens and gait may be unsteady.
- Kyphosis occurs—cervical vertebrae may be flexed; intervertebral discs narrow.
- Bodies of thoracic vertebrae compress slowly with aging leading to the hunchback appearance—loss of overall height results from disk shrinkage and kyphosis.
- Bone changes—loss of trabecular bones and bones become brittle.
- Osteoporosis occurs as a result of calcium loss from the bone and insufficient replacement.

- Osteoarthritis increases with age, equally affecting men and women. This condition results in physical stress on joints as a result of long-term mechanical, horizontal, chemical, and genetic factors.

### Psychosocial and Physiological Changes in Elderly Who Are Immobilized

- At risk for confusion, depression and disorientation—keep clock and calendar in room to help reorient to time and place.
- More susceptible to hazards of immobility—maintain own ADLs as much as possible and change position every 2 hours.

### Aging and Changes in Ability to Maintain Activity Levels

- As aging occurs, there is a decrease in the rate or speed of activity.

*(continued)*

# DEVELOPMENTAL CONSIDERATIONS (CONTINUED)

- Loss of muscle mass interferes with activities that require strength such as bending down, dressing, and reaching for objects.
- Dexterity decreases, leading to a change in performing manipulative skills.

## Nursing Care for Positioning Elderly Clients

- Ambulate within limitations of age.
- Alter position every 2 hours; align correctly.
- Prevent osteoporosis of long bones by providing exercises against resistance as ordered.
- Provide active and passive exercises—rest periods necessary and exercise paced throughout the day for the elderly.
- Provide range-of-motion exercises to all joints three times a day.
- Educate family that allowing the client to be sedentary is not helpful.
- Encourage walking, which is best single exercise for the elderly.

## The Elderly Can Suffer Impaired Mobility and Disability Due to Decreased Physical Function or Accidents

- Nearly 23% of older people living in the community have some degree of disability.
- Persons 85 and older constitute 27% of those who have impaired mobility.
- Impaired mobility can lead to many subsequent problems, including depression, negative self-image, dependent behavior, and loss of independence.
- Effects of disability can influence the individual's body image, physical appearance, and bodily sensations.
- Posture becomes more flexed and center of gravity shifts.

## Special Assessment Parameters Are Important for the Elderly

- Specific source of disability or impaired mobility
- Presence of accompanying disease state: arthritis, stroke, dementia, diabetes, heart failure, COPD
- Presence of pain
- Condition of skin
- Drug effects: sedation, incontinence, orthostatic hypotension
- Motivation for rehabilitation

- Nutritional status
- Best assistive aid for client
- Be aware of any vision problems your client may have, especially cataracts, glaucoma, or macular degeneration. Note poorly lighted areas in the home or dark areas in the corridors, throw rugs, uneven or uncarpeted areas adjoining carpeted areas, etc. which may cause the client to stumble or fall.
- Check your client's ability to be mobile—their gait, balance, posture, and whether the client shuffles or is able to pick up his or her feet. Check if the client leans forward and is therefore off balance. Poor or unsteady mobility is often a direct cause of falling.
- Assess the client's degree of muscle strength on both sides of body and/or loss of flexibility because as age increases, strength declines, resulting in a fall. Check the degree of range of motion to all joints before ambulating. Even a poor handgrip can be dangerous if the client is walking downstairs. If leg muscles are weak, it may be difficult to get off a bed or up from a chair and the client may lose his or her balance.
- Assess for certain medications the client is taking which may cause vertigo, poor balance, blurred vision, weakness, or even drowsiness. Review the medications for elderly clients, keeping in mind the fact that they may require only half the normal dose due to their age and inability to metabolize drugs. The use of alcohol may contribute to falls in the home environment, so if the client uses alcohol there should be client teaching that focuses on the potential danger.
- Chronic diseases such as osteoarthritis, Parkinson's, Alzheimer's, and diabetes with peripheral neuropathy can all contribute to falls. Clients who have these diseases may require special assessment and interventions to prevent falls.
- Most elderly clients are aware of the danger of falling and breaking a hip or a leg, so fear is usually present when they are moving or walking. Proper intervention and instructions with an assistive device (canes, walkers, wheelchairs, etc.) will help to allay these fears which may become so overpowering that they cause immobilization and depression. Even fear itself, with its concomitant caution, may result in a fall; if the nurse can work with the client to discuss fears about falling and specific behaviors to prevent falling, it would be very therapeutic.

## DEVELOPMENTAL CONSIDERATIONS (CONTINUED)

**Develop Nursing Care Plan to Meet Elderly Client's Needs**

- Focus on disability or impaired mobility.
- Establish supportive relationship.
- Teach activities of daily living. Determine activities that must be accomplished each day for individual to care for own needs and be as independent as possible.

- Use assistive devices until client is stable and able to ambulate independently.
- Increase activities as individual progresses and is able to assume activity.
- Give positive reinforcement for all effort expended.

# Oxygenation

Skill 7.1   Deep Breathing and Coughing   275

VARIATION:  Pursed-Lip Breathing   276

Skill 7.2   Collecting a Sputum Specimen   276

Skill 7.3   Obtaining Nose and Throat Specimens   277

VARIATION:  For a Throat Specimen   278

VARIATION:  For a Nasal Specimen   278

VARIATION:  Obtaining a Nasopharyngeal Culture   279

Skill 7.4   Oxygen Saturation (Using a Pulse Oximeter)   279

Skill 7.5   Using an Incentive Spirometer   280

VARIATION:  For a Flow-Oriented SMI   280

VARIATION:  For All Devices   281

Skill 7.6   Administering Oxygen by Cannula, Face Mask, or Face Tent   282

VARIATION:  Using a Cannula   282

VARIATION:  Using a Face Mask   283

VARIATION:  Face Tent   283

VARIATION:  Nasal Cannula   284

VARIATION:  Face Mask or Tent   284

Skill 7.7   Using an Oxygen Cylinder   284

Skill 7.8   Providing Oxygen via a Pediatric Tent   285

Skill 7.9   Measuring Peak Expiratory Flow   286

Skill 7.10   Preparing Client for Chest Physiotherapy (CPT)   287

Skill 7.11   Performing Chest Percussion   288

Skill 7.12   Performing Chest Vibration   288

Skill 7.13   Inserting an Oropharyngeal Airway   289

Skill 7.14   Inserting a Nasopharyngeal Airway (Nasal Trumpet)   290

Skill 7.15   Assisting with Endotracheal Intubation   291

Skill 7.16   Inflating a Tracheal Tube Cuff   293

Skill 7.17   Providing Care for Client with Endotracheal Tube   294

Skill 7.18   Extubating an Endotracheal Tube   294

Skill 7.19   Oropharyngeal, Nasopharyngeal and Nasotracheal Suctioning   295

Skill 7.20   Suctioning a Tracheostomy or Endrotracheal Tube   298

VARIATION:  Using a Ventilator to Provide Hyperventilation   300

VARIATION:  Closed Suction System (In-Line Catheter)   301

Skill 7.21   Providing Tracheostomy Care   302

VARIATION:  Using a Disposal Inner Cannula   305

Skill 7.22   Capping a Tracheostomy Tube with Speaking Valve   306

Skill 7.23 Caring for the Client on a
Mechanical Ventilator 307

Skill 7.24 Weaning a Client from a Ventilator 311

Skill 7.25 Assisting with Chest Tube Insertion 312

Skill 7.26 Maintaining Chest Tube Drainage 315

Skill 7.27 Chest Tube Removal 319

Skill 7.28 Clearing an Obstructed Airway 320

VARIATION: Chest Thrusts 321

Skill 7.29 Performing Rescue Breathing 324

Skill 7.30 Administering External Cardiac
Compressions 328

VARIATION: CPR Performed
by One Rescuer 330

VARIATION: CPR Performed
by Two Rescuers 330

Skill 7.31 Administering Automated External
Defibrillation 332

Most people in good health give little thought to their respiratory function. Changing position frequently, ambulating, and exercising usually maintain adequate ventilation and gas exchange. Many people tend to breathe in a shallow fashion and do not draw air into the lowest regions of the lungs, thus limiting potential gas exchange

Mounting evidence supports the use of slow, abdominal breathing to facilitate pain relief and to decrease blood pressure in clients with essential hypertension (Joseph et al., 2005). Deep, slow breathing also facilitates the beneficial "relaxation response" identified by Dr. Herbert Benson (1996).

# Skill 7.1   Deep Breathing and Coughing

## EVIDENCE-BASED NURSING PRACTICE

### Improving Oxygenation

Studies show that the $PO_2$ is lower when the client with unilateral lung disease is positioned on the diseased side. Since the dependent lung has greater blood flow, placing the healthy lung down improves oxygenation.

*Source:* Bridges, E. (2001). Ask the experts. *Critical Care Nurse*, 21(6), 66.

### Delegation

Unlicensed assistive personnel (UAP) can reinforce and assist clients in performing breathing exercises. However, it is the responsibility of the nurse to teach the client the breathing exercises, to evaluate the effectiveness of the teaching, and to assess the outcomes of the breathing exercises (e.g., ease of breathing, effectiveness of cough, breath sounds).

### Equipment

- None (although a pillow is optional for splinting an abdominal or thoracic incision)

### Preparation

Before starting to teach breathing exercises, determine if location of a surgical incision prevents deep breathing because of pain. If so, administer analgesic medication 30 minutes prior to implementing deep breathing exercises.

### Procedure

1. Prior to performing the procedure, introduce self and verify the client's identity using agency protocol. Explain to the client what you are going to do, why it is necessary, and how he or she can participate. Discuss how deep breathing and coughing will help keep the lungs expanded and clear of secretions, thus preventing respiratory complications.
2. Perform hand hygiene and observe other appropriate infection control procedures.
3. Provide for client privacy.
4. Prepare the client.
   - Assist the client to assume a comfortable semisitting position in bed or on a chair or a lying position in bed with one pillow. ➤*Rationale: To increase lung capacity and allow for deeper breathing.*
   - Have the client flex the knees. ➤*Rationale: To relax the muscles of the abdomen.*
   - Have the client place one or both hands on the abdomen just below the ribs. ➤*Rationale: This will help client to evaluate depth of inspiration through movement of abdomen.*
5. Perform abdominal breathing. Instruct the client to:
   - Breathe in deeply through the nose with the mouth closed, to stay relaxed, not to arch the back, and to concentrate on feeling the abdomen rise as far as possible. ➤*Rationale: When a person breathes in, the diaphragm contracts (drops), the lungs fill with air, and the abdomen rises or protrudes.*
   - Hold the breath for 3 to 5 seconds. ➤*Rationale: This helps keep the alveoli open.*

- Breathe out slowly.
- Perform relaxed diaphragmatic breathing as needed for respiratory status.

6. Perform controlled and huff coughing as the next step, if needed (e.g., if coughing is going to be beneficial to maintain or improve oxygenation).
   - For clients who have had thoracic or abdominal surgery, instruct them to place their hands or a pillow over the incisional site and to apply gentle pressure while deep breathing or coughing. ➤*Rationale: Helps decrease incisional strain and discomfort and facilitates effective coughing.*
   - Instruct the client to take three to four slow deep breaths, inhaling through the nose and exhaling through pursed lips as if gently blowing out a candle. ➤*Rationale: Increasing lung volume increases air flow through the small airways, expands the lungs, and helps mobilize secretions on expiration.* Limit the active deep breaths. ➤*Rationale: This helps avoid fatigue and hyperventilation.*
   - Ask the client to inhale deeply and hold his or her breath for a few seconds.
   - Instruct the client to cough twice while exhaling. This is controlled coughing. ➤*Rationale: The first cough loosens the mucus; the second expels the secretions.*
   - For huff coughing, the client leans forward and exhales with a series of "huff" sounds. ➤*Rationale: This helps keep the airways open while moving secretions up and out of the lungs.*
   - Allow the client to rest. Try to avoid prolonged episodes of coughing. ➤*Rationale: Prolonged episodes may cause fatigue and hypoxia.*
   - Instruct the client to perform several relaxed diaphragmatic breaths before the next cough effort.

7. Document the teaching and assessments for the exercises performed and the client's response.

### VARIATION: Pursed-Lip Breathing  ➔COPD

- Teach the client to inhale through the nose and then, pursing lips as if about to whistle, breathe out slowly and gently, making a slow "whooshing" sound without puffing out their cheeks. ➤*Rationale: This pursed-lip breathing creates a resistance to air flowing out of the lungs, increases pressure within the bronchi (main air passages), and minimizes collapse of smaller airways, a common problem for people with COPD.*
- Instruct the client to inhale deeply through the nose and count to 3.
- Have the client concentrate on tightening the abdominal muscles while breathing out slowly and evenly through pursed lips while counting to 7 or until the client cannot exhale any more. ➤*Rationale: Tightening the abdominal muscles and leaning forward helps compress the lungs and enhances effective exhalation.*
- Teach the client how to perform pursed-lip breathing while walking: Inhale while taking two steps, then exhale through pursed lips while taking the next four steps.
- Instruct the client to use this exercise whenever feeling short of breath and to increase gradually to 5 to 10 minutes four times a day. ➤*Rationale: Regular practice will help the client do this type of breathing without conscious effort.*

> ### CLINICAL ALERT
>
> Deep breathing is indicated, but coughing is contraindicated for the client post-eye, -ear, -brain, or -neck surgery, or if efforts are nonproductive.

## Skill 7.2   Collecting a Sputum Specimen

### Delegation

UAP can obtain a sputum specimen that is expectorated by a client. It is important to instruct the UAP about when to collect the specimen, how to position the client, and how to correctly collect the specimen. Obtaining a sputum specimen by use of pharyngeal suctioning, however, should be performed by the nurse because it is an invasive, sterile process and requires knowledge application and problem solving.

### Equipment

- Sterile specimen container with a cover
- Clean gloves (if assisting the client)
- Disinfectant and swabs, or liquid soap and water
- Paper towels
- Completed label
- Completed laboratory requisition
- Mouthwash

### Preparation

Determine the method of collection and gather the appropriate equipment.

### Procedure

1. Prior to performing the procedure, introduce self and verify the client's identity using agency protocol. Explain to the client what you are going to do, why it is necessary, and how he or she can participate. Discuss how the results will be used in plan-

ning further care or treatments. Give the client the following information and instructions:

- The purpose of the test, the difference between sputum and saliva, and how to provide the sputum specimen.
- Not to touch the inside of the sputum container.
- To expectorate the sputum directly into the sputum container.
- To keep the outside of the container free of sputum, if possible.
- How to hold a pillow firmly against an abdominal incision if the client finds it painful to cough.
- The amount of sputum required (usually, 1 to 2 tsp [4 to 10 mL] of sputum is sufficient for analysis).

2. Perform hand hygiene and observe other appropriate infection control procedures.
3. Provide for client privacy.
4. Provide necessary assistance to collect the specimen.

- Assist the client to a standing or a sitting position (e.g., high- or semi-Fowler's position or on the edge of a bed or in a chair). ➤Rationale: *These positions allow maximum lung ventilation and expansion.*
- Ask the client to hold the sputum cup on the outside, or, for a client who is not able to do so, put on gloves and hold the cup for the client.
- Ask the client to breathe deeply and then cough up secretions. ➤Rationale: *A deep inhalation provides sufficient air to force secretions out of the airways and into the pharynx.*
- Hold the sputum cup so that the client can expectorate into it, making sure that the sputum does not come in contact with the outside of the container. ➤Rationale: *Containing the sputum within the cup restricts the spread of microorganisms to others.*
- Assist the client to repeat coughing until a sufficient amount of sputum has been collected.
- Cover the container with the lid immediately after the sputum is in the container. ➤Rationale: *Covering the container prevents the inadvertent spread of microorganisms to others.*
- If spillage occurs on the outside of the container, clean the outer surface with a disinfectant. Some agencies recom-

mend washing the outside of all containers with liquid soap and water and then drying with a paper towel.
- Remove and discard the gloves. Perform hand hygiene.

5. Ensure client comfort and safety.

- Assess the client for respiratory difficulty and provide oxygen per the primary care provider's orders.
- Assist the client to rinse his or her mouth with a mouthwash as needed.
- Assist the client to a position of comfort that allows maximum lung expansion as required.

6. Label and transport the specimen to the laboratory.

- Ensure that the specimen label and the laboratory requisition contain the correct information. Attach the label and requisition securely to the specimen. ➤Rationale: *Inaccurate identification or information on the specimen container can lead to errors of diagnosis or therapy.*
- Arrange for the specimen to be sent to the laboratory immediately or refrigerated. ➤Rationale: *Bacterial cultures must be started immediately before any contaminating organisms can grow, multiply, and produce false results.*

7. Document all relevant information.

- Document the collection of the sputum specimen on the client's chart. Include the amount, color, consistency (e.g., thick, tenacious, watery), presence of hemoptysis (blood in the sputum), odor of the sputum, any measures needed to obtain the specimen (e.g., postural drainage), the general amount of sputum produced, any discomfort experienced by the client, and any interventions implemented to ensure adequate air exchange postprocedure (such as $O_2$ saturation monitoring or administration of $O_2$).

---

### DEVELOPMENTAL CONSIDERATIONS

**Elders**

- Elders may need encouragement to cough because a decreased cough reflex occurs with aging.
- Allow time for elders to rest and recover between coughs when obtaining a sputum specimen.

---

# Skill 7.3   Obtaining Nose and Throat Specimens

## Delegation

Obtaining nose and throat cultures is an invasive skill that requires the application of scientific knowledge and potential problem solving to ensure client safety. Therefore, the nurse needs to perform this skill and does not delegate it to UAP.

## Equipment

- Clean gloves
- Two sterile, cotton-tipped swabs in sterile culture tubes with transport medium
- Penlight
- Tongue blade (optional)

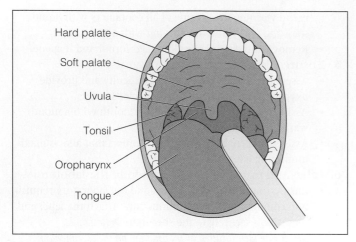

● Depressing the tongue to view the pharynx.

- Otoscope with a nasal speculum (optional)
- Container for the used nasal speculum
- Completed labels for each specimen container
- Completed laboratory requisition

## Preparation

Prepare the client and the equipment:

- Assist the client to a sitting position. ➤*Rationale: This is the most comfortable position for many people and the one in which the pharynx is most readily visible.*
- Put on gloves if the client's mucosa will be touched.
- Open the culture tube and place it on the sterile wrapper. ➤*Rationale: This prevents microorganisms from entering the tube.*
- Remove one sterile applicator and hold it carefully by the stick end keeping the remainder sterile. The swab end is kept from touching any objects that could contaminate it.

## Procedure

1. Prior to performing the procedure, introduce self and verify the client's identity using agency protocol. Explain to the client what you are going to do, why it is necessary, and how he or she can participate. Discuss how the results will be used in planning further care or treatments. Inform the client that he may gag while swabbing the throat or feel like sneezing during the swabbing of the nose; however, the procedure will take less than 1 minute.
2. Perform hand hygiene and observe other appropriate infection control procedures.
3. Provide for client privacy.
4. Collect the specimen.

## VARIATION: For a Throat Specimen

- Ask the client to tilt the head back, open the mouth, extend the tongue, and say "ah." ➤*Rationale: When the tongue is extended, the pharynx is exposed. Saying "ah" relaxes the throat muscles and helps minimize contraction of the constriction muscle of the pharynx (the gag reflex).*
- Use the penlight to illuminate the posterior pharynx while depressing the tongue with a tongue blade. Depress the anterior third of the tongue firmly without touching the throat. ➤*Rationale: Touching the throat stimulates the gag reflex. Check for inflamed areas.*
- Insert a swab into the mouth without touching any part of the mouth or tongue. ➤*Rationale: The swab should not pick up microorganisms in the mouth.*
- Gently and quickly, swab along the tonsils, making sure to contact any areas on the pharynx that are particularly erythematous (reddened) or that contain exudates (purulent drainage). ➤*Rationale: By moving the swab quickly, you can avoid initiating the gag reflex or causing discomfort. Erythematous areas and areas with exudate will likely have the most microorganisms. Rotating the swab where exudate is present may maximize the amount of specimen collected.*
- Remove the swab without touching the mouth or lips. ➤*Rationale: This prevents the swab from transmitting microorganisms to the mouth.*
- Insert the swab into the sterile tube without allowing it to touch the outside of the container. Push the tip of the swab into the liquid medium. Make sure the swab is placed in the correctly labeled tube. ➤*Rationale: Touching the outside of the tube could transmit microorganisms to it and then to others.*
- Crush the ampule of culture medium at the bottom of the tube.
- Place the top securely on the tube, taking care not to touch the inside of the cap. ➤*Rationale: Touching the inside of the cap could transmit additional microorganisms into the tube.*
- Repeat the above steps with the second swab.
- Discard the tongue blade in the waste container.
- Remove and discard gloves. Perform hand hygiene.

## VARIATION: For a Nasal Specimen

- Ask the client to blow her nose to clear her nasal passages. Check nostrils with penlight to check for patency.
- If using a nasal speculum, gently insert the lighted nasal speculum up one nostril.
- Insert the sterile swab carefully through the speculum, without touching the edges. ➤*Rationale: This prevents the swab from picking up microorganisms from the speculum. When working without a speculum, pass the swab along the septum and the floor of the nose.*
- When the area of mucosa that is reddened or contains exudate, is reached, rotate the swab quickly.
- Remove the swab without touching the speculum.

- Remove the nasal speculum if used.
- Insert the swab into the culture tube. Crush the ampule at the bottom of the tube and push the tip of the swab into the liquid medium.
- Repeat the above steps for the other nostril.

5. Label and transport the specimens to the laboratory.

- See Skill 7.2, step 6.

6. Document all relevant information.

- Record the collection of the nose and/or throat specimens on the client's chart. Include the assessments of the nasal mucosa and pharynx, and any discomfort the client experienced.

### VARIATION: Obtaining a Nasopharyngeal Culture

A nasopharyngeal culture uses the same steps as a nasal culture with the following exceptions: A special cotton-tipped swab on a flexible wire is used. While this swab is still in the package, bend the sterile swab in a curve and then open the package without contaminating the swab. Gently pass the swab through the more patent nostril about 8–10 cm (3 to 4 in.) into the nasopharynx.

---

**DEVELOPMENTAL CONSIDERATIONS**

**Infants**

- When taking a throat swab, avoid occluding an infant's nose because infants normally breathe only through the nose.

**Children**

- Have a parent stand the young child between the parent's legs with the child's back to the parent and the parent's arms gently but firmly around the child. As the parent tips the child's head back, ask the child to open wide and stick the tongue out. Assure the child that the procedure will be over quickly and may "tickle" but should not hurt.
- Cooperative children can be asked to put their hands under their buttocks, open their mouth, and laugh or pant like a dog (Bindler, Ball, London, & Ladewig, 2007).

---

# Skill 7.4   Oxygen Saturation (Using a Pulse Oximeter)

### Delegation

Application of the pulse oximeter sensor and recording of the $SpO_2$ value may be delegated to UAP. The interpretation of the oxygen saturation value and determination of appropriate responses are done by the nurse.

### Equipment

- Nail polish remover as needed
- Alcohol wipe
- Sheet or towel
- Pulse oximeter

Pulse oximeters with various types of sensors are available from several manufacturers. The oximeter unit consists of an inlet connection for the sensor cable, a faceplate that indicates (a) the oxygen saturation measurement (expressed as a percentage); and (b) the pulse rate. Cordless units are also available. A preset alarm system signals high and low $Sp_2$ measurements and a high and low pulse rate. The high and low $SpO_2$ levels are generally preset at 100% and 85%, respectively for adults. The high and low pulse rate alarms are usually present at 140 and 50 bpm for adults. These alarm limits can, however, be changed according to the manufacturer's directions.

---

**DEVELOPMENTAL CONSIDERATIONS**

**Infants**

- If an appropriate-sized finger or toe sensor is not available, consider using an earlobe or forehead sensor.
- The high and low $SpO_2$ alarm levels are generally preset at 95% and 80% for neonates.
- The high and low pulse rate alarms are usually preset at 200 and 100 for neonates.
- The oximeter may need to be taped, wrapped with an elastic bandage, or covered by a stocking to keep it in place.

**Children**

- Instruct the child that the sensor does not hurt. Disconnect the probe whenever possible to allow for movement.

**Elders**

- Use of vasoconstrictive medications, poor circulation, or thickened nails may make finger or toe sensors inaccurate.

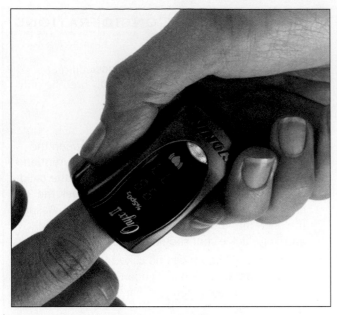

● Fingertip oximeter sensor (cordless).
(Courtesy of Nonin Medical, Inc.)

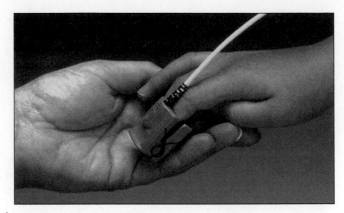

● Fingertip oximeter sensor (child).
(Courtesy of Nonin Medical)

## SETTING OF CARE

- Pulse oximetry is a quick, inexpensive, noninvasive method of assessing oxygenation. Like an automatic blood pressure cuff, it also provides a pulse rate reading. Use in the ambulatory or home setting whenever indicated.

- If the client requires frequent or continuous home monitoring, teach the client and family how to apply and maintain the equipment. Remind them to rotate the side periodically and assess for skin trauma.

# Skill 7.5   Using an Incentive Spirometer

*Prevent atelectasis*

*Exhale*
*seal*
*slow deep breath ↑ball 2-6 sec*
*∅ brisk ↓ val breath*

### Delegation

It is the responsibility of the nurse to teach the client how to use the incentive spirometer, assess the client's performance, and evaluate the outcomes of the therapy. UAP however, can reinforce and assist clients in using the incentive spirometer. The nurses should inform the UAP of the key points to using the incentive spirometer correctly.

### Equipment

- Flow-oriented or volume-oriented SMI
- Mouthpiece or breathing tube
- Label for mouthpiece
- Progress chart
- Nose clip (optional)

### Preparation

- Determine if the client has a disposable SMI at the bedside.
- This skill should not be performed immediately after a meal or other physically stressful activity.

### Procedure

1. Prior to performing the skill, introduce self and verify the client's identity using agency protocol. Explain to the client what you are going to do, why it is necessary, and how he or she can participate. Discuss how the results will be used in planning further care or treatments.
2. Perform hand hygiene and observe other appropriate infection control procedures.
3. Provide for client privacy.
4. Prepare the client.
   - Assist the client to an upright position in bed or on a chair. If the person is unable to assume a sitting position for a flow spirometer, have the person assume any position. ➤*Rationale: A sitting position facilitates maximum ventilation of the lungs.*

### VARIATION: For a Flow-Oriented SMI

5. Instruct the client to use the spirometer as follows:
   - Hold the spirometer in the upright position. ➤*Rationale: A tilted spirometer requires less effort to raise the balls or disks.*

- Exhale normally.
- Seal the lips tightly around the mouthpiece, take in a slow deep breath to elevate the balls and then hold the breath for 2 seconds initially, increasing to 6 seconds (optimum) to keep the balls elevated if possible. Instruct the client to *avoid* brisk low-volume breaths that snap the balls to the top of the chamber. The client may use a nose clip if the person has difficulty breathing only through the mouth. ➤*Rationale: A slow, deep breath ensures maximal ventilation. Greater lung expansion is achieved with a very slow inspiration than with a brisk shallow breath. Sustained elevation of the balls ensures adequate ventilation of the alveoli (lung air sacs).*
- Remove the mouthpiece and exhale normally.
- Cough productively, as needed, after using the spirometer. ➤*Rationale: Deep ventilation may loosen secretions and stimulate coughing. Effective coughing can facilitate the removal of the loose secretions.*
- Relax and take several normal breaths before using the spirometer again.
- Repeat the procedure to a total of 10 breaths, encouraging the client to take progressively deeper breaths up to the maximal goal.
- Repeat series of breaths once each hour while awake. ➤*Rationale: Practice increases inspiratory volume, maintains alveolar ventilation,and prevents atelectasis (collapse of the air sacs).*

*For a Volume-Oriented SMI*

6. Set the spirometer.
   - Set the spirometer to a "target" volume. ➤*Rationale: This provides an incentive and motivation for the client. Can start low and increase "target" after client success.*
7. Instruct the client to use the spirometer as follows:
   - Exhale normally.

- Seal the lips tightly around the mouthpiece and take in a slow, deep breath until the piston is elevated to the predetermined level. The piston level may be visible to the client to identify the volume obtained.
- Hold the breath for 6 seconds to ensure maximal alveolar ventilation.
- Remove the mouthpiece and exhale normally.
- Cough productively, as needed, after using the spirometer. ➤*Rationale: Deep ventilation may loosen secretions and stimulate coughing. Effective coughing can facilitate the removal of the loose secretions.*
- Relax and take several normal breaths before using the spirometer again.
- Repeat the procedure to a total of 10 breaths, encouraging the client to take progressively deeper breaths up to the maximal goal.
- Repeat series of breaths once each hour while awake. ➤*Rationale: Practice increases inspiratory volume, maintains alveolar ventilation, and prevents atelectasis.*
- Encourage the client to record the top volume achieved at each hour he or she performed the technique. ➤*Rationale: This facilitates cooperation of the client and assists in evaluating outcomes of the skill.*

### VARIATION: For All Devices

8. Clean the equipment.
   - Clean the mouthpiece with water and shake it dry. Label the mouthpiece and a disposable SMI with the client's name. A disposable SMI may be left at the bedside for the client to use as prescribed.
9. Document all relevant information.
   - Record the skill, including type of spirometer, number of breaths taken, volume or flow levels achieved, client response, and results of auscultation. Also include, when appropriate, client education and the ability of the client to perform the procedure without prompting.

### Documentation

Sample: 6/12/2009 1030 Coarse rales in RLL. Instructed on use of incentive spirometer. Able to use correctly and raise one ball for 3 seconds. Use of IS stimulated cough resulting in production of small amount light colored thick mucus. Encouraged to continue using IS each hour.
_____ S. Lee, RN

# Skill 7.6 Administering Oxygen by Cannula, Face Mask, or Face Tent

## Delegation

Initiating the administration of oxygen is considered similar to administering a medication and is not delegated to unlicensed assistive personnel (UAP). However, reapplying the oxygen delivery device may be performed by the UAP and many aspects of the client's response to oxygen therapy are observed during usual care and may be recorded by persons other than the nurse. Abnormal findings must be validated and interpreted by the nurse. The nurse is also responsible for ensuring that the correct delivery method is being use.

## Equipment

*Cannula*

- Oxygen supply with a flow meter and adapter
- Humidifier with distilled water or tap water according to agency protocol
- Nasal cannula and tubing
- Tape (optional)
- Padding for the elastic band (optional)

*Face Mask*

- Oxygen supply with a flow meter and adapter
- Humidifier with distilled water or tap water according to agency protocol
- Prescribed face mask of the appropriate size
- Padding for the elastic band

*Face Tent*

- Oxygen supply with a flow meter and adapter
- Humidifier with distilled water or tap water according to agency protocol
- Face tent of the appropriate size

## Preparation

- Determine the need for oxygen therapy, and verify the order for the therapy.
- Perform a respiratory assessment to develop baseline data if not already available.
- Prepare the client and support people.
- Assist the client to a semi-Fowler's position if possible. ▶*Rationale: This position permits easier chest expansion and hence easier breathing.*
- Explain that oxygen is not dangerous when safety precautions are observed. Inform the client and support people about the safety precautions connected with oxygen use.

## Procedure

1. Prior to performing the procedure, introduce self and verify the client's identity using agency protocol. Explain to the client what you are going to do,

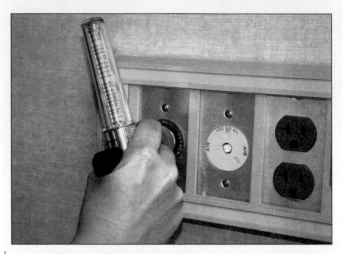
● Attach the flow meter to the wall outlet.

why it is necessary, and how he or she can participate. Discuss how the effects of the oxygen therapy will be used in planning further care or treatments.
2. Perform hand hygiene and observe other appropriate infection control procedures.
3. Provide for client privacy, if appropriate.
4. Set up the oxygen equipment and the humidifier.
   - Attach the flow meter to the wall outlet or tank. The flow meter should be in the OFF position.
   - If needed, fill the humidifier bottle with tap or distilled water, per agency policy. (This can be done before coming to the bedside.)
   - Attach the humidifier bottle to the base of the flow meter.
   - Attach the prescribed oxygen tubing and delivery device to the humidifier.
5. Turn on the oxygen at the prescribed rate, and ensure proper functioning.
   - Check that the oxygen is flowing freely through the tubing. There should be no kinks in the tubing, and the connections should be airtight. There should be bubbles in the humidifier as the oxygen flows through. You should feel the oxygen at the outlets of the cannula, mask, or tent.
   - Set the oxygen at the flow rate ordered.
6. Apply the appropriate oxygen delivery device.

## VARIATION: Using a Cannula

- Put the cannula with the outlet prongs curved downward, fitting into the nares, and the elastic band around the head or the tubing over the ears and under the chin.
- If the cannula will not stay in place, tape it at the sides of the face.
- Pad the tubing and band over the ears and cheekbones as needed.

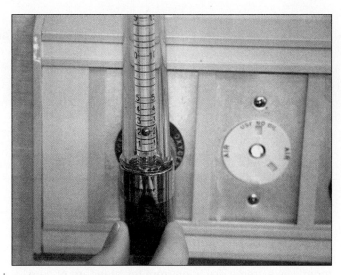

● This flow meter is set to deliver 2 L/min.

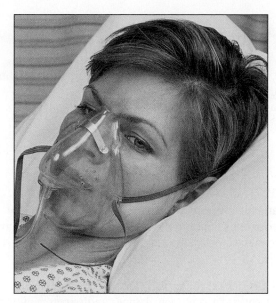

● A simple face mask.
(Photographer: Jenny Thomas)

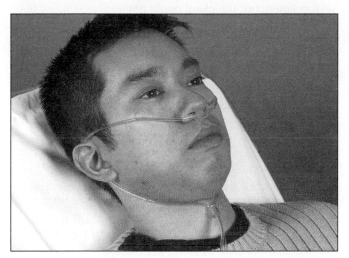

● A nasal cannula.

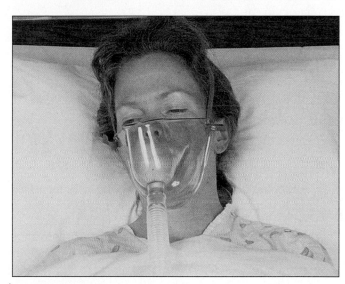

● An oxygen face tent.
(Photographer: Jenny Thomas)

## VARIATION: Using a Face Mask

- Guide the mask toward the client's face, and apply it from the nose downward.
- Fit the mask and metal nose bracket to the contours of the client's face. ➤*Rationale: The mask should mold to the face, so that very little oxygen escapes into the eyes or around the cheeks and chin.*
- Secure the elastic band around the client's head so that the mask is comfortable but snug.
- Pad the band behind the ears and over bony prominences. ➤*Rationale: Padding will prevent irritation from the mask.*

## VARIATION: Face Tent

- Place the tent over the client's face, and secure the ties around the head.

## CLINICAL ALERT

Oxygen is indicated for clients with COPD, but is used conservatively. High levels of oxygen can cause hypoventilation, $CO_2$ retention, may suppress breathing stimulus and lead to respiratory arrest due to $CO_2$ narcosis.

7. Assess the client regularly.
   - Assess the client's vital signs (including oxygen saturation), level of anxiety, color, and ease of respirations, and provide support while the client adjusts to the device.
   - Assess the client in 15 to 30 minutes, depending on the client's condition, and regularly thereafter.

## CLINICAL ALERT

- Avoid placing $SpO_2$ clip sensor on the thumb or edematous site. Wrap sensors can be used on the thumb or great toe.
- Avoid extremity with an intra-arterial catheter or noninvasive automatic BP cuff.

## CLINICAL ALERT

The anemic client may have a normal $SpO_2$ in spite of inadequate tissue oxygenation because available hemoglobin is maximally saturated with oxygen.

- Assess the client regularly for clinical signs of hypoxia, tachycardia, confusion, dyspnea, restlessness, and cyanosis. Review arterial blood gas results if they are available.

**VARIATION: Nasal Cannula**

- Assess the client's nares for encrustations and irritation. Apply a water-soluble lubricant as required to soothe the mucous membranes.
- Assess the top of the client's ears for any signs of irritation from the cannula strap. If present, padding with a gauze pad may help relieve the discomfort.

**VARIATION: Face Mask or Tent**

- Inspect the facial skin frequently for dampness or chafing, and dry and treat it as needed.
8. Inspect the equipment on a regular basis.
   - Check the liter flow and the level of water in the humidifier in 30 minutes and whenever providing care to the client.
   - Make sure that safety precautions are being followed.
9. Document findings in the client record using forms or checklists supplemented by narrative notes when appropriate.

## CLINICAL ALERT

Humidification of low-flow oxygen through nasal cannulae is not considered essential and is contraindicated because it supports bacterial growth.

## ▍ LEGAL ALERT

There was substantial evidence in medical malpractice action against a nurse to support award of punitive damages where the plaintiff's expert witness concluded that the nurse's conduct in disconnecting supplemental oxygen to the client during the client's transfer to another room was extreme deviation from the standard of care. Evidence was also present that the nurse disconnected oxygen despite pleadings from family members present who claimed that the client could not survive without his oxygen, and who requested that he be provided with a portable oxygen unit preparatory to the move. From this evidence, the jury could have found the nurse's conduct was grossly negligent and that she acted with disregard for consequences that were likely to follow. *Manning v. Twin Falls Clinic & Hosp., Inc.* (1992).

### Documentation

Sample: 9/16/09 0930 Returned from physical therapy c̄ c/o SOB. Resp. 26/min, shallow. P-92, BP 160/98, $SpO_2$ 92%. Skin warm, no cyanosis. Lung sounds clear, no retractions. $O_2$ per nasal cannula applied @ 3 L/min. _____ P. Isola, RN

9/16/09 1000 No further c/o SOB. Resp. 20/min, P 88, BP 152/92, $SpO_2$ 96%. $O_2$ per nasal cannula continues @ 3 L/min._____ P. Isola, RN

# Skill 7.7   Using an Oxygen Cylinder

### Equipment

- Steel cylinder portable oxygen tank
- Regulator/flow meter
- Oxygen delivery tubing

### Procedure

1. Place oxygen cylinder in carrier in secure upright position. ➤*Rationale: If cylinder of compressed air falls accidentally, unit becomes a missile with uncontrollable force and direction.*

- Attach regulator to cylinder neck, attach tubing, open cylinder release valve and adjust oxygen flow rate (L/min) as prescribed.
2. Using hexagon key, slowly turn cylinder release valve clockwise (left is loose) to crack tank open for a brief period, then close (right to tighten). ➤*Rationale: This action removes lint from system.*
3. Check pressure gauge on front of tank to determine amount of oxygen pressure in tank. ➤*Rationale: Full status is 2,200 PSI.*

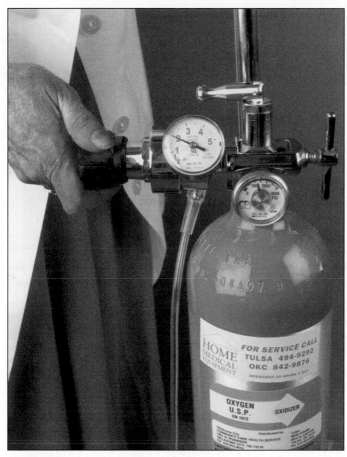

● Attach regulator to cylinder neck, attach tubing, open cylinder release valve and adjust oxygen flow rate (L/min) as prescribed.

## SIGNS AND SYMPTOMS OF HYPOXIA

### Early Symptoms

- Restlessness
- Headache
- Visual disturbances
- Confusion or change in behavior
- Tachypnea
- Tachycardia
- Hypertension
- Dyspnea
- Anxious face

### Advanced Symptoms

- Hypotension
- Bradycardia
- Metabolic acidosis (production of lactic acid)
- Cyanosis

### Chronic Hypoxia

- Polycythemia
- Clubbing of fingers and toes
- Peripheral edema
- Right-sided heart failure
- Chronic $PO_2$ less than 55 mm Hg; $O_2$ saturation less than 87%
- Elevated $Pco_2$ (respiratory acidosis)
- Elevated $Pco_2$ (respiratory acidosis)

4. Attach flow meter regulator unit over neck of cylinder, aligning pins with green "O" ring openings.
5. Use turn key to tighten regulator to cylinder neck.
6. Connect delivery tubing to "Christmas tree" adapter on regulator unit.

7. Open cylinder release valve using hexagon key on top of cylinder. ➤*Rationale: This allows oxygen flow.*
8. Slowly open regulator/flow meter and adjust to prescribed rate of oxygen delivery in liters per minute.

# Skill 7.8   Providing Oxygen via a Pediatric Tent

## Equipment

- Oxygen source
- Delivery tubing
- Disposable oxygen tent/canopy
- Oxygen blender
- Oxygen analyzer
- Sterile water for nebulizer
- Two bath blankets
- Ambient thermometer
- Pulse oximeter

## Preparation

1. Check physician's orders.
2. Gather equipment.
3. Explain purpose of tent to child and parents.
4. Provide favorite toy or blanket.
5. Perform hand hygiene.

## Procedure

*Setting Up Pediatric Tent*

1. Secure tent/canopy and place machine at head of empty bed/crib with control knobs on opposite side of working area.

## CLINICAL ALERT

Avoid use of friction-type toys or battery-operated devices when oxygen is in use.

2. Place thermometer in tent.
3. Connect oxygen regulator into oxygen source and select concentration.
4. Connect delivery tubing to canopy.
5. Plug in machine.
6. Set up humidifier/nebulizer and fill tray (at back of machine) with sterile water.
7. Pad crib frame that supports canopy with bath blankets. ➤*Rationale: Padding protects client from injury and absorbs excess moisture.*

*Monitoring Child in Tent*

8. Turn on oxygen to prescribed concentration (21–50%) and maintain temperature at 17.8°–21.2°C (64°–70°F).
9. Secure canopy by tucking in all sides under mattress. ➤*Rationale: To prevent oxygen leak at bottom of tent since oxygen is heavier than air.*
10. Monitor temperature regularly. ➤*Rationale: To determine if temperature goal is achieved.*
11. Analyze and record tent oxygen concentration, and check child's vital signs/oximetry as ordered.
12. Keep crib sides up for safety.

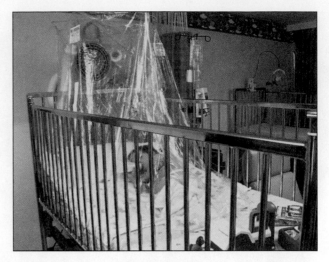

● The pediatric tent can be used for oxygen delivery, humidification, temperature control, or a combination of these.

13. Select toys that are washable, do not produce static electricity, and are appropriate to the child's age.
14. Check dampness of clothes and change PRN to prevent chilling.
15. Minimize number of times tent is opened to maintain desired $FIO_2$.

*Note:* Frequent linen changes may be necessary to prevent heat loss due to evaporation of moisture.

# Skill 7.9  Measuring Peak Expiratory Flow

### Delegation

PEFR measurement may be delegated to trained UAP. The nurse should double check any values found to be abnormal or significantly different from previous results and must interpret the findings. Modifications in the treatment regimen may not be initiated by UAP.

### Equipment

• Peak flow meter

### Procedure

1. Prior to performing the procedure, introduce self and verify the client's identity using agency protocol. Explain to the client what you are going to do, why it is necessary, and how he or she can participate. Discuss how the results will be used in planning further care or treatments.
2. Perform hand hygiene and observe other appropriate infection control procedures.
3. Provide for client privacy.
4. Position the client.

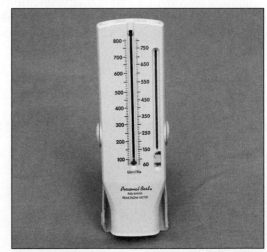

● Peak flow meter with marker in the zero position.

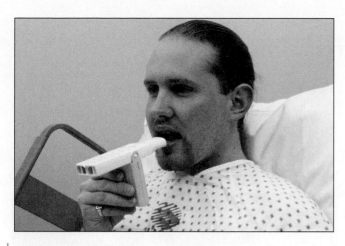

● PEFR measurement.

- If possible, the client should be sitting with the chest free from contact with the bed or chair. If not possible, place the client in semi-Fowler's or high-Fowler's position.
5. Reset the marker on the flow meter to the zero position.
6. Assist the client to use the flow meter.
   - Ask the client to take a deep breath in.
   - Client places the mouthpiece in the mouth with the teeth around the opening and lips forming a tight seal.
   - Have the client exhale as quickly and forcefully as possible. If you suspect the client is exhaling a significant amount of air through the nose, apply a nose clip.
7. Perform step 6 two more times, allowing the client to rest for 5 to 10 seconds in between. Record the highest level achieved.
8. Document findings in the client record using forms or checklists supplemented by narrative notes when appropriate.

# Skill 7.10   Preparing Client for Chest Physiotherapy (CPT)

## EVIDENCE-BASED NURSING PRACTICE

### Bronchial Hygiene Therapy

There is no firm scientific evidence that CPT measures are effective in preventing pulmonary complications. In order to justify continuation of postural drainage, the client must demonstrate one or more of the expected outcomes.

*Source:* Goodfellow, L. & Jones, M. (2002). Bronchial hygiene therapy. *American Journal of Nursing,* 102(1), 38.

## Equipment

- Hospital bed or other surface to place client in head-down position
- Gown or towel (optional)
- Tissues
- Container for sputum
- Clean gloves
- Stethoscope
- Pulse oximeter (if indicated)
- Mouthwash/oral hygiene product

## Procedure

1. Validate physician's order for CPT. ➤*Rationale: These procedures are tiring to clients, time consuming and contraindicated in cases of osteoporosis, pulmonary embolism, cardiac conditions, lung cancer, or other conditions not associated with excessive sputum production.*

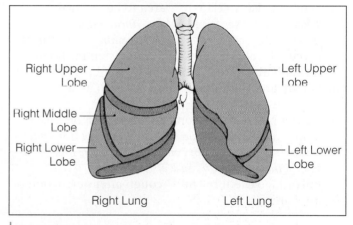

● Lobes of the lungs.

2. Perform hand hygiene.
3. Administer CPT before or at least 2 hours after meals to prevent vomiting.
4. Establish the location of lung segments if the entire lung field is to undergo CPT; the affected segment should be drained first. ➤*Rationale: Usually, the lower areas are the most affected.*
5. Provide privacy.
6. Prepare client by explaining CPT and purpose.
7. Auscultate chest for breath sounds and adventitious sounds prior to therapy.
8. Obtain pulse oximetry ($SpO_2$) if indicated before therapy.
9. Place towel over skin when performing CPT (optional).

# Skill 7.11   Performing Chest Percussion

### Equipment

See Skill 7.10, Preparing Client for CPT.

### Preparation

1. See Skill 7.10, Preparing Client for CPT.
2. Perform hand hygiene.

### Procedure

1. Cover area to be percussed with gown or cloth towel (optional).
2. Holding arms with elbows slightly flexed, cup your hands with thumbs and fingers closed. Keeping wrists loose and relaxed, rhythmically flex and extend wrists to clap over area to be drained. ➤*Rationale: This motion produces vibrations that loosen secretions for easier removal with coughing or suctioning.*
3. Percuss by alternating hands and listen for hollow sound with strikes.
4. Slowly and rhythmically percuss each area for 3–5 minutes.
5. Do not percuss over bony prominences, breasts, or tender areas. ➤*Rationale: Vibrations are not transmitted to the chest wall through bone or breast tissue and percussion in these areas can cause discomfort.*
6. Encourage client to "huff" cough after percussion of lung areas.

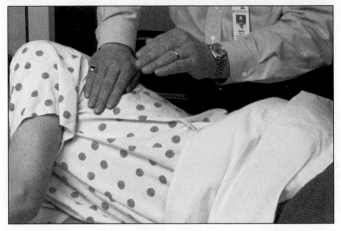

● Perform percussion and vibration with each position change.

7. Auscultate all lung areas for changes in breath sounds.
8. Don gloves, note character and measure quantity of sputum and discard.
9. Remove gloves and perform hand hygiene.
10. Offer oral hygiene.
11. Document procedure and client's response.

# Skill 7.12   Performing Chest Vibration

### Equipment

See Skill 7.10, Preparing Client for CPT.

### Preparation

1. See Skill 7.10, Preparing Client for CPT.
2. Perform hand hygiene.

### Procedure

1. Perform vibration following postural drainage and percussion in each position.
2. Cover area to be vibrated with gown or towel (optional).

3. Instruct client to breathe in through nose and exhale slowly through pursed lips.
4. Place your hands flat over area to be vibrated or place one hand on top of the other. Keep your arms and shoulders straight and wrists stiff.
5. Have client inhale deeply.
6. As client exhales through pursed lips, use moderate pressure to vibrate chest by quickly contracting and relaxing your arms and shoulders. ➤*Rationale: This increases the turbulence and velocity of exhaled air, loosens and mobilizes secretions from peripheral airways.*

7. Vibrate for 3 or 4 exhalations over the area.
8. Encourage clients to "huff" cough before changing positions.
   - Place hands flat over area to be vibrated, keeping wrists stiff.
9. Assess vital signs, pulse oximetry and auscultate breath sounds.
10. Don gloves.
11. Measure and note character of expectorated secretions, then discard.
12. Remove gloves and perform hand hygiene.
13. Provide oral hygiene.
14. Document procedure and client's response.

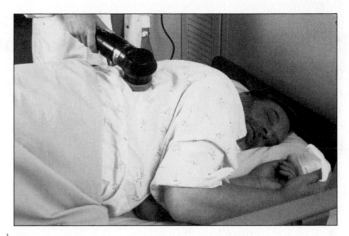

● Mechanical device is alternative to manual vibration.

# Skill 7.13   Inserting an Oropharyngeal Airway

## Equipment

Oropharyngeal tube
Tongue depressor
Clean gloves
Suction catheter
Suction source

## Procedure

1. Assure that client is unresponsive and has NO gag reflex. ▶*Rationale: Conscious client may vomit and aspirate or develop laryngospasm during tube insertion.*
2. Select appropriate size airway—length should be from corner of mouth to corner of ear tragus.
3. Perform hand hygiene; don gloves.
4. Gently open client's mouth with crossed finger technique, placing your thumb on client's lower teeth and index finger on the upper teeth and gently pushing them apart. You may need to use modified jaw thrust to insert tube.
5. Perform oral suctioning.
6. Hold tongue down with tongue depressor and advance airway to back of tongue OR advance airway upside down (curved upward) and, as airway passes uvula, rotate the airway 180°.
7. Check that concave curve fits over tongue. It should extend from the lips to the pharynx, displacing the tongue anteriorly. ▶*Rationale: Proper positioning helps prevent injury to lips, teeth, tongue, and posterior pharynx.*
8. Tape top and bottom of airway in position. ▶*Rationale: Stabilization of the tube prevents injuries.*
9. Position client on side to facilitate drainage.
10. Remove gloves, discard, and perform hand hygiene.
11. Observe position of airway and evaluate quality of client's spontaneous breathing.
12. Continue to monitor.

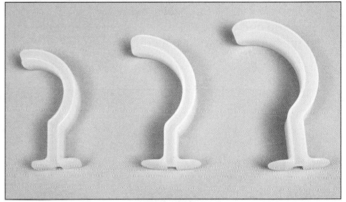

**A**

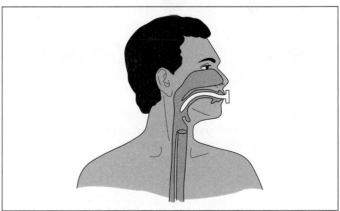

**B**

● **A**, Oropharyngeal airways; **B**, An oropharyngeal airway in place.

# Skill 7.14 Inserting a Nasopharyngeal Airway (Nasal Trumpet)

## Equipment

Flexible nasopharyngeal airway
Water-soluble lubricant
Clean gloves

## Procedure

1. Select appropriate size tube (length from tip of nose to earlobe and lumen slightly narrower than client's naris).
2. Perform hand hygiene; don gloves.
3. Lubricate entire length of tube.
4. Explain procedure to client.
5. Insert entire tube gently through naris, following anatomic line of nasal passage. If obstructed, try other naris.
6. Validate position by
   a. Feeling exhaled air through tube opening
   b. Inspecting for tube tip behind uvula.
7. Tape top and bottom of tube in position if necessary to prevent injury to lips, teeth, tongue, and posterior pharynx.

8. Position client on side to facilitate drainage of secretions.
9. Remove gloves, discard, and perform hand hygiene.
10. Continue to monitor position of airway and client's response.
11. Suction upper airway prn using clean technique.

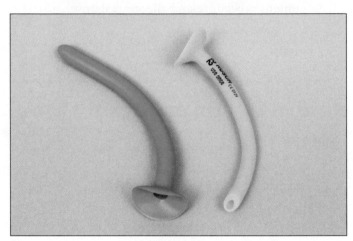

**A**

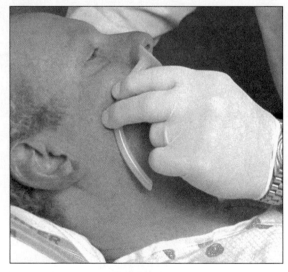

● Nasal trumpet protects airway from repeated trauma with upper airway (oropharyngeal) suctioning.

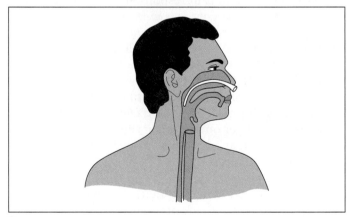

**B**

● **A**, Nasopharyngeal airways; **B**, A nasopharyngeal airway in place.

# Skill 7.15 Assisting with Endotracheal Intubation

## EVIDENCE-BASED NURSING PRACTICE

**Client's Response to Intubation**

Studies show that clients experience anger, worry, and fear at being unable to speak, especially in the first few days of intubation.

*Source:* Menzel, L. (1998). Factors related to the emotional responses of intubated patients to being unable to speak. *Heart & Lung, 27*(4), 245–251.

## Equipment

"Crash cart" (contains most needed supplies)

Laryngoscope with several blade sizes

Stylet to guide endotracheal tube (ONLY for oral intubation)

Endotracheal tubes

Water soluble lubricant

McGill forceps

Suction source

Oxygen source

Bag–valve–mask

Twill, adhesive tape, or Velcro holder

10-mL syringe for cuff inflation

Stethoscope

$CO_2$ detector (for airway placement validation)

Oral airway or bite block

Clean gloves, personal protective equipment including face shield

Established pulse oximetry and cardiac monitor if available

Wrist restraints (if ordered by physician)

Prepared sedative/neuromuscular blocking agent as ordered

Labeled container for client's dentures

*Note:* New noninvasive positive pressure ventilation methods using nasal pillows, nasal mask, oral mask or mouthpiece with special head gear provide an appropriate alternative to intubation for many clients with ventilatory insufficiency.

## Preparation

1. Determine that client has no protective airway reflexes.
2. Bring crash cart to client's doorway.
3. Check that all necessary equipment is functioning: (oxygen/suction source, and delivery systems, laryngoscope batteries).
4. Inflate and deflate airway cuff to determine if it is intact.
5. Perform hand hygiene and don gloves. Don personal protective equipment.
6. Insert stylet into tube (only for oral intubation), ensure that stylus does not extend beyond tube tip.
7. Lubricate tube.
8. Administer medication as ordered.
9. Remove client's dentures/bridgework and place in labeled container.
10. Review procedure for bag–valve–mask ventilation.

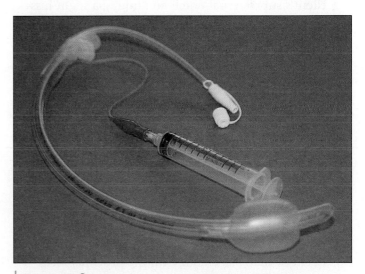

● CASS-ETT® has a lumen that opens above the tube cuff. Lumen (white tip) is connected to continuous suction to remove subglottic secretions that accumulate above the cuff in order to prevent pneumonia due to aspiration of these secretions.

## CLINICAL ALERT

The presence of an endotracheal tube bypasses defenses that normally protect the lower airways (filtration, humidification and hydration of inspired air and epiglottal closure). In addition, mucociliary transport of secretions and trapped pathogens is impaired. These alterations place intubated clients at risk for aspiration pneumonia.

## CLINICAL ALERT

While cuff pressures are typically maintained at 20–25mm Hg, an individual client's tracheal capillary pressure cannot be determined and excessive cuff pressure is the best predictor of tracheo-laryngeal injury.

## CLINICAL ALERT

Even if spontaneously breathing, the client should be pre-oxygenated with 100% $O_2$ for endotracheal tube placement. Ventilation must not be interrupted for over 30 seconds.

### Procedure

1. Don clean gloves and personal protective gear.
2. Place client in flat supine position with pillow under shoulders to hyperextend neck and help open airway. Position so that mouth, pharynx and trachea are aligned. ➤*Rationale: Proper positioning facilitates intubation.*
3. Restrain client's wrists only if necessary.
4. Premedicate client as ordered.
5. Preoxygenate client for several minutes, using bag–valve–mask. ➤*Rationale: To create an "oxygen reserve."*
6. Using thumb and index finger, apply cricoid pressure during tube insertion. ➤*Rationale: This facilitates tracheal placement and protects against aspiration of gastric contents.*
7. Maintain cricoid pressure while inflating cuff to "minimal leak" inflation by placing stethoscope at client's suprasternal notch and noting a slight hissing sound at peak of inspiration.
8. Attach bag–valve–mask, provide ventilation and look for chest to rise. ➤*Rationale: If chest does not rise, esophageal intubation is likely.*
9. Check tube placement using $CO_2$ detector. ➤*Rationale: Presence of $CO_2$ indicates tracheal intubation.*
10. Place stethoscope over epigastrium. ➤*Rationale: If gurgling is heard, and abdominal distention noted, esophageal placement is likely.*
11. Auscultate lung fields for bilateral breath sounds. ➤*Rationale: This ensures that accidental right main stem intubation has not occurred.*
12. Mark tube at level of client's front teeth and tape securely with twill or adhesive tape or velcro holder. ➤*Rationale: Secure taping prevents tube displacement.*
13. Recheck tube placement with the previous measures (steps 9–11).

## CLINICAL ALERT

Cricoid pressure may be used only if the client:
- Is nonresponsive
- Is not vomiting
- Does not have a cuffed tracheal tube in place

## CLINICAL ALERT

CDC guidelines recommend orotracheal over nasotracheal intubation to reduce the incidence of sinus infection.

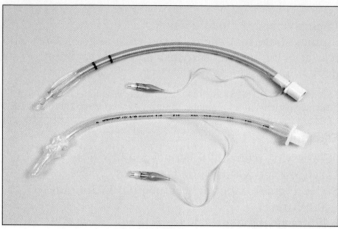

**A**

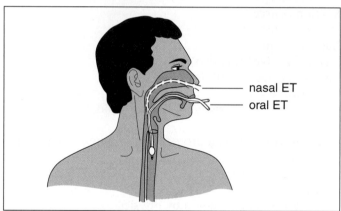

nasal ET
oral ET

**B**

● **A**, Endotracheal tubes (ET); **B**, An endotracheal tube in place.

14. Place bite block or oral airway if ET tube has been positioned orally.
15. Attach $O_2$ source to ET tube.
16. Discard disposable equipment, remove protective gear, gloves, and perform hand hygiene.
17. Position client in position as ordered.
18. Obtain chest x-ray to confirm tracheal placement of ET tube.
19. Place call bell and writing material within client's reach (as indicated).
20. Reposition and retape ET tube daily and prn.

# Skill 7.16   Inflating a Tracheal Tube Cuff

### Equipment

10-mL syringe
Suction equipment
Stethoscope
Clean gloves

*Note:* The foam cuff does not require injected air. Air enters the balloon when port is open.

### Procedure

1. Don clean gloves.
2. Attach 10-mL syringe to distal end of inflatable cuff port, making sure seal is tight.
3. Inflate cuff for a minimal leak or minimal occlusive volume detected by auscultating over the suprasternal notch for a hissing sound at peak of inspiration.
   ➤*Rationale: This provides an adequate seal without risking tracheal pressure necrosis.*
4. Ask client to speak—if voice is heard, inflation is inadequate for mechanical ventilation.
5. Connect ventilator or T-piece to tracheal tube opening if indicated.
6. Assess breath sounds every 2 hours. ➤*Rationale: Presence of bilateral breath sounds indicates proper tube position in trachea.*
7. Monitor cuff pressure regularly. ➤*Rationale: This may detect inadvertent cuff overinflation and prevent potential necrosis of tracheal tissue. Pressure is usually maintained at 20 to 25 mm Hg to prevent tracheal necrosis. However, an individual client's tracheal capillary pressure cannot be determined.*

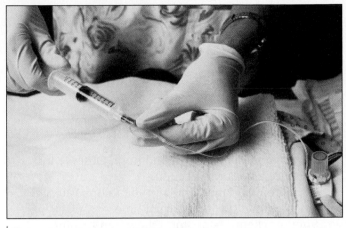

● Attach 10-mL syringe to inflate tube cuff.

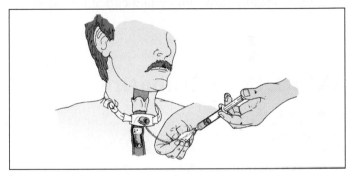

● Inflate tube cuff to minimal occlusive volume.

### CLINICAL ALERT

Low-pressure tracheal tube cuffs provide adequate blood flow to trachea, thus decreasing potential of tracheal tissue necrosis. These cuffs do not need periodic deflation.

### CLINICAL ALERT

Tracheal tube cuff inflation is essential for mechanically ventilated clients. Without cuff inflation, delivered air diverts out through the nose and mouth, and lungs are not ventilated.

# Skill 7.17 Providing Care for Client with Endotracheal Tube

### Procedure

1. Monitor breath sounds every 4 hours. Breath sounds should be heard equally throughout lung fields bilaterally.
2. Check marked points on tube at insertion level. ➤*Rationale: This determines if tube has moved.*
3. Inspect positioning and stabilization of tube. ➤*Rationale: A change of position can obstruct airway or cause erosion and necrosis of tissues.*
4. Inspect and clean mouth and nose. Observe for pressure areas or ulceration.
5. Reposition and tape oral ET tube to opposite side daily, noting tube depth each time.
6. Support client's head and tube when turning. ➤*Rationale: This prevents tube from becoming dislodged or airway from becoming obstructed.*
7. Place call bell within reach and provide alternative means of communication when cuffed tube is in place. ➤*Rationale: No air passes over larynx, so client is not able to summon help or communicate.*
8. Support client by spending extra time, using touch, and anticipating client's needs.
9. Ensure adequate hydration. ➤*Rationale: Artificial airways bypass the humidifying process of normal breathing.*
10. Provide suction toothbrushing every 12 hours, oral swabbing every 2 hours, and oropharyngeal subglottal suctioning every 6 hours. ➤*Rationale: This reduces oropharyngeal bacteria and helps prevent pulmonary infection.*

> **CLINICAL ALERT**
>
> Even with appropriate cuff inflation, intubated clients receiving gastric/enteral tube feedings are at high risk for aspiration.

# Skill 7.18 Extubating an Endotracheal Tube

### Equipment

Suction source
Oral suction catheter (or Yankauer)
Sterile suction catheter set
Clean gloves
Sterile gloves
Personal protective equipment
Oxygen source
Postextubation oxygen delivery device
Scissors or syringe for cuff deflation

### Preparation

1. Assess client's readiness for extubation.
2. Obtain vital signs.
3. Explain procedure to client.
4. Prepare postextubation oxygen administration device.
5. Place client in Fowler's position.

### Procedure

1. Perform hand hygiene and don clean gloves, and personal protective equipment.
2. Perform oral or nasopharyngeal suctioning.
3. Have client take several slow deep breaths. ➤*Rationale: This hyperoxygenates client in preparation for extubation.*

> **CLINICAL ALERT**
>
> Do not feed client orally immediately post-extubation. Seek consult for a feeding trial for clients at risk for aspiration.

4. Deflate tube cuff using syringe or cut pilot tubing.
5. Untie the tracheal tube.
6. Remove gloves, perform hand hygiene, and don sterile gloves.
7. Connect sterile catheter to suction source.
8. Insert sterile suction catheter into airway until resistance is met, then retract slightly.
9. Leave suction catheter in place.
10. Have client take a deep breath. ➤*Rationale: This dilates the vocal cords and makes removal easier and less traumatic.*
11. Apply suction while removing catheter and airway at the same time.
12. Immediately apply supplementary oxygen device.
13. Monitor client frequently at first, then regularly.
14. Dispose of equipment, remove gloves, protective gear, and perform hand hygiene.

# Skill 7.19 Oropharyngeal, Nasopharyngeal and Nasotracheal Suctioning

## Delegation

Oral suctioning using a Yankauer suction tube can be delegated to unlicensed assistive personnel (UAP) and to the client or family, if appropriate, because this is not a sterile procedure. The nurse needs to review the procedure and important points such as not applying suction during insertion of the tube to avoid trauma to the mucous membrane. Oropharyngeal suctioning uses a suction catheter and, although not a sterile procedure, should be performed by a nurse or respiratory therapist. Suctioning can stimulate the gag reflex, hypoxia, and dysrhythmias that may require problem solving. Nasopharyngeal and nasotracheal suctioning uses sterile technique and requires application of knowledge and problem solving and should be performed by the nurse or respiratory therapist.

## Equipment

*Oral and Nasopharyngeal/Nasotracheal Suctioning (using sterile technique)*

- Towel or moisture-resistant pad
- Portable or wall suction machine with tubing, collection receptacle, and suction pressure gauge
- Sterile disposable container for fluids
- Sterile normal saline or water
- Goggles or face shield, if appropriate
- Moisture-resistant disposal bag
- Sputum trap, if specimen is to be collected

*Oral and Oropharyngeal Suctioning (using clean technique)*

- Yankauer suction catheter or suction catheter kit
- Clean gloves

*Nasopharyngeal or Nasotracheal Suctioning (using sterile technique)*

- Sterile gloves
- Sterile suction catheter kit (#12 to #18 Fr for adults, #8 to #10 Fr for children, and #5 to #8 Fr for infants)
- Water-soluble lubricant
- Y-connector

## Procedure

1. Prior to performing the procedure, introduce self and verify the client's identity using agency protocol. Explain to the client what you are going to do, why it is necessary, and how he or she can participate. Inform the client that suctioning will relieve breathing difficulty and, although the procedure is painless, it is noisy and can cause discomfort by stimulating the cough, gag, or sneeze reflex. ▶*Rationale: Knowing that the procedure will alleviate breathing problems is often reassuring and will help the client to remain more calm.*

2. Perform hand hygiene and observe other appropriate infection control procedures.

3. Provide for client privacy.

4. Prepare the client.
   - Position a conscious person who has a functional gag reflex in the semi-Fowler's position with the head turned

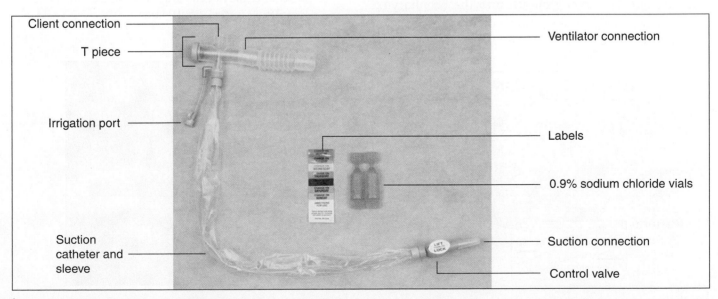

Client connection — 
T piece — 
Irrigation port — 
Suction catheter and sleeve — 

Ventilator connection — 
Labels — 
0.9% sodium chloride vials — 
Suction connection — 
Control valve — 

● A closed airway suction ("in-line") system.

to one side for oral suctioning or with the neck hyperextended for nasal suctioning. ➤*Rationale: These positions facilitate the insertion of the catheter and help prevent aspiration of secretions.*

- Position an unconscious client in the lateral position, facing you. ➤*Rationale: This position allows the tongue to fall forward, so that it will not obstruct the catheter on insertion. The lateral position also facilitates drainage of secretions from the pharynx and prevents the possibility of aspiration.*
- Place the towel or moisture-resistant pad over the pillow or under the chin.

5. Prepare the equipment.
   - Turn the suction device on and set to appropriate negative pressure on the suction gauge. The amount of negative pressure should be high enough to clear secretions but not too high. ➤*Rationale: Too high of a pressure can cause the catheter to adhere to the tracheal wall and cause irritation or trauma. A rule of thumb is to use the lowest amount of suction pressure needed to clear the secretions.* Wong (2007) suggests that the pressure should be limited to 60 to 100 mm Hg for a child and 40 to 80 mm Hg for a premature infant. Lemone and Burke (2008) and Moore (2003) recommend suction pressures between 80 and 120 mm Hg for adults.

*Oral and Oropharyngeal Suction*
- Apply clean gloves.
- Moisten the tip of the Yankauer or suction catheter with water or saline. ➤*Rationale: This reduces friction and eases insertion.*
- Pull the tongue forward, if necessary, using gauze.
- Do not apply suction (that is, leave your finger off the port) during insertion. ➤*Rationale: Applying suction during insertion causes trauma to the mucous membrane.*
- Advance the catheter about 10 to 15 cm (4 to 6 in.) along one side of the mouth into the oropharynx.

➤*Rationale: Directing the catheter along the side prevents gagging.*
- It may be necessary during oropharyngeal suctioning to apply suction to secretions that collect in the vestibule of the mouth and beneath the tongue.
- Remove and discard gloves. Perform hand hygiene.

*Nasopharyngeal and Nasotracheal Suction*
- Open the lubricant.
- Open the sterile suction package.
   a. Set up the cup or container, touching only the outside.
   b. Pour sterile water or saline into the container.
   c. Apply the sterile gloves, or apply an unsterile glove on the nondominant hand and then a sterile glove on the dominant hand. ➤*Rationale: The sterile gloved hand maintains the sterility of the suction catheter, and the unsterile glove holds the suction connecting tubing and prevents the transmission of the microorganisms to the nurse.*
- With your sterile gloved hand, pick up the sterile suction catheter and attach it to the suction connecting tubing being held in the nonsterile (nondominant) gloved hand.
- Test the pressure of the suction and the patency of the catheter by applying your sterile gloved finger or thumb to the port or open branch of the Y-connector (the suction control) to create suction.
- If needed, apply or increase supplemental oxygen.

6. Lubricate and introduce the catheter.
   - Lubricate the catheter tip with sterile water or saline. ➤*Rationale: This reduces friction and eases insertion.*
   - Remove oxygen with the nondominant hand, if appropriate.
   - *Without applying suction,* insert the catheter into either naris and advance it along the floor of the nasal cavity. ➤*Rationale: This avoids the nasal turbinates.*
   - Never force the catheter against an obstruction. If one nostril is obstructed, try the other.

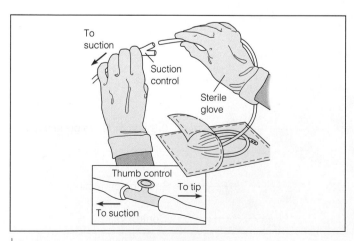
● Attaching the catheter to the suction unit.

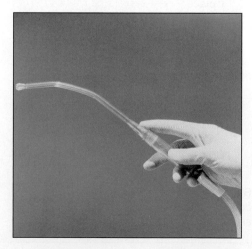
● Oral (Yankauer) suction tube.

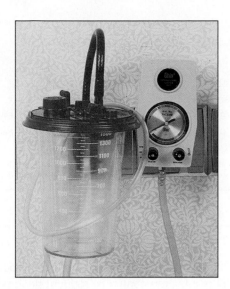

● A wall suction unit.
(Photographer: Jenny Thomas)

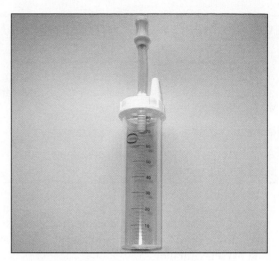

● A sputum collection trap.

7. Perform suctioning.
   - Apply your finger to the suction control port to start suction, and gently rotate the catheter. ➤*Rationale: Gentle rotation of the catheter ensures that all surfaces are reached and prevents trauma to any one area of the respiratory mucosa due to prolonged suction.*
   - Apply intermittent suction for 5 to 10 seconds while slowly withdrawing the catheter, then remove your finger from the control and remove the catheter. ➤*Rationale: Intermittent suction lessens the occurrence of trauma or irritation to the trachea and nasopharynx.*
   - A suction attempt should last only 10 to 15 seconds. During this time, the catheter is inserted, the suction applied and discontinued, and the catheter removed.
8. Rinse the catheter and repeat suctioning as above.
   - Rinse and flush the catheter and tubing with sterile water or saline.
   - Relubricate the catheter, and repeat suctioning until the air passage is clear.
   - Allow sufficient time between each suction for ventilation and oxygenation. Limit suctioning to 5 minutes total. ➤*Rationale: Applying suction for too long may cause secretions to increase or may decrease the client's oxygen supply.*
   - Encourage the client to breathe deeply and to cough between suctions. Use supplemental oxygen, if appropriate. ➤*Rationale: Coughing and deep breathing help carry secretions from the trachea and bronchi into the pharynx, where they can be reached with the suction catheter. Deep breathing and supplemental oxygen replenish oxygen that was decreased during the suctioning process.*
9. Obtain a specimen if required.
   - Use a sputum trap:

- Attach the suction catheter to the tubing of the sputum trap.
- Attach the suction tubing to the sputum trap airvent.
- Suction the client. The sputum trap will collect the mucus during suctioning.
- Remove the catheter from the client. Disconnect the sputum trap tubing from the suction catheter. Remove the suction tubing from the trap air vent.
- Connect the tubing of the sputum trap to the airvent. ➤*Rationale: This retains any microorganisms in the sputum trap.*
- Connect the suction catheter to the tubing.
- Flush the catheter to remove secretions from the tubing.
10. Promote client comfort.
    - Offer to assist the client with oral or nasal hygiene.
    - Assist the client to a position that facilitates breathing.
11. Dispose of equipment and ensure availability for the next suction.
    - Dispose of the catheter, gloves, water, and waste container.
      a. Rinse the suction tubing as needed by inserting the end of the tubing into the used water container.
      b. Wrap the catheter around your sterile gloved hand and hold the catheter as the glove is removed over it for disposal. Perform hand hygiene.
    - Empty and rinse the suction collection container as needed or indicated by protocol. Change the suction tubing and container daily.
    - Ensure that supplies are available for the next suctioning (suction kit, gloves, and water or normal saline).
12. Assess the effectiveness of suctioning.
    - Auscultate the client's breath sounds to ensure they are clear of secretions. Observe skin color, respiratory rate, heart rate, level of anxiety, and oxygen saturation levels.
13. Document relevant data.
    - Record the procedure: the amount, consistency, color, and odor of sputum (e.g., foamy, white mucus; thick, green-tinged mucus; or blood-tinged mucus) and the client's

---

## DEVELOPMENTAL CONSIDERATIONS

**Infants**

- A bulb syringe is used to remove secretions from an infant's nose or mouth. Care needs to be taken to avoid stimulating the gag reflex.

**Children**

- A catheter is used to remove secretions from an older child's mouth or nose.

**Elders**

- Elders often have cardiac and/or pulmonary disease, thus increasing their susceptibility to hypoxemia related to suctioning. Watch closely for signs of hypoxemia. If noted, stop suctioning and hyperoxygenate.

---

respiratory status before and after the procedure. This may include lung sounds, rate and character of breathing, and oxygen saturation.

- If the procedure is carried out frequently, it may be appropriate to record only once, at the end of the shift; however, the frequency of the suctioning must be recorded.

### Documentation

12/12/2009 0830 Producing large amounts of thick, tenacious white mucus to back of oral pharynx but unable to expectorate into tissue. Uses Yankauer suction tube as needed. SPO$_2$ sat increased from 89% before suctioning to 93% after suctioning. RR also decreased from 26 to 18–20 after suctioning. Lungs clear to auscultation. Continuous O$_2$ at 2 L/min via n/c. Will continue to reassess.
_____ L. Webb, RN

---

## SETTING OF CARE

- Teach clients and families that the most important aspect of infection control is frequent hand washing.
- Airway suctioning in the home is considered a clean procedure.
- The catheter or Yankauer should be flushed by suctioning recently boiled or distilled water to rinse away mucous, followed by the suctioning of air through the device to dry the internal surface and, thus, discourage bacterial growth. The outer surface of the device may be wiped with alcohol or hydrogen peroxide. The suction catheter or Yankauer should be allowed to dry and then be stored in a clean, dry area.
- Suction catheters treated in this manner described above may be reused. It is recommended that catheters be discarded after 24 hours. Yankauer suction tubes may be cleaned, boiled, and reused.

---

# Skill 7.20   Suctioning a Tracheostomy or Endotracheal Tube

### Delegation

Suctioning a tracheostomy or endotracheal tube is a sterile, invasive technique requiring application of scientific knowledge and problem solving. This skill is performed by a nurse or respiratory therapist and is not delegated to UAP.

### Equipment

- Resuscitation bag (Ambu bag) connected to 100% oxygen
- Sterile towel (optional)
- Equipment for suctioning (see Skill 7.19)
- Goggles and mask if necessary
- Gown (if necessary)
- Sterile gloves
- Moisture-resistant bag

### Preparation

- Determine if the client has been suctioned previously and, if so, review the documentation of the procedure. This information can be very helpful in preparing the nurse for both the physiologic and psychological impact of suctioning on the client.

### Procedure

1. Prior to performing the procedure, introduce self and verify the client's identity using agency protocol. Explain to the client what you are going to do, why it is necessary, and how he or she can participate. Inform the client that suctioning usually stimulates the cough reflex and that this assists in removing the secretions.

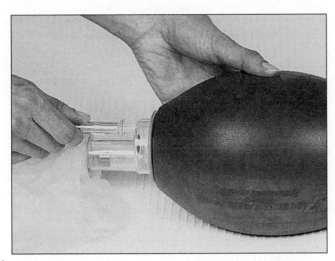

● Attaching the resuscitation apparatus to the oxygen source.
(Photographer: Jenny Thomas)

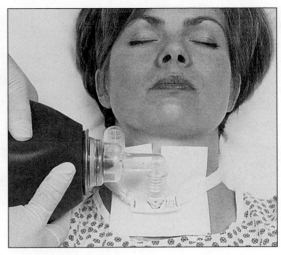

● Attaching the resuscitator to the tracheostomy.
(Photographer: Jenny Thomas)

2. Perform hand hygiene and observe other appropriate infection control procedures (e.g., gloves, goggles).
3. Provide for client privacy.
4. Prepare the client.
   • If not contraindicated, place the client in the semi-Fowler's position to promote deep breathing, maximum lung expansion, and productive coughing. ➤*Rationale: Deep breathing oxygenates the lungs, counteracts the hypoxic effects of suctioning, and may induce coughing. Coughing helps to loosen and move secretions.*
5. Prepare the equipment (open suction system). See Variation for Closed Suction System.
   • Attach the resuscitation apparatus to the oxygen source. Adjust the oxygen flow to 100%.
   • Open the sterile supplies:
     a. Suction kit or catheter
     b. Sterile basin/container
   • Pour sterile normal saline or water in sterile basin.
   • Place the sterile towel, if used, across the client's chest below the tracheostomy.
   • Turn on the suction, and set the pressure in accordance with agency policy. For a wall unit, a pressure setting between 80 and 120 mm Hg is normally used for adults, 60 and 100 mm Hg for children.
   • Apply goggles, mask, and gown if necessary.
   • Apply sterile gloves. Some agencies recommend putting a sterile glove on the dominant hand and an unsterile glove on the nondominant hand. ➤*Rationale: The sterile gloved hand maintains the sterility of the suction catheter, and the unsterile glove holds the suction connecting tubing and prevents the transmission of the microorganisms to the nurse.*
   • Holding the catheter in the dominant hand and the connector in the nondominant hand, attach the suction catheter to the suction tubing.

6. Flush and lubricate the catheter.
   • Using the dominant hand, place the catheter tip in the sterile saline solution.
   • Using the thumb of the nondominant hand, occlude the thumb control and suction a small amount of the sterile solution through the catheter. ➤*Rationale: This determines that the suction equipment is working properly and lubricates the outside and the lumen of the catheter. Lubrication eases insertion and reduces tissue trauma during insertion. Lubricating the lumen also helps prevent secretions from sticking to the inside of the catheter.*
7. If the client does not have copious secretions, hyperventilate the lungs with a resuscitation bag before suctioning.
   • Summon an assistant, if one is available, for this step.
   • Using your nondominant hand, turn on the oxygen to 12 to 15 L/min.
   • If the client is receiving oxygen, disconnect the oxygen source from the tracheostomy tube using your nondominant hand.
   • Attach the resuscitator to the tracheostomy or endotracheal tube.
   • Compress the Ambu bag three to five times, as the client inhales. This is best done by a second person who can use both hands to compress the bag, thus providing a greater inflation volume.
   • Observe the rise and fall of the client's chest to assess the adequacy of each ventilation.
   • Remove the resuscitation device and place it on the bed or the client's chest with the connector facing up.

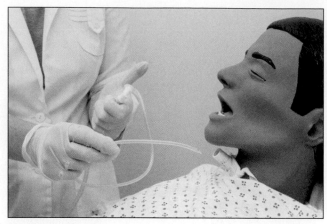

● Inserting the catheter into the trachea through the tracheostomy tube. *Note:* Suction is not being applied when inserting the catheter.

## VARIATION: Using a Ventilator to Provide Hyperventilation

If the client is on a ventilator, use the ventilator for hyperventilation and hyperoxygenation. Newer models have a mode that provides 100% oxygen for 2 minutes and then switches back to the previous oxygen setting as well as a manual breath or sigh button. ➤*Rationale: The use of ventilator settings provides more consistent delivery of oxygenation and hyperinflation than a resuscitation device.*

8. If the client has copious secretions, do not hyperventilate with a resuscitator. *Instead:*
   • Keep the regular oxygen delivery device on and increase the liter flow or adjust the FiO$_2$ to 100% for several breaths before suctioning. ➤*Rationale: Hyperventilating a client who has copious secretions can force the secretions deeper into the respiratory tract.*
9. Quickly but gently insert the catheter *without* applying any suction.
   • With your nondominant thumb off the suction port, quickly but gently insert the catheter into the trachea through the tracheostomy tube. ➤*Rationale: To prevent tissue trauma and oxygen loss, suction is not applied during insertion of the catheter.*
   • Insert the catheter about 12.5 cm (5 in.) for adults, less for children, or until the client coughs. If you feel resistance, withdraw the catheter about 1 to 2 cm (0.4 to 0.8 in.) before applying suction. ➤*Rationale: Resistance usually means that the catheter tip has reached the bifurcation of the trachea. Withdrawing the catheter prevents damaging the mucous membranes at the bifurcation.*
10. Perform suctioning.
    • Apply suction for 5 to 10 seconds by placing the nondominant thumb over the thumb port. ➤*Rationale: Suction time is restricted to a maximum of 10 seconds, preferably less, to minimize oxygen loss.*

• Rotate the catheter by rolling it between your thumb and forefinger while slowly withdrawing it. ➤*Rationale: This prevents tissue trauma by minimizing the suction time against any part of the trachea.*
• Withdraw the catheter completely, and release the suction.
• Hyperventilate the client.
• Suction again, if needed.

11. Reassess the client's oxygenation status and repeat suctioning.
    • Observe the client's respirations and skin color. Check the client's pulse if necessary, using your nondominant hand. If the client is on a cardiac monitor, assess the rate and rhythm.
    • Encourage the client to breathe deeply and to cough between suctions.
    • Allow 2 to 3 minutes with oxygen, as appropriate between suctions when possible. ➤*Rationale: This provides an opportunity for reoxygenation of the lungs.*
    • Flush the catheter and repeat suctioning until the air passage is clear and the breathing is relatively effortless and quiet.
    • After each suction, pick up the resuscitation bag with your nondominant hand and ventilate the client with no more than three breaths.

12. Dispose of equipment and ensure availability for the next suction.
    • Flush the catheter and suction tubing.
    • Turn off the suction and disconnect the catheter from the suction tubing.
    • Wrap the catheter around your sterile hand and peel the glove off so that it turns inside out over the catheter. Remove the other glove.
    • Discard the gloves and the catheter in the moisture-resistant bag. Perform hand hygiene.
    • Replenish the sterile fluid and supplies so that the suction is ready for use again. ➤*Rationale: Clients who require suctioning often require it quickly, so it is essential to leave the equipment at the bedside ready for use.*
    • Be sure that the ventilator and oxygen settings are returned to presuctioning settings. ➤*Rationale: On some ventilators this is automatic, but always check. It is very dangerous for clients to be left on 100% oxygen.*

13. Provide for client comfort and safety.
    • Assist the client to a comfortable, safe position that aids breathing. If the person is conscious, a semi-Fowler's position is frequently indicated. If the person is unconscious, Sims' position aids in the drainage of secretions from the mouth.

14. Document relevant data.
    • Record the suctioning, including the amount and description of suction returns, how client tolerated the procedure, and any other relevant assessments.

### Documentation

Sample: 12/13/2009 1000 Coarse crackles in RLL and LLL. Requires suctioning about every 1–2 hrs. Obtain large amount of pinkish tinged white thin mucus via ETT. Breath sounds clearer after suctioning. SPO$_2$ increases from 90% before suctioning to 95% after suctioning. Client signals when he wants to be suctioned.

_____C. Holmes, RN

### VARIATION: Closed Suction System (In-Line Catheter)

- If a catheter is not attached, apply clean gloves, aseptically open a new closed catheter set, and attach the ventilator connection on the T piece to the ventilator tubing. Attach the client connection to the endotracheal tube or tracheostomy.
- Attach one end of the suction connecting tubing to the suction connection port of the closed system and the other end of the connecting tubing to the suction device.
- Turn suction on, occlude or kink tubing, and depress the suction control valve (on the closed catheter system) to set suction to the appropriate level. Release the suction control valve.
- Use the ventilator to hyperoxygenate and hyperinflate the client's lungs.
- Unlock the suction control mechanism if required by the manufacturer.
- Advance the suction catheter enclosed in its plastic sheath with the dominant hand. Steady the T piece with the nondominant hand.
- Depress the suction control valve and apply intermittent suction for no more than 10 seconds and gently withdraw the catheter.
- Repeat as needed, remembering to provide hyperoxygenation and hyperinflation as needed.
- When completed suctioning, withdraw the catheter into its sleeve and close the access valve, if appropriate. ➤_Rationale: If the system does not have an access valve on the client connector, the nurse needs to observe for the potential of the catheter migrating into the airway and partially obstructing the artificial airway._
- Flush the catheter by instilling normal saline into the irrigation port and applying suction. Repeat until the catheter is clear.
- Close the irrigation port and close the suction valve.
- Remove and discard gloves. Perform hand hygiene.

### CLINICAL ALERT

Suction client's airway prn. Secretions are usually more copious following the irritation of intubation.

### DEVELOPMENTAL CONSIDERATIONS

**Infants and Children**

- An assistant or parent may be needed to gently hold the child and to keep hands out of the way. The assistant or parent should maintain the child's head in the midline position.

**Elders**

- Do a thorough lung assessment before and after suctioning to determine effectiveness of suctioning and to note any special problems.

### SETTING OF CARE

- Whenever possible, the client should be encouraged to clear the airway by coughing.
- Clients may need to learn to suction their secretions if they cannot cough effectively.
- Clean gloves should be used when endotracheal suctioning is performed in the home environment.
- The nurse needs to instruct the caregiver on how to determine the need for suctioning and the correct process and rationale underlying the practice of suctioning to avoid potential complications of suctioning.
- Stress the importance of adequate hydration: It thins secretions, which can aid in their removal by coughing or suctioning.

### CLINICAL ALERT

Suction catheter diameter should be no larger than one-half the inner diameter of the artificial airway. To determine catheter diameter size, multiply the artificial airway's diameter times 2 (e.g., for 8-mm tube, use a 16 French suction catheter).

If the calculated size falls between two suction catheter sizes (e.g., 7), select the smaller size catheter (e.g., size 6 rather than size 8) (Adirim, Smith, & Singh, 2006).

### CLINICAL ALERT

Hyperoxygenate the client before and after each time the airway is entered for suctioning, and wait 1 minute before suctioning again to prevent severe hypoxemia.

# Skill 7.21 Providing Tracheostomy Care

## Delegation

Tracheostomy care involves application of scientific knowledge, sterile technique, and problem solving, and therefore needs to be performed by a nurse or respiratory therapist.

## Equipment

- Sterile disposable tracheostomy cleaning kit or supplies including sterile containers, sterile nylon brush and/or pipe cleaners, sterile applicators
- Towel or drape to protect bed linens
- Sterile suction catheter kit (suction catheter and sterile container for solution)
- Sterile normal saline (Some agencies may use a mixture of hydrogen peroxide and sterile normal saline. Check agency protocol for soaking solution.)
- Sterile gloves (2 pairs—one pair is for suctioning if needed.)
- Clean gloves
- Moisture-proof bag
- Commercially prepared sterile tracheostomy dressing or sterile 4 × 4 gauze dressing
- Cotton twill ties
- Clean scissors

## Procedure

1. Prior to performing the procedure, introduce self and verify the client's identity using agency protocol. Explain to the client what you are going to do, why it is necessary, and how he or she can participate. Provide for a means of communication, such as eye blinking or raising a finger, to indicate pain or distress. Follow through by carefully observing the client throughout the procedure, offering periodic eye contact, caring touch, and verbal reassurance. Some clients respond well to a sense of efficiency and gentle humor, and nurses must decide when to use this approach.
2. Perform hand hygiene and observe other appropriate infection control procedures.
3. Provide for client privacy.
4. Prepare the client and the equipment.
   - Assist the client to a semi-Fowler's or Fowler's position to promote lung expansion.
   - Suction the tracheostomy tube, if needed.
   - If suctioning was required, allow the client to rest and restore oxygenation.
   - Open the tracheostomy kit or sterile basins.
   - Establish a sterile field.
   - Open other sterile supplies as needed including sterile applicators, suction kit, and tracheostomy dressing.

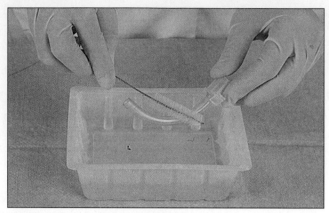

● Cleaning the inner cannula with a brush.
(Photographer: Elena Dorfman)

- Pour the soaking solution and sterile normal saline into separate containers.
- Apply clean gloves.
- Remove oxygen source.
- Unlock the inner cannula (if present) and remove it by gently pulling it out toward you in line with its curvature. Place the inner cannula in the soaking solution. ➤*Rationale: This moistens and loosens dried secretions.*
- Remove the soiled tracheostomy dressing. Place the soiled dressing in your gloved hand and peel the glove off so that it turns inside out over the dressing. Remove and discard gloves and the dressing. Perform hand hygiene.
- Apply sterile gloves. Keep your dominant hand sterile during the procedure.

5. Clean the inner cannula. (See Variation for using a disposable inner cannula.)
   - Remove the inner cannula from the soaking solution.
   - Clean the lumen and entire inner cannula thoroughly using the brush or pipe cleaners moistened with sterile normal saline. Inspect the cannula for cleanliness by holding it at eye level and looking through it into the light.
   - Rinse the inner cannula thoroughly in the sterile normal saline.
   - After rinsing, gently tap the cannula against the inside edge of the sterile saline container. Use a pipe cleaner folded in half to dry only the inside of the cannula; do not dry the outside. ➤*Rationale: This removes excess liquid from the cannula and prevents possible aspiration by the client, while leaving a film of moisture on the outer surface to lubricate the cannula for reinsertion.*

6. Replace the inner cannula, securing it in place.
   - Insert the inner cannula by grasping the outer flange and inserting the cannula in the direction of its curvature.

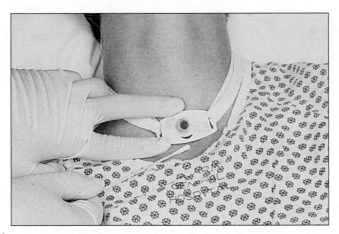

● Using an applicator stick to clean the tracheostomy site.
(Photographer: Jenny Thomas)

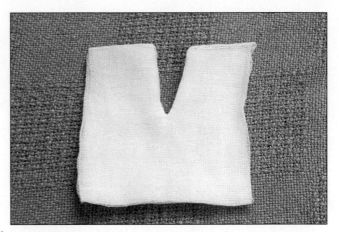

● A commercially prepared tracheostomy dressing of nonraveling material.

- Lock the cannula in place by turning the lock (if present) into position to secure the flange of the inner cannula to the outer cannula.

7. Clean the incision site and tube flange.
   - Using sterile applicators or gauze dressings moistened with normal saline, clean the incision site. Handle the sterile supplies with your dominant hand. Use each applicator or gauze dressing only once and then discard. ➤*Rationale: This avoids contaminating a clean area with a soiled gauze dressing or applicator.*
   - Hydrogen peroxide may be used (usually in a half-strength solution mixed with sterile normal saline; use a separate sterile container if this is necessary) to remove crusty secretions around the tracheostomy site. Do not use directly on the site. Check agency policy. Thoroughly rinse the cleaned area using gauze squares moistened with sterile normal saline. ➤*Rationale: Hydrogen peroxide can be irritating to the skin and inhibit healing if not thoroughly removed.*
   - Clean the flange of the tube in the same manner.
   - Thoroughly dry the client's skin and tube flanges with dry gauze squares.

8. Apply a sterile dressing.
   - Use a commercially prepared tracheostomy dressing or open and refold a nonraveling 4 × 4 gauze dressing into a V shape. Avoid using cotton-filled gauze squares or cutting the 4 × 4 gauze. ➤*Rationale: Cotton lint or gauze fibers can be aspirated by the client, potentially creating a tracheal abscess.*
   - Place the dressing under the flange of the tracheostomy tube.
   - While applying the dressing, ensure that the tracheostomy tube is securely supported. ➤*Rationale: Excessive movement of the tracheostomy tube irritates the trachea.*

9. Change the tracheostomy ties.
   - Change as needed to keep the skin clean and dry.

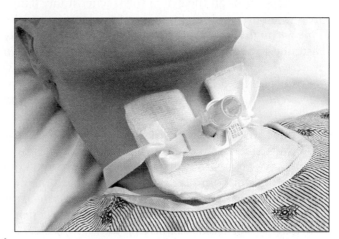

● A tracheostomy dressing placed under the flange of the tracheostomy tube.

- Twill tape and specially manufactured Velcro ties are available. Twill tape is inexpensive and readily available; however, it is easily soiled and can trap moisture that leads to irritation of the skin of the neck. Velcro ties are becoming more commonly used. They are wider, more comfortable, and cause less skin abrasion (American Thoracic Society, 2006).

*Two-Strip Method (Twill Tape)*
- Cut two unequal strips of twill tape, one approximately 25 cm (10 in.) long and the other about 50 cm (20 in.) long. ➤*Rationale: Cutting one tape longer than the other allows them to be fastened at the side of the neck for easy access and to avoid the pressure of a knot on the skin at the back of the neck.*
- Cut a 1-cm (0.5-in.) lengthwise slit approximately 2.5 cm (1 in.) from one end of each strip. To do this, fold the end of the tape back onto itself about 2.5 cm (1 in.), then cut a slit in the middle of the tape from its folded edge.

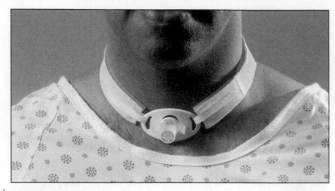

● A Velcro tracheostomy tie.
(Courtesy of Dale Medical)

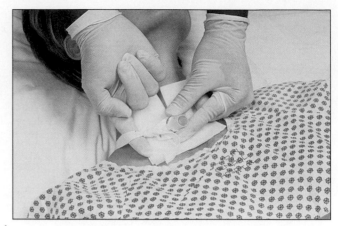

● Placing a finger underneath the tie tape before tying it.

• Leaving the old ties in place, thread the slit end of one clean tape through the eye of the tracheostomy flange from the bottom side; then thread the long end of the tape through the slit, pulling it tight until it is securely fastened to the flange. ➤*Rationale: Leaving the old ties in place while securing the clean ties prevents inadvertent dislodging of the tracheostomy tube. Securing tapes in this manner avoids the use of knots in the flange area, which can come untied or cause pressure and irritation.*

• If old ties are very soiled or it is difficult to thread new ties onto the tracheostomy flange with old ties in place, have an assistant put on a sterile glove and hold the tracheostomy in place while you replace the ties. ➤*Rationale: This is very important because movement of the tube during this procedure may cause irritation and stimulate coughing. Coughing can dislodge the tube if the ties are undone.*

• Repeat the process for the second tie.

• Ask the client to flex the neck. Slip the longer tape under the client's neck, place a finger between the tape and the client's neck, and tie the tapes together at the side of the neck. ➤*Rationale: Flexing the neck increases its circumference the way coughing does. Placing a finger under the tie prevents making the tie too tight, which could interfere with coughing or place pressure on the jugular veins.*

• Tie the ends of the tapes using square knots. Cut off any long ends, leaving approximately 1 to 2 cm (0.5 in.). ➤*Rationale: Square knots prevent slippage and loosening. Adequate ends beyond the knot prevent the knot from inadvertently untying.*

• Once the clean ties are secured, remove the soiled ties and discard.

*One-Strip Method (Twill Tape)*
• Cut a length of twill tape 2.5 times the length needed to go around the client's neck from one tube flange to the other.

• Thread one end of the tape into the slot on one side of the flange.

• Bring both ends of the tape together. Take them around the client's neck, keeping them flat and untwisted.

• Thread the end of the tape next to the client's neck through the slot from the back to the front.

• Have the client flex the neck. Tie the loose ends with a square knot at the side of the client's neck, allowing for slack by placing two fingers under the ties as with the two-strip method. Cut off long ends.

10. Tape and pad the tie knot.
   • Place a folded 4 × 4 gauze square under the tie knot, and apply tape over the knot. ➤*Rationale: This reduces skin irritation from the knot and prevents confusing the knot with the client's gown ties.*

11. Check the tightness of the ties.
   • Frequently check the tightness of the tracheostomy ties and position of the tracheostomy tube. ➤*Rationale: Swelling of the neck may cause the ties to become too tight, interfering with coughing and circulation. Ties can loosen in restless clients, allowing the tracheostomy tube to extrude from the stoma.*

12. Remove and discard sterile gloves. Perform hand hygiene.

13. Document all relevant information.
   • Record suctioning, tracheostomy care, and the dressing change, noting your assessments.

---

## CLINICAL ALERT

An obturator is kept at the bedside for emergency use. If the tracheostomy tube is inadvertently dislodged, it can be reinserted immediately using the obturator.

## DEVELOPMENTAL CONSIDERATIONS

### Infants and Children

- An assistant should always be present while tracheostomy care is performed.
- Always keep a sterile, packaged tracheostomy tube taped to the child's bed so that if the tube dislodges, a new one is available for immediate reintubation (Bindler, Ball, London, & Ladewig, 2007, p. 151).

### Elders

- Older adult skin is fragile and prone to breakdown. Care of the skin at the tracheostomy stoma is very important.

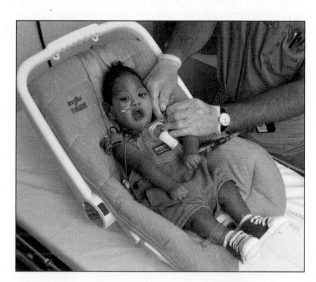

● Infant with a tracheostomy collar.

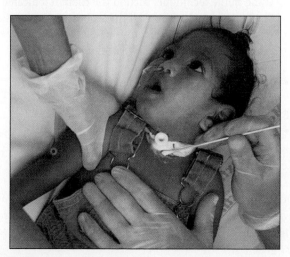

● Cleaning the tracheostomy tube.

## SETTING OF CARE

- For tracheostomies older than 1 month, clean technique (rather than sterile technique) is used for tracheostomy care.
- Stress the importance of good hand hygiene to the caregiver.
- Tap water may be used for rinsing the inner cannula.
- Teach the caregiver the tracheostomy care procedure and observe a return demonstration. Periodically reassess caregiver knowledge and/or tracheostomy care technique.
- Inform the caregiver of the signs and symptoms that may indicate an infection of the stoma site or lower airway.
- Names and telephone numbers of health care personnel who can be reached for emergencies or advice must be available to the client and/or caregiver.
- If the tracheostomy is permanent, provide contact information for available support groups.

## VARIATION: Using a Disposable Inner Cannula

- Check policy for frequency of changing the inner cannula because standards vary among institutions.
- Open a new cannula package.
- Using a gloved hand, unlock the current inner cannula (if present) and remove it by gently pulling it out toward you in line with its curvature.
- Check the cannula for amount and type of secretions and discard properly.
- Pick up the new inner cannula touching only the outer locking portion.
- Lock the cannula in place by turning the lock (if present).

## CLINICAL ALERT

When a child is admitted with a tracheostomy, talk with the parents about the method used for tracheostomy management at home. Develop a nursing care plan for tracheostomy management that integrates home management as well as teaching to enhance home management techniques.

## CLINICAL ALERT

Always keep a sterile packaged tracheostomy tube taped to the child's bed so that if the tube dislodges, a new one is available for immediate reintubation.

## Documentation

Sample: 12/11/2009 0900 Respirations 18–20/min. Lung sounds clear. Able to cough up secretions requiring little suctioning. Inner cannula changed. Trach dressing changed. Minimal amount of serosanguineous drainage present. Trach incision area pink to reddish in color 0.2 cm around entire opening. No broken skin noted in the reddened area. _____ J. Garcia, RN

> ### CLINICAL ALERT
>
> Remember that the child with an endotracheal tube or tracheostomy tube is unable to talk or cry. Implement other ways of communication. Picture boards with common activities or requests work for younger children. A tablet and pencil can be used by older children with normal motor skills.

---

# Skill 7.22   Capping a Tracheostomy Tube with Speaking Valve

### EVIDENCE-BASED NURSING PRACTICE

#### Use of a One-Way Speaking Valve

Subglottal air pressure is lost when a tracheostomy tube is in place. This reduction in air pressure is thought to be the primary mechanism responsible for aspiration in tracheostomized clients. Placement of a one-way speaking valve may restore this air pressure as well as improve laryngeal and pharyngeal sensation, may improve ability to expel material from the laryngeal vestibule either through throat clearing or coughing, and may improve swallow safety.

*Source:* Suiter, Debra, et al. (2003). Effects of cuff deflation and one-way tracheostomy speaking valve placement on swallow physiology. *Dysphagia, 18,* 284–292.

### Delegation

Capping a tracheostomy involves the application of scientific knowledge, assessment skills, and problem solving, and therefore needs to be performed by a nurse or a respiratory therapist.

### Equipment

- Suction apparatus
- Sterile suction catheters
- Sterile 10-mL syringe
- Clean gloves
- Sterile gloves
- Passy-Muir speaking valve and storage container

### Preparation

- Check the primary care provider's orders for speaking valve application. Check for other orders such as special monitoring or changes to ventilator settings, if appropriate. Determine the client's type of tracheostomy. Gather equipment.

### Procedure

1. Prior to performing the procedure, introduce self and verify the client's identity using agency protocol. Explain to the client what you are going to do, why it is necessary, and how he or she can participate.
2. Perform hand hygiene and observe other appropriate infection control procedures.
3. Provide for client privacy.
4. Position the client.
   - Assist the client to a Fowler's position if not contraindicated. ➤*Rationale: This position enhances lung expansion and may decrease fears about not being able to breathe.*
5. Suction the airways.
   - Using clean technique, suction the client's oropharynx if there are any secretions present. ➤*Rationale: This removes secretions that may be pooled above the cuff and avoids secretions entering lower airways when cuff is deflated.*
   - Ask client to cough. ➤*Rationale: This will also help clear secretions and allows the nurse to assess the client's cough reflex.*
   - Remove and discard clean gloves and used suction catheter. Perform hand hygiene.
   - Using sterile technique, suction the client if indicated. Suction the tracheostomy. If the secretions are excessive, report this finding to the nurse in charge or primary care provider to determine whether to proceed with the procedure.
   - Remove and discard sterile gloves and used suction catheter, if appropriate. Perform hand hygiene.
6. Prepare the tracheostomy tube.
   - Apply clean gloves.

*For a Fenestrated Uncuffed Tracheostomy Tube*
- Remove the inner cannula.

*For a Cuffed Tracheostomy Tube*
- Deflate the cuff. ➤*Rationale: The client will have no airway if the cuff remains inflated. Double-check the balloon of the cuff inflation tube because it will be deflated if the cuff is deflated.*

7. Evaluate the client's ability to exhale around the tracheostomy tube.
   - Place your stethoscope over the client's neck and listen for air movement during respirations (i.e., an air leak). ➤*Rationale: The client needs to maintain an open airway by being able to breathe around the tracheostomy tube.*
   - If no air leak is heard, notify the primary care provider. Do not place speaking valve on tracheostomy tube.
8. Place speaking valve cap over the hub of the tracheostomy tube.
   - Monitor the client closely, comparing the data with baseline assessments.
   - Assess for ability to speak.
   - If assessments deteriorate from baseline, remove the speaking valve.
9. Remove and discard gloves. Perform hand hygiene.
10. Apply clean gloves in preparation for removing speaking valve.

---

### CLINICAL ALERT

The speaking valve should be removed during sleep.

---

11. Remove the speaking valve.
    - The amount of time that the client is able to use the speaking valve will vary. ➤*Rationale: Some clients may need time to get used to the positive pressure that the valve produces in the trachea. Eventually, the different pressure will become more familiar to them* (Bier et al., 2004, p. 17).
12. Reinflate the cuff, if needed.
13. Remove and discard gloves. Perform hand hygiene.
14. Document all relevant information.
    - Document the amount, color, and consistency of the secretions; the amount of time the speaking valve was used, client's ability to speak and swallow, and client's tolerance of valve placement.

---

# Skill 7.23 Caring for the Client on a Mechanical Ventilator

## EVIDENCE-BASED NURSING PRACTICE

**Kinetic Rotation for Ventilatory Clients**

This study examined the effect to kinetic systematic mechanical rotation of clients with 40-degree turns for 17 hours per day on pulmonary function and prevention of ventilator-associated pneumonia. Of the 255 client enrollees (137 in the control group who were manually turned side to supine to side every 2 hours, and 118 kinetic therapy group), 21% of the kinetic therapy group could not tolerate bed rotation.

The study outcome supported benefits of kinetic therapy on pulmonary function, reduction of VAP, but no shorter duration of mechanical ventilation or hospitalization or improvement in survival.

The authors recommend kinetic therapy be used judiciously in clients who can tolerate it, especially neurologically depressed or sedated clients.

*Source:* Ahrens, Thomas, et al. (2004). Effect of kinetic therapy on pulmonary complications. *American Journal of Critical Care*, Vol. 13, No. 5, p. 376.

**Enteral Nutrition for Critically Ill Clients**

While enteral nutrition is usually preferred over parenteral nutrition in critically ill clients, this study found that repeated interruptions of enteral tube feedings for procedures results in significant underfeeding in 68% of these mechanically ventilated clients. Thirty-eight percent of clients received less than half of their calculated daily energy requirements, 30% received adequate nutritional intake and 1.7% was overfed due to additional kcalories received from concomitant administration of propofol.

*Source:* O'Leary-Kelley, Colleen (2005). Nutritional adequacy in patients receiving mechanical ventilation who are fed enterally. *American Journal of Critical Care*, Vol. 14, No. 3, p. 222.

**Delirium in Mechanically Ventilated Patients**

This study validated sensitivity, specificity, and inter-rater reliability of an instrument (CAM-ICU) for detection of delirium in mechanically ventilated patients. Delirium occurred in 83.3% of mechanically ventilated patients, 40% of whom were in a neutral level of sedation (neither agitated nor overly sedated), while they were in the ICU.

*Source:* Ely, E. W., et al. (2001, December). Delirium in mechanically ventilated patients. *Journal of the American Medical Association*, 286(21), 2703–2709.

## Delegation

Unlicensed assistive personnel (UAP) may provide basic care for clients on mechanical ventilation and collect routine data such as vital signs, but do not adjust ventilator settings or perform sterile procedures such as suctioning. They report any ventilator alarms, but do not assess the client or troubleshoot the system.

## Equipment

- Prescribed type of ventilator
- Oxygen source
- Bag-mask ventilator system (Ambu bag)
- Suctioning supplies
- Ventilator setting flow sheet and medical record forms or access to the electronic record system
- Stethoscope
- Pulse oximeter and other vital signs monitors
- End-tidal carbon dioxide ($ETCO_2$) colorimetric measuring device, or other system for measuring expired carbon dioxide level

## Preparation

- Review the manufacturer's manual for description of the ventilator controls and alarms if you are not adequately familiar with them.
- Review the client record for data indicating the changes that have been made in the client's ventilator settings over time and the client's tolerance of mechanical ventilation.

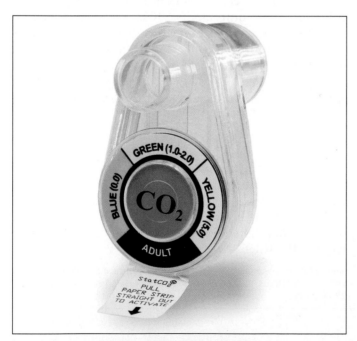

● $ETCO_2$ colorimetric measuring device.
(Courtesy of Mercury Medical)

## Procedure

1. Prior to performing ventilator or client care, introduce self and verify the client's identity using agency protocol. Explain to the client what you are going to do, why it is necessary, and how he or she can participate. Discuss how the results will be used in planning further care or treatments.
2. Perform hand hygiene and observe appropriate infection control procedures.
3. Provide for client privacy as needed.
4. Measure client temperature, pulse, blood pressure, and oxygen saturation using pulse oximetry. ➤*Rationale: Changes in these vital signs may indicate either client improvement or inadequate ventilation requiring adjustments in ventilator settings.*
5. If indicated, obtain ABGs. In some cases, these are ordered routinely and in other cases only if the client's condition warrants. Blood for ABGs may be drawn by the nurse, respiratory therapist, or laboratory technologist, depending on agency policy.
6. Confirm artificial airway tube placement by:
   - Auscultating lungs.
   - Measuring ETCO2. Readings of 2% to 5% at end-expiration indicate the tube is in the trachea.
   - Check ETT tube placement by examining the length markings along the tube. Normally, the lips will be at the marks between 20 to 22 cm.
   - Check to see when the most recent chest x-ray was done and what position was documented for the tube.
7. Check the tube cuff inflation by listening over the trachea at the end of inspiration. No airflow should be heard. Usually, the respiratory therapist checks cuff inflation. It can be measured using a manometer and is generally 20 to 25 cm $H_2O$. ➤*Rationale: Proper cuff inflation helps prevent VAP by ensuring that secretions that collect above the cuff cannot leak down into the lungs.*
8. Suction the client if indicated.
9. Once you have confirmed that the client's status does not require immediate intervention, examine the ventilator equipment and settings.
   - Tubing from the airway to the ventilator should be secured so it does not pull on the client's airway. This includes validating that there is adequate slack to allow the client to turn without pulling on the tubing.
   - Verify that ventilator settings are as ordered.
   - Verify that ventilator alarms are set correctly and are active.
   - Check for condensation in the tubing. Newer systems warm the tubing so that condensation is not generally a significant concern. If there is condensation in the tubing, empty it appropriately and discard. However, the closed system should not be opened unless absolutely necessary. Never empty fluid back into the humidifier, and use care

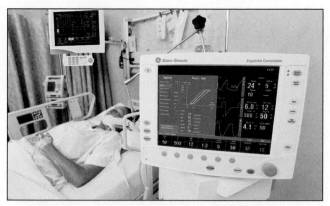

● Verify the ventilator settings and client data frequently.
(Courtesy of GE Healthcare, Madison, WI.)

that the fluid cannot run into the client's airway.
➤*Rationale: Liquid in the tubing may be contaminated.* Refill the humidifier if needed.

10. Provide thorough oral care every 2 hours. Brush the teeth using a toothbrush and toothpaste at least twice per day. ➤*Rationale: VAP can be reduced using this protocol* (Ross & Crumpler, 2007). Between brushings use toothette swabs and chlorhexidine or other antiseptic to swab the client's mouth in all reachable areas. Be certain to have suction ready in case it is needed or use toothettes that connect directly to suction.
    • Use a Yankauer (bulbous) suction tip to suction the mouth.
    • Some ETTs have a lumen above the cuff to allow for continuous suction of secretions that could collect there. If this is not the case, use a small suction catheter to reach deeply alongside the ETT and suction secretions that pool above the cuff.
    • If the client has an oral endotracheal airway, release the tape or holder, move and resecure the tube to the opposite side of the mouth every 24 hours. ➤*Rationale: This minimizes pressure on lips and oral mucosa.* Recheck that the tube is correctly positioned after such a move.
11. Administer medications as ordered to prevent complications of mechanical ventilation such as histamine receptor inhibitors to prevent gastric ulcers.
12. Institute actions to decrease complications such as deep venous thrombosis that may result from immobility related to the ventilator.
    • Perform range-of-motion exercises.
    • Assist the client to change positions at least every 2 hours, keeping the head of the bed elevated to 30 to 45 degrees.
    • Assist the client to stand, walk, or sit in a chair as tolerated. Often only clients with a stable tracheostomy are able to accomplish this.
    • Apply sequential compression devices to lower limbs according to agency policy.

• If the client has a tracheostomy and is able to eat, encourage adequate intake of fluids and dietary fiber to promote gastrointestinal motility. For clients with an ETT, enteral feedings through a gastric tube are preferred over parenteral nutrition.
• Administer prophylactic anticoagulant medications according to agency policy.
13. Establish an effective method of communicating with the intubated client who cannot speak.
    • Explain everything you are doing even if it appears the client cannot hear or understand.
    • If the client requires glasses, make them available.
    • If the client does not speak your language, provide a translator.
    • Ask yes/no questions when possible. Ask the client to nod the head if they agree. Hand signals can also be used. Be sure to allow adequate time for the client to respond.
    • Give the client a writing pad or slate if they are able to write.
    • Be sure that the call light or bell is with in reach at all times.
    • Acknowledge signs of frustration and attempt to determine and resolve the cause.
14. Administer pain or sedation medications as needed for comfort.
15. Document the ventilator settings and client parameters using checklists, flowcharts, and narrative notes as appropriate. Include results of settings changes, suctioning, activity, physical assessments, and laboratory data.

### Documentation

(Note that vital signs and ventilator settings would be recorded on flow sheets.)

10/1/09 1530 ETT remains in place and secured, ETCO$_2$ 3%. Lungs clear to auscultation. Oral care provided. No signs of oral trauma or infection. Skin warm, no cyanosis. Active ROM all extremities. Turned to left side, HOB @30 degrees. Skin dry & intact. No bowel sounds. Compression devices in place both calves. Indicates pain is 5 on scale of 0 to 10 by holding up fingers. Medicated IV with immediate reduction to pain level of 3. Family in to visit.

———————————————————————T. Kourza, RN

---

### CLINICAL ALERT

Many client/ventilator systems include heat moisture filters, which replace the need for external humidification of inspired gases. The use of these filters is only safe if pressure monitors are set properly so the machine can warn of impending heat moisture exchange filter occlusion.

## CLINICAL ALERT

In clients with reduced lung compliance (e.g., ARDS), tidal volume may be reduced to 6 mL/kg to prevent $Pco_2$) and reduced blood pH (7.2 lowest acceptable). Sedation and paralytic agents may be necessary to control ventilation in these clients.

## DEVELOPMENTAL CONSIDERATIONS

### Infants and Children

- Mechanical ventilation is used for children both in hospitals and in the home. Include the parents and other lay caregivers in all teaching and care instructions.
- When the child's condition is stable, provide age-appropriate activities such as play, art, and educational opportunities.

### Elders

- Older clients may be at greater risk for oxygen toxicity, especially if they have chronic lung conditions. As with all clients, the lowest effective oxygen concentration should be used.
- Provide reassurance and emotional support, recognizing that the need for ongoing mechanical ventilation may be viewed by the client or family as a sign of deteriorating health and movement toward death.

## SETTING OF CARE

Long-term mechanical ventilation in the home is commonplace in many communities.

- Teach caregivers all of the interventions, emergency, and safety measures needed to provide effective client assistance.
- Assist caregivers in contacting local emergency agencies to inform them that a ventilator-dependent client is in the home.
- Assist the client to determine if a backup power source is needed to run the ventilator should standard power be interrupted.
- Assist the client and family with community resources for obtaining needed equipment and disposal of biohazard waste. Ensure that they have extra supplies that might be needed in an emergency such as a bag and mask system.

# CULTURAL CONSIDERATIONS

Touch button voice systems are available that allow ventilated English or non-English-speaking clients to tap a touch screen that delivers preprogrammed audible words, phrases, or symbols to hold two-way communication with staff.

## CLINICAL ALERT

Paralytic agents have no effect on wakefulness or sensory perception, including perception of pain. With complete paralysis, pain might be manifested as increased heart rate, increased blood pressure, or sweating. Never assume that a client receiving a paralytic agent is asleep. Continually inform client about care, offer reassurance, and provide pain relief while the paralyzing effect of the drug persists.

## CLINICAL ALERT

Some "smart care" machines allow CPAP and PS plus an individualized weaning process based on present client parameters, including disease process. The machine gradually decreases the degree of support as long as the client remains in a breathing comfort zone. The machine then displays a message indicating it is appropriate to extubate the client.

## CLINICAL ALERT

The use of sedatives in mechanically ventilated clients prolongs its duration as well as length of hospitalization and ICU stay.

## PRACTICE GUIDELINES FOR PREVENTING VENTILATOR-ASSOCIATED PNEUMONIA

Preventing VAP is an important nursing goal. Clients who develop VAP have a significantly greater mortality rate than those clients who do not develop this infection. The IHI (2007) created the ventilator bundle—interventions that, when all are implemented simultaneously, can significantly reduce VAP. The bundle components are (a) elevating the head of the bed, (b) reducing sedation daily while assessing readiness to extubate, (c) prophylaxis for peptic ulcer disease, and (d) prophylaxis for deep venous thrombosis.

**Interventions to prevent or decrease VAP include the following:**

- Maintain rigorous hand hygiene.
- Maintain the head of the bed at 30 to 45 degrees unless contraindicated.
- Use oral (rather than nasal) endotracheal tubes if possible to reduce nasal or sinus colonization. Convert to a trachcostomy if long-term mechanical ventilation will be required.

- Provide oral care every 2 hours with tooth brushing twice a day and chlorhexidine rinses twice a day.
- Have the client be as physically active as possible: out of bed, performing weight-bearing and range-of-motion exercises.
- Do not change ventilator tubing or in-line suction catheter systems unless visibly soiled.
- Medicate for pain and anxiety. Treat pain first and then any remaining anxiety (Murray & Goodyear-Bruch, 2007).
- Maintain or enhance nutritional status. Gastric feedings should begin as soon as possible and be delivered through oral (rather than nasal) gastric tubes to reduce nasal or sinus colonization.
- Treat with appropriate antibiotics if VAP develops. The causative organisms could be *Streptococcus pneumoniae*, *Haemophilus influenzae*, *Pseudomonas*, *Klebsiella*, *Staphylococcus*, or *Enterobacter* species.

# Skill 7.24    Weaning the Client from a Ventilator

### Delegation

Adjusting ventilator settings is not delegated to UAP. If the UAP is caring for the client's basic needs, ensure that the UAP knows what data to gather and report to the nurse.

### Equipment

In addition to the existing ventilator equipment:
- Pulse oximeter
- Suctioning supplies
- Oxygen delivery system such as nasal cannula or mask for use after the endotracheal tube is removed

### Preparation

- Review the weaning protocol. In some cases, the primary care provider prescribes the incremental steps and settings to be used. In other cases, a standardized protocol may be used. The nurse will need to be knowledgeable about the decisions that need to be made at each step of the weaning process.
- If the client's condition permits, arrange for the client to sit in a chair during initial trials.

### Procedure

1. Prior to initiating weaning, introduce self and verify the client's identity using agency protocol. Explain to the client what you are going to do, why it is necessary, and how he or she can participate. Discuss how the results will be used in planning further care or treatments.
2. Perform hand hygiene and observe other appropriate infection control procedures.
3. Provide for client privacy as needed.
4. If the client has been on sedation, adjust the dose downward so the client is alert and can cooperate with instructions.
5. Position the client upright as much as possible.
   ▶*Rationale: This position promotes chest expansion.*
6. Suction the endotracheal tube above the cuff so that when the cuff is deflated, secretions do not fall into the airway.
7. Perform a spontaneous breathing trial according to agency policy. These may be performed for 5 to 15 minutes, up to four times per day (Astle & Smith, 2007). Several types of trials may be used.
   - *Pressure support:* Client controls the rate of respirations while the ventilator delivers positive pressure. The amount of pressure is decreased gradually (manually or by computer). Once the pressure is below 5 to 6 cm $H_2O$ without adverse reaction, the client is breathing independently and does not require ventilator support. This indicates that the endotracheal tube may be ready for removal.

- *SIMV:* The client breathes at his or her own rate, but the number of breaths delivered by the ventilator automatically is reduced gradually to zero.
- *Continuous positive airway pressure:* As the client breathes, a specific amount of pressure is kept in the airways at all times while the client breathes independently.
- *T-piece:* Less commonly used, the ventilator is removed and humidified oxygen is delivered into the endotracheal tube while the client breathes spontaneously.

8. Monitor the client's response to the breathing trial.
   - Mental status should not change.
   - Oxygen saturation >85% (or according to agency policy).
   - Blood gases within normal ranges for this client.
   - Pulse and BP within 20% of baseline.
   - Normal, symmetrical chest wall expansion; no use of accessory muscles.
   - Respirations rate, depth, and rhythm within normal range.
   - Minimal signs of anxiety.

9. If the client shows signs of distress, resume the previous ventilator settings.
   - Reassess vital signs.

---

**DEVELOPMENTAL CONSIDERATIONS**

**Elderly Clients in the Critical Care Unit Require More Intensive Observation and Consideration**

Aging is normally accompanied by a silent physiologic decline and diminished reserve in all body systems. These changes are not pathologic, but do make the elderly less adaptable to stress and illness. The elderly have a greater prevalence of chronic conditions that make them vulnerable to acute exacerbations. Over half of critical care clients are over the age of 65. Hospitalization is almost twice as long as that for clients under age 65 and survival is 81% compared to 98% in younger clients. However, quality of life post discharge from a critical care unit is not age related.

---

- Reassure the client that it may take a number of trials to achieve success.

10. Document the details of each trial. Include the ventilator settings, length of time of the trial, and all client data.

---

# Skill 7.25   Assisting with Chest Tube Insertion

## Delegation

Assisting the primary care provider with insertion of a chest tube is not delegated to unlicensed assistive personnel (UAP).

## Equipment

- Sterile chest tube tray that includes:
- Drapes
- 10-mL syringe
- Gauze sponges
- 22-gauge needle
- 25-gauge needle
- #11 blade scalpel
- Forceps
- Two rubber-tipped tube clamps
- Extra 4 × 4 gauze sponges or other occlusive bandage material
- Split drain sponges
- Chest tube and trocar or hemostat
- Suture materials
- Drainage system (water or dry seal)
- Suction source, if indicated

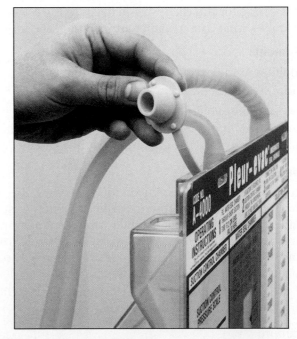

● Opening the water-seal filling port.

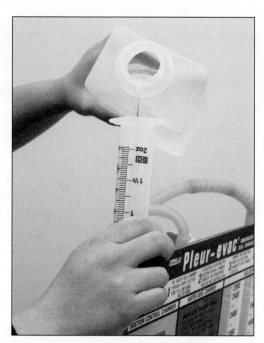

● Filling the water-seal chamber with sterile water.

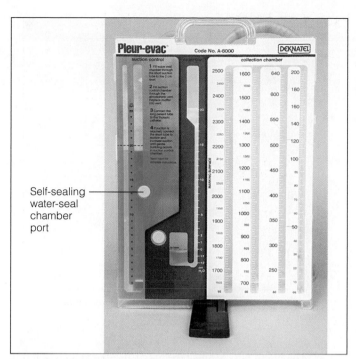

Self-sealing water-seal chamber port

● A three-chamber wet-suction/wet-seal disposable chest drainage system.

- Sterile gloves (for primary care provider and nurse)
- Local anesthetic vial
- Skin cleansing solution (e.g., povidone-iodine)
- Adhesive or foam tape
- Petrolatum gauze (optional)

### Preparation

- Although the primary care provider will have already done initial client and family teaching, the nurse reinforces key elements. Review the technique of chest tube insertion and its purpose with the client and family.
- Confirm with the primary care provider the desired types and numbers of equipment needed. Primary care providers have personal preferences for styles and sizes of chest tubes, and needs vary with the purpose of the tube.
- Premedicate the client for pain. Incorporate nonpharmacologic pain and stress-reducing strategies as much as possible.

### Procedure

1. Prior to performing the procedure, introduce self and verify the client's identity using agency protocol. Explain to the client what your role will be, why it is necessary, and how he or she can participate. Discuss how the results will be used in planning further care or treatments.
2. Perform hand hygiene and observe appropriate infection control procedures.
3. Provide for client privacy.
4. Position the client as directed by the primary care provider.
   - The client may be placed flat or in semi-Fowler's position. ➤*Rationale: The flat position is preferred for best access to the second or third intercostal space; a semi-Fowler's position is preferred for access into the sixth to eighth intercostal space.*
   - Turn the client laterally so that the area receiving the tube is facing upward.
5. Prepare for the insertion.
   - Open the chest tube tray and sterile gloves on the overbed table.
   - Assist the primary care provider to clean the insertion site.
   - Assist the primary care provider to draw up the local anesthetic.
6. Provide emotional support to the client during insertion. Monitor the client's condition and reaction to the procedure.
7. Dress the site. The primary care provider will usually place a purse-string suture to anchor the tube.
   - Apply sterile gloves and wrap the petrolatum gauze (if desired) around the chest tube at the insertion site.
   - Place drain gauze around the chest tube, one from the top and one from the bottom.
   - Place several additional gauze squares and tape or occlusive bandage materials over the drain gauze. These form an airtight seal at the insertion site.
8. Secure the tube.
   - Assist with connecting the chest tube to the valve or drainage system.

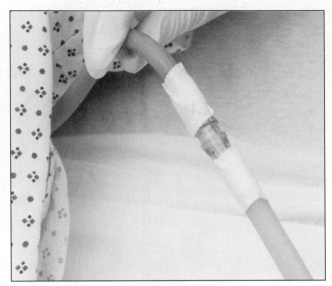

● Taped tubing connection with the connector exposed for observation of drainage.

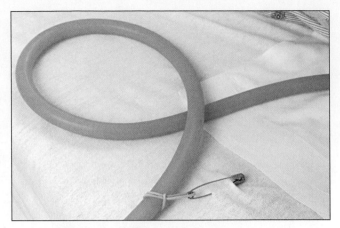

● Coiled drainage tubing secured on bed linen.

- Attach the longer tube from the collection chamber to the client's chest tube.
- Remove and discard gloves. Perform hand hygiene.
- Tape the chest tube to the client's skin.
- Tape all connections using spiral turns, but do not completely cover the collection tubing with tape. ➤*Rationale: Taping prevents inadvertent separation. Not covering all the collection tubing allows drainage to be seen.*
- Coil the drainage tubing and secure it to the linen, ensuring slack for the client to turn and move. ➤*Rationale: This prevents kinking of the tubing and impairment of drainage.*
- If suction is ordered, attach the remaining shorter tube from the suction chamber to the suction source, and turn it on. If wet suction is used, inspect the suction chamber for bubbling. Gentle bubbling indicates an appropriate suction level.
- If suction has not been ordered, keep the shorter rubber tube unclamped. This maintains negative or equal pressure in the system.

9. When all drainage connections are complete, ask the client to take a deep breath and hold it for a few seconds, then slowly exhale. These actions facilitate drainage from the pleural space and lung reexpansion.
10. Prepare the client for a chest x-ray to check for placement of the tube and lung expansion.
11. Ensure client safety.
    - Keep rubber-tipped chest tube clamps at the bedside. See Skill 7.26 for actions to take if the tube becomes discon-

nected from the drainage system or the system breaks or cracks.
    - Assess the client for signs of a new or worsening pneumothorax.
    - Assess the client for signs of subcutaneous emphysema (collection of gas under the skin). Palpate around the dressing site for crackling indicative of subcutaneous emphysema. ➤*Rationale: Subcutaneous emphysema can result from a poor seal at the chest tube insertion site. This is not an emergency but should be reported, documented, and monitored. It should reabsorb in a few days.*
    - Assess drainage and vital signs every 15 minutes for the first hour and then as ordered. Mark the collection chamber with a line and the date and time. Report bleeding or drainage greater than 100 mL/h.
12. Document the insertion in the client record using forms or checklists supplemented by narrative notes when appropriate. Include the name of the primary care provider, site of placement, type of tube, type of drainage system, characteristics of the immediate drainage, and other assessment findings.

**Documentation**

5/12/09 0130 32-Fr chest tube inserted into l chest by Dr. Novarty & connected to water-seal drainage unit. Suction at 20 cm H$_2$O. Immediately drained 120 mL straw-colored fluid. Moderate coughing after insertion, eased in 10 minutes. All connections taped, tubing taped to chest wall & attached to draw sheet. Tidaling c̄ respirations. Client instructed re: positioning & care of tube & collection device. Expresses understanding. VS 101 F, 100, 26, 170/94. _____ J. Lygas, RN

---

**CLINICAL ALERT**

Subcutaneous emphysema (air in tissue) may be felt around the chest tube insertion site, but should be reported if it extends beyond this.

---

**CLINICAL ALERT**

Strip and milk chest tubes only with physician's orders. Excessive negative pressure created by stripping and milking increases negative pressure in intrapleural space.

## MANAGING VENTILATOR-RELATED EVENTS

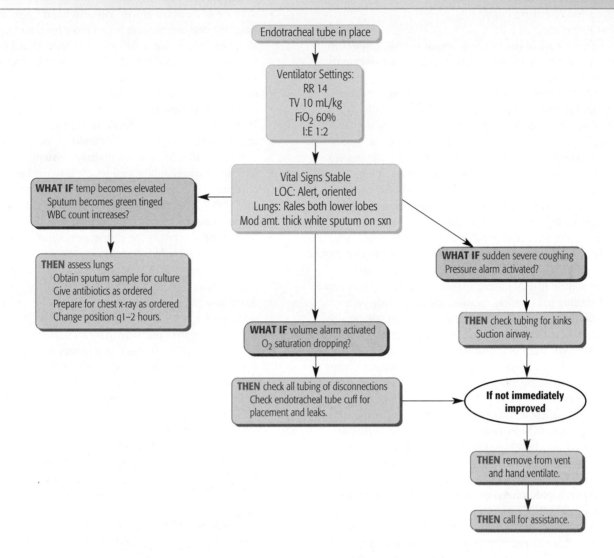

Endotracheal tube in place

Ventilator Settings:
RR 14
TV 10 mL/kg
FiO$_2$ 60%
I:E 1:2

Vital Signs Stable
LOC: Alert, oriented
Lungs: Rales both lower lobes
Mod amt. thick white sputum on sxn

**WHAT IF** temp becomes elevated
Sputum becomes green tinged
WBC count increases?

**THEN** assess lungs
Obtain sputum sample for culture
Give antibiotics as ordered
Prepare for chest x-ray as ordered
Change position q1–2 hours.

**WHAT IF** volume alarm activated
O$_2$ saturation dropping?

**THEN** check all tubing of disconnections
Check endotracheal tube cuff for
placement and leaks.

**WHAT IF** sudden severe coughing
Pressure alarm activated?

**THEN** check tubing for kinks
Suction airway.

**If not immediately improved**

**THEN** remove from vent
and hand ventilate.

**THEN** call for assistance.

# Skill 7.26   Maintaining Chest Tube Drainage

### Delegation

Care of chest tubes is not delegated to a UAP. However, aspects of the client's condition are observed during usual care and may be recorded by persons other than the nurse. Abnormal findings must be validated and interpreted by the nurse.

### Equipment

- Sterile gloves
- Two rubber-tipped tube clamps
- Petrolatum gauze (optional)
- 4 × 4 gauze sponges
- Split drain sponges
- Drainage system

- Skin cleansing solutions (e.g., povidone-iodine)
- Adhesive tape

### Preparation

- Determine when the last dressing change was performed.

### Procedure

1. Prior to performing the procedure, introduce self and verify the client's identity using agency protocol. Explain to the client what you are going to do, why it is necessary, and how he or she can participate. Discuss how the results will be used in planning further care or treatments.

2. Perform hand hygiene and observe other appropriate infection control procedures.

3. Provide for client privacy.

4. Assess the client.

   - Determine ease of respirations, breath sounds, respiratory rate and depth, oxygen saturation, and chest movements every 2 hours.

   - Observe the dressing site. Inspect the dressing for excessive and abnormal drainage, such as bleeding or foul-smelling discharge. Palpate around the dressing site for crackling indicative of subcutaneous emphysema. ➤*Rationale: Subcutaneous emphysema can result from inadequate seal (air leak) at the chest tube insertion site.*

   - Determine level of discomfort with and without activity. ➤*Rationale: Analgesics may need to be administered before the client moves or does deep-breathing and coughing exercises.*

   - Evaluate the impact of possible changes to the client's body image that occur when a person has tubes extending out from the body. It can be frightening, disorienting, there may be fear of pulling them out, or pulling on them and causing pain, or having someone else accidentally pull on them. A nurse who is sensitive to this will be able to offer a more comforting presence to the client.

5. Implement all necessary safety precautions.

   - Keep two 15- to 18-cm (6- to 7-in.) rubber-tipped clamps within reach at the bedside, to clamp the chest tube in an emergency.

   - Keep plain gauze 4 × 4s and one sterile petrolatum gauze within reach at the bedside to use with an air-occlusive material if the chest tube becomes dislodged.

   - Keep an extra drainage system unit available in the client's room. To change the drainage system, prepare the new system as described in Skill 7.25. If suction is being used, turn it off. Then:

     a. Clamp the chest tube close to the insertion site with two rubber-tipped clamps placed in opposite directions.

     b. Apply sterile gloves. Disconnect the original collection tubing and connect the new system immediately.

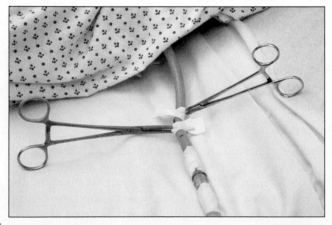

● Clamping a chest tube.

c. Reestablish the seals, remove the clamps, and reestablish suction as ordered.

- Remove and discard gloves. Perform hand hygiene.

- Keep the drainage system below chest level and upright at all times. ➤*Rationale: Keeping the unit below chest level prevents backflow of fluid from the drainage chamber into the pleural space. Keeping the unit upright maintains the water seal.*

6. Maintain the patency of the drainage system.

   - Check that all connections are secured with tape. ➤*Rationale: This ensures that the system is airtight.*

   - Inspect the drainage tubing for kinks or loops dangling below the entry level of the drainage system.

   - Coil the drainage tubing and secure it to the bed linen, ensuring enough slack for the client to turn and move (see Skill 7.25). ➤*Rationale: This prevents kinking of the tubing and impairment of the drainage system.*

   - Inspect the air vent in the system periodically to make sure it is not occluded. ➤*Rationale: A vent must be present to allow air to escape. Obstruction of the air vent causes an increased pressure in the system that could result in pneumothorax.*

   - Avoid any forceful manipulation of the tube, including milking (stripping) the chest tubing. Milking can create excessive negative pressure that can harm the pleural membranes and/or surrounding tissues (Coughlin & Parchinsky, 2006) and cause the client pain. No published research has shown that these previously used techniques prevented tube blockage or other complications (Wallen et al., 2007).

7. Assess fluid level fluctuations and bubbling in the drainage system.

   - Check for fluctuation (tidaling) of the fluid level in the water-seal chamber as the client breathes. Normally, fluctuations of 5 to 10 cm (2 to 4 in.) occur until the lung has reexpanded. ➤*Rationale: Fluctuations reflect the pressure changes in the pleural space during inhalation and exhalation. The fluid level rises when the client inhales and falls when the client exhales. The absence of fluctuations may indicate tubing obstruction from a kink, dependent loop, blood clot, or outside pressure (e.g., because the client is lying on the tubing), or may indicate that full lung reexpansion has occurred.*

   - In suction drainage systems, the fluid line remains constant. To check for fluctuation in suction systems, temporarily turn off the suction. Then observe the fluctuation.

   - Check for intermittent bubbling in the water of the water seal chamber. ➤*Rationale: Intermittent bubbling normally occurs when the system removes air from the pleural space, especially when the client takes a deep breath or coughs. Absence of bubbling may indicate that the drainage system is blocked or that the pleural space has healed and is sealed but this must be verified by x-ray. Continuous bubbling or a sudden change from an established pattern can indicate a break in the system (i.e., an air leak) and should be reported immediately.*

   - Check for gentle bubbling in the suction control chamber in wet systems. ➤*Rationale: Gentle bubbling indicates proper suction pressure.*

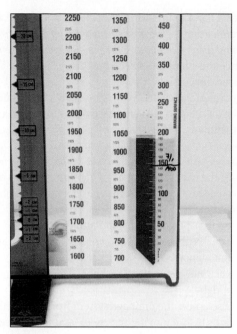

● Marking the date, time, and drainage level.

8. Assess the drainage.
   • Inspect the drainage in the collection container at least every 30 minutes during the first 2 hours after chest tube insertion and every 2 hours thereafter.
   • Every 8 hours, mark the time, date, and drainage level on a piece of adhesive tape affixed to the container, or mark it directly on a disposable container.
   • Note any sudden change in the amount or color of the drainage.
   • If drainage exceeds 100 mL/h or if a color change indicates hemorrhage, notify the primary care provider immediately.
9. Watch for dislodgement of the tubes, and remedy the problem promptly.
   • If the chest tube becomes disconnected from the drainage system, you must know whether there was bubbling in the water-seal chamber and air leak meter.
   a. If there has been no bubbling, there is probably no air leak from the lung and it is safe to clamp the tube while reestablishing the connections.
      1. Have the client exhale fully. Clamp the chest tube close to the insertion site with two rubber-tipped clamps placed in opposite directions. ➤*Rationale: Clamping the tube prevents external air from entering the pleural space. Two clamps ensure complete closure of the tube.*
      2. Apply sterile gloves. Quickly clean the ends of the tubing with an antiseptic, reconnect them, and tape them securely.
      3. Unclamp the tube as soon as possible.
      4. Remove and discard gloves. Perform hand hygiene.

   b. If there has been bubbling and an air leak from the lung, do not clamp the tube. ➤*Rationale: If air is leaking from the lung, clamping the tube will allow air buildup in the pleural space, which will rapidly result in a tension pneumothorax.*
      1. Apply sterile gloves. Quickly clean the ends of the tubing with an antiseptic, reconnect them, and tape them securely.
      2. Remove and discard gloves. Perform hand hygiene.
   c. Assess the client closely for respiratory distress (dyspnea, pallor, diaphoresis, blood-tinged sputum, or chest pain).
   d. Check vital signs every 10 minutes until stable.
   • If the chest tube becomes dislodged from the insertion site:
   a. Remove the dressing. If there is an air leak, immediately apply pressure with the petrolatum gauze, your hand (gloved if possible), or a towel but release it briefly every 30 seconds or if there are signs of respiratory distress. ➤*Rationale: If air is leaking from the lung, obstructing the insertion site will allow air buildup in the pleural space, which will rapidly result in a tension pneumothorax.*
   b. Notify the primary care provider immediately.
   c. Assess the client for respiratory distress every 10 to 15 minutes or as client condition indicates.
   • If the wet drainage system is accidentally tipped over:
   a. Immediately return it to the upright position. Check the water level in the water-seal and suction-control chambers.
   b. Ask the client to take several deep breaths. ➤*Rationale: Deep breaths help force air out of the pleural cavity that might have entered when the water seal was not intact.*
   c. Notify the primary care provider.
   d. Assess the client for respiratory distress.
10. If bubbling persists in the water-seal collection chamber or air leak chamber, determine its source. Continuous bubbling in the water-seal collection chamber normally occurs for only a few minutes after a chest tube is attached to drainage, because fluid and air initially rush out from the intrapleural space under high pressure.
   • To identify the source of an air leak, follow the next steps sequentially:
   a. Check the tubing connection sites. Tighten and retape any connection that seems loose. ➤*Rationale: The tubing connection sites are the most likely places for leaks to occur.*
   b. If bubbling continues, clamp the chest tube near the insertion site, and see whether the bubbling stops hile the client takes several deep breaths. ➤*Rationale: Clamping the chest will determine whether the leak is proximal or distal to the clamp. Chest tube clamping must be done only for a few seconds at a time.* ➤*Rationale: Clamping for long periods can aggravate an existing pneumothorax or lead to a recurrent pneumothorax.*
   c. If bubbling stops, proceed with the next step. The source of the air leak is above the clamp (i.e., between

the clamp and the client). It may be either at the insertion site or inside the client.

d. If bubbling continues, the source of the air leak is below the clamp (i.e., in the drainage system below the clamp). See next step.

- To determine whether the air leak is at the insertion site or internal (inside the client):
  a. With the tube unclamped, palpate gently around the insertion site. If the bubbling stops, the leak is at the insertion site. To remedy this situation, apply a petrolatum gauze and a 4 × 4 gauze around the insertion site, and secure these dressings with adhesive tape.
  b. If the leak is not at the insertion site, it is internal and may indicate a dislodged tube or a new pneumothorax. In this instance, leave the tube unclamped, notify the primary care provider, and monitor the client for signs of respiratory distress.
- To locate an air leak below the chest tube clamp:
  a. Move the clamp a few inches farther down and keep moving it downward a few inches at a time. Each time the clamp is moved, check the water-seal collection chamber for bubbling. ➤*Rationale: The bubbling will stop as soon as the clamp is placed between the air leak and the water-seal drainage.*
  b. Seal the leak when you locate it by applying tape to that portion of the drainage tube.
  c. If bubbling continues after the entire length of the tube is clamped, the air leak is in the drainage device. To remedy this situation, replace the drainage system according to agency protocol.

11. Take a specimen of the chest drainage as required.
- Specimens of chest drainage may be taken from a disposable chest drainage system through the resealable connecting tubing. If a specimen is required:
  a. Use a povidone-iodine swab to wipe the self-sealing tubing below the connection to the chest tube. Allow it to dry.
  b. Attach a sterile 18- or 20-gauge needle to a syringe, and insert the needle into the tubing, being careful not to pass all the way through the opposite side of the tubing.
  c. Aspirate the specimen, discard the needle in the appropriate container, cap and label the syringe, and send it to the laboratory with the appropriate requisition form.

12. Ensure essential client care.
- Encourage deep-breathing and coughing exercises every 2 hours, if indicated (this may be contraindicated in clients with a lobectomy). Premedicate the client for pain as needed. Have the client sit upright to perform the exercises, and splint the tube insertion site with a pillow or

with a hand to minimize discomfort. ➤*Rationale: Deep breathing and coughing help remove accumulations from the pleural space, facilitate drainage, and help the lung to reexpand.*
- While the client takes deep breaths, palpate the chest for thoracic excursion.
- Reposition the client every 2 hours. When the client is lying on the affected side, place rolled towels on either side of the tubing. ➤*Rationale: Frequent position changes promote drainage, prevent complications, and provide comfort. Rolled towels prevent occlusion of the chest tube by the client's weight.*
- Assist the client with range-of-motion exercises of the affected shoulder three times per day to maintain joint mobility.
- When transporting and ambulating the client:
  a. Attach rubber-tipped forceps to the client's gown for emergency use.
  b. Keep the water-seal unit below chest level and upright.
  c. Disconnect the drainage system from the suction apparatus before moving the client, and make sure the air vent is open. Or, if ordered, obtain a portable suction device.

13. Document findings in the client record using forms or checklists supplemented by narrative notes when appropriate. Record patency of chest tubes; type, amount, and color of drainage; presence of fluctuations; appearance of insertion site; laboratory specimens, if any were taken; respiratory assessments; client's vital signs and level of comfort; and all other nursing care provided to the client.

## DEVELOPMENTAL CONSIDERATIONS

**Elders**
- Coughing and deep-breathing exercises are particularly important because shallow breathing and decreased ability to cough may occur with aging.
- Encourage the client to take pain medication when needed. Elders may be reluctant to take pain medication.
- Use special care of the client's skin to the possibility of skin tears from tape and increased risk of skin breakdown over bony prominences as skin becomes thinner and less elastic.
- The older client is at increased risk for respiratory distress due to increased lung stiffness.

# Skill 7.27 Chest Tube Removal

## Delegation

Assisting with the removal of a chest tube is not delegated to UAP. However, many effects of the removal may be observed during usual care and may be recorded by persons other than the nurse. Abnormal findings must be validated and interpreted by the nurse.

## Equipment

- Clean gloves
- Sterile gloves
- Suture removal set with forceps and scissors
- Sterile petrolatum gauze
- 4 × 4 gauze sponges
- Adhesive tape
- Moisture-proof bag
- Linen-saver pad

## Preparation

- Ensure that the client has been informed that the chest tube will be removed and when. Clamp the tube, if ordered. Administer analgesics as ordered.

## Procedure

1. Prior to performing the procedure, introduce self and verify the client's identity using agency protocol. Explain to the client what you are going to do, why it is necessary, and how he or she can participate. Discuss how the results will be used in planning further care or treatments.
2. Perform hand hygiene and observe other appropriate infection control procedures.
3. Provide for client privacy.
4. Prepare the client:
   - Assist the client to a side-lying or semi-Fowler's position with the chest tube site exposed.
   - Place the linen-saver pad under the client, beneath the chest tube. ➤*Rationale: This protects the bed linens and provides a place for the chest tube after removal.*
   - Instruct the client on how to hold the breath during removal. Some experts recommend holding a full inhalation, others recommend holding a full exhalation

> **CLINICAL ALERT**
>
> The chest tube can be removed when drainage is less than 50–100 mL in 24 hours, or, if inserted for blood removal, drainage has become serous or sero serosanguineous and less than 100 mL in the past 8 hours.

(Coughlin & Parchinsky, 2006), and still others recommend the Valsalva maneuver—exhaling against the closed glottis (Roman & Mercado, 2006).

5. Prepare the sterile field and supplies. Have the petrolatum gauze opened and ready for quick application.
6. Remove the dressing around the chest tube.
   - Apply clean gloves and dispose of the dressing in the moisture-proof bag.
   - Remove and discard gloves. Perform hand hygiene.
7. Assist with removal of the tube.
   - Apply sterile gloves.
   - Assist the client with the breathing technique and provide emotional support during the primary care provider's removal of the sutures and tube.
   - Immediately apply the petrolatum gauze, and cover it with dry gauze and adhesive tape. ➤*Rationale: This forms an airtight bandage.*
   - Remove and discard gloves. Perform hand hygiene.
8. Assess and monitor the client's response to tube removal.
   - Obtain vital signs every 15 minutes for the first hour and, if stable, then as indicated.
   - Auscultate lung sounds every hour for the first 4 hours to determine that the lung is remaining inflated.
   - Observe for signs of pneumothorax.
9. Document the date and time of removal, any drainage noted, and the client's response to the procedure in the client record using forms or checklists supplemented by narrative notes when appropriate.
10. Prepare the client for a chest x-ray 1 to 2 hours after chest tube removal and possibly again in 12 to 24 hours.

## ASSESSING CHEST TUBE FUNCTIONING

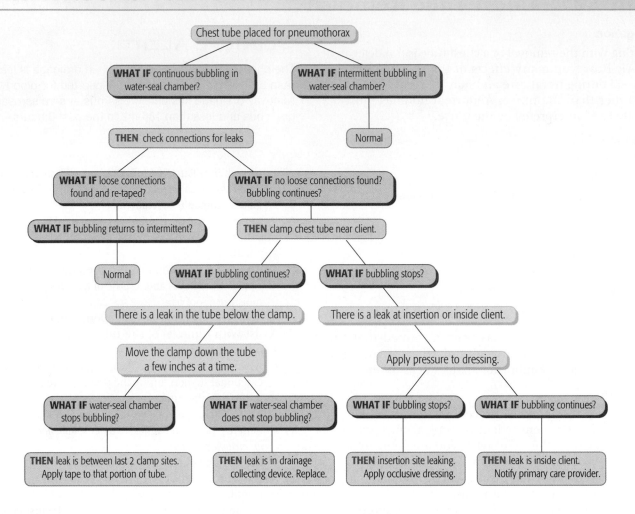

# Skill 7.28   Clearing an Obstructed Airway

### Delegation

Although unlicensed assistive personnel (UAP) cannot perform all aspects of a hospital code situation, they are trained in CPR and can perform obstructed airway techniques. If they are the first responders, UAP should initiate the intervention and not wait for a nurse.

### Equipment

- Standard precautions supplies, including gloves, masks, gowns, and protective eyewear, should always be easily accessible.

### Procedure

*Conscious Victim*

1. State your name and explain to the client that you are trained to help, what you are going to do, and how he or she can cooperate. Speak slowly, clearly, and with confidence.
2. Observe appropriate infection control procedures as much as possible.
3. Provide for client privacy. If another person is present and can cooperate, have that person get help. If family members are present, the nurse may request they leave for the moment.
4. Give abdominal thrusts (Heimlich maneuver).
   - Stand or kneel behind the victim, and wrap your arms around the victim's waist.
   - Make a fist with one hand, tuck the thumb inside the fist, and place the flexed thumb just above the victim's navel and below the xiphoid process. ➤*Rationale: A protruding thumb could inflict injury.*

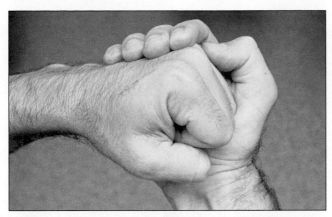

● The hand and fist position used for abdominal thrusts in a conscious victim.

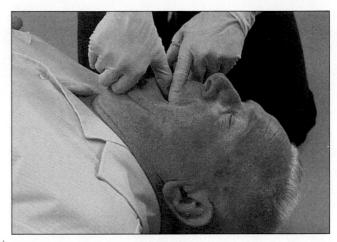

● The finger sweep maneuver.

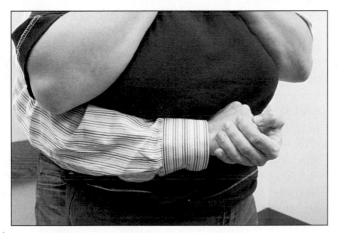

● The position to provide abdominal thrusts to a conscious victim.

- With the other hand, grasp the fist and press it into the victim's abdomen with a firm, quick upward thrust. Avoid tightening the arms around the rib cage.
- Deliver successive thrusts as separate and complete movements until the victim's airway clears or the victim becomes unconscious.
- If the victim becomes unconscious, lower the person carefully to the floor, supporting the head and neck to prevent injury.

*Unconscious Victim*

5. Activate the emergency response system using "911" or the agency arrest code.
6. Apply clean gloves and other personal protective equipment as soon as possible.
7. Open the airway.
   - Tilt the victim's head back, lift the chin. ➤*Rationale: This pulls the tongue away from the back of the throat.*
   - Remove an object if you see it:

a. If foreign material is visible in the mouth, it must be expediently removed. The finger sweep maneuver should be used only on unconscious persons and with extreme caution since the foreign material can be pushed back into the airway, causing increased obstruction.
b. To remove solid material, insert the index finger of your free hand along the inside of the person's cheek and deep into the throat. With your finger hooked, use a sweeping motion to try to dislodge and lift out the foreign object.
c. After removing the foreign object, clear out liquid material, such as mucus, blood, or emesis, with suction or using two fingers wrapped with a gauze pad.

8. Provide breaths.
   - If performing mouth-to-mouth breathing, insert a face shield into the victim's mouth, if available; apply a mask to the victim's face; *or,* pinch nose.
   - Give one 1-second breath and check for chest to rise.
   - If unable to ventilate, retilt the head and repeat breath.
   - If successful, give second 1-second breath.
9. If unsuccessful, proceed with full CPR, repeating ventilation attempts, chest compressions, and foreign object checks until the airway clears or the victim breathes.
   - In the hospital setting, a person trained in airway interventions will take over responsibility for clearing the airway.
   - When the emergency care is completed, remove and discard gloves and other personal protective equipment. Perform hand hygiene.

**VARIATION: Chest Thrusts**

Chest thrusts are to be administered only to women in advanced stages of pregnancy and markedly obese persons who cannot receive abdominal thrusts. See all steps above except substitute chest thrusts for the abdominal thrusts.

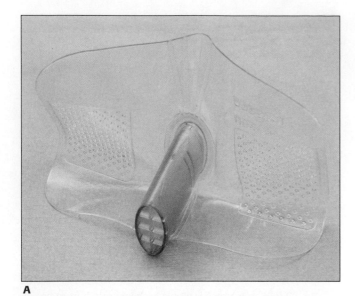

A

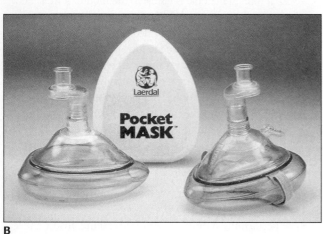

B

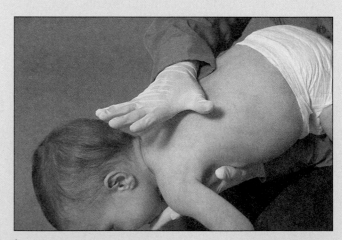

C

● Face masks: **A**, face shield; **B**, pocket mask with one-way valve; **C**, Ambu bag with face mask.

*To administer chest thrusts:*
- Place the thumb side of the fist on the middle of the breastbone, not on the xiphoid process.
- Grab the fist with the other hand and deliver a quick backward thrust.
- Repeat thrusts until the obstruction is relieved or the victim becomes unconscious. Chest thrusts to unconscious victims lying on the ground:
- Position the victim supine and kneel close to the side of the victim's trunk.
- Position the hands as for cardiac compression with the heel of the hand on the lower half of the sternum.
- Deliver five thrusts.
10. Document the date and time of the procedure, including the precipitating events and the client's response to the intervention.
- Describe the type of the procedure, the duration of breathlessness, and the type and size of any foreign object.
- Note vital signs, any complications, and type of follow-up care.

## DEVELOPMENTAL CONSIDERATIONS

### Infants

To administer a combination of back slaps and chest thrusts to infants:

1. Deliver back slaps.
   - Straddle the infant over your forearm with his or her head lower than the trunk.
   - Support the infant's head by firmly holding the jaw in the hand.
   - Rest your forearm on your thigh.
   - With the heel of the free hand, deliver five sharp slaps to the infant's back over the spine between the shoulder blades.
2. Deliver chest thrusts.
   - Turn the infant as a unit to the supine position:
   a. Place the free hand on the infant's back.
   b. While continuing to support the jaw, neck, and chest with the other hand, turn and place the

● Infant back slaps.

*(continued)*

## DEVELOPMENTAL CONSIDERATIONS (CONTINUED)

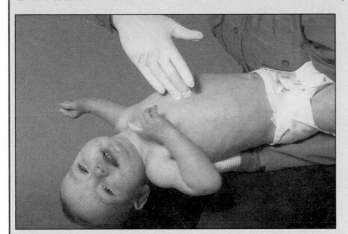

● Infant chest thrusts.

infant on the thigh with the baby's head lower than the trunk.

- Using two fingers, administer five chest thrusts over the sternum in the same location as external chest compression for cardiac massage, one finger-width below the nipple line, 1 second each.
- For a conscious infant, continue chest thrusts and back slaps until the airway is cleared or the infant becomes unconscious.
- If the infant is unconscious, begin CPR (see Skill 7.30).
  a. Assess the airway and give two breaths. If unable to ventilate, retilt the infant's head and try to give two breaths.
  b. If the air does not go in, then give chest compressions.
     Following the chest compressions, lift the jaw and tongue and check for foreign object. If an object is noted, sweep it out with finger.
  c. Repeat this sequence of breaths, foreign object checks, and chest compressions until the airway clears or the infant begins to breathe.

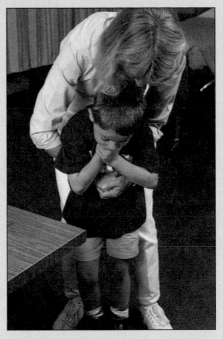

● Conscious child abdominal thrusts.

### Children

- For conscious children over age 1 who are choking, perform the Heimlich maneuver as for adults (Skill 7.28).

### Elders

- Older clients have a decreased gag reflex and, thus, may be more prone to choking. Preventive measures, such as adjusting the consistency of food, and close surveillance of clients with a history of choking may prevent an obstructed airway.
- Older clients can be injured by incorrect placement of the rescuer's hands. The sternum becomes more brittle with aging.

## SETTING OF CARE

- Stay with the individual and call the EMS.
- Any individual who receives intervention to treat an obstructed airway should seek immediate follow-up medical evaluation, even if the person remains conscious and the airway is cleared with abdominal thrusts.
- After removal of an airway obstruction at home, the client should receive a medical evaluation. The client may have aspirated foreign material, which can cause airway edema and infection.
- If the person becomes unconscious, activate the EMS.

### Family Role

- If a client has difficulty swallowing, teach the caregiver how to clear an obstructed airway.
- Young children are most likely to choke on objects such as small toys. Children do not understand the danger of placing objects in the mouth. Teach parents how to clear an obstructed airway and emphasize the importance of keeping small objects away from a young child.

# Skill 7.29 Performing Rescue Breathing

## Delegation

Although UAP cannot perform all aspects of a hospital code situation, they are trained in CPR and can perform rescue breathing techniques. If they are the first responders, UAP should initiate the intervention and not wait for a nurse.

## Equipment

- Standard precautions supplies, including gloves, masks, gowns, and protective eyewear, should always be easily accessible.
- Emergency equipment such as an Ambu bag and intubation equipment should be centrally located.
- Pocket face mask with one-way valve or mouth shields, or hand-compressible bag with mask with one-way valve (see Skill 7.28).

## Procedure

1. Determine that the client is unresponsive.
2. If victim does not respond, call a "code" or follow agency protocol to call for assistance. If another person is present and can cooperate, have that person go get help. Tell the person to return and let you know that help has been called.
3. Observe appropriate infection control procedures including applying clean gloves as much as possible.

4. Provide for client privacy. If family members are present, the nurse may request that they leave for the moment.
5. Position the client appropriately.
   - If the victim is lying on one side or face down, turn the client onto the back as a unit, while supporting the head and neck. Kneel beside the head.
6. Open the airway.
   - Use the head tilt–chin lift maneuver, or the jaw-thrust maneuver. A modified jaw thrust is used for victims with suspected neck injury. In unconscious victims, the tongue lacks sufficient muscle tone, falls to the back of the throat, and obstructs the pharynx. ➤*Rationale: Because the tongue is attached to the lower jaw, moving the lower jaw forward and tilting the head backward lifts the tongue away from the pharynx and opens the airway.*
   - If possible, insert an oropharyngeal (oral) airway. ➤*Rationale: This prevents the tongue from occluding the oropharynx.* Hold the airway with the curved end sideways and insert as far as possible into the mouth. Rotate the airway 90 degrees so the end is directed down the pharynx, gliding it over the tongue. The outer flange remains just outside the client's lips.

*Head Tilt–Chin Lift Maneuver*
- Place one hand palm downward on the forehead.
- Place the fingers of the other hand under the bony part of the lower jaw near the chin. The teeth should then be almost closed. The mouth should not be closed completely.

● The position of an unconscious person's tongue: **A**, airway occluded; **B**, airway open.

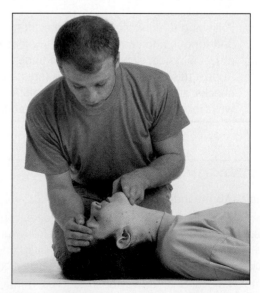

● Head tilt-chin lift maneuver.
(Susan Price © Dorling Kindersley)

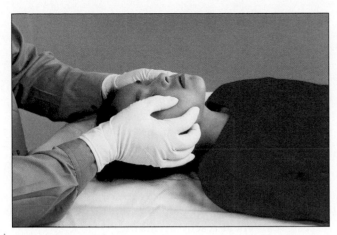

● Jaw-thrust maneuver.

- Simultaneously press down on the forehead with one hand, and lift the victim's chin upward with the other. Avoid pressing the fingers deeply into the soft tissues under the chin, because too much pressure can obstruct the airway.
- Open the victim's mouth by pressing the jaw downward with the thumb after tilting the head.
- Remove dentures if they cannot be maintained in place. However, dentures that can be maintained in place make a mouth-to-mouth seal easier should rescue breathing be required.

*Jaw-Thrust Maneuver*
- Kneel at the top of the victim's head.
- Grasp the angle of the mandible directly below the ear-lobe between your thumb and forefinger on each side of the victim's head.
- While tilting the head backward, lift the lower jaw until it juts forward and is higher than the upper jaw.
  - Rest your elbows on the surface on which the victim is lying.
  - Retract the lower lip with the thumbs prior to giving artificial respiration.
  - If the victim is suspected of having a spinal neck injury, do not hyperextend the neck.
7. Determine if the victim is breathing. This takes 5 to 10 seconds.
   - Place your ear and cheek close to the victim's mouth and nose.
   - Look at the chest and abdomen for rising and falling movement.
   - Listen for air escaping during exhalation.
   - Feel for air escaping against your cheek.
8. If no breathing is evident, provide rescue breathing. Mouth-to-Mouth Method
   - If available, insert a face shield (see Skill 7.28).
   - Maintain the open airway by using the head tilt–chin lift maneuver.

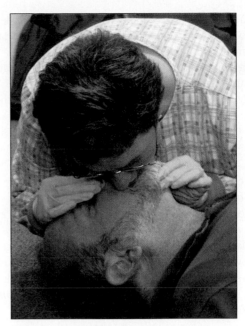

● Mouth-to-mouth rescue breathing.

- Pinch the victim's nostrils with the index finger and thumb of the hand on the victim's forehead. ➤*Rationale: Pinching closes the nostrils and prevents resuscitation air from escaping through them.*
- Take a deep breath, and place the mouth, opened widely, around the victim's mouth. Ensure an airtight seal.
- Give two full breaths (1 second per breath). Pause and take a breath after the first ventilation. ➤*Rationale: The 1-second time span allows adequate time to provide good chest expansion, and decreases the possibility of gastric distention. Excessive air volumes and rapid inspiratory flow rates can cause pharyngeal pressures that are great enough to open the esophagus, thus allowing air to enter the stomach.*
- Ensure adequate ventilation by observing the victim's chest rise and fall and by assessing the person's breathing as outlined in step 7.
- If the initial ventilation attempt is unsuccessful, reposition the victim's head and repeat the rescue breathing as above.
- If the victim still cannot be ventilated, proceed to clear the airway of any foreign bodies using the finger sweep, abdominal thrusts, or chest thrusts described earlier in Skill 7.28.

*Mouth-to-Nose Method*
This method can be used when there is an injury to the mouth or jaw or when the client is edentulous (tooth-less), making it difficult to achieve a tight seal over the mouth.
- Maintain the head tilt–chin lift position.
- Close the victim's mouth by pressing the palm of your hand against the victim's chin. The thumb of the same hand may be used to hold the bottom lip closed.

- Take a deep breath, and seal your lips around the victim's nose. Ensure a tight seal by making contact with the cheeks around the nose.
- Deliver two full breaths of 1 second each, and pause to inhale before delivering the second breath.
- Remove your mouth from the nose, and allow the victim to exhale passively. It may be necessary to separate the victim's lips or to open the mouth for exhaling, since the nasal passages may be obstructed during exhalation.

*Mouth-to-Mask Method*

- Remove the mask from its case and push out the dome.
- Connect the one-way valve to the mask port.
- Position yourself at the top of the victim's head, and open the airway using the jaw-thrust maneuver.
- Place the wider rim of the mask between the victim's lower lip and chin. Place the rest of the mask over the face using your thumbs on each side of the mask to hold it in place. ➤*Rationale: This keeps the mouth open under the mask.*

*Hand-Compressible Breathing Bag Method*

- Use one hand to secure the mask at the top and bottom and to hold the victim's jaw forward. Use the other hand to squeeze and release the bag.

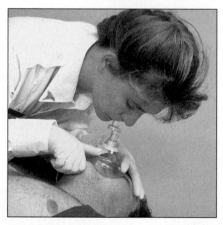

● Mouth-to-mask rescue breathing.

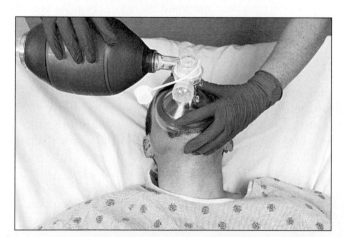

● Bag-to-mask breathing.

9. After delivering two successful breaths, determine the presence of a carotid pulse.
   - Take 5 to 10 seconds for this pulse check. Adequate time is needed since the victim's pulse may be very weak and rapid, irregular, or slow.
   - To palpate the carotid artery, first locate the larynx, and then slide your fingers alongside it into the groove between the larynx and the neck muscles on the same side you are. Use gentle pressure. ➤*Rationale: This avoids compressing the artery. The carotid pulse site is used because it is easy to reach and can often be palpated when more peripheral pulses, such as the radial, are imperceptible.*
10. If the carotid pulse is palpable, but breathing is not restored, repeat rescue breathing.
    - Inflate at the rate of 10 to 12 breaths per minute (1 breath every 5 to 6 seconds).
    - Blow slowly but enough to make the victim's chest rise.
    - If chest expansion fails to occur, ensure that the head is hyperextended and the jaw lifted upward, or check again for the presence of obstructive material, fluid, or vomitus.
    - After each inflation, move your mouth away from the victim's mouth by turning your head toward the victim's chest. ➤*Rationale: This movement allows the air to escape when the victim exhales. It also gives the nurse time to inhale and to watch for chest expansion.*
11. Reassess the carotid pulse after 12 inflations (1 minute) and every few minutes thereafter.
    - If you cannot locate the pulse, the victim's heart has stopped. Provide cardiac compression (see Skill 7.30).
12. When the emergency care is completed, remove and discard gloves and other standard precautions equipment. Perform hand hygiene.
13. Document the date and time of the arrest, including the precipitating events, the duration of breathlessness, and the client's response to the breathing.
    - Notify the primary care provider of the relevant events.

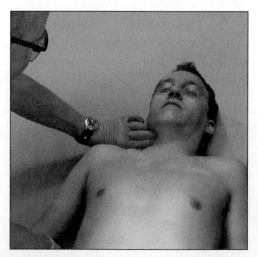

● Checking the carotid pulse.

## DEVELOPMENTAL CONSIDERATIONS

### Infants

- Airway obstruction by a foreign body is the most common cause of respiratory arrest in children.
- Acute epiglottitis can lead to upper airway obstruction in children. Symptoms usually occur suddenly and include drooling, difficulty swallowing, and a croaking sound with inspiration.

### Rescue Breathing

- Place one hand on the infant's forehead and tilt the head back gently. Do not hyperextend the neck because this can cause the soft trachea to collapse.
- The jaw-thrust maneuver can also be used if a neck injury is suspected.
- Assess breathing.
- When performing mouth-to-mouth breathing, cover both the mouth and nose of the infant.
- If an appropriate size mask and bag are available, they may be used. The mask should reach from the bridge of the nose to the chin but not cover the eyes.

- Following two successful breaths, check the brachial pulse.
- If breathing is absent but pulse is present, deliver 12 to 20 breaths per minute (1 breath every 3 to 5 seconds).

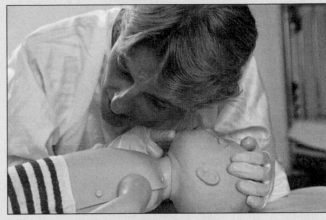

● Infant assessment of breathing.

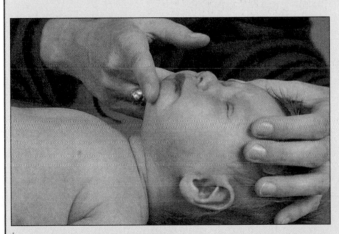

● Infant head tilt–chin lift maneuver.

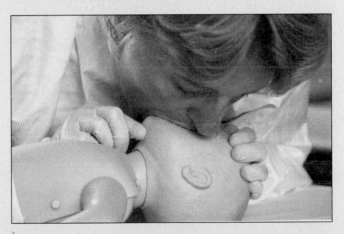

● Infant mouth-to-mouth rescue breathing.

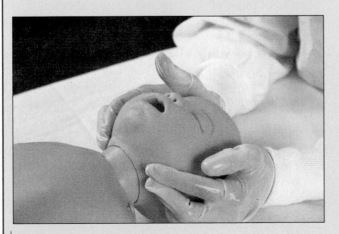

● Infant jaw-thrust maneuver.

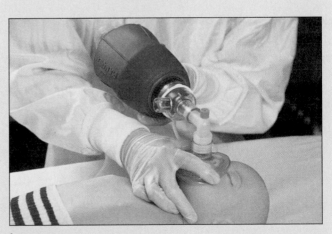

● Infant bag-to-mask breathing.

---

**SETTING OF CARE**

- If a client has cardiac or breathing problems, encourage the caregiver to learn CPR.
- Carry a pocket mask in the home care nursing bag at all times.
- Know how to activate the emergency medical system. In most cases of respiratory arrest the client will need oxygen, respiratory support, and ambulance transport to the emergency room.
- Assist the ambulance crew as needed and provide information about the client's history.

- Once the client is en route to the hospital, call the emergency room and give the report to the nurse in charge, including:
  - A brief health history.
  - Medications the client takes at home.
  - Findings prior to the respiratory arrest.
  - Duration of respiratory arrest and the client's response to resuscitation.
  - Vital signs.
- Provide emotional support to family members. If the client lives alone, contact family members, as needed.
- Notify the primary care provider.

---

# Skill 7.30   Administering External Cardiac Compressions

## EVIDENCE-BASED NURSING PRACTICE

### New Resuscitation Guidelines

A new form of cardiopulmonary resuscitation was developed at the University of Arizona Sarver Heart Center. Studies showed that this approach increased threefold the survival rate of the most common form of cardiac arrest. While still attaching the victim to the defibrillator, first responders did not wait for the device to analyze the heart rhythm, but started fast, forceful chest compressions. This new approach is valid only for cardiac arrest and is not recommended for the less common respiratory arrest seen in drowning or drug overdoses.

*Source:* University of Arizona press release, reported online by the *American Journal of Medicine,* April 10, 2006.

### Delegation

Although UAP cannot perform all aspects of a hospital code situation, they are trained in CPR and can perform external cardiac compression techniques. If they are the first responders, UAP should initiate the intervention and not wait for a nurse.

### Equipment

- Standard precautions supplies, including gloves, masks, gowns, and protective eyewear, should always be easily accessible.
- Emergency equipment such as an Ambu bag and defibrillation and intubation equipment should be centrally located.

- Pocket face mask with one-way valve or mouth shields, or hand-compressible Ambu bag with mask with one-way valve.
- A hard surface, such as a cardiac board or the floor, on which to place the victim.

### Procedure

1. Determine that the client is unresponsive.
2. If victim does not respond, call a "code" or follow agency protocol to call for assistance. If another person is present and can cooperate, have that person go get help. Tell the person to return and let you know that help has been called.
3. Observe appropriate infection control procedures including applying clean gloves as much as possible.
4. Provide for client privacy. If family members are present, the nurse may request they leave for the moment. Family members should be allowed the option of remaining in the room (AACN Practice Department, 2007). This option requires policies and procedures to be in place for a facilitator who can:
   - Explain the options to the family.
   - Support the family before, during, and after the event.
   - Support any family decisions not to be present.
   - Enforce contraindications for family presence such as extreme emotional behavior or interference with medical procedures.
5. Position the victim appropriately if not already done.
   - Place the victim supine on a firm surface. ➤*Rationale: Blood flow to the brain will be inadequate during CPR if the victim's head is positioned higher than the thorax. A hard surface facilitates compression of the heart between the sternum and the hard surface.*

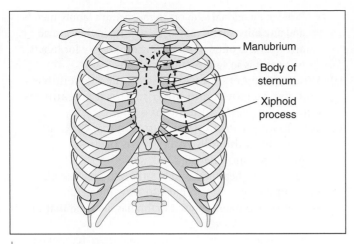

The sterum and ribs.

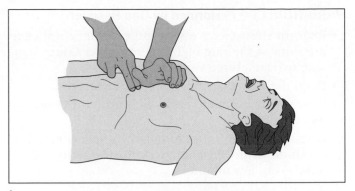

● Proper positioning of the hands during external cardiac compression.

- If the victim is in bed, place a cardiac board—preferably the full width of the bed—under the back. If necessary, place the victim on the floor.
- If the victim must be turned, turn the body as a unit while firmly supporting the head and neck so that the head does not roll, twist, or tilt backward or forward. ➤*Rationale: Turning the person as a unit prevents further injury (if present) to the neck or spine.*

6. Assess airway, breathing, and circulation.
7. Position the hands on the sternum. Proper hand placement is essential for effective cardiac compression. Position the hands as follows:
   - With the hand nearest the victim's legs, use your middle and index fingers to locate the lower margin of the rib cage.
   - Move the fingers up the rib cage to the notch where the lower ribs meet the sternum.
   - Place the heel of the other hand (nearest the person's head) along the lower half of the victim's sternum, close to the index finger that is next to the middle finger in the costal-sternal notch. ➤*Rationale: Proper positioning of the hands during cardiac compression prevents injury to underlying organs and the ribs. Compression directly over the xiphoid process can lacerate the victim's liver.*
   - Then place the first hand on top of the second hand so that both hands are parallel. The fingers may be extended or interlaced. Compression occurs only on the sternum and through the heels of the hands.
8. Administer cardiac compression.
   - Lock your elbows into position, straighten your arms, and position your shoulders directly over your hands.
   - For each compression, thrust straight down on the sternum. For an adult of normal size, depress the sternum 3.8 to 5.1 cm (1.5 to 2 in.). ➤*Rationale: The muscle force of both arms is needed for adequate cardiac compression of an adult. The weight of your shoulders and trunk supplies power for compression. Extension of the elbows ensures an adequate and even force throughout compression.*

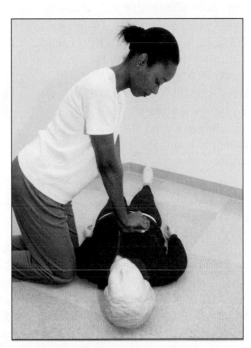

● Arm and hand position for external cardiac compression.

- Between compressions, completely release the compression pressure. However, do not lift your hands from the chest or change their position. ➤*Rationale: Releasing the pressure allows the sternum to return to its normal position and allows the heart chambers to fill with blood. Leaving the hands on the chest prevents taking a malposition between compressions and possibly injuring the person.*
- Provide external cardiac compressions at the rate of 100 per minute. Maintain the rhythm by counting "one and, two and," and so on. ➤*Rationale: The specified compression rate and rhythm simulate normal heart contractions.*
- Administer 30 external compressions and coordinate them with rescue breathing. See CPR performed by one rescuer or by two rescuers, next.

## VARIATION: CPR Performed by One Rescuer

- Perform chest compression: 30 external chest compressions at the rate of 100 per minute. Count "One and, two and, three and, . . ." up to 30.
- Open the airway and give two rescue breaths.
- Repeat four complete cycles of 30 compressions and two ventilations.
- Assess the victim's carotid pulse. If there is no pulse, continue with CPR and check for the return of the pulse every few minutes.

## VARIATION: CPR Performed by Two Rescuers

- One rescuer provides external cardiac compression and the other can provide rescue breathing, inflating the lungs once after every 15 compressions.
- Pause chest compressions for the two breaths unless an advanced airway (e.g., endotracheal tube) is in place. If an advanced airway is in place, give one ventilation every 6 to 8 seconds.
- Providers should switch positions after every five cycles, about 2 minutes.

9. When relieved from CPR:
   - Stand by to inform the team what has occurred and to assist as needed.

- Provide emotional support to the victim's family members and any others who may have witnessed the cardiac arrest. This is often a frightening experience for others because it is so sudden and so serious.

10. When the emergency care is completed, remove and discard gloves and other standard precautions equipment. Perform hand hygiene.

11. Terminating CPR. A rescuer terminates CPR only when one of the following events occurs:
    - Another trained individual takes over.
    - The victim's heartbeat and breathing are reestablished.
    - Adjunctive life support measures are initiated.
    - A physician states that the victim has died and that CPR is to be discontinued.
    - The rescuer becomes exhausted, and there is no one to take over.

12. Document the date and time of the arrest, including the precipitating events, the duration of respiratory and cardiac arrest and resuscitation efforts, and the client's response.
    - Record any advanced cardiac life support interventions such as defibrillation or initiation of intravenous therapy.
    - Document vital signs, rhythm strips, any complications, and type of follow-up care. Notify the primary care provider of the relevant events.

## DEVELOPMENTAL CONSIDERATIONS

### Infants

- Place the infant on a firm, flat surface if possible.
- Check carefully for airway obstruction in children with cardiac arrest. Cardiac arrest in children most often occurs after an initial respiratory arrest.
- To find the position for compressions, place your index finger on the sternum at the nipple line. Place your middle and ring fingers on the sternum next to your index finger, then lift your index finger.
- Compress the chest one-third to one-half the depth of the chest straight down using the pads of two fingers. Release the compression completely, keeping your fingers in the compression position while the other hand remains on the forehead, maintaining the open airway.
- Give compressions at a rate of 100 compressions/min with cycles of 30 compressions and two breaths.
- If two rescuers are present, instead of the two-finger technique described above, encircle the infant's chest with both hands, fingers behind the thorax and the thumbs over the lower half of the sternum for compression. In this fashion, the heart is compressed from both front and back, resulting in more effective CPR (Mutchner, 2007).

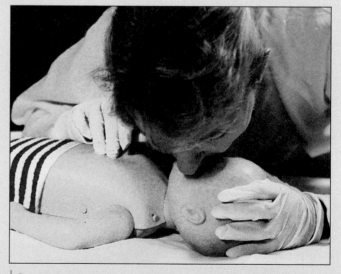

● CPR on an infant.

### Children (Ages 1 Year to Puberty)

- Check carefully for airway obstruction in children with cardiac arrest. Cardiac arrest in children most often occurs after an initial respiratory arrest.
- In children, to find the hand position for compressions, run your index and middle fingers up the ribs

## DEVELOPMENTAL CONSIDERATIONS (CONTINUED)

until you locate the sternal notch. With those two fingers on the lower end of the sternum, put the heel of the other hand on the sternum just above the location of the index finger.

- Use one or two hands for compressions, keeping the fingers off the chest. Compression depth is one-third to one-half the depth of the chest. Never lift the hands off the chest.

- CPR for a child is given at the following rate: 100 compressions/min with cycles of 30 compressions and two breaths for single rescuers and 15 compressions to 2 breaths for two-rescuer CPR (American Heart Association, 2006).

### Elders

- Older clients are most likely to be injured by incorrect placement of the rescuer's hands. The sternum becomes more brittle with aging.

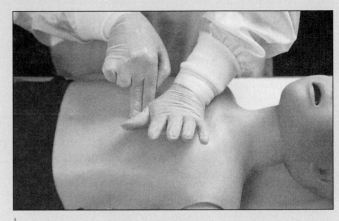

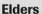 Locating the site for chest compressions on a child.

- The older client may have an advanced directive, or living will, expressing his or her wishes about life support.

## SETTING OF CARE

- Always carry a pocket mask in the home care nursing bag.

- Survey the scene for safety hazards, presence of bystanders, and other victims.

- Call for help or have another person call for EMS or 911.

- The person who calls the local EMS must be able to impart all of the following information:
  - Location of the emergency
  - Telephone number from which the call is being made
  - What happened
  - Number of people needing assistance
  - Condition of the victim(s)
  - What aid is being given
  - Any other information that is requested

- If the rescuer is alone, summon help and then perform CPR.

- Have a bystander elevate the lower extremities (optional). This may promote venous return and augment circulation during external cardiac compressions.

- If a second person identifies himself or herself as a trained EMS has been notified, the second rescuer offers to help with CPR.

- After activating the emergency response system, continue resuscitation until the ambulance arrives. Be prepared to give a report to the ambulance crew and assist them as needed.

- While the client is en route to the hospital, contact the emergency room and report the following to the nurse in charge:
  - A brief health history
  - Medications the client takes at home
  - Findings prior to the cardiopulmonary arrest
  - Duration of the cardiopulmonary arrest and the client's response to resuscitation

- Provide emotional support to family members. If the client is alone, contact family members or neighbors, as needed.

- Advise elderly clients to talk with the primary care provider about preparing an advanced directive for life support measures.

- Encourage caregivers or family members to learn CPR.

## CLINICAL ALERT

Begin compressions for a child with bradycardia (rate < 60) with signs of poor perfusion.

## CLINICAL ALERT

Compressions support blood flow to the heart, brain, and other organs. Coronary artery perfusion falls quickly when compressions are interrupted.

## CLINICAL ALERT

2005 Consensus Conference:

Chest compressions
- "Push hard and push fast"
- Allow chest to recoil completely

- Minimize interruptions
- Best compression–ventilation ratio–needs further studies.

# Skill 7.31  Administering Automated External Defibrillation

### Delegation

Any person who has been trained in its use can apply and activate the AED.

### Equipment

- AED with all components including the automatic override key, event documentation module or tape, electrodes and cables, and charged battery pack. Brands and models differ in their features.

### Procedure

1. Follow steps 1 through 9 of Skill 7.30. Traditional CPR must be performed until the AED can be attached.
2. Attach the AED.
   - Turn on the power of the AED.
   - Apply the electrode pads to dry skin: one in the upper right chest near the clavicle and the other in the lower left chest, below the nipple.
   - Attach the cables to the box if necessary.
3. Initiate rhythm analysis. Be sure no one is touching the client. The analysis may take 5 to 15 seconds. In most models, this also charges the AED.
4. Defibrillate as indicated.
   - Before delivering the shock, state loudly "Clear" and ensure that no one is touching the client.
   - Press the shock button and observe for the brief contraction of the client's muscles that indicates the shock has been delivered.
5. Resume CPR. The AED will automatically prompt to reanalyze the client in 2 to 3 minutes. Continue the

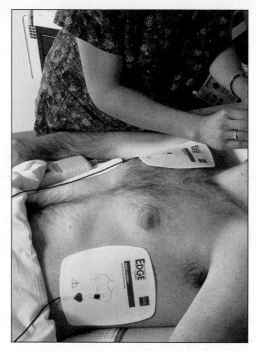

● Placement of AED electrode pads.

sequence of CPR and defibrillation until the AED specifies that no shock is indicated, the client converts to a functional rhythm (pulse is felt), or the code team takes over.

6. Document the events as in Skill 7.30 above including data provided by the AED. Attach electrocardiogram strips or other records made by the AED.

---

## DEVELOPMENTAL CONSIDERATIONS

### Infants

- AED is not recommended. VF is rare in infants and children, and the AED is usually not equipped to deliver the lower shock setting that would be needed.

### Children

- Follow the steps of adult AED use in children ages 1 through 8 or weighing at least 25 kg (55 lb).

- Use child-sized pads if available.
- Select a child shock dose on the AED if available. This may require turning a key or switch.
- For a child with an unwitnessed out-of-hospital arrest, perform five cycles (2 minutes) of CPR before using the AED.

## CLINICAL ALERT

AEDs should be used as soon as possible in the hospital setting; however, if four or five minutes have passed, the rescuer should provide five cycles of CPR (about 2 minutes) before attempting defibrillation on a child who has experienced an unwitnessed collapse outside of the hospital. The ventricular fibrillation waveform deteriorates rapidly within a few minutes of cardiac arrest as the heart consumes all available oxygen. Providing CPR initially will make the shock more likely to eliminate the VF, and the heart more likely to function following defibrillation.

*Source:* American Heart Association (2005–06, Winter). Currents in *Emergency Cardiovascular Care,* 16(3), 16.

## SETTING OF CARE

- Training in the use of an AED should be conducted in all health care facilities including clinics, long-term care facilities, and urgent care centers.
- AEDs can be used by trained lay rescuers.
- Use of the AED takes priority over CPR in witnessed arrest. The sequence of events is:
  - Confirm unresponsiveness, absence of breathing, and pulse.
  - Activate the EMS notification system (e.g., call 911).
  - Start CPR until the AED can be attached.
  - Defibrillate if indicated.
  - Resume CPR for five cycles.
- For an unwitnessed arrest, the sequence of events is:
  - Confirm unresponsiveness, absence of breathing, and pulse.
  - Activate the EMS notification system (e.g., call 911).
  - Perform CPR for five cycles.
  - Defibrillate with one shock.
  - Resume CPR without rechecking the rhythm (Mutchner, 2007).
- For a child with an unwitnessed arrest, perform five cycles (2 minutes) of CPR before using the AED.

## CLINICAL ALERT

The AutoPulse, an automated, noninvasive cardiac support pump, delivers chest compressions using a "hands-free" approach to restore blood flow faster and at a higher rate than manual resuscitation following a cardiac arrest.

## CLINICAL ALERT

The number of shocks an AED delivers and the energy level for each shock are preset by the manufacturer. Follow the AED voice and visual prompts. The shock sequence is usually completed three times if the client remain in fibrillation.

## DEVELOPMENTAL CONSIDERATIONS

THE PHYSIOLOGIC AGE CHANGES THAT OCCUR IN THE ELDERLY AFFECT THE RESPIRATORY SYSTEM.

- The respiratory muscles lose their strength and the rib cage becomes more rigid.
- The alveoli increase in size and decrease in number as well as become less elastic and more dilated.
- Gas exchange is reduced; the $PaO_2$ decreases 1 mm/year after age 60, so a reading of 77 mm Hg is not unusual in an elderly client.
- Skeletal alterations affect posture and may restrict lung expansion.

PULMONARY DISORDERS OCCUR MORE FREQUENTLY IN THE ELDERLY. COPD IS THE FOURTH LEADING CAUSE OF DEATH.

- Respiratory reserves are reduced with aging; the elderly are at greater risk for respiratory failure.
- Pneumonia may develop primarily or secondary to other conditions. Because it is a major cause of death in the elderly, pneumonia vaccine, influenza vaccine, and other preventive measures should be employed.

- Asthma may occur as a problem in the elderly who have never had the disease.
- Cancer of the lung is the leading cause of cancer death in the elderly.

IT IS IMPORTANT TO IMPLEMENT NURSING ACTIONS THAT SUPPORT THE RESPIRATORY SYSTEM IN THE ELDERLY.

- Deep breathing and exercise help promote ventilation.
- Hydration helps to liquefy secretions and reduce risk for infection.
- Monitor oxygen therapy closely with the elderly—note signs of hypoxia and decreased responsiveness due to possible carbon dioxide narcosis.
- The elderly are at risk for hypoxemia with bedrest ($PO_2$ may drop to 4 mm Hg even with a night's sleep). Position change, range of motion, and early mobilization all stimulate ventilation and must be encouraged in all clients.

# Perfusion

| | | |
|---|---|---|
| **Skill 8.1** | Using Digital Pressure | 335 |
| **Skill 8.2** | Using Pressure Dressing | 336 |
| **Skill 8.3** | Applying Antiemboli Stockings (Graduated Compression Stockings and Elastic Stockings) | 337 |
| **Skill 8.4** | Applying Pneumatic Compression Devices | 339 |
| **Skill 8.5** | Applying Sequential Compression Devices (SCDs) | 340 |
| **Skill 8.6** | Monitoring Clients on Telemetry | 343 |

| | | |
|---|---|---|
| **Skill 8.7** | Interpreting an ECG Strip | 345 |
| **Skill 8.8** | Recording a 12-Lead ECG | 350 |
| **Skill 8.9** | Monitoring Temporary Cardiac Pacing (Transvenous, Epicardial) | 352 |
| **Skill 8.10** | Assisting with Pacemaker Insertion | 353 |
| **Skill 8.11** | Maintaining Temporary Pacemaker Function | 355 |
| **Skill 8.12** | Providing Permanent Pacemaker Client Teaching | 356 |

Most people in good health give little thought to their cardiovascular function. Changing position frequently, ambulating, and exercising usually maintain adequate cardiovascular functioning. Immobility is detrimental to cardiovascular function.

Preventing venous stasis is an important intervention to reduce the risk of complications following surgery, trauma, or major medical problems. Antiemboli stockings and sequential compression devices are used to help prevent venous thromboembolism (VTE).

# Skill 8.1  Using Digital Pressure

## EXPECTED OUTCOMES

- Early detection of bleeding occurs, and loss of blood is minimized.
- Pressure dressing is applied and bleeding is controlled.
- Peripheral circulation is preserved.
- Vital signs within normal limits.

## Equipment

Towels or gauze dressing if available
Gloves

## Procedure

1. Perform hand hygiene and don gloves, sterile preferred.
2. Identify the closest artery proximal to the bleeding site. ➤*Rationale: The rapid loss of more than 25%–30% of the total blood volume leads to death.*
3. Apply direct pressure to artery, using your gloved finger.
4. If towels or 4 × 4 gauze pads are available, apply direct pressure to site of wound does not contain glass particles. ➤*Rationale: If pressure is placed on wound when glass is present, additional tissue damage can occur.*
5. Raise the affected limb above the level of the heart about 30°. ➤*Rationale: This decreases arterial blood flow to area and promotes venous return.*
6. Maintain direct pressure on site.
7. Maintain pressure for 5 minutes. ➤*Rationale: To promote clot formation.*
8. When bleeding has subsided, proceed to gently clean and address the wound.
9. To control nose bleeds (epistaxis), place client in sitting position, with head tilted forward. Pinch nose for 5 minutes. If ordered, apply ice pack to assist in vasoconstriction.
10. Remove gloves when bleeding subsides.
11. Perform hand hygiene immediately. ➤*Rationale: To protect yourself from possible contamination should any leakage have occurred through the gloves.*

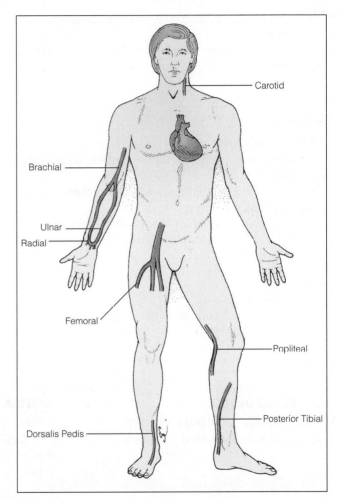

● Pulse sites that may be used to control bleeding.

## CLINICAL ALERT

Determine if individual is receiving medications or herbal therapies, which affect blood coagulation (e.g., coumadin). If so, increase time of applied pressure.

# Skill 8.2 Using Pressure Dressing

## EXPECTED OUTCOMES

- Early detection of bleeding occurs, and loss of blood is minimized.
- Pressure dressing is applied, and bleeding is controlled.
- Peripheral circulation is preserved.
- Vital signs within normal limits.

## Equipment

4 × 4 gauze pad
Sterile dressings—number and size depends on wound
Sterile gloves
Cleansing solution
Tape

## Preparation

1. Check physician's orders.
2. Assemble necessary supplies according to extent of wound.
3. If time permits, explain procedure to client and provide light and privacy.
4. Perform hand hygiene thoroughly if time permits.
5. Set up sterile field and prepare cleansing solution if time permits.

## Procedure

1. Put on sterile gloves.
2. Cleanse wound and apply dressing. Use several layers of 4 × 4 gauze pads.
3. Place tape tightly over entire dressing to provide an occlusive dressing. Do not completely circle an extremity or the body. ►*Rationale: To ensure that collateral blood flow is maintained.*
4. Check for pulses distal to pressure site.
5. Place all soiled material in biohazard bag.
6. Remove gloves and perform hand hygiene.
7. Monitor vital signs, and observe for signs of shock.
8. Continue to monitor extremity distal to pressure dressing for adequate circulation.
9. Position client for comfort.
10. Elevate extremity to prevent bleeding.
11. Monitor frequently for signs of bleeding and hemotoma.

*Note:* Hematomas feel spongy even under bandages.

## Documentation

- Size (in centimeters), location based on anatomical landmark, condition of wound
- Color, odor, amount of drainage
- Type and number of dressings used
- Approximate amount of blood loss
- Condition of dressing when removed (e.g., saturated with drainage)

| UNEXPECTED OUTCOMES | CRITICAL THINKING OPTIONS |
|---|---|
| Even with direct pressure and application of pressure dressing, bleeding continues. | • Reinforce pressure dressing<br>• Maintain IV infusion<br>• Notify physician, and be prepared to send client to surgery for wound closure<br>• Monitor closely for signs of shock<br>• Apply pressure to vessel above wound or, as a last resort, apply a tourniquet<br>• Place tourniquets proximal to site of hemorrhage to control bleeding if all other actions are unsuccessful |
| Wound edges do not approximate. | • Notify physician<br>• Be prepared to assist with wound closure or to send client to surgery |
| Glass particles are evident in wound. | • Irrigate wound profusely with sterile saline solution as ordered<br>• If large amount of glass or if glass is difficult to extract, notify physician, and be prepared to send client to surgery for wound cleansing and debridement<br>• Do not apply direct pressure or pressure dressing to wound containing glass |

# Skill 8.3 Applying Antiemboli Stockings (Graduated Compression Stockings and Elastic Stockings)

## EXPECTED OUTCOMES

- Compression stockings remain wrinkle-free and pressure is evenly distributed.
- Peripheral pulses are present during use of sequential stockings and elastic hosiery.
- Compression devices function properly.
- Client's skin remains intact while using compression stockings.

## Delegation

Unlicensed assistive personnel (UAP) frequently remove and apply antiemboli stockings as part of hygiene care. The nurse should stress the importance of removing and reapplying the stockings and reporting any changes in the client's skin to the nurse. The nurse is responsible for assessment of the skin.

## Equipment

- Single-use tape measure (to prevent cross-infection)
- Clean knee or thigh antiemboli stockings of appropriate size

## Preparation

Take measurements as needed to obtain the appropriate size stockings.

- Measure the length of both legs from the heel to the gluteal fold (for thigh-length stockings) or from the heel to the popliteal space or bend of the knee (for knee-length stockings).
- Measure the circumferences of each calf and each thigh at the widest point.
- Compare measurements to the size chart to obtain stockings of correct size. Obtain two sizes if there is a

## EVIDENCE-BASED NURSING PRACTICE

**Compression Stockings—Safe Practice Issues**

This study explored the use of graduated compression stockings and found that poorly fitting hose can be a direct cause of DVT and pressure ulcers on heels, top of foot, and due to tourniquet effect. Thigh-length hose are more difficult to apply and more apt to wrinkle and less comfortable. Clients also complain of stockings being painful, hot and itchy. It is important that nurses measure the client's legs for correct fit, assess extremities regularly, and encourage compliance through client education.

*Source:* Hayes, J., Lehman, C., Castoguay, P. (2002). Graduated compression stockings: Updating practice, improving compliance, *MED-SURG Nursing,* 11(4), 163.

significant difference. ➤*Rationale: Stockings that are too large for the client do not place adequate pressure on the legs to facilitate venous return, and may bunch, increasing the risk of pressure and skin irritation. Stockings that are too small may impede blood flow to the feet and cause skin breakdown.*

## Procedure

1. Prior to performing the procedure, introduce self and verify the client's identity using agency protocol. Explain to the client what you are going to do, why it is necessary, and how he or she can participate.
2. Perform hand hygiene and observe other appropriate infection control procedures.
3. Provide for client privacy.

## TABLE 8-1 MEASURING FOR GRADUATED COMPRESSION STOCKINGS (ELASTIC HOSIERY)

| Thigh-Hi Measuring | | Knee-Hi Measuring | |
|---|---|---|---|
| **Circumference** | **Length** | **Circumference** | **Length** |
| Measure mid-thigh circumference | Measure leg from bottom of heel to fold of buttocks | Measure calf at largest circumference | Measure leg from Achilles tendon to popliteal fold |

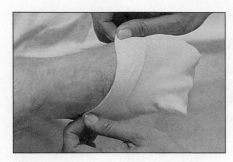

● Applying the inverted stocking over the toes.
Photographer: Elena Dorfman

4. Select an appropriate time to apply the stockings.
   - Apply stockings in the morning, if possible, before the client gets out of bed. ➤*Rationale: In sitting and standing positions, the veins can become distended so that edema occurs; the stockings should be applied before this occurs.*
   - Assist the client who has been ambulating to lie down and elevate legs for 15 to 30 minutes before applying the stockings. ➤*Rationale: This facilitates venous return, reduces swelling, and facilitates application of the stockings.*
5. Prepare the client.
   - Assist the client to a lying position in bed.
   - Wash and dry the legs as needed.
6. Apply the stockings.
   - Reach inside the stocking from the top, and grasping the heel, turn the upper portion of the stocking inside out so the foot portion is inside the stocking leg. ➤*Rationale: Firm elastic stockings are easier to fit over the foot and calf when inverted in this manner rather than bunching up the stocking.*
   - Ask the client to point the toes, then position the stocking on the client's foot. With the heel of the stocking down and stretching each side of the stocking, ease the stocking over the toes taking care to place the toe and heel portions of the stocking appropriately. ➤*Rationale: Pointing the toes makes application easier.*

## CLINICAL ALERT

Postoperative deep vein thrombosis of the lower extremity is often asymptomatic and in many, fatal pulmonary embolism is the first clinical sign of postoperative venous thromboembolism.

## DEVELOPMENTAL CONSIDERATIONS

### Children

- Antiemboli stocking are infrequently used on children.

### Elders

- Because the elastic is quite strong in antiemboli stockings, elders may need assistance with putting on the stockings. Clients with arthritis may need to have another person put the stockings on for them.
- Many elders have circulation problems and wear antiemboli stockings. It is important to check for wrinkles in the stockings and to see if the stocking has rolled down or twisted. If so, correct immediately. ➤*Rationale: The stockings must be evenly distributed over the limb to promote rather than hinder circulation.*
- Stockings should be removed once a day (check agency policy) so that a thorough assessment can be made of the legs and feet. ➤*Rationale: Redness and skin breakdown on the heels can occur quickly and go undetected if not thoroughly assessed on a regular basis.*
- Provide information about the importance of wearing the elastic stockings, how to wear them correctly, and how to take care of them.

## SETTING OF CARE

- Teach the client or caregiver how to apply the antiemboli stockings.
- Stress the importance of no wrinkles or rolling down of the stockings and the rationale.
- Instruct the client or caregiver to remove the stockings daily and inspect the skin on the legs.
- Provide instructions about the following: Laundering the stockings. They should be air dried because putting them in a dryer can affect the elasticity of the stockings. The need for two pairs of stockings to allow for one pair to be worn while the other is being laundered. Replacing the stockings when they lose their elasticity. Stockings are slippery if worn without slippers or shoes. If ambulatory, emphasize the need for footwear to prevent falling.

# Skill 8.4  Applying Pneumatic Compression Devices

## Equipment

Disposable leg sleeve(s) (Knee length or thigh length)
Tubing assembly
Compression controller (motor)
Measuring tape

## Preparation

1. Review physician's orders for type of disposable leg sleeve needed.
2. Identify client and explain that this device decreases the risk of developing deep-vein thrombosis (DVT) for clients following surgery or those on long-term bed rest. ➤*Rationale: This device counteracts blood stasis by increasing peak blood flow velocity. It helps to carry pooled blood from vein.*
3. Assess client for potential problems, contraindications for use of these devices. ➤*Rationale: Clients with ischemic conditions, massive edema of the leg, dermatitis, gangrene, on long-term bedrest, or with preexisting DVT within last six months are not candidates for these devices.*
4. Complete a neurovascular assessment. Include an evaluation of skin color, temperature, sensation, capillary refill, and presence and quality of pedal pulses. Document findings. ➤*Rationale: This assessment provides baseline data for evaluating neurovascular changes while devices are used.*
5. Assemble equipment. Read manufacturer's directions for connecting and operating compression controller.
6. Read directions for setting sleeve pressure (between 35 and 45 mm Hg). Maximum pressure should not exceed client's diastolic pressure.
7. Locate and identify the indicator lights on the controller for the ankle, calf, and thigh pressure. ➤*Rationale: Light is on when the pressure is applied to the three leg sleeves.*

## Procedure

1. Remove sleeve from plastic bag.
2. Unfold sleeve and follow directions to fit sleeve to client's leg. Leg is placed on white side (lining) of

> ## CLINICAL ALERT
>
> Follow hospital policy for amount of time alternating pneumatic compression devices are removed during the day. It is important to keep stockings on most of the day to prevent clot formation.

sleeve. Markings on the lining indicate the ankle and popliteal area.
3. Place client's leg on sleeve. Position back of knee over popliteal opening.
4. Starting at the side, wrap sleeve securely around client's leg.
5. Attach Velcro straps securely.
6. Check the fit by placing two fingers between client's leg and sleeve to determine if sleeve fits properly. Readjust Velcro as needed. ➤*Rationale: To ensure sleeve does not constrict circulation.*
7. Attach tubing and connect to plugs on leg sleeve by pushing ends firmly together.
8. Connect tubing assembly plug to controller at the tubing assembly connector site.
9. Ensure tubing is free of kinks or twists. ➤*Rationale: Kinks and twists can restrict airflow through system.*
10. Plug controller power cable into grounded electric outlet and attach unit to bedframe.
11. Turn controller power switch to ON. Monitor that alarms are audible.
12. Check that pressure indicator lights are functioning properly.
13. Monitor that compression cycles are correct.
14. Monitor neurovascular checks every 2–4 hours. Turn machine off immediately if the client complains or numbness or other signs of DVT.
15. Monitor client's tolerance of device.
16. Turn off machine at prescribed time intervals to assess skin and to provide skin care.
17. To remove sleeve, turn power switch OFF, disconnect tubing assembly from sleeve at connection site. Unwrap sleeve from leg.

# Skill 8.5 Applying Sequential Compression Devices (SCDs)

## Delegation

UAP often remove and reapply the SCD when performing hygiene care. The nurse should check that the UAP knows the correct application process for the SCD. Remind the UAP that the client should not have the SCD removed for long period of time because the purpose of the SCD is to promote circulation.

## Equipment

- Measuring tape
- SCD, including disposable sleeves, air pump, and tubing

## Procedure

1. Prior to performing the procedure, introduce self and verify the client's identity using agency protocol. Explain to the client what you are going to do, why it is necessary, and the procedure for applying the sequential compression device. ►*Rationale: The client's participation and comfort will be increased by understanding the reasons for applying the SCD.*

2. Perform hand hygiene and observe other appropriate infection control procedures.

3. Provide for client privacy and drape the client appropriately.

4. Prepare the client.
   - Place the client in a dorsal recumbent or semi-Fowler's position.
   - Measure the client's legs as recommended by the manufacturer if a thigh-length sleeve is required. ►*Rationale: Foot and knee-length sleeves come in just one size: the thigh circumference determines the size needed for a thigh-length sleeve.*

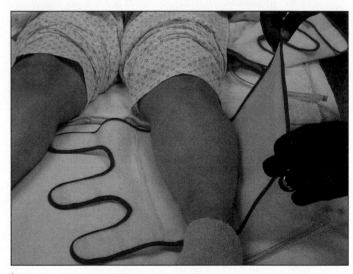

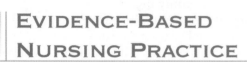 ● Place inflatable bladder directly behind client's calf.

## EVIDENCE-BASED NURSING PRACTICE

### Sequential Pneumatic Compression Devices

A study was conducted on 149 major trauma clients without lower limb injury, who were randomly assigned to either calf-thigh sequential pneumatic compression or plantar venous pneumatic compression devices. A total of 62 clients who received calf-thigh sequential pneumatic compression and 62 who received plantar venous intermittent pneumatic compression devices completed the trial. Thirteen clients randomized to plantar venous intermittent pneumatic compression (21.0%) and four clients randomized to calf-thigh sequential pneumatic compression (6.5%) had deep vein thrombosis. Seven of 13 clients with deep vein thrombosis after prophylaxis with plantar venous intermittent pneumatic compression had bilateral deep-vein thromboses, whereas all four clients with deep-vein thrombosis after prophylaxis with calf-thigh sequential pneumatic compression had unilateral deep-vein thrombosis. The conclusion is calf-thigh sequential pneumatic compression prevents deep-vein thrombosis more effectively than plantar venous intermittent pneumatic compression after major trauma without lower extremity injuries.

*Source:* Elliott, C., et al., (1999). Calf-thigh sequential pneumatic compression compared with plantar venous pneumatic compression to prevent deep-vein thrombosis after non-lower extremity trauma. *Journal of Trauma-Injury Infection and Critical Care,* 47(1), 25–32.

## DEVELOPMENTAL CONSIDERATIONS

### Children

- Because young children tend to be more active, the SCD is rarely necessary unless the child is immobile (e.g., comatose).

### Elders

- The SCD sleeves may become loose as clients move around in bed. Check that the sleeves are secure and properly positions.

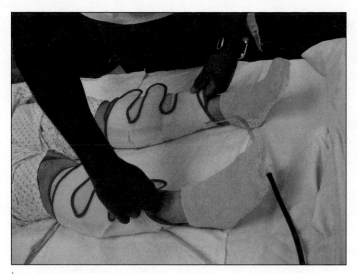

● Slip two fingers under wrap to ensure that it is not too tight.

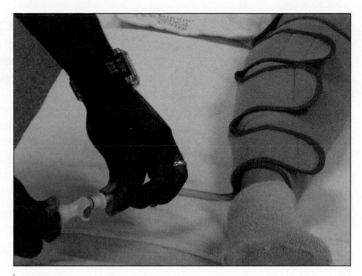

● Attach tubing from wrap to tubing connected to pump.

5. Apply the sequential compression sleeves.
   - Place a sleeve under each leg with the opening at the knee.
   - Wrap the sleeve securely around the leg, securing the Velcro tabs. Allow two fingers to fit between the leg and sleeve. ➤*Rationale: This amount of space ensures that the sleeve does not impair circulation when inflated.*
   - Grasp the loose portion of the stocking at the ankle and gently pull the stocking over the leg, turning it right side out in the process. If applying thigh-length stockings, stretch them over the knee until the top is below the gluteal fold.
   - Inspect the client's leg and stocking, smoothing any folds or creases. Ensure that the stocking is not rolled down or bunched at the top or ankle. Ensure that stocking is distributed evenly and that the heel is properly centered in the heel pocket. ➤*Rationale: Folds and creases can cause skin irritation under the stocking; bunching of the stocking can further impair venous return.*
   - Remove the stockings per agency policy, inspecting the legs and skin while the stockings are off.
   - Soiled stockings may be laundered by hand with warm water and mild soap. Hang to dry.

## CLINICAL ALERT

Contraindications to Use of Sequential Compression Devices

- Known or suspected acute DVT, phlebitis, severe atherosclerosis, or ischemic peripheral vascular disease.
- DVT within the last 6 months.
- Pulmonary embolism.
- Any condition where an increase in venous return to the heart might be detrimental.
- Local conditions such as dermatitis, gangrene, recent skin graft, infected leg wound or ulcer.

## EVIDENCE-BASED NURSING PRACTICE

**Recommend Bedrest for DVT?**

Recent prospective studies show that routine bed rest should not be recommended as part of standard care for clients with DVT. While elevation and rest of a swollen extremity provide some symptomatic relief, bed rest has been shown to increase the risk of clot propagation and does not decrease the rate of pulmonary embolism. Early ambulation may provide more rapid relief of pain and swelling.

*Source:* McRaw, S., & Ginsberg, J. (2004). Initial treatment of venous thromboembolism. *Supplement to Circulation: Journal of the American Heart Association,* 110(9), 1–3.

## SETTING OF CARE

- A sequential compression device may be used in the home. Inform the client or caregiver how to apply the device correctly and how to operate the system, including how to respond to the alarm.

| UNEXPECTED OUTCOMES | CRITICAL THINKING OPTIONS |
|---|---|
| Graduated Compression Stockings are not available. | • If ordered, use elastic (Ace) bandages. Anchor bandages on top of the foot and proceed up leg. Bandage should overlap one-third of bandage width; for a 4-inch width each turn overlaps by 1 1/2 inches. Ensure pressure is evenly distributed throughout bandage application.<br>• Assess that elastic bandages are tight enough for support but do not obstruct arterial flow. Assess neurovascular status 20 minutes after bandages applied and every 2–4 hours thereafter.<br>• While making each turn, place a finger between the bandage and skin with rotation to prevent bandage from becoming too tight. |
| Graduated Compression Stockings are loose and don't provide support. | • Remeasure legs and compare to chart to determine correct size.<br>• Hosiery may be old with no elasticity and should be discarded; ensure line drying rather than with electric dryer. |
| Graduated Compression Stockings do not provide support. | • Need to order different knit design and elastomeric yarn denier that will increase pressure. Pressure ranges from less than 15 mm Hg to 30–40 mm Hg at the ankle. Check physician's order for appropriate order. |
| for Compression Devices Client complains of numbness or tingling in leg. | • Remove devices immediately.<br>• Suggest use of foot pulse device as alternate.<br>• Complete neurovascular assessment.<br>• Notify physician of assessment findings. |
| Buildup of excess sleeve pressure (above 80 mm Hg). | • Check tubing for kinks or twists.<br>• Turn power switch to OFF position and then ON to restart system. |

Any disturbance in the rate or rhythm of the heartbeat is termed "dysrhythmia." Historically, the term "arrhythmia" has been used in the literature. Although the terms are often used interchangeably, dysrhythmia, which means a disturbance in cardiac rhythm, is more accurate. Dysrhythmias are classified according to their site of origin. The sites include: sinus, atrial, junctional, ventricular, and AV nodal tissue. A sinus dysrhythmia usually reflects a change in rate or rhythm. An atrial dysrhythmia results from a disturbance with the SA node or atria indicated by an abnormality in the P wave configuration. A junctional dysrhythmia occurs when there is a problem associated with the AV node as indicated by a change in the PR interval. A ventricular dysrhythmia results from a problem with the ventricle and is indicated by an abnormality in the configuration of the QRS complex. Although many dysrhythmias have no clinical manifestations, many others have serious consequences. A ventricular dysrhythmia is the most life-threatening because it compromises cardiac output.

### EXPECTED OUTCOMES
• ECG leads applied appropriately and without difficulty.
• Abnormal ECG findings interpreted accurately.
• Heart rate calculated correctly.
• Monitor wave forms are distinct and readable.

# Skill 8.6   Monitoring Clients on Telemetry

## Equipment

Telemetry transmitter box with 9-volt battery
Electrode pouch or gown with transmitter pocket
5-lead electrode cable and wires
Electrodes
Skin prep pad or alcohol swab

## Preparation

1. Gather equipment and perform hand hygiene.
2. Place a fresh 9-volt battery in the telemetry transmitter box.
3. Attach lead wire securely into transmitter box.
4. Explain procedure to client. Radio waves transmit the heart's electrical activity to a central monitoring station. This system allows the client to move around while his/her heart is constantly being monitored. Explain that the telemetry range is limited; therefore, client cannot wander out of the range, which is usually the nursing unit. If client goes off the unit, the nurse must be notified.
5. Instruct the client to notify the nurse if the electrode falls off.

## Procedure

1. Check the expiration date on the electrode packet.
   ➤*Rationale: To ensure electrode gel is moist.*
2. Determine appropriate lead to be monitored. Select 3- or 5-lead setup (depending on facility): 3 leads provide for choice of views (but no anterior view); 5 leads allow for 7 views, including anterior view.
3. Select electrode sites that are not over bony prominence, muscular area, joints, breasts, or skin creases.
   ➤*Rationale: Placing electrodes on these areas can lead to* artifact on the monitor screen. ➤*Note:* If client is overly obese, electrodes may have to be placed on the bones, since a large amount of adipose tissue results in poor image on the oscilloscope.
4. Assess skin site before placing electrode. Wipe skin areas using alcohol swab. Allow site to dry thoroughly before affixing electrode. ➤*Rationale: This removes oily substances and dead skin for better adherence of electrodes. Rub skin until slightly red.*
5. Attach lead wires to chest electrodes.
6. Apply electrodes to client's chest: peel off paper backing on electrode disc. Check that sponge pad in center of electrode is moist with conductive jelly. Place electrode on skin with adhesive side down. Press edges down to secure.

---

### ELECTRODE PLACEMENT

**White** to right shoulder (negative electrode)

**Black** to left shoulder (lead I positive electrode or $MCL_1$ negative electrode)

**Red** to left midclavicular upper abdominal area (lead II positive electrode)

**Brown** to fourth intercostal space, right sternal border ($MCL_1$ positive chest electrode), or left sternal border, or alternatively at left 5th intercostal space, midaxillary line ($V_6$ position)

**Green** to right abdomen or other convenient area (ground electrode)

*Note:* Limb leads and any one chest lead can be monitored using these electrode positions.

---

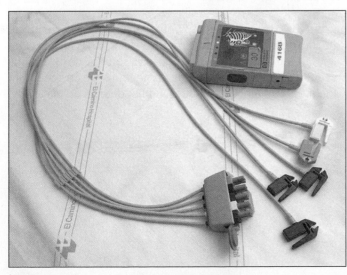

● Transmitter box, cable, and lead wires for telemetry.

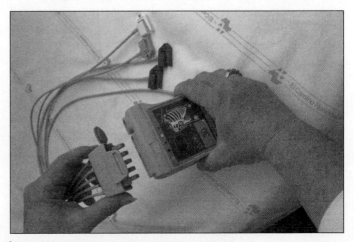

● Insert electrode cable into transmitter box.

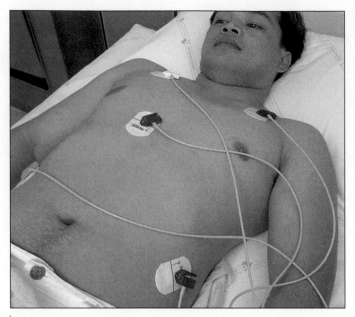

● Color-coded lead wires and placement of electrode for ECG monitoring.

7. Attach wire into transmitter box.
8. Have base station run an ECG strip to check clarity of transmission.
9. Set HIGH and LOW alarm limits on the monitor. Turn alarm buttons to ON per agency/unit protocol (e.g., 50 low, 100 high).
10. Assess skin surrounding the electrode for signs of irritation regularly.
11. Check lead placement at least once of shift unless notified by client or monitoring station that electrodes are not functioning properly.
12. Change electrodes at least every 3 days or if ECG strip indicates poor conduction of wave form.

## ELECTRODE SYSTEM FOR CARDIAC MONITORING

Three-, four-, or five-electrode systems are used in cardiac monitoring. The most popular method is the five-electrode system. This system allows the nurse to monitor any one of the six modified chest leads as well as the other leads without changing electrode placement.

- **Lead I:** Used to monitor atrial rhythms and hemiblocks. Depicts electrical current moving from right to left in the heart. Positive electrode placed on left arm or left side of chest, negative electrode placed on right arm or below right clavicle.

- **Lead II:** Used for routine monitoring and for detection of sinus node and atrial dysrhythmias. The positive electrode is placed below the rib at the left midclavicular line, and the negative electrode is placed below the right clavicle.

- **Lead III:** Used to detect changes associated with an inferior wall myocardial infarction. The positive electrode is placed on the left leg or lowest palpable rib on left midclavicular line. The negative electrode is placed below left clavicle.

- **$MCL_1$:** Used to assess ventricular dysrhythmias. The positive electrode is placed in the right sternal border at the fourth intercostal space. The negative electrode is placed below the left clavicle, and the ground electrode is placed on the right chest.

*See Table 8-2. Telemetry Electrode Placement.*

---

## TABLE 8–2 TELEMETRY ELECTRODE PLACEMENT

- **Lead I:** Records activity between a negative electrode (below right clavicle) and a positive electrode (below left clavicle). This lead looks at the heart's left lateral wall. Atrial arrhythmic activity is poorly identified.

- **Lead II:*** Records activity between a negative electrode (below right clavicle) and a positive electrode (midclavicular line on left flank). This lead looks at left inferior wall. It is used to diagnose supraventricular rhythms which arise from the atrial and junctional nodes. It best detects atrial activity.

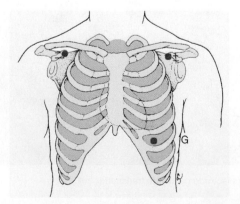

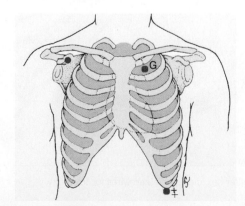

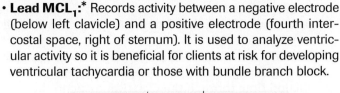

## TABLE 8–2 TELEMETRY ELECTRODE PLACEMENT *(CONTINUED)*

• **Lead III:** Records activity between a negative electrode (below left clavicle) and a positive electrode (lowest rib, left midclavicular line). It looks at left inferior wall.

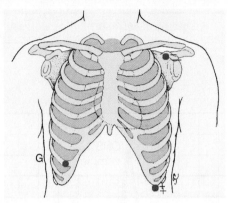

• **Lead MCL₁:*** Records activity between a negative electrode (below left clavicle) and a positive electrode (fourth intercostal space, right of sternum). It is used to analyze ventricular activity so it is beneficial for clients at risk for developing ventricular tachycardia or those with bundle branch block.

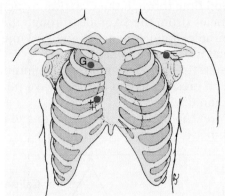

• **Lead MCL₆:** Records activity between a negative electrode (below left clavicle) and a positive electrode (fifth intercostal space, left midaxillary line). It monitors ventricular conduction changes much like MCL₁. Not as frequently used.

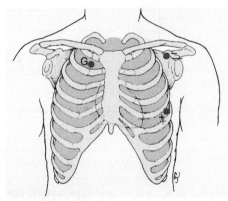

*Most popular leads for telemetry.

"G" indicates ground electrode—location may be anyplace on body; check facility protocol for placement.

# Skill 8.7    Interpreting an ECG Strip

## Equipment

Calipers (optional)
ECG rhythm strip

## Procedure

1. Assess ECG grid.
   a. Each small square represents 0.04 seconds (horizontal measurement).
   b. Each large block (5 small squares) represents 0.20 seconds.
   c. 15 large blocks represent 3 second.

2. Determine heart rate by calculating ventricular rate; normal is 50–100 per minute.
   a. Counter the number of R waves in a 6-second period (30 large blocks) and multiply this by 10 to obtain the heart rate.
   b. For true accuracy, count client's apical heart rate for 1 full minute.
3. Determine the regularity of ventricular rhythm (R waves should be equally spaced.)

4. Determine the P wave rate (Atrial depolarizations).
   a. There should be one P wave in front of each QRS complex.
   b. Note if there are more P waves or fewer P waves than QRS complexes.
5. Determine the regularity of the P waves; are they all equally spaced?
6. Measure the PR interval (beginning of the P wave to the beginning of the QRS complex); represents conduction time through the electrical tissue to the ventricles (from the SA node, through the AV Node, His bundle, bundle branches and Purkinje fibers); normal is 0.12 sec to 0.20 sec.
7. Measure the QRS duration from beginning of the Q wave, if present, to end of the S wave (normal is less than 0.12 sec).
8. Interpret the client's cardiac rhythm and place ECG rhythm sample strip in client's chart.

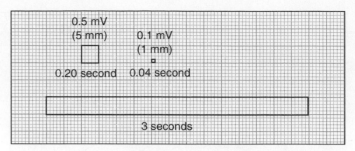

● ECG grid.

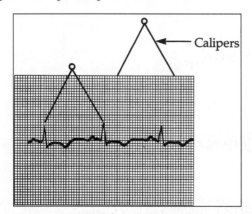

● Use calipers to measure heart rate.

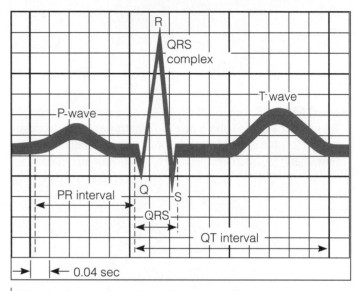

● It is important to determine configuration and location of wave pattern to interpret an ECG accurately.

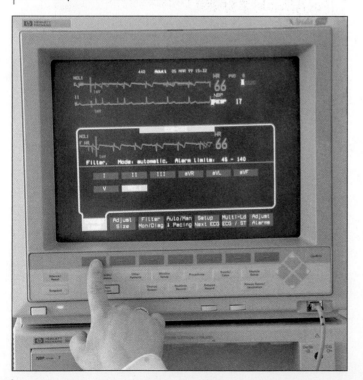

● ECG pattern and lead placement are depicted on oscilloscope.

### TABLE 8–3 NORMAL SINUS RHYTHM

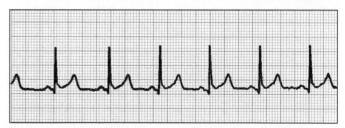

Regular configuration, uniform P wave precedes each QRS
Atrial rate 60–100
PR interval 0.12–0.2 seconds
QRS width <0.12 seconds
Ventricular rate 60–100

## TABLE 8–4 SELECTED CARDIAC RHYTHMS AND DYSRHYTHMIAS

### Sinus Tachycardia

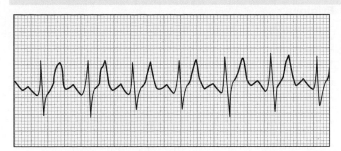

Regular rhythm >100/min
P waves—normal
Atrial rate—>100/min
PR interval—0.12–2.0
QRS complex width—0.06–0.08 usually normal

*Note:* A moderately faster heart rate can be a physiological normal variant.

#### Etiology
Underlying causes such as anxiety, fever, shock, drugs, exercise, electrolyte disturbances

#### Initial Treatment
Immediately initiate cardioversion if unstable
Treatment dependent on elimination of cause;
Anxiety measures
Pain relief
Antipyretics
$O_2$
Medications (sedatives, tranquilizers, anti-anxiety, etc.)
Calcium channel blockers and beta blockers

### Sinus Bradycardia

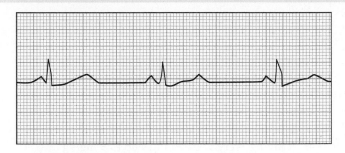

Regular rhythm <60/min
P waves—normal
Atrial rate—<60/minute
PR interval—0.20
QRS complex width—0.08 usually normal

*Note:* A slow heart rate can be physiologically normal for some clients.

#### Etiology
Drugs, altered metabolic states (hypothyroidism), cardiac diseases, athletes

#### Initial Treatment
Maintain patent airway; assist breathing as needed
Oxygen
IV
Atropine 0.5–1 mg bolus IV while awaiting pacer
May repeat to a total dose of 3 mg
Then, epinephrine (2–10 mg/min) or dopamine (2–10 mg/kg/min) infusion while awaiting pacer
Transcutaneous pacing

### Multifocal Premature Ventricular Contraction (PVCs)

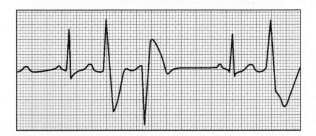

Irregular rhythm
P waves—none with premature beat, impulse originates in ventricle
Atrial rate—undetermined
PR interval—none with premature beat
QRS width—greater than 0.12 seconds for premature beat
Ventricular rate—varies

*Note:* Each PVC has different configuration as foci are from different areas of heart.

PVCs are result of increased automaticity of ventricular muscle cells.

### Ventricular Tachycardia

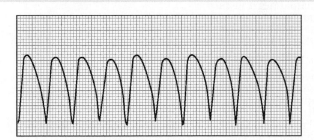

Regular rhythm
Atrial rate—cannot differentiate
PR interval—none
QRS width—greater than 0.12 seconds
Ventricular rate—130–250

*Note:* Ventricular tachycardia is a result of myocardial irritability and is life threatening.

*(continued)*

## TABLE 8–4 SELECTED CARDIAC RHYTHMS AND DYSRHYTHMIAS *(CONTINUED)*

**Etiology**

- Heart disease, MI
- Hypoxia
- Acidosis
- Electrolyte imbalances
- Myocardial ischemia
- Drug toxicity (especially digitalis)

**Initial Treatment**

- Oxygen
- Potassium or magnesium if electrolytes dictate
- Lidocaine bolus—1–1.5 mg/kg; may repeat doses of 0.5–0.75 mg/kg every 5–10 minutes up to 3 mg/kg
- Refractory to lidocaine: amiodarone or procainamide
- Continuous IV drip may be started
- Correct underlying cause

**Etiology**

- Acute MI
- Coronary artery disease, cardiomyopathy
- Electrolyte imbalance
- Drug intoxication (digitalis)

**Initial Treatment**

- Lidocaine 1.5 mg/kg bolus; may repeat in 3–5 minutes to maximum dose of 3 mg/kg
- Amiodarone 300 mg IV/IO can be followed by 150 mg IV/IO
- Cardioversion if cardiac output is compromised
- Pulseless ventricular tachycardia—follow treatment for ventricular fibrillation (epinephrine)

---

### Atrial Fibrillation

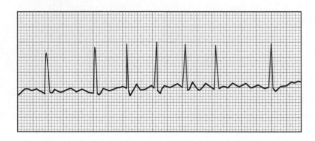

Irregularly irregular rhythm
Disorganized atrial activity—greater than 350 BPM
P waves—none identifiable
PR interval—not measured
QRS—variable
QRS complex: irregular

**Etiology**

Heart failure
Rheumatoid heart disease
Coronary heart disease
Hypertension
Hyperthyroidism

**Initial Treatment**

Cardioversion
Verapamil
Propranolol
Digitalis
Quinidine
Procainamide
Ibutilide
Amiodarone
Anticoagulant to reduce risk of clot formation and stroke

---

### Atrial Flutter

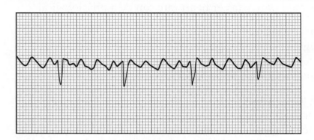

Regular or irregular rhythm (depending on block)
Atrial rate greater than 250 BPM
Ventricular rate can be irregular
PR interval—regular
P wave and PR interval cannot calculate
QRS complex—0.6 to 0.10 seconds

**Etiology**

Sympathetic nervous system stimulation
  (i.e., anxiety), caffeine, and alcohol intake
Thyrotoxins
Coronary heart disease; MI; pulmonary embolism

**Initial Treatment**

Cardioversion—preferred method
Digitalis
Calcium channel blocker (Cardizem) or beta-blocking
  agents to slow ventricular response
Followed by ibutilide, quinidine, procainamide

## TABLE 8–4 SELECTED CARDIAC RHYTHMS AND DYSRHYTHMIAS *(CONTINUED)*

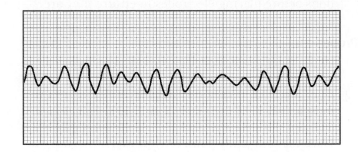

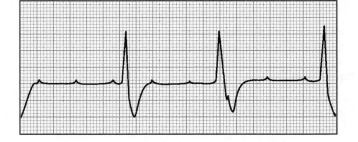

**Ventricular Fibrillation**

Irregular, totally chaotic rhythm
Atrial rate—cannot differentiate
PR interval—none
QRS width—fibrillating waves only
Ventricular rate—cannot differentiate

*Note:* Ineffective quivering of ventricles with no audible heartbeat, pulse, or respirations.

**Etiology**
• Myocardial ischemia, Acute MI
• Coronary artery disease
• Cardiomyopathy
• Acid-base imbalance
• Severe hypothemia
• Electrolyte imbalance

**Initial Treatment**
• Immediately defibrillate, shock
• CPR—5 cycles or about 2 minutes
• Ventricular fibrillation continues—give a vasopressor (epinephrine 1 mg IV push), repeat 3–5 minutes
• Defibrillate again and continue CPR
• Second-line drugs may be used, such as amiodarone (300 mg IV), lidocaine

**Third-Degree Heart Block**

Regular atrial and ventricular rhythm
Atrial rate—greater than ventricular rate
PR interval—varies
QRS width—less than 0.12 second if pacemaker cell in junction; greater than 0.12 seconds if cell in ventricle
Ventricular rate—40–60 if escape pacemaker is from junction; 20–40 if escape is from ventricle

*Note:* Electrical impulse originates in SA node but is blocked to the Purkinje fibers leading to decreased perfusion of vital organs.

**Etiology**
• Digitalis toxicity
• Myocardial infarction, anterior
• Organic heart disease

**Initial Treatment**
• Atropine bolus
• Transcutaneous pacing
• Dopamine or epinephrine
• Prepare for pacemaker insertion

## CLINICAL ALERT

Always assess client to determine if the abnormal rhythm is potentially life-threatening and emergency measures should be taken. Signs of hemodynamic instability include the following:

• Ongoing chest pain

• Shortness of breath

• Change in mental status

• SBP < 90mm Hg

• Heart rate > 150 per minute.

# Skill 8.8 Recording a 12-Lead ECG

## EXPECTED OUTCOMES

- ECG leads applied appropriately and without difficulty.
- Abnormal ECG findings interpreted accurately.
- Heart rate calculated correctly.
- Monitor wave forms are distinct and readable.

## Equipment

Electrodes
Skin prep pad or alcohol swab
ECG machine
Cable

## Preparation

1. Review physician's order for ECG and perform hand hygiene.
2. Identify client using two forms of ID and explain procedure. Reassure client that machine will not cause discomfort or electrocution.
3. Assess chest for placement of electrodes.
4. Determine if skin site care is necessary. If so, cleanse areas with skin prep pad or alcohol swab. Allow area to dry thoroughly before placing electrodes. ➤*Rationale: This will ensure a more secure fit for the electrodes and provide a better ECG tracing.*
5. Attach wires to electrodes before pressing onto client's chest. ➤*Rationale: This prevents pressure being applied to chest area. This is particularly necessary following open heart surgery or chest trauma.*

6. Check the color-coding on the manufacturer's directions before placing electrodes to ensure they are correct.

## Procedure

1. When placing electrodes, ensure lead wires are all going in the same direction.
2. Place electrodes on fleshy areas, avoiding bone and muscle. ➤*Rationale: To ensure good electrical conduction and clear ECG tracings.*
3. Place the four-limb leads, one on each limb, according to the color coding. Three standard leads will be recorded on the 12-lead ECG.
   a. Lead I: Right arm wrist (negative electrode) white; and left arm (positive electrode) black. Records activity between the two arms.
   b. Lead II: Right arm (negative electrode) and left leg ankle (positive electrode) red. Records activity between arm and leg.
   c. Lead III: Left arm (negative electrode) and left leg (positive electrode) green. Records activity between arm and leg.
4. Three augmented limb lead tracings are obtained on the ECG as follows.
   a. aVR: Records activity between the center of the heart and right arm.
   b. aVL: Records activity between the center of the heart and left arm.
   c. aVF: Records activity between the center of the heart and the left leg or foot.

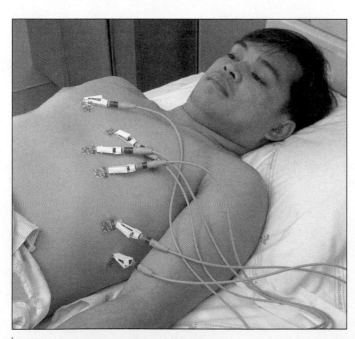

● Electrode placement for chest leads V$_1$–V$_6$.

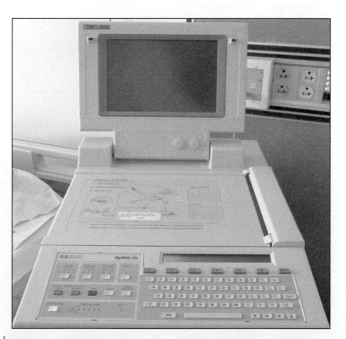

● Portable ECG machine for taking 12-lead tracing.

5. Place the chest leads as follows. (See figure.)
   a. V1: Fourth intercostal space, right sternal border. Records activity between the center of the heart and the fourth intercostals space; P wave is shown best here.
      (1) Palpate the jugular notch above sternum (feels like a depression).
      (2) Move finger down and palpate the manubrium of sternum (feels solid).
      (3) Continue to move finger down to the angle of Louis, which is at the top of the sternal body.
      (4) Move finger to the right of the angle of Louis to the second right rib.
      (5) Below the rib is the second intercostals space.
      (6) Move fingers down, palpating the next two ribs. Below the fourth rib and to the right of the sternal body is the fourth intercostals space. Place electrode in this area.
   b. V2: Fourth intercostal space, left sternal border.
   c. V3: Midway between V2 and V4, between 4th and 5th ICS.
   d. V4: Fifth intercostal space, left midclavicular line.

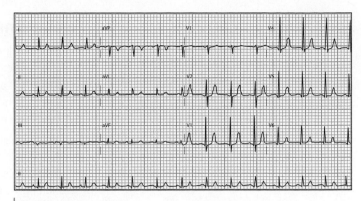

● Normal 12-lead ECG.

   e. V5: Fifth intercostal space, anterior axillary line, and mid-clavicular area.
   f. V6: Fifth intercostal space, left midaxillary line.
6. Begin taking the ECG according to manufacturer's directions on machine.
7. Place tracing copy on client's chart.
8. Remove electrodes; perform hand hygiene.

| UNEXPECTED OUTCOMES | CRITICAL THINKING OPTIONS |
|---|---|
| ECG is not clearly displayed on monitor. | • Ensure that electrodes are applied in correct position and are securely attached.<br>• Observe for electrical interference resulting in a 60-cycle interference on oscilloscope.<br>• Observe for excessive client activity resulting in artifact display on oscilloscope. |
| Electrodes do not adhere to skin, and interference appears on oscilloscope. | • Change placement of electrodes to another area. Shave area if needed for skin contact.<br>• Recleanse skin thoroughly using skin prep or alcohol and allow to dry. |
| Alarms ring without change in pattern. | • Check HIGH and LOW parameters. They may need to be changed.<br>• Check GAIN. It may be too low to sense pattern. |
| ECG pattern is abnormal. | • If client is asymptomatic, recheck lead placement.<br>• Check if pattern is a life-threatening arrhythmia (PVCs, ventricular tachycardia, ventricular fibrillation); if so, notify physician immediately.<br>• Increasing PVCs-notify Rapid Response Team.<br>• VT, VF—call code.<br>• Notify physician immediately. |
| Electrical interference appears on monitor. | • Check all other electric equipment in the immediate environment.<br>• Check for proper grounding of monitor.<br>• Change electrodes and cable; poor conduction may cause 60-cycle interference.<br>• Check that monitor is calibrated. |
| Electrodes cause skin irritation. | • Remove electrodes, cleanse site, and reapply electrodes on new site. |
| Chaotic rhythm appears on monitor. | • Check client's other assessment parameters to determine if clinical changes have occurred.<br>• Check electrode contact on skin, and ensure that wires are in contact with cable.<br>• Determine activity level of client. |

*(continued)*

| UNEXPECTED OUTCOMES *(cont.)* | CRITICAL THINKING OPTIONS *(cont.)* |
|---|---|
| High or low alarms on monitor continue to sound. | • Check for loose electrodes or try a different lead.<br>• Observe activity level of client.<br>• Check that alarm parameters on monitor are not set too close to client's pulse.<br>• Check client's position.<br>• Reposition electrodes, avoiding large muscle masses or bone. |
| Electrodes conduct poorly or diaphoretic client. | • Clean skin sites as usual; apply benzoin to the skin and let dry and apply electrodes.<br>• Clean skin sites as usual; apply spray deodorant to the skin, allow skin to dry, and apply electrodes. |
| Asystole displays on monitor. | • Check client's LOC and electrodes, wires, and cable connection.<br>• If the client has an arterial line, check for an arterial waveform in the absence of an ECG waveform. |

# Skill 8.9  Monitoring Temporary Cardiac Pacing (Transvenous, Epicardial)

## Equipment

Appropriate temporary pulse generator (select for single or dual chamber pacing)
9-volt battery for pulse generator (single or dual chamber)
Bridging cable for epicardial wires
Clean gloves
Established continuous cardiac monitoring—see telemetry monitoring skill

## Preparation

1. Validate that informed consent has been obtained for temporary pacing.
2. Identify client by checking two forms of client ID.
3. Explain rationale for temporary pacing and necessary restrictions/precautions, and provide reassurance of close continuous monitoring.
4. Perform hand hygiene.

## Procedure

### For Epicardial Pacing

1. Don clean gloves. ➤*Rationale: Gloves are worn to prevent microshock to client.*
2. Locate epicardial atrial pacing wires on right of client's sternum and ventricular pacing wires on left of client's sternum.
3. Securely connect lead wire electrode pins into connecting cable. ➤*Rationale: This promotes pacemaker impulse reception from and transmission to the myocardium.*
4. Connect cable to pulse generator (positive to positive, negative to negative). ➤*Rationale: Pacing stimulus goes from pulse generator to the negative terminal and back to pulse generator by the positive terminal.*

5. Remove protective cover to dial settings.
6. Select pacing mode (e.g., atrial, ventricular, AV synchronous, or demand).

### For Transvenous or Epicardial Pacing

1. Set dial at prescribed pacing rate (atrial and/or ventricular).
2. Set energy output (milliamperes or mA) on pulse generator to prescribed level (set for both atrial and ventricular pacing). ➤*Rationale: Energy output setting ensures that pacemaker stimulates the client's myocardium.*
3. Return plastic cover to protect generator dial settings and hang generator from pole at client's bedside.
4. Monitor pacemaker function for sensing (light indicates client's QRS complexes), capture (pacemaker spike is followed by QRS complex), and pacemaker rate.
5. Monitor client's heart rhythm, vital signs, and other responses to pacing, including femoral pulsation palpable with captured beats. ➤*Rationale: These demonstrate effectiveness of pacemaker support.*
6. Remove gloves and perform hand hygiene.
7. Evaluate electrode insertion/exit sites and dress according to agency protocol.

---

**CLINICAL ALERT**

Transvenous single chamber (ventricular) pacing is most commonly used as an emergency measure to support ventricular contraction and cardiac output. Epicardial leads provide either single chamber atrial pacing, single chamber ventricular pacing, or dual chamber pacing which is used to simulate normal pump function (atrial followed by ventricular stimulation/contraction).

# Skill 8.10   Assisting with Pacemaker Insertion

## Equipment

Emergency cart with defibrillator
External pacemaker pulse generator
Pacing catheter electrodes
ECG monitor
Client cable
Rubber glove
Sterile antiseptic solution
Sterile gloves, gown, and mask
Sterile towels
Lidocaine, 1%–2%
Alcohol wipes
Syringe
Needles
Suture with attached needle
Sterile 4 × 4 gauze pads
Tape
Cutdown tray
Gloves

## Preparation

1. Complete hand hygiene.
2. Provide sedation as necessary. Diazepam (Valium) or Versed is frequently used. Conscious sedation may be used.
3. Connect client to a continuous ECG monitor.
4. Place the client in a supine position with head flat or slightly lower than body.
5. If either the subclavian or external jugular vein is to be used, place a towel roll under the client's shoulders to provide better exposure of the insertion site.

## Procedure

1. Assist physician as needed.
   a. Physician dons mask, sterile gown, and gloves.
   b. Insertion site is cleansed with sterile antiseptic solution.
   c. Area is draped with sterile towels.
   d. Top of lidocaine is cleansed with alcohol wipe.
   e. Physician withdraws lidocaine, and skin is injected with 25-gauge needle.
   f. Insertion is accomplished (transvenous method via cutdown or percutaneously). Catheter electrode wires are positioned, and skin sutures are applied.
2. Continuously monitor the ECG and client status during the insertion.
3. Don gloves to prevent microshock to client.
4. Connect the pacing electrode to the appropriate outlet terminal (unipolar to negative and bipolar to both the positive and negative terminals).
5. Turn on power switch on external pacemaker.
6. Set rate according to physician's orders.

### ELECTRICAL SAFETY ALERT

- Use only grounded equipment; use common ground.
- Remove and tag any defective equipment.
- Maintain environmental humidity at 50%–60%.
- Do not roll equipment over electrical cords.
- Avoid placing wet articles on electrical equipment.
- Insulate exposed pacing electrodes at all times.
- Wear rubber gloves when handling pacing electrodes or terminals.
- Do not touch any electric equipment while handling wire or terminals.
- Discharge static electricity by touching faucets or other metal that communicates with ground.

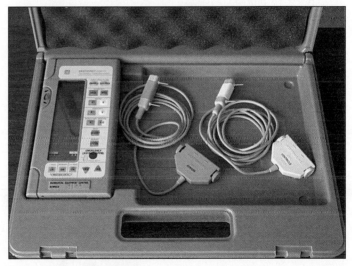

● Type of external pacemaker.

7. Set milliamperes (mA) by determining threshold. To do this, observe the ECG while slowly increasing the number of milliamperes from its lowest setting to a point where a QRS complex is detected following each stimulus.
8. Multiply the threshold level according to hospital policy (usually two to four times) to adjust the milliampere setting.
9. Set sensitivity mode according to physician's order (usually 1.5 mV).
10. Secure all connections. Put plastic cover back over pacemaker controls if required.

## REVISED NASPE/BPEG GENERIC CODE FOR ANTIBRADYCARDIA PACING*

| I | II | III | IV | V |
|---|---|---|---|---|
| Chamber(s) Paced | Chamber(s) Sensed | Response to Sensing | Rate Modulation | Multisite Pacing |
| 0 = None | O = None | O = None | O = None | O = None |
| A = Atrium | A = Atrium | T = Triggered | R = Rate modulation | A = Atrium |
| V = Ventricle | V = Ventricle | I = Inhibited | | V = Ventricle |
| D = Dual (A+V) | D = Dual (A+V) | D = Dual (T+I) | | D = Dual (A+V) |
| S = Single (A or V)† | S = Single (A or V)† | | | |

*This code differs from the 1987 version that listed programmability and antitachycardia functions. These functions are described in Bernstein, A. D., et al. (1993).

NASPE policy statement: The NASPE/BPEG defibrillator code. *Pacing and Clinical Electrophysiology*, 16, 1776–80.

†Manufacturer's designation only.

From Bernstein, A. D., et al. (2002). The revised NASPE/BPEG generic code for antibradycardia. adaptive-rate, and multisite pacing. *Pacing and Clinical Electrophysiology*, 25, 261.

11. Place external pacemaker and exposed wires in a rubber glove to ensure insulation against electric shock to client.
12. Apply sterile dressings to insertion site, and tape securely.
13. Obtain chest x-ray following insertion to validate lead placement if pacemaker not inserted using fluoroscopy.
14. Obtain 12-lead ECG.

### CLINICAL ALERT

Safety alert: When temporary transvenous pacemakers are used, the balloon air port is not to be used for IV access.

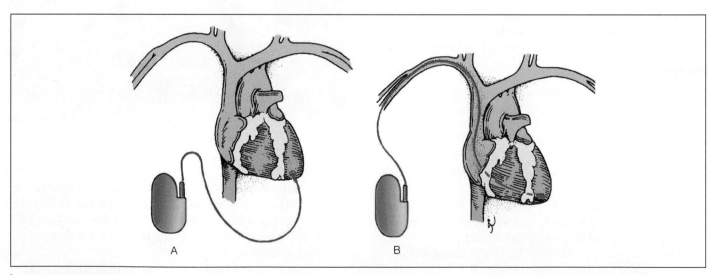

● Temporary pacemakers have two parts, the pulse generator and the electrode. The pulse generator is external to the body.
**A,** Epicardial ventricular pacemaker. **B,** Transvenous ventricular pacemaker.

# Skill 8.11 Maintaining Temporary Pacemaker Function

**Equipment**

Battery
Oscilloscope

**Procedure**

1. Observe for failure to sense.
   a. Observe the oscilloscope for presence of pacemaker artifact (spikes). Artifact before QRS complex in ventricular paced or preceding the P waves and QRS waves in AV sequential pacing.
   b. Check connections for secure, tight fit.
   c. Observe that pace–sense needle deflects to right, indicating pacing is occurring.
   d. Check sensitivity dial to determine if sensitivity threshold is set correctly.
2. Observe for failure to pace.
   a. Check that external generator is ON.
   b. Check battery to ensure it is functioning.
   c. Check lead connector sites.
   d. Check pace–sense indicator. (Absence of or slight deflection of the pace–sense indicator reveals battery failure.)
3. Observe for failure to capture.
   a. Observe for pacing artifact not followed by QRS complex. ➤*Rationale: This indicates a failure of the stimulus to trigger a ventricular response.*
   b. Check the setting of the mA, or output dial, to determine if setting should be increased. ➤*Rationale: The myocardial threshold may be altered as a result of disease or drugs.*
   c. Check all connector sites for secure, tight fit.
4. Observe that sutures are intact.
5. Assess insertion site for bleeding, hematoma formation, or infection.
6. Obtain chest x-ray post insertion.

7. Monitor client's response to therapy.
   a. Assess urine output. ➤*Rationale: Decreased urine output indicates poor cardiac output.*
   b. Observe for dyspnea, crackles, heart rate, decreased blood pressure.
   c. Monitor temperature.
   d. Observe client for signs of anxiety. Complete pacemaker teaching as necessary.
8. Obtain and analyze a strip for functioning of pacemaker.
9. Observe for battery failure.
10. Observe for electrical interference and development of microshocks.
    a. Ground all electrical equipment in close proximity to client.
    b. Cover exposed wires with nonconductive material.
    c. Wear gloves when handling generator/lead wires.
11. Complete pacemaker teaching as necessary.

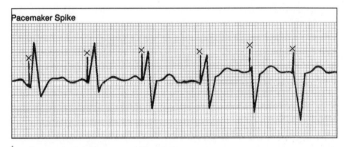

● ECG tracing showing pacemaker spike triggering ventricular depolarization (QRS).

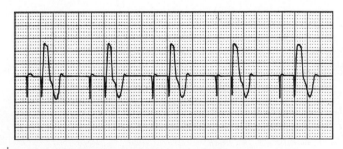

● ECG showing examples of pacemaker spikes.

# Skill 8.12 Providing Permanent Pacemaker Client Teaching

## EXPECTED OUTCOMES

- Client's cardiac rate is maintained through use of a pacemaker.
- Client is prepared psychologically and physically for insertion of the pacemaker.
- Pacemaker is inserted without complications.
- Heart rate and cardiac output improve.

## Equipment

Audiovisual aids
Written material

## Procedure

1. Ascertain what client already knows and understands.
2. Determine client's ability and level of interest in learning about pacemaker.
3. Recognize client's fears, and provide opportunity to talk about them.
4. Review facts: heart anatomy and physiology and pacemaker information. Use illustrations and audiovisual aids.
5. Clarify misconceptions and allay fears.
6. Provide rationale for any mobility restrictions.
7. Answer questions, and provide additional opportunities to discuss procedure.
8. Check pacemaker function regularly per instructions.

---

### PACEMAKER CLINICS

Many clients use telephone transmission of the generator's pulse rate to determine status of pacemaker function. Special equipment is used to transmit information concerning function of the pacemaker over the telephone to a receiving system in a pacemaker clinic. The equipment converts information to electronic signals that are permanently recorded on ECG strip. Physicians monitor client's records and can intervene quickly when abnormalities appear on ECG strip. This type of clinic is very common in outlying areas where clients are unable to go to a clinic easily.

---

9. Instruct client in clinical manifestations related to pacemaker failure and when to contact physician or pacemaker clinic.
10. Provide client with pacemaker information ID card (provided by manufacturer) and instruct to carry in wallet.
11. Suggest a Medical Alert band be worn at all times.

*Note:* Inform client of electromagnetic interference restrictions:
   a. No MRI; do not place cell phone or cardiovert over generator.
   b. Avoid airport hand wand, high-voltage areas, and diathermy.
   c. If dizziness experienced, move away from area.

| UNEXPECTED OUTCOME | CRITICAL THINKING OPTIONS |
|---|---|
| Temporary pacing is ineffective. | • Check for battery depletion and change if necessary (9-V batteries).<br>• Record rhythm strip and correlate to client's signs and symptoms.<br>• Monitor vital signs, mental status.<br>• Check sensitivity setting. (If too high, P or T wave may be sensed; if too low, fixed-rate pacing occurs.)<br>• Check mA setting (may be too high).<br>• Check pace indicator for movement.<br>• Check rate setting.<br>• Check all connections.<br>• Check catheter insertion site for swelling, hematoma. |
| Client does not understand function of pacemaker. | • If client is frightened, reassure him or her that a pacemaker is not dangerous.<br>• If client does not understand pacemaker or procedure, use illustrated learning aids.<br>• Allow time for questions and further explanations.<br>• Orient your teaching to the client's intellectual and interest level. |
| Electromagnetic interference occurs. | • Check all electric equipment for proper grounding. Use common ground.<br>• Remove unnecessary electric equipment from vicinity of client.<br>• Insulate generator terminals, and exposed electrodes in a rubber glove. |
| Inflammation occurs at insertion site. | • Provide daily site care using strict aseptic technique.<br>• Keep dressings dry at all times.<br>• Monitor vital signs.<br>• Instruct client to limit extremity movement. |
| Diaphragmatic pacing occurs. | • Observe for hiccoughs or muscle twitching.<br>• Change client's position.<br>• Decrease the amperage (mA).<br>• Notify physician that endocardial perforation may have occurred. |
| Failure to capture is suspected. | • Check client's heart rate. If heart rate less than the rate set on generator, and if pace indicator shows firing, suspect failure to capture.<br>• Check all connections.<br>• Anticipate that pacer wires are dislodged.<br>• Check battery.<br>• Change position of extremity.<br>• Turn client on left side; catheter may float back to epicardial wall.<br>• Increase amperage (mA) after checking threshold.<br>• Obtain chest x-ray and 12-lead ECG.<br>• Anticipate change of batteries, electrode terminals, or generator. |

# Reproduction

Skill 9.1  Maternal and Newborn Assessments  359

Skill 9.2  Assisting with a Pelvic Examination  372

Skill 9.3  Assessing Deep Tendon Reflexes and Clonus  373

Skill 9.4  Administration of Rh Immune Globulin (RhoGAM, HypRho-D)  374

Skill 9.5  Assisting during Amniocentesis  375

Skill 9.6  Assessment of Fetal Well-Being: Nonstress Test (NST)  376

Skill 9.7  Assessment of Fetal Well-Being: Contraction Stress Test (CST)  377

Skill 9.8  Assessment of Fetal Well-Being: Biophysical Profile (BPP)  378

Skill 9.9  Performing an Intrapartal Vaginal Examination  379

Skill 9.10  Assisting with Amniotomy (AROM: Artificial Rupture of Membranes)  381

Skill 9.11  Auscultating Fetal Heart Rate  381

Skill 9.12  External Electronic Fetal Monitoring  382

Skill 9.13  Internal Electronic Fetal Monitoring: Application of Fetal Scalp Electrode  384

Skill 9.14  Assisting with and Monitoring of Woman Undergoing Induction of Labor with Pitocin and Cervical Ripening Agents  385

Skill 9.15  Assisting with and Caring for the Woman with an Epidural during Labor  386

Skill 9.16  Care of the Woman with Prolapsed Cord  388

Skill 9.17  Assessing the Uterine Fundus Following Vaginal Birth  388

Skill 9.18  Evaluating the Lochia  389

Skill 9.19  Assessing Postpartum Perineal  391

Skill 9.20  Assisting with Breastfeeding after Childbirth  392

Skill 9.21  Performing Nasal Pharyngeal Suctioning  394

Skill 9.22  Suctioning an Infant with a Bulb Syringe  395

Skill 9.23  Assessing Newborn APGAR Scores  396

Skill 9.24  Thermoregulation of the Newborn  397

Skill 9.25  Umbilical Cord Clamp: Application, Care, and Removal  398

Skill 9.26  Assisting with Circumcision and Providing Circumcision Care  399

Skill 9.27  Initial Newborn Bath  400

Skill 9.28  The Infant Receiving Phototherapy  400

Nursing assessment of the obstetrical client is a major responsibility for any nurse whether she/he works in an office setting or in an acute care facility. The nurse midwife and nurse practitioners have become integral members of the interdisciplinary team that provides care for the family during the birthing process. More advanced practice nurses like the certified nurse midwife and the nurse practitioner have in-depth education and skill in performing assessment responsibilities with the physi-cian. While performing the physical assessment, the nurse should establish an environment in which the woman feels comfortable and free to discuss any concerns. The information collected during the antepartal (prenatal), intrapartal, postpartal, and newborn assessments can be used to identify needed areas for teaching and counseling. (Reference used (2004). Olds, London, Ladewig and Davidson *Maternity-Newborn Nursing & Women's Health Care 7 ed. Pearson/Prentice Hall.*)

# Skill 9.1   Maternal and Newborn Assessments

## TABLE 9–1   ANTEPARTAL ASSESSMENT

| | Normal Findings during Pregnancy | Abnormal Findings during Pregnancy |
|---|---|---|
| Take vital signs, blood pressure (BP), temperature, pulse, and respiration (TPR) | Temperature: 98–99°F; Pulse: 80–90 bpm (pulse rates can increase 10 beats; Respirations: 16–24 breaths/min (pregnancy may induce a mild form of hyperventilation and thoracic breathing; Blood Pressure (BP): 120/80 | Elevated temperature (infection) <br> Increased pulse rate: anxiety or excitement; cardiac disorder <br> Marked tachypnea: assess for respiratory distresss <br> Increased: possible anxiety (client should rest 20 to 30 minutes before you take BP again) <br> Rise of 30/15 above baseline data: sign of preeclampsia. Refer to Skill 9.3. <br> Decreased: sign of supine hypotensive syndrome. If lying on back, turn client on left side and take BP again. |
| Evaluate weight to assess maternal health and nutritional status and growth of fetus | Minimum weight gain during pregnancy: 24 lbs. <br> Underweight: 28–42 lbs. <br> Obese 15 lbs. or more <br> Normal weight gain: 25–35 to 40 lbs. | Inadequate weight gain; possible maternal malnutrition <br> Excessive weight gain: if sudden at onset, may indicate pregnancy induced hypertension; if gradual and continual may indicate overeating |
| Skin <br>   Color | Nail beds are pink; color of skin is consistent with racial background <br> *Striae* (reddish-purple lines) on breasts, hips, and thighs; After pregnancy, faint silvery-gray <br><br> *Spider nevi* common in pregnancy | Pallor—anemia; yellowish—liver disease or some form of jaundice <br> Dark skin persons with anemia may have bluish, reddish, mottled; dusty or pallor appearance of the palms and nail beds <br> Petechiae, multiple bruises, ecchymosis (hemorrhage; abuse) |
|   Condition <br><br><br>   Edema | Absence of edema (slight edema in lower extremities normal) <br> Usually no rashes <br><br><br> In lower extremities | Edema could be suggestive of pregnancy induced hypertension; <br> Presence of rash could indicate dermatitis; allergic reaction <br> Ulcerations could indicate varicose veins or decreased circulation <br> In upper extremities and face may indicate pregnancy induced hypertension |

*(continued)*

## TABLE 9-1 ANTEPARTAL ASSESSMENT (continued)

| | Normal Findings during Pregnancy | Abnormal Findings during Pregnancy |
|---|---|---|
| Nose, mouth, and neck | Nasal mucosa redder than oral; nasal mucosa edematous due to increased estrogen resulting in nasal stuffiness and nosebleeds; gingival tissue hypertrophy related to increase in estrogen | Pallor in mucosa may be anemia; edema in mucosa tissue may be inflammation or infection |
| Chest and lungs<br><br>Breasts and nipples<br>  Contour and size<br>  Presence of lumps<br>  Secretions | Should be no difference during pregnancy—refer to Ch 11 Assessment<br>Size increases noticeable during first 20 weeks; become modular; tingling sensation may be felt during first and third trimester; breasts feel heavy;<br>Darker pigmentation of nipple and aerola;<br>Colostrum secretions after 12 weeks;<br>Secondary areola appears at 20 weeks, characterized by series of washed-out spots surrounding primary areola;<br>Old striae marks may be present in multiparas | Refer to Ch 11, "Assessment," Skill 11.11<br>Redness, heat, tender, cracked or fissured nipples (infection); "pigskin" or orange peel appearance, nipple retraction, swelling, hardness (carcinoma)<br>Secretions, other than colostrum |
| Heart | Palpitations during pregnancy may occur due to sympathetic nervous system disturbance;<br>Short systolic murmurs that increase in held expiration are normal due to increased volume | Enlargement, thrills, thrusts, gross irregularity or skipped beats, gallop rhythm or extra sounds could indicate cardiac disease |
| Abdomen | Flat, rounded abdomen; progressive enlargement due to pregnancy;<br>*Linea nigra* (black line of pregnancy along midline of abdomen)<br>Primiparas: coincidentally with growth of fundus<br>Multiparas: after 13–15 weeks' gestation | |
| Fundal height in centimeters (fingerbreadths less accurate): measure from symphysis pubis to top of fundus | Fundus palpable slightly above symphysis pubis at 10–12 weeks<br>Halfway between symphysis and umbilicus at 16 weeks<br>Umbilicus at 20–22 weeks of fundus | |
| Fetal Heart Rate by quadrant, location, and rate. Refer to Skill 9.12. | 120–160<br>110–160 beats per minute<br>May be heard with Doppler at 10–12 weeks gestation; with fetoscope at 17–20 weeks | Decreased: indicates fetal distress with possible cord prolapse or cord compression<br>Accelerated: initial sign of fetal hypoxia<br>Absent: may indicate fetal demise |
| Fetal movement<br><br>Ballottement<br>Determine fetal position, using Leopold's maneuvers: Complete external palpations of the abdomen to determine fetal position, lie, presentation, and engagement<br>First maneuver: to determine part of fetus presenting into pelvis<br>Second maneuver: to locate the back, arms, and legs: fetal heart heard best over fetal back | Trained examiner should be able to feel fetal movement after 18th week<br>Tapping the uterus sharply during the 4th–5th month resulting in the fetus rising and then returning to the original position<br>Vertex presentation<br>Third maneuver: to determine part of fetus in fundus<br>Fourth maneuver: to determine degree of cephalic flexion and engagement | |

| Normal Findings during Pregnancy | Abnormal Findings during Pregnancy |
|---|---|

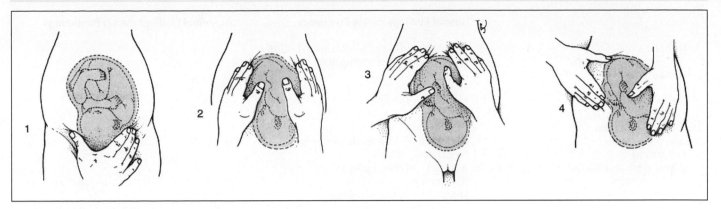

● Steps of Leopold's maneuvers.

| | Normal Findings during Pregnancy | Abnormal Findings during Pregnancy |
|---|---|---|
| Pelvis and Perineum<br>Refer to Skill 9.2 | <u>1–4 weeks gestation</u>: enlargement in anteroposterior diameter<br><u>4–8 weeks</u>: softening of cervix (Goodell's sign), softening or isthmus of uterus (Hegar's sign); cervix takes on bluish color (Chadwick's sign)<br>8–12 weeks: vagina and cervix appears bluish violet in color (Chadwick's sign)<br>External genital: in multiparas labia majora loose and pigmented; urinary and vaginal orifices visible and appropriately located<br>Vagina: in multiparas, vaginal folds smooth and flattened; may have episiotomy scar<br>Cervix: in multiparas, cervical os allows insertion of one fingertip | Absence of Goodell's sign: inflammatory condition, carcinoma |
| | Pelvic Measurements:<br>Internal measurements: Diagonal conjugate at least 11.5 cm<br>Obstetric conjugate estimated by subtracting 1.5–2 cm from diagonal conjugate<br>Mobility of coccyx; external intertuberosity diameter > 9 cm | Deviations in pelvic measurements may indicate that vaginal birth may not be possible<br>Disproportion of pubic arch<br><br>Fixed or malposition of coccyx |
| Reflexes<br>Refer to Skill 9.3 | Normal and symmetrical | Hyperactivity, clonus would be present in pregnancy induced hypertension |

## Assessment of Fetal Well Being

| | Normal Findings during Pregnancy | Abnormal Findings during Pregnancy |
|---|---|---|
| Evaluate lab findings<br>Complete Blood Count (CBC)<br>Hemoglobin (Hgb)<br>Hematocrit (HCT)<br><br>White Blood Cell Count (5,00–12,00/uL)<br>Red Blood Cell Count<br>Urinalysis: sugar, protein, albumin<br><br><br>Glucose | <br><br>12–16 g/dL<br>38%–47%; physiologic anemia (pseudoanemia) may occur<br>Elevations in pregnancy and labor are normal<br>No alteration<br>Normal color and specific gravity<br>Negative for protein, red blood cells, white blood cells, casts<br>Negative or small amount of glycosuria may occur in pregnancy | <br><br><br><br><br><br><br>Positive for sugar: may indicate subclinical or gestational diabetes<br>Proteinuria between 300 mg/L and 1 G (1+–2+ dipstick indicates mild pregnancy induced hypertension) |

*(continued)*

## TABLE 9–1 ANTEPARTAL ASSESSMENT (*continued*)

| | Normal Findings during Pregnancy | Abnormal Findings during Pregnancy |
|---|---|---|
| Rubella titer | Hemagglutination: inhibition (HAI) test –1:10 indicates immunity | |
| Hepatitis B screen | Negative | |
| HIV | Negative | |
| Syphilis test | Non reactive | |
| Gonorrhea culture | Negative | |
| Illicit drug screen | Negative | |
| Sickle cell screen | For those of African descent—negative | |
| Pap smear | Negative | |
| Blood type and Rh factor | A variety of blood groupings | |
| | Rh positive | If Rh negative, father's blood should be typed |
| | Does not require RhoGam | If Rh positive, titers should be followed; possible RhoGAM at termination of pregnancy. Refer to Skill 9.4. |
| Group B Streptococcus—Test Either cultured (35–37 weeks gestation) or new (2007) FDA approved IDI-Strep B provides results in one hour | Strep not present | If strep present, woman is given four hours of antibiotic treatment during labor (penicillin or ampicillin) |

**Assess for Signs of Labor**

| | | |
|---|---|---|
| Lightening and dropping (the descent of the presenting part into the pelvis) | Several days to 2 weeks before onset of labor | No lightening or dropping: may indicate disproportion between fetal presenting part and maternal pelvis |
| | Multipara: may not occur until onset of labor | |
| | Relief of shortness of breath and increase in frequency | |
| Assess for expulsion of mucus plug from the cervix; assess for bloody show | Usually expelled from cervix prior to onset of labor; Clear, pinkish, or blood-tinged vaginal discharge that occurs as cervix begins to dilate and efface | |
| Assess for ruptured membranes; Refer to Skill 9.11 | | |
| Time of rupture | Before, during, or after onset of labor | Breech presentation: frank meconium or meconium staining |
| Color of amniotic fluid | Clear, straw color | Greenish-brown: indicates meconium has passed from fetus, possible fetal distress |
| | | Yellow-stained: fetal hypoxia 36 hours or more prior to rupture of membrane of hemolytic disease |
| Quantity | Normal is 500 to 1000 mL rarely expelled at one time | Polyhydramnios—excessive amniotic fluid over 2000 mL |
| | | Observe newborn for congenital anomalies: craniospinal malformation, oro-gastriointestinal anomalies. |
| | | Down's syndrome, and congenital heart defects |
| | | Oligohydramnios—minimal amniotic fluid, less than 500 mL |
| | | Observe newborn for malformation of ear, genitourinary tract anomalies, and renal agenesis. |
| Odor of fluid | No odor | Odor may indicate infection: deliver within 24 hours |
| Assessment of Fetal Well Being | | Hypertensive disorder, Diabetes, Renal or Heart disease, are among conditions that may warrant diagnostic testing for fetal well being in the third trimester: |
| | | Amniocentesis: Refer to Skill 9.5 |
| | | Nonstress Testing (NST): Refer to Skill 9.6 |

| | Normal Findings during Pregnancy | Abnormal Findings during Pregnancy |
|---|---|---|
| | | Contraction Stress Test (CST): Refer to Skill 9.7<br>Biophysical Profile: Refer to Skill 9.8<br>Biophysical Profile Scoring: Refer to Skill 9.9 |
| Evaluate fundal height | Drop around 38th week: sign of fetus engaging in birth canal<br>Primipara: sudden drop<br>Multipara: slower, sometimes not until onset of labor | Large fundal growth: may indicate wrong dates, multiple pregnancy, hydatidiform mole, polyhydramnios, tumors<br>Small fundal growth: may indicate fetal demise, fetal anomaly, retarded fetal growth, abnormal presentation or lie, decreased amniotic fluid |

## TABLE 9–2  INTRAPARTAL ASSESSMENT

| | Normal Intrapartal Findings | Abnormal Intrapartal Findings |
|---|---|---|
| Take vital signs (TPR):<br>  Temperature<br>  Pulse | Temperature: 98–99°F;<br>Pulse: 80–90 bpm (pulse rates can increase 10 beats | Elevated temperature: infection<br>Increased pulse rates(excitement or anxiety; early shock; cardiac disease; drug use |
|   Respiration | Respirations: 16–24 breaths/min (pregnancy may induce a mild form of hyperventilation and thoracic breathing | Hyperventilation: anxiety/pain<br>Hyperventilation expected in transition phase<br>Decreased respirations with use of narcotics for pain<br>Marked tachypnea with respiration distress |
|   Blood pressure (BP) | Blood Pressure (BP)120/80 | Low BP with supine hypotension, hemorrhage, hypovolemia, shock, or drugs<br>High BP with pregnancy induced hypertension; pain |
| Pulse Oximeter<br>Fetal Heart Rate<br>Refer to Skill 9.12 | 95% or greater<br>120–160 | < 90% hypoxia, hypotension, hemorrhage |
| Weight | 25–35 lbs > than prepregnancy weight | > 35 lbs could be fluid retention, obesity, large infant, diabetes mellitus, pregnancy induced hypertension<br>< 15 lbs a small for gestation age infant, substance abuse, psychosocial problems |
| Fundus | 40 weeks just below xiphoid process | Uterine size not compatible with estimated date of birth: Small for gestational age (SGA); large for gestational age (LGA); hydramnios; multiple pregnancy; placental/fetal anomolies; malpresentations |
| Edema | Slight amount of dependent edema in lower extremities expected | Pitting edema of face, hands, legs, abdomen, sacral area indicative of pregnancy induced hypertension |
| Hydration | Normal skin turgor | Poor skin turgor with dehydration |

*(continued)*

## TABLE 9–2 INTRAPARTAL ASSESSMENT (*continued*)

| | Normal Intrapartal Findings | Abnormal Intrapartal Findings |
|---|---|---|
| Perineum | Same as antepartal | Varicosities of vulva, herpes lesions/ genital warts |
| Uterine contractions | Frequency: from start of one contraction to start of next<br>Duration: from beginning of contraction to time uterus begins to relax; 50–90 seconds<br>Intensity (strength of contraction): measured with monitoring device; Peak 25 mm Hg<br>End of labor may reach 50–75 mm Hg | Irregular contractions with long intervals between: indicates false labor<br>>90 second: uterine tetany; stop oxytocin if running<br><br>>75 mm Hg: uterine tetany or uterine rupture |
| Cervical dilatation (progressive cervical dilatation from size of fingertip to 10 cm; Refer to Skill 9.10 | First Stage: Latent phase (0–4 cm dilation); average 6.4 hrs<br>Active phase (4–8 cm)<br><br><br><br><br><br><br><br>Transition phase (8–10 cm): Length of time varies—may be 1–2 hours. Assess for bloody show<br>Observe for presence of nausea or vomiting<br>Evaluate urge to bear down; Beginning to bulge | Failure to dilate could be cervical rigidity, failure of presenting part to engage; cervical edema (pushing effort by woman before full dilatation and effacement of the cervix.<br>Prolonged time in any phase: may indicate poor fetal position, incomplete fetal flexion, cephalopelvic disproportion, or poor uterine contractions<br>Refer to Skill 9.15<br>Often uncontrolled Multipara: can cause precipitous delivery<br>"Panting" (can be controlled until safe delivery area established) |
| Cervical effacement (progressive thinning of cervix<br>Refer to Skill 9.10 | Occurs faster than dilatation; 0–100% | Failure to efface could be indicative of cervical rigidity, infections, scar tissue, failure of presenting part to engage; cephalopelvic disproportion |
| Fetal descent (progressive descent of fetal presenting part from station − 5 to + 4<br>Refer to Skill 9.10 | | |
| Membranes | Ruptured; if ruptured more than 12–24 hours before onset of labor | If not ruptured, doctor may perform amniotomy—refer to Skill 9.11 |
| Fetal status | Fetal heart rate (FHR) 110–160 bpm<br>Refer to Skill 9.11 Auscultation of Fetal Heart Rate | <110 or >160 may indicate fetal distress with cord compression or prolapse of cord; abnormal fetal patterns on fetal monitor (decreased variability, late decelerations, variable decelerations, absence of accelerations with fetal movement) |
| Evaluate fetal heart rate tracing<br>Refer to Skill 9.12 and Skill 9.13 | Short-term variability is present<br>Long-term variability ranges from 3–5 cycles/min | Absence of variability (no short term or long term present)<br>Severe variable decelerations (fetal heart rate <70 for longer than 30–45 seconds with decreasing variability) |

| | Normal Intrapartal Findings | Abnormal Intrapartal Findings |
|---|---|---|
| Deceleration | Early deceleration (10–20 beat drop) Recovery when acme contraction passes—often not serious | Monitor closely—distinguish from late deceleration (10–20 beat decrease with hypertonic contraction); leads to fetal distress |
| Variable deceleration; decrease in FHR, below 120/min | Mild; may be within normal parameters—continue to monitor | Cord compression—may result in fetal difficulty |
| Loss of beat-to-beat variation | If continues less than 15 minutes, no problem apparent | Late deceleration pattern occurs— monitor for hypertonic contraction; leads to total distress |
| Evaluate pain and anxiety | Medication required after dilated 4–5 cm unless using natural childbirth methods Refer to Skill 9.16 | Severe pain early in first stage of labor: inadequate prenatal teaching, back-ache due to position in bed, uterine tetany |
| Second Stage of Labor | Primipara: up to 2 hours Multipara: several minutes to 2 hours | >2 hours: increased risk of fetal brain damage and maternal exhaustion |
| Assess for presenting part | Vertex with ROA or LOA presentation | Occiput posterior, breech, face, or transverse lie |
| Assess caput (infant head) Multipara: move to delivery room when caput size of dime Primipara: move to delivery room when caput size of half dollar | Visible when bearing down during contraction | "Crowns" in room other than delivery room: delivery imminent (do not move client) |
| Assess fetal heart rate Bradycardia, drop of 20 beats/min below base line (less than 120 beats/min) Tachycardia, increase in FHR over 160 beats/min for 10 min | 120–160 bpm | Decreased: may indicate supine hypotensive syndrome (turn client on side and take again) Hemorrhage (check for other signs of bleeding: notify physician) Increased or decreased: may indicate fetal distress secondary to cord compression or prolapsed cord Refer to Skill 9.17 |
| Third stage (from delivery of baby to delivery of placenta) | Placental separation occurs within 30 minutes (usually 3–5 min) | Failure of placental separation Abnormality of uterus or cervix, weak, ineffectual uterine contraction, titanic contractions causing closure of cervix >3 hours: indicates retained placenta |
| Fourth stage (first hour postpartum) Assess vital signs every 15 minutes for 1 hour, every 30 minutes for 1 hour, every hour | | Mother in unstable condition (hemorrhage usual cause) Highest risk of hemorrhage in first postpartum hour |
| Temperature | | >37.5 degrees C: may indicate infection Slight elevation: due to dehydration from mouth breathing and NPO |
| Pulse | 60–100 bpm | Increased: may indicate pain or hemorrhage |
| Respirations | 12–20 breaths per minute | Increased: may indicate anxiety, pain, or posteclamptic condition |
| Blood pressure | 120–140/80 | Decreased: hemorrhage |
| Uterine assessment | Fundus firm, midline | Displaced to right indicates full bladder Refer to Skill 9.18 |
| Lochia assessment | Large amount, bright red | Excessive amounts may be caused by retained placental fragments |
| Comfort | Shivering response (tremors) | Refer to Skill 9.19 |
| APGAR scoring Refer to Table 9.3 and Skill 9.24 | Newborns who score 7–10 are considered free of immediate danger. | Newborns who score 4–6 are moderately depressed. Newborns who score 0–3 are severely depressed. |

## TABLE 9–3 POSTPARTAL (PP) MATERNAL ASSESSMENT

| | Normal PP Findings | Abnormal PP Assessment |
|---|---|---|
| Assess vital signs every hour for 4 hours, every 8 hours, and as needed | Pulse to normal range about third day | Decreased BP and increased pulse: probably postpartum hemorrhage<br>Elevated temperature >38 degrees C indicates possible infection<br>Temperature elevates when lactation occurs |
| Assess breasts and nipples daily<br>Refer to Skill 9.21 | Days 1–2: soft, intact, secreting colostrum<br>Days 2–3: engorged, tender, full, tight, painful<br><br>Day 3+: secreting milk<br>Increased pains as baby sucks: common in multiparas | Tenderness, heat, edema indicates engorgement<br>Sore or cracked (clean and dry nipples; decrease breastfeeding time; apply breast shield between feeding)<br>Milk does not "let down:" help client relax and decrease anxiety; give glass or wine or beer if not culturally, religiously, or otherwise contradicted<br>Reddened area could indicate mastitis<br>Palpable mass indicates mastitis<br>Engorgement indicates venous stasis |
| Nipples | Pigmented, intact, become erect when stimulated | Fissures, cracks, soreness can be caused by poor breastfeeding techniques; Inverted nipples will cause nipples not to erect when stimulated |
| Assess fundus every 15 minutes for 1 hour, every 8 hours for 48 hours, then daily<br>Refer to Skill 9.18 | Firm (like a grapefruit) in midline and at or slightly above umbilicus<br>Return to prepregnant size in 6 weeks: descending at rate of 1 fingerbreadth/day | Boggy fundus: immediately massage gently until firm; report to physician and observe closely; empty bladder; medicate with oxytocin if ordered<br>Fundus misplaced 1–2 fingerbreadths from midline: indicates full bladder (client must void or be catheterized) |
| Assess lochia every 15 minutes for 1 hour, every 8 hours for 48 hours, then daily<br>Refer to Skill 9.19 (in this document) | Scant to moderate amount, earthy odor, no clots | Clots indicates hemorrhage |
| Color | 1–3 days postpartum: dark red (rubra)<br>4–10 days postpartum: clear pink (serosa)<br>10–21 days postpartum: white, yellow brown (alba) | Failure to progress from rubra to serosa to alba indicates subinvolution |
| Quantity | Moderate amount, steadily decreases | No lochia: may indicate clot occluding cervical opening (support fundus; express clot) |
| Odor | None | Heavy bright red: indicates hemorrhage (massage fundus, give medication on order, notify physician<br>Spurts: may indicate cervical tear<br>Foul: may indicate infection |
| Assess perineum daily<br>Refer to Skill 9.20 | May have slight edema and bruising | Swelling or bruising: may indicate hematoma |
| Episiotomy | Episiotomy intact, no swelling, no discoloration | Redness, ecchymosis, discharge, or gaping stitches may indicate infection |
| Hemorrhoids | None present; could have a few small, nontender | Full, tender, red could indicate inflammation |

| | Normal PP Findings | Abnormal PP Assessment |
|---|---|---|
| Assess bladder every 4 hours | Voiding regularly (every 4 hours) with no pain; sufficient quantity | Not voiding: bladder may be full and displaced to one side, leading to increased lochia; inability to void could be urinary retention (catheterization may be necessary); symptoms of urgency, frequency, and dysuria could be infection |
| Assess bowels | Spontaneous bowel movement 2–3 days after delivery | Fear associated with pain from hemorrhoids, episiotomy or perineal trauma; no bowel movement could be constipation |
| Evaluate Rh-negative status | Client does not require RhoGAM | RhoGAM administered |
| Assess mother-infant bonding | Touching infant, talking to infant, talking about infant | Refuses to touch or hold infant |
| Assess extremities | Negative Homan's sign; no pain with palpation | Positive findings indicate thrombophlebitis |
| Evaluate Rh-negative status | Client does not require RhoGAM | RhoGAM administered |
| Material History: Definition of Terms<br>  Abortion: pregnancy loss before fetus is viable (usually <20 weeks or 500 g)<br>  Gravida: any pregnancy, including present one<br>  Primigravida: refers to first-time pregnancy | Multigravida: refers to second or any subsequent pregnancy<br>Para: past pregnancies that continued to viable age (20 weeks); infants may be alive or dead at birth<br>Primipara: refers to female who has delivered first viable infant; born either alive or dead | Nullipara: refers to female who has never carried pregnancy to viable age for fetus<br>Multipara: refers to female who has given birth to two or more viable infants; either alive or dead |

### TABLE 9–4 NEWBORN ASSESSMENT

| Assessment | Normal | Abnormal |
|---|---|---|
| Vital Signs<br>  Temperature<br>  Refer to Skill 9.25 | Rectal 97.8–99F; Axilla 97.5–99F | Elevated temperatures may be related to room too hot; too much clothing<br>Subnormal temperatures related to cold, sepsis, brainstem involvement<br>Differences of 2 degrees in either direction could indicate infection<br>Bradycardia indicative of severe asphysia or cardiac arrhythmia |
| Pulse | 120–160 bpm; will go higher if crying | Weak pulse related to decreased cardiac output<br>Tachycardia (>160) indicates infection, arrhythmia, central nervous system problems |
| Respirations | 30–60 breaths per min; transient tachypnea<br>Respiration movement irregular in rate and depth<br>Resonant chest (hollow sound on percussion)<br>Abdominal respirations | Tachypnea indicates pneumonia, respiratory distress syndrome (RDS)<br>Rapid, shallow breathing may occur if mother is given large doses of magnesium sulfate during labor for pregnancy induced hypertension (hypermagnesemia) |

*(continued)*

TABLE 9–4 **NEWBORN ASSESSMENT** (*continued*)

| Assessment | Normal | Abnormal |
|---|---|---|
| | | Respirations below 30 indicative of maternal anesthesia or analgesia during labor and delivery |
| | | Expiratory grunting, subcostal and substernal retractions, flaring of nostrils indicative of respiratory distress, apnea, or respiratory disorder |
| Blood pressure | At birth: 80–60/45–40; Day 10: 100/50 | Low BP indicates hypovolemia or shock |
| Assess cry | Lusty cry | Weak, groaning cry: possible neurological abnormality |
| | | High-pitched cry: newborn drug withdrawal (may occur 6–12 months after birth); hoarse or crowing inspirations; catlike cry: possible neurological or chromosomal abnormality |
| Assess weight | 5.5 lbs–8.14 lbs | < 8 lbs indicates Small for gestational age (SMA) or preterm |
| | | > 9 lbs indicates Large for gestation age (LGA) or infants born to diabetic mothers |
| | Normal weight loss during first 3 days up to 5–10% | Greater loss indicates feeding problems, decreased fluid intake, or losses due to meconium or urine |
| Skin Assessment<br>Refer to Skill 9.28<br>  Note skin color, pigmentation, turgor, and lesions | Pink | Cyanosis, pallor, beefy red |
| | Mongolian spots may occur over buttocks in dark skinned babies | Petechiae, ecchymoses, or purpuric spots: signs of possible hematologic disorder or clotting disorders |
| | Erythema | Impetigo (group A beta-hemolytic strep or staph |
| | Capillary hemangiomas on face or neck | Café au lait spots (patches of brown discoloration): possible sign of congenital neurological disorder |
| | | Raised capillary hemangiomas on areas other than face or neck |
| | Localized edema in presenting part | Edema of peritoneal wall |
| | | Poor skin turgor: indicates dehydration |
| | Cheesy white vernix | Yellow discolored vernix (meconium stained) |
| | Desquamation (peeling off) | |
| | Milia (small white pustules over nose and chin) | Impetigo neonatorum (small pustules with surrounding red areas) |
| | Jaundice after 24 hours; gone by second week | Jaundice at birth or within 12 hours |
| | Refer to Skill 9.29 | Dermal sinuses (opening to brain) |
| | | Holes along spinal column |
| | | Low hairline posteriorly: possible chromosomal abnormality |
| | | Sparse or spotty hair: congenital goiter or chromosomal abnormality |
| Note color of nails | Pink | Yellowing of nail beds (meconium stained) |
| Note muscle strength/tone | Strong/tremulous | Flaccid, convulsions, muscular twitching, hypertonicity |

| Assessment | Normal | Abnormal |
|---|---|---|
| Head and Neck Assessment<br>Note shape of head | Fontanels: anterior open until 18 months; posterior closed shortly after birth; is 3–4 cm long and 2–3 cm wide; diamond shaped<br>Posterior fontanel is 1–2 cm at birth and triangle shaped<br><br>Circumference is 1/4 size of body and 2 cm larger than the check circumference<br>Breech and cesarean newborn's heads are rounded and well shaped | Depressed fontanels indicate dehydration; closed or bulging indicate congenital anomalies; full or bulging indicate edema or increased ICP<br>Cephalohematoma that crosses the midline<br>Microcephaly and macrocephaly<br>Cephalohematoma trauma from birth lasts up to three weeks<br>Caput succedaneum occurring from a long labor and birth will disappear in about 1 week |
| Assess eyes | Slight edema of lids<br><br><br><br><br><br><br><br><br><br><br>Pupils equal and reactive to light by 3 weeks of age<br>Intermittent strabismus (occasional crossing of eyes)<br>Conjunctival or scleral hemorrhages<br>Symmetrical light reflex (light reflects off each eye in the same quadrant): sign of conjugate gaze<br>Blink reflex in response to light stimuli<br>Corneal reflex present<br>Vision: tracks objects to midline; fixed focus on objects at a distance; prefers faces and black and white to color<br>Cry usually tearless | Purulent discharge indicates infection<br>Lateral upward slope of eye with an inner epicanthal fold in infants not of Asian descent<br>Exophthalmos (bulging of eyeball): may be congenital anomaly, sign of congenital glaucoma or thyroid abnormality<br>Enophthalmos (recession of eyeball): may indicate damage to brain or cervical spine<br>Constricted pupil, unilateral dilated; unequal pupils due to CNS damage fixed pupil, nystagmus (rhythmic nonpurposeful movement of eyeball); continuous strabismus<br>Haziness of cornea<br>Absence of red reflex; asymmetrical light reflex<br>Blink reflex absent indicates CNS injury<br>Ulceration indicates herpes infection<br>Cataracts from congenital infection<br><br>Excessive tearing form plugged tear ducts; could be narcotic withdrawal |
| Note placement of ears, shape and position | The top of the ear should be on an imaginary line from the edge of the eye<br>Moro reflex with loud noises<br>Small, narrow, midline | Low-set ears: may indicate chromosomal or renal system abnormality<br>Unilateral Moro reflex indicates brachial palsy or fractured clavicle |
| Assess nose | Sneezes to clear nasal passageways<br>Nose breathers | Flat or broad bridge of nose seen in Down syndrome<br>Flaring nostrils indicates respiratory distress<br>Blockage of nares due to mucus or secretions<br>Refer to Skills 9.12 and 9.13<br>Thick, bloody nasal discharge if infection present |
| Assess mouth | Gag, swallowing, sucking reflexes present<br><br>Hard and soft palates intact<br><br>Esophagus intact; drooling in newborns | Absent of reflexes<br>Cleft lip, palate<br>Flat, white nonremovable spots (thrush)<br>Frequent vomiting: may indicate pyloric stenosis; esophageal atresia<br>Vomitus with bile: fecal vomiting<br>Profuse salivation: may indicate tracheoesophageal fistula |

*(continued)*

## TABLE 9–4 NEWBORN ASSESSMENT (*continued*)

| Assessment | Normal | Abnormal |
|---|---|---|
| | Tongue moves freely in all directions; pink color; noncoated | Lack of movement indicates neurologic damage<br>White cheesy coating indicates thrush |
| Assess neck | Short, straight, extra skin folds<br>Tonic neck reflex (Fencer's position) | Short neck in Turner syndrome<br>Distended neck veins<br>Fractured clavicle<br>Unusually short neck<br>Excess posterior cervical skin<br>Resistance to neck flexion |
| **Chest and Lung Assessment** | | |
| Assess chest | 2 cm smaller than head; wider than long; lower end of sternum may protrude<br>Bilateral expansion with no retractions | Funnel chest with congenital problems<br>Depressed sternum<br>Retractions, asymmetry of chest movements: indicates respiratory distress and possible pneumothorax |
| Assess lungs | Breath sounds louder in infants<br>Bronchial breath sounds bilaterally<br>Rales may indicate normal newborn atelectasis<br>Cough reflex absent until 2nd day | Thoracic breathing, unequal motion of chest, rapid grasping or grunting respirations, flaring nares<br>Deep sighing respirations<br>Grunt on expiration: possible respiratory distress |
| Breasts | Flat with symmetrical nipples<br>Engorgement occurs 3rd day; may have liquid discharge in full term newborns | Small for gestational age infants lack breast tissue |
| **Heart Assessment** | | |
| Assess the rate, rhythm, and murmurs of the heart | Rate: 100–160 at birth; stabilizes at 120–140<br>Regular rhythm<br>Murmurs: significance cannot usually be determined in newborn | Heart rate >200 or <100<br><br>Irregular rhythm<br>Dextrocardia, enlarged heart |
| **Abdomen and Gastrointestinal Tract Assessment** | | |
| Assess the abdomen | Prominent<br><br>No protrusion of umbilicus, however, protrusion may be seen in infants of African descent<br>Umbilical cord with one vein and two arteries; Soft granulation tissue at umbilicus; no bleeding; no bleeding Refer to Skill 9.26 | Distention of abdominal veins: possible portal vein obstruction<br>Umbilical hernia<br><br>One artery present in umbilical cord: may indicate other anomalies<br>Bleeding, redness or exudate indicates infection |
| Assess the gastrointestinal tract | Bowel sounds present<br>Liver 2 to 3 cm below right costal margin<br>Spleen tip palpable | Visible peristaltic waves<br>Increased pitch or frequency: intestinal obstruction<br>Decreased sounds: paralytic ileus<br>Distention of abdomen<br>Enlarged liver or spleen<br>Midline suprapubic mass: may indicate Hirschsprung's disease |
| Femoral pulses | Palpable<br>No bulges in inguinal area | Absent or diminished in coarctation of aorta<br>Inguinal hernia |
| **Genitourinary Tract Assessment** | | |
| Assess kidneys and bladder | May be able to palpate kidneys<br>Bladder percussed 1 to 4 cm above symphysis pubis<br>Voids at birth or within 3 hours | Enlarged kidney<br>Distended bladder; presence of any masses<br>Failure to void within 24–48 hours |

| Assessment | Normal | Abnormal |
|---|---|---|
| Assess the genitalia | Edema and bruising after delivery <br> Unusually large clitoris in females a short time after birth <br> Vaginal mucoid or bloody discharge may be present in the first week | Ambiguous genitalia (chromosomal abnormality) <br> Excessive vaginal bleeding indicates coagulation defect |
| Urethral orifice | Urethra opens on ventral surface of penile shaft <br> Refer to Skill 9.27 | Hypospadias (urethra opens on the inferior surface of the penis) <br> Epispadias (urethra opens on the dorsal surface of the penis) <br> Ulceration of urethral orifice <br> Hydroceles in males <br> Phimosis if still right after 3 months |
| Testes | Uncircumcised foreskin tight for 2 to 3 months <br> Testes in scrotal sac or inguinal canal | Enlarged testes indicates tumor <br> Small testes indicates Klinefelter syndrome or adrenal hyperplasia |
| **Spine and Extremities Assessment** | | |
| Assess the spine | Straight spine; slight lordosis; full term infant should hold head at 45-degree angle | Spina bifida, pilonidal sinus; scoliosis <br> Unable to hold head or floppy trunk indicates neurological problems |
| Assess extremities | Soft click with thigh rotation; should abduct to more than 60 degrees <br> Skin creases | Asymmetry of movement <br> Sharp click with thigh rotation: indicates possible congenital hip <br> Uneven major gluteal folds: indicates possible congenital hip <br> Polydactyly (extra digits on a hand or foot); syndactyly (webbing or fusion of fingers or toes) |
| | Feet in straight line; flat feet normal for first 3 months; some infants may have a positional clubfoot from position in utero | Talipes equinovarus (clubfoot) |
| Assess anus and rectum | Patent anus; passage of meconium within 48 hours after birth | Imperforate anus: no meconium |
| Reflexes | Rooting and sucking (turns in direction of stimulus to cheek or mouth—disappears about 4th–7th month <br> Palmar grasp (fingers grasp adult finger when palm is stimulated; goes away about 3rd to 4th month <br> Stepping (will step alternatively when held upright and one foot is touching a flat surface; disappears about 4 to 5 months <br> Babinski (fanning and extension of toes when sole of foot is stroked from heel across ball of foot; disappears at about 12 months | Poor sucking or fatigability in preterm <br> Absence of reflex in preterm, neurological involvement or depressed newborns <br> Neurological problems if response is asymmetrical <br> Neurological problems if response is asymmetrical <br><br> Low spinal cord defects if no response |

## TABLE 9–5 APGAR SCORING

| Sign | 0 | 1 | 2 |
|---|---|---|---|
| Heart rate | Absent | Slow (less than 100) | Over 100 |
| Respiratory effort | Absent | Slow, irregular | Good, crying |
| Muscle tone | Flaccid | Some flexion of extremities | Active motion |
| Reflex irritability | No response | Cry | Vigorous cry |
| Color | Blue, pale | Body pink, extremities blue | Completely pink |

APGAR scoring system is a method of evaluating a newborn's condition at 1 and 5 minutes after birth.
- Newborns who score 7–10 are considered free of immediate danger.
- Newborns who score 4–6 are moderately depressed.
- Newborns who score 0–3 are severely depressed.

Scores less than 7 at 5 minutes, repeat every 5 minutes for 20 minutes. Infant may be intubated unless 2 successive scores of 7 or more occur.

# Skill 9.2    Assisting with a Pelvic Examination

## Preparation

1. Ensure that the room is sufficiently warm by checking the room temperature and adjusting the thermostat if necessary. If overhead heat lamps are available, turn them on.
2. Explain the procedure to the woman. If she has never had a pelvic examination, show her the equipment to be used as part of the explanation. ➤Rationale: Explaining the procedure helps reduce anxiety and increase cooperation.
3. Ask the woman to empty her bladder and to remove clothing below the waist. ➤Rationale: An empty bladder promotes comfort during the internal examination.
4. Have padding on the stirrups. If stirrups are not padded, the woman may prefer to leave her shoes on during the procedure. ➤Rationale: Stirrups are usually padded to ease the pressure of the feet against the metal and to decrease the discomfort associated with the touch of the cold stirrups. If they are not padded, however, wearing shoes accomplishes the same purpose.
5. Give the woman a disposable drape or sheet to use during the exam. Ask her to sit at the end of the examining table with the drape opened across her lap.
6. Position the woman in the lithotomy position with her thighs flexed and adducted. Place her feet in the stirrups. Her buttocks should extend slightly beyond the edge of the examining table.
7. Drape the woman with the sheet, leaving a flap so that the perineum can be exposed. ➤Rationale: This position provides the exposure necessary to conduct the examination effectively. The drape helps preserve the woman's sense of dignity and privacy.

## Equipment

- Vaginal specula of various sizes, warmed with water or on a heating pad prior to insertion
- Sterile gloves
- Water-soluble lubricant
- Materials for Pap smear or ThinPrep Pap test and cultures
- Good light source

*Note:* Lubricant may alter the results of tests and cultures and is not used during the speculum examination. Its use is reserved for the bimanual examination.

## Procedure

Sterile Gloves

1. The examiner dons gloves for the procedure. Explain each part of the procedure as the certified nurse-midwife, nurse practitioner, or physician performs it.
2. Let the woman know that the examiner begins with an inspection of the external genitalia. The speculum is then inserted to allow visualization of the cervix and vaginal walls and to obtain specimens for testing. After the speculum is withdrawn, the exam-

### CLINICAL ALERT

With the examiner's consent (obtained beforehand), offer the woman a hand mirror so that she can watch all or part of the examination. This practice removes the "mystery" from the procedure and enables the woman to become familiar with the appearance of her body.

iner performs a bimanual examination of the internal organs using the fingers of one hand inserted in the woman's vagina while the other hand presses over the woman's uterus and ovaries. The final step of the procedure is generally a rectal examination.

3. Ask the woman to breathe slowly and regularly and to use any method she finds effective in helping her to remain relaxed.

4. Let her know when the examiner is ready to insert the speculum and ask her to bear down. ➤*Rationale: Relaxation helps decrease muscle tension. Bearing down helps open the vaginal orifice and relaxes the perineal muscles.*

5. After the speculum is withdrawn, lubricate the examiner's fingers prior to the bimanual examination. ➤*Rationale: Lubrication decreases friction and eases insertion of the examiner's fingers.*

6. After the examiner has completed the examination and moved away from the woman, move to the end of the examination table and face the woman. Cover her with the drape. Apply gentle pressure to her knees and encourage her to move toward the head of the table. Assist her to remove her feet from the stirrups, then offer your hand to her and assist her to sit up. ➤*Rationale: Assistance is important because the lithotomy position is an awkward one and many women, but especially those women who are pregnant, obese, or older, may find it difficult to get out of the stirrups.*

7. Provide her with tissues to wipe the lubricant from her perineum. ➤*Rationale: Vaginal secretions and lubricant may be discharged from the vagina when the woman sits upright.*

8. Provide the woman with privacy while she dresses. Be sure that she is not dizzy and that she is standing or sitting safely before leaving the room. ➤*Rationale: Lying supine may cause postural hypotension.*

# Skill 9.3   Assessing Deep Tendon Reflexes and Clonus

## Preparation

1. Explain the procedure, the indications for its use, and the information that will be obtained.

2. Most nurses check the patellar reflex and one other such as the biceps, triceps, or brachioradialis. ➤*Rationale: DTRs are assessed to gain information about CNS irritability secondary to preeclampsia and to assess the effects of magnesium sulfate if the woman is receiving it.*

## Equipment

• Percussion hammer

## Clinical Alert

If a percussion hammer is not available, you may use the side of your hand to elicit DTRs.

## Procedure

1. Elicit reflexes.
   • Patellar reflex. Position the woman with her legs hanging over the edge of the bed (feet should not be touching the floor). Briskly strike the patellar tendon, which is located just below the patella. Normal response is extension or a thrusting forward of the foot. ➤*Rationale: In an inpatient setting, the patellar reflex is often assessed while the woman lies supine. Flex her knees slightly and support them.*
   • Biceps reflex. Flex the woman's arm 45 degrees at the elbow and place your thumb on the biceps tendon. Allow your fingers to hold the biceps muscle. Strike your thumb in a slightly downward motion and assess the response. Normal response is flexion of the arm.

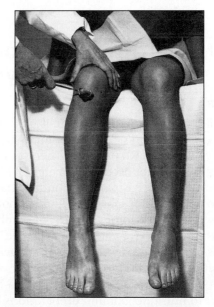
● Correct sitting position for eliciting the patellar reflex.

   • Triceps reflex. Flex the woman's arm up to 90 degrees and allow her hand to hang against the side of her body. Using the percussion hammer, strike the triceps tendon just above the elbow. Normal response is contraction of the muscle, which causes extension of the arm.
   • Brachioradialis reflex. Flex the woman's arm slightly and lay it on your forearm with her hand slightly pronated. Using the percussion hammer, strike the brachioradialis

tendon, which is found about 1 to 2 inches above the wrist. Normal response is pronation of the forearm and flexion of the elbow. ➤*Rationale: The correct position causes the muscle to be slightly stretched. Then when the tendon is stretched, with a tap the muscle should contract. Correct positioning and technique are essential to elicit the reflex.*

2. Grade reflexes. Reflexes are graded on a scale of 0 to 4+, as follows:

    4+ Hyperactive; very brisk, jerky, or clonic response; abnormal

    3+ Brisker than average; may not be abnormal

    2+ Average response; normal

    1+ Diminished response; low normal

    No response; abnormal

    ➤*Rationale: Normally reflexes are 1+ or 2+. With CNS irritation, hyperreflexia may be present; with high magnesium levels, reflexes may be diminished or absent.*

3. Assess for clonus. With the woman's knee flexed and the leg supported, vigorously dorsiflex the foot, maintain the dorsiflexion momentarily, and then release. With a normal response, the foot returns to its normal position of plantar flexion. Clonus is present if the foot "jerks" or taps against the examiner's hand. If so, record the number of taps or beats

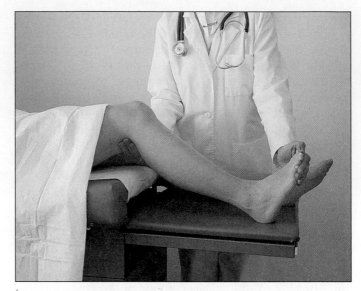

● To elicit clonus, sharply dorsiflex the foot.

of clonus. ➤*Rationale: Clonus occurs with more pronounced hyperreflexia and indicates CNS irritability.*

4. Report and record findings. For example: DTRs 21, no clonus or DTRs 41, 2 beats clonus.

---

# Skill 9.4    Administration of Rh Immune Globulin (RhoGAM, HypRho-D)

## Preparation

1. Confirm that Rh immune globulin is indicated by checking the woman's prenatal or intrapartal record to verify that she is Rh negative. Then confirm that sensitization has not occurred—maternal indirect Coombs' negative. Postpartally, confirm that the baby is Rh positive but not sensitized (direct Coombs' negative) and that the mother's indirect Coombs' is negative. Rh immune globulin is not indicated if the infant is Rh negative, too. ➤*Rationale: Rh immune globulin is only indicated for Rh-negative, unsensitized women.*

2. Confirm that the woman does not have a history of allergies to immune globulin preparations by checking entries on medication allergies in her chart and by asking her whether she has ever had any allergic reactions to medications, globulins, or blood products. ➤*Rationale: Rh immune globulin is made from the plasma portion of blood. Allergic reactions are possible.*

3. Explain the purpose and procedure. Have a consent form signed if required by agency policy. ➤*Rationale: Many agencies require separate consent for the administration of Rh immune globulin because it is a blood product. The woman should clearly understand the purpose of the Rh immune globulin, its rationale, the administration procedure, and any related risks. Generally*

the primary side effects are redness and tenderness at the injection site and allergic responses.

## Equipment

- Rh immune globulin, which is obtained from the blood bank or pharmacy according to agency protocol. Lot numbers for the drug and the crossmatch should be the same.
- Syringe and IM needle

## Procedure

1. Confirm the woman's identity and administer one vial of 300 mg Rh immune globulin IM in the deltoid muscle.

2. An immune globulin microdose is used after miscarriage, elective abortion, ectopic pregnancy, or molar pregnancy occurring within the first 12 weeks' gestation. Antepartally, the Rh immune globulin is generally given within 3 hours but not longer than 72 hours of the event.

3. If a larger bleed is suspected at birth (as in cases of severe abruptio placentae), additional doses may be administered at one time using multiple sites or at regular intervals as long as all doses are given within 72 hours of childbirth. ➤*Rationale: The normal 300-mcg*

*dose provides passive immunity following exposure of up to 15 mL of transfused RBCs or 30 mL of fetal blood.*

4. Provide opportunities for the woman to ask questions and express concerns. ➤*Rationale: Many women, especially primigravidas, are not aware of the risks for an Rh-positive fetus of a sensitized Rh-negative mother. They need to understand the importance of receiving Rh immune globulin for each pregnancy to ensure continued protection.*

5. Chart according to agency policy. Most agencies chart lot number, route, dose, and client education.

# Skill 9.5   Assisting during Amniocentesis

## Preparation

1. Explain the procedure and the indications for it and reassure the woman.

2. Determine whether an informed consent form has been signed. If not, verify that the woman's doctor has explained the procedure and ask her to sign a consent form. ➤*Rationale: It is the physician's responsibility to obtain informed consent. The woman's signature indicates her awareness of the risks and gives her consent to the procedure.*

## Equipment

- 22-gauge spinal needle with stylet
- 10- and 20-mL syringes
- 1% lidocaine (Xylocaine)
- Povidone-iodine (Betadine)
- Three 10-mL test tubes with tops (amber colored or covered with tape) ➤*Rationale: Amniotic fluid must be protected from the light to prevent breakdown of bilirubin.*

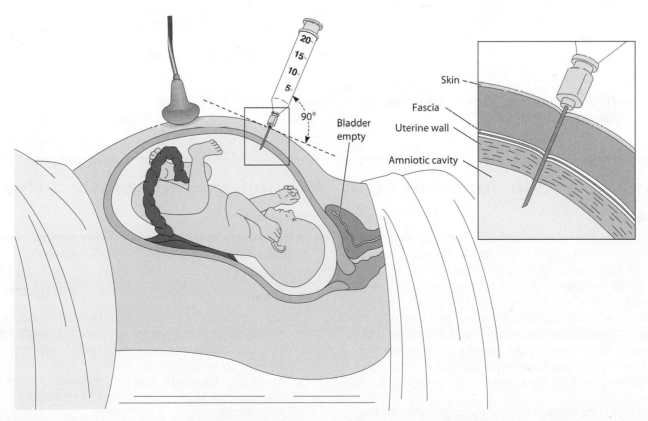

● Amniocentesis.

## Procedure

### Sterile Gloves

1. Obtain baseline vital signs, including maternal blood pressure (BP), pulse, respirations, temperature, and fetal heart rate (FHR) before the procedure begins.
2. Monitor BP, pulse, respirations, and FHR every 15 minutes during the procedure. ➤*Rationale: Baseline information is essential to detect any changes in maternal or fetal status that might be related to the procedure.*
3. The physician uses real-time ultrasound to determine the location of the placenta and to locate a pocket of amniotic fluid. Provide gel for the ultrasound and assist with the procedure as needed.
4. Cleanse the woman's abdomen. ➤*Rationale: Cleansing the abdomen prior to needle insertion helps decrease the risk of infection.*
5. The physician dons gloves, inserts the needle into the identified pocket of fluid, and withdraws a sample.
6. Obtain the test tubes from the physician. Label the tubes with the woman's correct identification and send to the lab with the appropriate lab slips.
7. Monitor the woman and reassess her vital signs.
   - Determine the woman's BP, pulse, respirations, and the FHR.
   - Palpate the woman's fundus to assess for uterine contractions.
   - Monitor her using an external fetal monitor for 20 to 30 minutes after the amniocentesis.
   - Determine a treatment course to counteract any supine hypotension and to increase venous return and cardiac output. ➤*Rationale: Monitoring maternal and fetal status postprocedure provides information about response to the procedure and helps detect any complications such as inadvertent fetal puncture.*

8. Assess the woman's blood type and determine any need for Rh immune globulin.
9. Administer Rh immune globulin if indicated. ➤*Rationale: To prevent Rh sensitization in an Rh-negative woman, Rh immune globulin is administered prophylactically following amniocentesis.*
10. Instruct the woman to report any of the following changes or symptoms to her primary caregiver:
    - Unusual fetal hyperactivity or, conversely, any lack of fetal movement
    - Vaginal discharge—either clear drainage or bleeding
    - Uterine contractions or abdominal pain
    - Fever or chills
    ➤*Rationale: These are signs of potential complications and require further evaluation.*
11. Encourage the woman to engage only in light activities for 24 hours and to increase her fluid intake. ➤*Rationale: Decreased maternal activity helps decrease uterine irritability and increase uteroplacental circulation. Increased fluid intake helps replace amniotic fluid through the uteroplacental circulation.*
12. Complete the client record. Record the type of procedure, the date and time, and the name of the physician who performed the procedure. Also record the maternal-fetal response, disposition of the specimen, and discharge teaching.

# Skill 9.6   Assessment of Fetal Well-Being: Nonstress Test (NST)

## Preparation

1. Identify the woman, comparing the name and medical record number appearing in the chart against identification arm band information.
2. Verify the correct procedure as ordered by the physician/CNM for the correct woman.
3. Explain the procedure, purpose, and implications of the procedure to the woman and her support person. The purpose of the nonstress test is to assess fetal well-being by monitoring fetal activity and concurrent fetal heart rate (FHR) response to fetal activity.
4. Allow time for and encourage any questions the woman and her support person may have. Reinforce any teaching as necessary.

## Equipment

- External fetal heart rate and contraction monitors (ultrasound transducer and tocodynamometer)
- Ultrasonic gel

## Procedure

1. Have the woman lie in a lateral position, comfortably with pillows for support if needed. ➤*Rationale: This position displaces the uterus to prevent compression of the vena cava and/or aorta.*
2. Apply fetal heart rate and contraction monitors as instructed in Skill 9.12 External Electronic Fetal Monitoring.
3. Monitor the fetal heart rate and any contraction activity for at least 20 minutes. Note any fetal

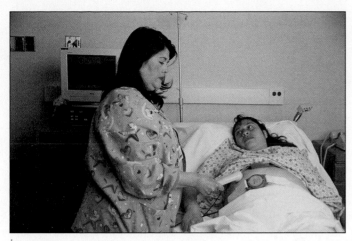

● Fetal acoustic stimulation testing.

movement. ➤*Rationale: Accelerations in fetal heart rate should occur in response to fetal movement and spontaneously.*

4. If there are no accelerations in 20 minutes, continue monitoring 20 more minutes. ➤*Rationale: The fetus*

*may be in a sleep cycle in which there are usually no heart rate accelerations.*

5. If there are no accelerations or fetal movement during the testing period, stimulation of the fetus may be necessary (acoustic stimulation, maternal intake of cold liquids).
6. The NST is considered "reactive" (normal) if there are two accelerations within a 20-minute period during a maximum of 60 minutes of testing. Each acceleration will peak at least 15 beats per minute (bpm) above the baseline and last at least 15 or more seconds at its base.
7. The NST is considered "nonreactive" if there are less than two accelerations as described above.
8. If the test is considered nonreactive (nonreassuring), further testing may be needed.

**Documentation**

Document the procedure, results, any intervention(s) needed, and any need for further testing in the woman's medical record and notify the ordering physician/CNM of the results of the NST per agency policy.

# Skill 9.7 Assessment of Fetal Well-Being: Contraction Stress Test (CST)

## Preparation

1. Identify the woman, comparing the name and medical record number appearing in the chart against identification arm band information.
2. Verify the correct procedure as ordered by the physician/CNM for the correct woman.
3. Explain the procedure, purpose, and implications of the procedure to the woman and support person. The purpose of the CST is to determine fetal heart rate response to contractions.
4. Ensure privacy.
5. Allow time for and encourage any questions the woman and her support person may have. Reinforce any teaching as necessary.

## Equipment

- External fetal heart rate and contraction monitors (ultrasound transducer and tocodynamometer)
- Ultrasonic gel

## Procedure

1. Position the woman in a semi-Fowler's or side-lying position. ➤*Rationale: The uterus should be displaced and not compressing the vena cava and/or aorta.*
2. Apply EFM transducers and obtain a minimum of 20-minute tracing.
3. Assess maternal vital signs.

4. Contact the physician before beginning the CST if any of the following are noted:
    a. Three or more palpable contractions that last 40 seconds or more (a spontaneous CST)
    b. A reactive nonstress test (a CST may not be needed)
    c. Late decelerations
5. Production of uterine contractions is conducted by either nipple stimulation or infusion of Pitocin intravenously.

**Nipple stimulation:** Instruct the woman to massage, roll, or lightly brush her fingertips across the nipple of one breast over her clothing for 2 minutes. Rest for 2 to 5 minutes. Repeat on the opposite breast. The complete cycle is repeated up to four times. Nipple stimulation should be stopped during a contraction, then started again after the contraction ends to avoid hyperstimulation of the uterus. Record each nipple stimulation on the monitor strip.

If no contractions occur, begin stimulation of both nipples for 2 minutes. Rest for 2 minutes. Repeat. Bilateral stimulation may be used for 10 minutes. Notify the physician if inadequate contractions are achieved after nipple stimulation cycles are completed.

The CST is complete when three contractions in 10 minutes have occurred. Contractions should be palpable and last 40 to 60 seconds.

When three contractions lasting 40 to 60 seconds occur in a 10-minute period, stop nipple stimulation and interpret the FHR pattern.

**Pitocin infusion (oxytocin challenge test):** Initiate intravenous Pitocin infusion per agency policy for Pitocin induction of labor. Stop Pitocin infusion when three palpable contractions have occurred in 10 minutes, lasting 40 to 60 seconds.

### Documentation

Document the procedure, results, and any intervention(s) needed in the woman's medical record and notify the ordering physician/CNM of the results of the NST per agency policy.

> ### TEST INTERPRETATION
>
> Negative (reassuring): No late decelerations.
>
> Positive (nonreassuring): Late decelerations occur with at least two of the three contractions.
>
> Suspicious (equivocal): Late deceleration occurs with one of three contractions.
>
> Hyperstimulation: Greater than five contractions in 10 minutes or contractions lasting longer than 90 seconds.

# Skill 9.8   Assessment of Fetal Well-Being: Biophysical Profile (BPP)

### Preparation

1. Identify the woman, comparing the name and medical record number appearing in the chart against identification arm band information.
2. Verify the correct procedure as ordered by the physician/CNM for the correct woman.
3. Explain the procedure, purpose, and implications of the procedure to the woman and her support person.
4. Allow time for and encourage any questions the woman and her support person may have. Reinforce any teaching as necessary.

### Equipment

- Ultrasound equipment
- Ultrasonic gel

### Procedure

This is performed by an ultrasonographer or RN who has had extensive education in ultrasonography for the purpose of obstetric ultrasound surveillance.

1. Ultrasound scanning is performed to assess for the following
   a. Fetal breathing movement
   b. Fetal movement
   c. Fetal tone (extension and flexion) of extremities
   d. Amniotic fluid volume
   e. Nonstress test
2. A nonstress test is performed using either an external fetal monitor or ultrasound equipment.
3. A score of 2 is given to each normal finding and a score of 0 is given to each abnormal finding for a maximum total score of 10. Scores of 8 to 10 are considered normal.

### Documentation

Document the procedure, results, and any intervention(s) needed in the woman's medical record and notify the ordering physician/CNM of the results of the BPP per agency policy.

### TABLE 9–6  CRITERIA FOR BIOPHYSICAL PROFILE SCORING

| Component | Normal (score = 2) | Abnormal (score = 0) |
|---|---|---|
| Fetal breathing movements | ≥ 1 episode of rhythmic breathing lasting ≥30 sec within 30 min | ≤ 30 sec of breathing in 30 min |
| Gross body movements | ≥ 3 discrete body or limb movements in 30 min (episodes of active continuous movement considered as single movement) | ≤ 2 movements in 30 min |
| Fetal tone | ≥ 1 episode of extension of a fetal extremity with return to flexion, or opening or closing of hand | No movements or extension/flexion |
| Amniotic fluid volume | Single vertical pocket >2 cm | Largest single vertical pocket ≤ 2 cm |
| Nonstress test | ≥ 2 accelerations of ≥ 15 beats/min for ≥ 15 sec in 20 min | 0 or 1 acceleration in 20 min |

# Skill 9.9 Performing an Intrapartal Vaginal Examination

## Preparation

1. Explain the procedure, the indications for the exam, what the exam may feel like, and that it may cause discomfort.
2. Assess for latex allergies.
3. Position the woman with her thighs flexed and abducted. Instruct her to put the heels of her feet together. Drape the woman with a sheet, leaving a flap to access the perineum. ➤*Rationale: This position provides access to the woman's perineum. The drape ensures privacy.*
4. Encourage the woman to relax her muscles and legs. ➤*Rationale: Relaxation decreases muscle tension and increases comfort.*
5. Inform the woman prior to touching her. Be gentle.

### BEFORE THE PROCEDURE Test for Fluid Leakage

If fluid leakage has been reported or noted, use Nitrazine test tape and a Q-tip with a slide for the fern test before performing the exam.

- The fern test is done by inserting the swab in the pool of fluid in the posterior vagina and then applying the fluid to a slide. ➤*Rationale: As long as lubricant has not been used, Nitrazine tape registers a change in pH if amniotic fluid is present.*

## Equipment

- Clean disposable gloves if membranes not ruptured
- Sterile gloves if membranes ruptured
- Lubricant
- Nitrazine test tape
- Slide
- Sterile cotton-tipped swab (Q-tip)

## Procedure

Clean Gloves (Sterile if membranes ruptured)

1. Pull glove on dominant hand. ➤*Rationale: A single glove is worn when membranes are intact. If a sterile exam is needed, both hands will be gloved with sterile gloves.*
2. Using your gloved hand, position the hand with the wrist straight and the elbow tilted downward. Insert your well-lubricated second and index fingers of the gloved hand gently into the vagina until they touch the cervix. Use care when positioning your hand. ➤*Rationale: This position allows the fingertips to point toward the umbilicus and find the cervix.*
3. If the woman verbalizes discomfort, acknowledge it and apologize. Pause for a moment and allow her to relax before progressing. ➤*Rationale: This validates the woman's discomfort and helps her feel more in control.*

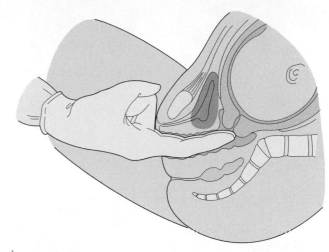

● To gauge cervical dilatation, place the index and middle fingers against the cervix and determine the size of the opening. Before labor begins, the cervix is long (approximately 2.5 cm), the sides feel thick, and the cervical canal is closed, so an examining finger cannot be inserted. During labor, the cervix begins to dilate, and the size of the opening progresses from 1 to 10 cm in diameter.

4. To determine the status of labor progress, perform the vaginal examination during and between contractions. ➤*Rationale: Cervical effacement, dilatation, and fetal station are affected by the presence of a contraction.*
5. Palpate for the opening, or a depression, in the cervix. Estimate the diameter of the depression to identify the amount of dilatation. ➤*Rationale: This allows determination of effacement and dilatation.*
6. Determine the status of the fetal membranes by observing for leakage of amniotic fluid. If fluid is expressed, test for amniotic fluid.
7. Palpate the presenting part. ➤*Rationale: Determining the presenting part is necessary to assess the position of the fetus and to evaluate fetal descent.*
8. Assess the fetal descent and station by identifying the position of the posterior fontanelle.
9. Record findings on the woman's chart and on the fetal monitor strip if a fetal monitor is being used.

> ### CLINICAL ALERT
>
> Use nonlatex gloves if the woman has a latex allergy.

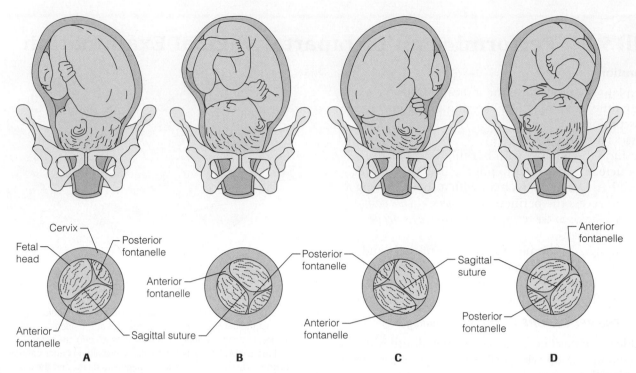

● Palpating the presenting part (portion of the fetus that enters the pelvis first). **A,** Left occiput anterior (LOA). The occiput (area over the occipital bone on the posterior part of the fetal head) is in the left anterior quadrant of the woman's pelvis. When the fetus is LOA, the posterior fontanelle (located just above the occipital bone and triangular in shape) is in the upper left quadrant of the maternal pelvis. **B,** Left occiput posterior (LOP). The posterior fontanelle is in the lower left quadrant of the maternal pelvis. **C,** Right occiput anterior (ROA). The posterior fontanelle is in the upper right quadrant of the maternal pelvis. **D,** Right occiput posterior (ROP). The posterior fontanelle is in the lower right quadrant of the maternal pelvis.

*Note:* The anterior fontanelle is diamond shaped. Because of the roundness of the fetal head, only a portion of the anterior fontanelle can be seen in each of the views, so it appears to be triangular in shape.

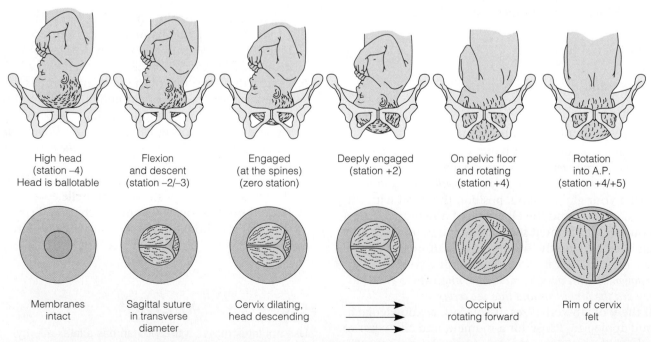

● The fetal head progressing through the pelvis. Bottom: The changes that will be detected on palpation of the occiput through the cervix while doing a vaginal examination.

*Note:* From Myles, M. F. (1975). Textbook for midwives (p. 246). Edinburgh, Scotland: Churchill-Livingstone.

# Skill 9.10    Assisting with Amniotomy (AROM: Artificial Rupture of Membranes)

## Preparation

1. Identify the woman, comparing the name and medical record number appearing in the chart against identification arm band information.
2. Verify the correct procedure for the correct woman.
3. Explain the procedure, purpose, and implications of the procedure to the woman and support person. *➤Rationale: Anticipatory guidance will decrease the woman's anxiety and facilitate cooperation during the procedure.*
4. Assist the woman to the lithotomy position, maintaining privacy. *➤Rationale: Proper positioning provides easier access to the cervix and enhances the woman's ability to relax.*
5. Assess FHR prior to, during, and following amniotomy. *➤Rationale: Rupturing the amniotic membranes changes the pressure inside the uterus and also causes risk of a prolapsed cord.*
6. Encourage and answer any questions the woman or her support person(s) may have at this time.

## Equipment

- Sterile vaginal exam glove
- Sterile amnio hook
- Sterile water-soluble lubricant
- Doppler or monitor (external or internal)
- Waterproof linen
- Towels

## Procedure

### Sterile Gloves

1. Using sterile technique, apply sterile lubricant to the MD's/CNM's sterile gloved hand, and open the package containing the amnio hook for the MD/CNM to grasp. *➤Rationale: Lubricant decreases friction between the gloved hand and vaginal wall during the procedure. Sterile technique is essential during amniotomy to prevent potential contamination and decrease the risks of maternal and fetal infection.*
2. Once the membranes are ruptured and fluid is seen, note the color, amount, and any odor if present. *➤Rationale: Amniotic fluid should be clear or slightly cloudy and without any odor. Meconium-stained or bloody amniotic fluid indicates or places the fetus at risk for complications. Foul-smelling fluid may indicate infection. Absent, decreased, or increased amounts of amniotic fluid may indicate fetal stress.*
3. Maternal temperature should be assessed every 2 hours or more frequently if febrile and/or MD/CNM ordered. *➤Rationale: A rise in maternal temperature might indicate an intrauterine infection (chorioamnionitis).*
4. Clean the perineum with a warm washcloth and change waterproof linen pads as needed. *➤Rationale: A dry underpad enhances maternal comfort.*
5. Assist the woman to a comfortable position.
6. Assess fetal heart rate immediately before and after the rupture of membranes. *➤Rationale: Fetal well-being must be confirmed prior to and after amniotomy to assess fetal tolerance to the procedure.*

## Documentation

Document date, time of ruptured membranes, color, amount and odor (if applicable), who performed the procedure, cervical exam results, fetal heart rate, and how the client tolerated the procedure.

# Skill 9.11    Auscultating Fetal Heart Rate

## Preparation

1. Explain the procedure, the indications for it, and the information that will be obtained.
2. Uncover the woman's abdomen.

## Equipment

- Doppler device

## Procedure

1. To use the Doppler:
   - Place ultrasonic gel on the diaphragm of the Doppler. Gel is used to maintain contact with the maternal abdomen and enhances conduction of sound.
   - Place the Doppler diaphragm on the woman's abdomen halfway between the umbilicus and symphysis and in the midline. You are most likely to hear the FHR in this area. Listen carefully for the sound of the fetal heartbeat
2. Check the woman's pulse against the fetal sounds you hear. If the rates are the same, reposition the Doppler and try again. *➤Rationale: If the rates are the same, you are probably hearing the maternal pulse and not the FHR.*
3. If the rates are not similar, count the FHR for 1 full minute. Note that the FHR has a double rhythm and only one sound is counted.

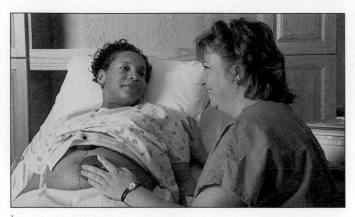

● When the fetal heartbeat is picked up by the electronic monitor, the sound can be heard by everyone in the room.

4. If you do not locate the FHR, move the Doppler laterally.
5. Auscultate the FHR between, during, and for 30 seconds following uterine contractions.

6. AWHONN (2003) frequency recommendations are as follows:
   • Low-risk women: Every 1 hour in the latent phase, every 30 minutes in the active phase, and every 15 minutes in the second stage.
   • High-risk women: Every 30 minutes in the latent phase, every 15 minutes in the active phase, and every 5 minutes in the second stage. ➤*Rationale: This evaluation provides the opportunity to assess the fetal status and response to labor.*
7. Document FHR data (rate and rhythm), characteristics of uterine activity, and any actions taken as a result of the FHR.

---

### CLINICAL ALERT

The FHR is heard most clearly through the fetal back. Locate the fetal back using Leopold's maneuvers.

---

## Skill 9.12  External Electronic Fetal Monitoring

### Preparation

Explain the procedure, the indications for it, and the information that will be obtained.

### Equipment

• Monitor
• Two elastic monitor belts
• Tocodynamometer ("toco")
• Ultrasound transducer
• Ultrasound gel

### Procedure

1. Turn on the monitor.
2. Place the two elastic belts around the woman's abdomen.

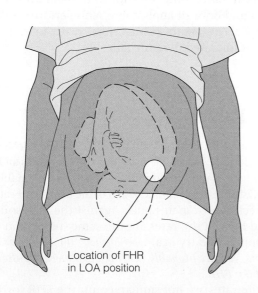

Location of FHR in LOA position

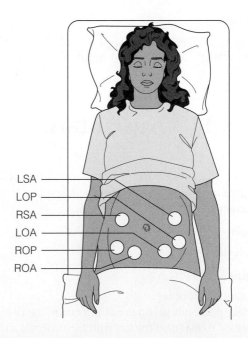

LSA
LOP
RSA
LOA
ROP
ROA

● Location of the FHR in relation to the more commonly seen fetal positions.

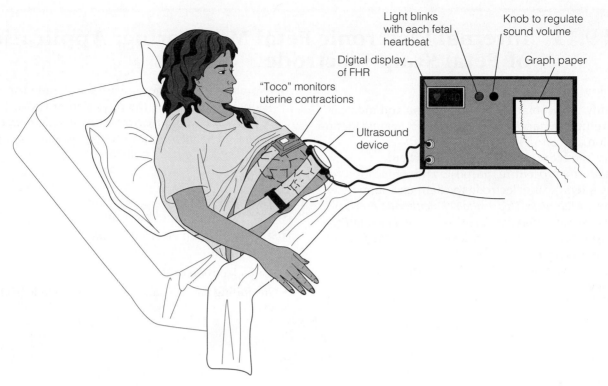

Light blinks with each fetal heartbeat

Knob to regulate sound volume

Digital display of FHR

Graph paper

"Toco" monitors uterine contractions

Ultrasound device

● External electronic fetal monitoring.

3. Place the toco over the uterine fundus off the midline on the area palpated to be most firm during contractions. Secure it with one of the elastic belts. ➤*Rationale: The uterine fundus is the area of greatest contractility.*

4. Note the UC tracing. The resting tone tracing (that is, without a UC) should be recording on the 10 or 15 mm Hg pressure line. Adjust the line to reflect that reading. ➤*Rationale: If the resting tone is set on the zero line, there often is a constant grinding noise.*

5. Apply the ultrasonic gel to the diaphragm of the ultrasound transducer. ➤*Rationale: Ultrasonic gel is used to maintain contact with the maternal abdomen.* The ultrasonic beam is directed toward the fetal heart.

6. Place the diaphragm on the maternal abdomen in the midline between the umbilicus and the symphysis pubis.

7. Listen for the FHR, which will have a whiplike sound. Move the diaphragm laterally if necessary to obtain a stronger sound.

8. When the FHR is located, attach the second elastic belt snugly to the transducer. ➤*Rationale: Firm contact is necessary to maintain a steady tracing.*

**CLINICAL ALERT**

Evaluating the FHR tracing provides information about fetal status and response to the stress of labor. The presence of reassuring characteristics is associated with good fetal outcomes. Rapid identification of nonreassuring characteristics allows prompt interventions and the opportunity to determine the fetal response to the interventions.

9. Place the following information on the beginning of the fetal monitor paper: date, time, woman's name, gravida, para, membrane status, and name of physician or certified nurse-midwife.

10. Ongoing documentation should provide information about FHR, including baseline rate in beats per minute (bpm), long-term variability (LTV), short-term variability (STV), response to uterine contractions (accelerations or decelerations), procedures performed, changes in position and the like, as well as any therapy initiated.

# Skill 9.13   Internal Electronic Fetal Monitoring: Application of Fetal Scalp Electrode

## Preparation

1. Identify the woman, comparing name and medical record number appearing in the chart against identification arm band information.
2. Verify correct procedure for correct client.
3. Explain the procedure, purpose, and implications of using a fetal scalp electrode to client and support person. ➤*Rationale: This method of monitoring provides more accurate continuous data than external monitoring because the signal is clearer and movement of the fetus or woman does not interrupt it.*
4. Assist the woman into lithotomy position, providing privacy.

5. Woman's membranes must have already ruptured spontaneously or by the physician or CNM.
   ➤*Rationale: Fetal scalp electrode cannot be applied to the scalp if the membranes are covering the scalp, and RNs are not allowed to rupture membranes.*

## Equipment

- Sterile exam glove
- Sterile water-soluble lubricant
- Spiral fetal scalp electrode apparatus
- Fetal monitor
- Scalp electrode cable
- Grounding pad (usually found in electrode packaging)

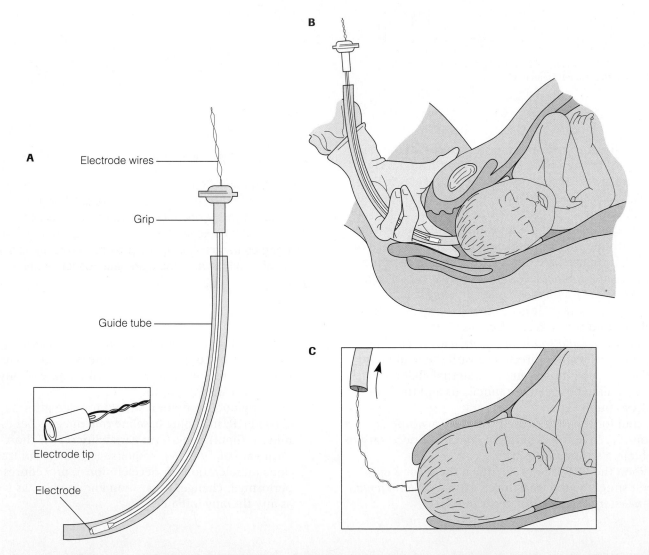

● Technique for internal, direct fetal monitoring. **A,** Spiral electrode. **B,** Attaching the spiral electrode to the scalp. **C,** Attached spiral electrode with the guide tube removed.

## Procedure

1. Using sterile technique, open lubricant package, don a sterile glove on the dominant hand, and apply lubricant to the glove with nondominant hand. ➤*Rationale: Sterile technique is essential to decrease the risk of intrauterine infection.*

2. Perform vaginal exam to determine dilatation and presentation of the fetus. Ensure presenting part is vertex. ➤*Rationale: The fetal scalp electrode is placed on the fetal occiput. To do so, the membranes must be ruptured, the cervix must be dilated at least 2 cm, the presenting part must be known, and it must be down against the cervix.*

3. Apply fetal scalp electrode according to package directions on a firm area of the fetal vertex, avoiding fontanelles, face, genitals, etc. This usually involves inserting the electrode within the firm plastic guide. Place end of the guide/electrode against firm area of the scalp, and rotate electrode end clockwise until resistance is met. Release the guide according to package directions and discard. ➤*Rationale: Care must be taken to avoid attaching the monitor to soft tissue, which could result in fetal trauma.*

4. Connect spiral electrode wire to a leg plate taped to mother's inner thigh with a grounding pad per package instructions. This in turn is attached to the electronic fetal monitor. ➤*Rationale: If the resting tone is set on the zero line, there often is a constant grinding noise.*

5. Verify fetal heart rate is tracing before discontinuing the intermittent or continuous external monitor.

6. To remove fetal scalp electrode, disconnect the electrode wire from the cable and rotate the lead counterclockwise. Once removed, visually examine the electrode to ensure it is intact. If unable to remove before going for a cesarean birth, tape electrode wire to the mother's thigh and notify the surgeon.

7. Document date and time of application and removal, including the condition of the electrode (intact).

---

# Skill 9.14 Assisting with and Monitoring of Woman Undergoing Induction of Labor with Pitocin and Cervical Ripening Agents

## Preparation

1. Identify the woman, comparing name and medical record number appearing in the chart against identification arm band information.

2. Obtain an order for the procedure, and have a written order in the chart.

3. Verify correct procedure as ordered by physician/CNM for the correct woman.

4. Explain the procedure, purpose, and implications of the procedure to the woman and her support person. ➤*Rationale: The mother and her family need to be aware that induction of labor may take longer than spontaneous labor. They also need to know there may be limitations on food intake and activity, continuous fetal monitoring, and frequent assessments due to the method of induction.*

5. Obtain informed consent per agency policy.

6. Obtain Pitocin premixed bag from pharmacy or mix 10 units Pitocin per 1000 mL secondary fluid. Obtain cervical ripening agent.

7. Allow time for and encourage any questions the woman and her support person may have. Reinforce any teaching as necessary.

## Equipment

- Fetal and contraction monitoring equipment (for Pitocin infusion)
- IV fluids (per agency policy, MD/CNM orders)
- IV administration sets (for Pitocin infusion)
- IV infusion pump (two if available) for Pitocin infusion
- Appropriate induction medications
- Sterile exam glove, sterile lubricant (cervical ripening)

## Procedure

### Oxytocin (Pitocin)

1. Apply fetal and contraction monitors per unit policy. Assess for reactive or reassuring fetal heart rate tracing. ➤*Rationale: A baseline of fetal well-being and uterine activity should be established before induction so that the nurse will recognize complications associated with oxytocin administrations, such as uterine hyperstimulation and fetal distress.*

2. Start IV infusion using aqueous solution at 125 mL/hr. ➤*Rationale: This is done to keep the woman hydrated and to have an intravenous line available when the oxytocin infusion is stopped.*

3. Assess maternal vital signs and hydration status. ➤*Rationale: Ongoing assessment of the woman's fluid balance (intake and output) is necessary because oxytocin has an antidiuretic effect.*

4. Attach secondary line to an infusion pump. ➤*Rationale: An intravenous infusion pump must be used during oxytocin induction to ensure that accurate volume and dosage of oxytocin are administered to the woman.*

5. Start Pitocin infusion per agency policy and increase accordingly. One suggested method is to begin at 1 to 2 mU/min and increase by 1 to 2 mU/min every 30 to 40 minutes.

6. Evaluate fetal heart rate pattern, contraction pattern, and maternal vital signs before each increase in Pitocin. ➤*Rationale: Accurate monitoring of uterine contraction frequency, duration, and intensity and uterine resting tone is essential to evaluate the effect of each oxytocin dosage level and determine the need to increase the infusion rate.*

7. Increase Pitocin rate until adequate labor is established and then maintain at the current rate. Decrease Pitocin if hyperstimulation occurs, per agency policy. ➤*Rationale: Since the half-life of oxytocin is very short (1 to 6 minutes), stopping an oxytocin infusion may quickly reverse the effects of excessive uterine activity and improve fetal oxygenation.*

### Misoprostol (Cytotec)

1. Monitor fetal heart rate and contractions per agency policy.
2. Have IV infusion or IV access established, per agency policy.
3. Have the woman empty her bladder prior to insertion of cervical ripening agent.
4. Perform sterile vaginal exam, establishing the cervix is "unfavorable" for induction using Pitocin only (1 cm or less, little to no effacement).
5. Remove glove, wash hands, don sterile glove, apply minimal lubricant, and insert two fingers (second and third digits) into the vagina with 25 micrograms (1/4 tablet) misoprostol at end of fingers. It is placed in the posterior vaginal fornix.
6. The woman should remain in bed for 30 minutes following insertion and then may be up to void.
7. This process may be repeated every 4 to 6 hours up to 24 hours. The physician/CNM should be notified if hyperstimulation occurs or if there is no onset of labor.
8. The fetal heart rate/contraction pattern should be evaluated for 3 hours following the insertion of misoprostol.
9. Monitor closely for uterine hyperstimulation.

### Dinoprostone (PGE2) (Cervidil or Prepidil)

Same procedures as for misoprostol except as follows:

1. Cervidil (10 mg): Administer as vaginal insert, × 1 dose. Monitor for 2 hours after insertion.
2. Prepidil (0.5 mg): Administer intracervically. Monitor for 1 to 2 hours. May repeat after 6 hours. No more than 3 doses in 24 hours. If hyperstimulation occurs, remove medication by gently pulling attached string out of vagina.

### Documentation

Document the procedures, results, vital signs, fetal heart rate/contraction patterns, and labor progress in the client's medical record, including date and times of administration of medication and any complications.

---

# Skill 9.15   Assisting with and Caring for the Woman with an Epidural during Labor

### Preparation

1. Identify the woman, using the name and medical record number and comparing the medical record with the identification arm band. Verify the correct procedure with the correct woman. Document informed consent by the woman. Ensure anesthesia personnel and/or the obstetrician explain possible side effects and complications.
2. Explain the procedure and interventions that may be required because of the epidural: continuous intravenous infusion, continuous fetal monitoring, complete bed rest, indwelling or intermittent urinary catheterization, frequent blood pressure assessments, and other interventions according to hospital policy. ➤*Rationale: The woman may be focused on pain relief and not aware of further interventions that will be required due to epidural infusion.*
3. Obtain the physician/CNM order for epidural.
4. Notify anesthesia personnel per hospital policy.
5. Throughout the procedure and following, allow time to answer any questions the woman or her support person may have. Follow up with further teaching regarding any matter that may have been unforeseen or out of the ordinary.

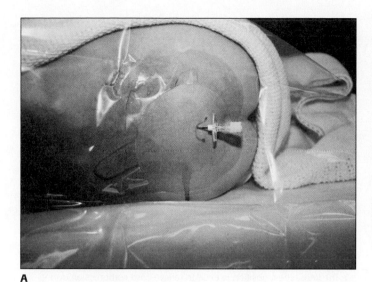
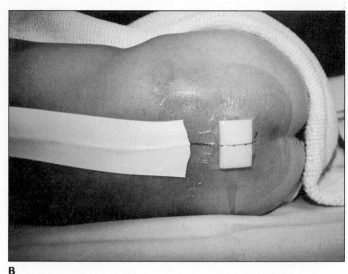

A                                                              B

● **A,** Epidural pain block being placed during surgery, and **B,** taped into place and wrapped securely. (Courtesy of Shriners Hospital for Children, Spokane, Washington.)

### Equipment

- Fetal and contraction monitoring equipment as ordered
- Intravenous fluid and apparatus as ordered and per hospital policy
- Epidural administration set
- Anesthetic medications per anesthesia department protocol, if certified registered nurse anesthetist (CRNA) or anesthesiologist does not provide it
- High-pressure volumetric pump if epidural will be a continuous infusion
- Ephedrine syringe, dosage according to hospital protocol

### Procedure

1. Obtain maternal baseline vital signs, fetal heart rate, and variability. The fetal heart rate tracing should show a reassuring tracing before starting the epidural process.
2. Administer an IV fluid bolus per hospital protocol before the epidural is begun (usually 500 to 1000 mL lactated Ringer's). ➤*Rationale: This is to avoid maternal hypotension associated with vasodilatation common with epidurals.*
3. Assist and support the woman in position per anesthesia personnel request (usually side-lying with knees flexed or sitting up on side of bed with back flexed). ➤*Rationale: This will assist the anesthesia personnel in locating the correct vertebrae between which to administer the epidural.*

4. Assess BP, heart rate, and fetal heart rate before and after test doses and frequently thereafter according to hospital policy, often every 5 minutes throughout the procedure and immediately following, then regularly according to hospital policy.
5. Have ephedrine at bedside in case of hypotensive or fetal bradycardia episode. Administer according to unit protocol and physician orders.
6. Assess the bladder for distention every 30 minutes. Catheterize with intermittent catheter if birth is imminent or indwelling if not. ➤*Rationale: A full bladder can slow the descent of the fetus, as well as risk damage to the bladder.*
7. Assess maternal position and body alignment frequently, changing position at least every hour.
8. Periodically assess the level of anesthesia and pain control. Notify anesthesia personnel as needed for changes in epidural infusion.
9. Change syringes as needed per hospital policy.
10. After birth, per hospital policy, a qualified RN may remove the epidural catheter.

### Documentation

Document the procedure throughout administration of the epidural and removal of the catheter. Document time of removal, condition of epidural puncture site, catheter condition (intact), any dressing applied (if applicable), and how the woman tolerated the procedure.

# Skill 9.16   Care of the Woman with Prolapsed Cord

### Preparation

This event is unexpected and an emergency. Preparation can only consist of calmly teaching the woman and her support person the rationale for interventions, what to expect, and the plan of care. Though difficult at times with this particular situation, privacy is to be maintained. Allow time for questions from the laboring woman, her support person, and any other family that may be present. Another RN may need to answer questions if the woman's RN is busy with the woman's care.

### Equipment

- Sterile exam glove
- Sterile lubricant
- Sterile gauze pad moistened with saline solution, if cord is outside of vagina
- Oxygen and mask
- Fetal monitor/Doppler

### Procedure

1. If the cord is visualized extending through the vagina, a sterile gauze moistened with sterile saline must be placed on the cord immediately to prevent the cord from drying. Do not handle the cord. ➤*Rationale: Handling the cord may cause it to spasm.*
2. Notify physician/CNM immediately.
3. Place the woman in the knee-chest position.
4. If the cord is palpated during vaginal exam (using sterile glove and lubricant), place two fingers on either side of the cord or both fingers on one side of the cord to avoid compressing it. Exert upward pressure against the presenting part to relieve pressure on the cord.
5. Continue assessing fetal heart rate to determine if interventions and position of fingers are successful in keeping fetal heart rate between 110 and 160 bpm.
6. Start oxygen via face mask at 10 L/min.

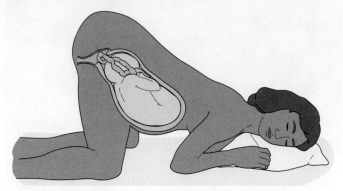

● The knee-chest position is used to relieve cord compression during cord prolapse emergency.

7. If fetal heart rate is not responding to knee-chest position and examiner's upward pressure on the fetal presenting part, place the mother in the knee-chest position. While changing the mother's position, examiner must keep fingers in the vagina to keep the presenting part off the cord.

Examiner must keep fingers on the presenting part until baby is born, usually via cesarean. This may require examiner to travel to the operating room (OR) on the bed with the mother to maintain the position of fingers and presenting part. The woman's position must be maintained until birth or arrival to OR and placement on the OR table. Though difficult, privacy should be maintained during transport to surgery. This may require extra personnel and sheets to cover the woman.

### Documentation

Document the course of events, interventions, and maternal and fetal response to interventions in the medical record per agency policy. If there is a poor fetal outcome, further quality assurance documentation may be necessary.

# Skill 9.17   Assessing the Uterine Fundus Following Vaginal Birth

### Preparation

1. Explain the procedure, the information it provides, and what it might feel like.
2. Ask the woman when she last voided. Ask her to void if it has been longer than 1 hour. ➤*Rationale: A full bladder can cause uterine atony.*

3. Have the woman lie flat in bed with her head on a pillow. If the procedure is uncomfortable, she may find that it helps to flex her legs. ➤*Rationale: The supine position prevents falsely high assessment of fundal height. Flexing the legs relaxes the abdominal muscles.*

## Equipment

- A clean perineal pad
- Clean gloves

## Procedure

1. Gently place one hand on the lower segment of the uterus for support. Using the fingertips of the other hand, massage in a circular motion down and into the abdomen to palpate until you locate the top of the fundus. ➤*Rationale: One hand stabilizes the uterus while the other hand locates the top of the fundus.*
2. Determine whether the fundus is firm. If it is, it will feel hard and round like a firm grapefruit in the abdomen. If it is not firm, massage the abdomen lightly until it becomes firm, then check for bleeding. ➤*Rationale: A firm fundus indicates that the uterine muscles are contracted and bleeding will not occur.*
3. Measure the top of the fundus in finger-breadths above, below, or at the fundus. ➤*Rationale: Fundal height gives information about the progress of involution.*
4. Determine the position of the fundus in relation to the midline of the body. If it is not in the midline, locate it and then evaluate the bladder for distention. ➤*Rationale: The fundus may deviate from the midline when the bladder is full because the enlarged bladder pushes the uterus aside.*
5. If the bladder is distended, use nursing measures to help the woman void. If she is not able to void after a specified period of time, catheterization may be necessary.
6. Measure urine output for the next few hours until normal elimination is established. ➤*Rationale: During the postpartum as diuresis occurs, the bladder may fill far more rapidly than normal, putting the woman at risk for uterine atony and hemorrhage.*

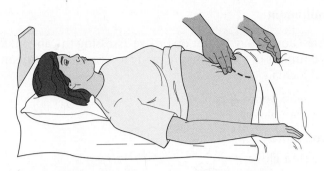

● Measuring the descent of the fundus in the woman with a vaginal birth. In this case the fundus is located two finger-breadths below the umbilicus.

7. Assess the lochia.
8. During the first few hours postpartum, if the fundus becomes boggy frequently or is located high above the umbilicus and the woman's bladder is empty, the uterine cavity may be filled with clots of blood. In this case, do the following:
   - Release the front of the perineal pad and lay it back so that you can see the perineum and the pad lying between the woman's legs.
   - Massage the uterine fundus until it is firm.
   - Keep one hand in position stabilizing the lower portion of the uterus. With the hand you used to massage the fundus, put steady pressure on the top of the now-firm fundus and see if you are able to express any clots. (Watch the pad between her legs for clots to pass from the vagina.) ➤*Rationale: If the woman's uterus is filled with blood, it acts as an irritant and the uterus will not remain contracted. When the muscle fibers relax, bleeding results, further aggravating the problem. Pushing on a uterus that is not firm is dangerous because it is possible to cause the uterus to invert, a true emergency.*
9. Provide the woman with a clean perineal pad.
10. Record findings. Fundal height is recorded in finger-breadths (e.g., "2 FB ↓U" or "1 FB ↑U").
11. If fundal massage was necessary, note that fact: "Uterus boggy →firm with light massage."
12. Communicate bogginess or heavy flow to primary provider.

### CLINICAL TIP

Gloves may be put on before assessing the abdomen and fundus or when you are ready to assess the perineum and lochia.

---

# Skill 9.18   Evaluating the Lochia

## Preparation

1. Explain why lochia occurs, why it is assessed, how it is assessed, and how it changes during the postpartum.
2. Ask the woman to void. ➤*Rationale: A full bladder can cause uterine atony and increase the amount of lochia.*
3. Complete the assessment of uterine fundal height and firmness. ➤*Rationale: In almost all cases, fundal*

*height and firmness are evaluated with an assessment of lochia. This practice provides a more thorough assessment.*

4. If she has not already done so for the fundal assessment, ask the woman to flex her legs. Then ask her to spread her legs apart. Use the bed sheet as a drape to preserve her modesty. ➤*Rationale: This position allows you to see the perineum and the perineal pad more effectively.*

## Equipment

*Note:* Gloves may be put on before assessing the abdomen and fundus or when you are ready to assess the perineum and lochia.

- Clean perineal pad
- Clean gloves

## Procedure

1. Don gloves.
2. Lower the perineal pad and observe the amount of lochia on the pad. Because women's pad-changing practices vary, ask her about the length of time the current pad has been in use, whether the amount is changed, and whether any clots were passed before this examination, such as during voiding. ➤*Rationale: During the first 1 to 3 days the woman's lochia should be rubra, which is dark red. A few small clots are normal and occur as a result of pooling of blood in the vagina when the woman is lying down. The passage of large clots is abnormal, and the cause should be investigated immediately.*
3. If the woman reports heavy bleeding or clots, ask her to put on a clean perineal pad and then reassess the pad in 1 hour. Also ask her to call you before flushing any clots she passes into the toilet during voiding.
4. When the uterine fundus is firm and stabilized with the nondominant hand, press down on it with the dominant hand while watching to see if any clots are expelled.
5. Determine the amount of lochia, using the following guide:
   - Heavy amount—Perineal pad has a stain larger than 6 inches in length within 1hour; 30 to 80 mL lochia.
   - Moderate amount—Perineal pad has a stain less than 6 inches in length within 1hour; 25 to 50 mL lochia.
   - Small amount—Perineal pad has a stain less than 4 inches in length after 1 hour; 10 to 25 mL lochia.
   - Scant amount—Perineal pad has a stain less than 1 inch in length after 1 hour or lochia is only on tissue when the woman wipes. ➤*Rationale: Lochia should never exceed a moderate amount such as 4 to 8 partially saturated perineal pads daily. Using a consistent standard for measuring lochia improves the accuracy of the information charted and conveyed to others.*
6. In most cases, a woman is discharged while her lochia is still rubra. Provide her with information about lochia serosa and lochia alba. ➤*Rationale: Accurate discharge information enables the woman to assess herself more accurately and enables her to judge better when to contact her caregiver.*
7. Record the findings specifically. For example, "Lochia moderate rubra, no clots passed."

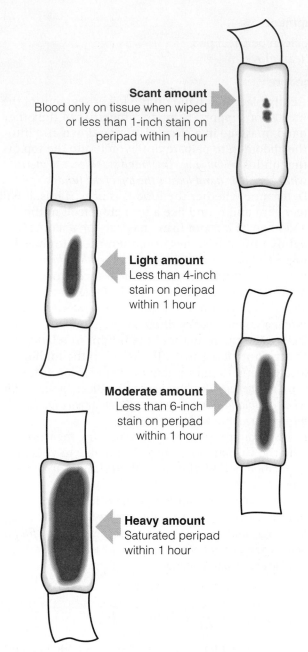

**Scant amount**
Blood only on tissue when wiped or less than 1-inch stain on peripad within 1 hour

**Light amount**
Less than 4-inch stain on peripad within 1 hour

**Moderate amount**
Less than 6-inch stain on peripad within 1 hour

**Heavy amount**
Saturated peripad within 1 hour

● Suggested guidelines for assessing lochia volume.

*Note:* From Jacobson, H. (1985, May–June). A standard for assessing lochia volume. *Maternal-Child Nursing.*

## CLINICAL ALERT

If blood loss exceeds the guide-lines given in this chapter, weigh the perineal pads and the chux pads to estimate the blood loss more accurately. Typically, 1 g 1 mL blood. Because blood can pool below the woman on the chux or peri pad, the pads are included in your assessment.

# Skill 9.19   Assessing Postpartum Perineal

## Preparation

1. Explain the purpose and the procedure for assessing the perineum during the postpartum period.
2. Complete the assessment of fundal height and lochia. ➤*Rationale: Typically, perineal assessment is the final step of the postpartum assessment.*
3. At this point in a postpartal assessment, the woman is lying on her back with her knees flexed. Her perineal pad has already been lifted away from her perineum to permit inspection of the lochia. If an episiotomy was performed or if the birth was difficult, the woman may be using an ice pack on her perineum to reduce swelling. The ice pack would also have been removed for inspection of the lochia.
4. Ask her to turn onto her side with her upper knee drawn forward and resting on the bed (Sims' position). ➤*Rationale: When the woman is supine, even with her knees flexed, it is very difficult to expose the posterior portion of the perineum. Thus, Sims' position makes it easiest to inspect the perineum and anal area.*

## Equipment

- Clean perineal pad, clean ice pack if desired/needed
- Small light source such as a penlight may be necessary
- Clean gloves

## Procedure

1. Use a systematic approach to assessment. ➤*Rationale: A systematic approach helps ensure that you do not overlook a significant finding.*
2. In evaluating the perineum, begin by asking the woman's perceptions. How does she describe her discomfort? Does it seem excessive to her? Has it become worse since the birth? Does it seem more severe than you would expect? (Note: Pain that seems disproportionately severe may indicate that the woman is developing a vulvar hematoma.) ➤*Rationale: Information from the client herself often helps identify developing problems.*
3. After talking with the woman, assess the condition of the tissue. To allow for full visualization, it may be helpful to ask the woman to lift the knee of her upper leg to expose her perineum more fully. In some cases it may help to use the nondominant hand to lift the buttocks and tissue. Note any swelling (edema), bruising (ecchymosis), and separation. ➤*Rationale: The tissue is often traumatized by the birth, and mild bruising is not unusual. However, excessive bruising may indicate that a hematoma is developing.*

4. Evaluate the episiotomy, if there is one, or any repaired laceration for its state of healing. Is it reddened? Note the edges of the incision. Are they well approximated? Tell the woman that you are going to palpate the incision gently, then do so. Note any areas of hardness. Note whether the incision is warmer to the touch than the surrounding tissue. ➤*Rationale: Gentle palpation should elicit minimal tenderness and there should be no redness, warmth, or areas of hardness, which suggest infection. Both bruising and infection interfere with normal healing. Typically, within 24 hours the edges of the incision should be "glued" together (well approximated).*
5. During the assessment be alert for odors. Typically the lochia has an earthy, but not unpleasant, smell that is easily identifiable. ➤*Rationale: A foul odor associated with drainage often indicates infection.*
6. Finally, assess for hemorrhoids. To visualize the anal area, lift the upper buttocks. If hemorrhoids are present, note the size, number, and pain or tenderness. ➤*Rationale: Hemorrhoids often develop during pregnancy or labor and can cause considerable discomfort. If hemorrhoids are present, the woman may benefit from available comfort measures.*
7. During the assessment, talk to the woman about the effectiveness of comfort measures being used. Provide teaching about care of the episiotomy, hemorrhoids, and the like. ➤*Rationale: Health teaching is an important part of nursing care. Many women*

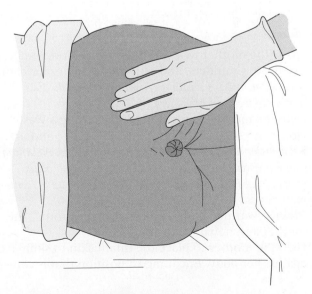

● Intact perineum with hemorrhoids. Note how the nurse's hand raises the upper buttocks to expose the anal area fully.

have concerns about the episiotomy and may not know, for example, that the suture used is dissolvable. This is an excellent time to provide information about good healthcare practices in both the short and long term.

8. Provide the woman with a clean perineal pad. Replenish the ice pack if necessary.

9. Record findings. For example: "Midline episiotomy; no edema, ecchymosis, or tenderness. Skin edges well approximated. Woman reports pain relief measures are controlling discomfort."

---

## CLINICAL ALERT

In evaluating the perineum, use the REEDA scale as a quick reminder of what to assess. Specifically:
R redness
E edema or swelling
E ecchymosis or bruising
D drainage
A approximation (how well the edges of an incision—the episiotomy—or a repaired laceration seem to be holding together)

---

# Skill 9.20   Assisting with Breastfeeding after Childbirth

Breastfeeding provides newborns and infants with immunologic, nutritional, and psychosocial advantages. It also promotes involution in women who have just given birth. Newborns who are put to breast soon after their birth benefit from the physical warmth of their mother's body, from the stimulation of sucking and swallowing, from replenishment of nutrients, and from the opportunity to interact intimately with their mother. As long as the mother is tolerating the birth well and her newborn is adjusting to extrauterine life without complication, breastfeeding can be promoted in the first 1 hour of life when the newborn is usually alert and ready to nurse.

### Preparation

1. Wash hands.

### Equipment

- None required

### Procedure

1. Assist the mother to a comfortable position. Support her head, shoulders, and arms as necessary for comfort. ➤*Rationale: A position of comfort allows the new mother to focus on breastfeeding.*

2. Help the mother to wash her hands using a washcloth with soap and water, then rinse well and dry. ➤*Rationale: Hands carry a variety of organisms, including Staphylococcus aureus, Escherichia coli, Streptococcus species, and Haemophilus influenzae, which are all common causes of mastitis, an infection of the breast.*

3. Provide warmed bath blankets to wrap around the mother and newborn together.

4. Help the mother to place the infant skin to skin against her body. Encourage a position that is comfortable for the mother. ➤*Rationale: The mother should hold the newborn in a way that feels natural and provides her with a free hand.*

5. Instruct the mother to use the thumb and first two fingers of her dominant hand to make a C-shape around her breast with the nipple in the center of the C-shape and to steadily support her breast. ➤*Rationale: This C-hold hand position enables the mother to position the breast correctly in the newborn's mouth.*

6. Help the mother to hold her newborn so that the mouth is in alignment with her breast at the level of the nipple. She then lightly tickles the infant's mouth with the nipple until the baby opens his or her mouth. She then brings the baby closely in to her breast. It is important that the baby takes the whole nipple into the mouth so that the gums are on the areola. Provide firm steady support as the newborn begins to suckle. If sucking does not begin, stroke the cheek gently to elicit suck-search response and then offer the breast again. Instruct the mother to be sure that the breast tissue does not occlude the newborn's nares. ➤*Rationale: The newborn's gums need to be positioned over the areola because this allows the baby's jaws to compress the milk ducts located directly beneath the areola as the newborn suckles.*

7. If the newborn is sufficiently responsive, have him or her suckle at both breasts. Initially some newborns suck well; others may simply lick or nuzzle the nipple. Reassure the mother that this is a positive interaction. ➤*Rationale: Even simple breast stimulation promotes the release of oxytocin, which aids uterine involution and lactation.*

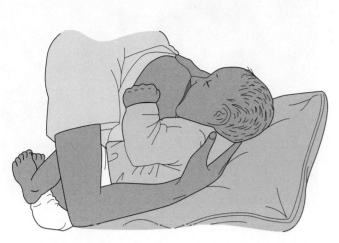

**A** Football hold
- Hold the baby's back and shoulders in the palm of your hand.
- Tuck the baby up under your arm, lining up the baby's lips with your nipple.
- Support the breast to guide it into the baby's mouth.
- Hold your breast until the baby nurses easily.

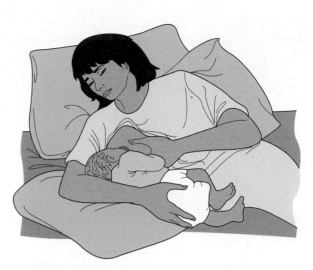

**B** Lying down
- Lie on your side with a pillow at your back and lay the baby so you are facing each other.
- To start, prop yourself up on your elbow and support your breast with the opposite hand.
- Pull the baby close to you, lining up the baby's mouth with your nipple.
- Once the baby is nursing well, lie back down. Hold your breast with the opposite hand.

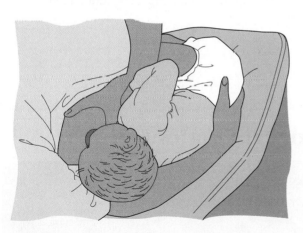

**C** Cradling
- Cradle the baby in the arm closest to the breast, with the baby's head in the crook of the arm.
- Have the baby's body facing you, tummy-to-tummy.
- Use your opposite hand to support the breast.

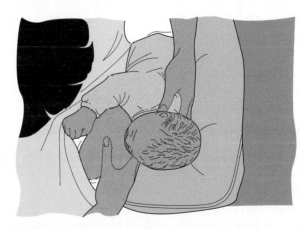

**D** Across the lap
- Lay your baby on pillows across your lap.
- Turn the baby facing you.
- Reach across your lap to support the baby's back and shoulders with the palm of your hand.
- Support your breast from underneath to guide it into the baby's mouth.

● Four common breastfeeding positions. **A,** Football hold. **B,** Lying down. **C,** Cradling. **D,** Across the lap.

*Source: Breastfeeding: A special relationship.* Breastfeeding Education Resources. 1-800-869-7892. Raleigh, NC. Copyright Lactation Consultants of NC.

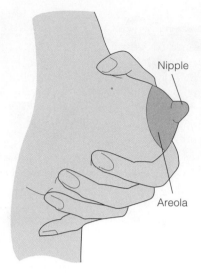

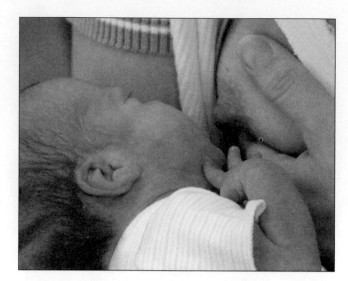

**A**

**B**

● **A,** C-hold hand position. **B,** Mother using C-hold.

*Source:* **A,** Courtesy Childbirth Graphics Ltd., Rochester, NY.

8. Document in the medical record the time and duration of the breastfeeding, the quality of the latch, and interaction between the mother and newborn. Note any difficulties such as flat or inverted nipples, and initiate referral to a lactation consultant.

---

**CLINICAL ALERT**

Be patient and allow the newborn and mother to experience breastfeeding in a relaxed way. Your calmness and support can help the mother feel confident and in control.

---

# Skill 9.21   Performing Nasal Pharyngeal Suctioning

### Preparation

1. Suction equipment is always available in the birthing area to clear secretions from the newborn's nose or oropharynx if respirations are depressed or if amniotic fluid was meconium stained.
2. Tighten the lid on the DeLee mucus trap or other suction device collection bottle. ➤*Rationale: This avoids spillage of secretions and prevents air from leaking out of the lid.*
3. Connect one end of the DeLee tubing to low suction.
4. Have blow-by oxygen available to be used with the DeLee mucus trap.

### Equipment

- DeLee mucus trap or other suction device
- Clean gloves

### Procedure

1. Don gloves.

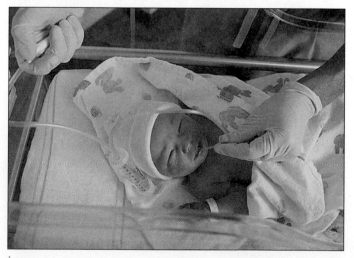

● DeLee mucus trap.

2. Without applying suction, insert the free end of the DeLee tubing 3 to 5 inches into the newborn's nose or mouth. ➤*Rationale: Applying suction while passing the tube would interfere with smooth passage of the tube.*

3. Place your thumb over the suction control and begin to apply suction. Continue to suction as you slowly remove the tube, rotating it slightly. ➤*Rationale: Suctioning during withdrawal removes fluid and avoids redepositing secretions in the newborn's nasopharynx.*

4. Continue to reinsert the tube and provide suction for as long as fluid is aspirated. ➤*Rationale: Excessive suctioning can cause vagal stimulation, which decreases the heart rate.*

5. If it is necessary to pass the tube into the newborn's stomach to remove meconium secretions that the newborn swallowed before birth, insert the tube through the newborn's mouth into the stomach. Apply suction and continue to suction as you withdraw the tube. ➤*Rationale: Because the newborn's nares are small and delicate, it is easier and faster to pass the suction tube through the mouth.*

6. Document the completion of the procedure and the amount and type of secretions. ➤*Rationale: This documentation provides a record of the intervention and the status of the infant at birth.*

# Skill 9.22    Suctioning an Infant with a Bulb Syringe

## Preparation

1. Verify the identity of the child. Explain the procedure to the child and parents.
2. Assess the child's respiratory status, including breath sounds, respiratory effort, and airway patency. Observe for excess secretions that the child is unable to manage by swallowing.
3. An assistant may be needed to gently position and hold the infant or child with the head in midline, and to keep the child's hands out of the way.
4. Turn on and set the wall suction to the pressure level ordered by the physician or suggested in the facility's procedure manual.

## Equipment

- Bulb syringe
- Normal saline nose drops
- Yankauer or tonsil tip suction catheter
- Normal saline solution
- Clean gloves

## Procedure

### Bulb Syringe

1. Place saline nose drops in the naris. ➤*Rationale: The nose drops loosen dried secretions.*
2. Deflate the bulb. Insert the tip of the bulb syringe into the infant's naris. ➤*Rationale: Deflating the bulb first prevents pushing the secretions back into the nasopharynx.*
3. Release the bulb and remove the syringe from the naris. Expel the secretions into the proper receptacle.
4. Assess the child's ability to breathe easily. Repeat the suctioning as necessary.
5. Document the procedure, character of secretions, and infant's response.

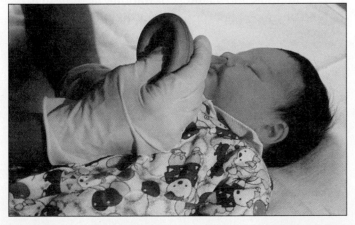
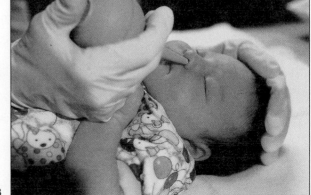

A                                                    B

● **A,** Insertion of a deflated bulb syringe. **B,** Removal of a reinflated bulb syringe.

### Yankauer

1. Insert the catheter tip into the mouth and turn on the suction.
2. Suction to remove secretions from the mouth and pharynx. Avoid causing a gag reflex. ➤*Rationale: The gag reflex may stimulate vomiting and compromise the airway.*
3. Rinse the catheter with normal saline.

4. Assess the child's respiratory status. Repeat suctioning if needed.
5. Document the procedures, character of secretions, and response of the child.

# Skill 9.23   Assessing Newborn APGAR Scores

## Preparation

1. Identify the person responsible to assign the Apgar score.
2. Preheat the radiant warmer to 36.5°C.
3. Prewarm blankets under the warmer.

## Equipment

- APGAR timer or digital timer that counts seconds or a timepiece with a second hand
- Infant warmer with ISC and probe preheated
- Clean gloves
- Stethoscope
- Sterile baby blanket

## Procedure

1. Don gloves. ➤*Rationale: A newborn infant is wet with amniotic fluid, vernix, and secretions. Consequently, universal precautions are indicated when handling the newborn until the initial bath is completed.*
2. Using the following five criteria, determine a score in each and assign an APGAR score at 1 minute.
    - Heart rate—Palpate the pulse at the base of the umbilical cord for 6 seconds and multiply by 10, or use the stethoscope to auscultate the heart rate. Score as follows:
        0—no heart rate detected
        1—heart rate below 100
        2—heart rate greater than 100
    - Respiratory effort—Observe respirations and cry. Score as follows:
        0—no respiratory effort or cry
        1—slow to breathe, weak cry
        2—robust cry, good respiratory effort

> ### CLINICAL ALERT
>
> Heart rate and respirations are the two most significant categories to evaluate.

- Muscle tone—Assess flexion of extremities and quality of muscle tone. Score as follows:
    0—flaccid
    1—some flexion of extremities
    2—active motion
- Reflex irritability—Assess response to noxious stimuli such as vitamin K injection. Score as follows:
    0—no response
    1—grimace
    2—cry
- Color—Assess skin color and score as follows:
    0—generally poor color, pale or cyanotic
    1—body is pink with some pallor or cyanosis over extremities, around mouth or eyes
    2—pink

➤*Rationale: Assessing these five parameters provides a quick indication of the newborn's adaptation to extrauterine life.* With practice, caregivers become skilled at assigning an accurate score. Repeat the score at 5 minutes and again at 10 minutes as indicated.

3. Document appropriately in the medical record.

# Skill 9.24 Thermoregulation of the Newborn

## Preparation

1. Prewarm the incubator or radiant warmer. Make sure warm towels and/or lightweight blankets are available.
2. Maintain the temperature of the birthing room at 22°C (71°F), with a relative humidity of 60% to 65%. ➤*Rationale: The change from a warm, moist intrauterine environment to a cool, dry drafty environment stresses the newborn's immature thermoregulation system.*

## Equipment

- Prewarmed towels or blankets
- Infant stocking cap
- Servocontrol probe
- Infant T-shirt and diaper
- Open crib
- Clean gloves

## Procedure

1. Don gloves. ➤*Rationale: Gloves are worn whenever there is the possibility of contact with body fluids—in this case, a newborn wet with amniotic fluid, vernix, and maternal blood.*
2. Place the newborn under the radiant warmer. Wipe the newborn free of blood, fluid, and excess vernix, especially from the head, using prewarmed towels. ➤*Rationale: The radiant warmer creates a heat-gaining environment. Drying is important to prevent the loss of body heat through evaporation.*
3. If the newborn is stable, wrap him or her in a prewarmed blanket, apply a stocking cap, and carry the newborn to the mother. The mother and her support person can hold and enjoy the newborn together. Alternatively, carry the newborn wrapped to the mother, loosen the blanket, and place the infant skin to skin on the mother's chest under a warmed blanket. ➤*Rationale: Use of a prewarmed blanket reduces convection heat loss and facilitates maternal-newborn contact without compromising the newborn's thermoregulation. Skin-to-skin contact with the mother or father helps maintain the newborn's temperature.*
4. After the newborn has spent time with the parents, return him or her to the radiant warmer. Leave the newborn uncovered (except for the cap and diaper) under the radiant warmer. ➤*Rationale: Radiant heat warms the outer skin surface, so the skin needs to be exposed.*
5. Tape a servocontrol probe on the newborn's anterior abdominal wall, with the metal side next to the skin. Do not place it over the ribs. Secure the probe

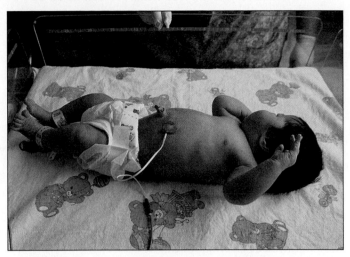

● Temperature monitoring for the newborn. A skin thermal sensor is placed on the newborn's abdomen, upper thigh, or arm and secured with porous tape or a foil-covered foam pad.

with porous tape or a foil-covered aluminum heat deflector patch. The figure below shows a newborn with a skin probe. Note that in this picture the newborn is no longer wearing a stocking cap.

6. Turn the heater to servocontrol mode so that the abdominal skin is maintained at 36.5°C to 37°C (97.5°F to 98.6°F).
7. Monitor the newborn's axillary and skin probe temperatures per agency protocol. ➤*Rationale: The temperature indicator on the radiant warmer continually displays the newborn's probe temperature. The axillary temperature is checked to ensure that the machine is accurately recording the newborn's temperature.*

---

## CLINICAL ALERT

Take action to help the newborn maintain a stable temperature:

- Keep the newborn's clothing and bedding dry.
- Double-wrap the newborn and put a stocking cap on him or her.
- Use the radiant warmer during procedures.
- Reduce the newborn's exposure to drafts.
- Warm objects that will be in contact with the newborn (e.g., stethoscopes).
- Encourage the mother to snuggle with the newborn under blankets or to breastfeed the newborn with hat and light cover on.

8. When the newborn's temperature reaches 37°C (98.6°F), add a T-shirt, double-wrap the infant (two blankets), and place the newborn in an open crib.
9. Recheck the newborn's temperature in 1 hour and regularly thereafter according to agency policy. ➤*Rationale: It is important to monitor the newborn's ability to maintain his or her own thermoregulation.*
10. If the newborn's temperature drops below 36.1°C (97°F), rewarm the infant gradually. Place the infant (unclothed except for a diaper) under the radiant

warmer with a servocontrol probe on the anterior abdominal wall. ➤*Rationale: Rapid heating can lead to hyperthermia, which is associated with apnea, insensible water loss, and increased metabolic rate.*
11. Recheck the newborn's temperature in 30 minutes, then hourly.
12. When the temperature reaches 37°C (98.6°F), dress the newborn, remove him or her from the radiant warmer, double-wrap, and place in an open crib. Check the temperature hourly until stable, then regularly according to agency policy.

# Skill 9.25 Umbilical Cord Clamp: Application, Care, and Removal

## Preparation

1. Obtain necessary supplies.

## Equipment

- Cord clamp
- Prescribed preparations; Triple dye, bacitracin ointment, or isopropyl alcohol for initial cordcare
- Cord clamp remover or scissors
- Gloves

## Procedure

### Cord Clamp Application

The goal of applying the cord clamp is to prevent bleeding and promote adaptation to the extrauterine circulation pattern.

1. Place a disposable clamp at the base of the cord about 1 inch distal to the skin demarcation line.
2. Secure the clamp by pressing until it clicks and locks.
3. Cut away excess cord distal to the disposable clamp.
4. Examine the cord and count the vessels.
5. Apply agency-specified antimicrobial agent over the base of the cord and on 1 inch of surrounding skin. ➤*Rationale: Antimicrobial ointments may be used for initial cord care in an attempt to minimize microorganisms and promote drying.*
6. Document status of the clamp and cord in the medical record.

### Routine Cord Care

The goal of routine cord care is to promote drying and sloughing of the cord and to prevent infection.

1. Apply diapers so that they are folded below the umbilical cord and do not dampen the cord with urine.
2. Change the diaper frequently to prevent urine from soaking the diaper and cord.
3. Keep the site clean and dry per agency protocol. ➤*Rationale: Wetness and moistness promote growth of microorganisms.*

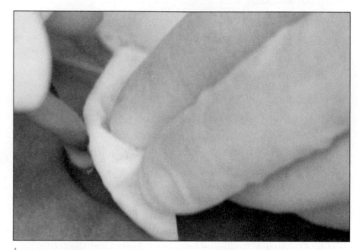

● The umbilical cord base is carefully cleaned.

4. Assess the cord for signs and symptoms of infection (foul smell, redness and drainage, localized heat and tenderness) or bleeding.
5. Document the condition of the cord in the medical record as part of routine assessment.

### Cord Clamp Removal

Cord clamps are removed once the site is dry and before discharge.

1. Verify that the stump is thoroughly dry.
2. Apply the cord clamp removal device or insert scissors into the loop at the base of the clamp.
3. Cut through the loop, directing the tool away from the cord and baby.
4. Observe for any oozing or bleeding.
5. Instruct parents regarding care of the site. Advise them to contact their primary care provider if bleeding, oozing, or odor is noticed.
6. Document the condition of the cord and teaching in the medical record.

# Skill 9.26 Assisting with Circumcision and Providing Circumcision Care

## Preparation

1. Obtain or verify parental consent.
2. Medicate the infant for pain.
3. Plan for distraction.
4. Plan for safe positioning.
5. Plan to prevent unnecessary heat loss.
6. Obtain necessary supplies.
7. Coordinate timing to avoid performing the procedure within 3 to 4 hours after feeding.

## Equipment

- Infant warmer
- Circ board
- Iodine skin prep
- Circ tray
- Analgesia medications
- Pacifier
- Sucrose solution
- Vaseline gauze
- Clean diaper
- Gloves

## Procedure

### Assisting with Circumcision

The goal of assisting with circumcision is to provide for the safety of the newborn and to relieve discomfort during the procedure.

1. Check the identity of the newborn, comparing the ID number on the infant bands with the number in the medical record with the circumcision order.
2. Confirm that consent has been obtained and documented properly.
3. Confirm that the newborn has been NPO for 3 hours or as ordered.
4. Have equipment and medications available for medicating the newborn for pain as ordered.
5. Secure the infant to the circ board using Velcro straps or other restraint devices.
6. Provide sucrose as ordered for comfort. Offer a pacifier for nonnutritive sucking.

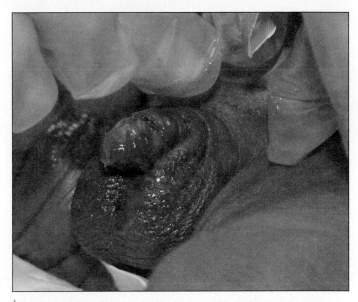

● Following circumcision, petroleum jelly may be applied to the site for the next few diaper changes.

### Care Following Circumcision

The goal of care following circumcision is to reduce trauma to the surgical site and to observe for signs of complications.

1. Apply petroleum gauze to the head of the penis.
   ➤*Rationale: Prevent the diaper from adhering to the surgical site and avoid trauma.*
2. Apply a clean diaper.
3. Assess the ability to void. Document urination following the procedure in the medical record.
   ➤*Rationale: Swelling or damage may obstruct the urethral opening.*
4. Return the newborn to his parents. Explain the procedure.
5. Teach parents to apply petroleum gauze to the site and use A&D ointment to prevent adherence of the diaper to the surgical site.
6. Monitor temperature.
7. Check the site hourly till discharge. Note any bleeding, discharge, temperature, or inability to void in the medical record.

# Skill 9.27 Initial Newborn Bath

## Preparation

1. The baby should be resting in a radiant warmer or an incubator.
2. Prewarm all baby blankets to be used.
3. Gather equipment and supplies.

## Equipment

- Clean gloves
- Warm water
- Washcloths
- Blankets or towels for drying

## Procedure

1. Assess newborn temperature. Once the newborn has demonstrated the ability to maintain a stable temperature greater than 36.6°F, a first bath can be given. ➤*Rationale: Temperature instability introduces a threat to newborn adaptation that can lead to serious complications, including respiratory distress, hypoglycemia, and acidosis. Preventing cold stress is an important goal for newborn care.*
2. Bathe the baby under the radiant warmer. If feasible, position the warmer close to a sink for a source of warm water. Alternatively, fill a basin with warm water. ➤*Rationale: The human newborn cannot maintain his or her temperature independently but requires protection against heat loss in the form of warm, dry blankets and hats, or an external heat source such as the warmth of the mother's body or a warmer.*
3. Using a clean, warm, wet washcloth, clean the eyes, washing from the inner to outer canthus of each eye, moving to a clean portion of the washcloth for each eye.
4. Wash the remainder of the face, cleaning the washcloth after each use.
5. A mild soap may be used for the remainder of the bath. Wash the folds of skin in the neck and axilla. Wash between the fingers and toes.
6. Wash the belly, extremities, and back. Wash the groin and diaper area. Dry the baby after each area is washed.
7. Complete cord care according to agency policy.
8. The hair and scalp can be washed using a mild shampoo, typically at a sink. To do so, wrap the baby in a warm blanket with arms tucked inside the blanket out of the way. Hold the infant in a football hold with head extended over the sink. Use the free, cupped hand to bring water from the faucet to the infant's head. Wet the scalp, apply a small quantity of shampoo, lather, and rinse, again using a cupped hand to bring water to the newborn's head. Dry the head thoroughly and apply a cap. (Note: The head may also be shampooed over a basin.) ➤*Rationale: The infant is wrapped for the shampoo to prevent excessive heat loss. Because significant heat loss can occur through the scalp, it is important to work quickly and to dry the head thoroughly. The cap helps retain heat.*
9. Repeat assessment of temperature. If the temperature is normal and stable, dress the newborn in a shirt, diaper, and cap. Wrap the baby and return to parents in an open crib. If the baby's axillary temperature is below 36.4°C (97.5°F), return the baby to the radiant warmer.
10. Document the bath, any significant findings, and temperature in the medical record.

### CLINICAL ALERT

Use only a small amount of soap. Excessive soap and lather can be difficult to rinse off.

### CLINICAL ALERT

Some nurses prefer to begin the bath with the shampoo.

# Skill 9.28 The Infant Receiving Phototherapy

## Preparation

1. Explain the purpose of phototherapy, the procedure itself (including the need to use eye patches), and possible side effects such as dehydration.
2. Note evidence of jaundice in the skin, sclera, and mucous membranes (in infants with darkly pigmented skin). Be sure that recent serum bilirubin levels are available. ➤*Rationale: The decision to use phototherapy is based on a careful assessment of the newborn's condition over a period of time. The most recent results prior to starting therapy serve as a baseline to evaluate the effectiveness of therapy.*

## Equipment

- Bank of phototherapy lights
- Eye patches
- Small scale to weigh diapers

## Procedure

1. Obtain vital signs, including the axillary temperature. ►*Rationale: This provides baseline data.*
2. Remove all of the infant's clothing except the diaper. ►*Rationale: Exposure of the newborn to high-intensity light (a bank of fluorescent lightbulbs or bulbs in the blue-white spectrum) decreases serum bilirubin levels in the skin by aiding biliary excretion of unconjugated bilirubin. Because the tissue absorbs the light, best results are obtained when there is maximum skin surface exposure.*
3. Apply eye coverings (eye patches or a bili mask) to the infant according to agency policy. ►*Rationale: Eye coverings are used because it is not known if phototherapy injures delicate eye structures, particularly the retina.*
4. Place the infant in an open crib or isolette (more commonly used in preterm infants and infants who are sicker) about 45 to 50 cm below the bank of phototherapy lights. Reposition every 2 hours. ►*Rationale: The isolette helps the infant maintain his or her temperature while undressed. Repositioning exposes different areas of skin to the lights, prevents the development of pressure areas on the skin, and varies the stimulation the infant receives.*
5. Monitor vital signs every 4 hours with axillary temperatures. ►*Rationale: Temperature assessment is indicated to detect hypothermia or hyperthermia. Deviation in pulse and respirations may indicate developing complications.*

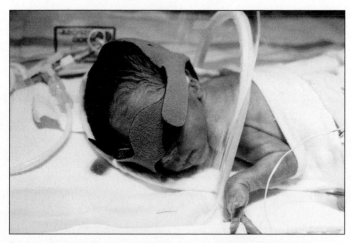

● Infant receiving phototherapy. The phototherapy light is positioned over the incubator or crib. Bilateral eye patches are always used during photo light therapy to protect the baby's eyes.

*Source:* Courtesy of Lisa Smith-Pedersen, RNC, MSN, NNP.

### CLINICAL ALERT

If the area of jaundice about the eyes begins to disappear, it is probable that the eye patches are allowing light to enter and better eye protection is needed.

6. Check the lights using a bilimeter to ensure safe effective treatment.
7. Cluster care activities.
8. Discontinue phototherapy and remove eye patches at least once per 8-hour shift. Also discontinue phototherapy and remove patches when feeding the infant and when the parents visit. ►*Rationale: Care activities are clustered to help ensure that the newborn has maximum time under the lights. Eye patches are removed to assess for signs of complications such as excessive pressure, discharge, or conjunctivitis. Patches are also removed to provide some social stimulation and to promote parental attachment.*
9. Maintain adequate fluid intake. Evaluate the need for IV fluids.
10. Monitor intake and output carefully. Weigh diapers before discarding. Record quantity and characteristics of each stool. ►*Rationale: Infants undergoing phototherapy treatment have increased water loss and loose stools as a result of bilirubin excretion. This increases their risk of dehydration.*
11. Assess specific gravity with each voiding. Weigh the newborn daily. ►*Rationale: Specific gravity provides one measure of urine concentration. Highly concentrated urine is associated with a dehydrated state. Weight loss is also a sign of developing dehydration in the newborn.*
12. Observe the infant for signs of perianal excoriation, and institute therapy if it develops. ►*Rationale: Perianal excoriation may develop because of the irritating effect of diarrhea stools.*
13. Ensure that serum bilirubin levels are drawn regularly according to orders or agency policy. Turn the phototherapy lights off while the blood is drawn. ►*Rationale: Serum bilirubin levels provide the most accurate indication of the effectiveness of phototherapy. They are generally drawn every 12 hours, but at least once daily. The phototherapy lights are turned off to ensure accurate serum bilirubin levels.*
14. Examine the newborn's skin regularly for signs of developing pressure areas, bronzing, maculopapular rash, and changes in degree of jaundice. ►*Rationale: Pressure areas may develop if the infant lies in one position for an extended period. A benign, transient bronze discoloration of the skin may occur with phototherapy when the infant has elevated direct serum bilirubin levels or liver disease. A maculopapular rash is another transient side effect of phototherapy that develops occasionally.*

15. Avoid using lotion or ointment on the exposed skin. ➤*Rationale: Lotion and ointments on a newborn receiving phototherapy may cause skin burns.*

16. Provide parents with opportunities to hold the newborn and assist in the infant's care. Answer their questions accurately and keep them informed of developments or changes. ➤*Rationale: A sick infant is a source of great anxiety for parents. Information helps them deal with their anxiety. Moreover, they have a right to be kept well informed of their baby's status so that they are able to make informed decisions as needed.*

*Note:* Phototherapy may also be provided using light-weight, fiberoptic blankets ("bili blankets"). The baby is wrapped in the blanket, which is plugged into an outlet. The eyes are not covered. With fiberoptic blankets the newborn is readily accessible for care, feedings, and diaper changes. The baby does not get overheated, and fluid and weight loss are not complications of this system. The infant is accessible to the parents, and the procedure seems less alarming to parents than standard phototherapy. A combination of a fiberoptic light source in the mattress under the baby and a standard phototherapy light source above is also used by some agencies. In addition, many agencies and pediatricians use fiberoptic blankets for home care.

# 10

# Tissue Integrity

**Skill 10.1** Performing a Dry Dressing Change 405

**Skill 10.2** Cleaning a Sutured Wound and Changing a Dressing on a Wound with a Drain 408

**Skill 10.3** Applying Wet-to-Moist Dressings 410

**Skill 10.4** Irrigating a Wound 412

**Skill 10.5** Applying an Abdominal Binder 413

**Skill 10.6** Using Alginates on Wounds 414

**Skill 10.7** Applying Bandages and Binders (Elastic Bandages) 416

**Skill 10.8** Maintaining Closed Wound Drainage 419

**Skill 10.9** Obtaining a Wound Drainage Specimen 420

VARIATION: Obtaining a Specimen for Anaerobic Culture Using a Sterile Syringe and Needle 422

**Skill 10.10** Assessing Ankle-Brachial Index (ABI) 422

**Skill 10.11** Changing a Dressing— Venous Ulcer 422

**Skill 10.12** Preventing Pressure Ulcers 426

**Skill 10.13** Providing Care for Clients with Pressure Ulcers 428

**Skill 10.14** Applying Transparent Film Dressing 429

**Skill 10.15** Using Hydrocolloid Dressing 431

**Skill 10.16** Using Electrical Stimulation 434

**Skill 10.17** Using Noncontact Normothermic Wound Therapy 435

**Skill 10.18** Using Negative Pressure Wound Therapy 437

**Skill 10.19** Applying a Transparent Wound Barrier 440

**Skill 10.20** Positioning and Exercising the Stump 442

**Skill 10.21** Shrinking/Molding the Stump 443

The skin serves a variety of functions, including protecting the individual from injury. Impaired skin integrity is not a frequent problem for most healthy people, but is a threat to elders and clients with restricted mobility, chronic illness, trauma, and those undergoing invasive procedures. When the skin or underlying tissues are damaged, the inflammatory process of the individual's immune response acts to eliminate any foreign material, if possible, and prepare the injured area for healing. This injury body area is called a **wound.** The nurse plays an important role in assessing client risk for developing wounds, in preventing wounds, and in treating various types of wounds.

### EXPECTED OUTCOMES

- Client's wounds do not become infected.
- Client's wound remains intact following staple and/or suture removal.
- Wound care is provided for contaminated wound and healing occurs.
- Drainage system functions without obstructions.
- Wound irrigation is completed using sufficient pressure to cleanse wound bed.
- Abdominal binder supports client's abdominal wound.
- Compression dressing applied to vascular ulcer site.
- Stage of pressure ulcer is accurately assessed.
- Pressure ulcer is treated effectively according to stage of ulcer formation.
- Pressure ulcer is healing within usual time frame.
- Skin remains free of breakdown in surrounding areas of pressure ulcer.
- Absence of additional pressure ulcer formation.

## EVIDENCE-BASED NURSING PRACTICE

**Maintaining a Moist Environment**

Dressings that promote a moist wound environment stimulate rapid wound healing. Saline soaks are not as effective as moisture-retentive dressings. The type of dressing used is dependent on the type of wound, whether infected or if debris is present, amount of exudates, cost, and client comfort.

*Source:* Joanne Briggs Institute for Evidence-Based Nursing & Midwifery. *www.joannabriggs.edu/au/procmana.html.*

**Pressure Relief in Surgical Clients**

Pressure ulcers can begin in the operating room. The occurrence of ulcers can be as high as 45% of surgical clients. There are many risk factors leading to ulcer development in as few as 2 1/2 hours. Risk factors include position client is placed in during procedure, necessity of positioning devices that place pressure on bony prominences. Medications that constrict blood vessels or lower blood pressure can also lead to pressure ulcers.

*Source:* Armstrong, D., Bortz, P. An integrative review of pressure relief in surgical patients. *American Organization of Operating Room Nurses Journal,* 74(3), 645.

### TABLE 10-1 TYPES OF WOUNDS

| Type | Cause | Description and Characteristics |
|---|---|---|
| Incision | Sharp instrument (e.g., knife or scalpel) | Open wound; deep or shallow |
| Contusion | Blow from a blunt instrument | Closed wound, skin appears ecchymotic (bruised) because of damaged blood vessels |
| Abrasion | Surface scrape, either unintentional (e.g., scraped knee from a fall) or intentional (e.g., dermal abrasion to remove pockmarks) | Open wound involving the skin |
| Puncture | Penetration of the skin and often the underlying tissues by a sharp instrument, either intentional or unintentional | Open wound |
| Laceration | Tissues torn apart, often from accidents (e.g., with machinery) | Open wound; edges are often jagged |
| Penetrating wound | Penetration of the skin and the underlying tissues, usually unintentional (e.g., from a bullet or metal fragments) | Open wound |

## EVIDENCE-BASED NURSING PRACTICE

### Pressure Ulcer Formation

There is an unresolved and inadequately explained issue of how a pressure ulcer progresses. Some clinicians believe the ulcer forms from top down and other theories have indicated that the pressure ulcer progresses from bottom up. There is limited research on this theory. Current literature indicates that the bottom-up theory is more appropriate, as the deeper tissues are involved in pressure ulcer formation. Latest opinion is that true pressure ulcers are an injury to soft tissue and muscle that occurs from pressure over bony prominences. It is recommended that further research be done.

*Source:* WOCN Society Response to NPUAP White Papers: Deep Tissue Injury, Stage I Pressure Ulcers, and Stage II Pressure Ulcers: 9th National NPUAP Conference, February 2005. Phyllis Bonham, Ph.D., MSN, RN, CWOCN, and Janet Ramundo, MSN, RN, FNP, CWOCN.

### Medieval Remedies

Medieval remedies, like maggots for bedsores, bee stings for MS, and leeches to improve blood flow after surgery, are enjoying a renaissance.

Leeches reemerged a while ago and now have a well-established role in plastic and reconstructive surgery.

Maggots are being considered more often for treatment of chronic wounds that do not heal. And bee venom is considered alternative medicine.

Maggots do a better job than more conservative therapy for pressure ulcer treatment. Physicians who use maggots in their practice say they like them because they work.

*Source:* Wound repair and regeneration. (2002, September). *Archives of Internal Medicine.*

## Skill 10.1   Performing a Dry Dressing Change

### Delegation

Due to the need for aseptic technique and assessment skills, most dressing changes are not delegated to UAP. In some states, UAP may apply dry dressings to clean, chronic wounds. UAP should observe an exposed wound or dressing during usual care and must report abnormal findings to the nurse. In some agencies, UAP may be permitted to reinforce the dressing (apply additional dry dressings over a saturated bandage), but this must be reported to the nurse as soon as possible. Assessment of the wound and abnormal findings must be validated and interpreted by the nurse.

### Equipment

- Clean OR Sterile gloves
- 4 × 4 gauze
- Hypoallergenic tape, tie tapes, or binder
- Bath blanket (if necessary)
- Moisture-proof bag
- Mask (optional)
- Acetone or another solution (if necessary to loosen adhesive)
- Sterile dressing set; if none is available, gather the following sterile items:
  - Drape or towel
  - Gauze squares
  - Container for the cleaning solution
  - Antimicrobial solution
  - Forceps

- Additional supplies required for the particular dressing (e.g., extra gauze dressings and ointment or powder, if ordered)

### Preparation

- Acquire assistance for changing a dressing on a restless or confused adult. ➤*Rationale: The person might move and contaminate the sterile field or the wound.*
- Make a cuff on the moisture-proof bag for disposal of the soiled dressings, and place the bag within reach. It can be taped to the bedclothes or bedside table. ➤*Rationale: Making a cuff keeps the outside of the bag free from contamination by the soiled dressings and prevents subsequent contamination of the nurse's hands or of sterile instrument tips when discarding dressings or sponges. Placement of the bag within reach prevents the nurse from reaching across the sterile field and the wound and potentially contaminating these areas.*

### Procedure

1. Prior to performing the procedure, introduce self and verify the client's identity using agency protocol. Explain to the client what you are going to do, why it is necessary, and how he or she can participate. Discuss how the results will be used in planning further care or treatments.
2. Perform hand hygiene and observe other appropriate infection control procedures.
3. Provide for client privacy. Assist the client to a comfortable position in which the wound can be readily exposed. Expose only the wound area, using a bath

blanket to cover the client, if necessary. ➤*Rationale: Undue exposure is physically and psychologically distressing to most people.*

4. If adhesive tape was used, remove it by holding down the skin and pulling the tape gently but firmly toward the wound. ➤*Rationale: Pressing down on the skin provides countertraction against the pulling motion. Tape is pulled toward the incision to prevent strain on the sutures or wound **and decrease the pain of tape removal.***

   • Use a solvent to loosen tape, if required. ➤*Rationale: Moistening the tape with acetone or a similar solvent lessens the discomfort of removal, particularly from hairy surfaces.*

   • **Remove soiled dressing** so that the underside is away from the client's face. ➤*Rationale: The appearance and odor of the drainage may be upsetting to the client.*

5. Dispose of soiled dressings in the moisture-proof bag without touching the outside of the bag. ➤*Rationale: Contamination of the outside of the bag is avoided to prevent the spread of microorganisms to the nurse and subsequently to others.*

6. Remove gloves, dispose of them in the moisture-proof bag, and perform hand hygiene.

7. Assess wound or incision for erythema, edema, or drainage. ➤*Rationale: Persistent drainage, edema, or temperature above 100.4 degrees F could indicate that a complication is occurring.*

8. Assess color of incision. (A healing incision looks pink or red.) ➤*Rationale: Redness that does not heal 48 hours after surgery may indicate impaired healing.*

9. Don clean gloves.

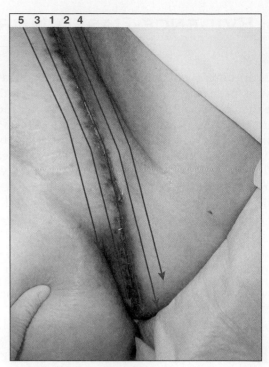

● Cleaning a wound from top to bottom.
(Courtesy of Cory Patrick Hartley, San Ramon Regional Medical Center, San Ramon, CA.)

10. Clean the wound if indicated.

   • Clean the wound, using a new pair of forceps, clean gloves, and moistened swabs.

   • Keep the forceps tips lower than the handles at all times. ➤*Rationale: This prevents their contamination by fluid traveling up to the handle and nurse's wrist and back to the tips.*

   • Clean with strokes from the top to the bottom, starting at the center and continuing to the outside.
   *or*

   • Clean outward from the wound. ➤*Rationale: The wound is cleaned from the least to the most contaminated area, for example, from the top of the incision, which is drier, to the bottom of the incision, where any drainage will collect and which is considered more contaminated, or from the center outward.*

## CLINICAL ALERT

Normal saline or Ringer's solution are widely advocated as fluids of choice for cleansing and irrigating wounds. Iodine and chlorhexidine are cytotoxic, particularly to fibroblasts. In severely infected wounds, antimicrobial irrigations may be used.

Providone iodine, hydrogen peroxide, Dakin's solution, and other agents are not used on acute wounds. They are drying agents and as such, the wound bed is dried, and the exudates and all its beneficial cells are removed from the area. Wounds maintained in a moist environment have a lower inflection rate then dry wounds.

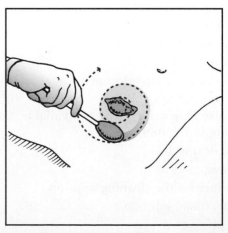

● Cleaning a wound from the center outward.

- Use a separate swab for each stroke, and discard each swab after use. ➤*Rationale: This prevents the introduction of microorganisms to other wound areas.*
- Repeat the cleaning process until all drainage is removed.

11. Place 4 × 4 gauze pads over wound or incision area, being careful not to touch wound or incision with gloves. ➤*Rationale:* Touching the wound or incision would contaminate the gloves. Reglove if that happens.

12. Remove and discard gloves. Perform hand hygiene.

13. Secure the dressing with tape, tie tapes, or a binder.
   - Place the tape so that the dressing cannot be folded back to expose the wound. Place strips at the ends of the dressing, and space tapes evenly in the middle.
   - Ensure that the tape is long and wide enough to adhere to the skin but not so long or wide that it loosens with activity.
   - Place the tape in the opposite direction from the body action, for example, across a body joint or crease, not lengthwise.
   - *Montgomery straps (tie tapes)* are commonly used for wounds requiring frequent dressing changes. ➤*Rationale: These straps prevent skin irritation and discomfort caused by removing the adhesive each time the dressing is changed.*

14. Document the dressing change and the client's response in the client record using forms or checklists supplemented by narrative notes when appropriate. Many agencies use a designated wound/skin documentation sheet.

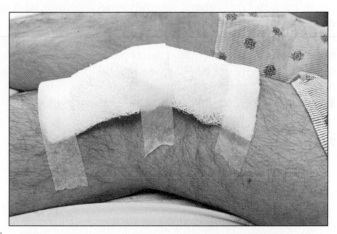

● Dressings over moving parts taped at right angle to the joint movement.

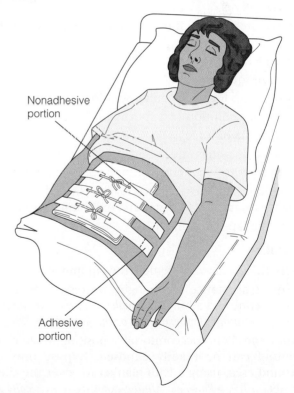

Nonadhesive portion

Adhesive portion

● Montgomery straps, or tie tapes, are used to secure large dressings that require frequent changing.

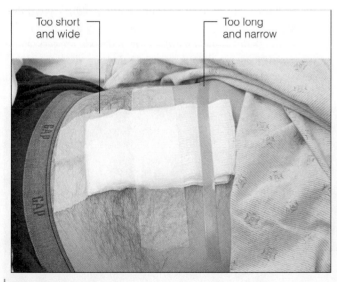

Too short and wide

Too long and narrow

● Taping the dressing.

# Skill 10.2  Cleaning a Sutured Wound and Changing a Dressing on a Wound with a Drain

## Delegation

Cleaning a newly sutured wound, especially one with a drain, requires application of knowledge, problem solving, and aseptic technique. As a result, this procedure is not delegated to UAP. The nurse can ask the UAP to report soiled dressings that need to be changed or if a dressing has become loose and needs to be reinforced. The nurse is responsible for the assessment and evaluation of the wound.

## Equipment

- Bath blanket (if necessary)
- Moisture-proof bag
- Mask (optional)
- Acetone or another solution (if necessary to loosen adhesive)
- Clean gloves
- Sterile gloves
- Sterile dressing set; if none is available, gather the following sterile items:
  - Drape or towel
  - Gauze squares
  - Container for the cleaning solution
  - Cleaning solution (e.g., normal saline)
  - Two pairs of forceps
  - Gauze dressings and surgipads
  - Applicators or tongue blades to apply ointments
- Additional supplies required for the particular dressing (e.g., extra gauze dressings and ointment, if ordered)
- Tape, tie tapes, or binder

## Preparation

Prepare the client and assemble the equipment.

- Acquire assistance for changing a dressing on a restless or confused adult. ➤*Rationale: The person might move and contaminate the sterile field or the wound.*
- Assist the client to a comfortable position in which the wound can be readily exposed. Expose only the wound area, using a bath blanket to cover the client, if necessary. ➤*Rationale: Undue exposure is physically and psychologically distressing to most people.*
- Make a cuff on the moisture-proof bag for disposal of the soiled dressings, and place the bag within reach. It can be taped to the bedclothes or bedside table. ➤*Rationale: Making a cuff helps keep the outside of the bag free from contamination by the soiled dressings and prevents subsequent contamination of the nurse's hands or of sterile*

instrument tips when discarding dressing or sponges. Placement of the bag within reach prevents the nurse from reaching across the sterile field and the wound and potentially contaminating these areas.

- Apply a face mask, if required. ➤*Rationale: Some agencies require that a mask be worn for surgical dressing changes to prevent contamination of the wound by droplet spray from the nurse's respiratory tract.*

## Procedure

1. Prior to performing the procedure, introduce self and verify the client's identity using agency protocol. Explain to the client what you are going to do, why it is necessary, and how he or she can participate. Discuss how the results will be used in planning further care or treatments.
2. Perform hand hygiene and observe other appropriate infection control procedures.
3. Provide for client privacy.
4. Remove binders and tape.
   - Remove binders, if used, and place them aside. Untie tie tapes, if used. Montgomery straps (tie tapes) are commonly used for wounds requiring frequent dressing changes. ➤*Rationale: These straps prevent skin irritation and discomfort caused by removing the adhesive each time the dressing is changed.*
   - If adhesive tape was used, remove it by holding down the skin and pulling the tape gently but firmly toward the wound. ➤*Rationale: Pressing down on the skin provides countertraction against the pulling motion. Tape is pulled toward the incision to prevent strain on the sutures or wound.*

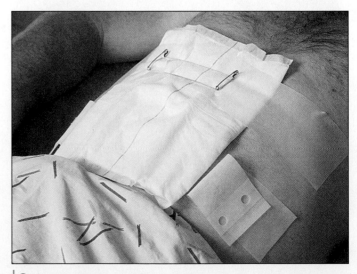

● Montgomery straps holding dressing.

- Use a solvent to loosen tape, if required. ➤*Rationale: Moistening the tape with acetone or a similar solvent lessens the discomfort of removal, particularly from hairy surfaces.*

5. Remove and dispose of soiled dressings appropriately.
   - Apply clean gloves, and remove the outer abdominal dressing or surgipad.
   - Lift the outer dressing so that the underside is *away* from the client's face. ➤*Rationale: The appearance and odor of the drainage may be upsetting to the client.*
   - Place the soiled dressing in the moisture-proof bag without touching the outside of the bag. ➤*Rationale: Contamination of the outside of the bag is avoided to prevent the spread of microorganisms to the nurse and subsequently to others.*
   - Remove the under dressings, taking care not to dislodge any drains. If the gauze sticks to the drain, support the drain with one hand and remove the gauze with the other.
   - Assess the location, type (color, consistency), and odor of wound drainage, and the number of gauzes saturated or the diameter of drainage collected on the dressings.
   - Discard the soiled dressings in the bag as before.
   - Remove and discard gloves in the moisture-proof bag. Perform hand hygiene.

6. Set up the sterile supplies.
   - Open the sterile dressing set, using surgical aseptic technique.
   - Place the sterile drape beside the wound.
   - Open the sterile cleaning solution, and pour it over the gauze sponges in the plastic container.
   - Apply sterile gloves.

7. Clean the wound, if indicated.
   - Clean the wound, using your gloved hands or forceps and gauze swabs moistened with cleaning solution.
   - If using forceps, keep the forceps tips lower than the handles at all times. ➤*Rationale: This prevents their contamination by fluid traveling up to the handle and nurse's wrist and back to the tips.*
   - Use the cleaning methods illustrated and described in or one recommended by agency protocol.
   - Use a separate swab for each stroke, and discard each swab after use. ➤*Rationale: This prevents the introduction of microorganisms to other wound areas.*
   - If a drain is present, clean it next, taking care to avoid reaching across the cleaned incision. Clean the skin around the drain site by swabbing in half or full circles from around the drain site outward, using separate swabs for each wipe.
   - Support and hold the drain erect while cleaning around it. Clean as many times as necessary to remove the drainage.
   - Dry the surrounding skin with dry gauze swabs as required. Do not dry the incision or wound itself. ➤*Rationale: Moisture facilitates wound healing.*

8. Apply dressings to the drain site and the incision.
   - Place a precut 4 × 4 gauze snugly around the drain, or open a 4 × 4 gauze to 4 × 8, fold it lengthwise to 2 × 8, and place the 2 × 8 gauze around the drain so that the ends overlap. ➤*Rationale: This dressing absorbs the drainage and helps prevent it from excoriating the skin. Using precut gauze or folding it as described, instead of cutting the gauze,*

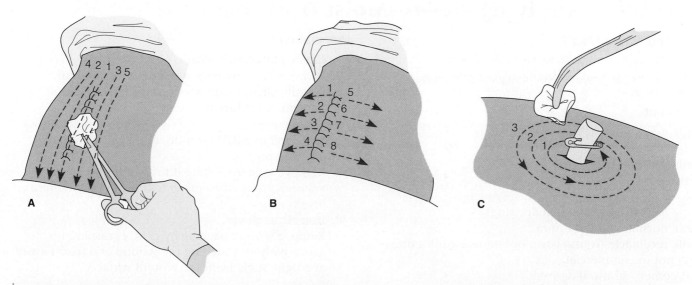

Methods of cleaning surgical wounds: **A,** cleaning the wound from top to bottom, starting at the center; **B,** cleaning a wound outward from the incision; **C,** cleaning around a Penrose drain site. For all methods, a clean sterile swab is used for each stroke.

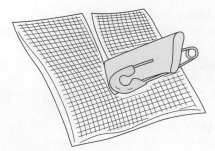

● Precut gauze in place around a Penrose drain.

*prevents any threads from coming loose and getting into the wound, where they could cause inflammation and provide a site for infection.*

- Apply the sterile dressings one at a time over the drain and the incision. Place the bulk of the dressings over the drain area and below the drain, depending on the client's usual position. ➤*Rationale: Layers of dressings are placed for best absorption of drainage, which flows by gravity.*
- Apply the final surgipad. Remove and discard gloves. Secure the dressing with tape or ties. Perform hard hygiene.

9. Document the procedure and all nursing assessments.

### Documentation

Sample: 3/21/2009 1100 Abdominal dressing changed. Small amount of serosanguineous drainage–size of a half dollar in middle of dressing. Incision approximated with slight redness at edges. Sutures intact.

——————————————————————— S. Jones, RN

---

## SETTING OF CARE

**Instruct caregivers to:**

- Provide pain medication approximately 30 minutes before the procedure if the wound care causes pain or discomfort.
- Wash hands thoroughly and dry prior to handling wound care supplies and providing wound care.
- Clean and wipe dry a flat surface for the sterile field.
- Keep pets out of the area when setting up for and performing sterile procedures.
- Acquire all needed supplies before starting a sterile procedure.
- Maintain sterile or clean technique as instructed.
- Handle all sterile supplies from the outside of the wrapper or the edges.
- Not touch the parts of supplies or equipment that will touch the client.
- Avoid skin injury by using paper tape or Montgomery straps instead of adhesive tape.
- Report any increasing wound drainage, pain, or redness, increasing swelling, or opening or gaping of wound edges.
- Place any soiled dressing materials in a waterproof bag and dispose of it according to public health recommendations.

---

# Skill 10.3  Applying Wet-to-Moist Dressings

### EXPECTED OUTCOMES

- Wound heals without complications.
- Sterile technique is maintained throughout procedure.

### Equipment

Sterile 4 × 8 noncotton gauze dressings
Semi-occlusive dressing, optional
Sterile gloves
Clean gloves
Tape
Plastic bag for contaminated dressings
Sterile normal saline solution
Sterile receptacle (round basin or emesis basin) if dressing not in commercial pack
Montgomery straps, if desired

### Preparation

1. Check physician's orders.
2. Perform hand hygiene and gather equipment.
3. Identify client using two forms of identification.
4. Explain procedure to client.
5. Provide privacy.
6. Raise bed to HIGH position, and lower side rail nearest you.
7. Remove tape by pulling it toward the wound. ➤*Rationale: This action prevents injury to newly formed tissue.*
8. Don clean gloves.
9. Remove wound packing by gently grasping the gauze without touching the wound and tear it away at a right angle from the wound surface.

➤*Rationale: Touching only the gauze prevents contamination of the wound.*

10. Place soiled dressings in disposable bag.
11. Remove gloves, and dispose of them in bag.
12. Perform hand hygiene.

**Procedure**

1. Open packages of dressings making sure sterility is maintained.
2. Pour normal saline solution over dressings.
3. Don sterile gloves.
4. Pick up sterile gauze dressings one at a time.
5. Fluff each dressing, and place over wound.
   ➤*Rationale: If packed tightly, dressing can prevent wound edges from contact with capillaries.*
6. Place gauze in the wound, covering all exposed surfaces. Press gauze lightly into depressions or cracks.
   ➤*Rationale: Necrotic tissue is more prevalent in these areas.*
7. Unfold a moist, sterile, 4 × 8 (ABD pad) dressing into a single layer and place it on top of wet dressings covering the wound area (not on skin).
8. Place a dry 4 × 8 pad over the dressing to hold it in place. Some protocols call for semi-occlusive dressing in place of pad.

## CLINICAL ALERT

Wet-to-dry dressings are used only to debride wounds, as they cause tissue damage. Maceration of healthy tissue can occur with dressings that are always wet. Dry dressings cause damage to granulating tissue if removed without first soaking the gauze.

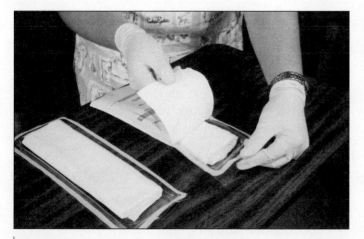

● Open sterile packages before beginning dressing change.

## CLINICAL ALERT

Heat lamps should not be used to treat pressure ulcers. Preferred wound care is to promote a clean, moist environment.

9. Remove gloves, and place in plastic bag.
10. Tape only the edges of the dressing. Montgomery tapes may be used to prevent excessive skin irritation and damage due to frequent dressing changes.
11. Position client for comfort. Lower bed, and raise side rail to UP position, if appropriate.
12. Discard soiled material in appropriate container.
13. Perform hand hygiene.
14. Observe wound for excessive drainage or drying out of dressing between dressing changes. Remoisten dressing if dry. ➤*Rationale: Unless excessive drainage occurs, or dressing dries out, dressings are usually changed every 8 hours.*
15. Provide client or family teaching regarding wound care, if appropriate.

*Note:* These dressings function as an osmotic dressing. Normal saline is isotonic. As water evaporates from saline dressing it becomes hypertonic and fluid from wound tissue is drained into dressing.

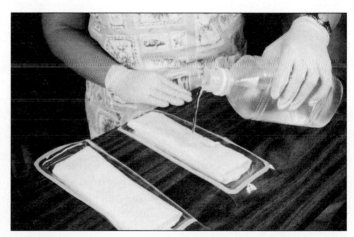

● Pour sterile saline solution over dressings to moisten.

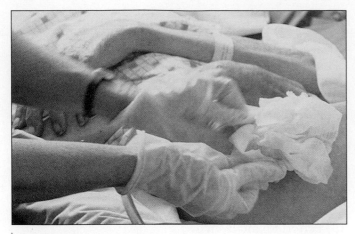

● Fluff dressings and apply over wound, covering all exposed surfaces.

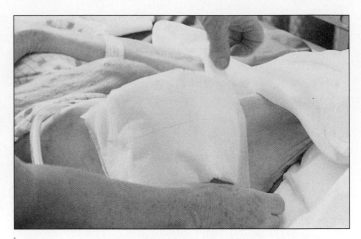

● Place moist ABD pad over dressings, then cover with dry pad.

| UNEXPECTED OUTCOMES | CRITICAL THINKING OPTIONS |
|---|---|
| Wound drainage increases. | • Decrease time between dressing changes. Change every 4 hours.<br>• Obtain order for culture and sensitivity to determine if different microorganisms are present or antibiotic medication is not sensitive to microorganisms. |
| Dressings dry between dressing changes. | • Moisten dressing with sterile normal saline before removing to prevent debridement of granulation tissue.<br>• Ensure that dressing is moist when applied to wound and cover with moist dressing.<br>• Moisten and change dressing more frequently.<br>• Semiocclusive dressing should be considered. |

# Skill 10.4   Irrigating a Wound

## Delegation

Due to the need for aseptic technique and assessment skills, wound irrigations are not delegated to UAP. However, UAP may observe the wound and dressing during usual care and must report abnormal findings to the nurse. Abnormal findings must be validated and interpreted by the nurse.

## Equipment

Although a wound may already be contaminated, sterile equipment is usually used during irrigation to prevent the possibility of adding new nonresident microorganisms to the site. In settings outside of hospitals, some reusable supplies such as irrigating syringes or basins may be cleaned and used again for a specific wound.

- Sterile dressing equipment and dressing materials
- Sterile irrigation set or individual supplies, including:
  - Sterile syringe (e.g., a 30- to 60-mL syringe) with a catheter of an appropriate size (e.g., #18 or #19) or an irrigating (catheter) tip syringe

- Sterile graduated container for irrigating solution
- Basin for collecting the used irrigating solution
- Moisture-proof sterile drape
- Moisture-proof bag
- Irrigating solution, usually 200 mL(6.5 oz) of solution warmed to body temperature, according to the agency's or primary care provider's choice
- Goggles, gown, and mask
- Clean gloves
- Sterile gloves

## Preparation

- Check that the irrigating fluid is at the proper temperature.

## Procedure

1. Prior to performing the procedure, introduce self and verify the client's identity using agency protocol. Explain to the client what you are going to do, why it is necessary, and how he or she can partici-

pate. Discuss how the results will be used in planning further care or treatments.

2. Perform hand hygiene and observe other appropriate infection control procedures.
3. Provide for client privacy.
4. Prepare the client.
   - Assist the client to a position in which the irrigating solution will flow by gravity from the upper end of the wound to the lower end and then into the basin.
   - Place the waterproof drape under the wounds and over the bed.
   - Apply clean gloves and remove and discard the old dressing.
5. Measure and assess the wound and drainage.
   - If indicated, clean the wound (see Skill 10.1, step 9).
   - Remove and discard gloves. Perform hand hygiene.
6. Prepare the equipment.
   - Open the sterile dressing set and supplies.
   - Pour the ordered solution into the solution container.
   - Position the basin below the wound to receive the irrigating fluid.
7. Irrigate the wound.
   - Apply clean gloves.
   - Instill a steady stream of irrigating solution into the wound. Make sure all areas of the wound are irrigated.
   - Use either a syringe with a catheter attached or with an irrigating tip to flush the wound.
   - If you are using a catheter to reach tracts or crevices, insert the catheter into the wound until resistance is met. Do not force the catheter. ➤*Rationale: Forcing the catheter can cause tissue damage.*
   - Continue irrigating until the solution becomes clear (no exudate is present).
   - Dry the area around the wound. ➤*Rationale: Moisture left on the skin promotes the growth of microorganisms and can cause skin irritation and breakdown.*
   - Remove and discard gloves. Perform hand hygiene.

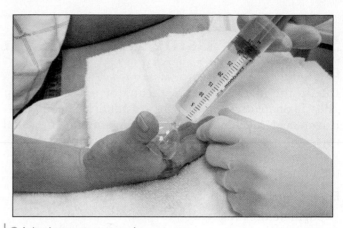

● Irrigating an open wound.

(Courtesy of Cory Patrick Hartley, San Ramon Regional Medical Center, San Ramon, CA.)

8. Assess and dress the wound.
   - Assess the appearance of the wound again, noting in particular the type and amount of exudate still present and the presence and extent of granulation tissue.
   - Using sterile technique, apply a sterile dressing to the wound based on the amount of drainage expected.
   - Remove and discard sterile gloves. Perform hand hygiene.
9. Document the irrigation and the client's response in the client record using forms or checklists supplemented by narrative notes when appropriate. Many agencies use a designated wound/skin documentation sheet.

### Documentation

Sample: 5/31/09 1000 Wound on (R) hip 3×3 cm, 6 mm deep, draining minimal amt. thick yellow. No odor. Skin around wound erythematous. Pain 0 on 0–10 scale. Irrigated c̄ NS until clear. Redressed c̄ sterile technique.

_____ N. Jamaghani, RN

# Skill 10.5   Applying an Abdominal Binder

### Equipment

Abdominal binder: woven-cotton, synthetic, or elasticized material. Most facilities use commercial Velcro binders. Safety pins for binders without Velcro closure

### Procedure

1. Perform hand hygiene.
2. Explain use of binder to client.
3. Place client in supine position.
4. Ask client to raise hips, and then slide the binder under client's hips at level of gluteal fold. Place top of binder at client's waist.
5. Bring ends of binder around client, and secure by pressing Velcro surfaces together. If using non-Velcro binder, secure binder with safety pins placed vertically along edges. Start pinning at bottom of binder and pin toward waist. ➤*Rationale: Pinning binder from bottom to waist provides uplifting support for abdominal muscles.*
6. Observe for wrinkles in binder. ➤*Rationale: Wrinkles can cause pressure areas especially over iliac crest.*
7. Assess client's ability to move freely, breathe deeply, and feel secure pressure over abdominal incision. ➤*Rationale: A binder that is too tight may compromise breathing or place pressure on incisional area.*
8. Assess effectiveness of binder every 4 hours, and rewrap every 8 hours if non-Velcro binder is used. Many clients use this binder only when ambulating.

# Skill 10.6   Using Alginates on Wounds

## Delegation

Due to the need for aseptic technique and assessment skills, alginate dressing changes are not delegated to UAP. However, UAP may observe the dressing during usual care and must report abnormal findings to the nurse. Abnormal findings must be validated and interpreted by the nurse.

## Equipment

- Alginate dressing
- Sterile dressing equipment and secondary dressing materials
- Solution for irrigation (e.g., sterile saline or water)
- Irrigating syringe
- Bowl
- Basin to collect irrigation
- Forceps or cotton-tipped applicators (optional)
- Moisture-proof bag
- Clean gloves
- Sterile gloves

## Procedure

1. Prior to performing the procedure, introduce self and verify the client's identity using agency protocol. Explain to the client what you are going to do, why it is necessary, and how he or she can participate. Discuss how the results will be used in planning further care or treatments.
2. Perform hand hygiene and observe other appropriate infection control procedures.
3. Prepare the client. Assist the client to a comfortable position in which the wound can be readily exposed.
4. Provide for client privacy. Expose only the wound area, using a bath blanket to cover the client, if necessary. ➤*Rationale: Undue exposure is physically and psychologically distressing to most people.*
5. Prepare the supplies.
   - Open the sterile dressing set and supplies.
   - Pour the ordered solution into the solution container.
   - Position the basin below the wound to receive the irrigating fluid.
6. Remove the existing dressing and alginate.
   - Apply clean gloves, remove and discard the outer secondary dressing in the moisture-proof bag.
   - If the previous alginate has absorbed drainage, it will be in gel form. Irrigate the wound with the prescribed solution until all of the dressing has been removed.
   - If the alginate dressing does not appear in gel form or does not remove easily with irrigation, either the secondary dressing is not maintaining a moist environment or

the wound is no longer producing enough exudate to warrant alginate dressing.
7. Assess the wound.
8. Clean the wound if indicated (see Skill 10.1, Step 9).
   - Remove and discard gloves. Perform hand hygiene.
9. Pack the wound with the alginate.
   - Apply sterile gloves.
   - Pack the alginate into all depressions and grooves of the wound. Cover all exposed surfaces.

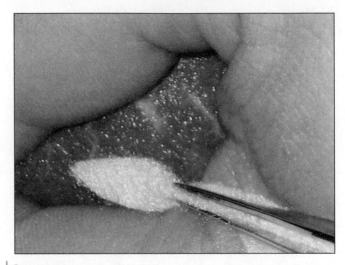

● Packing a wound with alginate.
(Courtesy of Cory Patrick Hartley, San Ramon Regional Medical Center, San Ramon, CA.)

---

**SETTING OF CARE**

- Discuss importance of adequate nutrition (especially fluids, protein, vitamins B and C, iron, and calories).
- Instruct in wound assessment and provide mechanism for documenting.
- Emphasize principles of asepsis, especially hand cleansing and proper methods of handling used dressings.
- Provide information about signs of wound infection and other complications to report.
- Reinforce appropriate aspects of pressure ulcer prevention.
- Demonstrate wound care techniques such as wound cleansing, dressing change.
- Discuss pain control measures, if needed.
- Verify how the client may bathe with the wound (i.e., does the wound need to be covered with a water-proof barrier or should it be cleansed in the shower?).
- Tap water may be used to cleanse wounds instead of normal saline (Fernandez, Griffiths, & Ussia, 2006).

10. Dress the wound.
    - Cover the alginate with petrolatum gauze, foam, or other secondary dressing that will keep the alginate in place and provide a moist wound environment.
    - Remove and discard gloves. Perform hand hygiene.

11. Document the dressing change and the client's response in the client record using forms or checklists supplemented by narrative notes when appropriate. Many agencies use a designated wound/skin documentation sheet.

## CLIENT TEACHING

Perform appropriate client teaching for promoting wound healing and maintenance of healthy skin.

### Maintaining Intact Skin

- Discuss relationship between adequate nutrition (especially fluids, protein, vitamins B and C, iron, and calories) and healthy skin.
- Demonstrate appropriate positions for pressure relief.
- Establish a turning or repositioning schedule.
- Demonstrate application of appropriate skin protection agents and devices.
- Instruct to report persistent reddened areas.
- Identify potential sources of skin trauma and means of avoidance.

### Wound Care

- Instruct family about hygiene and medical asepsis, hand cleansing before and after dressing changes, and using a clean area for storage of dressing supplies.
- Instruct the client and family on where to obtain needed supplies. Be sensitive to the cost of dressings (e.g., transparent barriers are costly) and suggest less expensive alternatives if necessary. Be creative in the use of household items for padding pressure areas.
- Instruct the client and family in proper disposal of contaminated dressings. All contaminated items should be double bagged in moisture-proof bags.

## DEVELOPMENTAL CONSIDERATIONS

### Infants

- The skin of infants is more fragile than that of older children and adults, and more susceptible to infection, shearing from friction, and burns.

### Children

- Staphylococcus and fungus are two major infectious agents affecting the skin of children. Abrasions or small lacerations, commonly experienced by children, provide an entry in the skin for these organisms. Minor wounds should be cleansed with warm, soapy water, and covered with a sterile bandage. Children should be instructed not to touch the wound.
- With more serious skin lesions, remind the child not to touch the wound, drains, or dressing. Cover with an appropriate bandage that will remain intact during the child's usual activities. Cover a transparent dressing with opaque material if viewing the site is distressing to the child. Restrain only when all alternatives have been tried and when absolutely necessary.
- For younger children, demonstrate wound care on a doll. Reassure that the wound will not be permanent and that nothing will fall out of the body.

### Elders

- Hold wrinkled skin taut during application of a transparent dressing. Obtain assistance if needed.
- Skin of elders is more fragile and can easily tear with removal of tape (especially adhesive tape). Use paper tape and tape remover as indicated, keeping tape use to the minimum required. Use extreme caution during tape removal. If possible, use conforming gauze bandage (e.g., Elastomull, Kerlix Lite, or Kling) to hold dressing in place.
- Elders who are in long-term care facilities often have the following factors: immobility, malnutrition, and incontinence, all of which increase the risk for development of skin breakdown.
- Skin breakdown can occur as quickly as within 2 hours, so assessments should be done with each repositioning of the client.
- A thorough assessment of a client's heels should be done every shift. The skin can break down quickly from friction of movement in bed. Whenever possible, heels should be suspended off the mattress using pillows or other mechanisms.

# Skill 10.7   Applying Bandages and Binders (Elastic Bandages)

## Delegation

Application of binders can be delegated to UAP or family members/caregivers after the nurse has performed initial assessment that these persons can perform this skill safely. Application of bandages over wounds may be taught to clients or family members/caregivers for home care purposes.

## Equipment

- Clean bandage or binder of the appropriate material and size **(Elastic bandage)**
- Padding, such as abdominal pads or gauze squares
- Tape, clips, or Velcro

## Procedure

1. Prior to performing the procedure, introduce self and verify the client's identity using agency protocol. Explain to the client what you are going to do, why it is necessary, and how he or she can participate. Discuss how the results will be used in planning further care or treatments.
2. Perform hand hygiene and observe other appropriate infection control procedures.
3. Provide for client privacy.
4. Position and prepare the client appropriately.
   - Provide the client with a chair or bed, and arrange support for the area to be bandaged. For example, if a hand needs to be bandaged, ask the client to place the elbow on a table, so that the hand does not have to be held up unsupported. ➤*Rationale: Because bandaging takes time, holding up a body part without support can fatigue the client.*
   - Make sure that the area to be bandaged is clean and dry. Wash and dry the area if necessary. Perform wound care as indicated. ➤*Rationale: Washing and drying remove microorganisms, which flourish in dark, warm, moist areas.*
   - Align the part to be bandaged with slight flexion of the joints, unless this is contraindicated. ➤*Rationale: Slight flexion places less strain on the ligaments and muscles of the joint.*
5. Apply the bandage. Apply the beginning of the bandage to the most distal part of the body to be bandaged first. ➤*Rationale: Wrapping from distal to proximal facilitates venous return and diminishes swelling.*

### Circular Turns

- Hold the bandage in your dominant hand, keeping the roll uppermost, and unroll the bandage about 8 cm (3 in.). This length of unrolled bandage allows good control for placement and tension.
- Hold the end down with the thumb of the other hand.
- Encircle the body part two times with the first wraps, then make sure that each layer overlaps one-half to

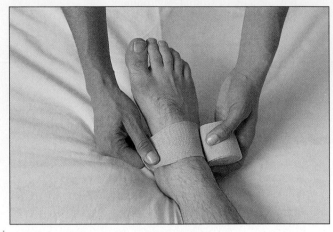

● Starting a bandage with circular turns.

two-thirds of the previous layer. This provides even support to the area.

- The bandage should be firm, but not too tight. Ask the client if the bandage feels comfortable. A tight bandage can interfere with blood circulation, whereas a loose bandage does not provide adequate protection.
- Secure the end of the bandage with tape or clips if there is no Velcro fastener.

### Spiral Turns

- Make two circular turns. ➤*Rationale: Two circular turns anchor the bandage.*
- Continue spiral turns at about a 30-degree angle, each turn overlapping the preceding one by two-thirds the width of the bandage.
- Terminate the bandage with two circular turns, and secure the end as described for circular turns.

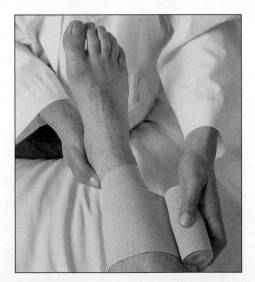

● Applying spiral turns.

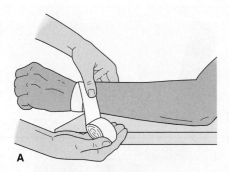
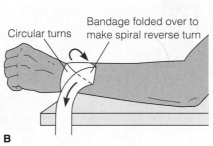
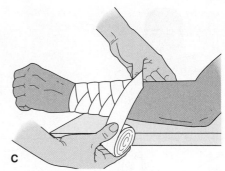

Circular turns

Bandage folded over to make spiral reverse turn

**A** **B** **C**

● Applying spiral reverse turns.

### Spiral Reverse Turns

- Anchor the bandage with two circular turns, and bring the bandage upward at about a 30-degree angle.
- Place the thumb of your free hand on the upper edge of the bandage. ►*Rationale: The thumb will hold the bandage while it is folded on itself.*
- Unroll the bandage about 15 cm (6 in.), and then turn your hand so that the bandage falls over itself.
- Continue the bandage around the limb, overlapping each previous turn by two-thirds the width of the bandage. Make each bandage turn at the same position on the limb so that the turns of the bandage will be aligned.
- Terminate the bandage with two circular turns, and secure the end as described for circular turns.

### Recurrent Turns

- Anchor the bandage with two circular turns.
- Fold the bandage back on itself, hold it with the thumb of the other hand, and bring it centrally over the distal end to be bandaged.
- Bring the bandage back over the end to the right of the center bandage but overlapping it by two-thirds the width of the bandage.

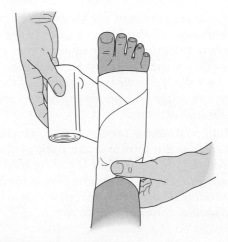

● Completing a recurrent bandage.

- Bring the bandage back on the left side, also overlapping the first turn by two-thirds the width of the bandage.
- Continue this pattern of alternating right and left until the area is covered. Overlap the preceding turn by two-thirds the bandage width each time.
- Terminate the bandage with two circular turns. Secure the end appropriately.

### Figure-Eight Turns

- Anchor the bandage with two circular turns.
- Carry the bandage above the joint, around it, and then below it, making a figure eight.

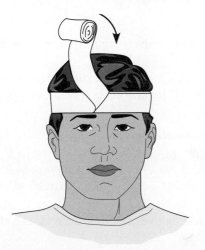

● Starting a recurrent bandage.

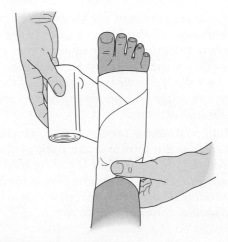

● Applying a figure-eight bandage.

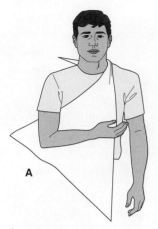
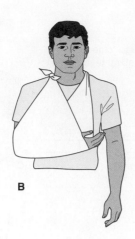

A triangle arm sling.

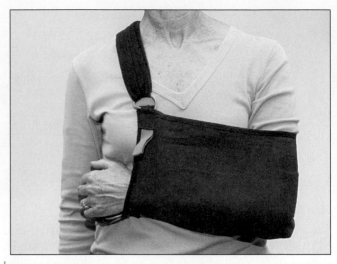

A commercial arm sling.

- Continue above and below the joint, overlapping the previous turn by two-thirds the width of the bandage.
- Terminate the bandage above the joint with two circular turns, and then secure the end appropriately.

### Arm Sling

- Ask the client to flex the elbow to an 80-degree angle or less, depending on the purpose. The thumb should be facing upward or inward toward the body. ➤*Rationale: An 80-degree angle is sufficient to support the forearm, to prevent swelling of the hand, and to relieve pressure on the shoulder joint (e.g.,to support the paralyzed arm of a stroke client whose shoulder might otherwise become dislocated). A more acute angle is preferred if there is swelling of the hand (see how to apply a sling for maximum hand elevation, below).*
- If a triangle is used, place one end of the unfolded binder over the shoulder of the uninjured side so that the binder falls down the front of the chest of the client with the point of the triangle (apex) under the elbow of the injured side.
- Take the upper corner, and carry it around the neck until it hangs over the shoulder on the injured side.
- Bring the lower corner of the binder up over the arm to the shoulder of the injured side. Using a square knot, secure this corner to the upper corner at the side of the neck on the injured side. ➤*Rationale: A square knot will not slip. Tying the knot at the side of the neck prevents pressure on the bony prominences of the vertebral column at the back of the neck.*
- If a commercial sling is used, it may also include a second strap that goes around the back of the client's chest from the finger end of the sling to the elbow. ➤*Rationale: This strap holds the arm close to the body at all times, providing shoulder immobilization such as is used following a shoulder dislocation or surgery.*

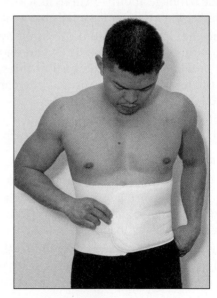

A straight abdominal binder.

- Make sure the wrist is supported. ➤*Rationale: This maintains alignment.*
- Remove the sling periodically to inspect the skin for indications of irritation, especially around the site of the knot.

### Straight Abdominal Binder

- Place the binder smoothly around the body. ➤*Rationale: A binder placed too high interferes with respiration; one placed too low interferes with elimination and walking.*
- Apply padding over the iliac crests if the client is thin.

- Bring the ends around the client, overlap them, and secure them with clips or Velcro.
- Document the application of the bandage or binder and the client's response in the client record using forms or checklists supplemented by narrative notes when appropriate.

## Documentation

Sample: 6/3/09 1900 c/o severe sharp and cramping pain in shoulder when moving it. Commercial sling c̄ shoulder immobilizer applied to l arm c̄ elbow flexed 60°. Upper extremity warm, no wounds or lesions, peripheral pulses strong, brisk capillary refill. Able to move fingers and wrist s̄ pain. Client verbalizes understanding of need to request assistance c̄ ADLs.

_____ L. Morris, RN

### DEVELOPMENTAL CONSIDERATIONS

**Children**

- Allow the child to help with the procedure by holding supplies, opening boxes, counting turns, and so on.
- If a young client is apprehensive, demonstrate the procedure on a doll or stuffed animal.
- Encourage the child to decorate his bandage.
- Teach the caregivers to apply bandages and binders safely.

**Elders**

- Older clients may need extra support during the procedure, especially if arthritis, contractures, or tremors are present.
- Avoid constricting the client's circulation with a tight bandage or binder. Observe skin and bony prominences frequently for signs of impaired circulation. The risk for skin breakdown increases with age.

### EVIDENCE BASED NURSING PRACTICE

**Treatment of Ambulatory Venous Ulcer Patients and Warming Therapy**

This was a limited study but other studies indicate the same type of findings. Five clients with a mean age of 65 and pressure ulcers for more than 8 months were treated with warm-up therapy along with zippered compression stockings for 2 weeks. These clients were monitored for 12 weeks. The therapy consisted of warm therapy three times a day for 1 hour each at a temperature of 38-degrees Celsius. The results indicated that four of five clients increased granulation tittue and decreased pain. Four of five clients were completely healed during the 12-week follow-up.

_Source:_ Cherry, G. C., & Wilson, Dphil J. (1999, September). The treatment of ambulatory venous ulcer patients and warming therapy. _Ostomy/Wound Management_ 45(9), 65–70.

### SETTING OF CARE

- Assess the client or caregiver's ability and willingness to perform the bandaging procedure.
- Ensure that the client has the proper supplies and knows how to obtain replacement supplies.
- The client should have two binders so that there is one to wear while the other is being washed. Bandages and binders should be washed inside a mesh laundry bag to keep them from becoming twisted and to prevent Velcro or hooks from catching on other laundry.
- Instruct the client's caregiver to:
  a. Cleanse hands thoroughly before handling dressing supplies and applying the bandage.
  b. Report skin breakdown, redness, pain, or pallor of the affected area.
  c. Check for adequate peripheral circulation after applying the bandage.

# Skill 10.8  Maintaining Closed Wound Drainage

## Delegation

Assessment of the wound, wound drainage, and patency of the wound suction require application of knowledge and problem solving and is the responsibility of the nurse and is not delegated to UAP. The UAP, however, can empty the drainage unit, measure the drainage, and record the amount on the intake and output record. The nurse must ensure that the UAP knows how to empty the unit without contaminating it.

## Equipment

- Clean gloves
- Calibrated drainage receptacle
- Moisture-proof pad
- Alcohol sponge
- Closed wound drainage system (e.g., Hemovac or Jackson–Pratt)

## Preparation

- Determine the type and placement of the client's closed wound drainage.

## Procedure

1. Prior to performing the procedure, introduce self and verify the client's identity using agency protocol. Explain to the client what you are going to do, why it is necessary, and how he or she can participate. Discuss how the results will be used in planning further care or treatments.
2. Perform hand hygiene and observe other appropriate infection control procedures.
3. Provide for client privacy.

---

### SETTING OF CARE

- Schedule regular nursing visits to teach wound care and to observe the drainage site.
- Teach the client or a caregiver to empty, measure, and record the drainage at least once daily.
- Instruct the caregiver to observe the wound daily for signs of infection, such as redness, edema, tenderness, or purulent drainage. The client's temperature should be measured twice daily. ➤*Rationale: Elevated temperature can indicate infection.*
- Ensure that the client has the proper supplies and knows how to obtain new items as needed.
- Notify the primary care provider of excess drainage, signs of infection, or occlusion of the tube.
- Determine when the primary care provider plans to remove the drain, and help the client keep the appointment.

---

4. Empty the drainage unit.
   - Apply clean gloves.
   - Place the Hemovac or Jackson–Pratt unit on the waterproof pad.
   - Open the plug of the drainage unit.
   - Invert the unit and empty it into the collecting receptacle.
5. Reestablish suction.

### Hemovac

- Place the unit on a solid, flat surface with port open.
- Place palm of hand on unit and press the top and the bottom together.
- While holding the top and bottom together, cleanse the opening and plug with alcohol swab.
- Replace the drainage plug before releasing hand pressure. ➤*Rationale: This reestablishes the vacuum necessary for the closed drainage system to work.*

### Jackson–Pratt

- Compress the bulb with the port open.
- While maintaining tight compression on the bulb, cleanse the ends of the emptying port.
- Insert the plug into the emptying port. ➤*Rationale: This reestablishes the vacuum necessary for the closed drainage system to work.*
6. Secure the unit to the client's gown or position suction unit on the bed.
   - Ensure that the unit is below the level of the wound. ➤*Rationale: This facilitates drainage.*
7. Remove and discard gloves. Perform hand hygiene.
8. Document all relevant information.
   - Record the emptying of the drainage unit and the nursing assessments.
   - Record the amount and type of drainage on the intake and output record.

---

# Skill 10.9   Obtaining a Wound Drainage Specimen

## Delegation

Obtaining a wound culture is an invasive procedure that requires the application of sterile technique, knowledge of wound healing, and potential problem solving to ensure client safety. Therefore, the nurse needs to perform this skill and does not delegate it to UAP.

## Equipment

- Clean gloves
- Protective eyewear, if appropriate
- Sterile gloves
- Moisture-resistant bag
- Sterile dressing set

- Normal saline and irrigating syringe
- Culture tube with swab and culture medium (aerobic and anaerobic tubes are available) or sterile syringe with needle for anaerobic culture
- Completed labels for each container
- Completed requisition to accompany the specimens to the laboratory

## Preparation

Check the medical orders to determine if the specimen is to be collected for an **aerobic** (growing only in the presence of oxygen) or **anaerobic** (growing only in the absence of oxygen) culture. Aerobic organisms are generally found on the surface of the wound, whereas anaerobic organisms would be found in deep wounds, tunnels, and cavities. Administer an analgesic 30 minutes before the procedure if the client is complaining of pain at the wound site to prevent unnecessary discomfort during the procedure.

### Procedure

1. Prior to performing the procedure, introduce self and verify the client's identity using agency protocol. Explain to the client what you are going to do, why it is necessary, and how he or she can participate. Discuss how the results will be used in planning further care or treatments.
2. Perform hand hygiene and observe other appropriate infection control procedures.
3. Provide for client privacy.
4. Remove any moist outer dressings that cover the wound.
   - Apply clean gloves.
   - Remove the outer dressing, and observe any drainage on the dressing. Hold the dressing so that the client does not see the drainage. ➤*Rationale: The appearance of the drainage could upset the client.*
   - Determine the amount, color, consistency, and odor of the drainage. For example, "one 4 × 4 gauze saturated with yellow-greenish, thick, malodorous drainage."
   - Discard the dressing in the moisture-resistant bag. Handle it carefully so that the dressing does not touch the outside of the bag. ➤*Rationale: Touching the outside of the bag will contaminate it.*
   - Remove and discard gloves. Perform hand hygiene.
5. Open the sterile dressing set using sterile technique.
   - See Skills 4.17, 4.18, and 4.19.
6. Assess the wound.
   - Apply sterile gloves.
   - Assess the appearance of the tissues in and around the wound and the drainage. Infection can cause reddened tissues with a thick discharge, which may be foul-smelling, whitish, or colored.
7. Cleanse the wound.
   - Using gauze swabs or irrigation, cleanse the wound with normal saline until all visible exudates have been removed. See Skill 10.4 on page 412.
   - After cleansing, apply a sterile gauze pad to the wound. ➤*Rationale: This absorbs excess saline.*
   - If a topical antimicrobial ointment or cream is being used to treat the wound, use a swab to remove it. ➤*Rationale: Residual antiseptic must be removed prior to culture.*
   - Remove and discard sterile gloves.
8. Obtain the aerobic culture.
   - Apply clean gloves.
   - Open a specimen tube and place the cap upside down on a firm, dry surface so that the inside will not become contaminated, or if the swab is attached to the lid, twist the

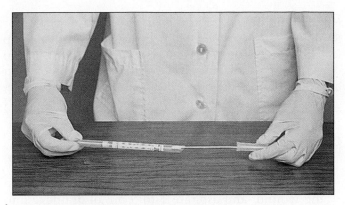

A culturette tube for a wound specimen.

cap to loosen the swab. Hold the tube in one hand and take out the swab in the other.
   - Rotate the swab back and forth over clean areas of granulation tissue from the sides or base of the wound. ➤*Rationale: Microorganisms most likely to be responsible for a wound infection reside in viable tissue.*
   - Do not collect pus or pooled exudates to culture. ➤*Rationale: These secretions contain a mixture of contaminants that are not the same as those causing the infection.*
   - Avoid touching the swab to intact skin at the wound edges. ➤*Rationale: This prevents the introduction of superficial skin organisms into the culture.*
   - Return the swab to the culture tube, taking care not to touch the top or the outside of the tube. ➤*Rationale: The outside of the container must remain free of pathogenic microorganisms to prevent their spread to others.*
   - Crush the inner ampule containing the medium for organism growth at the bottom of the tube. ➤*Rationale: This ensures that the swab with the specimen is surrounded by culture medium.*
   - Twist the cap to secure.
   - If a specimen is required from another site, repeat the steps. Specify the exact site (e.g., inferior drain site or lower aspect of incision) on the label of each container. Be sure to put each swab in the appropriately labeled tube.
9. Dress the wound.
   - Apply any ordered medication to the wound.
   - Cover the wound with a sterile moist transparent wound dressing. See Skill 10.19 on page 440.
   - Remove and discard gloves. Perform hand hygiene.
10. Arrange for the specimen to be transported to the laboratory immediately. Be sure to include the completed requisition.
11. Document all relevant information.
   - Record on the client's chart the taking of the specimen and source.
   - Include the date and time; the appearance of the wound; the color, consistency, amount, and odor of any drainage; the type of culture collected; and any discomfort experienced by the client.

**Documentation**

Sample: 5/27/09 1000 Obtained specimen from (R) hip for anaerobic culture. Pressure ulcer 3 × 3 cm, 6 mm deep, minimal amt. thick, yellow drainage. No odor. Skin around wound reddened. Rates pain at 0 on 0–10 scale.
———————————————————————— N. Jamaghani, RN

**VARIATION: Obtaining a Specimen for Anaerobic Culture Using a Sterile Syringe and Needle**

- Apply clean gloves.
- Insert a sterile 10-mL syringe (without needle) into the wound, and aspirate 1 to 5 mL of drainage into the syringe.

- Attach the needle to the syringe, and expel all air from the syringe and needle.
- Immediately inject the drainage into the anaerobic culture tube.

  *or*

  Use an anaerobic culture swab system in which the swab is immediately placed into a tube filled with an oxygen-free gas or gel environment.
- Label the tube appropriately.
- Remove and discard gloves. Perform hand hygiene.
- Send the tube of drainage to the laboratory immediately. Do not refrigerate the specimen.

# Skill 10.10  Assessing Ankle-Brachial Index (ABI)

**Equipment**

Sphygmomanometer (2 cuffs, one arm and one leg)
Doppler, handheld

**Procedure**

1. Review chart to determine if client has diabetes. ►*Rationale: The ABI may not be reliable in these clients because arterial calcification causes false readings (high).* The ABI is used to indirectly assess lower extremity peripheral blood flow.
2. Explain procedure to client.
3. Place client in supine position. Instruct to lie quietly for 5 minutes.
4. Place cuff above elbow, apply ultrasound gel to brachial pulse area.
5. Hold ultrasound probe at 45° angle. ►*Rationale: This position opposes direction of brachial artery blood flow.*
6. Inflate cuff pressure and slowly deflate pressure until systolic pulse sound is heard.
7. Obtain blood pressure readings in both arms. Use the higher systolic pressure as the brachial pressure in the ratio.
8. Wrap leg cuff around leg 5 cm above ankle's medial malleolus.
9. Place Doppler probe at a 45° angle to dorsalis pedis or posterior tibial artery.
10. Inflate cuff until Doppler sound stops.
11. Deflate cuff slowly while maintaining Doppler probe in place over artery.
12. Obtain two readings of posterior tibial or dorsalis pedis measurements and select highest value to be used in ABI calculation.
13. Divide ankle systolic pressure by brachial systolic pressure to obtain Ankle-Brachial Index (ABI). Normally, ankle pressure is equal to or slightly higher then brachial pressure.
14. Review ABI guidelines to determine severity of arterial insufficiency.
15. Document findings in nurses' notes and place note on chart for physician.

| ABI GUIDELINES | |
| --- | --- |
| 1.0–1.2 ABI | Normal–No arterial insufficiency |
| 0.8–1.0 ABI | Mild insufficiency |
| 0.5–0.8 ABI | Moderate insufficiency |
| <0.5 ABI | Severe insufficiency |
| <0.3 ABI | Limb threatening |

# Skill 10.11  Changing a Dressing—Venous Ulcer

**Equipment**

Cleansing solution
Normal saline solution
Sterile 4 × 4 dressings
Moisture-retentive dressings (hydrocolloid, transparent film or foam for light-to-moderate drainage)

Absorbent dressings (foams, alginates, and absorptive dressings) for moderate to heavy exudate
Compression dressing
Clean gloves
Sterile gloves

Biohazard bag
Scissors
Absorbent pad

### Preparation

1. Perform hand hygiene.
2. Gather equipment.
3. Explain procedure to client.
4. Provide privacy for client.
5. Raise bed to HIGH position and lower side rails.
6. Open sterile packages, and arrange on over-bed table.
7. Place absorbent pad under wound.

### Procedure

1. Don clean gloves.
2. Remove compression bandage and old dressing, and place in biohazard bag. Compression dressings may be left in place for 3–7 days depending on amount of drainage and type of dressing.
3. Assess and measure wound. ➤*Rationale: This determines effectiveness of treatment.*
4. Cleanse off debris by pouring cleansing solution over wound.
5. Rinse wound with sterile normal saline.

---

## CLINICAL ALERT

The wound bed should be kept moist to promote granulation and reepithelialization and to reduce pain. Ointments provide the most occlusive moisturizer because they contain oil and water.

---

6. Debride wound, if ordered, using one of the following methods:
   a. Autolytic: Applying occlusive dressings that assist in maintaining a moist wound environment, therefore promoting reepithelialization. ➤*Rationale: Autolytic uses body's own enzymes and moisture to rehydrate, moisten, and slough tissue.*
   b. Chemical: Apply enzyme debriding agents (accuzyme, collagenase, papain, etc.).

*Note:* The major disadvantage of this method is that viable tissue is removed with necrotic tissue.

   c. Mechanical: Apply wet-to-dry dressings, use hydrotherapy, irrigation.

7. Dry wound using sterile 4 × 4 dressings. Place in biohazard bag.
8. Remove gloves, and don sterile gloves.

---

## CLINICAL ALERT

Use of semiocclusive dressings reduces incidence of wound infections by more than 50%. They maintain a moist environment, reduce airborne bacteria, and provide a mechanical barrier for bacterial entry.

---

## CLINICAL ALERT

### Compression Therapy

#### Inelastic System

An Unna boot is frequently used to control edema in lower extremities. An inelastic bandaging system is applied to the lower extremity. As it dries it becomes rigid and when calf muscles press against the rigid bandage it pumps blood more effectively. This system can be used for both mobile and immobile clients. As edema subsides the boot becomes less effective.

#### Elastic Therapy

Graduated compression and multilayer compression stockings and compression pumps are more effective in increasing venous return. Both mobile and immobile clients can use these stockings, although it is more difficult for the client who is mobile. The stockings are available in different pressures.

---

## ARTERIAL ULCERS

### Assessment

- Assess arterial flow; dorsalis pedis, femerol, popliteal, or posterior tibial.
- Use Doppler to assess pulses if necessary.
- Assess Ankle-Brachial Index; below 0.5 indicates severe arterial insufficiency.
- Assess temperature of skin.
- Observe color of extremities.
- Assess for presence of pain when client resting.

### Treatment

- Debridement.
- Pain control.
- Occlusive dressings: reduce pain, protect the wound from infection, control exudates, enhance autolytic debridement, maintain moist wound environment.
- Secure dressing with gauze; do not use tape as skin is fragile and tears easily.
- Management of disease process, i.e. BP, eliminate smoking, control blood glucose.
- Surgical intervention to improve circulation.
- Vacuum compression therapy.
- Hyperbaric oxygen therapy.

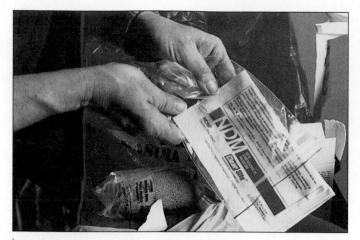

❶ Obtain appropriate wound dressing kit, if available.

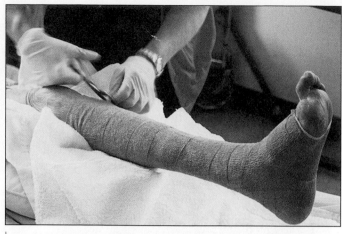

❷ Remove compression dressing, being careful not to cut skin.

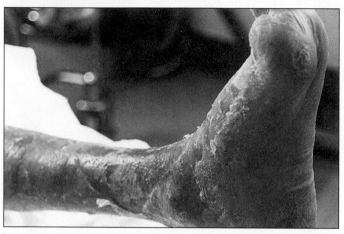

❸ Assess wound healing and evaluate progress (Stage II).

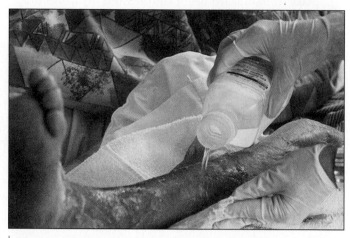

❹ Pour normal saline solution over wound to clean off debris.

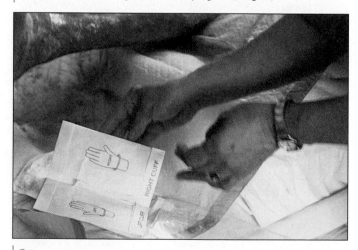

❺ Don sterile gloves before cleaning wound with 4 × 4 gauze pads.

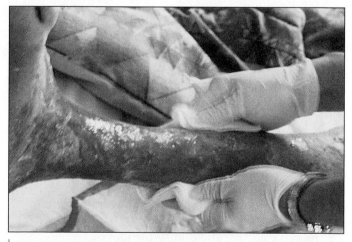

❻ Dry with 4 × 4 gauze pad after cleansing.

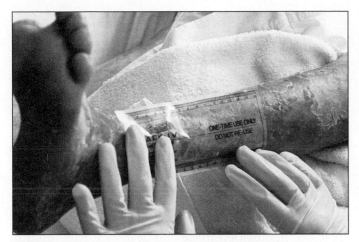

⑦Measure wound to evaluate effectiveness of treatment.

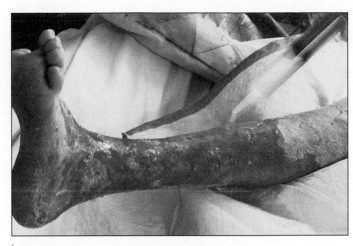

⑧Apply medicated moisturizer on wound, if ordered

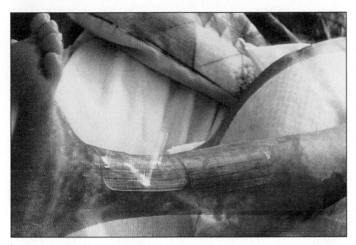

⑨Apply moisture-retentive dressing over wound site.

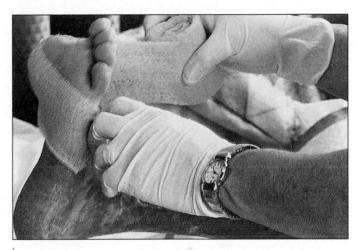

⑩ Apply compression dressing for venous or lymphatic conditions.

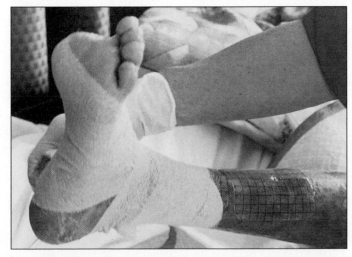

⑪ Cover entire area with compression dressing.

9. Apply medicated moisturizer over wound, if ordered. ►*Rationale: This keeps wound area moist.*
10. Remove backing on moisture-retentive dressing, and place over open wound site. These dressings prevent entry of bacteria from surface of dressing.
11. Palpate arterial system; dorsalis pedis, posterior, or tibial pulse. If pulses are nonpalpable obtain an Ankle-Brachial Index (ABI).
12. Apply compression dressing if ABI is greater than 0.6. ►*Rationale: Effective compression bandages generate 40–70 mm Hg pressure. If arterial insufficiency is present another ulcer can occur.*

*Note:* Medicinal maggots were originally used in the 1930s. In the past 10 years they have been reintroduced, now used to debride or eliminate necrotic tissue and remove pathogenic bacteria. There is evidence from recent studies that they may accelerate wound healing by promoting the formation of granulation tissue. The larvae feed on dead tissue, cellular debris, and exudates from necrotic wounds through extracorporeal digestion. This treatment has proven to be effective in clients with venous ulcers, diabetic ulcers, and arterial ulcers.

13. Reposition leg in elevated position. Leg should be elevated 18 cm above heart for 2 to 4 hours during the day and night. ➤*Rationale: This prevents edema and venous stasis, and promotes healing.*
14. Remove gloves, and place in biohazard bag. Place all used supplies in bag.
15. Place biohazard bag in appropriate receptacle.
16. Perform hand hygiene.
17. Lower bed and raise side rails.
18. Assess peripheral circulation every 4 hours. ➤*Rationale: This ensures compression dressing is not too tight.*

## EVIDENCE-BASED CLINICAL PRACTICE

**Treatment of Ambulatory Venous Ulcer Patients and Warming Therapy**

This is a limited study but other studies indicate the same type of findings. Five clients with a mean age of 65 and pressure ulcers for more than 8 months were treated with warm-up therapy along with zippered compression stockings for 2 weeks. These clients were monitored for 12 weeks. The therapy consisted of warm therapy three times a day for 1 hour each at a temperature of 38-degrees C. The results indicated that four of five clients increased granulation tissue and decreased pain. Four of five clients were completely healed during the 12-week follow-up.

*Source:* Cherry, G. C. & Wilson, Dphil J. (1999, September). The treatment of ambulatory venous ulcer patients and warming therapy. *Ostomy/Wound Management* 45(9), 65–70.

# Skill 10.12   Preventing Pressure Ulcers

### EXPECTED OUTCOMES

- State of pressure ulcer is accurately accessed.
- Pressure ulcer is treated effectively according to stage of ulcer formation.
- Pressure ulcer is healing within usual time frame.
- Skin remains free of breakdown in surrounding areas of pressure ulcer.
- Absence of additional pressure ulcer formation.

### Procedure

1. Inspect skin at least daily, particularly over bony prominences. Heels and sacrum are most common areas for skin breakdown. Use Braden or Norton scale for assessment. Document assessment findings.
2. Individualize client's bathing schedule. Daily baths are not essential. ➤*Rationale: Daily cleansing can destroy the skin's natural barrier, making it more susceptible to external irritants.*
   a. Avoid hot bath water. ➤*Rationale: Tepid water prevents injury to skin.*
   b. Use mild cleansing agents to minimize dryness.
   c. Cleanse skin immediately if urine, fecal incontinence, or wound drainage seeps onto skin.
   d. Provide humidity to prevent drying of skin.
   e. Use cream or thin layer of cornstarch to protect skin.

3. Avoid massaging bony prominences. ➤*Rationale: Massaging can lead to deep tissue trauma.*
   a. Keep bony prominences from direct contact with one another.
   b. Use pillow, foam wedges, or other positioning devices.
   c. Use elbow pads and heel elevators.
4. Promote adequate dietary intake of protein, calories, and nutrients. Protein should be approximately 1.2 to 1.5 g/kg body weight daily. ➤*Rationale: Adequate protein intake in addition to vitamins and minerals help prevent pressure ulcer formation.*
5. Ensure adequate fluid intake. ➤*Rationale: Prevent dehydration which is a risk factor for pressure ulcer formation.*
6. Reposition bedridden client every 1–2 hours.
   a. Do not position directly on trochanter.
   b. Do not turn more than 30° angle.

### CLINICAL ALERT

Be alert to altered skin integrity when pressure is reduced in one anatomical area by turning and repositioning, as the newer location may be placed at risk for pressure ulcer formation.

c. Raise heels off bed by placing pillows under legs; allow heels to hang over edges.

d. Use trapeze or turning sheet to reposition client.

7. Encourage mobility or range-of-motion exercises. ➤*Rationale: Range-of-motion exercises promote activity and reduce effects of pressure on tissue.*

8. Minimize force and friction on skin when turning or moving client. Use turning sheets or Hoyer lift.

9. Maintain head of bed at lowest degree of elevation consistent with medical problem. Below 30° if possible.

10. Place at-risk clients on pressure-reducing devices, in both bed and chair, such as foam, static-air, alternating gel, water mattress, or air fluidized mattress.

11. Encourage chair-fast clients to shift position every 15 minutes.

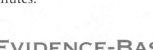

## EVIDENCE-BASED NURSING PRACTICE

**Pressure Ulcer Formation**

There is an unresolved and inadequately explained issue of how a pressure ulcer progresses. Some clinicians believe the ulcer forms from top down and other theories have indicated that the pressure ulcer progresses from bottom up. There is limited research on this theory. Current literature indicates that the bottom-up theory is more appropriate, as the deeper tissues are involved in pressure ulcer formation. Latest opinion is that true pressure ulcers are an injury to soft tissue and muscle that occurs from pressure over bony prominences. It is recommended that further research be done.

*Source:* WOCN Society Response to NPUAP White Papers: Deep Tissue Injury, Stage I Pressure Ulcers, and Stage II Pressure Ulcers: 9th National NPUAP Conference, February 2005. Phyllis Bonham, Ph.D., MSN, RN, CWOCN, and Janet Ramundo, MSN, RN, FNP, CWOCN.

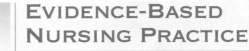

## EVIDENCE-BASED NURSING PRACTICE

**Pressure Relief in Surgical Clients**

Pressure ulcers can begin in the operating room. The occurrence of ulcers can be as high as 45% of surgical clients. There are many risk factors leading to ulcer development in as few as 2 1/2 hours. Risk factors include position client is placed in during procedure, necessity of positioning devices that place pressure on bony prominences. Medications that constrict blood vessels or lower blood pressure can also lead to pressure ulcers.

*Source:* Armstrong, D., Bortz, P. An integrative review of pressure relief in surgical patients. *American Organization of Operating Room Nurses Journal,* 74(3), 645.

## CLINICAL ALERT

Air-fluidized beds and low-air-loss beds are recommended to manage pressure ulcers, especially in clients with large or multiple ulcers.

### Air-Fluidized

Warm, pressurized air circulates through beads in the bed and creates support surface. Polyester sheet allows for moisture and air to pass through, keeping skin dry.

Treatment can take several months. Use of this bed is very expensive.

### Low-Air-Loss

Head and foot of bed can be elevated. Bed is a modified standard bed frame, lighter and more portable than air-fluidized bed. Bed circulates cool air.

Urine and feces do not pass through fabric on the bed.

Bed is portable and lighter.

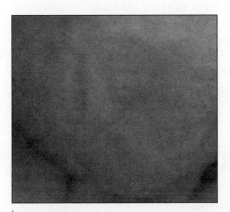

● Stage I pressure ulcer.

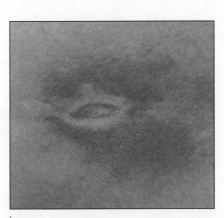

● Stage II pressure ulcer.

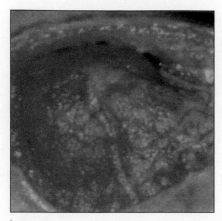

● Stage III pressure ulcer.

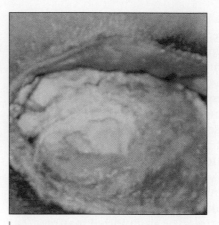

● Stage IV pressure ulcer.

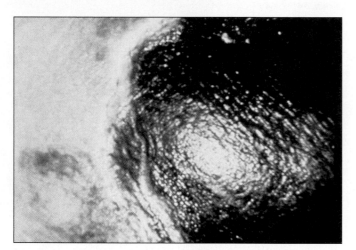

● Eschar must be removed by debridement before staging is done.

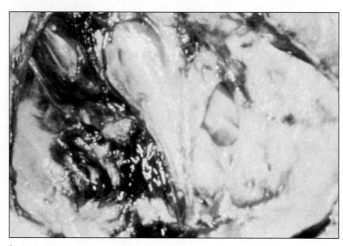

● Clinical signs of infection.

# Skill 10.13   Providing Care for Clients with Pressure Ulcers

## Procedure

1. Monitor client's overall condition daily. ➤*Rationale: Clients who are dying will have the tendency to develop new skin breakdown (skin failure) as other organs fail.* Existing pressure ulcers of lesser Staging I and II almost always worsen over time and become at least Stage III.
2. Differentiate type of ulcer, pressure versus nonpressure.
3. Determine stage of ulcer.
4. Monitor and assess ulcer characteristics daily:
   a. Observe dressing to determine if dry, intact, and not leaking.
   b. Observe ulcer bed, if appropriate, and document findings.
5. Assess pain level of client and provide adequate pain relief.
6. Photograph ulcer according to facility policy. ➤*Rationale: To determine progress of ulcer healing.*
7. Monitor progress toward healing and for potential complications.

a. Measure pressure ulcer size weekly using a Pressure Ulcer Scale. Usual healing time is 2 to 4 weeks.
b. If healing is not progressing or has not healed in usual time frame, reevaluate treatment plan and client's condition.
8. Maintain turning and positioning schedule to promote healing and prevent additional ulcer formation.
9. Complete a nutritional assessment. Positive nitrogen balance and protein intake are necessary for healing.
10. Complete a psychosocial assessment to determine client's adherence to pressure ulcer treatment regimens.

### CLINICAL ALERT

Clients near the end of life have the right to refuse ulcer care. However, "Do Not Resuscitate" orders do not relieve the staff from providing quality pressure ulcer prevention or treatment.

11. Complete dressing change according to facility policy and type of dressing used. Follow manufacturer's guidelines for dressing change. ➤*Rationale: Dressing changes are based on a combination of factors, such as manufacturer suggested use, pressure ulcer characteristics, and goals for healing.*

# Skill 10.14  Applying Transparent Film Dressing

## Equipment

Sterile normal saline
Transparent dressing (e.g., Op-Site, Tegaderm, Bioclusive)
Sterile 4 × 4 gauze pads
Scissors
Hypoallergenic tape
Clean gloves
Plasticizing agent (e.g., skin prep [optional])

## Preparation

1. Check physician's orders and client care plan.
2. Check type of dressing ordered. ➤*Rationale: These dressings are very important in preventing pressure ulcers; they prevent friction and shear over bony prominences when moving clients.*
3. Gather supplies.
4. Obtain appropriately sized transparent dressing. Dressing can be applied to flat surface. (Coccyx area cannot be treated with this type of dressing.)
5. Perform hand hygiene.
6. Identify client using two types of identification and explain procedure to client.
7. Provide privacy.

## Procedure

1. Raise bed to HIGH position, and lower side rail on working side of bed.
2. Don clean gloves.
3. Remove old dressing, "walk off" dressing from one edge to the other, and discard in appropriate receptacle.
4. Wash pressure ulcer with sterile gauze pads moistened with sterile normal saline.
5. Dry thoroughly with sterile gauze pad.
6. Measure wound using pliable device. ➤*Rationale: Comparison of measurement assists in determining effectiveness of treatment.*
7. Apply plasticizing agent (skin prep, skin gel) over surrounding tissue if ordered. ➤*Rationale: Do not apply directly on ulcer area because the agent contains alcohol,*

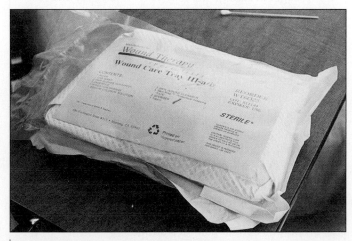

● Dressing carts may be used to keep supplies closer to client area.  ● Obtain specific dressing tray for ordered treatment.

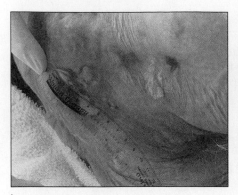

● Assess size of wound to determine appropriate size of transparent dressing.

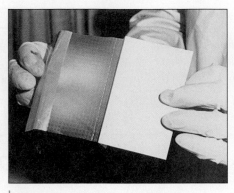

● Remove backing from Op-Site dressing before applying.

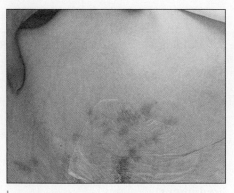

● Apply transparent adhesive dressing over wound.

*which burns the ulcer area.* Alternate Treatment: If skin is irritated, apply No Sting Barrier Film Spray to area surrounding tissue. ➤*Rationale: To protect/prevent skin breakdown.*

8. Loosen transparent dressing from one side of backing paper.
9. "Walk on" dressing: Start at one edge of site and gently lay the dressing down, keeping it free of wrinkles. Allow at least a 1 1/2-inch margin of dressing beyond ulcer margin. ➤*Rationale: This ensures coverage of entire wound area.*
10. Cut off tabs if using Op-Site after wound is completely covered.
11. Tape edges with hypoallergenic tape. ➤*Rationale: This assists in preventing frequent dressing changes due to loose dressings.* These dressings can remain in place for 1 week.
12. Remove gloves, and discard in appropriate receptacle.
13. Position client for comfort.
14. Lower bed, and raise side rails.
15. Remove and discard equipment.
16. Perform hand hygiene.

## USING HYDROGEL DRESSINGS

• Hydrogel dressings contain 95% water; they are very absorbent and dehydrate easily when not covered with a secondary dressing.

• Dressings cannot absorb much exudate; they should be used for dry wounds such as skin tears, surgical wounds, and radiation therapy burns.

• Dressings are nonadhesive, can be transparent and conform to wound surfaces.

• Sterile aqueous hydrogen fiber is used to fill cavity with gel; also used to fill dead space in large wounds. Do not overfill wounds to prevent tissue damage.

• Hydrogel sheets are placed in direct contact with wound bed and margins; air bubbles and plastic covering on sheet must be removed. The unique cooling properties soothe painful wounds.

---

**SAMPLE PRESSURE ULCER ASSESSMENT GUIDE**

Patient Name: _____     Date: _____ Time: _____

**Ulcer 1:**
Site _____
Stage[a] _____
Size (cm)
  Length _____
  Width _____
  Depth _____

**Ulcer 2:**
Site _____
Stage[a] _____
Size (cm)
  Length _____
  Width _____
  Depth _____

| | Ulcer 1 | | | Ulcer 2 | |
|---|---|---|---|---|---|
| Sinus Tract | | | Sinus Tract | | |
| Tunneling | | | Tunneling | | |
| Undermining | | | Undermining | | |
| Necrotic Tissue | | | Necrotic Tissue | | |
|   Slough | | |   Slough | | |
|   Eschar | | |   Eschar | | |
| Exudate | | | Exudate | | |
|   Serous | | |   Serous | | |
|   Serosanguineous | | |   Serosanguineous | | |
|   Purulent | | |   Purulent | | |
| Granulation | | | Granulation | | |
| Epithelialization | | | Epithelialization | | |
| Pain | | | Pain | | |

**Surrounding Skin:**

| | | | | | |
|---|---|---|---|---|---|
| Erythema | | | Erythema | | |
| Maceration | | | Maceration | | |
| Induration | | | Induration | | |

Description of Ulcer(s): _____
_____

Indicate Ulcer Sites:

Anterior     Posterior
(Attach a color photo of the pressure ulcer[s] [Optional])

[a]Classification of pressure ulcers:
*Stage I:* Nonblanchable erythema of intact skin, the heralding lesion of skin ulceration. In individuals with darker skin, discoloration of the skin, warmth, edema, induration, or hardness may also be indicators.
*Stage II:* Partial thickness skin loss involving epidermis, dermis, or both.
*Stage III:* Full thickness skin loss involving damage to or necrosis of subcutaneous tissue that may extend down to, but not through, underlying fascia. The ulcer presents clinically as a deep crater with or without undermining adjacent tissue.
*Stage IV:* Full thickness skin loss with extensive destruction, tissue necrosis, or damage to muscle, bone, or supporting structures (e.g., tendon or joint capsule).

*Source:* Pressure Ulcer Treatment: Quick Reference Guide for Clinicians, No. 15. U.S. Department of Health and Human Services, AHCPR.

# Skill 10.15 Using Hydrocolloid Dressing

## Equipment

Sterile normal saline
Hydrocolloid dressing (e.g., DuoDERM, Restore, Ultec, Comfeel Plus)
Hydrogel if needed (ClearSite, Aquasorb)
Sterile 4 × 4 gauze pads
Hypoallergenic tape
Clean gloves
Skin prep, optional

*Note:* These dressings promote a moist wound environment, aid in autolytic debridement, and have no toxic components. They are waterproof and bacteria proof.

## Procedure

1. Select dressing size to ensure coverage 1 1/4-inch beyond ulcer margin. (Dressing available in 4 × 4 to 8 × 8 sizes.) ➤*Rationale: This ensures complete covering of wound.* Use for small ulcers and in Stage II and III.

*Note:* These dressings can be used for nondressing wounds (i.e., postsurgical incisions, abrasions, blisters, and early stage pressure ulcers).

2. Perform hand hygiene and don clean gloves.
3. Cleanse skin with gauze pad moistened with sterile normal saline and pat dry with gauze pad.
4. Measure wound using pliable device.
5. Apply skin prep to surrounding skin to protect, if ordered.
6. Fill ulcer area with Hydrogel if ordered—usually used with Stage III or IV pressure ulcer of the hip when exudate is present. Do not overfill with gel. ➤*Rationale: Facilitates autolytic debridement of devitalized tissue.*
7. Warm dressing by holding in hands. ➤*Rationale: To increase activity of adhesive.*
8. Remove silicone release paper backing from dressing. Minimize finger contact with adhesive surface. ➤*Rationale: Dressing is sterile and contamination should be avoided.*
9. Center dressing over affected area. Gently roll dressing over pressure ulcer—do not stretch dressing. ➤*Rationale: Stretching the dressing may cause wrinkling of dressing which allows air to enter wound.*
10. Placing dressing 1/3 above wound and 2/3 below wound maximizes time between dressing changes. ➤*Rationale: Increases absorption capacity of dressing.*
11. Mold the dressing gently to skin, and hold down with hand for approximately 1 minute.

12. Apply skin prep to area that is to be covered by tape if ordered. Allow to dry. Do not apply skin prep under hydrocolloid dressing. ➤*Rationale: Hydrocolloid dressings are placed over broken skin; skin prep may cause damage to skin.*
13. Picture-frame sides of hydrocolloid dressing with silk or hypoallergenic tape.
14. Check dressing each shift for impaired integrity.
15. Change dressing at first sign of impaired integrity. Dressings should not be left on longer than 7 days. Usually left in place for 3–4 days.

*Note:* DuoDERM is removed when exudate seeps from edges of dressing or white blister appears under dressing. Comfeel Plus is changed when dressing becomes transparent or there is leakage.

---

**NUTRITIONAL ASSESSMENT OF CLIENT WITH PRESSURE ULCER(S)**

Client Name: _____ Date: _____ Time _____

To be filled out for all clients at risk on initial evaluation and every 12 weeks thereafter, as indicated. Trends will document the efficacy of nutritional support therapy.

**Protein Compartments**

Somatic:
Current Weight (kg)          _____
Previous Weight (kg)          _____    ( _____date)
Percent Change in Weight     _____

Height (cm)                  _____
Height/Weight
Current Body Mass Index (BM)  _____    [wt/(ht)²]
Previous BMI                  _____    ( _____date)
Percent Change in BMI        _____

Visceral:
Serum Albumin               _____
   (Normal ≥ 3.5 mg/dL)
Total Lymphocyte Count (TLC)  _____    (optional)
   (White Blood Cell count x percent Lymphocytes/100)

Guide to TLC:
• Immune competence          ≥ 1,800 mm³
• Immunity partly impaired    < 1,800 but ≥ 900 mm³
• Anergy                     < 900 mm³

**State of Hydration**

24-Hour Intake _____ mL     24-Hour Output _____ mL

Note: Thirst, tongue dryness in non-mouth-breathers, and tenting of cervical skin may indicate dehydration. Jugular vein distention may indicate overhydration.

**Estimated Nutritional Requirement**

Estimated Nonprotein Calories (NPC) _____ /kg     Estimated Protein _____ (g/kg)
Actual NPC                          _____ /kg     Actual Protein    _____ (g/kg)

**Recommendations/Plan**

1.
2.
3.
4.

*Source:* Pressure Ulcer Treatment: Quick Reference Guide for Clinicians, No. 15. U.S. Department of Health and Human Services, AHCPR.

### TABLE 10–2 ADDITIONAL MOIST WOUND DRESSINGS

| Type of Alternative | Use | Outcome of Treatment | Considerations |
|---|---|---|---|
| Hydrogel Sheet | • Interacts with aqueous solutions<br>• Used with minor wounds with light to moderate drainage<br>• Absorbs minimal to heavy exudates<br>• Nonadherent | Softens necrotic tissue<br>Creates moist environment | Use outer dressing to prevent wound from drying out.<br>Change dressing every 1–2 days. |
| Impregnated Loose Forms | • Absorbs minimal to moderate exudates<br>• Nonadherent | Conforms to irregular surfaces<br>Eliminates dead space<br>Creates moist environment | Requires outer dressing<br>Change daily |
| Alginate | • Absorbs heavy exudates<br>• Converts to gel when comes in contact with wound drainage<br>• Easily removed from wound<br>• Nonadherent | Maintains moist environment<br>Promotes fast healing of wound | Not to be used on dry wounds |
| Foams<br>  Hydrophilic<br><br><br><br>  Hydrophobic | • Absorbs minimal to heavy exudates<br>• Nonadherent<br><br><br>• Softens necrotic tissue. | Maintains moist environment<br>Decreases tissue trauma when removed. Increases time between dressing changes. | Requires external dressing |
| Medical Hydrolysate of Collagen | • Soluble and degrades in wound site<br>• Absorbs wound exudates<br>• Is interactive with wound site to provide mechanical protection against physical and bacterial insult | Absorbs up to 30 times own weight<br>Used in stage I–IV pressure ulcers<br>Accelerates tissue remodeling and reduces scarring | Cover with nonstick dressing<br>Soak dressing in warm water before removing |

16. Remove dressing by pressing hand down on adjacent skin surface while carefully lifting edge of dressing from skin. Continue lifting dressing around periphery until all edges are released, then lift dressing carefully away from wound.

*Note:* Although frequently listed as wound care alternatives, topical disinfectant agents such as iodine and silver sulfadiazine are very controversial in wound care. Iodine is cytotoxic to fibroblasts and can impair wound healing. Silver solutions are sometimes used to prevent bacterial colonization in infection prone areas. They do not eliminate existing infections.

17. Remove gloves and perform hand hygiene.
18. Record stage, size, and appearance of ulcer; date; and reason for removal of hydrocolloid dressing.

### CLINICAL ALERT

Hydrocolloid dressings are occlusive, thus, do not allow water, bacteria, or oxygen into the wound. They are not used if the wound or surrounding skin is infected. They have limited use with wounds with heavy exudates.

## TABLE 10-3  COMPARISONS OF MOISTURE-RETENTIVE DRESSINGS

|  | **Transparent** | **Hydrocolloid** |
|---|---|---|
| Common Brands | Tegaderm<br>Op-Site<br>Bioclusive | Tegasorb<br>DuoDERM<br>Comfeel<br>Restore |
| Characteristics | Sterile<br>Semipermeable membranes with hypoallergenic adhesive<br>Permeable to oxygen and moisture vapor<br>Allows oxygen exchange<br>Impermeable to bacteria, prevents contamination | Impermeable to oxygen<br>Dressing gel maintains moist environment that promotes autolysis<br>Impermeable to external bacteria and contamination<br>Minimally to moderately absorptive |
| Function | Provides moist environment<br><br>Promotes autolysis and protects newly formed tissue<br>Assists with debridement | Dressing contains hydroactive particles that absorb exudate to form a hydrated gel over wound<br>When dressing removed, gel separates from dressing, which protects newly formed tissue |
| Use | Easy assessment of wound; dressing is transparent<br>Nondraining or minimally draining wounds only, nonabsorbable<br>Pressure ulcers, stage I and some stage II<br>Minor burns, lacerations | Absorbs exudate while preserving moist environment needed for autolysis of slough<br>Irrigate gel with saline to allow for assessing wound<br>Pressure ulcers, some stage III and some clean stage IV<br>Wounds with mild or moderate exudate<br>Wounds with necrosis or slough |
| Contraindications | Infected wounds<br>Wounds with fragile surrounding skin | Wounds that need frequent assessment, not transparent<br>Wounds with heavy exudate |

## UNEXPECTED OUTCOMES

Client does not have sufficient exercise; appetite decreased.

Client's wound does not heal with traditional types of treatments.

Skin is exposed to moisture.

Nutritional or hydration deficit occurs.

Shearing and friction secondarily related to immobility or reduced activity.

## CRITICAL THINKING OPTIONS

- Encourage small, frequent feedings.
- Offer high calorie drinks like eggnog or Isocal.

- In client care conference discuss the following:
  - Is everyone following same treatment?
  - Are causative agents preventing healing?
  - Should treatment be adjusted or changed?
  - Would use of a support surface be effective?
  - Is surgical debridement and grafting necessary for healing?

- Establish bowel or bladder program and select absorbent products for wound care that wick the moisture from skin.
- Cleanse skin with pH-balanced cleansers avoiding friction and dry skin after each incontinence and dry thoroughly.
- Apply skin barrier product.
- Consider use of fecal management system or urinary catheter.

- Monitor nutritional and fluid intake accurately.
- Obtain order for vitamin supplements if client is not already on vitamins.
- Increase protein intake by supplementing with high protein drinks.

- Keep head of bed in lowest position possible to prevent client from sliding down in bed.
- Use lifting devices to move client up in bed or out of bed to prevent friction on skin.
- Instruct client on use of trapeze to assist in repositioning.

# Skill 10.16    Using Electrical Stimulation

## EXPECTED OUTCOMES

- Granulation tissue is evident using adjunctive therapy.
- Periwound area remains healthy without evidence of maceration.
- Moist wound environment is maintained.
- Pain is reduced with adjunctive therapy.
- Wound progresses through usual phases with electrical stimulation.
- Wound healing occurs faster with radiant heat dressing.
- Exudate is removed and wound healing occurs using negative pressure wound therapy.

## Equipment

Normal saline solution
Bag for soiled dressings
Gauze pads
2 sterile basins
Hydrogel sheets
Electrode
Bandage tape
Alligator clip
Stimulator
2 pair clean gloves
Sterile gloves

## Preparation

1. Determine if client is candidate for electrical stimulation.
2. Determine phase of wound healing. ➤*Rationale: This determines the correct treatment protocol.*
3. Set the stimulator settings according to manufacturer's directions, based on client's phase in wound healing. The settings include: polarity, pulse rate, intensity, duration, and frequency.
4. Explain procedure to client.
5. Gather equipment.
6. Perform hand hygiene.
7. Provide privacy.

## Procedure

1. Raise bed to high position, lower side rails as needed.
2. Place client in position to enable staff to work with wound area and equipment. (Placement depends on wound site.)
3. Place supplies on over-bed table, near working area.
4. Open all supply packages, maintaining sterility.
5. Pour sterile normal saline into one basin.
6. Don clean gloves.
7. Place disposal bag near wound. ➤*Rationale: For ease in disposing of soiled dressings.*
8. Remove dressing carefully to avoid interfering with granulation tissue.
9. Remove clean gloves; place in disposal bag. Don sterile gloves.
10. Place sterile basin next to wound to catch irrigation solution as wound is cleansed.
11. Pour sterile normal saline into wound to cleanse wound. ➤*Rationale: To remove exudates, slough, and petrolatum products. Current will not be conducted into wound tissue if petrolatum products remain in the wound.*
12. Remove excess irrigation solution using sterile gauze pads.
13. Place fluffed gauze pads into normal saline solution, squeeze out excess liquid.
14. Fill wound cavity with gauze including any undermined/tunneled spaces. Pack gently.
15. Place surface (active) electrode in wound bed, over gauze packing. ➤*Rationale: This transfers electrical energy into wound bed, producing positive effects on necessary components for wound healing (i.e., blood flow, oxygen uptake, DNA, and protein synthesis).*
16. Cover with dry gauze pad.
17. Tape dry pad securely.
18. Connect alligator clip to foil.
19. Connect to stimulator lead.
20. Place a wet washcloth over area where dispersive electrode will be placed.
21. Select a dispersive pad that is larger than the sum of areas of active electrodes and wound packing.
22. Place dispersive electrode proximal to wound, over soft tissue, avoiding bony prominences. *Note:* The greater the separation between two electrodes, the deeper the current path. Larger separation space is used to treat deep and undermined wounds. Closer separation space is used for shallow or partial thickness wounds. Ensure electrodes do not touch.
23. Ensure all edges of electrode are in good contact with skin. Hold electrode in place with nylon elasticized strap.

24. Place client in position of comfort. Electrical stimulation treatments usually last 60 minutes.
25. Remove gloves and discard.
26. Perform hand hygiene.
27. Don clean gloves.
28. Remove electrode from wound following treatment.
29. Remove saline soaked gauze and cover wound with occlusive dressing.

*Note:* Hydrogel sheets or amorphous hydrogel impregnated gauze can be used to conduct current. If hydrogel gauze is the conductor, it is changed BID.

---

### CANDIDATES FOR ELECTRICAL STIMULATION

- Pressure ulcers, stage I–IV
- Diabetic ulcers
- Venous ulcers, ischemic ulcer
- Traumatic wounds
- Surgical wounds
- Wound flap
- Donor site, burn wound

---

# Skill 10.17  Using Noncontact Normothermic Wound Therapy

## Equipment

Warming cover (latex free)
Warming card
Temperature control unit (TCU)
AC adapter
Wound measuring guide
Sterile normal saline solution
Skin scalant
Carrying pouch
Sterile normal saline
Skin sealant
Gauze pads
Moisture proof pad
Sterile basin and irrigating syringe
Sterile gloves
Clean gloves
Disposable bag

## Preparation

1. Check physician's orders and client care plan.
2. Gather equipment. Select appropriate sized wound cover and warming card after measuring wound.
3. Check that temperature control unit's battery is charged; if not, recharge with battery pack or wall outlet power source.
4. Explain procedure to client.
5. Provide privacy for client.
6. Perform hand hygiene.

## Procedure

1. Place equipment on over-bed table.
2. Open sterile normal saline bottle, gauze pads, and basin with irrigating syringe.
3. Place disposable bag near wound site.
4. Position client for easy access to wound.
5. Remove compression stockings, if used.
6. Don clean gloves.
7. Remove old dressing and place in disposal bag.
8. Remove clean gloves and discard into disposal bag. Don sterile gloves.
9. Fill irrigating syringe with normal saline. *►Rationale: Using the syringe will increase pressure in wound to assist with removing debris and slough.*
10. Place moisture-proof pad or sterile basin under wound site.
11. Irrigate wound using the prescribed amount of irrigating solution.
12. Cleanse the surrounding skin with normal saline.
13. Dry periwound skin area.
14. Apply scalant to periwound area. *►Rationale: This protects periwound area from exudates.*
15. Select wound cover size that is appropriate size for wound. *►Rationale: To ensure that there is adequate healthy periwound skin between edge of foam and wound.*
16. Hold wound cover near edges only. Pull away 1/2 of wound cover liner.
17. Place wound cover over wound, so wound can be seen through window. Do not stretch wound cover over skin while applying. *►Rationale: Damage can occur to skin.*
18. Check for holes in wound cover, wrinkling, and folding of its edges. *►Rationale: Wound cover will not be a barrier if this occurs.*
19. Press adhesive portion of cover to skin.
20. Pull away other half of wound cover liner and press adhesive portion to skin.
21. Gently smooth adhesive portion of wound cover with your fingertips to ensure adhesive sticks to skin.

## CLINICAL ALERT

This warming treatment is done three times a day for 1 hour each treatment. Ensure that there is at least 1 hour between treatments. You can expect a significant increase in exudate for at least 7–10 days. This is considered a normal consequence of wound healing process.

The wound cover is sterile and protects wound from contamination and trauma. The cover maintains a moist and warm wound, which creates a healing environment. The cover is a thin shell with a window and a foam frame. The shell has an adhesive border, is water resistant and can be cleaned. It is flexible and moves with the client. The foam cover absorbs excess exudates to protect periwound area from maceration. The foam frame keeps the pocket above the wound surface, so warming card is not in contact with the wound. The window is in the center of the cover and contains a pocket for the warming card.

22. Instruct the client that wound cover is worn 24 hours per day and requires no additional dressing.
23. Attach wound cover to Warm-Up® therapy system.
24. Remove gloves and discard into disposal bag.
25. Perform hand hygiene.

### For Using Warm-Up® Therapy System

1. Select appropriate size warming card based on size of wound cover.
2. Plug warming card into gray socket on temperature control unit (TCU).
3. Insert warming card into wound cover pocket. (Warming card is used throughout warming therapy and is only for one client; it can be cleaned with damp cloth and clean water, if needed. Do not apply the warming card directly to the periwound area. Always cover the card with the wound cover. ➤*Rationale: Thermal injury can occur.*
4. Turn off TCU.
5. Select mode of power (can use battery or AC adapter wall outlet).
6. Check that battery has sufficient charge for therapy session, usually one hour.
    a. If battery needs charging; plug AC adapter into TCU, then plug the AC adapter into wall outlet.
    b. Charge TCU until amber light on AC adapter flashes rapidly. It takes up to two hours to fully charge battery.
7. Plug AC adapter into black socket on the TCU, if using the TUC with the AC adapter. Plug AC adapter into wall outlet.
8. Position TCU and warming card cable to allow client some movement. Instruct client not to lie on any electronic component, cable, cord, or wound cover.

## CLINICAL ALERT

Do not use compression therapy while warming card and TCU are in place. Client injury could occur.

9. Press the ON button to begin therapy. Follow physician orders for length of time for therapy. The unit will automatically turn off after two hours of continuous use.
10. Shut off TCU and remove warming card by grasping edge of card and sliding it out of wound cover pocket. Place card in plastic pouch for storage between treatments. DO NOT REMOVE WOUND COVER. ➤*Rationale: Wound cover is replaced if drainage occurs, the cover comes loose, the periwound area becomes macerated, or it has been in place 72 hours.*
11. Replace compression therapy if ordered.

### For Changing Wound Cover

1. Check wound cover to ensure it needs to be changed.
2. Gather equipment for new wound cover.
3. Explain procedure to client.
4. Perform hand hygiene.
5. Follow steps in Skill 10.17 "Using Noncontact Normothermic Wound Therapy, Preparation."
6. Don clean gloves.

## LEGAL ALERT

Wound care practitioners are at risk for litigation. Clients who experience wounds frequently believe it is because of neglect by health care workers. Wound care practitioners may face liability for

- Negligence
- Violations of Medicare and Medicaid fraud and abuse prohibitions
- Abandonment for terminating services to clients

To prove negligence, a client must show that the provider owed the client a duty, breached the duty owed the client, and the breach of duty must result in injury or damage to the client. Owing a duty of reasonable care to a client incorporates the standards of wound care. Breaching a duty occurs when the health-care practitioner does something that should not have been done. To be charged with causing injury the client would need to prove that injuries occurred as a result of practitioner error.

*Source:* Thomas Hess, C. *Clinical Guide: Wound Care,* 4th ed. Springhouse, 2002, p.109–114.

# Skill 10.18   Using Negative Pressure Wound Therapy

## EXPECTED OUTCOMES

- Granulation tissue is evident using adjunctive therapy.
- Periwound area remains healthy without evidence of maceration.
- Moist wound environment is maintained.
- Pain is reduced with adjunctive therapy.
- Wound progresses through usual phases with electrical stimulation.
- Wound healing occurs faster with radiant heat dressing.
- Exudate is removed and wound healing occurs using negative wound therapy.

## Equipment

Skin prep agent, optional
Razor, optional
Clean gloves
Sterile gloves
V.A.C.® device
Disposal bag
Sterile scissor
Equipment
Foam, Black or White V.A.C.® kit
Gauze pads
Sterile normal saline
Irrigating syringe
Moisture proof pad or sterile basin

## Preparation

1. Evaluate if client is candidate for V.A.C.® therapy: nutritionally stable, able to use device 22 hours each day, uses a pressure support surface if wound is over

## EVIDENCE-BASED NURSING PRACTICE

**Vacuum-Assisted Closure for Sternal Wounds:**
**A First-Line Therapeutic Management Approach**

A retrospective review of 103 clients was completed at one institution. The clients underwent vacuum-assisted closure therapy after median sternotomy between June 1999 and March 2004. The clients' wounds were classified as sterile wounds, superficial sternal infections, and mediastinitis. The wound closure device was applied sterilely to all wounds over a layer of Acticoat. The results indicated that vacuum-assisted closure was utilized in the treatment of 103 clients with sternal wounds. (67 males and 36 females). The median age was 52 years (3 months to 91 years). Client comorbidities included diabetes, chronic obstructive pulmonary disease, end stage renal disease, immunosuppression and other conditions. The therapy was utilized for 11 days per client. Sixty-eight of the clients had definitive chest closure with open reduction internal fixation and/or flap closure. The remaining 32 percent of the clients had no definitive closure method. The overall mortality rate was 28 percent, although none of the 4 deaths were directly related to the use of the therapy. The conclusion indicated that vacuum-assisted closure therapy has been shown to decrease wound edema, decrease time to definitive closure, and reduce wound bacterial colony counts.

*Source:* Agarwal, JP, et al. Vacuum-assisted Closure for Sternal Wounds: A First-line Therapeutic Management Approach. *Plastic Reconstructive Surgery* (2005, September 15), 116(4); 1035–40.

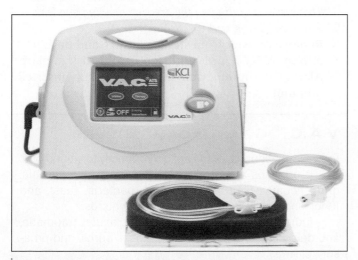

● V.A.C.®-ATS machine is placed on level surface or hangs on foot of bed. (Courtesy of Kinetic Concepts, Inc. San Antonio, TX.)

bony prominence. ➤*Rationale: If therapy turned off longer than 2 hours, dressing must be removed and replaced with traditional dressing.*

2. Assess wound to determine if therapy can be implemented.
   a. Wound surrounded by at least 2 cm of intact periwound tissue to maintain airtight seal.
   b. Wound open enough to insert foam dressing that touches all edges.
   c. Wound debrided.
   d. Sufficient circulation to assist in healing process.
3. Select correct foam dressing according to size and type of wound. Black foam has larger pores and is used to stimulate granulation tissue and wound

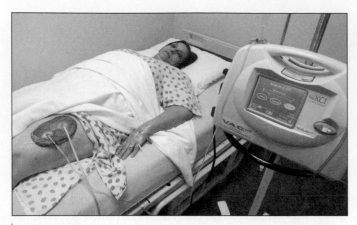

● Functioning.

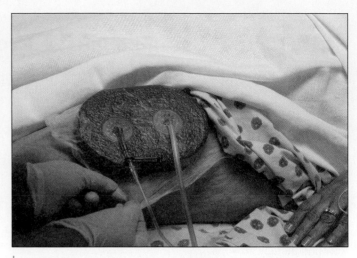

● Releasing.

contraction. White (soft) foam is used when granulation tissue needs to be restricted or client cannot tolerate pain associated with Black foam. White foam is used with superficial wounds, shallow chronic ulcers, and tunneling or undermining wounds.

4. Gather equipment and supplies.
5. Provide privacy.
6. Explain procedure to client and determine his willingness to use this therapy.
7. Perform hand hygiene.

**Procedure**

1. Place disposal bag near wound.
2. Open supplies and place on over-bed table. Open kit maintaining sterility.
3. Draw up normal saline irrigating solution in syringe.
4. Don clean gloves.
5. Place moisture proof pad or sterile basin under wound. ➤*Rationale: Protects skin and bed during irrigation.*
6. Clean wound using aggressive irrigation. If debridement is to be done, only a trained professional can perform the skill. Notify the appropriate person. ➤*Rationale: Devitalized tissue should be removed as areas of soft or stringy slough delays the healing process.*
7. Remove gloves and place in disposal bag.
8. Don sterile gloves.
9. Dry wound and prepare periwound tissue with skin preparation agent if necessary. ➤*Rationale: To promote an airtight seal.*
10. Cut the V.A.C.®foam to fit the shape and entire wound cavity, including tunneling or undermined areas. White foam is used for tunneled wounds.
11. Size and trim drape to cover foam dressing, leaving a 3.5 cm border per wound skin.
12. Gently place the foam into wound ensuring entire wound is covered.

## CLINICAL ALERT

Do not pack foam into any areas of the wound. Forcing foam dressings in a compressed manner into any wound may lead to risk of adverse health issues.

13. Apply tubing to foam. Tubing can be laid on top of foam or placed inside foam dressing. Keep tubing away from bony prominences.
14. Cover foam and 3.5 cm per wound area with drape. Do not stretch drape or compress foam with drape. ➤*Rationale: This ensures a tight seal without causing tension or a shearing force on periwound tissue.*
15. Lift tubing and place on drape that has been bunched up to protect skin from pressure of tube.
16. Secure tubing with additional piece of drape or tape several centimeters away from dressing. ➤*Rationale: This prevents pulling on the dressing, leading to a leak.*
17. Remove gloves and discard.
18. Remove canister from sterile package and push it into the V.A.C.® unit until you hear it click in place. Alarm will sound if canister is not properly inserted into unit.

## V.A.C.® GRANUFOAM® SILVER

Provides continuous delivery of silver directly to wound bed.

It provides a protective barrier to reduce aerobic, gram-negative, and gram-positive bacteria, yeast, and fungi, and it may reduce infections in wounds.

Indicated for client with chronic, acute, traumatic, and dehisced wounds, partial thickness burns, and pressure ulcers.

19. Connect dressing tubing to canister tubing.
20. Open both clamps, one on dressing tubing and one on canister tubing.
21. Place V.A.C.® unit on level surface or hang from footboard.
22. Press power button ON.
23. Adjust V.A.C.® unit settings according to physician's orders or Guidelines for Treating Wound Types in the Reference Manual. Target pressure should be set for 5 minutes on and 2 minutes off (intermittent therapies on machine). Intensity of setting sets the negative pressure.
24. Assess dressing in 1 minute. ➤*Rationale: The dressing should collapse unless air leak is present.*
25. Dressing changes must be completed every 48 hours unless wound is infected, then change every 12–24 hours.

**Procedure for Removing Dressing**

1. Perform hand hygiene.
2. Don clean gloves.
3. Raise tube connector above level of pump unit.
4. Tighten clamp on dressing tube.
5. Separate canister tube and dressing tubes by disconnecting the connector.
6. Allow pump unit to pull exudates in canister tube into canister; then tighten clamps on canister tube.
7. Press Therapy ON/OFF to deactivate pump.

8. Stretch drape horizontally and slowly pull up from skin. Gently remove it from skin. Do not peel it off skin.
9. Discard disposable equipment including gloves in appropriate bag or container.
10. Perform hand hygiene.

*Note:* Dressing changes are completed every 48 hrs; if infected, every 12 hours.

**Procedure for Disconnecting V.A.C.® Unit**

1. Turn the unit to OFF.
2. Clamp both clamps on tubing.
3. Press quick release connector to separate dressing tubing from canister tubing.
4. Cover ends of tubing with gauze and secure.

**Procedure for Reconnecting V.A.C.® Unit**

1. Remove gauze from ends of tubing.
2. Connect tubing.
3. Unclamp clamps.
4. Press V.A.C.® green power button to ON.
5. Select NO at new client prompt. Unit will resume previous settings.
6. Press therapy to ON.

**Procedure for Changing Canister**

1. Don clean gloves.
2. Assess that canister unit is full. Unit will alarm when full.
3. Tighten clamps on canister tubing from dressing tubing.
4. Pull back on release knob on V.A.C.® unit at same time as you pull canister from slot.
5. Put canister in biohazard disposable bag and place in designated area for disposal.
6. Dispose of gloves.
7. Perform hand hygiene.

*Note:* Average length of treatment is 4–6 weeks. Home systems are available as well.

| UNEXPECTED OUTCOMES | CRITICAL THINKING OPTIONS |
|---|---|
| Warm-Up® Therapy system shows heat light is on and low battery light is flashing. | • Charge battery.<br>• Use TCU and AC adapter together. |
| Fault light is flashing and an alarm is sounding on TCU. | • Reconnect warming card, it may be disconnected.<br>• Warming card or cable could be bent or damaged. Replace warming card.<br>• TCU is broken. Turn TCU on and off. If light continues and alarm continues, turn off TCU and obtain new unit. |
| Nothing lights up on TCU panel. | • TCU is not on or battery is low. Turn unit ON or charge battery. |
| Wound is too large for V.A.C.® kit. | • Use more than 1 foam piece.<br>• Place pieces so they touch each other.<br>• Use only one tubing to one of the pieces. |
| Periwound skin is fragile. | • Use skin prep prior to applying drape.<br>• Frame wound with skin barrier or DuoDERM.<br>• Cut drape large enough to enclose foam dressing and skin barrier layer. |
| Dressing does not collapse following V.A.C.® application. | • Listen for whistling sound indicating a leak in the system.<br>• Gently press around tubing, check for wrinkles or drape not covering correctly.<br>• Most leaks occur around tubing.<br>• Use excess drape to patch over leak. |
| Foam is not collapsed in wound bed. | • Ensure therapy is ON. Ensure clamps are open and tubing is not kinked.<br>• Check for leaks and patch. |
| Audible alarm sounds on VAC system and therapy is stopped. | • Check for blockage in tubing and replace as needed.<br>• If problem continues after tubing is replaced, notify company that produces the system. |
| Dressing adheres to wound with negative pressure system. | • Instill sterile water or normal saline into dressing, let sit for 15–20 minutes, then gently remove dressing from wound. |

# Skill 10.19   Applying a Transparent Wound Barrier

**Delegation**

Due to the need for aseptic technique and assessment skills, most dressing changes are not delegated to UAP. In some states, UAP may apply dry dressings to clean, chronic wounds. UAP should observe an exposed wound or dressing during usual care and must report abnormal findings to the nurse. In some agencies, UAP may be permitted to reinforce the dressing (apply additional dry dressings over a saturated bandage), but this must be reported to the nurse as soon as possible. Assessment of the wound and abnormal findings must be validated and interpreted by the nurse.

**Equipment**

• Clean gloves
• Sterile gloves (optional)
• Alcohol or acetone
• Moisture-proof bag
• Sterile gauze and the wound-cleaning agents specified by the primary care provider or agency (e.g., sterile saline)
• Wound barrier dressing
• Scissors
• Paper tape

## Preparation

- Review the order regarding frequency and type of dressing change, and determine agency protocol about solutions used to clean the wound and whether clean or sterile technique is to be used. Many agencies recommend clean rather than sterile technique for chronic wounds such as a pressure ulcer. If possible, schedule the dressing change at a time convenient for the client. Some dressing changes require only a few minutes and others can take much longer.

## Procedure

1. Prior to performing the procedure, introduce self and verify the client's identity using agency protocol. Explain to the client what you are going to do, why it is necessary, and how he or she can participate. Discuss how the results will be used in planning further care or treatments.
2. Perform hand hygiene and observe other appropriate infection control procedures.
3. Provide for client privacy. Assist the client to a comfortable position in which the wound can be readily exposed. Expose only the wound area, using a bath blanket to cover the client, if necessary. ➤*Rationale: Undue exposure is physically and psychologically distressing to most people.*
4. Remove the existing dressing (see Skill 10.1, steps 5 through 7).
5. Assess the wound.
6. Thoroughly clean the skin area around the wound.
   - Apply clean gloves.
   - Clean the skin well with normal saline or a mild cleansing agent. Always rinse the adjacent skin well before applying a dressing.
   - Clip the hair about 5 cm (2 in.) around the wound area if indicated.
   - Remove gloves and dispose of them in the moisture-proof bag. Perform hand hygiene.
7. Clean the wound if indicated.
   - Apply clean or sterile gloves in accordance with agency protocol.
   - Clean the wound with the prescribed solution.
   - Dry the surrounding skin with dry gauze.
8. Apply the wound barrier.
   - Review the instructions on the barrier package. Remove part of the paper backing on the dressing.

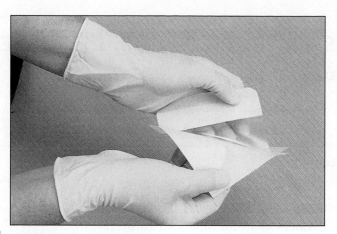

● Transparent wound dressing.

### Transparent Wound Dressing

- Apply the dressing at one edge of the wound site, allowing at least 2.5-cm (1-in.) coverage of the skin surrounding the wound.
- Gently lay or press the barrier over the wound. Keep it free of wrinkles, but avoid stretching it too tightly. ➤*Rationale: A stretched dressing restricts mobility and can pull loose easily.*
- Remove and discard gloves. Perform hand hygiene.
9. Reinforce the dressing only if absolutely needed.
   - Apply paper or other porous tape to "window frame" the edges of the dressing.
10. Assess the wound at least daily.
    - Determine the extent of serous fluid accumulation under the dressing, wound healing, and the need to repair the dressing.
    - If excessive serum has accumulated, consider replacing the transparent wound barrier with a more absorbent type of dressing, such as hydrocolloid.
    - If the dressing is leaking, remove it and apply another dressing.
11. Document the dressing change and the client's response in the client record using forms or checklists supplemented by narrative notes when appropriate. Many agencies use a designated wound/skin documentation sheet.

# Skill 10.20  Positioning and Exercising the Stump

## EXPECTED OUTCOMES
- Stump wound heals without complications.
- Stump maintains functional alignment.
- Stump is prepared for prosthesis use.

## Equipment

Pillows

## Preparation

1. Check chart for physician's orders.
2. Identify client and explain purpose of positioning and exercising.
3. Provide privacy.
4. Perform hand hygiene.

## Procedure

### For Preoperative Care

1. Evaluate nutritional status and request nutritional consult if indicated. ➤Rationale: Adequate protein is necessary to promote wound healing.
2. Recruit assistance of OT, PT, and social worker for early multidisciplinary care planning. A prosthetist explains future prosthetic care to the client and possibly organizes amputee peer visit, as this helps lessen anxiety about living with an amputation.
3. Explain importance of exercises to client. Tell client that because flexor muscles are stronger than extensors, stump will be permanently flexed and abducted unless the client practices extension and adduction exercises. ➤Rationale: Exercises increase muscle strength and improve mobility of amputated extremity. Both are necessary for optimal ambulation with a prosthesis.
4. Teach client quadriceps-setting exercises with a below-the-knee amputation.
   a. Extend leg and try to push back of knee into bed; try to move patella proximally.
   b. Contract quadriceps and hold contraction for 10 seconds.
   c. Repeat this procedure four or five times.
   d. Repeat the exercise at least four times a day.
5. Teach use of ambulatory aids. ➤Rationale: Prepares client for post-surgery mobility.
6. Explain phantom limb sensation; the client may continue to "feel" the lost limb post surgery.
7. Counsel families, for they also mourn the loss of a visible body part. ➤Rationale: They too need psychological support and education about rehabilitation and necessary skills for self-care.

> ## CLINICAL ALERT
>
> Keep a tourniquet nearby in the event of excessive stump incision bleeding.

> ## CLINICAL ALERT
>
> Adequate pain management in the preoperative period can reduce the occurrence of phantom limb pain postoperatively.

### For Postoperative Care

1. Monitor for complications: hemorrhage, infection, unrelieved pain, wound that will not heal.
2. Assess for excessive wound drainage. Keep tourniquet at bedside. ➤Rationale: If excessive bleeding occurs, tourniquet must be applied, as hemorrhage is a potentially life-threatening complication.
3. Administer ordered pain medication and continually assess to determine if pain is controlled.
4. Do not place stump on pillow, but elevate foot of bed for first 24 hours ONLY to reduce stump edema and pain. ➤Rationale: Elevation on a pillow can promote flexion contracture of stump.
5. Turn client to prone or supine position for at least 1 hour every 4 hours. ➤Rationale: This promotes hip extension and helps counteract possible flexion contracture formation.
6. Avoid dependent positioning of stump. ➤Rationale: To prevent edema and discomfort. Edema may be present for up to 4 months after amputation.
7. While washing the stump, tap and massage the stump skin toward the incision line. ➤Rationale: To prevent development of painful adhesions.
8. Teach stump extension exercises.
   a. Lie in a prone position with foot hanging over the end of the bed.
   b. Keep stump next to intact leg to extend stump and to contract gluteal muscles.
   c. Hold the contraction for 10 seconds.
   d. Repeat this exercise at least four times a day.
9. Teach adduction exercise.
   a. Place a pillow between the client's thighs.
   b. Squeeze the pillow for 10 seconds and then relax for 10 seconds.
   c. Repeat this exercise at least four times a day.
10. Have the client keep track of time spent with the stump flexed and then spend an equal amount of time with the stump extended.
11. Encourage appropriate use of trapeze: Use both hands to pull up with trapeze; place foot flat on mattress to lift body. Do not use heel to push in the mattress. ➤Rationale: Pushing with the heel can lead to pressure ulcers.
12. After stump incision heals, have client begin to bear weight on stump, initially pressing into padded surface (pillow on chair seat). ➤Rationale: To reduce pain and help prepare the stump for prosthesis.

# Skill 10.21   Shrinking/Molding the Stump

## Equipment

Two elastic bandages: 4 inches for below-the-knee
   amputation (BKA), 6 inches for above-the-knee
   amputation (AKA)
Tape or safety pins
Commercial stump shrinker (sheath)

## Preparation

1. Review client's chart to determine date and type of
   amputation.
2. Gather equipment.
3. Identify client using two forms of ID and explain
   rationale for procedure.
4. Perform hand hygiene.
5. Provide privacy.

## Procedure

1. Wash stump with soap and water and allow to dry
   for at least 10 minutes before bandaging. Do not use
   lotions, powders, or alcohol.
2. Inspect and encourage client to assess stump for circulatory status, pressure areas, wound healing, and
   edema.
3. Explain that purpose of wrap is to form a conical
   AKA stump to prepare for prosthesis use.

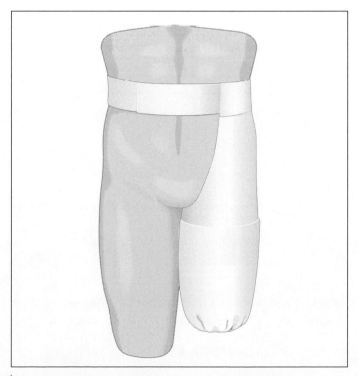

● "Commercial shrinkers" may be used for above-the-knee
amputations (AKA).

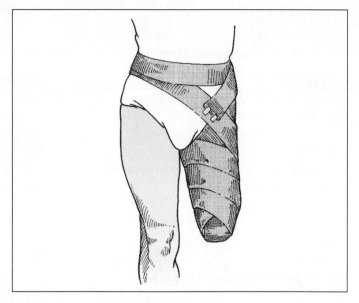

● Compression bandage may be used following amputation to mold
and shrink stump in preparation for prosthesis.

4. Explain that wrap is to be worn at all times except
   during bathing or when wearing a prosthesis.
5. Start by placing bandage end outer surface on distal
   stump. ➤*Rationale: The pressure gradient of the bandage
   should be greatest at the distal stump.*
6. Wrap bandage medially and diagonally around
   stump. Have client assist by holding turns. Stretch
   bandages to two-thirds of the limit of the elastic.
7. Continue to wrap smoothly up the stump with medially directed spirals or figure eight turns (not circular). Progress up the stump and well into groin area.
   ➤*Rationale: Circular turns constrict circulation. Medial turns
   help correct stump tendency toward abduction.*
8. Finish bandaging with a "spica" turn over and around
   the client's pelvis, then back down to stump. ➤*Rationale:
   Large "spica" turn prevents bandage slipping.*
9. Secure the bandage with tape or (cautiously) with
   safety pins. Do not use bandage clips. ➤*Rationale: Clips
   can pierce the skin, or easily come loose.*
10. Reapply elastic bandage every 4–6 hours, or when
    loose. ➤*Rationale: It must never be in place for more than
    12 hours without being rewrapped.*

## CLINICAL ALERT

Amputees use more energy in ambulation than nonam-
putees. The elderly with an AKA must put forth an effort
100% above normal to walk at a slow rate. The longer the
residual limb, the less energy the client must expend for
ambulation.

11. If client has a stump "shrinker sheath," roll down and stretch the sheath using plastic ring. Fit onto stump end and apply, making sure there are no wrinkles.

12. Teach client home care of residual limb and prosthesis (washing; assessing for redness, pressure points, irritation, swelling skin breakdown; socket, stump, socks, liners, mechanical parts, etc.).

| UNEXPECTED OUTCOMES | CRITICAL THINKING OPTIONS |
| --- | --- |
| Client sits in chair most of day and keeps stump elevated on a pillow while in bed. | • Discuss hip and knee contracture complications that occur with prolonged flexion positioning of the stump.<br>• Review and reinforce exercises that promote stump adduction and extension to prevent contractures and facilitate prosthesis use. |
| Stump edema occurs in spite of compression bandage application. | • Evaluate wrapping procedure.<br>• Ensure that wraps are applied with pressure greater at distal stump and reapplied several times a day.<br>• Instruct client to avoid prolonged dependent positioning of stump.<br>• Consult prosthetist for possible rigid shrinker use.<br>• Apply shrinker before client gets out of bed. |
| Client expresses fear of losing other leg. | • Teach client to care for the remaining extremity.<br>• Inspect for lesions, wash and dry daily, use lotion for dry skin (not between toes), keep nails trimmed straight across, avoid mechanical, chemical, or thermal injury, wear shoes that are wide and deep enough for toes.<br>• Avoid smoking and exercise daily.<br>• Consult podiatrist for individual foot care or shoe orthotic adaptations, especially if diabetic.<br>• Consult physician for management of diabetes or atherosclerosis. |

# Assessments

Skill 11.1    Assessing Appearance
              and Mental Status                    448

Skill 11.2    Assessing the Skin                   451

Skill 11.3    Assessing the Hair                   456

Skill 11.4    Assessing the Nails                  457

Skill 11.5    Assessing the Skull and Face         459

Skill 11.6    Assessing the Eyes and Vision        460

Skill 11.7    Assessing the Ears and Hearing       466

Skill 11.8    Assessing the Nose and Sinuses       469

Skill 11.9    Assessing the Mouth and
              Oropharynx                            471

Skill 11.10   Assessing the Neck                   475

Skill 11.11   Assessing the Thorax and Lungs       477

Skill 11.12   Assessing the Heart and Central
              Vessels                               484

Skill 11.13   Assessing the Peripheral Vascular
              System                                487

Skill 11.14   Assessing the Breasts and Axillae    489

Skill 11.15   Assessing the Abdomen                494

Skill 11.16   Assessing the Musculoskeletal
              System                                498

Skill 11.17   Assessing the Neurologic System      501

Skill 11.18   Assessing the Female Genitals
              and Inguinal Area                     510

Skill 11.19   Assessing the Male Genitalia
              and Inguinal Area                     512

Skill 11.20   Assessing the Anus                   515

Skill 11.21   Assessing the Client in Pain         516
              VARIATION: Daily Pain Diary          519
              VARIATION: Child Pain
              Assessment                            519

Skill 11.22   Assessing Body Temperature           522
              VARIATION: Measuring an Infant
              or Child's Temperature                523

Skill 11.23   Assessing an Apical-Radial Pulse     529

Skill 11.24   Assessing an Apical Pulse            531

Skill 11.25   Assessing Peripheral Pulses          533

Skill 11.26   Assessing Respirations               535

Skill 11.27   Assessing Blood Pressure             537

Skill 11.28   Assessing Pulse Oximeter             543

Skill 11.29   Measuring Length                     544

Skill 11.30   Measuring Height                     545

Skill 11.31   Measuring Weight                     546

Skill 11.32   Measuring Body Mass Index            546

Skill 11.33   Measuring Head Circumference         547

Skill 11.34   Measuring Chest Circumference        547

Skill 11.35   Measuring Abdominal Girth            548

Skill 11.36   Assessing the Heart Rate             548

Skill 11.37   Assessing the Respiratory Rate       549

**Skill 11.38**  Assessing Blood Pressure          549

**Skill 11.39**  Assessing a Child's Body
Temperature                                         551

**Skill 11.40**  Glasgow Coma Scale                553

**Skill 11.41**  Neurovascular Assessment          554

**Skill 11.42**  Intracranial Pressure Monitoring
and Daily Care                                     554

**Skill 11.43**  Assessing Visual Acuity           555

**Skill 11.44**  Assessing Hearing Acuity          557

Health assessment, the collection and interpretation of data regarding the client's previous and current health status, is one of the most important professional responsibilities of the registered nurse. Vigilance in performing relevant assessment techniques, determining the meaning of the findings, and taking appropriate action based on the evaluation of the data are central aspects of effective nursing care and cannot be delegated to those without the requisite skills and knowledge.

In order for the process of assessment to be more client focused than nurse focused, we must guide our intentions. Rather than viewing this process as simply gathering information and data, the nurse should view it as a process of discovery in which the nurse and client identify patterns, accessing what is already known to the client. The nurse uses listening skills to hear clients' stories and beliefs about what is going on inside their bodies and to seek clarification and verification. The nurse may also use intuitive skills to enhance the pattern recognition process.

It is essential for the nurse to access information about the client's spiritual health and well being along with physical health. Accrediting organizations specify that a spiritual assessment be conducted on all clients. The assessment need not take much time, and many resources are available to assist nurses in spiritual assessment and care (Dossey, Keegan & Guzzetta, 2005; Young & Koopsen, 2005).

Although the nurse is able to perform a comprehensive assessment of each individual body system, more commonly the generalist nurse performs a brief screening assessment of all systems (sometimes referred to as a head-to-toe assessment) when first encountering the client and then more detailed focused assessments of particular systems as indicated by the client's condition. Independent clinical judgment drives the selection of those components for which an assessment is indicated. Box 11–1 presents the order generally followed in performing a head-to-toe assessment. This order provides a systematic approach and includes all vital areas to assess while minimizing positioning changes for both nurse and client. Advance practice nurses such as nurse practition-

ers may perform much more in-depth assessments of selected systems.

The traditional vital signs are body temperature, pulse, respirations, and blood pressure. Many agencies such as the Veterans Administration, American Pain Society, and the Joint Commission on Accreditation of Healthcare Organizations have designated pain as a fifth vital sign. Pain assessment is covered in Chapter 1. In addition, the effectiveness of respirations and circulation is commonly measured noninvasively through pulse oximetry (See Chapter 7 Oxygenation) at the same time as other vital signs. These signs, which should be looked at both individually and collectively, enable nurses to monitor the functions of the body. Vital signs reflect changes that otherwise might not be observed. Monitoring a client's vital signs should not be an automatic or routine procedure; it should be a thoughtful, scientific assessment. Vital signs should be evaluated with reference to the client's present and prior health status and compared to accepted standards. If findings appear inconsistent with those anticipated, they should immediately be rechecked. Vital signs normally vary with the client's age.

---

### TIMES TO ASSESS VITAL SIGNS

- On admission to a health care agency to obtain baseline data.

- When a client has a change in health status or reports symptoms such as chest pain or feeling hot or faint.

- Before and after surgery or an invasive procedure.

- Before and/or after the administration of a medication that could affect the respiratory or cardiovascular systems, for example, before giving a digitalis preparation.

- Before and after any nursing intervention that could affect the vital signs (e.g., ambulating a client who has been on bed rest).

## BOX 11-1 HEAD-TO-TOE FRAMEWORK

### General Survey Including Vital Signs

Areas below are assessed including determination of current complaints and inspection. Palpation, percussion, and auscultation are used if indicated.

- Head
  - Hair and face
  - Eyes and vision
  - Ears and hearing
  - Nose
  - Mouth and oropharynx
- Neck
  - Muscles
  - Lymph nodes
  - Trachea
  - Thyroid gland
  - Carotid arteries
  - Neck veins
- Upper extremities
  - Skin and nails
  - Muscle strength and tone
  - Joint range of motion
- Brachial and radial pulses
- Sensation
- Chest and back
  - Skin
  - Thorax shape and size
  - Lungs
  - Heart
  - Spinal column
  - Breasts and axillae
- Abdomen
  - Skin
  - Abdominal sounds
  - Femoral pulses
- External genitals
- Anus
- Lower extremities
  - Skin and toenails
  - Gait and balance
  - Joint range of motion
  - Popliteal, posterior tibial, and dorsalis pedis pulses

# CULTURAL CONSIDERATIONS

Here are a few examples of different cultural norms in nonverbal communication. Cultural norms will vary within a culture, and from generation to generation. Therefore, it is extremely important to observe carefully, ask your client about preferences, and not make assumptions. Your assessment and care will benefit greatly from this awareness of differences.

### Eye Contact

Keep in Mind—Eye contact and the handshake have different meanings for different cultures. For example, some Native American communities consider direct eye contact an invasion of privacy and a firm handshake aggressive. Many Asian cultures avoid eye contact as a sign of respect for the other individual. The nurse of Western European descent might believe that a client who avoids direct eye contact is somewhat suspicious, and that a weak handshake signifies disinterest. In some Middle Eastern and Latin countries, direct eye contact is common and accepted.

*Nursing Implications*—Be careful not to assume things about your client based on the norms for your own cultural group. For example, if you value eye contact as a sign of interest, you may incorrectly assume your client is disinterested if he or she does not maintain eye contact. In fact, the client may be trying to show respect for you.

Observing your client with family and other individuals is a helpful way to learn about his or her usual pattern of eye contact.

### Touch and Personal Space

Keep in Mind—Americans tend to keep a certain amount of space between themselves and others, typically 3 feet, and use touch sparingly. French people typically feel comfortable standing very close to others and are comfortable touching. Cultural groups such as Orthodox Jews and Chinese Americans may consider excessive touching, especially from the opposite sex, offensive.

*Nursing Implications*—Note patterns of touch between family members, or individuals of the same culture. Just as with eye contact, it may be difficult for you to change your habits of touch and personal space. However, if you sense unease in your clients, reevaluate your actions to be more sensitive to their comfort level. When in doubt, ask your client if he or she feels comfortable in the situation.

### Use of Body Language

Keep in Mind—Body language can easily be misinterpreted during the assessment, so pay careful attention to the assumptions you are making based on your own cultural norms. For example, many Americans typically nod

*(continued)*

## CULTURAL CONSIDERATIONS (CONTINUED)

to indicate agreement or approval. Asian people may nod to be polite, but this may not actually indicate agreement.

*Nursing Implications*—Make sure that you are not relying solely on nonverbal clues to determine if your client understands or agrees with you. Instead of asking, "Did you understand how we will test your blood?" and relying on a nod for affirmation, you might ask, "Can you explain how we will test your blood?" Also try to follow up on your questions so that you actually hear a verbal "yes" or a "no" response.

# Skill 11.1  Assessing Appearance and Mental Status

## Procedure

1. Prior to performing the procedure, introduce self and verify the client's identity using agency protocol. Explain to the client what you are going to do, why it is necessary, and how he or she can participate. Discuss how the results will be used in planning further care or treatments.
2. Perform hand hygiene and observe appropriate infection control procedures.
3. Provide for client privacy.

| Assessment | Normal Findings | Deviations from Normal |
|---|---|---|
| 4. Observe body build, height, and weight in relation to the client's age, lifestyle, and health. | Proportionate, varies with lifestyle | Excessively thin or obese |
| 5. Observe client's posture and gait, standing, sitting, and walking. | Relaxed, erect posture; coordinated movement | Tense, slouched, bent posture; uncoordinated movement; tremors, unbalanced gait |
| 6. Observe client's overall hygiene and grooming. Relate these to the person's activities prior to the assessment. | Clean, neat | Dirty, unkempt |
| 7. Note body and breath odor in relation to activity level. | No body odor or minor body odor relative to work or exercise; no breath odor | Foul body odor; ammonia odor; acetone breath odor; foul breath |
| 8. Observe for signs of distress in posture or facial expression. | No apparent distress | Bending over because of abdominal pain, wincing, frowning, or labored breathing |
| 9. Note obvious signs of health or illness (e.g., in skin color or breathing). | Well developed, well nourished, intact skin, easy breathing | Pallor, (paleness) weakness, lesions, cough |
| 10. Assess the client's attitude (frame of mind). | Cooperative, able to follow instructions | Negative, hostile, withdrawn, anxious |
| 11. Note the client's affect/mood; assess the appropriateness of the client's responses. | Appropriate to situation | Inappropriate to situation, sudden mood changes, paranoia |
| 12. Listen for speech quantity (amount and pace) and quality (loudness, clarity, inflection). | Understandable, moderate pace; clear tone and inflection | Rapid or slow pace; overly loud or soft |
| 13. Listen for relevance and organization of thoughts. | Logical sequence, relevant answers, has sense of reality | Illogical sequence, flight of ideas, confusion, generalizations, vague |
| 14. Document findings in the client record using handwritten or electronic forms and checklists supplemented by narrative notes when appropriate. | | |

## ADMISSION DATA

Date 4-16-09 Time 3:15 p.m. Primary Language English
Arrived Via: ☐ Wheelchair ☐ Stretcher ☑ Ambulatory
From: ☐ Admitting ☐ ER ☑ Home ☐ Nursing Home ☐ Other
Admitting M.D. R. Katz      Time Notified 5 p.m.

### ORIENTATION TO UNIT

|  | YES | NO |  | YES | NO |
|---|---|---|---|---|---|
| Arm Band Correct | ☑ | ☐ | Visiting Hours | ☑ | ☐ |
| Allergy Band | ☑ | ☐ | Smoking Policy | ☑ | ☐ |
| Telephone | ☑ | ☐ | TV, Lights, Bed Controls, |  |  |
| Electrical Policy | ☑ | ☐ | Call Lights, Side Rails | ☑ | ☐ |
| Educational Mat'l | ☑ | ☐ | Nurses Station | ☑ | ☐ |
| (TV Brochure) | ☑ | ☐ |  |  |  |

Family M.D. R. Katz
Weight 125 lb. Height 5 ft. 2 in. BP:R — L 122/80
Temp. 103F Pulse 92, weak Resp 28, shallow
Source Providing Information ☑ Patient ☐ Other
Unable to Obtain History ☐
Reason for Admission (Onset, Duration, Pt.'s Perception) "Chest cold" X 2 weeks S.O.B on exertion. "Lung pain, fever," "Dr. says I have pneumonia."

## ALLERGIES & REACTIONS

Drugs Penicillin
Food/Other
Signs & Symptoms rash, nausea
Blood Reaction ☐ Yes ☑ No Dyes/Shellfish ☐ Yes ☑ No

## MEDICATIONS

| Current Meds | Dose/Freq. | Last Dose |
|---|---|---|
| Synthroid | 0.1 mg. daily | 4-16, 8 a.m. |

Disposition of Meds: ☒ Home ☐ Pharmacy ☐ Safe *At Bedside

## MEDICAL HISTORY

☑ No Major Problems      ☐ Gastro
☐ Cardiac                ☐ Arthritis
☐ Hyper/Hypotension      ☐ Stroke
☐ Diabetes               ☐ Seizures
☐ Cancer                 ☐ Glaucoma
☐ Respiratory            ☑ Other Childbirth - 2006

| Surgery/Procedures | Date |
|---|---|
| Appendectomy | 1996 |
| Partial thyroidectomy | 2003 |

## SPECIAL ASSISTIVE DEVICES

☐ Wheelchair    ☐ Contacts     ☐ Venous        ☐ Dentures
☐ Braces        ☐ Hearing Aid  Access          ☐ Partial
☐ Cane/Crutches ☐ Prosthesis   Device          ☐ Upper
☐ Walker        ☐ Glasses      ☐ Epidural Catheter ☐ Lower
☐ Other  None

## VALUABLES

Patient informed Hospital not responsible for personal belongings.
Valuables Disposition: ☐ Patient ☐ Safe ☐ Given to
Patient/SO Signature  None

## PSYCHOSOCIAL HISTORY

Recent Stress None
Coping Mechanism Not assessed because of fatigue
Support System Husband, coworkers, friends
Calm: ☑ Yes ☐ No
Anxious: ☐ Yes ☐ No Facial muscles tense; trembling
Religion Catholic. Would want Last Rites
Tobacco Use: ☐ Yes ☑ No
Alcohol Use: ☐ Yes ☑ No
Drug Use: ☐ Yes ☑ No

## NEUROLOGICAL

Oriented: ☑ Person ☑ Place ☑ Time ☐ Confused ☐ Sedated
☐ Alert ☐ Restless ☑ Lethargic ☐ Comatose
Pupils: ☑ Equal ☐ Unequal ☑ Reactive ☐ Sluggish
☐ Other 3mm.
Extremity Strength: ☑ Equal ☐ Unequal
Speech: ☑ Clear ☐ Slurred ☐ Other

## MUSCULO-SKELETAL

Normal ROM of Extremities ☑ Yes ☐ No
☑ Weakness ☐ Paralysis ☐ Contractures ☐ Joint Swelling ☑ Pain
☐ Other ↓ related to fatigue    when coughing

## RESPIRATORY

Pattern: ☐ Even ☐ Uneven ☑ Shallow ☑ Dyspnea
☑ Other diminished breath sounds
Breathing Sounds: ☐ Clear ☑ Other inspiratory crackles
Secretions: ☐ None ☑ Other pink, thick sputum
Cough: ☐ None ☑ Productive ☐ Nonproductive

## CARDIOVASCULAR

Pulses: Apical Rate 92-W ☑ Reg. ☐ Irregular ☐ Pacemaker
S = Strong W = Weak A = Absent D = Doppler
Radial R 92 L — Pedal R — L —
Edema: ☑ Absent ☐ Present Site
Perfusion: ☐ Warm ☐ Dry ☑ Diaphoretic ☐ Cool (Hot)

## GASTROINTESTINAL

Oral Mucosa ☐ Normal ☑ Other pale and dry
Bowel Sounds: ☑ Normal ☐ Other Abd. soft
Wt. Change: ☐ ☑ N/V Stool Frequency/Character 1/day; soft
Last B/M 4-15-09 ☐ Ostomy (type)
Equip.

## GENITOURINARY

Urine: Last Voided This morning
☐ Normal ☐ Anuria ☐ Hematuria ☐ Dysuria ☐ Incontinent
☒ Other ↓ amount & frequency since ill
☐ Catheter (type) ___ Other
LMP 4-1-09 ☐ Vaginal/Penile Discharge
Other

## SELF CARE

Need Assist with: ☐ Ambulating ☐ Elimination
☐ Meals ☒ Hygiene ☐ Dressing
while fatigued

Amanda Aquilini [F. age 27]
#4637651      DOB 11-02-81

✳️ **NORTH BROWARD HOSPITAL DISTRICT**
**NURSING ADMINISTRATION ASSESSMENT**

Nursing assessment form.

*(continued)*

Nursing assessment form *(continued)*.

## NUTRITION

**General Appearance:** ☑ Well Nourished ☐ Emaciated
☐ Other

**Appetite:** ☐ Good ☐ Fair ☑ Poor -x2 days
**Diet** Liquid   **Meal Pattern** 3/day
☐ Feeds Self ☐ Assist ☐ Total Feed

## SKIN ASSESSMENT

**Color:** ☐ Normal ☐ Flushed ☑ Pale ☐ Dusky ☐ Cyanotic
☐ Jaundiced ☑ Other  Cheeks flushed, hot
**General Description** Surgical scars:
RLQ abdomen; anterior neck

**Note Cultures Obtained** _____

### PRESSURE SORE ™ AT RISK SCREENING CRITERIA

**OVERALL SKIN CONDITION**
Grade
| | |
|---|---|
| 0 | Turgor (elasticity adequate, skin warm and moist) |
| ✓ 1 | Poor turgor, skin cold & dry |
| 2 | Areas mottled, red or denuded |
| 3 | Existing skin ulcer/lesions |

**BOWEL AND BLADDER CONTROL**
Grade
| | |
|---|---|
| ✓ 0 | Always able to ask for bedpan |
| 1 | Incontinence of urine |
| 2 | Incontinence of feces |
| 3 | Totally incontinent Confined to bed |

**REHABILITATIVE STATE**
Grade
| | |
|---|---|
| 0 | Fully ambulatory |
| ✓ 1 | Ambulated with assistance |
| 2 | Chair to bed ambulation only |
| 3 | Confined to bed |
| 4 | Immobile in bed |

**NUTRITIONAL STATE**
Grade
| | |
|---|---|
| 0 | Eats all |
| ✓ 1 | Eats very little |
| 2 | Refuses food often |
| 3 | Tube feeding |
| 4 | Intravenous feeding |

**MENTAL STATE**
Grade
| | |
|---|---|
| ✓ 0 | Alert and clear |
| 1 | Confused |
| 2 | Disoriented/senile |
| 3 | Stuporous |
| 4 | Unconcious |

**CHRONIC DISEASE STATUS**
(i.e. COPD, ASCVD. Peripheral Vascular Disease, Diabetes, or Renal Disease, Cancer, Motor or Sensory Deficits, Elderly, Other)
Grade
| | |
|---|---|
| ✓ 0 | Absent |
| 1 | One Present |
| 2 | Two Present |
| 3 | Three or more Present |

**TOTAL** _____   Refer to Skin Care Protocol

## FALLS SCREENING

If one or more of the following are checked institute fall precautions/plan of care
☐ History of Falls ☐ Unsteady Gait ☐ Confusion/Disorientation ☐ Dizziness

If two or more of the following are checked institute fall precautions/plan of care
☐ Age over 80
☐ Impaired vision
☐ Multiple Diagnoses
☐ Inability to understand or follow directions
☐ Utilizes cane, walker, w/c
☐ Impaired hearing
☐ Sleeplessness
☐ Urgency/frequency in elimination
☐ Medication/Sedative /Diuretic etc.

| NURSE SIGNATURE/TITLE | DATE | TIME |
|---|---|---|
| Mary Medina, RN | 4-16-09 | 3:30pm |
| NURSE SIGNATURE/TITLE | DATE | TIME |

## EDUCATION/DISCHARGE PLANNING

1. What do you know about your present illness? "Dr. says I have pneumonia." "I will have an I.V."
2. What information do you want or need about your illness?
3. Would you like family/SO involved in your care? Husband, Michael
4. How long do you expect to be in the hospital? "1-2 days"
5. What concerns do you have about leaving the hospital? _____

### CHECK APPROPRIATE BOX

Will patient need post discharge assistance with ADLs/physical functioning? ☐ Yes ☑ No ☐ Unknown

Does patient have family capable of and willing to provide assistance post discharge?
☑ Yes ☐ No ☐ Unknown ☐ No family

Is assistance needed beyond that which family can provide?
☐ Yes ☑ No ☐ Unknown

Previous admission in the last six months?
☐ Yes ☑ No ☐ Unknown

**Patient lives with** Husband and 1 child
**Planned discharge to** Home
**Comments:** Fatigue and anxiety may have interfered with learning. Re-teach anything covered at admission, later.

**Social Services Notified** ☐ Yes ☑ No

### NARRATIVE NOTES

S--c/o sharp chest pain when coughing and dyspnea on exertion. States unable to carry out regular daily exercise for past week. Coughing relieved "if I sit up and sit still." Nausea associated with coughing. Having occasional "chills." Occasionally becomes frightened, stating, "I can't breathe." Well groomed but "too tired to put on make-up." Assesses own supports as "good" (eg, relationship c husband). Is "worried" about daughter. States husband will be out of town until tomorrow. Left 8-year-old daughter with neighbor. Concerned too about her work (is attorney). "I'll never get caught up." Had water at noon—no food today.
O--Chest expansion < 3cm, no nasal flaring or use of accessory muscles. Breath sounds and insp. crackles in ® upper and lower chest. Capillary refill 5 seconds.

✿✿ **NORTH BROWARD HOSPITAL DISTRICT**
**NURSING ADMINISTRATION ASSESSMENT**

## DEVELOPMENTAL CONSIDERATIONS

### Infants

- Observation of children's behavior can provide important data for the general survey, including physical development, neuromuscular function, and social and interactional skills.
- It may be helpful to have parents hold older infants and very young children for part of the assessment.
- Measure height of children under age 2 in the supine position with knees fully extended.
- Weigh without clothing.
- Include measurement of head circumference until age 2. Standardized growth charts include head circumference up to age 3.

### Children

- Anxiety in preschool-age children can be decreased by letting them handle and become familiar with examination equipment.

- School-age children may be very modest and shy about exposing parts of the body.
- Adolescents should be examined without parents present unless the adolescent requests their presence.
- Weigh children without shoes and with as little clothing as possible.

### Elders (Over Age 65)

- Allow extra time for clients to answer questions.
- Adapt questioning techniques as appropriate for clients with hearing or visual limitations.
- Elders with osteoporosis can lose several inches in height. Be sure to document height and ask if they are aware of becoming shorter in height.
- When asking about weight loss, be specific about amount and time frame, for example, "Have you lost more than five pounds in the last two months?"

# Skill 11.2  Assessing the Skin

### Delegation

Due to the substantial knowledge and skill required, assessment of the skin is not delegated to UAP. However, the skin is observed during usual care and UAP should record their findings. Abnormal findings must be validated and interpreted by the nurse.

### Equipment

- Millimeter ruler
- Clean gloves
- Magnifying glass

### Procedure

1. Prior to performing the procedure, introduce self and verify the client's identity using agency protocol. Explain to the client what you are going to do, why it is necessary, and how he or she can participate. Discuss how the results will be used in planning further care or treatments.
2. Perform hand hygiene and observe appropriate infection control procedures.
3. Provide for client privacy.

4. Inquire if the client has any history of the following: pain or itching; presence and spread of lesions, bruises, abrasions, pigmented spots; previous experience with skin problems; associated clinical signs; family history; presence of problems in other family members; related systemic conditions; use of medications, lotions, home remedies; excessively dry or moist feel to the skin; tendency to bruise easily; association of the problem with season of year, stress, occupation, medications, recent travel, housing, and so on; recent contact with allergens (e.g., metal paint).

## CLINICAL ALERT

If possible and the client agrees, take a digital or instant photograph of significant skin lesions for the client record. Include a measuring guide (ruler or tape) in the picture to demonstrate lesion size.

| Assessment | Normal Findings | Deviations from Normal |
|---|---|---|
| 5. Inspect skin color (best assessed under natural light and on areas not exposed to the sun). | Varies from light to deep brown or black; from light pink to ruddy pink; from yellow overtones to olive | Pallor, cyanosis, jaundice, erythema |
| 6. Inspect uniformity of skin color. | Generally uniform except in areas exposed to the sun; areas of lighter pigmentation (palms, lips, nail beds) in dark-skinned people | Areas of either hyperpigmentation or hypopigmentation |
| 7. Assess edema, if present (i.e., location, color, temperature, shape, and the degree to which the skin remains indented or pitted when pressed by a finger). Measuring the circumference of the extremity with a millimeter tape may be useful for future comparison. | No edema | See the scale for describing edema |
| 8. Inspect, palpate, and describe skin lesions. Apply gloves if lesions are open or draining. Palpate lesions to determine shape and texture. Describe lesions according to location, distribution, color, configuration, size, shape, type, or structure (see Table 11–1). Use the millimeter ruler to measure lesions. If gloves were applied, remove and discard gloves. Perform hand hygiene. | Freckles, pigmented birthmarks that have not changed since childhood, and some long-standing vascular birthmarks such as strawberry or port-wine hemangiomas, some flat and raised nevi (moles); no abrasions or other lesions | Various interruptions in skin integrity; irregular, multicolored, or raised nevi, some pigmented birthmarks such as melanocystic nevi, and some vascular birthmarks such as cavernous hemangiomas. Even these deviations from normal may not be dangerous or require treatment. Assessment by an advanced-level practitioner is required |
| 9. Observe and palpate skin moisture. | Moisture in skin folds and the axillae (varies with environmental temperature and humidity, body temperature, and activity) | Excessive moisture (e.g., in hyperthermia); excessive dryness (e.g., in dehydration) |
| 10. Palpate skin temperature. Compare the two feet and the two hands, using the backs of your fingers. | Uniform; within normal range | Generalized hyperthermia (e.g., in fever); generalized hypothermia (e.g., in shock); localized hyperthermia (e.g., in infection); localized hypothermia (e.g., in arteriosclerosis |
| 11. Note skin turgor (fullness or elasticity) by lifting and pinching the skin on an extremity. | When pinched, skin springs back to previous state; may be slower in elders | Skin stays pinched or tented or moves back slowly (e.g., in dehydration). Count in seconds how long the skin remains tented |
| 12. Document findings in the client record using forms or checklists supplemented by narrative notes when appropriate. Draw location of skin lesions on body surface diagrams. | | |

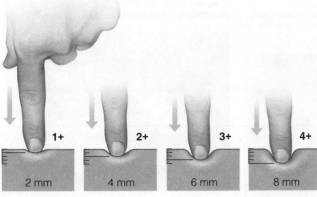

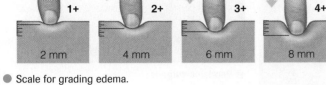

● Scale for grading edema.

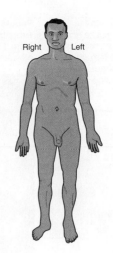 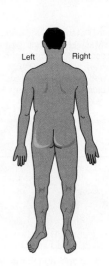

Right  Left   Left  Right

● Diagram for charting skin lesions.

## TABLE 11-1 SECONDARY SKIN LESIONS

Atrophy

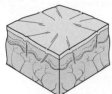

A translucent, dry, paper-like, sometimes wrinkled skin surface resulting from thinning or wasting of the skin due to loss of collagen and elastin.
*Examples:* Striae, aged skin.

Ulcer

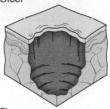

Deep, irregularly shaped area of skin loss extending into the dermis or subcutaneous tissue. May bleed. May leave scar.
*Examples:* Pressure ulcers, stasis ulcers, chancres.

Erosion

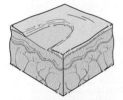

Wearing away of the superficial epidermis causing a moist, shallow depression. Because erosions do not extend into the dermis, they heal without scarring.
*Examples:* Scratch marks, ruptured vesicles.

Fissure

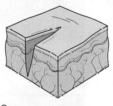

Linear crack with sharp edges, extending into the dermis.
*Examples:* Cracks at the corners of the mouth or in the hands, athlete's foot.

Lichenification

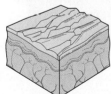

Rough, thickened, hardened area of epidermis resulting from chronic irritation such as scratching or rubbing.
*Example:* Chronic dermatitis.

Scar

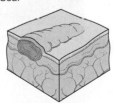

Flat, irregular area of connective tissue left after a lesion or wound has healed. New scars may be red or purple; older scars may be silvery or white.
*Examples:* Healed surgical wound or injury, healed acne.

Scales

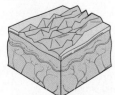

Shedding flakes of greasy, keratinized skin tissue. Color may be white, gray, or silver. Texture may vary from fine to thick.
*Examples:* Dry skin, dandruff, psoriasis, and eczema.

Keloid

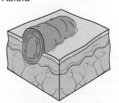

Elevated, irregular, darkened area of excess scar tissue caused by excessive collagen formation during healing. Extends beyond the site of the original injury. Higher incidence in people of African descent.
*Examples:* Keloid from ear piercing or surgery.
Linear erosion.
*Examples:* Scratches, some chemical burns.

Crust

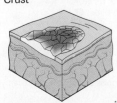

Dry blood, serum, or pus left on the skin surface when vesicles or pustules burst. Can be red-brown, orange, or yellow. Large crusts that adhere to the skin surface are called scabs.
*Examples:* Eczema, impetigo, herpes, or scabs following abrasion.

Excoriation

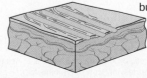

**Macule, Patch** Flat, unelevated change in color. Macules are 1 mm to 1 cm in size and circumscribed. Examples: freckles, measles, petechiae, flat moles. Patches are larger than 1 cm and may have an irregular shape. Examples: port wine birthmark, vitiligo (white patches), rubella. ❶

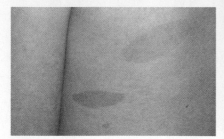

❶ **Multiple café-au-lait macules**

**Nodule, Tumor** Elevated, solid, hard mass that extends deeper into the dermis than a papule. Nodules have a circumscribed border and are 0.5 to 2 cm. Examples: squamous cell carcinoma, fibroma. Tumors are larger than 2 cm and may have an irregular border. Examples: malignant melanoma, hemangioma. ❹

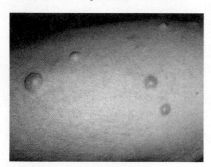

❹ **Peripheral neurofibromas**

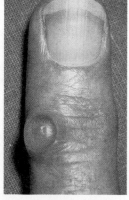

❼ **Digital mucous cyst**

**Papule** Circumscribed, solid elevation of skin. Papules are less than 1 cm. Examples: warts, acne, pimples, elevated moles. ❷

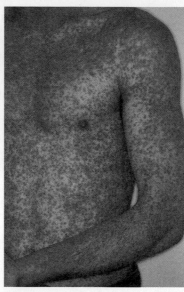

❷ **Papular drug eruption** (Courtesy Scott D. Bennion, MD.)

**Pustule** Vesicle or bulla filled with pus. Examples: acne vulgaris, impetigo. ❺

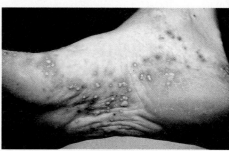

❺ **Chronic pustular psoriasis**

**Cyst** A 1-cm or larger, elevated, encapsulated, fluid-filled or semisolid mass arising from the subcutaneous tissue or dermis. Examples: sebaceous and epidermoid cysts, chalazion of the eyelid. ❼

**Plaque** Plaques are larger than 1 cm. Examples: psoriasis, rubeola. ❸

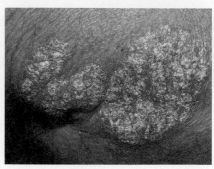

❸ **Psoriasis vulgaris**

**Vesicle, Bulla** A circumscribed, round or oval, thin translucent mass filled with serous fluid or blood.
Vesicles are less than 0.5 cm. Examples: herpes simplex, early chicken pox, small burn blister.
Bullae are larger than 0.5 cm. Examples: large blister, second-degree burn, herpes simplex. ❻

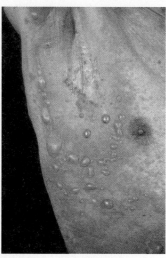

❻ **Bullous pemphigoid**

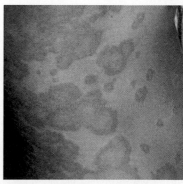

**Wheal** A reddened, localized collection of edema fluid; irregular in shape. Size varies. Examples: hives, mosquito bites. ❽

❽ **Allergic wheals, urticaria**

❙● Primary skin lesions: 1, macule, patch; 2, papule; 3, plaque; 4, nodule, tumor; 5, pustule; 6, vesicle, bulla; 7, cyst; 8, wheal.

*Note:* 1–7 from *Dermatology Secrets in Color*, 2nd ed., by J. E. Fitzpatrick and J. L. Aeling, 2001, Philadelphia: Hanley & Belfus; 8 reprinted with permission from the American Academy of Dermatology. All rights reserved. 2 courtesy of Scott D. Bennion, MD.

# DEVELOPMENTAL CONSIDERATIONS

## Infants

- *Physiologic* jaundice may appear in newborns 2 to 3 days after birth and usually lasts about 1 week. Pathologic jaundice, or that which indicates a disease, appears within 24 hours of birth and may last more than 8 days.
- Newborns may have milia (whiteheads), tiny white nodules over the nose and face, and vernix caseosa (white cheesy, greasy material on the skin).
- Premature infants may have lanugo, a fine downy hair covering their shoulders and back.
- In dark-skinned infants, areas of hyperpigmentation may be found especially on the back, in the sacral area.
- Diaper dermatitis (a rash in the groin area) may be seen in infants.
- If a rash is present, inquire in detail about immunization history.
- Assess skin turgor by pinching the skin on the abdomen.

## Children

- Children normally have minor skin lesions (e.g., bruising or abrasions) on arms and legs due to their high activity level. Lesions on other parts of the body may be signs of disease or abuse, and a thorough history should be taken.
- Secondary skin lesions may occur frequently as children scratch or expose a primary lesion to microbes.
- With puberty, oil glands become more productive, and children may develop acne. Most persons 12 to 24 years have some acne.
- In dark-skinned children, areas of hyperpigmentation may be found on the back, especially in the sacral area.
- If a rash is present, inquire in detail about immunization history.

## Elders

- Changes in white skin occur at an earlier age than in black skin.
- The skin loses its elasticity and develops wrinkles. Wrinkles first appear on the skin of the face and neck, which are abundant in collagen and elastic fibers.
- The skin appears thin and translucent because of loss of dermis and subcutaneous fat.
- The skin is dry and flaky because sebaceous and sweat glands are less active. Dry skin is more prominent over the extremities.
- The skin takes longer to return to its natural shape after being pinched between the thumb and finger. This is called tenting.
- Due to the normal loss of peripheral skin turgor in elders, assess for hydration by checking skin turgor over the sternum or clavicle.
- Flat tan to brown-colored macules, referred to as senile lentigines or melanotic freckles, are normally apparent on the back of the hand and other skin areas that are exposed to the sun. These macules may be as large as 1 to 2 cm.
- Warty lesions (seborrheic keratosis) with irregularly shaped borders and a scaly surface often occur on the face, shoulders, and trunk. These benign lesions begin as yellowish to tan and progress to a dark brown or black.
- Vitiligo tends to increase with age and is thought to result from an autoimmune response.
- Cutaneous tags (acrochordons) are most commonly seen in the neck and axillary regions. These skin lesions vary in size and are soft, often flesh colored, and pedicled.
- Visible, bright red, fine dilated blood vessels commonly occur as a result of the thinning of the dermis and the loss of support for the blood vessel walls.
- Pink to slightly red lesions with indistinct borders (actinic keratoses) may appear at about age 50, often on the face, ears, backs of the hands, and arms. They may become malignant if untreated.

## SETTING OF CARE

- When making a home visit, take a penlight or examination lamp with you in case the home has inadequate lighting.
- If skin lesions are suggestive of physical abuse, follow state regulations for follow-up and reporting. Signs of abuse may include a pattern of bruises, unusual location of burns, or lesions that are not easily explainable. If lesions are present in adults or verbal-age children, conduct the interview and assessment in private.
- Document lesions by taking a photo (if client consents). Another method that can be used is to lay clean double-thick clear plastic (such as a grocery bag) over the lesion or wound and trace the shape with a permanent marker. Cut away and dispose of the bottom layer that came in contact with the client and place the top layer in the client record. Use this method only if contact with the plastic does not contaminate the wound.
- Type or structure. Skin lesions are classified as primary (those that appear initially in response to some change in the external or internal environment of the skin) and secondary (those that do not appear initially but result from modifications such as chronicity, trauma, or infection of the primary lesion). For example, a vesicle (primary lesion) may rupture and cause an erosion (secondary lesion).
- Size, shape, and texture. Note size in millimeters and whether the lesion is circumscribed or irregular; round or oval shaped; flat, elevated, or depressed; solid, soft, or hard; rough or thickened; fluid filled or has flakes.
- Color. There may be no discoloration, one color (e.g., red, brown, or black), several colors, as with ecchymosis (a bruise), in which an initial dark red or blue color fades to a yellow color. When color changes are limited to the edges of a lesion, they are described as circumscribed; when spread over a large area, they are described as diffuse.
- Distribution. Distribution is described according to the location of the lesions on the body and symmetry or asymmetry of findings in comparable body areas.
- Configuration. Configuration refers to the arrangement of lesions in relation to each other. Configurations of lesions may be annular (arranged in a circle), may be clustered together or grouped, may be linear (arranged in a line), may be arc or bow shaped, may be merged together or indiscrete, may follow the course of cutaneous nerves, or may be meshed in the form of a network.

# Skill 11.3   Assessing the Hair

### Delegation

Assessment of the hair is not delegated to UAP. However, many aspects are observed during usual care and may be recorded by persons other than the nurse. Abnormal findings must be validated and interpreted by the nurse.

### Equipment

- Clean gloves

### Procedure

1. Prior to performing the procedure, introduce self and verify the client's identity using agency proto-
col. Explain to the client what you are going to do, why it is necessary, and how he or she can participate. Discuss how the results will be used in planning further care or treatments.
2. Perform hand hygiene, apply gloves, and observe other appropriate infection control procedures.
3. Provide for client privacy.
4. Inquire if the client has any history of the following: recent use of hair dyes, rinses, or curling or straightening preparations; chemotherapy; and the presence of acute or chronic conditions.

| Assessment | Normal Findings | Deviations from Normal |
|---|---|---|
| 5. Inspect the evenness of growth over the scalp. | Evenly distributed hair | Patches of hair loss (i.e., alopecia |
| 6. Inspect hair thickness or thinness. | Thick hair | Very thin hair |
| 7. Inspect hair texture and oiliness. | Silky, resilient hair | Brittle hair, excessively oily or dry hair |
| 8. Note presence of infections or infestations by parting the hair in several areas, checking behind the ears and along the hairline at the neck. | No infection or infestation | Flaking, sores, lice, nits (louse eggs), and ringworm |
| 9. Inspect amount of body hair. | Variable | Hirsutism (abnormal hairiness); naturally absent or sparse leg hair |
| 10. Remove and discard gloves. Perform hand hygiene. | | |
| 11. Document findings in the client record using forms or checklists supplemented by narrative notes when appropriate. | | |

## DEVELOPMENTAL CONSIDERATIONS

### Infants

- There is a wide variation of normal hair distribution in infants, which can range from very little or none to a great deal of body and scalp hair.

### Children

- As puberty approaches, axillary and pubic hair will appear (see Box 11–2 later in this chapter).

### Elders

- There may be loss of scalp, pubic, and axillary hair.
- Hairs of the eyebrows, ears, and nostrils become bristle-like and coarse.

## SETTING OF CARE

- When making a home visit, ask to see the products the client usually uses on the hair. Assist the client to determine if the products are appropriate for the client's type of hair and scalp (e.g., for dry or oily hair). Provide education regarding hygiene of the hair and scalp.
- When making a home visit, examine the equipment that the client uses on the hair. Provide client teaching regarding appropriate combs and brushes and regarding safety in using electric hair styling appliances such as hair dryers.

# Skill 11.4   Assessing the Nails

**Delegation**

Due to the substantial knowledge required, assessment of the nails is not delegated to UAP. However, many nail characteristics are observed during usual care and may be recorded by persons other than the nurse. Abnormal findings must be validated and interpreted by the nurse.

**Procedure**

1. Prior to performing the procedure, introduce self and verify the client's identity using agency protocol. Explain to the client what you are going to do, why it is necessary, and how he or she can partici-

pate. Discuss how the results will be used in planning further care or treatments. In most situations, clients with artificial nails or polish on fingernails or toenails are not required to remove these for assessment. If the assessment cannot be conducted due to the presence of polish or artificial nails, document this in the record.

2. Observe appropriate infection control procedures.
3. Provide for client privacy.
4. Inquire if the client has any history of the following: presence of diabetes mellitus, peripheral circulatory disease, previous injury, or severe illness.

| Assessment | Normal Findings | Deviations from Normal |
|---|---|---|
| 5. Inspect fingernail plate shape to determine its curvature and angle. | Convex curvature; angle of nail plate about 160° (see **A**) | Spoon nail (see **B**); clubbing (180° or greater) (see **C** and **D**) |
| 6. Inspect fingernail and toenail texture. | Smooth texture | Excessive thickness or thinness or presence of grooves or furrows; Beau's lines (see **E**); discolored or detached nail—often due to fungus or injury |
| 7. Inspect fingernail and toenail bed color. | Highly vascular and pink in light-skinned clients; dark-skinned clients may have brown or black pigmentation in longitudinal streaks | Bluish or purplish tint (may reflect cyanosis); pallor (may reflect poor arterial circulation) |
| 8. Inspect tissues surrounding nails. | Intact epidermis | Hangnails; paronychia (inflammation) |
| 9. Perform blanch test of capillary refill. Press two or more nails between your thumb and index finger; look for blanching and return of pink color to nail bed. Count in seconds the time for the color to return completely. | Prompt return of pink or usual color (generally less than 2 seconds) | Delayed return of pink or usual color (may indicate circulatory impairment) |
| 10. Document findings in the client record using forms or checklists supplemented by narrative notes when appropriate. | | |

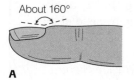
About 160°

A

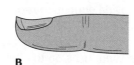

B

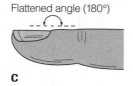
Flattened angle (180°)

C

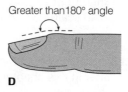
Greater than180° angle

D

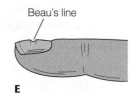
Beau's line

E

● **A,** A normal nail, showing the convex shape and the nail plate angle of about 160 degrees; **B,** a spoon-shaped nail, which may be seen in clients with iron deficiency anemia; **C,** early clubbing; **D,** late clubbing (may be caused by long-term oxygen lack); **E,** Beau's line on nail (may result from severe injury or illness).

## DEVELOPMENTAL CONSIDERATIONS

### Infants

- Newborns nails grow very quickly, are extremely thin, and tear easily.

### Children

- Bent, bruised, or ingrown toenails may indicate that shoes are too tight.
- Nail biting should be discussed with an adult family member because it may be a symptom of stress.

### Elders

- The nails grow more slowly and thicken.
- Longitudinal bands commonly develop, and the nails tend to split.
- Bands across the nails may indicate protein deficiency; white spots, zinc deficiency; and spoon-shaped nails, iron deficiency.
- Toenail fungus is more common and difficult to eliminate (although not dangerous to health).

# Skill 11.5   Assessing the Skull and Face

## Delegation

Due to the substantial knowledge and skill required, assessment of the skull and face is not delegated to UAP. However, many aspects of the skull and face are observed during usual care and may be recorded by persons other than the nurse. Abnormal findings must be validated and interpreted by the nurse.

## Procedure

1. Prior to performing the procedure, introduce self and verify the client's identity using agency protocol. Explain to the client what you are going to do, why it is necessary, and how he or she can partici-pate. Discuss how the results will be used in planning further care or treatments.
2. Perform hand hygiene and observe appropriate infection control procedures.
3. Provide for client privacy.
4. Inquire if the client has any history of the following: past problems with lumps or bumps, itching, scaling, or dandruff; history of loss of consciousness, dizziness, seizures, headache, facial pain, or injury; when and how any lumps occurred; length of time any other problem existed; any known cause of problem; associated symptoms, treatment, and recurrences.

| Assessment | Normal Findings | Deviations from Normal |
|---|---|---|
| 5. Inspect the skull for size, shape, and symmetry. | Rounded (normocephalic and symmetric, with frontal, parietal, and occipital prominences); smooth skull contour | Lack of symmetry; increased skull size with more prominent nose and forehead; longer mandible (may indicate excessive growth hormone or increased bone thickness) |
| 6. Inspect the facial features (e.g., symmetry of structures and of the distribution of hair). | Symmetric or slightly asymmetric facial features, palpebral fissures equal in size, symmetric nasolabial folds | Increased facial hair, low hair line, thinning of eyebrows, asymmetric features, exophthalmos, myxedema facies, moon face |
| 7. Inspect the eyes for edema and hollowness. | No edema | Periorbital edema; sunken eyes |
| 8. Note symmetry of facial movements. Ask the client to elevate the eyebrows, frown, or lower the eyebrows, close the eyes tightly, puff the cheeks, and smile and show the teeth. | Symmetric facial movements | Asymmetric facial movements (e.g., eye on affected side cannot close completely); drooping of lower eyelid and mouth; involuntary facial movements (i.e., tics or tremors) |
| 9. Document findings in the client record using forms or checklists supplemented by narrative notes when appropriate. | | |

## DEVELOPMENTAL CONSIDERATIONS

**Infants**

- Newborns delivered vaginally can have elongated, molded heads, which take on more rounded shapes after a week or two. Infants born by cesarean section tend to have smooth, rounded heads.
- The posterior fontanel (soft spot) is about 1 cm in size and usually closes by 8 weeks. The anterior fontanel is larger, about 2 to 3 cm in size. It closes by 18 months.
- Newborns can lift their heads slightly and turn them from side to side. Voluntary head control is well established by 4 to 6 months.

# Skill 11.6   Assessing the Eyes and Vision

## Delegation

Due to the substantial knowledge and skill required, assessment of the eyes and vision is not delegated to UAP. However, many aspects of eye function are observed during usual care and may be recorded by persons other than the nurse. Abnormal findings must be validated and interpreted by the nurse.

## Equipment

- Millimeter ruler
- Penlight
- Snellen or E chart
- Opaque card

## Procedure

1. Prior to performing the procedure, introduce self and verify the client's identity using agency protocol. Explain to the client what you are going to do, why it is necessary, and how he or she can participate. Discuss how the results will be used in planning further care or treatments.
2. Perform hand hygiene, and observe appropriate infection control procedures.
3. Provide for client privacy.
4. Inquire if the client has any history of the following: family history of diabetes, hypertension, blood dyscrasia, or eye disease, injury, or surgery; client's last visit to an ophthalmologist; current use of eye medications; use of contact lenses or eyeglasses; hygienic practices for corrective lenses; current symptoms of eye problems (e.g., changes in visual acuity, blurring of vision, tearing, spots, photophobia, itching, or pain).

| Assessment | Normal Findings | Deviations from Normal |
|---|---|---|
| **External Eye Structures** | | |
| 5. Inspect the eyebrows for hair distribution, alignment, skin quality, and movement (ask client to raise and lower the eyebrows). | Hair evenly distributed; skin intact<br>Eyebrows symmetrically aligned; equal movement | Loss of hair; scaling and flakiness of skin<br>Unequal alignment and movement of eyebrows |
| 6. Inspect the eyelashes for evenness of distribution and direction of curl. | Equally distributed; curled slightly outward | Turned inward |
| 7. Inspect the eyelids for surface characteristics (e.g., skin quality and texture), position in relation to the cornea, ability to blink, and frequency of blinking. Inspect the lower eyelids while the client's eyes are closed. | Skin intact; no discharge; no discoloration<br>Lids close symmetrically<br>Approximately 15 to 20 involuntary blinks per minute; bilateral blinking<br>When lids open, no visible sclera above corneas, and upper and lower borders of cornea are slightly covered | Redness, swelling, flaking, crusting, plaques, discharge, nodules, lesions<br>Lids close asymmetrically, incompletely, or painfully<br>Rapid, monocular, absent, or infrequent blinking<br>Ptosis, ectropion, or entropion; rim of sclera visible between lid and iris |

| Assessment | Normal Findings | Deviations from Normal |
|---|---|---|
| 8. Inspect the bulbar conjunctiva (that lying over the sclera) for color, texture, and the presence of lesions. | Transparent; capillaries sometimes evident; sclera appears white (darker or yellowish and with small brown macules in dark-skinned clients) | Jaundiced sclera (e.g., in liver disease); excessively pale sclera (e.g., in anemia); reddened sclera (e.g., marijuana use, rheumatoid disease); lesions or nodules (may indicate damage by mechanical, chemical, allergenic, or bacterial agents) |
| 9. Inspect the cornea for clarity and texture. Ask the client to look straight ahead. Hold a penlight at an oblique angle to the eye, and move the light slowly across the corneal surface. | Transparent, shiny, and smooth; details of the iris are visible<br>In older people, a thin, grayish white ring around the margin, called arcus senilis, may be evident | Opaque; surface not smooth (may be the result of trauma or abrasion)<br>Arcus senilis in clients under age 40 |
| 10. Inspect the pupils for color, shape, and symmetry of size. Pupil charts are available in some agencies. See below for variations in pupil diameters. | Black in color; equal in size; normally 3 to 7 mm in diameter; round, smooth border, iris flat and round | Cloudiness, mydriasis, miosis, anisocoria; bulging of iris toward cornea; pupils less than 3 or greater than 7 mm in normal light conditions; unequal pupil size |

1 2 3  4  5  6  7  8  9  10

● Variations in pupil diameters in millimeters.

| | | |
|---|---|---|
| 11. Assess each pupil's direct and consensual reaction to light to determine the function of the third (oculomotor) cranial nerve.<br>• Partially darken the room.<br>• Ask the client to look straight ahead.<br>• Using a penlight and approaching from the side, shine a light on the pupil.<br>• Observe the response of the illuminated pupil. It should constrict (direct response).<br>• Shine the light on the pupil again, and observe the response of the other pupil. It should also constrict (consensual response). | Illuminated pupil constricts (direct response)<br>Nonilluminated pupil constricts (consensual response) | Neither pupil constricts<br>Unequal responses<br>Absent responses |
| 12. Assess each pupil's reaction to accommodation.<br>• Hold an object (a penlight or pencil) about 10 cm (4 in.) from the bridge of the client's nose.<br>• Ask the client to look first at the top of the object and then at a distant object (e.g., the far wall) behind the penlight. Alternate the gaze from the near to the far object.<br>• Observe the pupil response. The pupils should constrict when looking at the near object and dilate when looking at the far object. | Pupils constrict when looking at near object; pupils dilate when looking at far object; pupils converge when near object is moved toward nose | One or both pupils fail to constrict, dilate, or converge |

*(continued)*

| Assessment | Normal Findings | Deviations from Normal |
|---|---|---|

### External Eye Structures *(continued)*

- Next, move the penlight or pencil toward the client's nose. The pupils should converge. To record normal assessment of the pupils, use the abbreviation **PERRLA** (pupils equally round and react to light and accommodation).

### Visual Fields

13. Assess peripheral visual fields to determine function of the retina and neuronal visual pathways to the brain and second (optic) cranial nerve.
    - Have the client sit directly facing you at a distance of 60 to 90 cm (2 to 3 ft).
    - Ask the client to cover the right eye with a card and look directly at your nose.
    - Cover or close your eye directly opposite the client's covered eye (i.e., your left eye), and look directly at the client's nose.
    - Hold an object (e.g., a penlight or pencil) in your fingers, extend your arm, and move the object into the visual field from various points in the periphery. The object should be at an equal distance from the client and yourself. Ask the client to tell you when the moving object is first spotted.
      a. To test the temporal field of the left eye, extend and move your right arm in from the client's right periphery.
      b. To test the upward field of the left eye, extend and move the right arm down from the upward periphery.
      c. To test the downward field of the left eye, extend and move the right arm up from the lower periphery.
      d. To test the nasal field of the left eye, extend and move your left arm in from the periphery.

    - Repeat the above steps for the right eye, reversing the process.

**Normal Findings:**

When looking straight ahead, client can see objects in the periphery

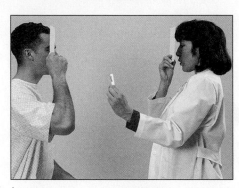

● Assessing the client's left peripheral vision field.

Temporally, peripheral objects can be seen at right angles (90 degrees) to the central point of vision

The upward field of vision is normally 50 degrees because the orbital ridge is in the way

The downward field of vision is normally 70 degrees because the cheekbone is in the way

The nasal field of vision is normally 50 degrees away from the central point of vision because the nose is in the way

**Deviations from Normal:**

Visual field smaller than normal (possible glaucoma); one-half vision in one of both eyes (possible nerve damage)

| Assessment | Normal Findings | Deviations from Normal |
|---|---|---|
| **Extraocular Muscle Tests** | | |
| 14. Assess six ocular movements to determine eye alignment and coordination. These can be performed on clients over 6 months of age.<br>• Stand directly in front of the client and hold the penlight at a comfortable distance, such as 30 cm (1 ft) in front of the client's eyes.<br>• Ask the client to hold the head in a fixed position facing you and to follow the movements of the penlight with the eyes only.<br>• Move the penlight in a slow, orderly manner through the six cardinal fields of gaze, that is, from the center of the eye along the lines of the arrows in and back to the center.<br>• Stop the movement of the penlight periodically so that nystagmus can be detected. | Both eyes coordinated, move in unison, with parallel alignment<br><br>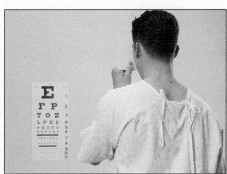<br><br>**1** Superior rectus (CN III)   **6** Inferior oblique (CN III)   **1** Superior rectus (CN III)<br>**2** Lateral rectus (CN VI)   **5** Medial rectus (CN III)   **2** Lateral rectus (CN VI)<br>**3** Inferior rectus (CN III)   **4** Superior oblique (CN IV)   **3** Inferior rectus (CN III)<br><br>● The six muscles that govern eye movement. | Eye movements not coordinated or parallel; one or both eyes fail to follow a penlight in specific directions, e.g., **strabismus** (cross-eye).<br>**Nystagmus** (rapid involuntary rhythmic eye movement) other than at end point may indicate neurologic impairment |
| 15. Assess for location of light reflex by shining penlight on pupil in corneal surface (Hirschberg test). | Light falls symmetrically on both pupils (e.g., at "6 o'clock" on both pupils) | Light falls off center on one eye (indicates misalignment) |
| 16. Have client fixate on a near or far object. Cover one eye and observe for movement in the uncovered eye (cover test). | Uncovered eye does not move | If misalignment is present, when dominant eye is covered, the uncovered eye will move to focus on object |
| **Visual Acuity** | | |
| 17. Assess near vision by providing adequate lighting and asking the client to read from a magazine or newspaper held at a distance of 36 cm (14 in.). If the client normally wears corrective lenses, the glasses or lenses should be worn during the test. | Able to read newsprint | Difficulty reading newsprint unless due to aging process |
| 18. Assess distance vision by asking the client to wear corrective lenses, unless they are used for reading only, i.e., for distances of only 36 cm (12 to 14 in.).<br>• Ask the client to stand or sit 6 m (20 ft) from a Snellen or character chart, cover the eye not being tested, and identify the letters or characters on the chart.<br>• Take three readings: right eye, left eye, both eyes.<br>• Record the readings of each eye and both eyes (i.e., the smallest line from which the person is able to read one-half or more of the letters). | 20/20 vision on Snellen-type chart<br><br>● Testing distance vision. | Denominator of 40 or more on Snellen-type chart with corrective lenses |

*(continued)*

| Assessment | Normal Findings | Deviations from Normal |
|---|---|---|
| **Visual Acuity _(continued)_**<br><br>At the end of each line of the chart are standardized numbers (fractions). The top line is 20/200. The numerator (top number) is always 20, the distance the person stands from the chart. The denominator (bottom number) is the distance from which the normal eye can read the chart. Therefore, a person who has 20/40 vision can see at 20 feet from the chart what a normal-sighted person can see at 40 feet from the chart. Visual acuity is recorded as "s—c" (without correction), or "c—c" (with correction). You can also indicate how many letters were misread in the line, e.g., "visual acuity 20/40-2 c—c" indicates that two letters were misread in the 20/40 line by a client wearing corrective lenses. | | |
| 19. If the client is unable to see even the top line (20/200) of the Snellen-type chart, perform one or more of the following functional vision tests.<br><br>**Light Perception**<br>Shine a penlight into the client's eye from a lateral position, and then turn the light off. Ask the client to tell you when the light is on or off.<br><br>**Hand Movements**<br>Hold your hand 30 cm (1 ft) from the client's face and move it slowly back and forth, stopping it periodically. Ask the client to tell you when your hand stops moving.<br><br>**Counting Fingers**<br>Hold up some of your fingers 30 cm (1 ft) from the client's face, and ask the client to count your fingers. | | Functional vision only (e.g., light perception, hand movements, counting fingers at 30 cm [1 ft]) |
| 20. Document findings in the client record using forms or checklists supplemented by narrative notes when appropriate. | | |

## DEVELOPMENTAL CONSIDERATIONS

### Infants

- Infants 4 weeks of age should gaze at and follow objects.
- Ability to focus with both eyes should be present by 6 months of age.
- Infants do not have tears until about 3 months of age.
- Visual acuity is about 20/300 at 4 months and progressively improves.

### Children

- Epicanthal folds, common in persons of Asian heredity, may cover the medial canthus and cause eyes to appear misaligned. Epicanthal folds may also be seen in young children of any race before the bridge of the nose begins to elevate.
- Preschool children's acuity can be checked with picture cards or the E chart. Acuity should approach 20/20 by 6 years of age.
- Always perform the acuity test with glasses on if a child has a prescription to wear lenses.
- Children should be tested for color vision deficit. From 8% to 10% of Caucasian males and from 0.5% to 1% of Caucasian females have this deficit; it is much less common in non-Caucasian children. The Ishihara or Hardy-Rand-Rittler test can be used.

### Elders

*Visual Acuity*

- Visual acuity decreases as the lens of the eye ages and becomes more opaque and loses elasticity.
- The ability of the iris to accommodate to darkness and dim light diminishes.
- Peripheral vision diminishes.

- The adaptation to light (glare) and dark decreases.
- Accommodation to far objects often improves, but accommodation to near objects decreases.
- Color vision declines; older people are less able to perceive purple colors and to discriminate pastel colors.
- Many elders wear corrective lenses; they are most likely to have hyperopia. Visual changes are due to loss of elasticity (presbyopia) and diminishing transparency of the lens.

*External Eye Structures*

- The skin around the orbit of the eye may darken.
- The eyeball may appear sunken because of the decrease in orbital fat.
- Skin folds of the upper lids may seem more prominent, and the lower lids may sag.
- The eyes may appear dry and dull because of the decrease in tear production from the lacrimal glands.
- A thin, grayish white arc or ring (arcus senilis) appears around part or all of the cornea. It results from an accumulation of a lipid substance on the cornea. The cornea tends to cloud with age.
- The iris may appear pale with brown discolorations as a result of pigment degeneration.
- The conjunctiva of the eye may appear paler than that of younger adults and may take on a slightly yellow appearance because of the deposition of fat.
- Pupil reaction to light and accommodation is normally symmetrically equal but may be less brisk.
- The pupils can appear smaller in size, unequal, and irregular in shape because of sclerotic changes in the iris.

## SETTING OF CARE

- When making a home visit, take your equipment and charts with you. Also include a tape measure to lay out the 20 feet for distance vision testing.
- Use the assessment as an opportunity to reinforce proper eye care and the need for regular vision testing.

# Skill 11.7 Assessing the Ears and Hearing

## Delegation

Assessment of the ears and hearing is not delegated to UAP. However, many aspects of ear function are observed during usual care and may be recorded by persons other than the nurse. Abnormal findings must be validated and interpreted by the nurse.

## Equipment

- Otoscope with several sizes of ear specula

## Procedure

1. Prior to performing the procedure, introduce self and verify the client's identity using agency protocol. Explain to the client what you are going to do, why it is necessary, and how he or she can partici-pate. Discuss how the results will be used in planning further care or treatments.
2. Perform hand hygiene and observe appropriate infection control procedures.
3. Provide for client privacy.
4. Inquire if the client has any history of the following: family history of hearing problems or loss; presence of ear problems or pain; medication history, especially if there are complaints of ringing in ears (tinnitus); hearing difficulty (its onset, factors contributing to it, and how it interferes with activities of daily living); use of a corrective hearing device (when and from whom it was obtained).
5. Position the client comfortably, seated if possible.

| Assessment | Normal Findings | Deviations from Normal |
|---|---|---|
| **Auricles** | | |
| 6. Inspect the auricles for color, symmetry of size, and position. To inspect position, note the level at which the superior aspect of the auricle attaches to the head in relation to the eye. | Color same as facial skin <br><br> Symmetrical <br> Auricle aligned with outer canthus of eye, about 10° from vertical | Bluish color of earlobes (e.g., cyanosis); pallor (e.g., frostbite); excessive redness (inflammation or fever) <br> Asymmetry <br> Low-set ears (associated with a congenital abnormality, such as Down syndrome) |

Normal alignment      Low-set ears and deviation in alignment

● Alignment of ears.

| | | |
|---|---|---|
| 7. Palpate the auricles for texture, elasticity, and areas of tenderness. <br> • Gently pull the auricle upward, downward, and backward. <br> • Fold the pinna forward (it should recoil). <br> • Push in on the tragus. <br> • Apply pressure to the mastoid process. | Mobile, firm, and not tender; pinna recoils after it is folded | Lesions (e.g., cysts); flaky, scaly skin (e.g., seborrhea); tenderness when moved or pressed (may indicate inflammation or infection of external ear) |

| Assessment | Normal Findings | Deviations from Normal |
|---|---|---|

**External Ear Canal and Tympanic Membrane**

8. Inspect the external ear canal for cerumen, skin lesions, pus, and blood.

Distal third contains hair follicles and glands

Dry cerumen, grayish-tan color; or sticky, wet cerumen in various shades of brown

Redness and discharge
Scaling
Excessive cerumen obstructing canal

---

9. Inspect the tympanic membrane for color and gloss using an otoscope.
   - Attach a speculum to the otoscope. Use the largest diameter that will fit the ear canal without causing discomfort. ➤*Rationale: This achieves maximum vision of the entire ear canal and tympanic membrane.*
   - Tip the client's head away from you, and straighten the ear canal. For an adult, straighten the ear canal by pulling the pinna up and back. ➤*Rationale: Straightening the ear canal facilitates vision of the ear canal and the tympanic membrane.*
   - Hold the otoscope either (a) right side up, with your fingers between the otoscope handle and the client's head, or (b) upside down, with your fingers and the ulnar surface of your hand against the client's head. ➤*Rationale: These positions stabilize the head and protect the eardrum and canal from injury if a quick head movement occurs.*
   - Gently insert the tip of the otoscope into the ear canal, avoiding pressure by the speculum against either side of the ear canal. ➤*Rationale: The inner two-thirds of the ear canal is bony; if the speculum is pressed against either side, the client will experience discomfort.*

Pearly gray color, semitransparent.

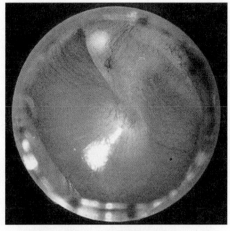

● Normal tympanic membrane.

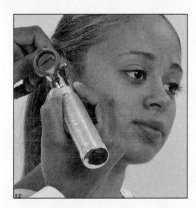

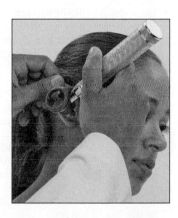

● Inserting an otoscope.

Pink to red, some opacity
Yellow-amber
White
Blue or deep red
Dull surface

---

**Gross Hearing Acuity Tests**

10. Assess client's response to normal voice tones. If client has difficulty hearing the normal voice, proceed with the following tests.

Normal voice tones audible

Normal voice tones not audible (e.g., requests nurse to repeat words or statements, leans toward the speaker, turns the head, cups the ears, or speaks in loud tone of voice)

*(continued)*

| Assessment | Normal Findings | Deviations from Normal |
|---|---|---|
| **Gross Hearing Acuity Tests (continued)** | | |
| 10A. *Watch tick test.* Perform the watch tick test. The ticking of a watch has a higher pitch than the human voice.<br>• Have the client occlude one ear. Out of the client's sight, place a ticking watch 2 to 3 cm (1 to 2 in.) from the unoccluded ear.<br>• Ask what the client can hear.<br>• Repeat with the other ear. | Able to hear ticking in both ears | Unable to hear ticking in one or both ears |
| 10B. *Tuning fork tests.* Perform Weber's test to assess bone conduction by examining the lateralization (sideward transmission) of sounds.<br>• Hold the tuning fork at its base. Activate it by tapping the fork gently against the back of your hand near the knuckles or by stroking the fork between your thumb and index fingers. It should be made to ring softly.<br>• Place the base of the vibrating fork on top of the client's head and ask where the client hears the noise.<br>• Hold the handle of the activated tuning fork on the mastoid process of one ear, **A** until the client states that the vibration can no longer be heard.<br>• Immediately hold the still vibrating fork prongs in front of the client's ear canal. Push aside the client's hair if necessary. Ask whether the client now hears the sound. Sound conducted by air is heard more readily than sound conducted by bone. The tuning fork vibrations conducted by air are normally heard longer. | Sound is heard in both ears or is localized at the center of the head (Weber negative)<br>Air-conducted (AC) hearing is greater than bone-conducted (BC) hearing, i.e., AC > BC (positive Rinne)<br><br><br>● Placing the base of the tuning fork on the client's skull (Weber's test). | Sound is heard better in impaired ear, indicating a bone-conductive hearing loss; or sound is heard better in ear without a problem, indicating a sensorineural disturbance (Weber positive)<br>Bone conduction time is equal to or longer than the air conduction time, i.e., BC > AC or BC = AC (negative Rinne; indicates a conductive hearing loss)<br><br><br>**A**<br><br>**B**<br>● Rinne test tuning fork placement. **A**, Base of the tuning fork on the mastoid process; **B**, tuning fork prongs placed in front of the client's ear. |
| 11. Document findings in the client record using forms or checklists supplemented by narrative notes when appropriate. | | |

## DEVELOPMENTAL CONSIDERATIONS

### Infants

To assess gross hearing, ring a bell from behind the infant or have the parent call the child's name to check for a response. Newborns will quiet to the sound and may open their eyes wider. By 3 to 4 months of age, the child will turn head and eyes toward the sound.

- All newborns should be assessed for hearing using auditory brain response testing prior to discharge from the hospital.

### Children

- To inspect the external canal and tympanic membrane in children less than 3 years old, pull the pinna down and back. Insert the otoscopic speculum only 1/4 to 1/2 inch.

- Perform routine hearing checks and follow up on abnormal results. In addition to congenital or infection-related causes of hearing loss, noise-induced hearing loss is becoming more common in adolescents and young adults as a result of exposure to loud music and prolonged use of headsets at loud volumes (Daniel, 2007). Teach that music loud enough to prevent hearing a normal conversation can damage hearing.

### Elders

- The skin of the ear may appear dry and be less resilient because of the loss of connective tissue.

- Increased coarse and wire-like hair growth occurs along the helix, antihelix, and tragus.

- The pinna increases in both width and length, and the earlobe elongates.

- Earwax is drier.

- The tympanic membrane is more translucent and less flexible. The intensity of the light reflex may diminish slightly.

- Sensorineural hearing loss occurs.

- Generalized hearing loss (presbycusis) occurs in all frequencies, although the first symptom is the loss of high-frequency sounds: the f, s, sh, and ph sounds. To such persons, conversation can be distorted and result in what appears to be inappropriate or confused behavior.

## SETTING OF CARE

- Ensure that the examination is conducted in a quiet place. In particular, elders will have difficulty accurately reporting results of hearing tests if there is excessive outside noise.

- If necessary, ask the adult present with an infant or child to assist in holding the child still during the examination.

# Skill 11.8   Assessing the Nose and Sinuses

### Delegation

Assessment of the nose and sinuses is not delegated to UAP. However, many aspects of nasal function are observed during usual care and may be recorded by persons other than the nurse. Abnormal findings must be validated and interpreted by the nurse.

### Equipment

- Nasal speculum
- Flashlight/penlight

### Procedure

1. Prior to performing the procedure, introduce self and verify the client's identity using agency proto-col. Explain to the client what you are going to do, why it is necessary, and how he or she can participate. Discuss how the results will be used in planning further care or treatments.
2. Perform hand hygiene and observe appropriate infection control procedures.
3. Provide for client privacy.
4. Inquire if the client has any history of the following: allergies, difficulty breathing through the nose, sinus infections, injuries to nose or face, nosebleeds; medications taken; changes in sense of smell.
5. Position the client comfortably, seated if possible.

| Assessment | Normal Findings | Deviations from Normal |
|---|---|---|
| **Nose** | | |
| 6. Inspect the external nose for any deviations in shape, size, or color and flaring or discharge from the nares. | Symmetric and straight<br>No discharge or flaring<br>Uniform color | Asymmetric<br>Discharge from nares<br>Localized areas of redness or presence of skin lesions |
| 7. Lightly palpate the external nose to determine any areas of tenderness, masses, and displacements of bone and cartilage. | Not tender; no lesions | Tenderness on palpation; presence of lesions |
| 8. Determine patency of both nasal cavities. Ask the client to close the mouth, exert pressure on one naris, and breathe through the opposite naris. Repeat the procedure to assess patency of the opposite naris. | Air moves freely as the client breathes through the nares | Air movement is restricted in one or both nares |
| 9. Inspect the nasal cavities using a flashlight or a nasal speculum.<br>• Hold the speculum in your right hand to inspect the client's left nostril and your left hand to inspect the client's right nostril.<br>• Tip the client's head back.<br>• Facing the client, insert the tip of the closed speculum (blades together) about 1 cm or up to the point at which the blade widens. Care must be taken to avoid pressure on the sensitive nasal septum.<br>• Stabilize the speculum with your index finger against the side of the nose. Use the other hand to position the head and then to hold the light.<br>• Open the speculum as much as possible and inspect the floor of the nose (vestibule), the anterior portion of the septum, the middle meatus, and the middle turbinates. The posterior turbinate is rarely visualized because of its position.<br>• Inspect the lining of the nares and the integrity and the position of the nasal septum. | <br>● Using a nasal speculum to inspect the nasal passages.<br><br>● The inferior and middle turbinates of the nasal passage. | |
| 10. Observe for the presence of redness, swelling, growths, and discharge.<br>Mucosa red, edematous<br>Abnormal discharge (e.g., pus) | Mucosa pink<br>Clear, watery discharge<br>No lesions | Mucosa red, edematous<br>Abnormal discharge (e.g., pus)<br>Presence of lesions (e.g., polyps) |
| 11. Inspect the nasal septum between the nasal chambers. | Nasal septum intact and in midline | Septum deviated to the right or to the left or septum eroded |

| Assessment | Normal Findings | Deviations from Normal |
|---|---|---|
| **Facial Sinuses** | | |
| 12. Palpate the maxillary and frontal sinuses for tenderness. | Not tender | Tenderness in one or more sinuses |
| 13. Document findings in the client record using forms or checklists supplemented by narrative notes when appropriate. | | |

---

## DEVELOPMENTAL CONSIDERATIONS

### Infants

- A speculum is usually not necessary to examine the septum, turbinates, and vestibule. Instead, push the tip of the nose upward with the thumb and shine a light into the nares.
- Ethmoid and maxillary sinuses are present at birth; frontal sinuses begin to develop by 1 to 2 years of age; and sphenoid sinuses develop later in childhood. Infants and young children have fewer sinus problems than older children and adolescents.

### Children

- A speculum is usually not necessary to examine the septum, turbinates, and vestibule, and it might cause the child to be apprehensive. Instead, push the tip of the nose upward with the thumb and shine a light into the nares.

- Ethmoid sinuses continue to develop until age 12. Sinus problems in children under this age are rare.
- Cough and runny nose are the most common signs of sinusitis in preadolescent children.
- Adolescents may have headaches, facial tenderness, and swelling, similar to the signs seen in adults.

### Elders

- The sense of smell markedly diminishes because of a decrease in the number of olfactory nerve fibers and atrophy of the remaining fibers. Elders are less able to identify and discriminate odors.
- Nosebleeds may result from hypertensive disease or other arterial vessel changes.

---

# Skill 11.9   Assessing the Mouth and Oropharynx

### Delegation

Assessment of the mouth and oropharynx is not delegated to UAP. However, many aspects of mouth function are observed during usual care and may be recorded by persons other than the nurse. Abnormal findings must be validated and interpreted by the nurse.

### Equipment

- Clean gloves
- Tongue depressor
- 2 × 2 gauze pads
- Penlight

### Procedure

1. Prior to performing the procedure, introduce self and verify the client's identity using agency protocol. Explain to the client what you are going to do, why it is necessary, and how he or she can participate. Discuss how the results will be used in planning further care or treatments.
2. Perform hand hygiene and observe appropriate infection control procedures.
3. Provide for client privacy.
4. Inquire if the client has any history of the following: routine pattern of dental care, last visit to dentist; length of time ulcers or other lesions have been present; denture discomfort; medications client is receiving.
5. Position the client comfortably, seated if possible.

| Assessment | Normal Findings | Deviations from Normal |
|---|---|---|
| **Lips and Buccal Mucosa** | | |
| 6. Inspect the outer lips for symmetry of contour, color, and texture. Ask the client to purse the lips as if to whistle. | Uniform pink color (darker, e.g., bluish hue, in Mediterranean groups and dark-skinned clients)<br>Soft, moist, smooth texture<br>Symmetry of contour<br>Ability to purse lips | Pallor; cyanosis<br>Blisters; generalized or localized swelling; fissures, crusts, or scales (may result from excessive moisture, nutritional deficiency, or fluid deficit)<br>Inability to purse lips (may indicate facial nerve damage) |
| 7. Inspect the inner lips and buccal mucosa for color, moisture, texture, and the presence of lesions.<br>• Apply clean gloves.<br>• Ask the client to relax the mouth, and, for better visualization, pull the lip outward and away from the teeth.<br>• Grasp the lip on each side between the thumb and index finger. | Uniform pink color (freckled brown pigmentation in dark-skinned clients)<br>Moist, smooth, soft, glistening, and elastic texture (drier oral mucosa in elders due to decreased salivation)<br><br>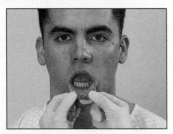<br>● Inspecting the mucosa of the lower lip. | Pallor; leukoplakia (white patches), red, bleeding<br>Excessive dryness<br>Mucosal cysts; irritations from dentures; abrasions, ulcerations; nodules |
| **Teeth and Gums** | | |
| 8. Inspect the teeth and gums while examining the inner lips and buccal mucosa.<br>• Ask the client to open the mouth. Using a tongue depressor, retract the cheek. View the surface buccal mucosa from top to bottom and back to front. A flashlight or penlight will help illuminate the surface. Repeat the procedure for the other side.<br>• Examine the back teeth. For proper vision of the molars, use the index fingers of both hands to retract the cheek. Ask the client to relax the lips and first close, then open, the jaw. ▶Rationale: *Closing the jaw assists in observation of tooth alignment and loss of teeth; opening the jaw assists in observation of dental fillings and caries.* Observe the number of teeth, tooth color, the state of fillings, dental caries, and tartar along the base of the teeth. Note the presence and fit of partial or complete dentures.<br>• Inspect the gums around the molars. Observe for bleeding, color, retraction (pulling away from the teeth), edema, and lesions. | 32 adult teeth<br>Smooth, white, shiny tooth enamel<br>Pink gums (bluish or brown patches in dark-skinned clients)<br>Moist, firm texture to gums<br>No retraction of gums (pulling away from the teeth)<br><br>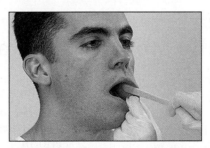<br>● Inspecting the buccal mucosa using a tongue depressor. | Missing teeth; ill-fitting dentures<br>Brown or black discoloration of the enamel (may indicate staining or the presence of caries)<br>Excessively red gums<br>Spongy texture; bleeding; tenderness (may indicate periodontal disease)<br>Receding, atrophied gums; swelling that partially covers the teeth<br><br>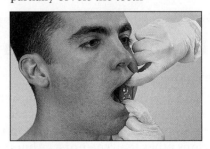<br>● Inspecting the back teeth. |

| Assessment | Normal Findings | Deviations from Normal |
|---|---|---|
| 9. Inspect the dentures. Ask the client to remove complete or partial dentures. Inspect their condition, noting in particular broken or worn areas. | Smooth, intact dentures | Ill-fitting dentures; irritated and excoriated area under dentures |

**Tongue/Floor of the Mouth**

| Assessment | Normal Findings | Deviations from Normal |
|---|---|---|
| 10. Inspect the surface of the tongue for position, color, and texture. Ask the client to protrude the tongue. | Central position<br>Pink color (some brown pigmentation on tongue borders in dark-skinned clients); moist; slightly rough; thin whitish coating<br>Smooth, lateral margins; no lesions<br>Raised papillae (taste buds) | Deviated from center (may indicate damage to hypoglossal [twelfth cranial] nerve); excessive trembling<br>Smooth red tongue (may indicate iron, vitamin B12, or vitamin B3 deficiency)<br>Dry, furry tongue (associated with fluid deficit), white coating (may be oral yeast infection)<br>Nodes, ulcerations, discolorations (white or red areas); areas of tenderness |
| 11. Inspect tongue movement. Ask the client to roll the tongue upward and move it from side to side. | Moves freely; no tenderness | Restricted mobility |
| 12. Inspect the base of the tongue, the mouth floor, and the frenulum. Ask the client to place the tip of the tongue against the roof of the mouth. | Smooth tongue base with prominent veins | Swelling, ulceration |

**Palates and Uvula**

| Assessment | Normal Findings | Deviations from Normal |
|---|---|---|
| 13. Inspect the hard and soft palate for color, shape, texture, and the presence of bony prominences. Ask the client to open the mouth wide and tilt the head backward. Then, depress tongue with a tongue depressor as necessary, and use a penlight for appropriate visualization. | Light pink, smooth, soft palate<br>Lighter pink hard palate, more irregular texture | Discoloration (e.g., jaundice or pallor)<br>Palates the same color<br>Irritations<br>Exostoses (bony growths) growing from the hard palate |
| 14. Inspect the uvula for position and mobility while examining the palates. To observe the uvula, ask the client to say "ah" so that the soft palate rises. | Positioned in midline of soft palate | Deviation to one side from tumor or trauma; immobility (may indicate damage to trigeminal [fifth cranial] nerve or vagus [tenth cranial] nerve) |

**Oropharynx and Tonsils**

| Assessment | Normal Findings | Deviations from Normal |
|---|---|---|
| 15. Inspect the oropharynx for color and texture. Inspect one side at a time to avoid eliciting the gag reflex. To expose one side of the oropharynx, press a tongue depressor against the tongue on the same side about halfway back while the client tilts the head back and opens the mouth wide. Use a penlight for illumination, if needed. | Pink and smooth posterior wall | Reddened or edematous; presence of lesions, plaques, or drainage |
| 16. Inspect the tonsils (behind the fauces [throat]) for color, discharge, and size. | Pink and smooth<br>No discharge | Inflamed<br>Presence of discharge |

*(continued)*

| Assessment | Normal Findings | Deviations from Normal |
|---|---|---|
| **Oropharynx and Tonsils** *(continued)* | | |
| 17. Remove and discard gloves. Perform hand hygiene. | Of normal size or not visible | Swollen |
| 18. Document findings in the client record using forms or checklists supplemented by narrative notes when appropriate. | • *Grade 1 (normal):* The tonsils are behind the tonsillar pillars (the soft structures supporting the soft palate). | • *Grade 2:* The tonsils are between the pillars and the uvula.<br>• *Grade 3:* The tonsils touch the uvula.<br>• *Grade 4:* One or both tonsils extend to the midline of the oropharynx. |

## CLIENT TEACHING

- Although clients may be sensitive to discussion of their personal hygiene practices, use the assessment as an opportunity to provide teaching regarding appropriate oral and dental care for the entire family. Refer clients to a dentist if indicated.

## DEVELOPMENTAL CONSIDERATIONS

### Infants

- Inspect the palate and uvula for a cleft. A bifid (forked) uvula may indicate an undetected cleft palate (i.e., a cleft in the cartilage that is covered by skin).
- Newborns may have a pearly white nodule on their gums, which resolves without treatment.
- The first teeth erupt at about 6 to 7 months of age. Assess for dental hygiene; parents should cleanse the infant's teeth daily with a soft cloth or soft toothbrush.
- Fluoride supplements should be given by 6 months if the child's drinking water contains less than 0.3 parts per million (ppm) fluoride.
- Children should see a dentist by 1 year of age.

### Children

- Tooth development should be appropriate for age.
- White spots on the teeth may indicate excessive fluoride ingestion.
- Drooling is common up to 2 years of age.
- The tonsils are normally larger in children than in adults and commonly extend beyond the palatine arch until the age of 11 or 12 years.

### Elders

- The oral mucosa may be drier than that of younger persons because of decreased salivary gland activity. Decreased salivation occurs in elderly people taking prescribed medications such as antidepressants, antihistamines, decongestants, diuretics, antihypertensives, tranquilizers, antispasmodics, and antineoplastics. Extreme dryness is associated with dehydration.
- Some receding of the gums occurs, giving an appearance of increased toothiness.
- Taste sensations diminish. Sweet and salty tastes are lost first. Elderly persons may add more salt and sugar to food than they did when they were younger. Diminished taste sensation is due to atrophy of the taste buds and a decreased sense of smell. It indicates diminished function of the fifth and seventh cranial nerves.
- Tiny purple or bluish black swollen areas (varicosities) under the tongue, known as caviar spots, are not uncommon.
- The teeth may show signs of staining, erosion, chipping, and abrasions due to loss of dentin.
- Tooth loss occurs as a result of dental disease but is preventable with good dental hygiene.
- The gag reflex may be slightly sluggish.
- Elders who are homebound or are in long-term care facilities often have teeth or dentures in need of repair, due to the difficulty of obtaining dental care in these situations. Do a thorough assessment of missing teeth and those in need of repair, whether they are natural teeth or dentures.

# Skill 11.10   Assessing the Neck

## Delegation

Assessment of the neck is not delegated to UAP. However, many aspects of the neck are observed during usual care and may be recorded by persons other than the nurse. Abnormal findings must be validated and interpreted by the nurse.

## Procedure

1. Prior to performing the procedure, introduce self and verify the client's identity using agency protocol. Explain to the client what you are going to do, why it is necessary, and how he or she can participate. Discuss how the results will be used in planning further care or treatments.
2. Perform hand hygiene and observe appropriate infection control procedures.
3. Provide for client privacy.
4. Inquire if the client has any history of the following: problems with neck lumps; neck pain or stiffness; when and how any lumps occurred; previous diagnoses of thyroid problems; and other treatments provided (e.g., surgery, radiation).

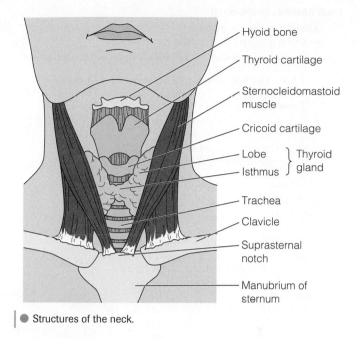

- Hyoid bone
- Thyroid cartilage
- Sternocleidomastoid muscle
- Cricoid cartilage
- Lobe } Thyroid
- Isthmus } gland
- Trachea
- Clavicle
- Suprasternal notch
- Manubrium of sternum

● Structures of the neck.

| Assessment | Normal Findings | Deviations from Normal |
|---|---|---|
| **Neck Muscles** | | |
| 5. Inspect the neck muscles (sternocleidomastoid and trapezius) for abnormal swellings or masses. Ask the client to hold the head erect. | Muscles equal in size; head centered | Unilateral neck swelling; head tilted to one side (indicates presence of masses, injury, muscle weakness, shortening of sternocleidomastoid muscle, scars) |
| 6. Observe head movement. Ask client to:<br>• Move the chin to the chest. ➤Rationale: This determines function of the sternocleidomastoid muscle.<br>• Move the head back so that the chin points upward. ➤Rationale: This determines function of the trapezius muscle.<br>• Move the head so that the ear is moved toward the shoulder on each side. ➤Rationale: This determines function of the sternocleidomastoid muscle.<br>• Turn the head to the right and to the left. ➤Rationale: This determines function of the sternocleidomastoid muscle. | Coordinated, smooth movements with no discomfort<br>Head flexes 45°<br>Head hyperextends 60°<br>Head laterally flexes 40°<br>Head laterally rotates 70° | Muscle tremor, spasm, or stiffness<br>Limited range of motion; painful movements; involuntary movements (e.g., up-and-down nodding movements associated with Parkinson's disease)<br>Head hyperextends less than 60°<br>Head laterally flexes less than 40°<br>Head laterally rotates less than 70° |

*(continued)*

| Assessment | Normal Findings | Deviations from Normal |
|---|---|---|
| **Neck Muscles** *(continued)* | | |
| 7. Assess muscle strength. | | |
| • Ask the client to turn the head to one side against the resistance of your hand. Repeat with the other side. ➤*Rationale: This determines the strength of the sternocleidomastoid muscle.* | Equal strength | Unequal strength |
| • Ask the client to shrug the shoulders against the resistance of your hands. ➤*Rationale: This determines the strength of the trapezius muscles.* | Equal strength | Unequal strength |
| **Lymph Nodes** | | |
| 8. Palpate the entire neck for enlarged lymph nodes. | Not palpable | Enlarged, palpable, possibly tender (associated with infection and tumors) |
| • Face the client, and bend the client's head forward slightly or toward the side being examined. ➤*Rationale: This relaxes the soft tissue and muscles.* | | |
| • Palpate the nodes using the pads of the fingers. Move the fingertips in a gentle rotating motion. | | |
| • When examining the submental and submandibular nodes, place the fingertips under the mandible on the side nearest the palpating hand, and pull the skin and subcutaneous tissue laterally over the mandibular surface so that the tissue rolls over the nodes. | | |
| • When palpating the supraclavicular nodes, have the client bend the head forward to relax the tissues of the anterior neck and to relax the shoulders so that the clavicles drop. Use your hand nearest the side to be examined when facing the client (i.e., your left hand for the client's right nodes). Use your free hand to flex the client's head forward if necessary. Hook your index and third fingers over the clavicle lateral to the sternocleidomastoid muscle. | | |
| • When palpating the anterior cervical nodes and posterior cervical nodes, move your fingertips slowly in a forward circular motion against the sternocleidomastoid and trapezius muscles, respectively. | | |
| • To palpate the deep cervical nodes, bend or hook your fingers around the sternocleidomastoid muscle. | | |

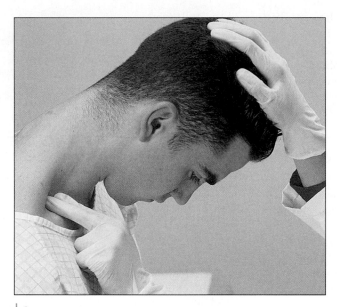

● Palpating the supraclavicular lymph nodes.

| Assessment | Normal Findings | Deviations from Normal |
|---|---|---|
| **Trachea** | | |
| 9. Palpate the trachea for lateral deviation. Place your fingertip or thumb on the trachea in the suprasternal notch (see figure on page 479), and then move your finger laterally to the left and the right in spaces bordered by the clavicle, the anterior aspect of the sternocleidomastoid muscle, and the trachea. | Central placement in midline of neck; spaces are equal on both sides | Deviation to one side, indicating possible neck tumor; thyroid enlargement; enlarged lymph nodes |
| 10. Document findings in the client record using forms or checklists supplemented by narrative notes when appropriate. | | |

---

## DEVELOPMENTAL CONSIDERATIONS

### Infants and Children

- Examine the neck while the infant or child is lying supine. Lift the head and turn it from side to side to determine neck mobility.

- An infant's neck is normally short, lengthening by about age 3 years. This makes palpation of the trachea difficult.

---

# Skill 11.11  Assessing the Thorax and Lungs

## Delegation

Assessment of the thorax and lungs is not delegated to UAP. However, many aspects of breathing are observed during usual care and may be recorded by persons other than the nurse. Abnormal findings must be validated and interpreted by the nurse.

## Equipment

- Stethoscope
- Skin marker/pencil
- Centimeter ruler

## Procedure

1. Prior to performing the procedure, introduce self and verify the client's identity using agency protocol. Explain to the client what you are going to do, why it is necessary, and how he or she can participate. Discuss how the results will be used in planning further care or treatments.

2. Perform hand hygiene and observe appropriate infection control procedures.

3. Provide for client privacy. In women, drape the anterior thorax when it is not being examined.

4. Inquire if the client has any history of the following: family history of illness, including cancer, allergies, tuberculosis; lifestyle habits such as smoking and occupational hazards (e.g., inhaling fumes); medications being taken; current problems (e.g., swellings, coughs, wheezing, pain).

| Assessment | Normal Findings | Deviations from Normal |
|---|---|---|
| **Posterior Thorax** | | |
| 5. Inspect the shape and symmetry of the thorax from posterior and lateral views. Compare the anteroposterior diameter to the transverse diameter. | Anteroposterior to transverse diameter in ratio of 1:2<br>Thorax symmetric | Barrel chest; increased anteroposterior to transverse diameter<br>Thorax asymmetric |
| 6. Inspect the spinal alignment for deformities. Have the client stand. From a lateral position, observe the three normal curvatures: cervical, thoracic, and lumbar. | Spine vertically aligned | Exaggerated spinal curvatures (kyphosis, lordosis) |
| • To assess for lateral deviation of the spine (scoliosis), observe the standing client from the rear. Have the client bend forward at the waist and observe from behind. | Spinal column is straight, right and left shoulders and hips are at same height. | Spinal column deviates to one side, often accentuated when bending over. Shoulders or hips not even (level) |
| 7. Palpate the posterior thorax. | | |
| • For clients who have no respiratory complaints, rapidly assess the temperature and integrity of all thorax skin. | Skin intact; uniform temperature | Skin lesions; areas of hyperthermia |
| • For clients who do have respiratory complaints, palpate all areas for bulges, tenderness, or abnormal movements. Avoid deep palpation for painful areas, especially if a fractured rib is suspected. In such a case, deep palpation could lead to displacement of the bone fragment against the lungs. | Thorax intact; no tenderness; no masses | Lumps, bulges; depressions; areas of tenderness; movable structures (e.g., rib) |
| 8. Palpate the posterior thorax for respiratory excursion (thoracic expansion). Place the palms of both your hands over the lower thorax with your thumbs adjacent to the spine and your fingers stretched laterally. Ask the client to take a deep breath while you observe the movement of your hands and any lag in movement. | Full and symmetric thorax expansion (i.e., when the client takes a deep breath, your thumbs should move apart an equal distance and at the same time; normally the thumbs separate 3 to 5 cm [1½ to 2 in.] during deep inspiration) | Asymmetric and/or decreased thorax expansion |

● Position of the nurse's hands when assessing posterior respiratory excursion on the posterior thorax.

| Assessment | Normal Findings | Deviations from Normal |
|---|---|---|
| 9. Palpate the thorax for vocal (tactile) **fremitus**, the faintly perceptible vibration felt through the chest wall when the client speaks. <br> • Place the palmar surfaces of your fingertips or the ulnar aspect of your hand or closed fist on the posterior thorax, starting near the apex of the lungs, *position A)*. <br> • Ask the client to repeat such words as "blue moon" or "one, two, three." <br> • Repeat the two steps, moving your hands sequentially to the base of the lungs, through positions B–E in. <br> • Compare the fremitus on both lungs and between the apex and the base of each lung, using either one hand and moving it from one side of the client to the corresponding area on the other side *or* using two hands that are placed simultaneously on the corresponding areas of each side of the thorax. | Bilateral symmetry of vocal fremitus <br> Fremitus is heard most clearly at the apex of the lungs <br> Low-pitched voices of males are more readily palpated than higher pitched voices of females <br><br> 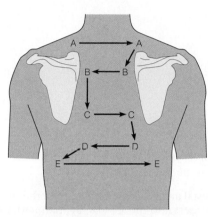<br> ● Areas and sequence for palpating tactile fremitus on the posterior chest. | Decreased or absent fremitus (associated with pneumothorax) <br> Increased fremitus (associated with consolidated lung tissue, as in pneumonia) |
| 10. Percuss the thorax. Percussion of the thorax is performed to determine whether underlying lung tissue is filled with air, liquid, or solid material and to determine the positions and boundaries of certain organs. Because percussion penetrates to a depth of 5 to 7 cm (2 to 3 in.), it detects superficial rather than deep lesions. <br> • Ask the client to bend the head and fold the arms forward across the chest. ▸*Rationale: This separates the scapula and exposes more lung tissue to percussion.* <br> • Percuss in the intercostal spaces at about 5 cm (2 in.) intervals in a systematic sequence. <br> • Compare one side of the lung with the other. <br> • Percuss the lateral thorax every few inches, starting at the axilla and working down to the eighth rib. | Percussion notes resonate, except over scapula <br> Lowest point of resonance is at the diaphragm (i.e., at the level of the 8th to 10th rib posteriorly) <br> *Note:* Percussion on a rib normally elicits dullness. <br><br> 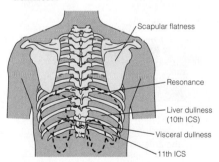<br> ● Normal percussion sounds on the posterior chest. | Asymmetry in percussion <br> Areas of dullness or flatness over lung tissue (associated with fluid, consolidation of lung tissue, or a mass) <br><br> 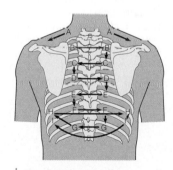<br> ● Sequence for posterior chest percussion. |

*(continued)*

| Assessment | Normal Findings | Deviations from Normal |
|---|---|---|
| **Posterior Thorax (continued)** | | |
| 11. Auscultate the thorax using the diaphragm of the stethoscope. ➤Rationale: *The diaphragm of the stethoscope is best for transmitting the high-pitched breath sounds.*<br>• Use the systematic zigzag procedure used in percussion.<br>• Ask the client to take slow, deep breaths through the mouth. Listen at each point to the breath sounds during a complete inspiration and expiration.<br>• Compare findings at each point with the corresponding point on the opposite side of the thorax. | Vesicular and bronchovesicular breath sounds (see Table 11–2) | Adventitious breath sounds (e.g., crackles, gurgles, friction rub, wheeze; see Table 11–3)<br>Absence of breath sounds |
| 12. Inspect breathing patterns (e.g., respiratory rate and rhythm). | Quiet, rhythmic, and effortless respirations | See Table 11–10 for altered breathing patterns and sounds |
| 13. Inspect the costal angle (angle formed by the intersection of the costal margins) and the angle at which the ribs enter the spine. | Costal angle is less than 90°, and the ribs insert into the spine at approximately a 45° angle | Costal angle is widened (associated with chronic obstructive pulmonary disease) |
| 14. Palpate the anterior thorax (see posterior thorax palpation). | | |
| 15. Palpate the anterior thorax for respiratory excursion.<br>• Place the palms of both your hands on the lower thorax, with your fingers laterally along the lower rib cage and your thumbs along the costal margins.<br>• Ask the client to take a deep breath while you observe the movement of your hands. | Full symmetric excursion; thumbs normally separate 3 to 5 cm (1½ to 2 in.) 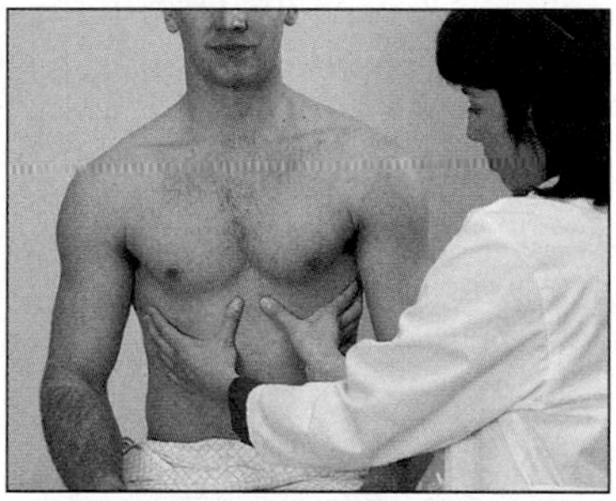<br><br>● Position of the nurse's hands when assessing respiratory excursion on the anterior thorax. | Asymmetric and/or decreased respiratory excursion |
| 16. Palpate tactile fremitus in the same manner as for the posterior thorax and using the sequence shown in the illustration to the right. If the breasts are large and cannot be retracted adequately for palpation, this part of the examination is usually omitted. | Same as posterior vocal fremitus; fremitus is normally decreased over heart and breast tissue 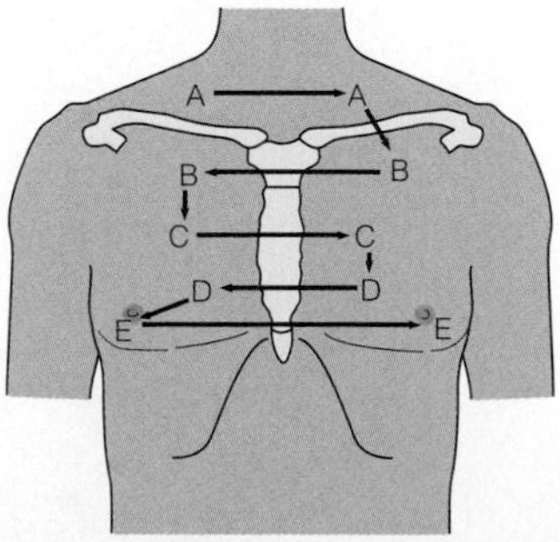<br><br>● Areas and sequence for palpating tactile fremitus on the anterior chest. | Same as posterior fremitus |

| Assessment | Normal Findings | Deviations from Normal |
|---|---|---|
| 17. Percuss the anterior thorax systematically.<br>• Begin above the clavicles in the supraclavicular space, and proceed downward to the diaphragm.<br>• Compare one side of the lung to the other.<br>• Displace female breast to facilitate percussion of the lungs. | Percussion notes resonate down to the sixth rib at the level of the diaphragm but are flat over areas of heavy muscle and bone, dull on areas over the heart and the liver, and tympanic over the underlying stomach. | Asymmetry in percussion notes<br>Areas of dullness or flatness over lung tissue |

● *Sequence for anterior chest percussion.*

● *Normal percussion sounds on the anterior chest.*

| Assessment | Normal Findings | Deviations from Normal |
|---|---|---|
| 18. Auscultate the trachea. | Bronchial and tubular breath sounds (see Table 11–2 on page 487) | Adventitious breath sounds (see Table 11–3 on page 487) |
| 19. Auscultate the anterior thorax. Use the sequence used in percussion, beginning over the bronchi between the sternum and the clavicles. | Bronchovesicular and vesicular breath sounds (see Table 11–2) | Adventitious breath sounds (see Table 11–3) |
| 20. Document findings in the client record using forms or checklists supplemented by narrative notes when appropriate. | | |

## Documentation

Sample: 6/10/09 0830 Lungs clear to auscultation except for fine crackles both lower lobes, lessened after coughing. Rarely moves in bed. Assisted to a chair. Reviewed deep breathing exercises. Effective return demonstration. _____ N. Schmidt, RN

## DEVELOPMENTAL CONSIDERATIONS

### Infants

- The thorax is rounded; that is, the diameter from the front to the back (anteroposterior) is equal to the transverse diameter. It is also cylindrical, having a nearly equal diameter at the top and the base. This makes it harder for infants to expand their thoracic space.

- To assess tactile fremitus, place your hand over the crying infant's thorax.

- Infants tend to breathe using their diaphragm; assess rate and rhythm by watching the abdomen, rather than the thorax, rise and fall.

- The right bronchial branch is short and angles downward as it leaves the trachea, making it easy for small objects to be inhaled. Sudden onset of cough or other signs of respiratory distress may indicate that the infant has inhaled a foreign object.

### Children

- By about 6 years of age, the anteroposterior diameter has decreased in proportion to the transverse diameter, with a 1:2 ratio present.

- Children tend to breathe more abdominally than thoracically up to age 6.

*(continued)*

## DEVELOPMENTAL CONSIDERATIONS (CONTINUED)

- During the rapid growth spurts of adolescence, spinal curvature and rotation (scoliosis) may appear. Children should be assessed for scoliosis by age 12 and annually until their growth slows. Curvature greater than 10% should be referred for further medical evaluation.

### Elders

- The thoracic curvature may be accentuated (kyphosis) because of osteoporosis and changes in cartilage, resulting in collapse of the vertebrae. This can also compromise and decrease normal respiratory effort.

- Kyphosis and osteoporosis alter the size of the chest cavity as the ribs move downward and forward.

- The anteroposterior diameter of the thorax widens, giving the person a barrel-chested appearance. This is due to loss of skeletal muscle strength in the thorax and diaphragm and constant lung inflation from excessive expiratory pressure on the alveoli.

- Breathing rate and rhythm are unchanged at rest; the rate normally increases with exercise but may take longer to return to the preexercise rate.

- Inspiratory muscles become less powerful, and the inspiratory reserve volume decreases. A decrease in depth of respiration is therefore apparent.

- Expiration may require the use of accessory muscles. The expiratory reserve volume significantly

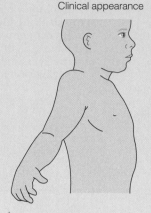
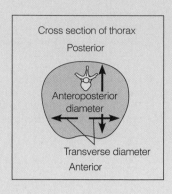

Clinical appearance

Cross section of thorax
Posterior

Anteroposterior diameter

Transverse diameter

Anterior

● Configurations of the child's thorax showing anteroposterior diameter and transverse diameter.

increases because of the increased amount of air remaining in the lungs at the end of a normal breath.

- Deflation of the lung is incomplete.

- Small airways lose their cartilaginous support and elastic recoil; as a result, they tend to close, particularly in basal or dependent portions of the lung.

- Elastic tissue of the alveoli loses its stretchability and changes to fibrous tissue. Exertional capacity decreases.

- Cilia in the airways decrease in number and are less effective in removing mucus; elderly clients are therefore at greater risk for pulmonary infections.

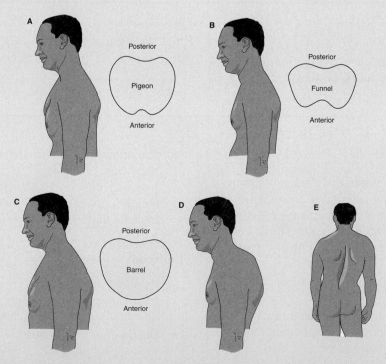

Posterior

Pigeon

Anterior

Posterior

Funnel

Anterior

Posterior

Barrel

Anterior

● Chest deformities: **A**, pigeon chest; **B**, funnel chest; **C**, barrel chest; **D**, kyphosis; **E**, scoliosis.

## TABLE 11–2  NORMAL BREATH SOUNDS

| Type | Description | Location | Characteristics |
|---|---|---|---|
| Vesicular | Soft-intensity, low-pitched, "gentle sighing" sounds created by air moving through smaller airways (bronchioles and alveoli) | Over peripheral lung; best heard at base of lungs | Best heard on inspiration, which is about 2.5 times longer than the expiratory phase (5:2 ratio) |
| Bronchovesicular | Moderate-intensity and moderate-pitched "blowing" sounds created by air moving through larger airways (bronchi) | Between the scapulae and lateral to the sternum at the first and second intercostal spaces | Equal inspiratory and expiratory phases (1:1 ratio) |
| Bronchial (tubular) | High-pitched, loud, "harsh" sounds created by air moving through the trachea | Anteriorly over the trachea; not normally heard over lung tissue | Louder than vesicular sounds; have a short inspiratory phase and long expiratory phase (1:2 ratio) |

## TABLE 11–3  ADVENTITIOUS BREATH SOUNDS

| Name | Description | Cause | Location |
|---|---|---|---|
| Crackles (rales) | Fine, short, interrupted crackling sounds; alveolar rales are high pitched. Sound can be simulated by rolling a lock of hair near the ear. Best heard on inspiration but can be heard on both inspiration and expiration. May not be cleared by coughing. | Air passing through fluid or mucus in any air passage | Most commonly heard in the bases of the lower lung lobes |
| Gurgles (rhonchi) | Continuous, low-pitched, coarse, gurgling, harsh, louder sounds with a moaning or snoring quality. Best heard on expiration but can be heard on both inspiration and expiration. May be altered by coughing. | Air passing through narrowed air passages as a result of secretions, swelling, tumors | Loud sounds can be heard over most lung areas but predominate over the trachea and bronchi |
| Friction rub | Superficial grating or creaking sounds heard during inspiration and expiration. Not relieved by coughing. | Rubbing together of inflamed pleural surfaces | Heard most often in areas of greatest thoracic expansion (e.g., lower anterior and lateral thorax) |
| Wheeze | Continuous, high-pitched, squeaky musical sounds. Best heard on expiration. Not usually altered by coughing. | Air passing through a constricted bronchus as a result of secretions, swelling, tumors | Heard over all lung fields |

# Skill 11.12   Assessing the Heart and Central Vessels

## Delegation

Assessment of the heart and central vessels is not delegated to UAP. However, many aspects of cardiac function are observed during normal findings and must be validated and interpreted by the nurse.

## Equipment

- Stethoscope
- Centimeter ruler

## Procedure

1. Prior to performing the procedure, introduce self and verify the client's identity using agency protocol. Explain to the client what you are going to do, why it is necessary, and how he or she can participate. Discuss how the results will be used in planning further care or treatments.
2. Perform hand hygiene and observe appropriate infection control procedures.
3. Provide for client privacy.
4. Inquire if the client has any history of the following: family history of incidence of heart disease, high cholesterol levels, high blood pressure, stroke, obesity, congenital heart disease, arterial disease, hypertension, and rheumatic fever and age at which event occurred; client's past history of rheumatic fever, heart murmur, heart attack, varicosities, or heart failure; present symptoms indicative of heart disease (e.g., fatigue, dyspnea, orthopnea, edema, cough, chest pain, palpitations, syncope, hypertension, wheezing, hemoptysis); presence of diseases that affect heart (e.g., obesity, diabetes, lung disease, endocrine disorders); lifestyle habits that are risk factors for cardiac disease (e.g., smoking, alcohol intake, eating and exercise patterns, areas and degree of stress perceived).

| Assessment | Normal Findings | Deviations from Normal |
|---|---|---|
| 5. Simultaneously inspect and palpate the precordium for the presence of abnormal pulsations, lifts, or heaves. Locate the valve areas of the heart:<br>• Locate the angle of Louis. It is felt as a prominence on the sternum.<br>• Move your fingertips down each side of the angle until you can feel the second intercostal spaces. The client's right second intercostal space is the aortic area, and the left second intercostal space is the pulmonic area.<br>• From the pulmonic area, move your fingertips down three left intercostal spaces along the side of the sternum. The left fifth intercostal space close to the sternum is the tricuspid or right ventricular area.<br>• From the tricuspid area, move your fingertips laterally 5 to 7 cm (2 to 3 in.) to the left midclavicular line (LMCL). This is the apical or mitral area, or point of maximal impulse (PMI). If you have difficulty locating the PMI, have the client roll onto the left side to move the apex closer to the chest wall. | 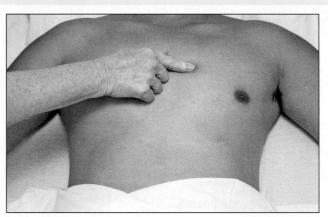<br>● The second intercostal space.<br><br>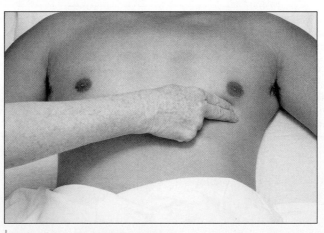<br>● The fifth intercostal space, MCL. | |

| Assessment | Normal Findings | Deviations from Normal |
|---|---|---|
| • Inspect and palpate the aortic and pulmonic areas, observing them at an angle and to the side, to note the presence or absence of pulsations. Observing these areas at an angle increases the likelihood of seeing pulsations. | No pulsations | Pulsations |
| • Inspect and palpate the tricuspid area for pulsations and heaves or lifts. | No pulsations<br>No lift or heave | Pulsations<br>Diffuse lift or heave, indicating enlarged or overactive right ventricle |
| • Inspect and palpate the apical area for pulsation, noting its specific location (it may be displaced laterally or lower) and diameter. If displaced laterally, record the distance between the apex and the MCL in centimeters. | Pulsations visible in 50% of adults and palpable in most PMI in fifth LICS at or medial to MCL<br>Diameter of 1 to 2 cm (1/3 to 1/2 in.)<br>No lift or heave | Diffuse lift or heave, indicating enlarged or overactive right ventricle<br>PMI displaced laterally or lower (indicates enlarged heart)<br>Diameter over 2 cm (1/2 in.); indicates enlarged heart or aneurysm<br>Diffuse lift or heave lateral to apex; indicates enlargement or overactivity of left ventricle |
| • Inspect and palpate the epigastric area at the base of the sternum for abdominal aortic pulsations. | Aortic pulsations | Bounding abdominal pulsations (e.g., aortic aneurysm) |
| 6. Auscultate the heart in all four anatomic sites: aortic, pulmonic, tricuspid, and apical (mitral). Auscultation need not be limited to these areas; the nurse may need to move the stethoscope to find the most audible sounds for each client. | $S_1$: Usually heard at all sites<br>Usually louder at apical area<br>$S_2$: Usually heard at all sites<br>Usually louder at base of heart | Increased or decreased intensity<br>Varying intensity with different beats<br>Increased intensity at aortic area<br>Increased intensity at pulmonic area |
| • Eliminate all sources of room noise. ➤*Rationale: Heart sounds are of low intensity, and other noise hinders the nurse's ability to hear them.* | *Systole:* silent interval; slightly shorter duration than diastole at normal heart rate (60 to 90 beats per minute [bpm]) | Sharp-sounding ejection clicks<br>$S_3$ in older adults<br>$S_4$ may be a sign of hypertension |
| • Keep the client in a supine position with head elevated 30° to 45°.<br>• Use both the diaphragm and the bell to listen to all areas.<br>• In every area of auscultation, distinguish both $S_1$ and $S_2$ sounds.<br>• When auscultating, concentrate on one particular sound at a time in each area: the first heart sound, followed by systole, then the second heart sound, then diastole. Systole and diastole are normally silent intervals.<br>• Later, reexamine the heart while the client is in the upright sitting position. ➤*Rationale: Certain sounds are more audible in certain positions.* | *Diastole:* silent interval; slightly longer duration than systole at normal heart rates<br>$S_3$ in children and young adults<br>$S_4$ in many older adults | |

**Carotid Arteries**

| Assessment | Normal Findings | Deviations from Normal |
|---|---|---|
| 7. Palpate the carotid artery, using extreme caution.<br>• Palpate only one carotid artery at a time. ➤*Rationale: This ensures adequate blood flow through the other artery to the brain.* | Symmetric pulse volumes<br>Full pulsations, thrusting quality<br>Quality remains same when client breathes, turns head, and changes from sitting to supine position<br>Elastic arterial wall | Asymmetric volumes (possible stenosis or thrombosis)<br>Decreased pulsations (may indicate impaired left cardiac output)<br>Increased pulsations<br>Thickening, hard, rigid, beaded, inelastic walls (indicate arteriosclerosis) |

*(continued)*

| Assessment | Normal Findings | Deviations from Normal |
|---|---|---|
| **Carotid Arteries** *(continued)* | | |
| • Avoid exerting too much pressure and massaging the area. ➤*Rationale: Pressure can occlude the artery, and carotid sinus massage can precipitate bradycardia. The carotid sinus is a small dilation at the beginning of the internal carotid artery just above the bifurcation of the common carotid artery, in the upper third of the neck.* <br> • Ask the client to turn the head slightly toward the side being examined. This makes the carotid artery more accessible. | | |
| 8. Auscultate the carotid artery. <br> • Turn the client's head slightly away from the side being examined. ➤*Rationale: This facilitates the placement of the stethoscope.* <br> • Auscultate the carotid artery on one side and then the other. <br> • Listen for the presence of a bruit. If you hear a bruit, gently palpate the artery to determine the presence of a thrill. | No sound heard on auscultation | Presence of bruit in one or both arteries (suggests occlusive artery disease) |
| **Jugular Veins** | | |
| 9. Inspect the jugular veins for distention while the client is placed in a semi-Fowler's position (15° to 45° angle), with the head supported on a small pillow. | Veins not visible (indicating right side of heart is functioning normally) | Veins visibly distended (indicating advanced cardiopulmonary disease) |
| 10. If jugular distention is present, assess the jugular venous pressure (JVP). <br> • Locate the highest visible point of distention of the internal jugular vein. Although either the internal or the external jugular vein can be used, the internal jugular vein is more reliable. ➤*Rationale: The external jugular vein is more easily affected by obstruction or kinking at the base of the neck.* <br> • Measure the vertical height of this point in centimeters from the sternal angle, the point at which the clavicles meet. <br> • Repeat the preceding steps on the other side. | Level of the highest visible point of distention <br><br> The vertical distance between the sternal angle and the highest level of jugular distention <br><br> Level of the sternal angle <br><br> External jugular vein <br><br> Internal jugular vein <br><br> 30° – 45° <br><br> ● Assessing the highest point of distention of the jugular vein. | Bilateral measurements above 3 to 4 cm are considered elevated (may indicate right-sided heart failure) <br> Unilateral distention (may be caused by local obstruction) |
| 11. Document findings in the client record using forms or checklists supplemented by narrative notes when appropriate. | | |

## DEVELOPMENTAL CONSIDERATIONS

### Infants

- Physiologic splitting of the second heart sound ($S_2$) may be heard when the child takes a deep breath and the aortic valve closes a split second before the pulmonic valve. If splitting of $S_2$ is heard during normal respirations, it is abnormal and may indicate an atrial-septal defect, pulmonary stenosis, or another heart problem.
- Infants may normally have sinus arrhythmia that is related to respiration. The heart rate slows during expiration and increases when the child breathes in.
- Murmurs may be heard in newborns as the structures of fetal circulation, especially the ductus arteriosus, close.

### Children

- Heart sounds may be louder because of the thinner chest wall.
- A third heart sound ($S_3$), caused as the ventricles fill, is best heard at the apex and is present in about one-third of all children.

- The PMI is higher and more medial in children under 8 years old.

### Elders

- If no disease is present, heart size remains the same size throughout life.
- Cardiac output and strength of contraction decrease, thus lessening the older person's activity tolerance.
- The heart rate returns to its resting rate more slowly after exertion than it did when the individual was younger.
- $S_4$ heart sound is considered normal in older adults.
- Extra systoles commonly occur. Ten or more extra systoles per minute are considered abnormal.
- Sudden emotional and physical stress may result in cardiac arrhythmias and heart failure.

# Skill 11.13   Assessing the Peripheral Vascular System

### Delegation

Due to the substantial knowledge and skill required, assessment of the peripheral vascular system is not delegated to UAP. However, many aspects of the vascular system are observed during usual care

### Procedure

1. Prior to performing the procedure, introduce self and verify the client's identity using agency protocol. Explain to the client what you are going to do, why it is necessary, and how he or she can partici-

pate. Discuss how the results will be used in planning further care or treatments.
2. Perform hand hygiene and observe appropriate infection control procedures.
3. Provide for client privacy.
4. Inquire if the client has any history of the following: past history of heart disorders, varicosities, arterial disease, and hypertension; lifestyle habits such as exercise patterns, activity patterns and tolerance, smoking, and use of alcohol.

| Assessment | Normal Findings | Deviations from Normal |
|---|---|---|
| **Peripheral Pulses** | | |
| 5. Palpate the peripheral pulses on both sides of the client's body individually, simultaneously (except the carotid pulse), and systematically to determine the symmetry of pulse volume. If you have difficulty palpating some of the peripheral pulses, use a Doppler ultrasound probe. | Symmetric pulse volumes<br>Full pulsations | Asymmetric volumes (indicate impaired circulation)<br>Absence of pulsation (indicates arterial spasm or occlusion)<br>Decreased, weak, thready pulsations (indicate impaired cardiac output)<br>Increased pulse volume (may indicate hypertension, high cardiac output, or circulatory overload) |

*(continued)*

| Assessment | Normal Findings | Deviations from Normal |
|---|---|---|
| **Peripheral Veins**<br>6. Inspect the peripheral veins in the arms and legs for the presence and/or appearance of superficial veins when limbs are dependent and when limbs are elevated. | In dependent position, presence of distention and nodular bulges at calves<br>When limbs elevated, veins collapse (veins may appear tortuous or distended in older people) | Distended veins in the thigh and/or lower leg or on posterolateral part of calf from knee to ankle |
| 7. Assess the peripheral leg veins for signs of phlebitis.<br>• Inspect the calves for redness and swelling over vein sites.<br>• Palpate the calves for firmness or tension of the muscles, the presence of edema over the dorsum of the foot, and areas of localized warmth. ➤*Rationale: Palpation augments inspection findings, particularly for greater pigmented people in whom redness may not be visible.*<br>• Push the calves from side to side to test for tenderness.<br>• Firmly dorsiflex the client's foot while supporting the entire leg in extension (Homans' test), or have the person stand or walk. | Limbs not tender<br>Symmetric in size | Tenderness on palpation<br>Pain in calf muscles with forceful dorsiflexion of the foot (positive Homans' test)<br>Warmth and redness over vein<br>Swelling of one calf or leg<br>No one sign or symptom consistently confirms or excludes presence of phlebitis or a deep venous thrombosis. Pain, tenderness, and swelling are the most predictive (Merli, 2006) |
| **Peripheral Perfusion**<br>8. Inspect the skin of the hands and feet for color, temperature, edema, and skin changes. | Skin color pink<br>Skin temperature not excessively warm or cold<br>No edema<br>Skin texture resilient and moist | Cyanotic (venous insufficiency)<br>Pallor that increases with limb elevation<br>Dependent rubor, a dusky red color when limb is lowered (arterial insufficiency)<br>Brown pigmentation around ankles (arterial or chronic venous insufficiency)<br>Cool skin (arterial insufficiency)<br>Marked edema (venous insufficiency)<br>Mild edema (arterial insufficiency)<br>Skin thin and shiny or thick, waxy, shiny, and fragile, with reduced hair and/or ulceration (venous or arterial insufficiency) |
| 9. Assess the adequacy of arterial flow if arterial insufficiency is suspected. | | |
| **Capillary Refill Test**<br>• Squeeze the client's fingernail and toenail between your fingers sufficiently to cause blanching (about 5 seconds).<br>• Release the pressure, and observe how quickly normal color returns. Color normally returns immediately (less than 2 seconds). | Immediate return of color | Delayed return of color (arterial insufficiency) |
| **Other Assessments**<br>• Inspect the fingernails for changes indicative of circulatory impairment. See the section on assessment of nails, earlier in this chapter.<br>• See also peripheral pulse assessment, earlier. | | |
| 10. Document findings in the client record using forms or checklists supplemented by narrative notes when appropriate. | | |

## CLIENT TEACHING

- Use the assessment as an opportunity to provide teaching regarding appropriate care of the extremities in those at high risk for or with actual vascular impairment. Educate clients and families regarding skin and nail care, exercise, and positioning to promote circulation.

## Documentation

Sample: 6/10/09 0830 Legs mottled red bilaterally toes to mid-calf. States "actually looks a bit better." Capillary refill 4 seconds in toes on both feet. Pedal pulses present but weak. Homans' test negative. c/o pain in calves after walking 100 feet.

_____ N. Schmidt, RN

## DEVELOPMENTAL CONSIDERATIONS

### Infants

- Screen for coarctation of the aorta by palpating the peripheral pulses and comparing the strength of the femoral pulses with the radial pulses and apical pulse. If coarctation is present, femoral pulses will be diminished and radial pulses will be stronger.

### Children

- Changes in the peripheral vasculature, such as bruising, petechiae, and purpura, can indicate serious systemic diseases in children (e.g., leukemia, meningococcemia).

### Elders

- The overall effectiveness of blood vessels decreases as smooth muscle cells are replaced by connective tissue. The lower extremities are more likely to show signs of arterial and venous impairment because of the more distal and dependent position.
- Peripheral vascular assessment should always include upper and lower extremities' temperature, color, pulses, edema, skin integrity, and sensation.

Any differences in symmetry of these findings should be noted.

- Proximal arteries become thinner and dilate.
- Peripheral arteries become thicker and dilate less effectively because of arteriosclerotic changes in the vessel walls.
- Blood vessels lengthen and become more tortuous and prominent. Varicosities occur more frequently.
- In some instances, arteries may be palpated more easily because of the loss of supportive surrounding tissues. Often, however, the most distal pulses of the lower extremities are more difficult to palpate because of decreased arterial perfusion.
- Systolic and diastolic blood pressures increase, but the increase in the systolic pressure is greater. As a result, the pulse pressure widens. Any client with a blood pressure reading above 140/90 should be referred for follow-up assessments.
- Peripheral edema is frequently observed and is most commonly the result of chronic venous insufficiency or low protein levels in the blood (hypoproteinemia).

# Skill 11.14 Assessing the Breasts and Axillae

## Delegation

Assessment of the breasts and axillae is not delegated to UAP. However, persons other than the nurse may record aspects observed during usual care. Abnormal findings must be validated and interpreted by the nurse.

## Equipment

- Centimeter ruler

## Procedure

1. Prior to performing the procedure, introduce self and verify the client's identity using agency protocol. Explain to the client what you are going to do, why it is necessary, and how he or she can participate. Inquire whether the client has ever had a clinical breast exam previously. Discuss how the results will be used in planning further care or treatments.

2. Perform hand hygiene and observe appropriate infection control procedures.
3. Provide for client privacy.
4. Inquire if the client has a history of breast masses and what was done about them; pain or tenderness in the breasts and relation to the woman's menstrual cycle; discharge from the nipple; medication history (some medications, e.g., oral contraceptives, steroids, digitalis, and diuretics, may cause nipple discharge; estrogen replacement therapy may be associated with the development of cysts or cancer); risk factors that may be associated with development of breast cancer (e.g., mother, sister, aunt with breast cancer; alcohol consumption, high-fat diet, obesity, use of oral contraceptives, menarche before age 12, menopause after age 55, age 30 or more at first pregnancy). Inquire if the client performs breast self-examination; technique used and when performed in relation to the menstrual cycle.

| Assessment | Normal Findings | Deviations from Normal |
|---|---|---|
| 5. Inspect the breasts for size, symmetry, and contour or shape while the client is in a sitting position. | *Females:* Rounded shape; slightly unequal in size; generally symmetric<br>*Males:* Breasts even with the chest wall; if obese, may be similar in shape to female breasts | Recent change in breast size; swellings; marked asymmetry |
| 6. Inspect the skin of the breast for localized discolorations or hyperpigmentation, retraction or dimpling, localized hypervascular areas, swelling, or edema. | Skin uniform in color (same in appearance as skin of abdomen or back)<br><br>Skin smooth and intact<br>Diffuse symmetric horizontal or vertical vascular pattern in light-skinned people<br>Striae (stretch marks); moles and nevi | Localized discolorations or Hyperpigmentation<br>Retraction or dimpling (result of scar tissue or an invasive tumor)<br>Unilateral, localized hypervascular areas (associated with increased blood flow)<br>Swelling or edema appearing as pig skin or orange peel due to exaggeration of the pores |

● A lesion causing retraction of the skin.

7. Emphasize any retraction by having the client:
   • Raise the arms above the head.
   • Push the hands together, with elbows flexed.
   • Press the hands down on the hips.

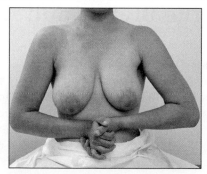

● Pushing the hands together to accentuate retraction of breast tissue.

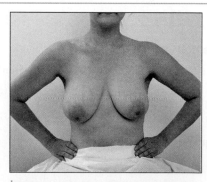

● Pressing the hands down on the hips to accentuate retraction of the breast tissue.

| Assessment | Normal Findings | Deviations from Normal |
|---|---|---|
| 8. Inspect the areola area for size, shape, symmetry, color, surface characteristics, and any masses or lesions. | Round or oval and bilaterally the same<br>Color varies widely, from light pink to dark brown<br>Irregular placement of sebaceous glands on the surface of the areola (Montgomery's tubercles) | Any asymmetry, mass, or lesion |
| 9. Inspect the nipples for size, shape, position, color, discharge, and lesions. | Round, everted, and equal in size; similar in color; soft and smooth; both nipples point in same direction (out in young women and men, downward in older women)<br>No discharge, except from pregnant or breast-feeding females<br>Inversion of one or both nipples that is present from puberty | Asymmetrical size and color<br>Presence of discharge, crusts, or cracks<br>Recent inversion of one or both nipples |
| 10. Palpate the axillary, subclavicular, and supraclavicular lymph nodes while the client sits with the arms abducted and supported on the nurse's forearm. For palpation of clavicular lymph nodes, see page 476. Use the flat surfaces of all fingertips to palpate the four areas of the axilla:<br>• The edge of the greater pectoral muscle along the anterior axillary line<br>• The thoracic wall in the midaxillary area<br>• The upper part of the humerus<br>• The anterior edge of the latissimus dorsi muscle along the posterior axillary line. | No tenderness, masses, or nodules<br>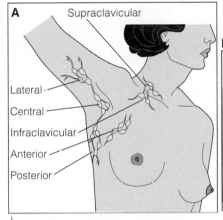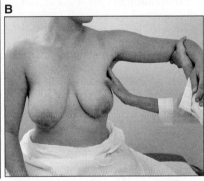<br>● Location and palpation of the lymph nodes that drain the lateral breast: **A,** lymph nodes; **B,** palpating the axilla. | Tenderness, masses, or nodules |
| 11. Palpate the breast for masses, tenderness, and any discharge from the nipples. Palpation of the breast is generally performed while the client is supine. ▶*Rationale: In the supine position, the breasts flatten evenly against the chest wall, facilitating palpation.* For clients who have a past history of breast masses, who are at high risk for breast cancer, or who have pendulous breasts, examination in both a supine and a sitting position is recommended.<br>• If the client reports a breast lump, start with the "normal" breast to obtain baseline data that will serve as a comparison to the involved breast.<br>• To enhance flattening of the breast, instruct the client to abduct the arm and place her hand behind her head. Then place a small pillow or rolled towel under the client's shoulder. | No tenderness, masses, nodules, or nipple discharge<br>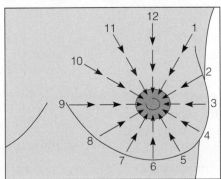<br>● Hands-of-the-clock or spokes-on-a-wheel pattern of breast palpation. | Tenderness, masses, nodules, or nipple discharge<br>If you detect a mass, record the following data:<br>• *Location:* the exact location relative to the quadrants and axillary tail, or the clock and the distance from the nipple in centimeters<br>• *Size:* the length, width, and thickness of the mass in centimeters. If you are able to determine the discrete edges, record this fact<br>• *Shape:* whether the mass is round, oval, lobulated, indistinct, or irregular<br>• *Consistency:* whether the mass is hard or soft<br>• *Mobility:* whether the mass is movable or fixed<br>• *Skin over the lump:* whether it is reddened, dimpled, or retracted<br>• *Nipple:* whether it is displaced or retracted<br>• *Tenderness:* whether palpation is painful |

*(continued)*

| Assessment | Normal Findings | Deviations from Normal |
|---|---|---|
| • For palpation, use the palmar surface of the middle three fingertips (held together) and make a gentle rotary motion on the breast.<br>• Choose one of three patterns for palpation:<br>  a. Hands-of-the-clock or spokes-on-a-wheel<br>  b. Concentric circles<br>  c. Vertical strips pattern<br>• Start at one point for palpation, and move systematically to the end point to ensure that all breast surfaces are assessed.<br>• Pay particular attention to the upper outer quadrant area and the tail of Spence. | 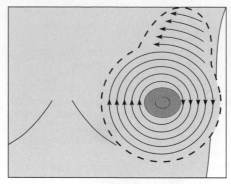<br>● Concentric circles pattern of breast palpation. | 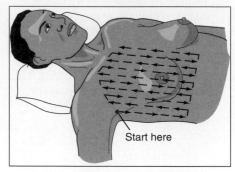<br>● Vertical strips pattern for breast palpation. |
| 12. Palpate the areola and the nipples for masses. Compress each nipple to determine the presence of any discharge. If discharge is present, milk the breast along its radius to identify the discharge-producing lobe. Assess any discharge for amount, color, consistency, and odor. Note also any tenderness on palpation. | No tenderness, masses, nodules, or nipple discharge | Tenderness, masses, nodules, or nipple discharge |
| 13. Teach the client the technique of breast self-examination (BSE). | | |
| 14. Document findings in the client record using forms or checklists supplemented by narrative notes when appropriate. | | |

## CLIENT TEACHING

Instruct the client to perform the following steps.

### Inspection Before a Mirror

Look for any change in size or shape; lumps or thickenings; any rashes or other skin irritations; dimpled or puckered skin; any discharge or change in the nipples (e.g., position or asymmetry). Inspect the breasts in all of the following positions:

• Stand and face the mirror with your arm relaxed at your sides or hands resting on the hips; then turn to the right and the left for a side view (look for any flattening in the side view).

• Bend forward from the waist with arms raised over the head.

• Stand straight with the arms raised over the head and move the arms slowly up and down at the sides. (Look for free movement of the breasts over the chest wall.)

• Press your hands firmly together at chin level while the elbows are raised to shoulder level.

### Palpation: Lying Position

• Place a pillow under your right shoulder and place the right hand behind your head. This position distributes breast tissue more evenly on the chest.

• Use the finger pads (tips) of the three middle fingers (held together) on your left hand to feel for lumps.

## CLIENT TEACHING (CONTINUED)

- Press the breast tissue against the chest wall firmly enough to know how your breast feels. A ridge of firm tissue in the lower curve of each breast is normal.
- Use small circular motions along one arrow in your chosen pattern. Then move your fingers about 2 cm and feel along the next arrow. Repeat this action as many times as necessary until the entire breast is covered.
- Bring your arm down to your side and feel under your armpit, where breast tissue is also located.
- Repeat the exam on your left breast, using the finger pads of your right hand.

**Palpation: Standing or Sitting**

- Repeat the examination of both breasts while upright with one arm behind your head. This position makes it easier to check the area where a large percentage of breast cancers are found, the upper outer part of the breast and toward the armpit.
- Optional: Do the upright BSE in the shower. Soapy hands glide more easily over wet skin. Report any changes to your health care provider promptly.

## DEVELOPMENTAL CONSIDERATIONS

### Infants

- Newborns, both boys and girls, up to 2 weeks of age may have breast enlargement and white discharge from the nipples (witch's milk).
- Supernumerary ("extra") nipples infrequently are present along the mammary chain; these may be associated with renal anomalies.

### Children

- Female breast development begins between 9 and 13 years of age and occurs in five stages (Tanner stages). One breast may develop more rapidly than the other, but at the end of development, they are more or less the same size.
  Stage 1  Prepubertal with no noticeable change
  Stage 2  Breast bud with elevation of nipple and enlargement of the areola
  Stage 3  Enlargement of the breast and areola with no separation of contour
  Stage 4  Projection of the areola and nipple
  Stage 5  Recession of the areola by about age 14 or 15, leaving only the nipple projecting
- Boys may develop breast buds and have slight enlargement of the areola in early adolescence. Further enlargement of breast tissue (gynecomastia) can occur. This growth is transient, usually lasting about 2 years, resolving completely by late puberty.

- Axillary hair usually appears in Tanner stages 3 or 4 and is related to adrenal rather than gonadal changes.

### Pregnant Females

- Breast, areola, and nipple size increase.
- The areolae and nipples darken; nipples may become more erect; areolae contain small, scattered, elevated Montgomery's glands.
- Superficial veins become more prominent, and jagged linear stretch marks may develop.
- A thick yellow fluid (colostrum) may be expressed from the nipples after the first trimester.

### Elders

- In the postmenopausal female, breasts change in shape and often appear pendulous or flaccid; they lack the firmness they had in younger years.
- The presence of breast lesions may be detected more readily because of the decrease in connective tissue.
- General breast size remains the same. Although glandular tissue atrophies, the amount of fat in breasts (predominantly in the lower quadrants) increases in most women.

# Skill 11.15   Assessing the Abdomen

## Delegation

Assessment of the abdomen is not delegated to UAP. However, signs and symptoms of problems may be observed during usual care be validated and interpreted by the nurse.

## Equipment

- Examining light
- Tape measure (metal or unstretchable cloth)
- Water-soluble skin-marking pencil
- Stethoscope

## Procedure

1. Prior to performing the procedure, introduce self and verify the client's identity using agency protocol. Explain to the client what you are going to do, why it is necessary, and how he or she can participate. Discuss how the results will be used in planning further care or treatments.
2. Perform hand hygiene and observe appropriate infection control procedures.
3. Provide for client privacy.
4. Inquire if the client has any history of the following: incidence of abdominal pain; its location, onset, sequence, and chronology; its quality (description); its frequency; associated symptoms (e.g., nausea, vomiting, diarrhea); bowel habits; incidence of constipation or diarrhea (have client describe what client means by these terms); change in appetite, food intolerances, and foods ingested in last 24 hours; specific signs and symptoms (e.g., heartburn, flatulence and/or belching, difficulty swallowing, hematemesis [vomiting blood], blood or mucus in stools, and aggravating and alleviating factors); previous problems and treatment (e.g., stomach ulcer, gallbladder surgery, history of jaundice).
5. Assist the client to a supine position, with the arms placed comfortably at the sides. Place small pillows beneath the knees and the head to reduce tension in the abdominal muscles. Expose the client's abdomen only from the chest to the pubic area to avoid chilling and shivering, which can tense the abdominal muscles.

| Assessment | Normal Findings | Deviations from Normal |
|---|---|---|
| 6. Inspect the abdomen for skin integrity (refer to the discussion of skin assessment, earlier in this chapter). | Unblemished skin<br>Uniform color<br>Silver-white striae (stretch marks) or surgical scars | Presence of rash or other lesions<br>Tense, glistening skin (may indicate ascites, edema)<br>Purple striae (associated with Cushing's disease or rapid weight gain and loss) |
| 7. Inspect the abdomen for contour and symmetry:<br>• Observe the abdominal contour (profile line from the rib margin to the pubic bone) while standing at the client's side when the client is supine. | Flat, rounded (convex), or scaphoid (concave) | Distended |
| • Ask the client to take a deep breath and to hold it. ▶*Rationale: This makes an enlarged liver or spleen more obvious.* | No evidence of enlargement of liver or spleen | Evidence of enlargement of liver or spleen |
| • Assess the symmetry of contour while standing at the foot of the bed.<br>• If distention is present, measure the abdominal girth by placing a tape around the abdomen at the level of the umbilicus. If girth will be measured repeatedly, use an indelible skin marker to outline the upper and lower margins of the tape placement for consistency of future measurements. | Symmetric contour<br><br>● Measuring abdominal girth. | Asymmetric contour, e.g., localized protrusions around umbilicus, inguinal ligaments, or scars (possible hernia or tumor) |

| Assessment | Normal Findings | Deviations from Normal |
|---|---|---|
| 8. Observe abdominal movements associated with respiration, peristalsis, or aortic pulsations. | Symmetric movements caused by respiration<br>Visible peristalsis in very lean people<br>Aortic pulsations in thin persons at epigastric area | Limited movement due to pain or disease process<br>Visible peristalsis in nonlean clients (possible bowel obstruction)<br>Marked aortic pulsations |
| 9. Observe the vascular pattern. | No visible vascular pattern | Visible venous pattern (dilated veins) is associated with liver disease, ascites, and venocaval obstruction |

### Auscultation of the Abdomen

| | | |
|---|---|---|
| 10. Auscultate the abdomen for bowel sounds, vascular sounds, and peritoneal friction rubs. Warm the hands and the stethoscope diaphragm and bell. ➤*Rationale: Cold hands and a cold stethoscope may cause the client to contract the abdominal muscles, and these contractions may be heard during auscultation.* | Audible bowel sounds<br>Absence of arterial bruits<br>Absence of friction rub<br><br>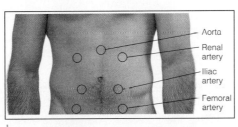<br>● Auscultating the abdomen for bowel sounds. | Hypoactive, i.e., extremely soft and infrequent (e.g., one per minute). Hypoactive sounds indicate decreased motility and are usually associated with manipulation of the bowel during surgery, inflammation, paralytic ileus, or late bowel obstruction<br>Hyperactive/increased, i.e., high-pitched, loud, rushing sounds that occur frequently (e.g., every 3 seconds); also known as borborygmi |

### For Bowel Sounds

| | | |
|---|---|---|
| • Use the diaphragm. ➤*Rationale: Intestinal sounds are relatively high pitched and best transmitted by the diaphragm. Light pressure with the stethoscope is adequate.* | 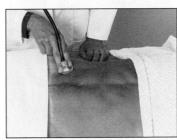<br>Aorta<br>Renal artery<br>Iliac artery<br>Femoral artery<br>● Sites for auscultating the abdomen. | Hyperactive sounds indicate increased intestinal motility and are usually associated with diarrhea, an early bowel obstruction, or the use of laxatives<br>True absence of sounds (none heard in 3 to 5 minutes) indicates a cessation of intestinal motility |

### For Vascular Sounds

- Use the bell of the stethoscope over the aorta, renal arteries, iliac arteries, and femoral arteries.
- Listen for bruits.

### Peritoneal Friction Rubs

| | | |
|---|---|---|
| • Peritoneal friction rubs are rough, grating sounds like two pieces of leather rubbing together. Friction rubs may be caused by inflammation, infection, or abnormal growths.<br>• To auscultate the splenic site, place the stethoscope over the left lower rib cage in the anterior axillary line, and ask the client to take a deep breath. A deep breath may accentuate the sound of a friction rub area.<br>• To auscultate the liver site, place the stethoscope over the lower right rib cage. | | Loud bruit over aortic area (possible aneurysm)<br>Bruit over renal or iliac arteries |

*(continued)*

| Assessment | Normal Findings | Deviations from Normal |
|---|---|---|

### Percussion of the Abdomen

11. Percuss several areas in each of the four quadrants to determine presence of tympany (gas in stomach and intestines) and dullness (decrease, absence, or flatness of resonance over solid masses or fluid). Use a systematic pattern: Begin in the lower right quadrant, proceed to the upper right quadrant, the upper left quadrant, and the lower left quadrant.

Tympany over the stomach and gas-filled bowels; dullness, especially over the liver and spleen, or a full bladder

Large dull areas (associated with presence of fluid or a tumor)

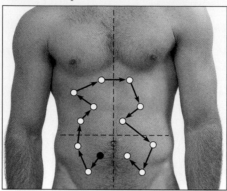

● Systematic percussion sites for all four abdominal quadrants.

### Palpation of the Abdomen

12. Perform light palpation first to detect areas of tenderness and/or muscle guarding. Systematically explore all four quadrants. Ensure that the client's position is appropriate for relaxation of the abdominal muscles, and warm the hands. ➤*Rationale: Cold hands can elicit muscle tension and thus impede palpatory evaluation.*

No tenderness; relaxed abdomen with smooth, consistent tension

Tenderness and hypersensitivity
Superficial masses
Localized areas of increased tension

### Light Palpation

- Hold the palm of your hand slightly above the client's abdomen, with your fingers parallel to the abdomen.
- Depress the abdominal wall lightly, about 1 cm or to the depth of the subcutaneous tissue, with the pads of your fingers.
- Move the finger pads in a slight circular motion.
- Note areas of tenderness or superficial pain, masses, and muscle guarding. To determine areas of tenderness, ask the client to tell you about them and watch for changes in the client's facial expressions.
- If the client is excessively ticklish, begin by pressing your hand on top of the client's hand while pressing lightly. Then slide your hand off the client's and onto the abdomen to continue the examination.

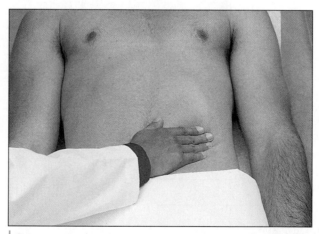

● Light palpation of the abdomen.

| Assessment | Normal Findings | Deviations from Normal |
|---|---|---|
| **Palpation of the Bladder**<br>13. Palpate the area above the pubic symphysis if the client's history indicates possible urinary retention. | Not palpable<br>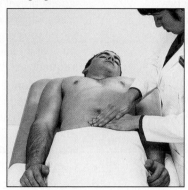<br>● Palpating the bladder. | Distended and palpable as smooth, round, tense mass (indicates urinary retention) |

14. Document findings in the client record using forms or checklists supplemented by narrative notes when appropriate.

## Documentation

Sample: 6/10/09 0945 c/o "gassy" pain lower right quadrant. No bowel movement × 48 hrs. Ate 75% regular diet yesterday. Abdomen flat. Active bowel sounds all 4 quadrants. Tympany above umbilicus, dull below. No masses felt on palpation. 30 mL Milk of Magnesia given.

N. Schmidt, RN

## SETTING OF CARE

- Be sure you have the required equipment on a home visit, including a tape measure and skin-marking pen.
- Use pillows to position the client.
- Undressing the client to perform a complete abdominal examination may not be necessary. Focus the assessment on areas indicated by the history and present complaint.

## DEVELOPMENTAL CONSIDERATIONS

### Infants

- Internal organs of newborns and infants are proportionately larger than those of older children and adults, so their abdomens are rounded and tend to protrude.
- Umbilical hernias may be present at birth.

### Children

- Toddlers have a characteristic "pot belly" appearance, which can persist until age 3 to 4 years.
- Late preschool and school-age children are leaner than toddlers and have a flat abdomen.
- Peristaltic waves may be more visible than in adults.
- Children may not be able to pinpoint areas of tenderness; by observing facial expressions the examiner can determine areas of maximum tenderness.

- If the child is ticklish, guarding, or fearful, use a task that requires concentration (such as squeezing the hands together) to distract the child, or have the child place his or her hands on yours as you palpate the abdomen, "helping" you to do the exam.

### Elders

- The rounded abdomens of elders are due to an increase in adipose tissue and a decrease in muscle tone.
- The abdominal wall is slacker and thinner, making palpation easier and more accurate than in younger clients. Muscle wasting and loss of fibroconnective tissue occur.
- The pain threshold in elders is often higher; major abdominal problems such as appendicitis or other acute emergencies may therefore go undetected.

*(continued)*

## DEVELOPMENTAL CONSIDERATIONS (CONTINUED)

- Gastrointestinal pain needs to be differentiated from cardiac pain. Gastrointestinal pain may be located in the thorax or abdomen, whereas cardiac pain is usually located in the thorax. However, these relationships are not absolute because cardiac abnormalities may present as gastrointestinal complaints, especially in women. Factors aggravating gastrointestinal pain are usually related to either ingestion or lack of food intake; gastrointestinal pain is usually relieved by antacids, food, or assuming an upright position. Common factors that can aggravate cardiac pain are activity or anxiety. Rest or nitroglycerin relieves cardiac pain.

- Stool passes through the intestines at a slower rate in elders, and the perception of stimuli that produce the urge to defecate often diminishes.

- Fecal incontinence may occur in confused or neurologically impaired older adults.

- Many elders erroneously believe that the absence of a daily bowel movement signifies constipation. When assessing for constipation, the nurse must consider the client's diet, activity, medications, and characteristics and ease of passage of feces as well as the frequency of bowel movements.

- The incidence of colon cancer is higher among elders than younger adults. Symptoms include a change in bowel function, rectal bleeding, and weight loss. Changes in bowel function, however, are associated with many factors, such as diet, exercise, and medications.

- Decreased absorption of oral medications often occurs with aging.

- In the liver, impaired metabolism of some drugs may occur with aging.

## Skill 11.16   Assessing the Musculoskeletal System

### Delegation

Assessment of the musculoskeletal system is not delegated to UAP. However, many aspects of its functioning are observed during usual care and may be recorded by persons other than the nurse. Abnormal findings must be validated and interpreted by the nurse.

### Equipment

- Goniometer
- Tape measure

### Procedure

1. Prior to performing the procedure, introduce self and verify the client's identity using agency protocol. Explain to the client what you are going to do, why it is necessary, and how he or she can participate. Discuss how the results will be used in planning further care or treatments.
2. Perform hand hygiene and observe appropriate infection control procedures.
3. Provide for client privacy.
4. Inquire if the client has any history of the following: presence of muscle or joint pain: onset, location, character, associated phenomena (e.g., redness and swelling of joints), and aggravating and alleviating factors; limitations to movement or inability to perform activities of daily living; previous sports injuries; loss of function without pain.

### SETTING OF CARE

- When making a home visit, observe the client in natural movement around the living area. To assess children, have them remove their clothes down to the underwear.

- A complete examination of joints, bone, and muscles may not be necessary. Focus the assessment on areas indicated by the history and present complaint.

| Assessment | Normal Findings | Deviations from Normal |
|---|---|---|
| 5. Inspect the muscles for size. Compare the muscles on one side of the body (e.g., of the arm, thigh, and calf) to the same muscle on the other side. For any discrepancies, measure the muscles with a tape. | Equal size on both sides of body | Atrophy (a decrease in size) or hypertrophy (an increase in size)<br>Asymmetry |
| 6. Inspect the muscles and tendons for contractures (shortening). | No contractures | Malpositition of body part, e.g., foot drop (foot flexed downward) |
| 7. Inspect the muscles for tremors, for example, by having the client hold the arms out in front of the body. | No tremors | Presence of tremor |
| 8. Test muscle strength. Compare the right side with the left side.<br>*Sternocleidomastoid:* Client turns the head to one side against the resistance of your hand. Repeat with the other side.<br>*Trapezius:* Client shrugs the shoulders against the resistance of your hands.<br>*Deltoid:* Client holds arm up and resists while you try to push it down.<br>*Biceps:* Client fully extends each arm and tries to flex it while you attempt to hold arm in extension.<br>*Triceps:* Client flexes each arm and then tries to extend it against your attempt to keep arm in flexion.<br>*Wrist and finger muscles:* Client spreads the fingers and resists as you attempt to push the fingers together.<br>*Grip strength:* Client grasps your index and middle fingers while you try to pull the fingers out.<br>*Hip muscles:* Client is supine, both legs extended; client raises one leg at a time while you attempt to hold it down.<br>*Hip abduction:* Client is supine, both legs extended. Place your hands on the lateral surface of each knee; client spreads the legs apart against your resistance.<br>*Hip adduction:* Client is in same position as for hip abduction. Place your hands between the knees; client brings the legs together against your resistance.<br>*Hamstrings:* Client is supine, both knees bent. Client resists while you attempt to straighten the legs.<br>*Quadriceps:* Client is supine, knee partially extended; client resists while you attempt to flex the knee.<br>*Muscles of the ankles and feet:* Client resists while you attempt to dorsiflex the foot and again resists while you attempt to flex the foot. | Equal strength on each body side 25% or less of normal strength | **Grading Muscle Strength**<br>**0:** 0% of normal strength; complete paralysis<br>**1:** 10% of normal strength; no movement, contraction of muscle is palpable or visible<br>**2:** 25% of normal strength; full muscle movement against gravity, with support<br>**3:** 50% of normal strength; normal movement against gravity<br>**4:** 75% of normal strength; normal full movement against gravity and against minimal resistance<br>**5:** 100% of normal strength; normal full movement against gravity and against full resistance |

*(continued)*

| Assessment | Normal Findings | Deviations from Normal |
|---|---|---|
| **Bones** | | |
| 9. Inspect the skeleton for structure. | No deformities | Bones misaligned |
| 10. Palpate the bones to locate any areas of edema or tenderness. | No tenderness or swelling | Presence of tenderness or swelling (may indicate fracture, neoplasms, or osteoporosis) |
| **Joints** | | |
| 11. Inspect the joint for swelling. Palpate each joint for tenderness, smoothness of movement, swelling, crepitation, and presence of nodules. | No swelling<br>No tenderness, swelling, crepitation or nodules<br>Joints move smoothly | One or more swollen joints<br>Presence of tenderness, swelling, crepitation, or nodules |
| 12. Assess joint range of motion.<br>• Ask the client to move selected body parts. The amount of joint movement can be measured by a **goniometer,** a device that measures the angle of the joint in degrees. | Varies to some degree in accordance with person's genetic makeup and degree of physical activity<br><br>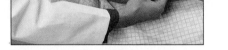<br>● A goniometer used to measure joint angle. | Limited range of motion in one or more joints |
| 13. Document findings in the client record using forms or checklists supplemented by narrative notes when appropriate. | | |

## DEVELOPMENTAL CONSIDERATIONS

### Infants

- Palpate the clavicles of newborns. A mass and crepitus may indicate a fracture experienced during vaginal delivery. The newborn may also have limited movement of the arm and shoulder on the affected side.
- When the arms and legs of newborns are pulled to extension and released, newborns naturally return to the flexed fetal position.
- Check muscle strength by holding the infant lightly under the arms with feet placed lightly on a table. Infants should not fall through the hands and should be able to bear body weight on their legs if normal muscle strength is present.
- Check infants for developmental dysplasia of the hip (congenital dislocation) by examining for asymmetric gluteal folds, asymmetric abduction of the legs (Ortolani and Barlow tests), or apparent shortening of the femur.
- Infants should be able to sit without support by 8 months of age, crawl by 7 to 10 months, and walk by 12 to 15 months.
- Observe for symmetry of muscle mass, strength, and function.

### Children

- Pronation and "toeing in" of the feet are common in children between 12 and 30 months of age.
- Genu varum (bowleg) is normal in children for about 1 year after beginning to walk.
- Genu valgus (knock-knee) is normal in preschool and early school-age children.

## DEVELOPMENTAL CONSIDERATIONS (CONTINUED)

- Lordosis (swayback) is common in children before age 5.
- Observe the child in normal activities to determine motor function.
- During the rapid growth spurts of adolescence, spinal curvature and rotation (scoliosis) may appear. Children should be assessed for scoliosis by age 12 and annually until their growth slows. Curvature greater than 10% should be referred for further medical evaluation.
- Muscle mass increases in adolescence, especially as children engage in strenuous physical activity, and requires increased nutritional intake.
- Children are at risk for injury related to physical activity and should be assessed for nutritional status, physical conditioning, and safety precautions in order to prevent injury.

- Adolescent girls who participate in strenuous athletic activities are at risk for delayed menses, osteoporosis, and eating disorders; assessment should include a history of these factors.

**Elders**

- Muscle mass decreases progressively with age, but there are wide variations among different individuals.
- The decrease in speed, strength, resistance to fatigue, reaction time, and coordination in the older person is due to a decrease in nerve conduction and muscle tone.
- The bones become more fragile and osteoporosis leads to a loss of total bone mass. As a result, elders are predisposed to fractures and compressed vertebrae.
- In most elders, osteoarthritic changes in the joints can be observed.
- Note any surgical scars from joint replacement surgeries.

# Skill 11.17   Assessing the Neurologic System

## Delegation

Due to the substantial knowledge and skill required, assessment of the neurologic system is not delegated to UAP. However, many aspects of neurologic behavior are observed during usual care and may be recorded by persons other than the nurse. Abnormal findings must be validated and interpreted by the nurse.

## Equipment (Depending on Components of Examination)

- Percussion hammer
- Wisps of cotton to assess light-touch sensation
- Sterile safety pin for tactile discrimination

## Procedure

1. Prior to performing the procedure, introduce self and verify the client's identity using agency protocol. Explain to the client what you are going to do, why it is necessary, and how he or she can participate. Discuss how the results will be used in planning further care or treatments.
2. Perform hand hygiene and observe appropriate infection control procedures.
3. Provide for client privacy.
4. Inquire if the client has any history of the following: presence of pain in the head, back, or extremities, as well as onset and aggravating and alleviating factors; disorientation to time, place, or person; speech dis-

order; history of loss of consciousness, fainting, convulsions, trauma, tingling or numbness, tremors or tics, limping, paralysis, uncontrolled muscle movements, loss of memory, mood swings, or problems with smell, vision, taste, touch, or hearing.

### CLINICAL ALERT

All questions and tests used in a neurologic examination must be age, language, education level, and culturally appropriate. Individualize questions and tests before using them.

## Language

5. If the client displays difficulty speaking:
   - Point to common objects and ask the client to name them.
   - Ask the client to read some words and to match the printed and written words with pictures.
   - Ask the client to respond to simple verbal and written commands, for example, "point to your toes" or "raise your left arm."

## Orientation

6. Determine the client's orientation to *time, place,* and *person* by tactful questioning. Ask the client the time of day, date, day of the week, city and state of residence, duration of illness, and names of family members. Ask the client why he or she is seeing a

health care provider. Orientation is lost gradually, and early disorientation may be very subtle. "Why" questions may elicit a more accurate clinical picture of the client's orientation status than questions directed to time, place, and person. To evaluate the response, you must know the correct answer.

More direct questioning may be necessary for some people, for example, "Where are you now?" "What day is it today?" Most people readily accept these questions if initially the nurse asks, "Do you get confused at times?" If the client cannot answer these questions regarding place and time accurately, also include assessment of the *self* by asking the client to state his or her full name.

## Memory

7. Listen for lapses in memory. Ask the client about difficulty with memory. If problems are apparent, three categories of memory are tested: immediate recall, recent memory, and remote memory.

   *To assess immediate recall:*
   - Ask the client to repeat a series of three digits (e.g., 7–4–3), spoken slowly.
   - Gradually increase the number of digits (e.g., 7–4–3–5, 7–4–3–5–6, and 7–4–3–5–6–7), until the client fails to repeat the series correctly.
   - Start again with a series of three digits, but this time ask the client to repeat them backward. The average person can repeat a series of five to eight digits in sequence and four to six digits in reverse order.

   *To assess recent memory:*
   - Ask the client to recall the recent events of the day, such as how the client got to the clinic. This information must be validated, however.
   - Ask the client to recall information given early in the interview (e.g., the name of a doctor).
   - Provide the client with three facts to recall (e.g., a color, an object, and an address), and ask the client to repeat all three. Later in the interview, ask the client to recall all three items.

   *To assess remote memory,* ask the client to describe a previous illness or surgery (e.g., 5 years ago) or a birthday or anniversary. Generally remote memory will be intact until late in neurologic pathology. It is least useful to assess for acute neurologic problems.

## Attention Span and Calculation

8. Test the ability to concentrate or maintain *attention span* by asking the client to recite the alphabet or to count backward from 100. Test the ability to calculate by asking the client to subtract 7 or 3 progressively from 100, that is, 100, 93, 86, 79, or 100, 97, 94, 91 (referred to as *serial sevens* or *serial threes*). Normally, an adult can complete the serial sevens test in about 90 seconds with three or fewer errors. Because educational level, language, or cultural differences affect calculating ability, this test may be inappropriate for some people.

## Level of Consciousness

9. Apply the Glasgow Coma Scale (Table 11–4): eye response, motor response, and verbal response. An assessment totaling 15 points indicates the client is alert and completely oriented. A comatose client scores 7 or less.

## Cranial Nerves

10. For the specific functions and assessment methods of each cranial nerve, see Table 11–5. Test each

---

### TABLE 11–4 LEVELS OF CONSCIOUSNESS: GLASGOW COMA SCALE

| Faculty Measured | Response | Score |
|---|---|---|
| Eye opening | Spontaneous | 4 |
| | To verbal command | 3 |
| | To pain | 2 |
| | No response | 1 |
| Motor response | To verbal command | 6 |
| | To localized pain | 5 |
| | Flexes and withdraws | 4 |
| | Flexes abnormally | 3 |
| | Extends abnormally | 2 |
| | No response | 1 |
| Verbal response | Oriented, converses | 5 |
| | Disoriented, converses | 4 |
| | Uses inappropriate words | 3 |
| | Makes incomprehensible sounds | 2 |
| | No response | 1 |

## TABLE 11–5 CRANIAL NERVE FUNCTIONS AND ASSESSMENT METHODS

| Cranial Nerve | Name | Type | Function | Assessment Method |
|---|---|---|---|---|
| I | Olfactory | Sensory | Smell | Ask client to close eyes and identify different mild aromas, such as coffee, vanilla, peanut butter, orange/lemon, chocolate. |
| II | Optic | Sensory | Vision and visual fields | Ask client to read Snellen-type chart; check visual fields by confrontation; and conduct an ophthalmoscopic examination (see Skill 11.6). |
| III | Oculomotor | Motor | Extraocular eye movement (EOM); movement of sphincter of pupil; movement of ciliary muscles of lens | Assess six ocular movements and pupil reaction (see Skill 11.6). |
| IV | Trochlear | Motor | EOM; specifically, moves eyeball downward and laterally | Assess six ocular movements (see Skill 11.6). |
| V | Trigeminal Ophthalmic branch | Sensory | Sensation of cornea, skin of face, and nasal mucosa | While client looks upward, lightly touch the lateral sclera of the eye with sterile gauze to elicit blink reflex. To test light sensation, have client close eyes, wipe a wisp of cotton over client's forehead and paranasal sinuses. |
|  | Maxillary branch | Sensory | Sensation of skin of face and anterior oral cavity (tongue and teeth) | Assess skin sensation as for ophthalmic branch above. |
|  | Mandibular branch | Motor and sensory | Muscles of mastication; sensation of skin of face | Ask client to clench teeth. |
| VI | Abducens | Motor | EOM; moves eyeball laterally | Assess directions of gaze. |
| VII | Facial | Motor and sensory | Facial expression; taste (anterior two-thirds of tongue) | Ask client to smile, raise the eyebrows, frown, puff out cheeks, close eyes tightly. Ask client to identify various tastes placed on tip and sides of tongue: sugar (sweet), salt, lemon juice (sour), and quinine (bitter); identify areas of taste. |
| VIII | Auditory Vestibular branch Cochlear branch | Sensory Sensory | Equilibrium Hearing | Romberg test. Assess client's ability to hear spoken word and vibrations of tuning fork. |
| IX | Glossopharyngeal | Motor and sensory | Swallowing ability, tongue movement, taste (posterior tongue) | Apply tastes on posterior tongue for identification. Ask client to move tongue from side to side and up and down. |
| X | Vagus | Motor and sensory | Sensation of pharynx and larynx; swallowing; vocal cord movement | Assessed with cranial nerve IX; assess client's speech for hoarseness. |
| XI | Accessory | Motor | Head movement; shrugging of shoulders | Ask client to shrug shoulders against resistance from your hands and turn head to side against resistance from your hand (repeat for other side). |
| XII | Hypoglossal | Motor | Protrusion of tongue; moves tongue up and down and side to side | Ask client to protrude tongue at midline, then move it side to side. |

nerve not already evaluated in another component of the health assessment. A quick way to remember which cranial nerves are assessed in the face is shown in the figure to the right.

## Reflexes

11. Generalist nurses do not commonly assess each of the deep tendon reflexes except for the plantar (Babinski) reflex, indicative of possible spinal cord injury. Reflexes are reported using the scale below, comparing one side of the body with the other to evaluate the symmetry of response.

> 0 No reflex response
> +1 Minimal activity (hypoactive)
> +2 Normal response
> +3 More active than normal
> +4 Maximal activity (hyperactive)

## Babinski Reflex

- Use a moderately sharp object, such as the handle of the percussion hammer, a key, or an applicator stick.
- Stroke the lateral border of the sole of the client's foot, starting at the heel, continuing to the ball of the foot, and then proceeding across the ball of the foot toward the big toe.
- Observe the response. Normally, all five toes bend downward; this reaction is called a negative Babinski. In an abnormal (positive) Babinski response, the toes spread outward and the big toe moves upward.

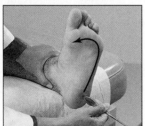

● Testing plantar (Babinski) reflexes.

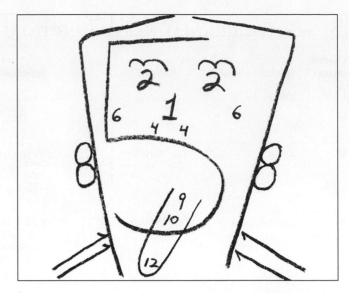

● Cranial nerves by the numbers: The next time you're trying to remember the locations and functions of the cranial nerves, picture this drawing. All twelve cranial nerves are represented, though some may be a little harder to spot than others. For example, the shoulders are formed by the number "11" because cranial nerve XI controls neck and shoulder movement. If you immediately recognize that the sides of the face and the top of the head are formed by the number "7," you're well on your way to using this memory device.

*Source:* © 2006, HealthCom Media. All rights reserved. From *American Nurse Today*, November 2006, Vol 1 No. (2), pg. 21–22 www.americannursetoday.com.

## Motor Function

| Assessment | Normal Findings | Deviations from Normal |
|---|---|---|
| 12. *Gross Motor and Balance Tests:* Generally, the Romberg test and one other gross motor function and balance tests are used. | | |
| **Walking Gait** | | |
| Ask the client to walk across the room and back, and assess the client's gait. | Has upright posture and steady gait with opposing arm swing; walks unaided, maintaining balance | Has poor posture and unsteady, irregular, staggering gait with wide stance; bends legs only from hips; has rigid or no arm movements |

| Assessment | Normal Findings | Deviations from Normal |
|---|---|---|
| **Romberg Test**<br><br>Ask the client to stand with feet together and arms resting at the sides, first with eyes open, then closed. Stand close during this test. ➤*Rationale: This prevents the client from falling.* | *Negative Romberg:* may sway slightly but is able to maintain upright posture and foot stance | *Positive Romberg:* cannot maintain foot stance; moves the feet apart to maintain stance<br>If client cannot maintain balance with the eyes shut, client may have sensory ataxia (lack of coordination of the voluntary muscles)<br>If balance cannot be maintained whether the eyes are open or shut, client may have cerebellar ataxia |
| **Standing on One Foot with Eyes Closed**<br><br>Ask the client to close the eyes and stand on one foot. Repeat on the other foot. Stand close to the client during this test. | Maintains stance for at least 5 seconds | Cannot maintain stance for 5 seconds |
| **Heel–Toe Walking**<br><br>Ask the client to walk a straight line, placing the heel of one foot directly in front of the toes of the other foot. | Maintains heel–toe walking along a straight line | Assumes a wider foot gait to stay upright |

● Heel–toe walking test.

| Assessment | Normal Findings | Deviations from Normal |
|---|---|---|
| **Toe or Heel Walking**<br><br>Ask the client to walk several steps on the toes and then on the heels. | Able to walk several steps on toes or heels | Cannot maintain balance on toes and heels |

*(continued)*

| Assessment | Normal Findings | Deviations from Normal |
|---|---|---|
| 13. *Fine Motor Tests for the Upper Extremities:* | | |

**Finger-to-Nose Test**

| Assessment | Normal Findings | Deviations from Normal |
|---|---|---|
| Ask the client to abduct and extend the arms at shoulder height and then rapidly touch the nose alternately with one index finger and then the other. The client repeats the test with the eyes closed if the test is performed easily. | Repeatedly and rhythmically touches the nose | Misses the nose or gives slow response |

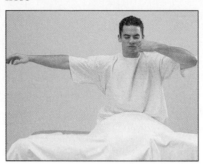

● Finger-to-nose test.

**Alternating Supination and Pronation of Hands on Knees**

| Assessment | Normal Findings | Deviations from Normal |
|---|---|---|
| Ask the client to pat both knees with the palms of both hands and then with the backs of the hands alternately at an ever-increasing rate. | Can alternately supinate and pronate hands at rapid pace | Performs with slow, clumsy movements and irregular timing; has difficulty alternating from supination to pronation |

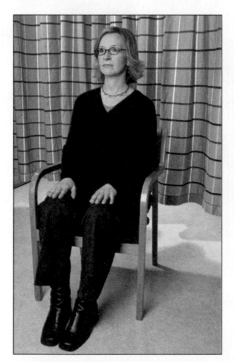 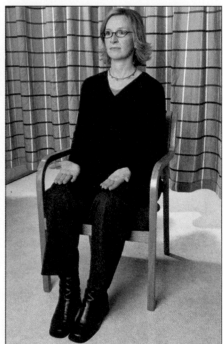

● Alternating supination and pronation of hands on knees test.

| Assessment | Normal Findings | Deviations from Normal |
|---|---|---|

### Finger to Nose and to the Nurse's Finger

Ask the client to touch the nose and then your index finger, held at a distance of about 45 cm (18 in.), at a rapid and increasing rate.

Performs with coordination and rapidity

Misses the finger and moves slowly

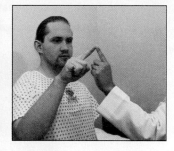

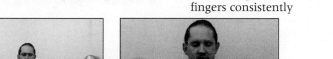

● Finger-to-nose and to the nurse's finger test.

### Fingers to Fingers

Ask the client to spread the arms broadly at shoulder height and then bring the fingers together at the midline, first with the eyes open and then closed, first slowly and then rapidly.

Performs with accuracy and rapidity

Moves slowly and is unable to touch fingers consistently

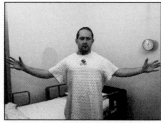

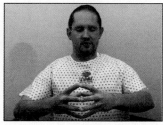

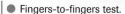

● Fingers-to-fingers test.

### Fingers to Thumb (Same Hand)

Ask the client to touch each finger of one hand to the thumb of the same hand as rapidly as possible.

Rapidly touches each finger to thumb with each hand

Cannot coordinate this fine discrete movement with either one or both hands

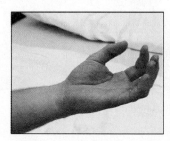

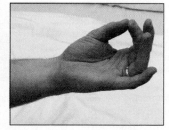

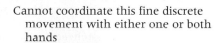

● Fingers-to-thumb (same hand) test.

14. *Fine Motor Tests for the Lower Extremities:* Ask the client to lie supine to perform these tests.

*(continued)*

| Assessment | Normal Findings | Deviations from Normal |
|---|---|---|

**Heel Down Opposite Shin**

Ask the client to place the heel of one foot just below the opposite knee and run the heel down the shin to the foot. Repeat with the other foot. The client may also use a sitting position for this test.

Demonstrates bilateral equal coordination

Has tremors or is awkward; heel moves off shin

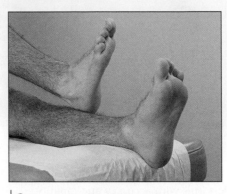

● Heel down opposite shin test.

15. *Light-Touch Sensation:* Compare the light-touch sensation of symmetric areas of the body. ➤*Rationale: Sensitivity to touch varies among different skin areas.*
   - Ask the client to close the eyes and to respond by saying "yes" or "now" whenever the client feels the cotton wisp touching the skin.
   - With a wisp of cotton, lightly touch one specific spot and then the same spot on the other side of the body.
   - Test areas on the forehead, cheek, hand, lower arm, abdomen, foot, and lower leg. Check a distal area of the limb first (i.e., the hand before the arm and the foot before the leg). ➤*Rationale: The sensory nerve may be assumed to be intact if sensation is felt at its most distal part.*
   - If areas of sensory dysfunction are found, determine the boundaries of sensation by testing responses about every 2.5 cm (1 in.) in the area. Make a sketch of the sensory loss area for recording purposes.

Light tickling or touch sensation

Loss of sensation (**anesthesia**); more than normal sensation (**hyperesthesia**); less than normal sensation (**hypoesthesia**); or an abnormal sensation such as burning, pain, or an electric shock (**paresthesia**)

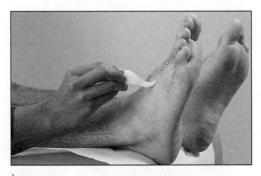

● Assessing light-touch sensation.

16. *Pain Sensation*
   Assess pain sensation as follows:
   - Ask the client to close the eyes and to say "sharp," "dull," or "don't know" when the sharp or dull end of a safety pin is felt.
   - Alternately, use the sharp and dull end to lightly prick designated anatomic areas at random (e.g., hand, forearm, foot, lower leg, abdomen). The face is not tested in this manner.

Able to discriminate "sharp" and "dull" sensations

Areas of reduced, heightened, or absent sensation (map them out for recording purposes)

| Assessment | Normal Findings | Deviations from Normal |
|---|---|---|
| • Allow at least 2 seconds between each test to prevent summation effects of stimuli, i.e., several successive stimuli perceived as one stimulus. | | |
| 17. *Position or Kinesthetic Sensation:* Commonly, the middle fingers and the large toes are tested for the kinesthetic sensation (sense of position).<br>• To test the fingers, support the client's arm and hand with one hand. To test the toes, place the client's heels on the examining table.<br>• Ask the client to close the eyes.<br>• Grasp a middle finger or a big toe firmly between your thumb and index finger, and exert the same pressure on both sides of the finger or toe while moving it.<br>• Move the finger or toe until it is up, down, or straight out, and ask the client to identify the position.<br>• Use a series of brisk up-and-down movements before bringing the finger or toe suddenly to rest in one of the three positions. | Can readily determine the position of fingers and toes<br><br>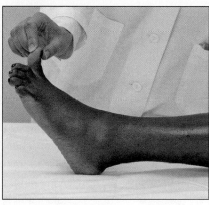<br>● Position or kinesthetic sensation. | Unable to determine the position of one or more fingers or toes |
| 18. Document findings in the client record using forms or checklists supplemented by narrative notes when appropriate. Describe any abnormal findings in objective terms, for example, "When asked to count backwards by threes, client made seven errors and completed the task in 4 minutes." | | |

## DEVELOPMENTAL CONSIDERATIONS

### Infants

- Reflexes commonly tested in newborns include the following:
  - Rooting: Stroke the side of the face near mouth; infant opens mouth and turns to the side that is stroked.
  - Sucking: Place nipple or finger 3 to 4 cm into mouth; infant sucks vigorously.
  - Tonic neck: Place infant supine, turn head to one side; arm on side to which head is turned extends; on opposite side, arm curls up (fencer's pose).
  - Palmar grasp: Place finger in infant's palm and press; infant curls fingers around.
- Stepping: Hold infant as if weight bearing on surface; infant steps along, one foot at a time.
- Moro: Present loud noise or unexpected movement; infant spreads arms and legs, extends fingers, then flexes and brings hands together; may cry.
- Most of these reflexes disappear between 4 and 6 months of age.

### Children

- Present the procedures as games whenever possible.
- Positive Babinski reflex is abnormal after the child ambulates or at age 2.

*(continued)*

## DEVELOPMENTAL CONSIDERATIONS (CONTINUED)

- For children under age 5, the Denver Developmental Screening Test II provides a comprehensive neurologic evaluation—particularly for motor function.
- Note the child's ability to understand and follow directions.
- Assess immediate recall or recent memory by using names of cartoon characters. Normal recall in children is one less than age in years.
- Assess for signs of hyperactivity or abnormally short attention span.
- Children should be able to walk backward by age 2, balance on one foot for 5 seconds by age 4, heel–toe walk by age 5, and heel–toe walk backward by age 6.
- The Romberg test is appropriate over age 3.

### Elders

- A full neurologic assessment can be lengthy. Conduct in several sessions if indicated, and cease the tests if the client is noticeably fatigued.
- A decline in mental status is not a normal result of aging. Changes are more the result of physical or psychologic disorders (e.g., fever, fluid and electrolyte imbalances, medications). Acute, abrupt-onset mental status changes are usually caused by delirium. These changes are often reversible with treatment. Chronic subtle insidious mental health changes are usually caused by dementia and are usually irreversible.
- Intelligence and learning ability are unaltered with age. Many factors, however, inhibit learning (e.g., anxiety, illness, pain, cultural barrier).
- Short-term memory is often less efficient. Long-term memory is usually unaltered.

- Because old age is often associated with loss of support persons, depression is a common disorder. Mood changes, weight loss, anorexia, constipation, and early morning awakening may be symptoms of depression.
- The stress of being in unfamiliar situations can cause confusion in elders.
- As a person ages, reflex responses may become less intense.
- Because elders tire more easily than younger clients, a total neurologic assessment is often done at a different time from the other parts of the physical assessment.
- Although there is a progressive decrease in the number of functioning neurons in the central nervous system and in the sense organs, elders usually function well because of the abundant reserves in the number of brain cells.
- Impulse transmission and reaction to stimuli are slower.
- Many elders have some impairment of hearing, vision, smell, temperature and pain sensation, memory, and mental endurance.
- Coordination changes, including a reduced speed of fine finger movements. Standing balance remains intact, and Romberg's test remains negative.
- Reflex responses may slightly increase or decrease. Many show loss of Achilles reflex, and the plantar reflex may be difficult to elicit.
- When testing sensory function, the nurse needs to give elders time to respond. Normally, elders have unaltered perception of light touch and superficial pain, decreased perception of deep pain, and decreased perception of temperature stimuli. Many also reveal a decrease or absence of position sense in the large toes.

# Skill 11.18  Assessing the Female Genitals and Inguinal Area

## Delegation

Due to the substantial knowledge and skill required, assessment of the female genitals and inguinal lymph nodes is not delegated to UAP. However, persons other than the nurse may record any aspect of the genital system that is observed during usual care. Abnormal findings must be validated and interpreted by the nurse.

## Equipment

- Clean gloves
- Drape
- Supplemental lighting, if needed

## Procedure

1. Prior to performing the procedure, introduce self and verify the client's identity using agency protocol. Explain to the client what you are going to do, why it is necessary, and how she can participate. Discuss how the results will be used in planning further care or treatments.
2. Perform hand hygiene, apply gloves, and observe appropriate infection control procedures.
3. Provide for client privacy. Request the presence of another woman if desired, required by agency policy, or requested by the client.

4. Inquire regarding the following: age of onset of menstruation, date of last menstrual period (LMP), regularity of cycle, duration, amount of daily flow, and whether menstruation is painful; incidence of pain during intercourse; vaginal discharge; number of pregnancies, number of live births, labor or delivery complications; urgency and frequency of urination at night; blood in urine, painful urination, incontinence; history of sexually transmitted infection, past and present.

5. Cover the pelvic area with a sheet or drape at all times when not actually being examined. Position the client supine.

| Assessment | Normal Findings | Deviations from Normal |
|---|---|---|
| 6. Inspect the distribution, amount, and characteristics of pubic hair. | There are wide variations; generally kinky in the menstruating adult, thinner and straighter after menopause<br>Distributed in the shape of an inverse triangle | Scant pubic hair (may indicate hormonal problem)<br>Hair growth should not extend over the abdomen |
| 7. Inspect the skin of the pubic area for parasites, inflammation, swelling, and lesions. To assess pubic skin adequately, separate the labia majora and labia minora. | Pubic skin intact, no lesions<br>Skin of vulva area slightly darker than the rest of the body<br>Minimal odor<br>Labia round, full, and relatively symmetric in adult females | Lice, lesions, scars, fissures, swelling, erythema, excoriations, varicosities, or leukoplakia<br>Malodorous discharge; thin, friable labia; protruding uterus |
| 8. Palpate the inguinal lymph nodes. Use the pads of the fingers in a rotary motion, noting any enlargement or tenderness. | No enlargement or tenderness.<br><br>Superior or horizontal group<br>Inferior or vertical group<br>● Lymph nodes of the groin area. | Enlargement and tenderness |
| 9. Remove and discard gloves. Perform hand hygiene. | | |
| 10. Document findings in the client record using forms or checklists supplemented by narrative notes when appropriate. | | |

## DEVELOPMENTAL CONSIDERATIONS

### Infants

- Infants can be held in a supine position on the parent's lap with the knees supported in a flexed position and separated.
- In newborns, because of maternal estrogen, the labia and clitoris may be edematous and enlarged, and there may be a small amount of white or bloody vaginal discharge.
- Assess the mons and inguinal area for swelling or tenderness that may indicate presence of an inguinal hernia.

### Children

- Ensure that you have the parent or guardian's approval to perform the examination and then tell the child what you are going to do. Preschool children are taught not to allow others to touch their "private parts."

*(continued)*

## DEVELOPMENTAL CONSIDERATIONS (CONTINUED)

- Girls should be assessed for Tanner staging of pubertal development (see Box 11–2).
- Girls should be referred to a primary care provider for a Papanicolaou (Pap) test if sexually active, or by age 18 years.
- The clitoris is a common site for syphilitic chancres in younger females.

### Elders

- Labia are atrophied and flatter in older females.
- The clitoris is a potential site for cancerous lesions in older females.
- The vulva atrophies as a result of a reduction in vascularity, elasticity, adipose tissue, and estrogen levels. Because the vulva is more fragile, it is more easily irritated.

- The vaginal environment becomes drier and more alkaline, resulting in an alteration of the type of flora present and a predisposition to vaginitis. Dyspareunia (difficult or painful intercourse) is also a common occurrence.
- The cervix and uterus decrease in size.
- The fallopian tubes and ovaries atrophy.
- Ovulation and estrogen production cease.
- Vaginal bleeding unrelated to estrogen therapy is abnormal in older women.
- Prolapse of the uterus can occur in older females, especially those who have had multiple pregnancies.

## BOX 11–2 FIVE STAGES OF PUBIC HAIR DEVELOPMENT IN FEMALES

*Stage 1:* Preadolescence. No pubic hair except for fine body hair.

*Stage 2:* Usually occurs at ages 11 and 12. Sparse, long, slightly pigmented curly hair develops along the labia.

*Stage 3:* Usually occurs at ages 12 and 13. Hair becomes darker in color and curlier and develops over the pubic symphysis.

*Stage 4:* Usually occurs between ages 13 and 14. Hair assumes the texture and curl of the adult but is not as thick and does not appear on the thighs.

*Stage 5:* Sexual maturity. Hair assumes adult appearance and appears on the inner aspect of the upper thighs.

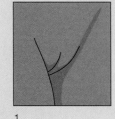 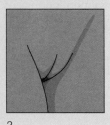
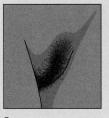 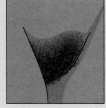 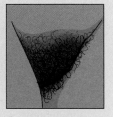

● Stages of female pubic hair development.

# Skill 11.19 Assessing the Male Genitalia and Inguinal Area

### Delegation

Due to the substantial knowledge and skill required, assessment of the male genitals and inguinal area is not delegated to UAP. However, persons other than the nurse may record any aspect of the genital system that is observed during usual care. Abnormal findings must be validated and interpreted by the nurse.

### Equipment

- Clean gloves

### Procedure

1. Prior to performing the procedure, introduce self and verify the client's identity using agency protocol. Explain to the client what you are going to do, why it is necessary, and how he can participate. Discuss how the results will be used in planning further care or treatments.

2. Perform hand hygiene, apply gloves, and observe appropriate infection control procedures.
3. Provide for client privacy. Request the presence of another person if desired, required by agency policy, or requested by the client.
4. Inquire if the client has any history of the following: usual voiding patterns and changes, bladder control, urinary incontinence, frequency, urgency, abdominal pain; symptoms of sexually transmitted infection; swellings that could indicate presence of hernia; family history of nephritis, malignancy of the prostate, or malignancy of the kidney.
5. Cover the pelvic area with a sheet or drape at all times when not actually being examined.

| Assessment | Normal Findings | Deviations from Normal |
|---|---|---|
| **Pubic Hair** | | |
| 6. Inspect the distribution, amount, and characteristics of pubic hair. | Triangular distribution, often spreading up the abdomen | Scant amount or absence of hair |
| **Penis** | | |
| 7. Inspect the penile shaft and glans penis for lesions, nodules, swellings, and inflammation. | Penile skin intact<br>Appears slightly wrinkled and varies in color as widely as other body skin<br>Foreskin easily retractable from the glans penis<br>Small amount of thick white smegma between the glans and foreskin | Presence of lesions, nodules, swellings, or inflammation |
| 8. Inspect the urethral meatus for swelling, inflammation, and discharge.<br>• Compress or ask the client to compress the glans slightly to open the urethral meatus to inspect it for discharge. | Pink and slitlike appearance<br>Positioned at the tip of the penis | Inflammation; discharge<br>Variation in meatal locations (e.g., hypospadias, on the underside of the penile shaft, and epispadias, on the upper side of the penile shaft) |
| **Scrotum** | | |
| 9. Inspect the scrotum for appearance, general size, and symmetry.<br>• To facilitate inspection of the scrotum during a physical examination, ask the client to hold the penis out of the way.<br>• Inspect all skin surfaces by spreading the rugated surface skin and lifting the scrotum as needed to observe posterior surfaces. | Scrotal skin is darker in color than that of the rest of the body and is loose<br>Size varies with temperature changes (the dartos muscles contract when the area is cold and relax when the area is warm)<br>Scrotum appears asymmetric (left testis is usually lower than right testis) | Discolorations; any tightening of skin (may indicate edema or mass)<br>Marked asymmetry in size |
| **Inguinal Area** | | |
| 10. Inspect both inguinal areas for bulges while the client is standing, if possible.<br>• First, have the client remain at rest.<br>• Next, have the client hold his breath and strain or bear down as though having a bowel movement. Bearing down may make the hernia more visible. | No swelling or bulges | Swelling or bulge (possible inguinal or femoral hernia) |
| 11. Remove and discard gloves. Perform hand hygiene. | | |
| 12. Document findings in the client record using forms or checklists supplemented by narrative notes when appropriate. | | |

# DEVELOPMENTAL CONSIDERATIONS

## Infants

- The foreskin of the uncircumcised infant is normally tight at birth and should not be retracted. It will gradually loosen as the baby grows and is usually fully retractable by 2 to 3 years of age. Assess for cleanliness, redness, or irritation.
- Assess for placement of the urethral meatus.
- Palpate the scrotum to determine if the testes are descended; in the newborn and infant, the testes may retract into the inguinal canal, especially with stimulation of the cremasteric reflex.
- Assess the inguinal area for swelling or tenderness that may indicate presence of an inguinal hernia.

## Children

- Ensure that you have the parent or guardian's approval to perform the examination and then tell the child what you are going to do. Preschool children are taught not to allow others to touch their "private parts."

- In young boys, the cremasteric reflex can cause the testes to ascend into the inguinal canal. If possible have the boy sit cross-legged; this stretches the muscle and decreases the reflex.
- Table 11–6 shows the five Tanner stages of development of pubic hair, penis, and testes/scrotum.

## Elders

- The penis decreases in size with age; the size and firmness of the testes decrease.
- Testosterone is produced in smaller amounts.
- More time and direct physical stimulation are required for an older man to achieve an erection, but he can maintain the erection for a longer period before ejaculation than he could at a younger age.
- Seminal fluid is reduced in amount and viscosity.
- Urinary frequency, nocturia, dribbling, and problems with beginning and ending the stream are usually the result of prostatic enlargement.

## TABLE 11–6 TANNER STAGES OF MALE PUBIC HAIR AND EXTERNAL GENITAL DEVELOPMENT (12 TO 16 YEARS)

| Stage | Pubic Hair | Penis | Testes/Scrotum |
|---|---|---|---|
| | None, except for body hair like that on the abdomen | Size is relative to body size, as in childhood | Size is relative to body size, as in childhood |
| | Scant, long, slightly pigmented at base of penis | Slight enlargement occurs | Becomes reddened in color and enlarged |
| | Darker, begins to curl and becomes more coarse; extends over pubic symphysis | Elongation occurs | Continuing enlargement |
| | Continues to darken and thicken; extends on the sides, above and below | Increase in both breadth and length; glans develops | Continuing enlargement; color darkens |
| | Adult distribution that extends to inner thighs, umbilicus, and anus | Adult appearance | Adult appearance |

# Skill 11.20   Assessing the Anus

## Delegation

Assessment of the anus is not delegated to UAP. However, the condition of the anal area may be observed during usual care and may be recorded by persons other than the nurse. Abnormal findings must be validated and interpreted by the nurse.

## Equipment

- Clean gloves

## Procedure

1. Prior to performing the procedure, introduce self and verify the client's identity using agency protocol. Explain to the client what you are going to do, why it is necessary, and how he or she can participate. Discuss how the results will be used in planning further care or treatments.
2. Perform hand hygiene, apply gloves, and observe appropriate infection control procedures for all rectal examinations.
3. Provide for client privacy. Drape the client appropriately to prevent undue exposure of body parts.
4. Inquire if the client has any history of the following: bright blood in stools, tarry black stools, diarrhea, constipation, abdominal pain, excessive gas, hemorrhoids, or rectal pain; family history of colorectal cancer; when last stool specimen for occult blood was performed and the results; and for males, if not obtained during the genitourinary examination, signs or symptoms of prostate enlargement (e.g., slow urinary stream, hesitance, frequency, dribbling, and nocturia).
5. Position the client in a left lateral or Sims' position with the upper leg acutely flexed. A dorsal recumbent position with hips externally rotated and knees flexed may also be used. For males, a standing position while the client bends over the examining table may also be used.

| Assessment | Normal Findings | Deviations from Normal |
|---|---|---|
| 6. Inspect the anus and surrounding tissue for color, integrity, and skin lesions. Then, ask the client to bear down as though defecating. Bearing down creates slight pressure on the skin that may accentuate rectal fissures, rectal prolapse, polyps, or internal hemorrhoids. Describe the location of all abnormal findings in terms of a clock, with the 12 o'clock position toward the pubic symphysis. | Intact perianal skin; usually slightly more pigmented than the skin of the buttocks<br>Anal skin is normally more pigmented, coarser, and moister than perianal skin and is usually hairless | Presence of fissures (cracks), ulcers, excoriations, inflammations, abscesses, protruding hemorrhoids (dilated veins seen as reddened protrusions of the skin), lumps or tumors, fistula openings, or rectal prolapse (varying degrees of protrusion of the rectal mucous membrane through the anus) |
| 7. Remove and discard gloves. Perform hand hygiene. | | |
| 8. Document findings in the client record using forms or checklists supplemented by narrative notes when appropriate. | | |

## DEVELOPMENTAL CONSIDERATIONS

### Infants

- Lightly touching the anus should result in a brief anal contraction ("wink" reflex).

### Children

- Erythema and scratch marks around the anus may indicate a pinworm parasite. Children with this condition may be disturbed by itching during sleep.

### Elders

- Chronic constipation and straining at stool cause an increase in the frequency of hemorrhoids and rectal prolapse.

# Skill 11.21   Assessing the Client in Pain

## Delegation

The nurse is responsible for the initial and regular reassessment of pain. As the fifth vital sign, it may be that unlicensed assistive personnel (UAP) most frequently assess clients for pain if they are responsible for vital signs. After the assessment and in collaboration with the client, the nurse can discuss and delegate the performance of appropriate comfort measures to UAP. For example, the UAP may reposition the client at regular intervals, give the client a back massage, or provide rest periods. Emphasize to the UAP the importance of reporting any changes in the client's pain to the nurse.

## Equipment

- Pain assessment flow sheet (see figure on following page)
- Pain rating scale

## Preparation

- Identify those factors that may cause the client to be in pain. For example, does the client have a prior history of low back pain or diabetic neuropathy? Has the client had a major surgical procedure? Has the client experienced recent trauma? Note the client's baseline vital signs.

## Procedure

1. Prior to performing the procedure, introduce self and verify the client's identity using agency protocol. Explain to the client what you are going to do, why it is necessary, and how he or she can participate. Discuss how the results will be used in planning further care or treatments.
2. Perform hand hygiene and observe other appropriate infection control procedures.
3. Provide for client privacy.
4. Assess client's perception of pain. For clients experiencing acute or severe pain, the nurse may focus on the first three aspects of the assessment—determining location, intensity, and quality—and quickly follow with an intervention. Clients with less severe or chronic pain can usually provide a more detailed description and the nurse can obtain a comprehensive pain assessment.
   - *Location.* Ask the client to place a mark on the figure on the pain assessment flow sheet or form with figure, if appropriate. If there is more than one area of pain, use letters (e.g., A, B, C) to differentiate between the various

sites. If the client is unable or unwilling to mark the figure, ask the client to tell you where the pain is located. Follow up by asking the client to point to the painful site with one finger. ➤*Rationale: This will help verify if the verbal description and the location are the same.*
   - *Intensity.* Ask the client to rate the pain using the appropriate scale per agency policy.
   - *Quality.* Ask the client, "What words would you use to describe your pain?" ➤*Rationale: Although this question may be difficult for the client to answer, the assessment is most accurate when the client provides the description.*
   - *Onset, duration, and recurrence.* This assessment can include such questions as "How long have you been having pain?" "Have you noticed any activity (e.g., swallowing, eating, stress, urinating, exertion) that increases or decreases the pain?" "How long does the pain last?" "How often does the pain occur?" "Is the pain better or worse at certain times of the day or night?"
   - *Manner of expressing pain.* Observe for behavioral cues such as grimacing, crying, or a change in body posture. ➤*Rationale: Learning how a client expresses pain is particularly important for the client who cannot communicate or is very young, very old, or unable to hear.*
   - *Precipitating factors.* Ask what causes or increases the pain. ➤*Rationale: Knowledge of those activities can both help prevent the pain from occurring and, sometimes, help determine the cause.*
   - *Alleviating factors.* Ask questions such as "What makes the pain go away or lessen?" "What methods of relief have you tried?" "How long did you use them?" "How effective were they?" ➤*Rationale: Asking these questions can assist the nurse and the client to determine if some of the methods (such as listening to music or relaxation) can continue to be used while at the health care facility.*
   - *Associated symptoms.* Ask if there are any other symptoms (e.g., nausea, vomiting, dizziness) that occur prior to, with, or after the pain. ➤*Rationale: These symptoms may relate to the onset of the pain or may result from the presence of the pain.*
   - *Effects of pain.* Explore the client's feelings and the effect the pain has on the client's life. This is particularly important for the client with chronic pain. ➤*Rationale: Assessing the areas of sleep, appetite, physical activity, relationships, emotions, and concentration provides the nurse with information about the level of the client's functioning on a daily basis.*
   - *Other comments.* Ask if there is any other information that would be helpful for the primary care providers and nurses to know. Emphasize that you want to work with the client and family to get the best control of the pain.

Sunrise Hospital and Medical Center & Sunrise Children's Hospital
**Pain Management Flow Sheet**

SR-1420 (6/00)

***Monitoring Guidelines outlined on back of form**

**Patient's stated pain level goal:__________**

**Mode of Administration**

**A**-PO opioid and nonopioid medications
**B**-PCA Infuser Basal with Patient Control
**C**-Continuous Infusion
**D**-Epidural Infuser Continuous Basal Only
**E**-Epidural Infuser Basal & Patient Control
**F**-Intermittent IV/IM Injection
**G**-Transdermal opioids
**H**-On-QPump
**I**-Per Rectum

**Level of Pain Assessment Scales**

**Faces Pain Rating Scale**

0 ............2..............4..............6............8.............10

1-10 Pain Scale

0 - - - - - - - - - - - - - - - - 10

No pain or pain relieved — Worst pain imaginable

**0-10 Sum Scale**

**A. Vocal**
**0** = Positive/ETT
**1** = Whimpers
**2** = Crying
**3** = Screaming

**C. Facial**
**0** = Smiling
**1** = Neutral
**2** = Frown/grimace
**3** = Clenched teeth

**B. Body Movement**
**0** = Moves easily
**1** = Neutral shifting
**2** = Tense/flailing limbs

**D. Touching (localizing)**
**0** = Notouching
**1** = Reaching/patting
**2** = Grabbing

**Location of Pain:**

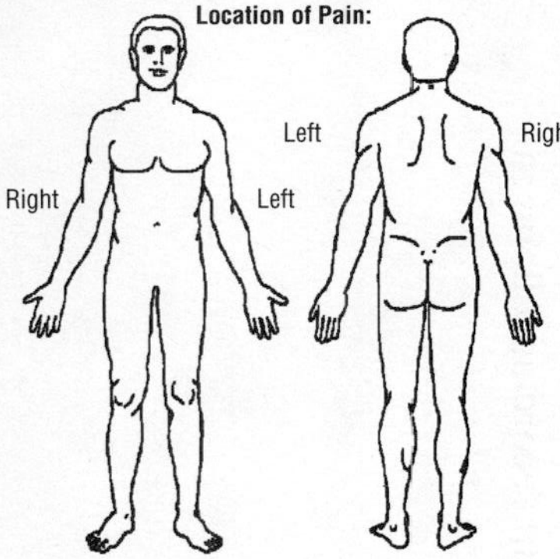
Right
Left
Left
Right

**A** = No pain
**B-Z** = Use letters to mark location of pain on graph

**Frequency of Pain:**
**0** = Occasional **F** = Frequent **C** = Constant

**Type of Pain**
**A** = Burning **D** = Sharp **G** = Isolated
**B** = Stabbing **E** = Shooting **H** = Other
**C** = Radiating **F** = Dull

| | | | | | | | | | | | | | | | | | | |
|---|---|---|---|---|---|---|---|---|---|---|---|---|---|---|---|---|---|---|
| **Date** | | | | | | | | | | | | | | | | | | |
| **Time** | | | | | | | | | | | | | | | | | | |
| **Initials** | | | | | | | | | | | | | | | | | | |
| Mode of Admin | | | | | | | | | | | | | | | | | | |
| Level of Pain | | | | | | | | | | | | | | | | | | |
| Location of Pain | | | | | | | | | | | | | | | | | | |
| Frequency of Pain | | | | | | | | | | | | | | | | | | |
| Type of Pain | | | | | | | | | | | | | | | | | | |
| Arousal Score | | | | | | | | | | | | | | | | | | |
| Non-Pharm. Intervent. | | | | | | | | | | | | | | | | | | |
| Analgesia Order | | | | | | | | | | | | | | | | | | |
| Reason for Order | | | | | | | | | | | | | | | | | | |
| Side Effects | | | | | | | | | | | | | | | | | | |
| Adverse Effects **(Y/N)** | | | | | | | | | | | | | | | | | | |
| Sensory Function **Epidural Only** | | | | | | | | | | | | | | | | | | |
| Motor Function **Epidural Only** | | | | | | | | | | | | | | | | | | |
| Neuro Score **Epidural Only** | | | | | | | | | | | | | | | | | | |
| Catheter Site **Epidural Only** | | | | | | | | | | | | | | | | | | |
| Cath Integrity **Epidural Only** | | | | | | | | | | | | | | | | | | |
| $O_2$ Saturation | | | | | | | | | | | | | | | | | | |
| Respirations | | | | | | | | | | | | | | | | | | |
| Pulse | | | | | | | | | | | | | | | | | | |
| Blood Pressure | | | | | | | | | | | | | | | | | | |
| See Nursing Notes **(Y/N)** | | | | | | | | | | | | | | | | | | |

| **Initials** | **Signature** |
|---|---|
| | |
| | |
| | |
| | |
| | |

Patient Identification Label

**Arousal Score:**
**0** = Alert **1** = Medically sedated/ETT
**2** = Drowsy **3** = Somnolent
**4** = Asleep

**Non-Pharmacologic Interventions L**
**C** = Cold **P** = Pacifier
**D** = Distraction **PO** = Positioning
**H** = Heat **R** = Relaxation
**HO** = Holding **RO** = Rocking
**I** = Imagery **S** = SecurityObject
**M** = Massage **T** = TensUnit
**MU** = Music **O** = Other

**Analgesia Order:**
**1** = Increase in dosage/rate
**2** = Decrease in doseage/rate
**3** = Extra bolus
**4** = PRN medication for break-through pain
**5** = Discontinue

**Reason for Analgesia Order:**
**1** = Unrelieved pain
**2** = Decreased arousal/neuroscore
**3** = Side effects (Seebelow)
**4** = Discontinue therapy/change to oral route
**5** = Adverse drug reactions
**(Document all adverse drug reactions in Nsg notes and complete an ADR report)**

**Side Effects:** **0** = None
**A** = Anxiety **N** = Nausea
**C** = Confused **R** = Respiratory Depression
**Co** = Constipation **U** = Urinary Rentention
**I** = Itching **V** = Vomiting

**Sensory Function Epidural Only**
**0** = Moves all extremities well
**1** = Unable to move all extremities well

**Motor Function Epidural Only**
**0** = Able to feel tactile pressure
**1** = Unable to feel tactile pressure

**Neuro Score: Epidural Only**
**0** = No numbness, no weakness
**1** = Medically sedated/ETT
**2** = Numbness with out weakness
**3** = Numbness and weakness

**Catheter Site: Epidural Only**
**1** = No redness, drainage, inflammation or swelling
**2** = Red, inflamed
**3** = Visable clear drainage
**4** = Visable purulent drainage
**5** = Visable serosanguinous/sanguinous drainage
**6** = Swelling

**Catheter Integrity Upon Removal: Epidural Only**
**1** = Catheter tip visually intact
**2** = Catheter NOT visually intact-See Nsg Notes

● Pain Management Flow Sheet. Children's Hospital.

*Note:* From Aprille Ciaverella, RN, and Lori Townsend, RN, at Sunrise Hospital and Medical Center and Sunrise Children's Hospital, Las Vegas, Nevada.

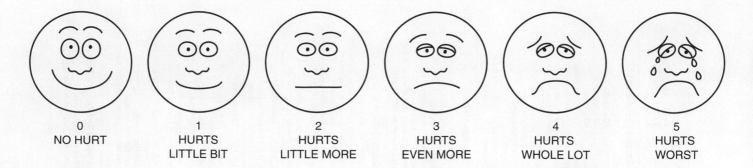

| 0 | 1 | 2 | 3 | 4 | 5 |
|---|---|---|---|---|---|
| NO HURT | HURTS LITTLE BIT | HURTS LITTLE MORE | HURTS EVEN MORE | HURTS WHOLE LOT | HURTS WORST |

Explain to the person that each face is for a person who feels happy because he has no pain (hurt) or sad because he has some or a lot of pain. Face 0 is very happy because he doesn't hurt at all. Face 1 hurts just a little bit. Face 2 hurts a little more. Face 3 hurts even more. Face 4 hurts a whole lot. Face 5 hurts as much as you can imagine, although you don't have to be crying to feel this bad. Ask the person to choose the face that best describes how he is feeling.

Rating scale is recommended for persons age 3 years and older.

**Brief word instructions:** Point to each face using the words to describe the pain intensity. Ask the child to choose the face that best describes own pain and record the appropriate number.

● The FACES rating scale.

*Note:* From Hockenberry, M., & Wilson D. (2007). *Wong's Nursing Care of Infants and Children*, 8th ed. (p. 210). St. Louis, MO: Mosby. Copyrighted by Mosby Elsevier, Inc.

5. Assess physiologic response to pain. Note blood pressure, pulse rate, respiratory rate, skin color, and presence of diaphoresis. ➤*Rationale: Signs of sympathetic nervous system stimulation (fight or flight) may be present with acute pain; however, clients with chronic pain may not have physical signs because of CNS adaptation.*

6. Assess affected body part, if appropriate. ➤*Rationale: Additional assessment may provide additional information about the pain and possible intervention.*

7. Document findings of the pain assessment and include the intervention(s) and the client's response to the interventions. ➤*Rationale: Thorough assessment and documentation assists the nurse to gain insights into the nature and pattern of the client's pain and ensures continuity of care. Maintaining a pain management flow sheet (see figure on previous page) will clarify and communicate each client's pain experience to enhance effective pain relief efforts. In settings where a pain management flow sheet is not used, data can be documented in the client record as follows in* "Documentation."

### Documentation

Sample: 7/22/09 0900 Admitted for elective foot surgery. c/o dull, throbbing, continuous pain in right cheek and jaw area radiating to right shoulder. Rates pain at 6/10. States pain began 6 months ago. Holding jaw throughout interview, became teary when describing negative effects on sleep, mood, and daily functioning. Associates onset with stress at work, and states she has been clenching her teeth throughout the day and grinding her teeth during sleep. States pain seems worse today with anxiety about surgery. Reports that Advil and heating pad relieve pain temporarily. Given moist heat pack to use now and relaxation breathing demonstrated with client participation.

_____ M. Blaszko, RN

7/22/09 0930 Rates pain at 1/10. Referrals to TMJ specialist and counseling made. Discussed maintaining a daily pain diary to identify patterns and to share with primary care provider.

_____ M. Blaszko, RN

## SETTING OF CARE

Address the following:

**Client**

- Level of knowledge: Pharmacologic and nonpharmacologic pain relief measures selected; adverse effects and measures to counteract these effects; warning signs to report to primary care provider.
- Self-care abilities for analgesic administration: Ability to use analgesics appropriately; physical dexterity to take pills or to administer intravenous medications and to store medications safely; ability to obtain prescriptions or over-the-counter medications at the pharmacy.

**Family**

- Caregiver availability, skills, and willingness: Primary and secondary persons able and willing to assist

with pain management; shopping if the client has restricted activity; ability to comprehend selected therapies (e.g., infusion pumps, imagery, massage, positioning, and relaxation techniques) and perform them or assist the client with them as needed.
- Family role changes and coping: Effect on financial status, parenting and spousal roles, sexuality, social roles.

**Community**

- Resources: Availability of and familiarity with resources such as supplies, home health aide, or financial assistance.

---

## VARIATION: Daily Pain Diary

For clients who experience chronic pain, a daily diary may illuminate pain patterns and factors that exacerbate or mediate the pain experience. In home care, the family or other caregiver can be taught to complete the diary. The record can include:

- Time or onset of pain and activity or situation preceding pain
- Relevant data (e.g., weather conditions the client deems significant)
- Physical pain character (quality) and intensity level (1–10)
- Emotions experienced and intensity level (0–10)
- Use of analgesics or other relief measures
- Duration of pain
- Time spent in relief activities and effectiveness of these activities

## VARIATION: Child Pain Assessment

Pain is considered the fifth vital sign, and every child has the right to be assessed for pain and receive pain management. The goal of pain assessment is to provide accurate information about the location and intensity of pain and its effects on the child's functioning. Various pain scales have been developed to assess pain in children. Some

pain assessment scales rely on the nurse's observation of the child's behavior if the child is nonverbal. Other scales depend on the child's report of pain intensity.

### Neonatal Infant Pain Scale (NIPS)

- Use in preterm and term infants up to 6 weeks after birth.
- Observe the infant's facial expression, cry quality, breathing pattern, arm and leg position, and state of arousal.

### FLACC Pain Scale

- This scale is designed to measure acute pain in infants and young children following surgery or while sleeping.
- FLACC is an acronym for the five categories that are assessed: Face, Legs, Activity, Cry, and Consolability.
- Use until the child is able to self-report pain with another pain scale.

### Oucher Scale

- Use in children between 3 and 7 years of age. Select the scale that matches the child's ethnic background—Caucasian, African American, or Hispanic.
- The child selects the face that matches his or her level of pain. The older child can select a number between 0 and 10.

## TABLE 11-7 NEONATAL INFANT PAIN SCALE (NIPS)

| Characteristic | Scoring Criteria |
| --- | --- |
| **Facial Expression** | |
| 0 = Relaxed muscles<br>1 = Grimace | • Restful face with neutral expression<br>• Tight facial muscles; furrowed brow, chin, and jaw (Note: At low gestational ages, infants may have no facial expression.) |
| **Cry** | |
| 0 = No cry<br>1 = Whimper<br>2 = Vigorous cry | • Quiet, not crying<br>• Mild moaning, intermittent cry<br>• Loud screaming, rising, shrill, and continuous (Note: Silent cry may be scored if infant is intubated, as indicated by obvious facial movements.) |
| **Breathing Patterns** | |
| 0 = Relaxed<br>1 = Change in breathing | • Relaxed, usual breathing pattern maintained<br>• Change in breathing, irregular, faster than usual, gagging, or holding breath |
| **Arm Movements** | |
| 0 = Relaxed/restrained<br>1 = Flexed/extended | • Relaxed, no muscle rigidity, occasional random (with soft restraints) movements of arms<br>• Tense, straight arms; rigid; or rapid extension and flexion |
| **Leg Movements** | |
| 0 = Relaxed/restrained<br>1 = Flexed/extended | • Relaxed, no muscle rigidity, occasional random (with soft restraints) movements of legs<br>• Tense, straight legs; rigid; or rapid extension and flexion |
| **State of Arousal** | |
| 0 = Sleeping/awake<br>1 = Fussy | • Quiet, peaceful, sleeping; or alert and settled<br>• Alert and restless or thrashing; fussy |

*Source:* From Lawrence, J., Alcock, D., McGrath, P., et al. (1993). The development of a tool to assess neonatal pain. *Neonatal Network,* 12(6), 61.

## TABLE 11–8 FLACC BEHAVIORAL PAIN ASSESSMENT SCALE

| Categories | Scoring | | |
| --- | --- | --- | --- |
| | **0** | **1** | **2** |
| **Face** | No particular expression or smile | Occasional grimace or frown; withdrawn, disinterested | Frequent to constant frown, clenched jaw, quivering chin |
| **Legs** | Normal position or relaxed | Uneasy, restless, tense | Kicking or legs drawn up |
| **Activity** | Lying quietly, normal position, moves easily | Squirming, shifting back and forth, tense | Arched, rigid, or jerking |
| **Cry** | No cry (awake or asleep) | Moans or whimpers, occasional complaint | Crying steadily, screams or sobs; frequent complaints |
| **Consolability** | Content, relaxed | Reassured by occasional touching, hugging, or being talked to; distractable | Difficult to console or comfort |

### How to Use the FLACC

**In patients who are awake:** observe for 1 to 5 minutes or longer. Observe legs and body uncovered. Reposition patient or observe activity. Assess body for tenseness and tone. Initiate consoling interventions if needed.

**In patients who are asleep:** observe for 5 minutes or longer. Observe body and legs uncovered. If possible, reposition the patient. Touch the body and assess for tenseness and tone.

#### Face
- Score 0 if the patient has a relaxed face, makes eye contact, shows interest in surroundings.
- Score 1 if the patient has a worried facial expression, with eyebrows lowered, eyes partially closed, cheeks raised, mouth pursed.
- Score 2 if the patient has deep furrows in the forehead, closed eyes, an open mouth, deep lines around nose and lips.

#### Legs
- Score 0 if the muscle tone and motion in the limbs are normal.
- Score 1 if patient has increased tone, rigidity, or tension; if there is intermittent flexion or extension of the limbs.
- Score 2 if patient has hypertonicity, the legs are pulled tight, there is exaggerated flexion or extension of the limbs, tremors.

#### Activity
- Score 0 if the patient moves easily and freely, normal activity or restrictions.
- Score 1 if the patient shifts positions, appears hesitant to move, demonstrates guarding, a tense torso, pressure on a body part.
- Score 2 if the patient is in a fixed position, rocking; demonstrates side-to-side head movement or rubbing of a body part.

#### Cry
- Score 0 if the patient has no cry or moan, awake or asleep.
- Score 1 if the patient has occasional moans, cries, whimpers, sighs.
- Score 2 if the patient has frequent or continuous moans, cries, grunts.

#### Consolability
- Score 0 if the patient is calm and does not require consoling.
- Score 1 if the patient responds to comfort by touching or talking in 30 seconds to 1 minute.
- Score 2 if the patient requires constant comforting or is inconsolable.

Whenever feasible, behavioral measurement of pain should be used in conjunction with self-report. When self-report is not possible, interpretation of pain behaviors and decisions regarding treatment of pain require careful consideration of the context in which the pain behaviors are observed.

### Interpreting the Behavioral Score

Each category is scored on the 0–2 scale, which results in a total score of 0–10.

| | |
| --- | --- |
| **0** = Relaxed and comfortable | **4–6** = Moderate pain |
| **1–3** = Mild discomfort | **7–10** = Severe discomfort or pain or both |

*From* Merkel, S. I., Voepel-Lewis, T., Shayevitz, J. R., & Malviya, S. (1997). The FLACC: A behavioral scale for scoring postoperative pain in young children. *Pediatric Nursing, 23*(3), 293–297. The FLACC scale was developed by Sandra Merkel, MS, RN, Terri Voepel-Lewis, MS, RN, and Shobha Malviya, MD, at C. S. Mott Children's Hospital, University of Michigan Health System, Ann Arbor, MI. Used with permission.

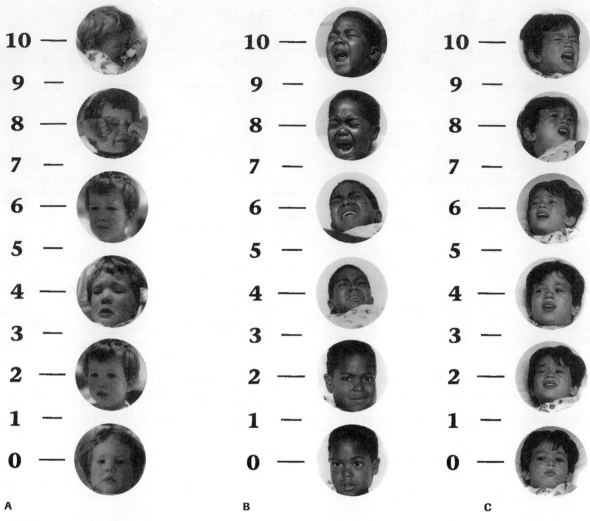

● Oucher Scale 3–7 years.

*In the form presented in this book, the Ocher is for educational purposes only and cannot be used for patient care.

**A.** The Caucasian version of the Oucher, developed and copyrighted by Judith E. Beyer, RN, Ph.D., 1983.

**B.** The African American version of the Oucher, developed and copy righted by Mary J. Denyes, RN, Ph.D., and Antonio M. Villarruel, RN, Ph.D., 1990. Cornelia P. Porter, RN, Ph.D., and Charlotta Marshall, RN, MSN, contributed to the development of the scale.

**C.** The Hispanic version of the Oucher, developed and copyrighted by Antonio M. Villarruel, RN, Ph.D., and Mary J. Denyes, RN, Ph.D., 1990. http://www.oucher.org.

# Skill 11.22 Assessing Body Temperature

## Delegation

Routine measurement of the client's temperature can be delegated to unlicensed assistive personnel (UAP)—or to family members/caregivers in nonhospital settings. The nurse must explain the appropriate type of thermometer and site to be used and ensure that the person knows when to report an abnormal temperature and how to record the finding. The interpretation of an abnormal temperature and determination of appropriate responses are done by the nurse.

## Equipment

- Thermometer
- Thermometer sheath or cover
- Water-soluble lubricant for a rectal temperature
- Clean gloves for a rectal temperature
- Towel for axillary temperature
- Tissues/wipes

## Preparation

Check that all equipment is functioning normally.

## CLINICAL ALERT

Be sure to record the temperature from an electronic thermometer before replacing the probe into the charging unit. With many models, replacing the probe erases the temperature from the display.

## Procedure

1. Prior to performing the procedure, introduce self and verify the client's identity using agency protocol. Explain to the client what you are going to do, why it is necessary, and how he or she can participate. Discuss how the results will be used in planning further care or treatments.
2. Perform hand hygiene and observe appropriate infection control procedures. Apply gloves if performing a rectal temperature.
3. Provide for client privacy.
4. Place the client in the appropriate position (e.g., lateral or Sims' position for inserting a rectal thermometer).
5. Place the thermometer (see Box 11–3 on page 531).
   • Apply a protective sheath or probe cover if appropriate.
   • Lubricate a rectal thermometer.
6. Wait the appropriate amount of time. Electronic and tympanic thermometers will indicate that the reading is complete by means of a light or tone. Check package instructions for length of time to wait prior to reading chemical dot or tape thermometers.
7. Remove the thermometer and discard the cover or wipe with a tissue if necessary. If gloves were applied, remove and discard gloves. Perform hand hygiene.
8. Read the temperature and record it on your worksheet. If the temperature is obviously too high, too low, or inconsistent with the client's condition, recheck it with a thermometer known to be functioning properly.
9. Wash the thermometer if necessary and return it to the storage location.
10. Document the temperature in the client record. A rectal temperature may be recorded with an "R" next to the value or with the mark on a graphic sheet circled. An axillary temperature may be recorded with "AX" or marked on a graphic sheet with an X.

## VARIATION: Measuring an Infant or Child's Temperature

### Equipment

Digital or electronic thermometer with disposable probe cover
Water-soluble lubricant
Gloves, if necessary

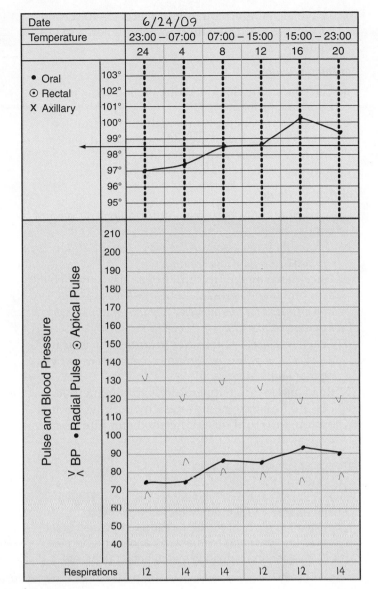

Vital signs graphic record.

## Procedure

1. Determine appropriate thermometer and route for child. ▶*Rationale:* Oral route is appropriate for child over 3 years of age and electronic, nonbreakable thermometer is preferred.
2. Perform hand hygiene and identify client with two forms of ID.
3. Explain procedure at child's level of understanding.
4. Remove probe from cover or attach probe tip to electronic thermometer.

### For Oral Route (only for child 3 years or older)

a. Place probe under child's tongue, one side or the other.
b. Have child close mouth and either hold thermometer in place or monitor while taking temperature.

c. Leave digital thermometer in place 45–90 seconds or remove electronic thermometer when audible signal occurs.

### For Rectal Route

a. Place infant or child in prone or side-lying position.
b. Lubricate probe.
c. Insert thermometer ¼ to ½ inch into rectum for infant—½ to 1 inch for child, and hold in place.
d. Turn on scanner and follow directions.
e. Remove probe when tone or beep is heard.

### For Axillary Route

a. Assist infant or child to a comfortable position and expose axilla.
b. Dry axilla if necessary. ➤*Rationale: A moist axillary area can produce a false low reading.*
c. Place thermometer in center of axilla. Lower child's arm down and across the chest. ➤*Rationale: This position ensures that thermometer remains in contact with large vessels of axilla.*
d. Leave in place 1–2 minutes or until tone is heard. ➤*Rationale: Axillary temperature readings take longer to register than oral or rectal.*
5. Read and record temperature, indicate method.
6. Discard probe cover into trash by pushing ejection button, or return digital thermometer into its case.

> ## CLINICAL ALERT
>
> Only use client's own dedicated electronic thermometer (including rectal and oral) if diagnosis includes *Clostridium difficile*—associated diarrhea because of the potential for spreading the bacteria and increasing the risk of transmitting a nosocomial infection to others.

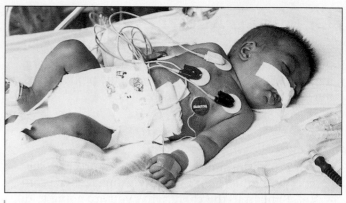

● The axillary method is often used for children who are unconscious, have seizures, or have a structural abnormality.

> ## CLINICAL ALERT
>
> Do not use ear thermometer in infected or draining ear, or if adjacent lesion or incision exists.

> ## CLINICAL ALERT
>
> Temperature assessment is the single most important infection control monitoring criterion for nosocomial infections and fever of unknown origin.

> ## CLINICAL ALERT
>
> The temperature of an unconscious client is never taken by mouth. The rectal or tympanic method is preferred.

## EVIDENCE-BASED NURSING PRACTICE

**Correct Technique for Taking a Tympanic Temperature**

Studies on the correct technique for taking a tympanic temperature indicated that the ear tug (pulling the pinna upward and backward for an adult and down and backward for a child) is essential for an accurate reading. Eliminating this step will not allow the thermometer to be directly at the tympanic membrane.

*Source: Best Practice,* Vital signs (1999), vol. 3, no. 3, p. 5. http://www.joannabriggs.edu.au.

> ### REDUCING MERCURY IN HOSPITALS
>
> A survey of American hospitals released in late September, 2005, indicated that 97% of hospitals have taken steps to reduce or eliminate mercury. 72% of hospitals have inventoried and replaced mercury-containing devices or labeled them for proper handling.
>
> *Source:* Survey conducted by American Hospital Association, Health Care Without Harm, and U.S. Environmental Protection Agency.

## CLINICAL ALERT

Temperature varies with the time of day: It is highest between 5 and 7 P.M. and lowest between 2 and 6 A.M. This variation is termed circadian thermal rhythm. A consistent method of body temperature measurement should be used so that readings are comparable.

## LEGAL ALERT

**Nurse's Negligence**

The client had transthoracic vagotomy after which the doctor ordered vital signs every 15 minutes x 1 hour and every hour for 10 hours Vital signs were recorded 4 times for 1 day. The next day the client's temperature was 102 degrees F and it remained there until the next day when it was 105 degrees F. The nurse administered aspirin when it rose to 106 degrees F. The nurse then contacted the doctor who found signs of serious wound infection. The client suffered organic brain syndrome as a direct result of the continued high temperature. The court found that the nurses breached standard of care then they failed to notify the doctor of the client's high temperature.

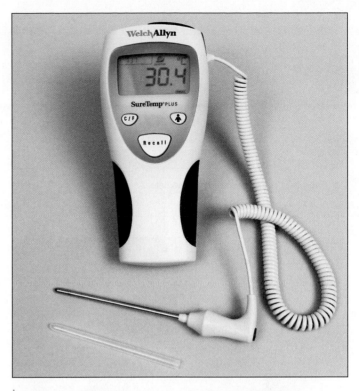

● An electronic thermometer. Note the probe and probe cover.

### TABLE 11-9 ADVANTAGES AND DISADVANTAGES OF SITES FOR BODY TEMPERATURE MEASUREMENT

| Site | Advantages | Disadvantages |
|---|---|---|
| Oral | Accessible and convenient | Thermometers can break if bitten. Inaccurate if client has just ingested hot or cold food or fluid or smoked. Could injure the mouth following oral surgery. |
| Rectal | Reliable measurement | Inconvenient and more unpleasant for clients; difficult for client who cannot turn to the side. Could injure the rectum following rectal surgery. Presence of stool may interfere with thermometer placement. If the stool is soft, the thermometer may be embedded in stool rather than against the wall of the rectum. |
| Axillary | Safe and noninvasive | The thermometer must be left in place a long time to obtain an accurate measurement. |
| Tympanic membrane | Readily accessible; reflects the core temperature; very fast. | Can be uncomfortable and involves risk of injuring the membrane if the probe is inserted too far. Repeated measurements may vary. Right and left measurements can differ. Presence of cerumen can affect the reading. |
| Temporal artery | Safe and noninvasive; very fast. | Requires electronic equipment that may be expensive or unavailable; variation in technique needed if the client has perspiration on the forehead. |

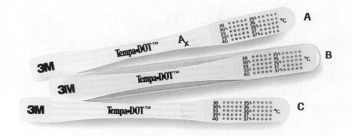

● One-piece home electronic thermometer.

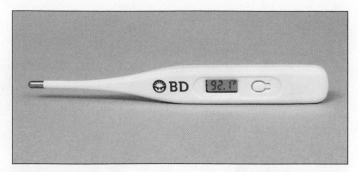

● A temperature-sensitive skin tape.

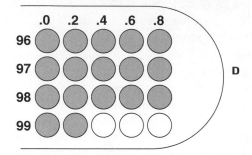

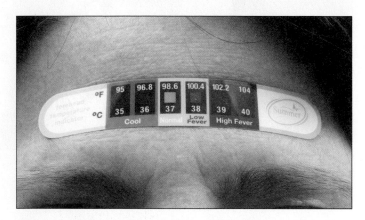

● Chemical dot thermometers; **A,** axillary (note the "Ax" in the stem); **B,** rectal (note the plastic cover); **C,** oral; **D,** an enlargement showing a reading of 99.2 degrees F.

(Courtesy of 3M Medical Division-3M Health Care.)

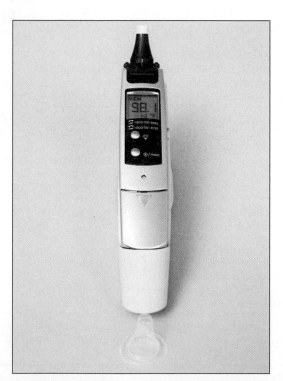

● An infrared tympanic thermometer used to measure the tympanic membrane temperature.

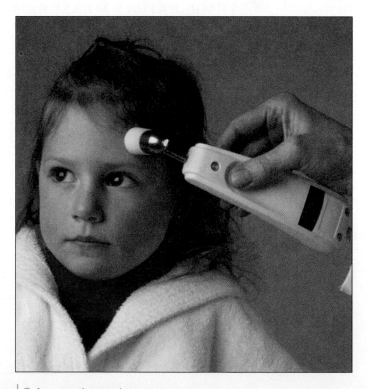

● A temporal artery thermometer.

# BOX 11–3 HEAD-TO-TOE FRAMEWORK

**Oral**    Place the bulb on either side of the frenulum.

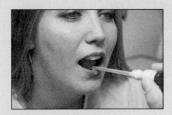

● Oral thermometer placement.

**Rectal**    Apply clean gloves.
Instruct the client to take a slow deep breath during insertion.
Never force the thermometer if resistance is felt.
Insert 3.5 cm (1.5 in.) in adults.

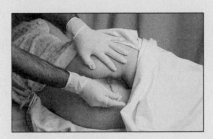

● Inserting a rectal thermometer.

**Axillary**    Pat the axilla dry if very moist.
The bulb is placed in the center of the axilla.

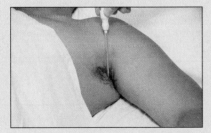

● Placing the bulb of the thermometer in the center of the axilla.

**Tympanic membrane**    Pull the pinna slightly upward and backward. Point the probe slightly anteriorly, toward the eardrum.
Insert the probe slowly using a circular motion until snug.

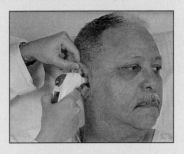

● Pull the pinna of the ear up and back while inserting the tympanic thermometer.

**Temporal artery**    Brush hair aside if covering the temporal artery area. With the probe flush on the center of the forehead, depress the red button; keep depressed. Slowly slide the probe midline across the forehead to the hair line, not down the side of the face. Lift the probe from the forehead and touch on the neck just behind the earlobe. Release the button.

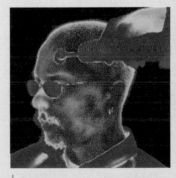 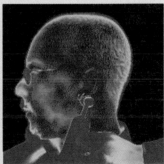

● Positioning a temporal artery thermometer.

## DEVELOPMENTAL CONSIDERATIONS

### Infants

- The body temperature of newborns is extremely labile, and newborns must be kept warm and dry to prevent hypothermia.
- Using the axillary site, you need to hold the infant's arm against the chest to keep the thermometer in place.
- The axillary route may not be as accurate as other routes for detecting fevers in children (El Radhi & Patel, 2006).
- The tympanic route is fast and convenient. Place the infant supine and stabilize the head. Pull the pinna straight back and slightly downward. Remember that the pinna is pulled upward for children over 3 years of age and adults but downward for children younger than 3. Direct the probe tip anteriorly and insert far enough to seal the canal. The tip will not touch the tympanic membrane.
- Avoid the tympanic route in a child with active ear infections or tympanic membrane drainage tubes.
- The tympanic membrane route may be more accurate in determining temperature in febrile infants (Nimah, Bshesh, Callahan, & Jacobs, 2006).
- When using a temporal artery thermometer, touching only the forehead or behind the ear is needed.
- The rectal route is least desirable in infants.

### Children

- Tympanic or temporal artery sites are preferred.
- For the tympanic route, have an adult hold the child in his or her lap with the child's head held gently against the adult for support. Pull the pinna straight back and upward for children over age 3.
- Avoid the tympanic route in a child with active ear infections or tympanic membrane drainage tubes.
- The oral route may be used for children over age 3, but nonbreakable, electronic thermometers are recommended.
- For a rectal temperature, place the child prone across your lap or in a side-lying position with the knees flexed. Insert the thermometer 1 inch into the rectum.

### Elders

- Elders' temperatures tend to be lower than those of middle-aged adults.
- Elders' temperatures are strongly influenced by both environmental and internal temperature changes. Their thermoregulation control processes are not as efficient as when they were younger, and they are at higher risk for both hypothermia and hyperthermia.
- Elders can develop significant buildup of ear cerumen that may interfere with tympanic thermometer readings.
- Elders are more likely to have hemorrhoids. Inspect the anus before taking a rectal temperature.
- Elders' temperatures may not be a valid indication of the seriousness of the pathology of a disease. They may have pneumonia or a urinary tract infection and have only a slight temperature elevation. Other symptoms, such as confusion and restlessness, may be displayed and need follow-up to determine if there is an underlying process.

## CLIENT TEACHING CONSIDERATIONS

- Teach the client accurate use and reading of the type of thermometer to be used. Examine the thermometer used by the client in the home for safety and proper functioning. Facilitate the replacement of mercury thermometers with nonmercury ones.
- Observe the client/caregiver taking and reading a temperature. Reinforce the importance of reporting the site and type of thermometer used and the value of using the same thermometer consistently.
- Discuss means of keeping the thermometer clean, such as warm water and soap, and avoiding cross-contamination.
- Instruct the client or family member to notify the health care provider if the temperature is higher than a specified level, for example, 38.5°C (101.3°F).
- Check that the client knows how to record the temperature. Provide a recording chart/table if indicated.
- Discuss environmental control modifications that should be taken during illness or extreme climate conditions (e.g., heating, air conditioning, appropriate clothing and bedding).

## SETTING OF CARE

- Ensure that the client has water-soluble lubricant if using a rectal thermometer.
- When making a home visit, take a thermometer with you in case the client does not own a functional thermometer.
- Consider whether environmental conditions such as lack of heat or air conditioning are affecting the client's temperature or temperature measurement.
- Pacifier thermometers are being used more in the home setting for children under 2 years old. The manufacturer's instructions must be followed carefully since many require adding 0.5 degree F in order to estimate rectal temperature (Braun, 2006).

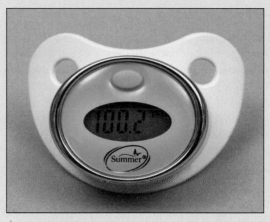

● A pacifier thermometer.

# Skill 11.23   Assessing an Apical-Radial Pulse

## Delegation

UAP are generally not responsible for assessing apical-radial pulses.

## Equipment

- Watch with a second hand or indicator
- Stethoscope
- Antiseptic wipes

## Preparation

If using the two-nurse technique, ensure that the other nurse is available at this time.

## Procedure

1. Prior to performing the procedure, introduce self and verify the client's identity using agency protocol. Explain to the client what you are going to do, why it is necessary, and how he or she can participate. Discuss how the results will be used in planning further care or treatments.
2. Perform hand hygiene and observe appropriate infection control procedures.
3. Provide for client privacy.
4. Position the client appropriately. Assist the client to a comfortable supine or sitting position. Expose the area of the chest over the apex of the heart. If previous measurements were taken, determine what position the client assumed, and use the same position. ➤*Rationale: This ensures an accurate comparative measurement.*
5. Locate the apical and radial pulse sites. In the two-nurse technique, one nurse locates the apical impulse with the stethoscope while the other nurse palpates the radial pulse site (see Skills 11.24 and 11.25).

6. Count the apical and radial pulse rates.

### VARIATION: Two-Nurse Technique

- Place the watch where both nurses can see it. The nurse who is taking the radial pulse may hold the watch.
- Decide on a time to begin counting. A time when the second hand is on 12, 3, 6, or 9 or an even number on digital clocks is usually selected. The nurse taking the radial pulse says "Start" at the same time. ➤*Rationale: This ensures that simultaneous counts are taken.*
- Each nurse counts the pulse rate for 60 seconds. Both nurses end the count when the nurse taking the radial pulse says "Stop." ➤*Rationale: A full 60-second count is necessary for accurate assessment of any discrepancies between the two pulse sites.*
- The nurse who assesses the apical rate also assesses the apical pulse rhythm and volume (i.e., whether the heartbeat is strong or weak). If the pulse is irregular, note whether the irregular beats come at random or at predictable times.
- The nurse assessing the radial pulse rate also assesses the radial pulse rhythm and volume.

### VARIATION: One-Nurse Technique

- Assess the apical pulse for 60 seconds.
- Assess the radial pulse for 60 seconds.
7. Document the apical and radial (AR) pulse rates, rhythm, volume, and any pulse deficit in the client record. Also record related data such as variation in pulse rate compared to normal for the client and other pertinent observations, such as pallor, cyanosis, or dyspnea.

## DEVELOPMENTAL CONSIDERATIONS

### Infants

- Use the apical pulse for the heart rate of newborns, infants, and children 2 to 3 years old to establish baseline data for subsequent evaluation, to determine whether the cardiac rate is within normal range, and to determine if the rhythm is regular.
- Place a baby in a supine position, and offer a pacifier if the baby is crying or restless. Crying and physical activity will increase the pulse rate. For this reason, take the apical pulse rate of infants and small children before assessing body temperatures.
- Locate the apical pulse in the fourth intercostal space, lateral to the midclavicular line during infancy.
- Brachial, popliteal, and femoral pulses may be palpated. Due to a normally low blood pressure and rapid heart rate, infants' other distal pulses may be difficult to feel.
- Newborn infants may have heart murmurs that are not pathologic, but reflect functional incomplete closure of fetal heart structures (ductus arteriosus or foramen ovale).

### Children

- To take a peripheral pulse, position the child comfortably in the adult's arms, or have the adult remain close by. This may decrease anxiety and yield more accurate results.

- To assess the apical pulse, assist a young child to a comfortable supine or sitting position.
- Demonstrate the procedure to the child using a stuffed animal or doll, and allow the child to handle the stethoscope before beginning the procedure. This will decrease anxiety and promote cooperation.
- The apex of the heart is normally located in the fourth intercostal space in young children; fifth intercostal space in children 7 years of age and over.
- Locate the apical impulse along the fourth intercostal space, between the MCL and the anterior axillary line.
- Count the pulse prior to other uncomfortable procedures so that the rate is not artificially elevated by the discomfort.

### Elders

- If the client has severe hand or arm tremors, the radial pulse may be difficult to count.
- Cardiac changes in elders, such as decrease in cardiac output, sclerotic changes to heart valves, and dysrhythmias often indicate that obtaining an apical pulse will be more accurate.
- Elders often have decreased peripheral circulation so that pedal pulses should also be checked for regularity, volume, and symmetry.
- The pulse returns to baseline after exercise more slowly than with other age groups.

## CLIENT TEACHING

- Teach the client/family to monitor the pulse prior to taking medications that affect the heart rate. Tell them to report any notable changes in heart rate or rhythm (regularity) to the health care provider.
- Inform the client/family of activities known to significantly affect pulse rate such as emotional stress, exercise, ingesting caffeine, and sleep. Clients sensitive to pulse rate changes should consider whether any of these activities should be modified in order to stabilize the pulse.

## SETTING OF CARE

- Ensure that all users are familiar with using an electronic pulse-measuring device if indicated.
- Some clients require lengthy monitoring of the pulse and cardiac pattern (electrocardiogram). A special device, often referred to as a Holter monitor, is used for this type of monitoring. It is usually applied in an office or clinic setting and the client wears the portable recorder for 24 hours. Other portable devices used for recording episodic arrhythmias include cardiac event monitors. The client activates the device during times when symptoms appear and then the recorded data can be transmitted to a central location through a telephone.

# Skill 11.24  Assessing an Apical Pulse

## Delegation

Due to the degree of skill and knowledge required, UAP are generally not responsible for assessing apical pulses.

## Equipment

- Watch with a second hand or indicator
- Stethoscope
- Antiseptic wipes
- If a DUS, the transducer probe, the stethoscope head-set, transmission gel, and tissues/wipes

## Preparation

If using the DUS, check that the equipment is functioning normally.

## Procedure

1. Prior to performing the procedure, introduce self and verify the client's identity using agency protocol. Explain to the client what you are going to do, why it is necessary, and how he or she can participate. Discuss how the results will be used in planning further care or treatments.
2. Perform hand hygiene and observe appropriate infection control procedures.
3. Provide for client privacy.
4. Position the client appropriately in a comfortable supine position or in a sitting position. Expose the area of the chest over the apex of the heart.
5. Locate the apical impulse. This is the point over the apex of the heart where the apical pulse can be most clearly heard.

Location of apical pulse for a child under 4 years, a child 4 to 6 years and an adult.

- Palpate the angle of Louis (the angle between the manubrium, the top of the sternum, and the body of the sternum). It is palpated just below the suprasternal notch and is felt as a prominence.
- Slide your index finger just to the left of the sternum, and palpate the second intercostal space.

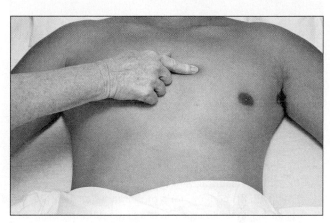

● Palpating the point of maximal impulse PMI: Second intercostal space.

- Place your middle or next finger in the third intercostal space, and continue palpating downward until you locate the fifth intercostal space.

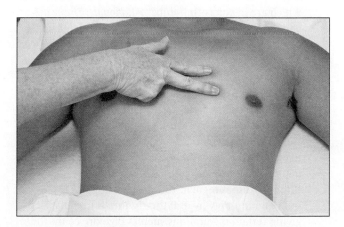

● Third intercostal space.

- Move your index finger laterally along the fifth intercostal space toward the midclavicular line (MCL). Normally, the apical impulse is palpable at or just medial to the MCL.

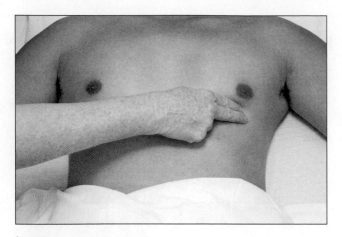

● Fifth intercostals space: MCL.

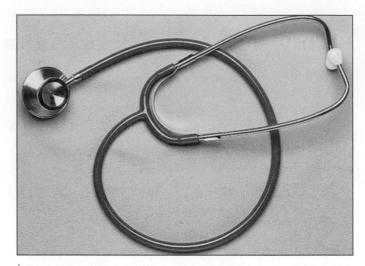

● Stethoscope with both a bell and diaphragm.

6. Auscultate and count heartbeats.
   • Use antiseptic wipes to clean the earpieces and diaphragm of the stethoscope if their cleanliness is in doubt. ➤*Rationale: The diaphragm needs to be cleaned and disinfected if soiled with body substances.*
   • Warm the diaphragm of the stethoscope by holding it in the palm of the hand for a moment. ➤*Rationale: The metal of the diaphragm is usually cold and can startle the client when placed immediately on the chest.*
   • Insert the earpieces of the stethoscope into your ears in the direction of the ear canals, or slightly forward, *to facilitate hearing.*
   • Tap your finger lightly on the diaphragm. ➤*Rationale: This is to be sure it is the active side of the stethoscope head.* If necessary, rotate the head to select the diaphragm side.
   • Place the diaphragm of the stethoscope over the apical impulse and listen for the normal $S_1$ and $S_2$ heart sounds, which are heard as "lub-dub." ➤*Rationale: The heartbeat is normally loudest over the apex of the heart.* Each lub-dub is counted as one heartbeat. ➤*Rationale: The two heart sounds are produced by closure of the heart valves. The S1 heart sound (lub) occurs when the atrioventricular valves close after the ventricles have been sufficiently filled. The $S_2$ heart sound (dub) occurs when the semilunar valves close after the ventricles empty.*
   • If you have difficulty hearing the apical pulse, ask the supine client to roll onto the left side or the sitting client to lean slightly forward. ➤*Rationale: This positioning moves the apex of the heart closer to the chest wall.*
   • If the rhythm is regular, count the heartbeats for 30 seconds and multiply by 2. If the rhythm is irregular or for giving certain medications such as digoxin, count the beats for 60 seconds. ➤*Rationale: A 60-second count provides a more accurate assessment of an irregular pulse than a 30-second count.*

7. Assess the rhythm and the strength of the heartbeat.
   • Assess the rhythm of the heartbeat by noting the pattern of intervals between the beats. A normal pulse has equal time periods between beats.

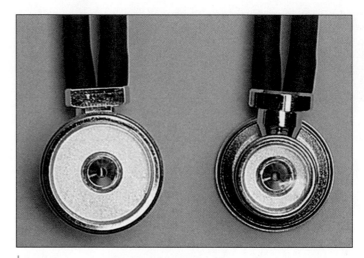

● Close-up of a diaphragm (left) and a bell (right).

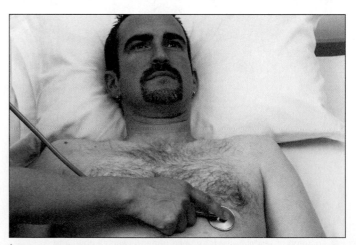

● Taking an apical pulse using the diaphragm of the stethoscope. Note how the diaphragm is held against the chess.

- Assess the strength (volume) of the heartbeat. Normally, the heartbeats are equal in strength and can be described as strong or weak.

8. Document the apical pulse rate and rhythm and nursing actions in the client record. Also record pertinent related data such as variation in pulse rate compared to normal for the client and abnormal skin color and skin temperature.

## Documentation

Sample: 2/24/09 1000 Radial pulse 116 & irregular. Had been 82 & regular at 0600. T, R, & BP within client's usual range. C/o slight dizziness. Skin warm & dry. Apical pulse 120, irregular, with slight pause after q 3rd beat. MD notified & ECG ordered.

_____ G. Chapman, RN

# Skill 11.25   Assessing Peripheral Pulses

## Delegation

Measurement of the client's radial or brachial pulse can be delegated to UAP or family members/caregivers in nonhospital settings. Reports of abnormal pulse rates or rhythms require reassessment by the nurse, who also determines appropriate action if the abnormality is confirmed. UAP are generally not delegated these techniques due to the skill required in locating and interpreting peripheral pulses other than the radial or brachial artery and in using Doppler ultrasound devices.

## Equipment

- Watch with a second hand or indicator
- If using a Doppler ultrasound stethoscope (DUS), the transducer probe, the stethoscope headset, transmission gel, and tissues/wipes

## Procedure

1. Prior to performing the procedure, introduce self and verify the client's identity using agency protocol. Explain to the client what you are going to do, why it is necessary, and how he or she can participate. Discuss how the results will be used in planning further care or treatments.

2. Perform hand hygiene and observe appropriate infection control procedures.
3. Provide for client privacy.
4. Select the pulse point. Normally, the radial pulse is taken, unless it cannot be exposed or circulation to another body area is to be assessed.
5. Assist the client to a comfortable resting position. When the radial pulse is assessed, with the palm facing downward, the client's arm can rest alongside the body or the forearm can rest at a 90-degree angle across the chest. For the client who can sit, the forearm can rest across the thigh, with the palm of the hand facing downward or inward.
6. Palpate and count the pulse. Place two or three middle fingertips lightly and squarely over the pulse point. ▸*Rationale: Using the thumb is contraindicated because the nurse's thumb has a pulse that could be mistaken for the client's pulse.*
   - Count for 15 seconds and multiply by 4. Record the pulse in beats per minute on your worksheet. If taking a client's pulse for the first time, when obtaining baseline data, or if the pulse is irregular, count for a full minute. If an irregular pulse is found, also take the apical pulse.
7. Assess the pulse rhythm and volume.

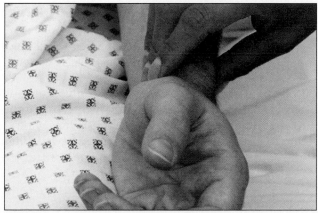

● **A,** radial

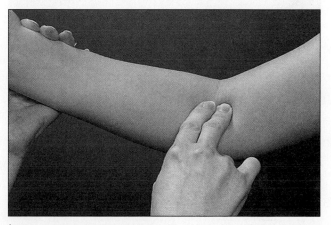

● **B,** brachial

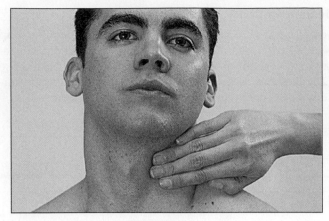

● **C,** carotid

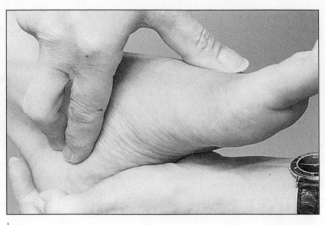

● **F,** posterior tibial

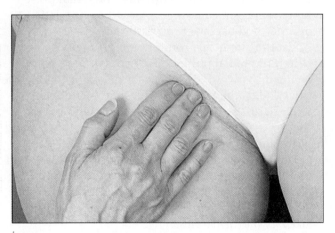

● **D,** femoral

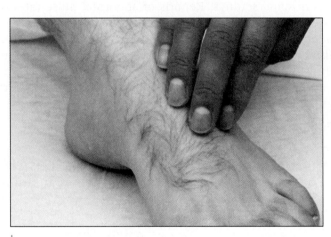

● **G,** pedal (dorsalis pedis)

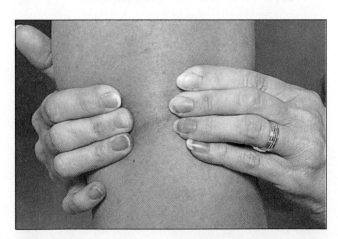

● **E,** popliteal

- Assess the pulse rhythm by noting the pattern of the intervals between the beats. A normal pulse has equal time periods between beats. If this is an initial assessment, assess for 1 minute.
- Assess the pulse volume. A normal pulse can be felt with moderate pressure, and the pressure is equal with each beat. A forceful pulse volume is full; an easily obliterated pulse is weak. Record the rhythm and volume on your worksheet.
8. Document the pulse rate, rhythm, and volume and your actions in the client record. Also record in the nurse's notes pertinent related data such as variation in pulse rate compared to normal for the client and abnormal skin color and skin temperature.

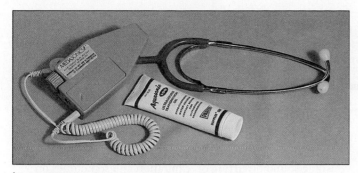

● A Doppler ultrasound stethoscope (DUS)

## VARIATION: Using a DUS

- If used, plug the stethoscope headset into one of the two output jacks located next to the volume control. DUS units may have two jacks so that a second person can listen to the signals.
- Apply transmission gel either to the probe at the narrow end of the plastic case housing the transducer, or to the client's skin. ➤*Rationale: Ultrasound beams do not travel well through air. The gel makes an airtight seal, which then promotes optimal ultrasound wave transmission.*
- Press the "on" button.
- Hold the probe against the skin over the pulse site. Use a light pressure, and keep the probe in contact with the skin. ➤*Rationale: Too much pressure can stop the blood flow and obliterate the signal.*
- Adjust the volume if necessary. Distinguish artery sounds from vein sounds. The artery sound (signal) is distinctively pulsating and has a pumping quality. The venous sound is intermittent and varies with respirations. Both artery and vein sounds are heard simultaneously through the DUS because major arteries and veins are situated close together throughout the body. If arterial sounds cannot be easily heard, reposition the probe.

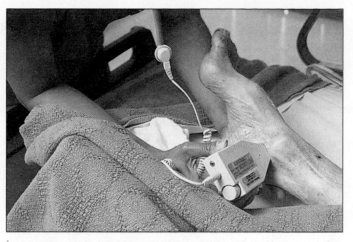

● Using a DUS to assess the posterior tibial pulse.

- After assessing the pulse, remove all gel from the probe to prevent damage to the surface. Clean the transducer with water-based solution. ➤*Rationale: Alcohol or other disinfectants may damage the face of the transducer. Remove all gel from the client.*

## EVIDENCE-BASED NURSING PRACTICE

### Pulse Rate Measurement

Studies have indicated that the accuracy of pulse rate measurement is influenced by the number of counted seconds (counting the pulse for 60 second is more accurate than 15 or 30 seconds). However, clinical significance of the result is not clear, so length of count period may be of limited significance.

*Source: Best practice,* Vital Signs (1999), vol. 3, no. 3, p. 2. http://www.joannabriggs.edu.au.

# Skill 11.26    Assessing Respirations

## EVIDENCE-BASED NURSING PRACTICE

### Accuracy in Counting Respirations

One study found that counting respirations for 15 second versus a full minute produced a significant difference in the rate; thus, the conclusion is respirations should be counted for a full minute.

*Source: Best Practice,* Vital Signs (1999), vol. 3, no. 3, p. 2. http://www.joannabriggs.edu.au.

### Delegation

Counting and observing respirations may be delegated to UAP. The follow-up assessment, interpretation of abnormal respirations, and determination of appropriate responses are done by the nurse.

### Equipment

Watch with a second hand or indicator

## TABLE 11–10 ALTERED BREATHING PATTERNS AND SOUNDS

| Breathing Patterns | Breath Sounds |
|---|---|
| **Rate** <br> • *Tachypnea*—quick, shallow breaths <br> • *Bradypnea*—abnormally slow breathing <br> • *Apnea*—cessation of breathing <br><br> **Volume** <br> • *Hyperventilation*—overexpansion of the lungs characterized by rapid and deep breaths <br> • *Hypoventilation*—underexpansion of the lungs, characterized by shallow respirations <br><br> **Rhythm** <br> • *Cheyne-Stokes breathing*—rhythmic waxing and waning of respirations, from very deep to very shallow breathing and temporary apnea <br><br> **Ease or Effort** <br> • *Dyspnea*—difficult and labored breathing during which the individual has a persistent, unsatisfied need for air and feels distressed <br> • *Orthopnea*—ability to breathe only in upright sitting or standing positions | **Audible without Amplification** <br> • *Stridor*—a shrill, harsh sound heard during inspiration with laryngeal obstruction <br> • *Stertor*—snoring or sonorous respiration, usually due to a partial obstruction of the upper airway <br> • *Wheeze*—continuous, high-pitched musical squeak or whistling sound occurring on expiration and sometimes on inspiration when air moves through a narrowed or partially obstructed airway <br> • *Bubbling*—gurgling sounds heard as air passes through moist secretions in the respiratory tract <br><br> **Chest Movements** <br> • *Intercostal retraction*—indrawing between the ribs <br> • *Substernal retraction*—indrawing beneath the breastbone <br> • *Suprasternal retraction*—indrawing above the clavicles <br><br> **Secretions and Coughing** <br> • *Hemoptysis*—the presence of blood in the sputum <br> • *Productive cough*—a cough accompanied by expectorated secretions <br> • *Nonproductive cough*—a dry, harsh cough without secretions |

## Preparation

For a routine assessment of respirations, determine the client's activity schedule and choose a suitable time to monitor the respirations. A client who has been exercising will need to rest for a few minutes to permit the accelerated respiratory rate to return to normal.

## Procedure

1. Prior to performing the procedure, introduce self and verify the client's identity using agency protocol. Explain to the client what you are going to do, why it is necessary, and how he or she can participate. Discuss how the results will be used in planning further care or treatments.
2. Perform hand hygiene and observe appropriate infection control procedures.
3. Provide for client privacy.
4. Observe or palpate and count the respiratory rate.
   • The client's awareness that the nurse is counting the respiratory rate could cause the client to purposefully alter the respiratory pattern. If you anticipate this, place a hand against the client's chest to feel the chest movements with breathing, or place the client's arm across the chest and observe the chest movements while supposedly taking the radial pulse.

   • Count the respiratory rate for 30 seconds if the respirations are regular. Count for 60 seconds if they are irregular. An inhalation and an exhalation count as one respiration.
5. Observe the depth, rhythm, and character of respirations.
   • Observe the respirations for depth by watching the movement of the chest. ➤*Rationale: During deep respirations, a large volume of air is exchanged; during shallow respirations, a small volume is exchanged.*
   • Observe the respirations for regular or irregular rhythm. ➤*Rationale: Normally, respirations are evenly spaced.*
   • Observe the character of respirations—the sound they produce and the effort they require. ➤*Rationale: Normally, respirations are silent and effortless.*
6. Document the respiratory rate, depth, rhythm, and character on the appropriate record.

## Documentation

Sample: 5/17/09 1320 Respirations irregular, varying from 18–34/min. in past hour. Shallower resp. during tachypnea. Slight wheezing noted. Resp. therapist called to provide treatment.

_____ D. Katano, RN

## DEVELOPMENTAL CONSIDERATIONS

### Infants

- An infant or child who is crying will have an abnormal respiratory rate and rhythm and needs to be quieted before respirations can be accurately assessed.

- Infants use their diaphragms for inhalation and exhalation. If necessary, place your hand gently on the infant's abdomen to feel the rapid rise and fall during respirations.

- Most newborns are complete nose breathers, and nasal obstruction can be life threatening.

- Some newborns display "periodic breathing" in which they pause for a few seconds between respirations. This condition can be normal, but parents should be alert to prolonged or frequent pauses (apnea) that require medical attention.

- Compared to adults, infants have fewer alveoli and their airways have a smaller diameter. As a result, infants' respiratory rate and effort of breathing will increase with respiratory infections.

### Children

- Because young children are diaphragmatic breathers, observe the rise and fall of the abdomen. If necessary, place your hand gently on the abdomen to feel the rapid rise and fall during respirations.

- Count respirations prior to other uncomfortable procedures so that the respiratory rate is not artificially elevated by the discomfort.

### Elders

- Ask the client to remain quiet, or count respirations after taking the pulse.

- Elders experience anatomic and physiologic changes that cause the respiratory system to be less efficient. Any changes in rate or type of breathing should be reported immediately.

## SETTING OF CARE

- Monitor respiratory rate following the administration of respiratory depressants such as morphine.

- Assess the home setting for factors that could interfere with breathing such as exhaust, gas, or paint fumes or persons who smoke.

- If the client has just come in from another room, allow the client to rest a minute or two before counting respirations.

- Have an adult hold a child gently to reduce movement while counting respirations.

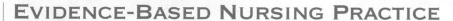

# Skill 11.27   Assessing Blood Pressure

## EVIDENCE-BASED NURSING PRACTICE

**Effect of Music on Vital Signs**

The impact of music (Mendelson's classical violin) on vital signs was studied on a pulmonary medical unit. The results showed a trend toward a decrease in systolic and diastolic blood pressure as well as a decrease in heart rate.

*Source:* Burgner, Kathleen (2005, June 27). Musical intervention. *Advance for Nurses,* 2, 21–23.

**Forearm Blood Pressure**

Statistical analysis has shown that blood pressure taken in the upper arm vs. the forearm varies by 14–20 mm Hg. The two pressures are therefore not interchangeable. If the appropriate cuff size is not available and the forearm has to be used, document the site used.

*Source:* Schell, K., Bradley, E., et al. (2005). Clinical comparison of automatic, noninvasive blood pressure in the forearm and upper arm. *Am J Crit Care,* 14(3), 232.

**Stethoscope Accuracy in Measuring Blood Pressure**

Studies indicate that when measuring blood pressure, accuracy is much higher when using the bell (rather than the diaphragm) of the stethoscope.

*Source:* Best Practice, Vital signs (1999), vol. 3, no. 3, p. 3. http://www.joannabriggs.edu.au.

*(continued)*

## EVIDENCE-BASED NURSING PRACTICE (CONTINUED)

**Body Position Influence on Blood Pressure**

When the client's arm was placed above or below the level of the heart, BP changed by as much as 20 points mm Hg. Therefore, it is recommended that clients sit with their arm supported horizontally at heart level.

Studies show that when hypertensive clients crossed their legs while having their BP taken, the systolic readings rose by 9.45 points mm Hg and the diastolic rose by 3.7 points mm Hg. Clients should have their feet on the floor during a BP measurement.

*Source: Best Practice,* Vital signs (1999), vol. 3, no. 3, p. 3. http://www.joannabriggs.edu.au. Fitzpatrick, F., Ortiz, L., et al. (1999). *Nursing Research* 48(2), 105.

### CLINICAL ALERT

The American Heart Association recommends routine use of the bell of the stethoscope for blood pressure (Korotkoff's sounds) auscultation.

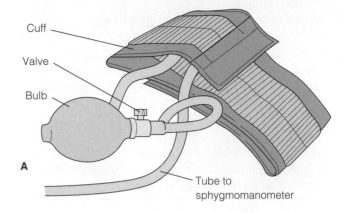

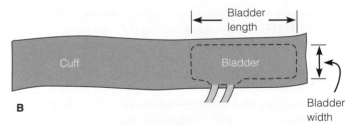

● **A,** Blood pressure cuff and bulb; **B,** the bladder inside the cuff.

### Delegation

Blood pressure measurement may be delegated to UAP. The interpretation of abnormal blood pressure readings and determination of appropriate responses are done by the nurse.

### Equipment

- Stethoscope or DUS
- Blood pressure cuff

The blood pressure cuff consists of a rubber bag that can be inflated with air called the bladder. It is covered with cloth and has two tubes attached to it. One tube connects to a rubber bulb that inflates the bladder. A small valve on the side of this bulb traps and releases the air in the bladder. The other tube is attached to a sphygmomanometer.

Blood pressure cuffs come in various sizes (newborn, infant, child, small adult, adult, large adult, thigh) because the bladder must be the correct width and length for the client's arm. The width should be 40% of the circumference, or 20% wider than the diameter of the midpoint, of the limb on which it is used. The arm circumference, not the age of the client, should always be used to determine bladder size. Lay the cuff lengthwise at the midpoint of the upper arm, and hold the outermost side of the bladder edge laterally on the arm. With the other hand, wrap the width of the cuff around the arm, and ensure that the width is 40% of the arm circumference.

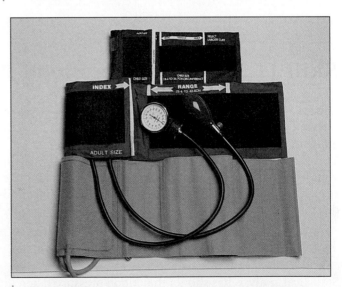

● Three standard cuff sizes: a small cuff for an infant, small child, or frail adult; a normal adult-size cuff; and a large cuff for measuring the blood pressure on the leg or arm of an obese client.

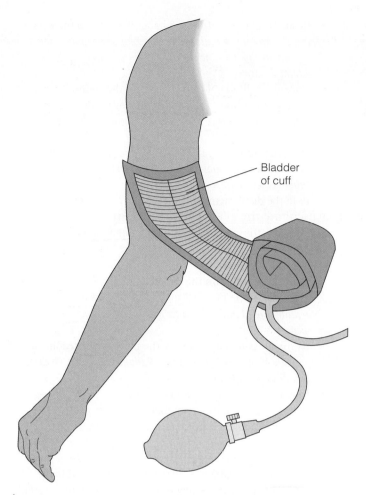

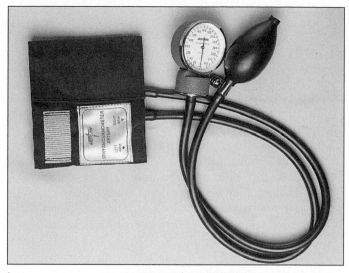

● Blood pressure equipment: an aneroid sphygmomanometer and cuff.

● Determining that the bladder of a blood pressure cuff is 40% of the arm circumference or 20% wider than the diameter of the midpoint of the limb.

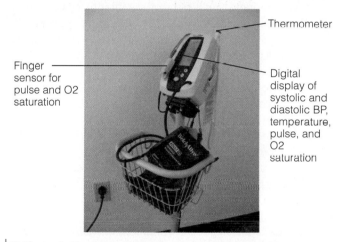

● Electronic blood pressure monitors register blood pressures.

The length of the bladder also affects the accuracy of measurement. The bladder should be sufficiently long to cover at least two-thirds of the limb's circumference.

Blood pressure cuffs are made of nondistensible material so that an even pressure is exerted around the limb. Most cuffs are held in place by hooks, snaps, or Velcro. Others have a cloth bandage that is long enough to encircle the limb several times; this type is closed by tucking the end of the bandage into one of the bandage folds.

### Sphygmomanometer

The sphygmomanometer indicates the pressure of the air within the bladder. The aneroid sphygmomanometer is a calibrated dial with a needle that points to the calibrations.

The pumping action to inflate the blood pressure cuff can be used as a prompt for self-care. As the nurse inflates a manual cuff, taking a few slow and complete breaths will help the nurse remain calm and focused, and to really tune into the whole person as vital signs are accessed.

Many agencies use digital (electronic) sphygmomanometers, which eliminate the need to listen for the sounds of the client's systolic and diastolic blood pressures through a stethoscope. Electronic blood pressure devices should be calibrated periodically to check accuracy. All health care facilities should have manual blood pressure equipment available as backup.

### Preparation

1. Ensure that the equipment is intact and functioning properly. Check for leaks in the tubing of the sphygmomanometer.
2. Make sure that the client has not smoked or ingested caffeine within 30 minutes prior to measurement. ►*Rationale: Smoking constricts blood vessels, and caffeine increases the pulse rate. Both of these cause a temporary increase in blood pressure.*

## Procedure

1. Prior to performing the procedure, introduce self and verify the client's identity using agency protocol. Explain to the client what you are going to do, why it is necessary, and how he or she can participate. Discuss how the results will be used in planning further care or treatments.
2. Perform hand hygiene and observe appropriate infection control procedures.
3. Provide for client privacy.
4. Position the client appropriately.
   - The adult client should be sitting unless otherwise specified. Both feet should be flat on the floor. ➤*Rationale: Legs crossed at the knee result in elevated systolic and diastolic blood pressures* (Pickering et al., 2005).
   - The elbow should be slightly flexed with the palm of the hand facing up and the forearm supported at heart level. Readings in any other position should be specified. The blood pressure is normally similar in sitting, standing, and lying positions, but it can vary significantly by position in certain persons. ➤*Rationale: The blood pressure increases when the arm is below heart level and decreases when the arm is above heart level*(Pickering et al., 2005).
   - Expose the upper arm.
5. Wrap the deflated cuff evenly around the upper arm. Locate the brachial artery. Apply the center of the bladder directly over the artery. ➤*Rationale: The bladder inside the cuff must be directly over the artery to be compressed if the reading is to be accurate.*
   - For an adult, place the lower border of the cuff approximately 2.5 cm (1 in.) above the antecubital space.
6. If this is the client's initial examination, perform a preliminary palpatory determination of systolic pressure. ➤*Rationale: The initial estimate tells the nurse the maximal pressure to which the sphygmomanometer needs to be elevated in subsequent determinations. It also prevents underestimation of the systolic pressure or overestimation of the diastolic pressure should an auscultatory gap occur.*
   - Palpate the brachial artery with the fingertips.
   - Close the valve on the bulb.
   - Pump up the cuff until you no longer feel the brachial pulse. At that pressure the blood cannot flow through the artery. Note the pressure on the sphygmomanometer at which the pulse is no longer felt. ➤*Rationale: This gives an estimate of the systolic pressure.*
   - Release the pressure completely in the cuff, and wait 1 to 2 minutes before making further measurements. ➤*Rationale: A waiting period gives the blood trapped in the veins time to be released. Otherwise, false high systolic readings will occur.*
7. Position the stethoscope appropriately.
   - Cleanse the earpieces with antiseptic wipe.
   - Insert the ear attachments of the stethoscope in your ears so that they tilt slightly forward. ➤*Rationale: Sounds are heard more clearly when the ear attachments follow the direction of the ear canal.*
   - Ensure that the stethoscope hangs freely from the ears to the diaphragm. ➤*Rationale: If the stethoscope tubing rubs against an object, the noise can block the sounds of the blood within the artery.*
   - Place the bell side of the amplifier of the stethoscope over the brachial pulse site. ➤*Rationale: Because the blood pressure is a low-frequency sound, it is best heard with the bell-shaped diaphragm.*
   - Place the stethoscope directly on the skin, not on clothing over the site. ➤*Rationale: This is to avoid noise made from rubbing the amplifier against cloth.*
   - Hold the diaphragm with the thumb and index finger.
8. Auscultate the client's blood pressure.
   - Pump up the cuff until the sphygmomanometer reads 30 mm Hg above the point where the brachial pulse disappeared.
   - Release the valve on the cuff carefully so that the pressure decreases at the rate of 2 to 3 mm Hg per second. ➤*Rationale: If the rate is faster or slower, an error in measurement may occur.*
   - As the pressure falls, identify the manometer reading at Korotkoff phases 1,4, and 5. ➤*Rationale: There is no clinical Significance to phases 2 and 3* (Pickering et al., 2005).
   - Deflate the cuff rapidly and completely.
   - Wait 1 to 2 minutes before making further determinations. ➤*Rationale: This permits blood trapped in the veins to be released.*
   - Repeat the above steps to confirm the accuracy of the reading—especially if it falls outside the normal range (although this may not be routine procedure for hospitalized or well clients). If there is greater than a 5 mm Hg difference between the two readings, additional measurements may be taken and the results averaged (Pickering et al., 2005).
9. If this is the client's initial examination, repeat the procedure on the client's other arm. There should be a difference of no more than 10 mm Hg between the arms. The arm found to have the higher pressure should be used for subsequent examinations.

### VARIATION: Obtaining a Blood Pressure by the Palpation Method

If it is not possible to use a stethoscope to obtain the blood pressure or if Korotkoff's sounds cannot be heard, palpate the radial or brachial pulse site as the cuff pressure is released. The manometer reading at the point where the pulse reappears is an estimate of the systolic blood pressure.

### VARIATION: Taking a Thigh Blood Pressure

- Help the client to assume a prone position. If the client cannot assume this position, measure the blood pressure while the client is in a supine position with the knee slightly flexed. Slight flexing of the knee will facilitate placing the stethoscope on the popliteal space.

- Expose the thigh, taking care not to expose the client unduly.
- Locate the popliteal artery.
- Wrap the cuff evenly around the midthigh with the compression bladder over the posterior aspect of the thigh and the bottom edge above the knee. ➤*Rationale: The bladder must be directly over the posterior popliteal artery if the reading is to be accurate.*
- If this is the client's initial examination, perform a preliminary palpatory determination of systolic pressure while palpating the popliteal artery.
- In adults, the systolic pressure in the popliteal artery is often 20 to 30 mm Hg higher than that in the brachial artery; the diastolic pressure is usually the same.

## VARIATION: Using an Electronic Indirect Blood Pressure Monitoring Device

- Place the blood pressure cuff on the extremity according to the manufacturer's guidelines.
- Turn on the blood pressure switch.
- If appropriate, set the device for the desired number of minutes between blood pressure determinations.
- When the device has determined the blood pressure reading, note the digital results.

- Electronic/automatic blood pressure cuffs can be left in place for many hours. Remove the cuff and check skin condition periodically.

10. Remove the cuff from the client's arm.
11. Wipe the cuff with an approved disinfectant. ➤*Rationale: Cuffs can become significantly contaminated.* Many institutions use disposable blood pressure cuffs. The client uses a disposable cuff for the length of stay and then it is discarded. ➤*Rationale: This decreases the risk of spreading infection by sharing cuffs.*
12. Document and report pertinent assessment data according to agency policy. Record two pressures in the form "130/80" where "130" is the systolic (phase 1) and "80" is the diastolic (phase 5) pressure. Record three pressures in the form "130/90/0," where "130" is the systolic, "90" is the first diastolic (phase 4), and sounds are audible even after the cuff is completely deflated (Pickering et al., 2005). Use the abbreviations RA or RL for right arm or right leg and LA or LL for left arm or left leg. Record a difference of greater than 10 mm Hg between the two arms or legs.

## DEVELOPMENTAL CONSIDERATIONS

### Infants

- Use a pediatric stethoscope with a small diaphragm.
- The lower edge of the blood pressure cuff can be closer to the antecubital space of an infant.
- Use the palpation method if auscultation with a stethoscope or DUS is unsuccessful.
- Arm and thigh pressures are equivalent in children under 1 year of age.
- The systolic blood pressure of a newborn ranges between 50 and 80 mm Hg; the diastolic between 25 and 55 mm Hg (D'Amico & Barbarito, 2007).
- One quick way to determine the normal systolic blood pressure of a child is to use the following formula: Normal systolic BP = 80 + (2 × child's age in years)

### Children

- Blood pressure should be measured in all children over 3 years of age and in children less than 3 years of age with certain medical conditions (e.g., congenital heart disease, renal malformation, medications that affect blood pressure).
- Explain each step of the process and what it will feel like. Demonstrate on a doll.
- Use the palpation technique for children under 3 years old.

- Cuff bladder width should be 40% and length should be 80% to 100% of the arm circumference.
- Take the blood pressure prior to other uncomfortable procedures so that the blood pressure is not artificially elevated by the discomfort.
- In children, the diastolic pressure is considered to be the onset of phase 4, where the sounds become muffled.
- In children, the thigh pressure is about 10 mm Hg higher than the arm.

### Elders

- Skin may be very fragile. Do not allow cuff pressure to remain high any longer than necessary.
- Determine if the client is taking antihypertensives and, if so, when the last dose was taken.
- Medications that cause vasodilation (antihypertensive medications) along with the loss of baroreceptor efficiency in the elderly place them at increased risk for having orthostatic hypotension (significant fall in blood pressure when changing from supine to sitting or standing). Measuring blood pressure while the client is in the lying, sitting, and standing positions—and noting any changes—can determine this.
- If the client has arm contractures, assess the blood pressure by palpation, with the arm in a relaxed position. If this is not possible, take a thigh blood pressure.

## TABLE 11-11 SELECTED SOURCES OF ERROR IN BLOOD PRESSURE ASSESSMENT

| Error | Effect |
| --- | --- |
| Bladder cuff too narrow | Erroneously high |
| Bladder cuff too wide | Erroneously low |
| Arm unsupported | Erroneously high |
| Insufficient rest before the assessment | Erroneously high |
| Repeating assessment too quickly | Erroneously high systolic or low diastolic readings |
| Cuff wrapped too loosely or unevenly | Erroneously high |
| Deflating cuff too quickly | Erroneously low systolic and high diastolic readings |
| Deflating cuff too slowly | Erroneously high diastolic reading |
| Failure to use the same arm consistently | Inconsistent measurements |
| Arm above level of the heart | Erroneously low |
| Assessing immediately after a meal or while client smokes or has pain | Erroneously high |
| Failure to identify auscultatory gap | Erroneously low systolic pressure and erroneously low diastolic pressure |

## CLIENT TEACHING

- Explain to the client and family what the equipment actually does and the information it provides.

- Instruct clients with automatic blood pressure devices such as the type often used in emergency departments to keep the elbow extended when the cuff inflates.

## SETTING OF CARE

- If the client takes blood pressure readings at home, the nurse should use the same equipment or calibrate it against a system known to be accurate.
- Observe the client or family member taking the blood pressure and provide feedback if further instruction is needed.
- Home blood pressure measurement done by the client or family can be more accurate than blood pressure measured in a clinic or office setting. This is because so-called "white coat" hypertension can occur, which is an elevation in blood pressure due to mild anxiety associated with the health care provider's presence—who historically wore a white laboratory coat (Smith, 2005).
- If the client is in a chair or low bed, position yourself so that you maintain the client's arm at heart level and you can read the sphygmomanometer at eye level.

## CULTURAL CONSIDERATIONS

Many cultures believe that certain substances protect one's health. For example, Italians, Greeks, and Native Americans believe that garlic or onions eaten raw or worn on the body will prevent illness such as high blood pressure. If a client wishes to include these items in his or her diet or wear them, the nursing staff should respect this practice, since it is an important cultural tradition for many groups.

# Skill 11.28   Assessing Pulse Oximeter

## Delegation

Application of the pulse oximeter sensor and recording of the $SpO_2$ value may be delegated to UAP. The interpretation of the oxygen saturation value and determination of appropriate responses are done by the nurse.

## Equipment

- Nail polish remover as needed
- Alcohol wipe
- Sheet or towel
- Pulse oximeter

Pulse oximeters with various types of sensors are available from several manufacturers. The *oximeter unit* consists of an inlet connection for the sensor cable, a faceplate that indicates (a) the oxygen saturation measurement (expressed as a percentage); and (b) the pulse rate. Cordless units are also available. A preset alarm system signals high and low $SpO_2$ measurements and a high and low pulse rate. The high and low $SpO_2$ levels are generally preset at 100% and 85%, respectively for adults. The high and low pulse rate alarms are usually preset at 140 and 50 bpm for adults. These alarms limits can, however, be changed according to the manufacturer's directions.

## Preparation

Check that the oximeter equipment is functioning normally.

## Procedure

1. Prior to performing the procedure, introduce self and verify the client's identity using agency protocol. Explain to the client what you are going to do, why it is necessary, and how he or she can participate. Discuss how the results will be used in planning further care or treatments.
2. Perform hand hygiene and observe appropriate infection control procedures.
3. Provide for client privacy.
4. Choose a sensor appropriate for the client's weight, size, and desired location. Because weight limits of sensors overlap, a pediatric sensor could be used for a small adult.
   - If the client is allergic to adhesive, use a clip or sensor without adhesive. If using an extremity, assess the proximal pulse and capillary refill at the point closest to the site.
   - If the client has low tissue perfusion due to peripheral vascular disease or therapy using vasoconstrictive medications, use a nasal sensor or a reflectance sensor on the forehead. Avoid using lower extremities that have compromised circulation and extremities that are used for infusions or other invasive monitoring.

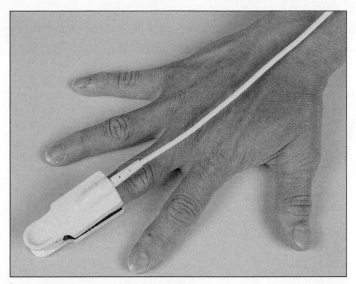

● Fingertip oximeter sensor (cordless).

(Courtesy of Nonin Medical Inc.)

5. Prepare the site.
   - Clean the site with an alcohol wipe before applying the sensor.
   - It may be necessary to remove a female client's dark nail polish. ➤*Rationale: It can interfere with accurate measurements.*
   - Alternatively, position the sensor on the side of the finger rather than perpendicular to the nail bed (Rajkumar, Karmarkar, & Knott, 2006).
6. Apply the sensor, and connect it to the pulse oximeter.
   - Make sure the LED and photodetector are accurately aligned, that is, opposite each other on either side of the finger, toe, nose, or earlobe. Many sensors have markings to facilitate correct alignment of the LEDs and photodetector.
   - Attach the sensor cable to the connection outlet on the oximeter. Turn on the machine according to the manufacturer's directions. Appropriate connection will be confirmed by an audible beep indicating each arterial pulsation. Some devices have a wheel that can be turned clockwise to increase the pulse volume and counterclockwise to decrease it.
   - Ensure that the bar of light or waveform on the face of the oximeter fluctuates with each pulsation.
7. Set and turn on the alarm when using continuous monitoring.
   - Check the preset alarm limits for high and low oxygen saturation and high and low pulse rates. Change these alarm limits according to the manufacturer's directions as

indicated. Ensure that the audio and visual alarms are on before you leave the client. Atone will be heard and a number will blink on the faceplate.

8. Ensure client safety.
   - Inspect and/or move or change the location of an adhesive toe or finger sensor every 4 hours and a spring-tension sensor every 2 hours.
   - Inspect the sensor site tissues for irritation from adhesive sensors.

9. Ensure the accuracy of measurement.
   - Minimize motion artifacts by using an adhesive sensor, or immobilize the client's monitoring site. ➤*Rationale: Movement of the client's finger or toe may be misinterpreted by the oximeter as arterial pulsations.*

   - If indicated, cover the sensor with a sheet or towel to block large amounts of light from external sources (e.g., sunlight, procedure lamps, or bilirubin lights in the nursery). ➤*Rationale: Bright room light may be sensed by the photodetector and alter the SpO$_2$ value.*
   - Compare the pulse rate indicated by the oximeter to the radial pulse periodically. ➤*Rationale: A large discrepancy between the two values may indicate oximeter malfunction.*

10. Document the oxygen saturation on the appropriate record at designated intervals.

### Physical Assessments for the Child

(For physical assessment of the newborn, see Chapter 9, "Reproduction.")

---

## DEVELOPMENTAL CONSIDERATIONS

### Infants

- If an appropriate-sized finger or toe sensor is not available, consider using an earlobe or forehead sensor.
- The high and low SpO$_2$ alarm levels are generally preset at 95% and 80% for neonates.
- The high and low pulse rate alarms are usually preset at 200 and 100 for neonates.
- The oximeter may need to be taped, wrapped with an elastic bandage, or covered by a stocking to keep it in place.

### Children

- Instruct the child that the sensor does not hurt. Disconnect the probe whenever possible to allow for movement.

### Elders

- Use of vasoconstrictive medications, poor circulation, or thickened nails may make finger or toe sensors inaccurate.

---

## SETTING OF CARE

- Pulse oximetry is a quick, inexpensive, noninvasive method of assessing oxygenation. Like an automatic blood pressure cuff, it also provides a pulse rate reading. Use in the ambulatory or home setting whenever indicated.

- If the client requires frequent or continuous home monitoring, teach the client and family how to apply and maintain the equipment. Remind them to rotate the site periodically and assess for skin trauma.

---

# Skill 11.29 Measuring Length

### Preparation

Have the parent remove any hat or shoes the infant is wearing.

### Equipment

Measuring board or other length-measuring device.

### Procedure

1. When using a measuring board, place the infant's head against the top of the board.

2. Use the parent or an assistant to hold the infant's head in the midline, and gently push down on the knees until the legs are straight. ➤*Rationale: Because of the normally flexed posture of the infant, the body must be extended to obtain an accurate measurement.*

3. Position the heels of the feet on the footboard, and record the length to the nearest 0.5 cm or ¼ inch.

4. Repeat the measurement for accuracy. If a difference between the two readings is found, take the average reading for documentation.

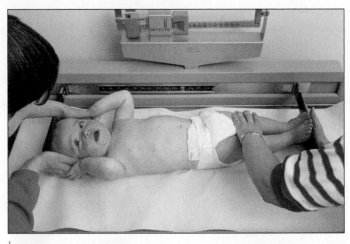

● Measuring an infant's length.

5. Plot the measurement for the child's age on the standardized growth curve.

*Note:* If such a measuring device is not available, place the infant on a paper sheet stabilizing the infant in the same manner as when using the board. Make one mark at the vertex of the head and another at the heel. Then measure the distance between the two marks. Record the length in centimeters or inches.

# Skill 11.30  Measuring Height

### Preparation

Have the child remove shoes and hat.

### Equipment

Stadiometer or platform scale with stature-measuring device.

### Procedure

1. With shoes removed, have the child stand straight with the back to the wall. The head should be held erect and in the midline position.
2. The shoulders, buttocks, and heels should touch the wall. The outer canthus of the eyes should be on the same horizontal plane as the external auditory canals. ▶*Rationale: Positioning the head properly helps ensure consistency in placement of the headpiece on the crown of the head.*
3. Move the headpiece down to touch the crown.
4. Make the height reading to the nearest 0.5 cm of 1/4 inch.
5. Plot the measurement for the child's age on the standardized growth curve.

*Note:* In the older child and adolescent, height is often measured using a platform scale with an attached stature-measuring device. Have the child stand erect facing forward. Move the stature-measuring device to the top of the head. Have the child step off the scale, and read the height in centimeters or inches.

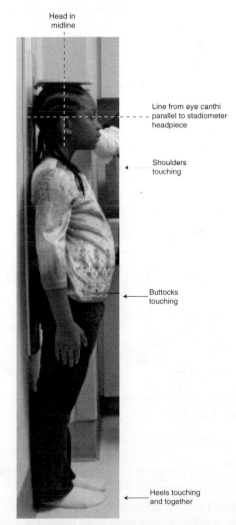

● Measuring a child's height. Position the head in an erect and midline position while the shoulders, buttocks, and heels touch the wall. Move the headpiece down to touch the crown.

# Skill 11.31  Measuring Weight

### Equipment
Infant scale for infants
Paper
Standing scale for older children

### Preparation
1. Check the balance of the scale before using it.
2. Have the parent or assistant remove all of the infant's clothing and diaper. Weigh toddlers in their underclothes. Weigh older children in their street clothes with heavy clothing and shoes removed. Infants with acute diarrheal disease or chronic health problem may need to be weighed nude for accuracy. ►*Rationale: It is important to try to minimize the amount of clothing worn by children when being weighed to improve comparisons with previous weights taken.*
3. Clean the infant scale tray between uses. Place a paper cover over the scale tray.

### Procedure
1. Place the infant on the scale and keep a hand close. ►*Rationale: Infants move quickly and it is essential to protect them from falling.*
2. Distract the infant, and take the reading when the infant stops moving. ►*Rationale: It takes a few second of inactivity for the scale to settle on the infant's actual weight.*
3. Record the weight in the nearest 10 g or 1/2 oz.
4. Plot the measurement for the child's exact age in months on the standardized growth curve.

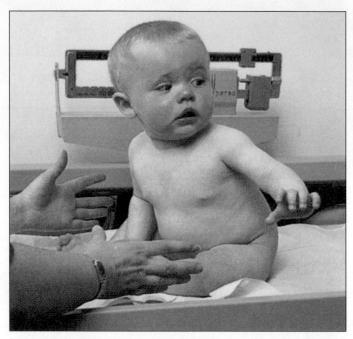

● A platform scale is used to weigh an infant.

### For Older Children
The older child can be weighed on a standing scale.
1. Provide privacy for the older child and adolescent.
2. Have the child stand still on the scale.
3. Move the weights until the scale is balanced for the child's weight.
4. Record the weight to the nearest 0.1 kg or 1/4 lb.

# Skill 11.32  Measuring Body Mass Index

The body mass index (BMI) uses a formula of kg per $m^2$ to assess nutritional status and total body weight relative to height. The child's BMI can be easily determined after plotting the length and weight, or height and weight, on the standardized growth curves. ►*Rationale: Tracking the change in BMI can often provide clues to nutritional problems, including obesity, health promotion issues, or illness.*

---

### CLINICAL TIP

In order to calculate body mass index (BMI), follow these steps:
1. Be sure that weight is in kilograms. If it is in pounds, divide that number by 2.2 to get kg.
2. Change height measurement to meters. Since 1 meter = 39.37 inches (or 0.0254 meters = 1 inches), you need to multiply the child's height in inches to obtain heights in meters.
3. Now square the number of meters.
4. You are ready to calculate BMI. Divide kg of weight by height in meters squared. If a child weighs 26.5 pounds, covert to kgC 26.5 pounds = 12 kg. The child's height is 34.5 inches of 0.8763 meters. Then meters$^2$ = 0.7679. So the BMI = 15.63.
5. An online BMI calculator is available at http:.www.cdc.gov/growthcharts.

# Skill 11.33 Measuring Head Circumference

**Preparation**

Remove any hat, hair binders, or barrettes the infant is wearing.

**Equipment**

Disposable, nonstretching measuring tape with centimeter and millimeter markings

**Procedure**

1. Wrap the tape around the head at the supraorbital prominence above the eyebrows, above the ears, and around the occipital prominence. Take care to prevent the tape from slipping or causing a paper cut. ➤*Rationale: This is usually the point of largest circumference of the head.*
2. Record the circumference to the nearest 0.5 cm or 1/8 inch. Repeat the measurement to confirm the reading.
3. Plot the measurement for the child's exact age in months on the standardized growth curve.

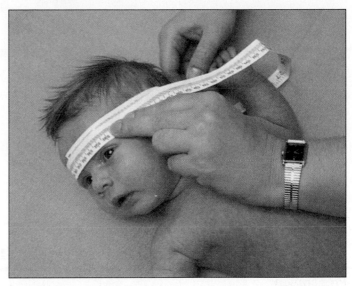

● Measuring head circumference.

# Skill 11.34 Measuring Chest Circumference

**Preparation**

Remove all clothing from the child's chest.

**Equipment**

Disposable, nonstretching measuring tape with centimeter and millimeter markings

**Procedure**

1. Wrap the tape measure around the chest, placed just under the axilla and at the nipple line.
2. Record the circumference measurement to the nearest 0.5 cm or 1/8 inch.
3. Compare the chest circumference to the head circumference measurement. ➤*Rationale: The head and chest circumference will be approximately equal until after 1 year of age, when the chest circumference begins to surpass head circumference.*

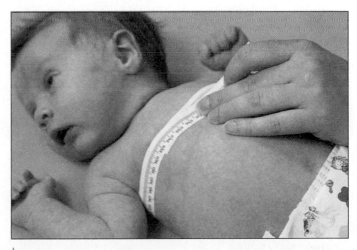

● Measuring chest circumference.

# Skill 11.35 Measuring Abdominal Girth

## Preparation

Remove all clothing from the abdomen.

## Equipment

Disposable, nonstretching measuring tape with centimeter and millimeter markings.

## Procedure

1. Wrap the tape around the abdomen at the level of the umbilicus, taking care to prevent a paper cut.

2. In the measurement is taken at another location on the abdomen, place ink marks at the location of the measurement. ➤*Rationale: This action will enable you to another nurse to make a future measurement at the same location.*

3. Record the measurement to the nearest 0.5 cm or 1/2 inch. Compare the reading to those taken previously to determine a change in size.

# Skill 11.36 Assessing the Heart Rate

## Preparation

- Move clothing away from the anterior chest.
- Give the infant a pacifier or other distraction to get a resting pulse rate.

## Equipment

Stethoscope

## Procedure

1. Place the cleaned stethoscope on the anterior chest at the fifth intercostals space in a midclavicular position. ➤*Rationale: The apical heart rate is preferred in infants and young children, and it is also used for older children when the condition warrants it. In infants and children, it is difficult to palpate the pulse in an extremity consistently enough to count the rate.*

2. Each "lub-dub" sound is one beat. Count the beats for 1 full minute, or count for 30 seconds and multiply by 2.

3. While auscultating the heart rate, note if the rhythm is regular or irregular.

    Pulse rates may be palpated in children over 3 years of age. Sites commonly used include the brachial, radial, femoral, and dorsal pedis. In addition, the pulse rhythm, strength, and amplitude may be checked.

    - Note if the rhythm is regular or irregular.
    - Compare the distal and proximal pulses in an extremity for strength.
    - Record if the pulsation is normal, bounding, or thready. The range of normal heart rates by age is listed in the table to the right.

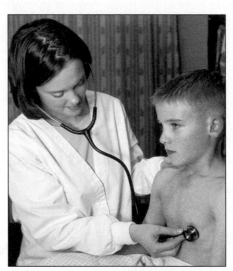

● Assessing the apical heart rate.

TABLE 11–12 **NORMAL HEART RATES FOR CHILDREN AT DIFFERENT AGES**

| Age | Heart Rate Range (beats/min) | Average Heart Rate (beats/min) |
|---|---|---|
| Newborns | 100–170 | 120 |
| Infants to 2 years | 80–130 | 110 |
| 2–6 years | 70–120 | 100 |
| 6–10 years | 70–110 | 90 |
| 10–16 years | 60–100 | 85 |

# Skill 11.37 Assessing the Respiratory Rate

The procedure for measuring a child's respiratory rate is essentially the same as for an adult. However, keep in mind these points:

- Observe the abdomen rather than the chest rise and fall in an infant and young child. ➤*Rationale: Since an infant's and young child's respirations are diaphragmatic, the abdomen moves more than the chest with breathing.*
- Abdominal movement in a child will be irregular.
- Count breaths for 1 full minute, or count for 30 second and multiply by 2.

The range of normal respiratory rates based on age is listed in the Table below.

**TABLE 11–13 NORMAL RESPIRATORY RATE CHANGES FOR EACH AGE GROUP**

| Age | Respiratory Rate per Minute |
|---|---|
| Newborn | 30–80 |
| 1 year | 20–40 |
| 3 years | 20–30 |
| 6 years | 16–22 |
| 10 years | 16–20 |
| 17 years | 12–20 |

# Skill 11.38 Assessing Blood Pressure

## Preparation

- To select the proper cuff size, compare the cuff to the size of the child's upper arm or thigh.
- The bladder of the cuff should cover about 80% of the circumference of the extremity used.
- The bladder width should cover about two thirds of the upper arm or thigh. ➤*Rationale: If the bladder is too small, the blood pressure reading will be falsely high; if it is too large, the pressure will be falsely low.*

## Equipment

- Various sizes blood pressure cuffs
- Electronic blood pressure monitor
- Sphygmomanometer and stethoscope
- Blood pressure values by age, sex, and height percentiles

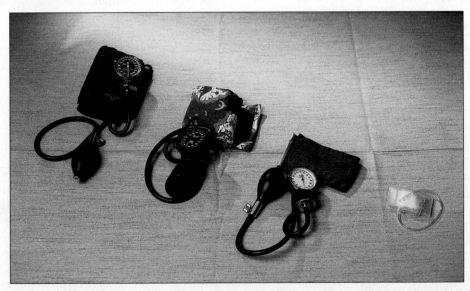

● Blood pressure cuffs are available in various types and sizes for pediatric patients.

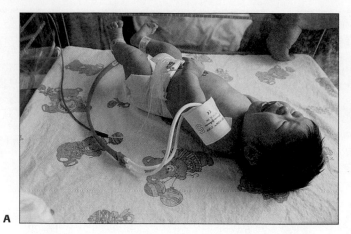

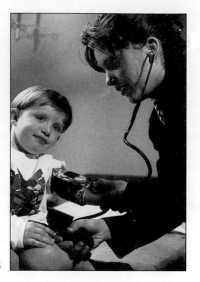

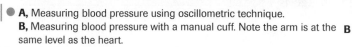

● **A,** Measuring blood pressure using oscillometric technique.
**B,** Measuring blood pressure with a manual cuff. Note the arm is at the **B**
same level as the heart.
(A, courtesy of Photographer: Elena Dorfman.)

## VARIATION: Oscillometry

### Procedure

Electronic equipment is often used to obtain the systolic blood pressure for infants and young children. With this technique, a transducer uses pressure oscillations received and transmitted by the blood pressure cuff to estimate the blood pressure and mean arterial pressure (Stebor, 2005).

1. Place the cuff around the desired extremity directly against the skin.
2. Place the arm at heart level with muscles relaxed.
3. Activate the equipment according to the manufacturer's recommendations.
4. Pressure is recorded as the number over "D."
5. Document the blood pressure reading and compare values for age, sex, and height percentile. Children with a blood pressure reading over the 90th percentile for age, sex, and height percentiles should be referred for management of the elevated blood pressure.

---

### CLINICAL ALERT

To choose the appropriate cuff size for a newborn, measure the newborn's limb circumference with a measuring take around the midpoint of the limb used. If the blood pressure cuff has marks to determine fit, use these lines to ensure that the cuff is not too small. The cuff width should not extend to or beyond any joint on the limb used. Make sure the artery mark on the cuff is placed over the brachial artery (Stebor, 2005).

## VARIATION: Manual Sphygmomanometer

### Procedure

1. Wrap the cuff snugly around the desired extremity directly against the skin.
2. Hold the arm at heart level.
3. Palpate for the pulse, and place the stethoscope over the pulse area.
4. Close the air escape valve. Pump the cuff with the bulb until the gauge rises and no beat is auscultated. Continue pumping until the gauge rises another 20 to 30 mm.
5. Slowly release the air through the valve at 2 to 3 mm/sec while watching the falling gauge.
6. Note the number at which the first return of a pulse is heard; this is the systolic pressure.
7. Continuing releasing the air to determine the diastolic pressure: If the child is less than 12 years, a muffled sound will be heard. Record this as the diastolic pressure. If the child is older than 12 years, all sound will disappear at the diastolic pressure.
8. Blood pressure is read as systolic over diastolic pressure.
9. Document the blood pressure reading and compare to values for age, sex, and height percentile.

### VARIATION: Blood Pressure by Palpation

If the pulsation cannot be auscultated, blood pressure can still be measured by palpation. Wrap the cuff around the desired extremity, close the air valve, and palpate for the pulse. Keeping your fingers on the pulse, pump the cuff with the bulb until the pulse is no longer felt. Slowly open the air valve, watching the gauge, and note the number at which the pulse is again palpated. This is the palpated systolic blood pressure read as the number over "P."

# Skill 11.39  Assessing a Child's Body Temperature

Body temperature can be measured in two scales: Fahrenheit or centigrade. Follow the manufacturer's guidelines for the use of electronic thermometers.

The four routes for measuring body temperature are oral, rectal, axillary, and tympanic.

### VARIATION: Oral Route

The oral route may be used for the child over 3 years of age who is able to cooperate by holding the thermometer with the mouth closed. The expected temperature is 37°C (98.6°F).

### Preparation

- Assess the cooperation of the child to hold the thermometer in the mouth, under the tongue with the mouth closed.

### Equipment

- An electronic nonbreakable probe is preferred.

### Procedure

1. Cover the oral probe with the protective sheath.
2. Place the oral probe or an electronic thermometer under the tongue, and have the child close his or her mouth.
3. Turn on the scanner and follow the manufacturer's recommendations. It will sound a tone or beep when finished. Remove the probe.
4. Read and record the temperature.

### VARIATION: Rectal Route

The rectal route should be used only when no other route is possible, due to the potential for rectal perforation and because most children view this as an intrusive procedure. The rectal temperature is one degree higher than the oral temperature, 37.6°C (99.7°F). The rectal temper-ature is a close approximation of core body temperature (Craig, Lancaster, Taylor et al., 2002).

### Preparation

- Place the infant or child prone on a bed or the parent's lap; turn the older child on the side.

### Equipment

- Electronic thermometer with sheath
- Water-soluble lubricant

### Procedure Clean Gloves

1. Cover the tip of the electronic thermometer protective sheath with a water-soluble lubricant.
2. For the infant, place the tip 1/4 to 1/2 inch into the rectum. For the child, place the tip 1 inch into the rectum. ▸*Rationale: This reduces the risk of rectal perforation.*
3. Turn on the scanner and follow the manufacturer's recommendations. It will tone or beep when finished. Remove the probe.
4. Read and record the temperature.

### VARIATION: Axillary Route

The axillary route is often used for newborns and for children who are seizure-prone, unconscious, or immunosuppressed, or who have a structural abnormality that precludes an alternative route. The axillary temperature is generally 0.6°C (1°F) lower than the oral temperature. Current research indicates that the axillary temperature difference between oral and rectal routes increases when the child's body temperature increases (Falzon, Grech, Caruana et al., 2003). Therefore, the axillary route is not as accurate as other methods for identifying children with fevers.

### Procedure

1. The electronic thermometer with protective sheath is held in place in the axilla, with the child's arm pressed close to his or her side.

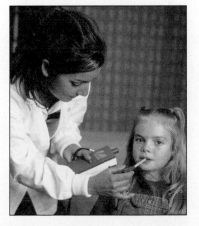

● Measuring the oral temperature.

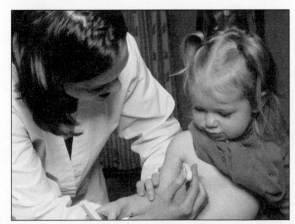

● Measuring the axillary temperature.

2. Turn on the scanner and follow the manufacturer's recommendations. It will sound a tone or beep when finished. Remove the probe.
3. Read and record the temperature.

### VARIATION: Tympanic Route

The tympanic route is a convenient and fast method for taking temperatures in infants and children. Infrared technology provides a rapid reading. The ear temperature reflects the body temperature because the tympanic membrane shares its blood supply with the hypothalamus. The tympanic thermometer is easy to use, provides a rapid reading, and is noninvasive in nature. However, because of inaccuracies in measurement by this route, the tympanic temperature reading should not be used as an approximation of rectal temperature when a precise reading is important for treatment decisions (Craig, Lancaster, Taylor et al., 2002).

### Preparation

1. Place the infant in a supine position on a flat surface. Stabilize the infant's head, and turn the infant's head 90 degrees for easy access.
2. Position the child on the parent's or assistant's lap with head secured.

### Equipment

• Tympanic thermometer with clean disposable probe

### Procedure for Child Younger than 1 Year

1. If using the child's right ear, hold the thermometer in your right hand. For the child's left ear, hold the thermometer in your left hand.
2. Pull the pinna of the ear straight back and downward. Approach the ear from behind to direct the tip anteriorly to make sure the thermometer tip is aimed toward the tympanic membrane. ➤*Rationale: The tip must be aimed at the tympanic membrane to ensure accuracy.*

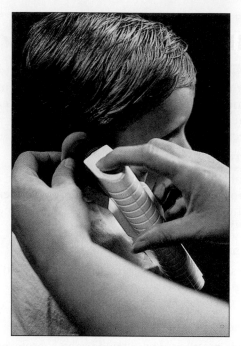

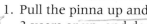 Position for inserting a thermometer when the tympanic route is used. The pinna is pulled up and back to straighten the ear canal in this young child.

3. Place the probe in the ear as far as possible to seal the canal. Turn on the scanner.
4. Leave the probe in the ear according to the manufacturer's recommendations.
5. Remove the probe, and read and record the temperature.

### Procedure for Child Older than 1 Year

1. Pull the pinna up and back in children over about 3 years or up, and downward under that age.
2. Place the probe and continue as described previously for the child younger than 1 year.
3. Read and record the temperature.

# Skill 11.40   Glasgow Coma Scale

**Procedure**

1. When the child has had an injury to the head or has altered consciousness, assess each of the three categories of the Glasgow Coma Scale according to the criteria in the table.
2. Note the time and score for each category. Total the scores for all three categories to get the Glasgow Coma Score. A score of 15 is the maximum and indicates the best level of neurologic functioning.
3. Repeat the test at regular intervals. ➤*Rationale: Since the test provides a numeric score for altered consciousness, regular measurements help detect subtle changes in the child's condition.*
4. Document the score and time performed.

### TABLE 11–14  GLASGOW COMA SCALE FOR ASSESSMENT OF COMA IN INFANTS AND CHILDREN

| Category | Score | Infant and Young Child Criteria |
|---|---|---|
| Eye opening | 4 | Spontaneous opening |
| | 3 | To loud noise |
| | 2 | To pain |
| | 1 | No response |
| Verbal response | 5 | Smiles, coos, cries to appropriate stimuli |
| | 4 | Irritable; cries |
| | 3 | Inappropriate crying |
| | 2 | Grunts, moans |
| | 1 | No response |
| Motor response | 6 | Spontaneous movement |
| | 5 | Withdraws to touch |
| | 4 | Withdraws to pain |
| | 3 | Abnormal flexion (decorticate) |
| | 2 | Abnormal extension (decerebrate) |
| | 1 | No response |

Add the score from each category to get the total. The maximum score is 15, indicating the best level of neurological functioning. The minimum is 3, indicating total neurologic unresponsiveness.

James, H. E. (1986). Neurologic evaluation and support in the child with acute brain insult. *Pediatric Annals,* 15(1), 17.

# Skill 11.41  Neurovascular Assessment

## Procedure

1. Assess the swelling in the extremity associated with the injury. ➤*Rationale: The swelling associated with the injury may constrict blood flow to the distal extremity and pinch the nerves, especially when constriction is present, such as a cast.*

2. Assess the extremity distal to the injury for color and temperature and compare to the other extremity.

3. Assess the capillary refill time by pressing on a finger or toe for a couple of seconds, until the skin is blanched. Count how long it takes for blood or color to return to the area pressed. It should take 2 seconds or less.

4. Assess the extremity for pain and sensation (numbness, tingling, pins and needles sensation) and compare to the other extremity.

5. Consider all the findings simultaneously to complete the neurovascular assessment.

6. The presence of most or all of the following indicates significantly impaired circulation and pressure or injury to the nerve that needs emergency intervention:
   - Pallor or cyanosis
   - Capillary refill time greater than 4 seconds
   - Cool or cold temperature
   - Moderate or severe pain
   - Numbness, tingling, or pins and needles sensation

7. Document the assessment, and repeat it frequently, especially if one or two findings are present. ➤*Rationale: If the circulatory and neurologic constriction is not detected and promptly relieved, permanent damage to the distal extremity may result.*

# Skill 11.42  Intracranial Pressure Monitoring and Daily Care

## Preparation

1. Review the patient's chart related to indications for intracranial pressure monitoring.

2. Review the physician's orders for monitoring and drainage parameters.

3. Verify the identity of the child.

4. Assess the child and family's understanding of the need for intracranial pressure monitoring. Provide explanations to the child and family.

## Equipment

ICP transducer system and monitor

## Procedure Sterile Gloves

1. Assess the system and all connections for leaks and kinked tubing. Maintain the sterility of the equipment. ➤*Rationale: Patency of the system helps prevent infection and allows for CSF drainage.*

2. Ensure that the fluid-filled transducer system is placed and maintained at the level of the foramen of Monro, the line between the top of the ear and the outer canthus of the eye. Balance the ICP transducer to zero for calibration according to hospital guidelines and when the child's position changes. ➤*Rationale: This ensures the accuracy of pressure readings and waveforms by the transducer system.*

3. ICP monitoring is usually continuous. Document ICP and CPP at the frequency ordered by the physician or by hospital protocol. Monitor and print ICP waveforms.

4. Assess the child's responsiveness, vital signs, and neurologic status. Assess for signs of ICP. ➤*Rationale: Patients with brain injuries are at risk for seizures and cerebral edema, which further compromise CPP.*

| TABLE 11–15 ICP WAVEFORMS AND IMPLICATIONS | | |
|---|---|---|
| **Waveform** | **Pressure mm Hg** | **Implications** |
| A | 50–100 | Symptoms related to cerebral dysfunction, changes in vital signs, respiratory pattern, motor function, headache, and emesis |
| B | 20–50 | Decreasing level of consciousness, agitation, varying respiratory pattern |
| C | 4–20 | No clinical significance |
| Normal | 4–15 | Normal |

| TABLE 11-16 | SIGNS OF INCREASED INTRACRANIAL PRESSURE | |
|---|---|
| **Timing of Signs** | **Signs** |
| Early signs | Headache<br>Visual disturbances, diplopia<br>Nausea and vomiting<br>Dizziness or vertigo<br>Slight change in vital signs<br>Pupils not as reactive or equal<br>Sunsetting eyes<br>Seizures<br>Slight change in level of consciousness |
| Additional signs in infants | Bulging fontanelle<br>Wide sutures, increased head circumference<br>Dilated scalp veins<br>High-pitched, catlike cry |
| Late signs | Significant decrease in level of consciousness<br>Cushing's triad<br>• Increased systolic blood pressure and widened pulse pressure<br>• Bradycardia<br>• Irregular respirations<br>Fixed and dilated pupils |

5. Assess pain and comfort level. Administer sedation and pain medication as prescribed. ➤*Rationale: Patients may experience pain at the catheter insertion site and pain from increased ICP. Medications promote the child's comfort and help reduce elevations in ICP.*

6. Assess the insertion site for bleeding, CSF leakage, and signs and symptoms of infection.
7. If the system is draining CSF, assess the output for color, amount, and quality per unit protocol.
8. Maintain the child's position with the head at midline with the remainder of the body and the head of the bed elevated 15 to 30 degrees. ➤*Rationale: This position prevents compression of blood vessels in the neck and obstruction of venous blood flows.*
9. Monitor patient neurologic status during nursing care and continue or stop depending on patient response. Document care and patient response. ➤*Rationale: Some environmental stimuli, the voice, and nursing care procedures may have an effect on ICP and brain compliance* (Johnson, 1999). Poor brain compliance is evidenced by: deterioration in clinical signs, increase in ICP greater than 10 mm Hg above baseline longer than 3 minutes, and wide amplitude waveform and/or the appearance of plateau waves.
10. Document the ICP reading, CPP, waveforms, and the child's neurologic status.

## CLINICAL ALERT

Cerebral perfusion pressure (CPP) is calculated by subtracting the ICP from the mean arterial pressure. Normal CPP is 60 to 150 mm Hg. Normal ICP is 5 to 15 mm Hg.

# Skill 11.43   Assessing Visual Acuity

Vision acuity screening should begin at about 3 years of age, when the child can cooperate with the procedure. Several procedures may be used to screen visual acuity in children.

Most states have law regulating the ages or grades at which children must have vision screening performed, and what passing standards are accepted. Check your state laws or codes for guidelines.

### VARIATION: Snellen Letter Chart

The Snellen letter (alphabet) chart is the most commonly used assessment tool for visual acuity. It consists of lines of letters in decreasing size.

• Most charts are designed for reading from a distance of 20 feet. When the child reads the line designated "20 feet" while standing 20 feet away, vision is 20/20. If, however, the child can only read the line labeled "40 feet" while standing 20 feet away, vision is 20/40.

• Charts are also available that can be used at a distance of 10 feet. A child who stands 10 feet from this chart and reads the 10-foot line (10/10) has vision equivalent to that of 20/20 when using the 20-foot chart.

### VARIATION: HOTV, Snellen E, or Picture Chart

For toddlers and children who have not yet mastered the alphabet, the HOTV, Snellen E or picture chart may be used, positioned either 10 or 20 feet away.

• The HOTV test uses a chart with the letters H, O, T, and V used in random order on lines in decreasing size. The child either names the letters or points to them on a card held close by. The procedure followed is the same as with the Snellen test, but because children can point to the letters on the chart in front of them, they do not need to know the alphabet. The HOTV test can also be used after a practice session with children who do not speak English.

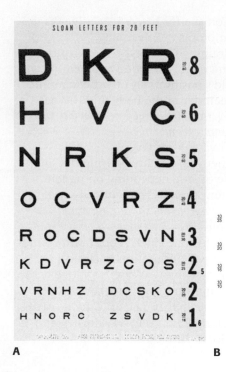

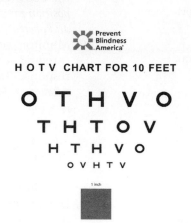

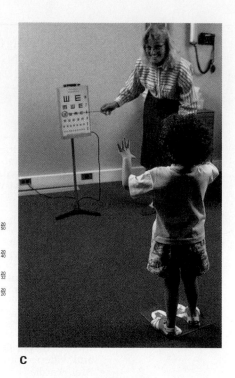

**A**             **B**                     **C**

● Visual acuity charts. **A,** Snellen letter chart. **B,** HOTV chart. **C,** Snellen E chart. A and B courtesy of the National Society to Prevent Blindness.

- In the Snellen E chart, the capital letter E is shown facing in different directions. The child is asked to point in the direction of the "legs" of the E. Another option is to give the child a paper with an E on it and have the child turn it in the direction the E is pointing on the chart.
- The picture chart has commonly identified silhouettes (e.g., house, apple, umbrella). The child is asked to identify the pictures.

### Preparation

1. The procedure is explained to the child and parent. With a young child, make a game of identifying the letter, direction of the E, or the picture. Practice with the child before starting, providing positive feedback for correct responses. ➤*Rationale: This ensures that the child understands the directions for the test to improve the chances of an accurate screening test result.*
2. Place the chart at the child's eye level and ensure that it is well lit.

### Equipment

- Screening chart
- Card or other item to cover one eye

### Procedure

1. Place the heels of the child at the 20-foot mark (or 10-foot mark if using that chart).
2. Assess each eye separately and then both together. If the child wears glasses, check the vision both with and without glasses. If the child is wearing contacts, leave them in and note that the results were with contacts. ➤*Rationale: It is important to detect significant differences in visual acuity of the eyes of children under 5 years.* When one eye has poorer vision than the other, the brain may decide to stop using the eye with poor vision, leading to further vision deterioration. Corrective lenses are required to enable the child to use both eyes and to preserve vision.
3. While one eye is being tested, use the child's hand, a patch, or a piece of cardboard to cover the other eye. Tell the child to keep the covered eye open during the testing. Use a different eye cover for each child to minimize the spread of infection among children.
4. Observe for squinting, moving the head forward (to be closer to the chart), excessive blinking, or tearing during the examination. ➤*Rationale: These may be signs that the child has a vision problem.*

5. Document the last line the child can read correctly (i.e., the last line in which the child reads more than half the symbols on the line). Refer to Table 11–17 for expected visual acuity by age.

6. When a child's vision is not within the passing standards range for age, the child should be retested in 1 to 2 weeks. If the results are still unsatisfactory, make the appropriate referral to the child's pediatrician or other healthcare provider, an ophthalmologist, or an optometrist.

**TABLE 11–17 PASSING STANDARDS FOR VISUAL ACUITY TESTING BASED ON AGE**

| Age | Visual Activity |
| --- | --- |
| 3–4 years | 20/40 |
| 5 years | 20/30 |
| 6 years | 20/20 |

# Skill 11.44   Assessing Hearing Acuity

It is important to perform hearing acuity screening to ensure that the child is able to hear for speech and language development to occur. Newborn and infant hearing screening is performed using evoked otoacoustic emission and auditory brainstem response. Several procedures may be used to screen hearing acuity in children. Various conditions during childhood, such as frequent ear infections, could result in a hearing loss.

## VARIATION: Pure Tone Audiometry

### Preparation

1. When screening a large group of children, such as in a school, the machine may be taken to the classroom for demonstration and practice.

2. Check the transmission of sound to be sure both earphones work properly.

3. Explain the procedure in terms the child can understand. Show the earphones. Turn the sound loud enough for the child to hear and practice raising a hand in response to the sound. ➤*Rationale: This action helps ensure that accurate results from the screening test are obtained.*

4. If a soundproof room is not available, the audiometer should be set up in a quiet environment. ➤*Rationale: It is important to reduce exposure to other sources of sound that could interfere with the child's response to the audiometer's sounds.*

## CLINICAL ALERT

The sounds of the audiometer are delivered at hertz levels, or the frequency of sound in cycles per second. Lower numbers indicate lower sounds, such as speech tones. Higher numbers indicate higher sounds, such as heard in music. The decibels, loudness of the sounds, can also be controlled by the audiometer.

5. Clean the earphones with alcohol swabs between children. ➤*Rationale: This practice removes most microorganisms for infection control between children.*

### Equipment

- Calibrated audiometer
- Scoring sheet
- Alcohol swabs

### Procedure

1. Position the child so that his or her back is toward the machine and faced away from the tester. ➤*Rationale: This position ensures that the child cannot see the examiner press the lever to present the sound, and cannot receive visual cues from the examiner's face when the sound is presented.*

2. Place the headset on the child's head and adjust for a proper fit. Note the right and left indicators on the earphones.

3. Follow directions for using the audiometer. Deliver sounds and watch for the child to raise a hand when heard. The sound cue is given to the child using a random order when testing the ears. ➤*Rationale: This action ensures that the child cannot anticipate the sound and potentially cause an inaccurate interpretation of the screening test.*

4. Test each ear at the following pitches: 500, 1000, 2000, and 4000 Hz at increasing levels of loudness (decibels).

5. If the child does not pass the screening with both ears, retest the child in 2 weeks. If the child still does not pass, refer for further evaluation. ➤*Rationale: The child with an upper respiratory infection may not hear well and needs time for the infection to improve. Continued failure of the screening may indicate a hearing problem.*

6. Document the results of the hearing test.

| TABLE 11–18 | PASSING STANDARDS FOR HEARING ACUITY WITH PURE TONE AUDIOMETER |
| --- | --- |
| **Hertz** | **Decibels** |
| 500 | 20–25 |
| 1000 | 20–25 |
| 2000 | 20–25 |
| 4000 | 25 |

## DEVELOPMENTAL CONSIDERATIONS

If the young child does not seem to understand what to do once screening begins, remove the headphones and practice more. Have blocks ready and instruct the child to place a block in a basket when hearing the sound. Turn up the decibel level slightly and practice until the child understands. Then turn the decibel level back to the appropriate screening level.

## VARIATION: Tympanometry

Tympanometry provides an estimate of middle ear pressure and an indirect measure of tympanic membrane compliance (movement). Older infants and children can be tested. Abnormal findings often indicate fluid accumulation in the middle ear that prevents the efficient transmission of sound to the inner ear. This can result in hearing loss over time.

## SETTING OF CARE

Each state has specific laws mandating when children attending school should be screened for hearing acuity, and the hertz and decibel levels to be included. Consult your state school code for guidance about local requirements.

### Preparation

• Explain the procedure to the child and parents and the need for the child to hold still.

### Equipment

• Calibrated tympanometer
• Disposable earpiece
• Graph paper

### Procedure

1. Encourage the child to hold still during the test. The infant and young child may need assistance in holding still. ➤*Rationale: Lack of movement reduces the chance of pain or injury from the earpiece in the auditory canal.*
2. Gently insert the earpiece with the tympanometer probe into the auditory canal until the canal is sealed and airtight. ➤*Rationale: The canal must be sealed tight to get an accurate measurement of the pressure it takes to move the tympanic membrane.*
3. Turn on the tympanometer according to manufacturer instructions and emit the tone. The pressure is measured by the probe and plots it on a graph.
4. Repeat the procedure in the other ear.
5. Insert the printout into the child's medical record and document the results of the test.

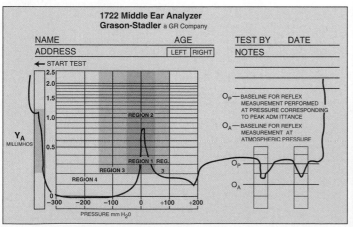

**A**

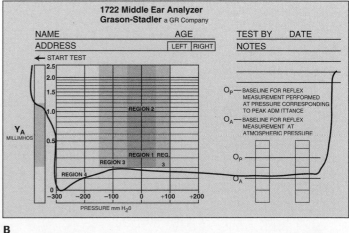

**B**

● **A,** This tympanogram demonstrates normal hearing as evidenced by the curve showing the tympanic membrane's movement when a sound wave is emitted into the ear canal. Mobility is between 0.2 mL and 1 mL, the normal range. **B,** In contrast, note the flat pattern in the second tympanogram, which shows very restricted mobility of the tympanic membrane in response to sound.

# 12

# Caring Interventions

Skill 12.1    Changing an Unoccupied Bed    562

Skill 12.2    Changing an Occupied Bed    567

Skill 12.3    Providing Morning Care    570

Skill 12.4    Bathing an Adult or Pediatric Client    571

Skill 12.5    Providing Evening Care    581

Skill 12.6    Providing a Back Massage    581

Skill 12.7    Brushing and Flossing the Teeth    583

Skill 12.8    Providing Special Oral Care for the Unconscious or Debilitated Client    587

Skill 12.9    Shaving a Male Client    589

Skill 12.10    Providing Hair Care    590

Skill 12.11    Shampooing Hair    591

Skill 12.12    Identifying the Presence of Lice and Nits (Lice Eggs)    592

Skill 12.13    Removing Lice and Nits    593

Skill 12.14    Providing Nail Care    595

Skill 12.15    Providing Foot Care    595

Skill 12.16    Providing Routine Eye Care    598

Skill 12.17    Providing Eye Care for Comatose Client    598

Skill 12.18    Providing Postoperative Socket Care    599

Skill 12.19    Removing and Cleaning an Artificial Eye (Ocular Prosthesis)    599

Skill 12.20    Removing and Cleaning Contact Lenses    600

Skill 12.21    Removing, Cleaning, and Inserting a Hearing Aid    601

Skill 12.22    Providing Perineal-Genital Care    603

Skill 12.23    Assisting an Adult to Eat    605

Skill 12.24    Serving a Food Tray    607

Skill 12.25    Assisting the Dysphagic Client to Eat    607

Skill 12.26    Preparing for Medication Administration    609

Skill 12.27    Converting Dosage Systems    610

Skill 12.28    Calculating Dosages    611

Skill 12.29    Using the Narcotic Control System    611

Skill 12.30    Using an Automated Dispensing System    613

Skill 12.31    Administering Medication Protocol    614

Skill 12.32    Administering Oral Medications    616

Skill 12.33    Administering Medications by Enteral Tube    619

Skill 12.34    Administering Sublingual Medications    621

Skill 12.35    Administering Ophthalmic Medications    622

Skill 12.36    Administering Otic Medications    624

Skill 12.37    Administering Nasal Medications    625

Skill 12.38    Administering Metered-Dose Inhaler Medications    626

Skill 12.39    Administering Dry Powder Inhaled (DPI) Medications    628

Skill 12.40    Administering Medication by Nonpressurized (Nebulized) Aerosol (NPA)    629

Skill 12.41    Administering Vaginal Medications    630

Skill 12.42    Administering Rectal Medications    631

Skill 12.43    Preparing Injections    633

Skill 12.44    Administering Intradermal Injections    637

Skill 12.45    Administering Subcutaneous Injections    638

Skill 12.46    Preparing Insulin Injections    640

Skill 12.47    Teaching Client to Use Insulin Delivery System—Insulin Pen    643

Skill 12.48    Teaching Use of Insulin Pump    644

Skill 12.49    Administering Suncutaneous Anticoagulates (Heparin, LMWH, Arixtra)    646

Skill 12.50    Administering Intramuscular (IM) Injections    647

Skill 12.51    Using Z-Track Method    651

Skill 12.52    Adding Medications to Intravenous Fluid Containers    654

Skill 12.53    Administering Intermittent Intravenous Medication Using a Secondary Set    656

Skill 12.54    Administering Intravenous Medications Using IV Push    658

Skill 12.55    Managing Pain with a PCA Pump    660

Skill 12.56    Administering Blood Transfusions    661

Skill 12.57    Administering Blood Components    663

Skill 12.58    Managing Central Lines    663

Skill 12.59    Changing a Central Line Dressing    665

Skill 12.60    Working with Implanted Vascular Access Devices    667

Skill 12.61    HOME SETTING: Bathing Client in the Home    670

Skill 12.62    HOME SETTING: Transferring Client to Tub or Shower    670

Skill 12.63    HOME SETTING: Adapting Bedmaking to the Home    671

Skill 12.64    HOME SETTING: Providing Wound Care    671

Skill 12.65    HOME SETTING: Removing Lice    671

Skill 12.66    HOME SETTING: Administering Medications    672

Skill 12.67    HOME SETTING: Sterilizing Nondisposable Medication Equipment    673

Because people are usually confined to bed when ill, often for a long period, the bed becomes an important element in the client's life. A place that is clean, safe, and comfortable contributes to the client's ability to rest and sleep and to a sense of well-being. From a holistic perspective, bed-making can be viewed as the preparation of a healing space. When performed with caring intention for benefit of the client occupying the space during their healing journey, the environment will be affected in positive ways.

Basic furniture in a health care facility includes the bed, bedside cabinet, overbed table, one or more chairs, and a storage space for clothing. Most bed units also have a call light, light fixtures, electric outlets, and hygienic equipment in the bedside cabinet. Three types of equipment often installed in an acute care facility are a suction outlet for several kinds of suction, an oxygen outlet for most oxygen equipment, and a sphygmomanometer to measure the client's blood pressure. Some long-term care agencies also permit clients to have personal furniture, such as a television, a chair, and lamps, at the bedside. In the home a client often has personal and medical equipment near the bed.

**Personal hygiene** is the self-care by which people attend to such functions as bathing, toileting, general body hygiene, and grooming. Hygiene is a highly personal matter determined by various factors, including individual and cultural values and practices. It involves care of the skin, hair, nails, teeth, oral and nasal cavities, eyes, ears, and perineal-genital areas.

It is important for nurses to know exactly how much assistance a client needs for hygienic care. Clients may require help after urinating or defecating, after vomiting, and whenever they become soiled, for example, from wound drainage or from profuse perspiration. In addition, culture-specific beliefs and practices influence hygienic care. Table 12–1 lists factors that influence hygienic practices.

Nurses commonly use the following terms to describe the various types of hygienic care:

- Early morning care is provided to clients as they awaken in the morning. This care consists of providing a urinal or bedpan to the client confined to bed, washing the face and hands, and giving oral care.
- Morning care is often provided after clients have breakfast, although it may be provided before breakfast. It usually includes providing for elimination needs, a bath or shower, perineal care, and oral, nail, and hair care. Making the client's bed is part of morning care.
- Hour of sleep (HS) care is provided to clients before they retire for the night. It usually involves providing for elimination needs, washing face and hands, giving oral care, and possibly giving a back massage. Some clients prefer bathing in the evening. If possible, the nurse needs to accommodate the client's routine schedule for personal hygiene.
- As-needed (prn) care is provided as required by the client. For example, a client who is diaphoretic (sweating profusely) may need bathing and a change of clothes and linen frequently.

## MASSAGE

Massage is a comfort measure that can aid relaxation, promote circulation of blood and lymph, decrease muscle tension, and ease anxiety (Melancon & Miller, 2005). The physical contact between nurse and client can convey caring in powerful ways that transcend words. By increasing superficial circulation as well as neurological distraction, pain intensity can be directly reduced as a result of massage. The use of creams, oils, aromatherapy, or liniments may amplify therapeutic potential. Massage is contraindicated in areas of skin breakdown, suspected clots, or infections.

Research demonstrates that back massage has the ability to elicit a relaxation response. Other findings suggest that a simple 3-minute back rub can enhance client comfort and relaxation and have a positive effect on cardiovascular parameters such as blood pressure, heart rate, and respiratory rate (McNamara, Burnham, Smith, & Carroll, 2003). Back massage can improve the quality of sleep among clients who are critically ill and diffuse agitated behaviors in individuals with Alzheimer's disease. For those with cancer, massage can be helpful for relaxation and pain management as long as care is taken to avoid bruising (in the presence of clotting issues), fractures (with metastatic disease in bones), and pain or infection (with open wounds). Simply lightening the amount of pressure applied can address these concerns (Corbin, 2005). Other research has demonstrated reduction in nausea associated with cancer treatment (Billhult, Bergbom, & Stener-Victorin, 2007), and reduction in pain intensity in women in labor (Chang, Chen, & Huang, 2006).

Evidence for using massage therapy with infants is mounting. For example, studies have supported the use of massage for improving sleep and weight gain in premature and low-birthweight infants (Field, Diego, Hernandez-Reif, Deeds, & Figuereido, 2006; Kelmanson & Adulas, 2006).

Ironically, nurses in acute care settings seldom use this basic nursing skill. The intensity of the acute care environment and the time demands of high-technology nursing may be contributing factors leading to the disappearance of the back massage. Nurses, however, need to reconsider this simple, effective, traditional skill when

## TABLE 12–1 FACTORS THAT INFLUENCE INDIVIDUAL HYGIENIC PRACTICES

| Factor | Variables |
| --- | --- |
| Culture | North American culture places a high value on cleanliness. Many North Americans bathe or shower once or twice a day, whereas people from some other cultures bathe once a week. Some cultures consider privacy essential for bathing, whereas others practice communal bathing. Body odor is offensive in some cultures and accepted as normal in others. |
| Religion | Ceremonial washings are practiced by some religions. |
| Environment | Finances may affect the availability of facilities for bathing. For example, homeless people may not have warm water available; soap, shampoo, shaving lotion, and deodorants may be too expensive for people who have limited resources. |
| Developmental level | Children learn hygiene in the home. Practices vary according to the individual's age; for example, preschoolers can carry out most tasks independently with encouragement. |
| Health and energy | Ill people may not have the motivation or energy to attend to hygiene. Some clients who have neuromuscular impairments may be unable to perform hygienic care. |
| Personal preferences | Some people prefer a shower to a tub bath. People have different preferences regarding the time of bathing (e.g., morning versus evening). |

research indicates the positive client outcomes. Interestingly, a randomized, controlled study demonstrated both physical and psychological stress reduction in nurses who received a 15-minute weekly back massage (Bost, 2006). Skill 12.6 provides guidelines for giving a back massage.

Perineal-genital care is also referred to as **perineal care** or **peri-care**. Perineal care as part of the bed bath is embarrassing for many clients. Nurses also may find it embarrassing initially, particularly with clients of the opposite sex. Most clients who require a bed bath from the nurse are able to clean their own perineal area with minimal assistance. The nurse may need to hand a moistened washcloth and soap to the client, rinse the washcloth, and provide a towel.

Because some clients are unfamiliar with terminology for the genitals and perineum, it may be difficult for nurses to explain what is expected. Most clients, however, understand what is meant if the nurse simply says, "I'll give you a washcloth to finish your bath." Older clients may be familiar with the term *private parts*. Whatever expression the nurse uses, it needs to be one that the client understands and one that is comfortable for the nurse to use.

The nurse needs to provide perineal care efficiently and matter-of-factly. Nurses should wear gloves while providing this care for the comfort of the client and to protect themselves from infection. Skill 12.22 explains how to provide perineal–genital care.

Good oral hygiene includes daily stimulation of the gums, mechanical brushing and flossing of the teeth, flushing of the mouth, and regular checkups by a dentist. The nurse is often in a position to help people maintain oral hygiene by helping or teaching them to clean their teeth and oral cavity, by inspecting whether clients (especially children) have done so, or by actually providing mouth care to clients who are ill or incapacitated. The nurse can also be instrumental in identifying problems that require the intervention of a dentist or oral surgeon and arranging a referral.

The appearance of the hair often reflects a person's feelings of self-concept and sociocultural well-being.

Becoming familiar with hair care needs and practices that may be different from our own is an important aspect of providing competent nursing care to all clients. People who feel ill may not groom their hair as before. A dirty scalp and hair are itchy and uncomfortable, and can have an odor. The hair may also reflect state of health (e.g., excessive coarseness and dryness may be associated with endocrine disorders such as hypothyroidism). The box below lists common hair problems.

Each person has particular ways of caring for hair. Many dark-skinned people need to oil their hair daily because it tends to be dry. Oil prevents the hair from breaking and the scalp from drying. A wide-toothed comb is usually used because finer combs pull and break the hair. Some people brush their hair vigorously before retiring; others comb their hair frequently.

---

**COMMON HAIR PROBLEMS**

- Alopecia (hair loss)—can be caused by chemotherapeutic agents and radiation of the head.
- Dandruff—a diffuse scaling of the scalp. Often accompanied by itching. Can usually be treated effectively with a commercial shampoo.
- Pediculosis (lice)—there are three common kinds:
  - Head lice (Pediculus capitis): Found on the scalp and tend to stay hidden in the hairs.
  - Body lice (Pediculus corporis): Tend to cling to clothing so that when a client undresses, the lice may not be in evidence on the body. These lice suck blood from the person and lay their eggs on the clothing.
  - Crab lice (Pediculus pubis): Stay hidden in pubic hair.
- Scabies—a contagious skin infestation by the itch mite. The mites cause intense itching that is more pronounced at night.

---

# Skill 12.1   Changing an Unoccupied Bed

## EXPECTED OUTCOMES
- Bed remains clean, dry, and free of wrinkles.
- Client's skin is free of irritation.
- Nurse does not experience stress on back during bathing and bedmaking.

## Delegation
Bed-making is usually delegated to unlicensed assistive personnel (UAP). If appropriate, inform the UAP of the proper disposal method for linens that contain drainage. Ask the UAP to inform you immediately if any tubes or

dressings become dislodged or removed. Stress the importance of the call light being readily available while the client is out of bed.

## Equipment

- Clean gloves, if needed
- Two flat sheets or one fitted and one flat sheet
- Cloth drawsheet (optional)
- One blanket
- One bedspread
- Incontinent pads (optional)
- Pillowcase(s) for the head pillow(s)
- Plastic laundry bag or portable linen hamper, if available

## Preparation

- Determine what linens the client may already have in the room *to avoid stockpiling of unnecessary extra linens.*

## Procedure

1. If the client is in bed, prior to performing the procedure, introduce self and verify the client's identity using agency protocol. Explain to the client what you are going to do, why it is necessary, and how he or she can participate.
2. Perform hand hygiene and observe other appropriate infection control procedures.
3. Provide for client privacy.
4. Place the fresh linen on the client's chair or overbed table; do not use another client's bed. ➤*Rationale: This prevents cross contamination (the movement of microorganisms from one client to another) via soiled linen.*
5. Assess and assist the client out of bed using assistive devices (e.g., cane, walker, safety belt) as appropriate. ➤*Rationale: This ensures client safety.*
   - Make sure that this is an appropriate and convenient time for the client to be out of bed.
   - Assist the client to a comfortable chair.
6. Raise the bed to a comfortable working height.
7. Apply clean gloves if linens and equipment have been soiled with secretions and/or excretions.
8. Strip the bed.
   - Check bed linens for any items belonging to the client, and detach the call bell or any drainage tubes from the bed linen.
   - Loosen all bedding systematically, starting at the head of the bed on the far side and moving around the bed up to the head of the bed on the near side. ➤*Rationale: Moving around the bed systematically prevents stretching and reaching and possible muscle strain.*
   - Remove the pillowcases, if soiled, and place the pillows on the bedside chair near the foot of the bed.
   - Fold reusable linens, such as the bedspread and top sheet on the bed, into fourths. First, fold the linen in half by

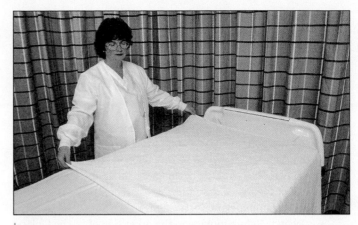

● Fold reusable linens into fourths when removing them from the bed.

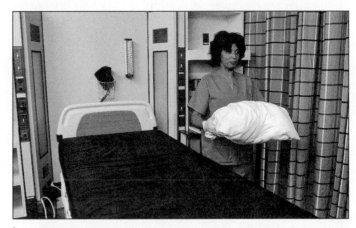

● Roll soiled linen inside the bottom sheet and hold away from the body.

bringing the top edge even with the bottom edge, and then grasp it at the center of the middle fold and bottom edges. ➤*Rationale: Folding linens saves time and energy when reapplying the linens on the bed and keeps them clean.*
   - Remove the incontinent pad and discard it if soiled.
   - Roll all soiled linen inside the bottom sheet, hold it away from your uniform, and place it directly into the linen hamper, not on the floor. ➤*Rationale: These actions are essential to prevent the transmission of microorganisms to the nurse and others.*
   - Grasp the mattress securely, using the lugs if present, and move the mattress up to the head of the bed.
   - Remove and discard gloves if used. Perform hand hygiene.
9. Apply the bottom sheet and drawsheet.
   - Place the folded bottom sheet with its center fold on the center of the bed. Make sure the sheet is hem side down for a smooth foundation. Spread the sheet out over the mattress, and allow a sufficient amount of sheet at the top to tuck under the mattress. ➤*Rationale: The top of the sheet needs to be well tucked under to remain securely in place,*

*especially when the head of the bed is elevated.* Place the sheet along the edge of the mattress at the foot of the bed and do not tuck it in (unless it is a contour or fitted sheet).

- Miter the sheet at the top corner on the near side and tuck the sheet under the mattress, working from the head of the bed to the foot.
- If a drawsheet is used, place it over the bottom sheet so that the centerfold is at the centerline of the bed and the top and bottom edges extend from the middle of where the client's back would be on the bed to the area where the mid-thigh or knee would be. Fanfold the uppermost half of the folded drawsheet at the center or far edge of the bed and tuck in the near edge.
- *Optional:* Before moving to the other side of the bed, place the top linens on the bed hem side up, unfold them, tuck them in, and miter the bottom corners. ►*Rationale: Completing one entire side of the bed at a time saves time and energy.*

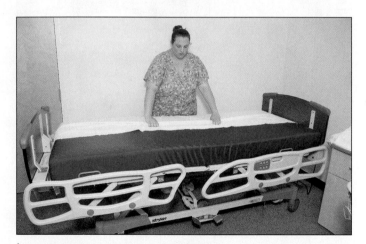

● Placing the bottom sheet on the bed.

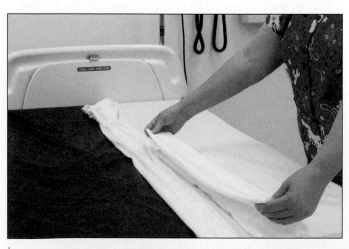

● Placing a clean drawsheet on the bed.

10. Move to the other side and secure the bottom linens.
    - Tuck in the bottom sheet under the head of the mattress, pull the sheet firmly, and miter the corner of the sheet.
    - Pull the remainder of the sheet firmly so that there are no wrinkles. ►*Rationale: Wrinkles can cause discomfort for the client and breakdown of skin. Tuck the sheet in at the side.*
    - Tuck in the drawsheet, if appropriate.

11. Apply or complete the top sheet, blanket, and spread.
    - Place the top sheet, hem side up, on the bed so that its centerfold is at the center of the bed and the top edge is even with the top edge of the mattress.
    - Unfold the sheet over the bed.
    - *Optional:* Make a vertical or a horizontal toe pleat in the sheet. A toe pleat provides additional room for the client's feet and helps prevent foot drop.
      a. *Vertical toe pleat:* Make a fold in the sheet 5 to 10 cm (2 to 4 in.) perpendicular to the foot of the bed.
      b. *Horizontal toe pleat:* Make a fold in the sheet 5 to 10 cm (2 to 4 in.) across the bed near the foot.
      Loosening the top covers around the feet after the client is in bed is another way to provide additional space.
    - Follow the same procedure for the blanket and the spread, but place the top edges about 15 cm (6 in.) from the head of the bed to allow a cuff of sheet to be folded over them.

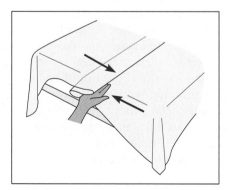

● A vertical toe pleat.

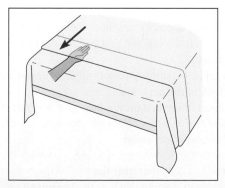

● A horizontal toe pleat: Make a fold in the sheet 5 to 10 cm (2 to 4 in.) across the bed near the foot.

- Tuck in the sheet, blanket, and spread at the foot of the bed, and miter the corner, using all three layers of linen. Leave the sides of the top sheet, blanket, and spread hanging freely unless toe pleats were provided.
- Fold the top of the top sheet down over the spread, providing a cuff. ➤*Rationale: The cuff of sheet makes it easier for the client to pull the covers up.*
- Move to the other side of the bed and secure the top bedding in the same manner.

12. Put clean pillowcases on the pillows as required.
- Grasp the closed end of the pillowcase at the center with one hand.
- Gather up the sides of the pillowcase and place them over the hand grasping the case. Then grasp the center of one short side of the pillow through the pillowcase.
- With the free hand, pull the pillowcase over the pillow.
- Adjust the pillowcase so that the pillow fits into the corners of the case and the seams are straight. ➤*Rationale: A smoothly fitting pillowcase is more comfortable than a wrinkled one.*
- Place the pillows appropriately at the head of the bed.

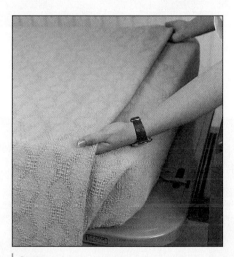

● Pleat top linen to allow space for feet.

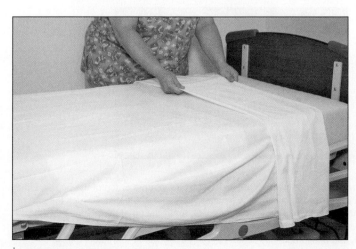

● Making a cuff of the top linens.

13. Provide for client comfort and safety.
- Attach the call light so that the client can conveniently reach it. Some call lights have clamps that attach to the sheet or pillowcase. Others are attached by a safety pin. Most beds now have a call light button on the side rail.
- If the bed is currently being used by a client, either fold back the top covers at one side or fanfold them down to the end of the bed. ➤*Rationale: This makes it easier for the client to get into the bed.*
- Place the bedside cabinet and the overbed table so that they are available to the client.
- Leave the bed in the high position if the client is returning by stretcher, or place in the low position if the client is returning to bed after being up ambulating or sitting in a chair.

14. Document and report pertinent data.
- Bed-making is not normally recorded.
- Record any nursing assessments, such as the client's physical status and pulse and respiratory rates before and after being out of bed, as indicated.

## VARIATION: Making a Surgical Bed

A **surgical bed** is used for the client who is having surgery and will return to bed for the postoperative phase. When making a surgical bed, the linens are horizontally fanfolded to facilitate transfer of the client into the bed. In some agencies, the client is brought back to the unit on a stretcher and transferred to the bed in the room. In other agencies, the client's bed is brought to the surgery suite and the client is transferred there. In the latter situation, the bed needs to be made with clean linens as soon as the client goes to surgery so that it can be taken to the operating room when needed.

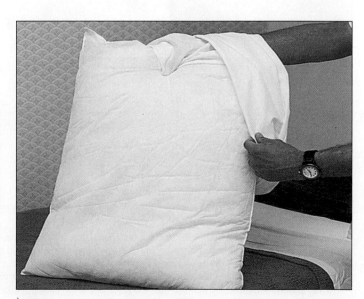

● Method for putting a clean pillowcase on a pillow.

- Strip the bed.
- Place and leave the pillows on the bedside chair. ►*Rationale: Pillows are left on a chair to facilitate transferring the client into the bed.*
- Apply the bottom linens as for an unoccupied bed. Place a bath blanket on the foundation of the bed if this is agency practice. ►*Rationale: A flannel bath blanket provides additional warmth.*
- Place the top covers (sheet, blanket, and bedspread) on the bed as you would for an unoccupied bed. Do not tuck them in, miter the corners, or make a toe pleat.
- Make a cuff at the top of the bed as you would for an unoccupied bed. Fold the top linens up from the bottom.
- On the side of the bed where the client will be transferred, fold up the two outer corners of the top linens so they meet in the middle of the bed forming a triangle.
- Pick up the apex or point of the triangle and fanfold the top linens lengthwise to the side of the bed opposite from where the client will enter the bed. ►*Rationale: This facilitates the client's transfer into the bed.*

- Leave the bed in high position with the side rails down. ►*Rationale: The high position facilitates the transfer of the client.*
- Lock the wheels of the bed if the bed is not to be moved. ►*Rationale: Locking the wheels keeps the bed from rolling when the client is transferred from the stretcher to the bed.*

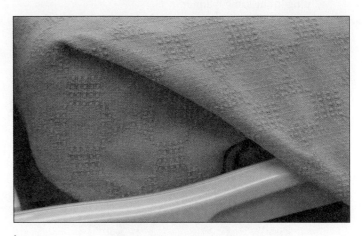

● Mitered corners help keep bed linens secure.

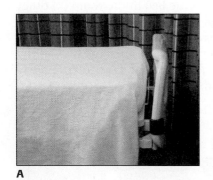
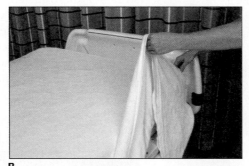
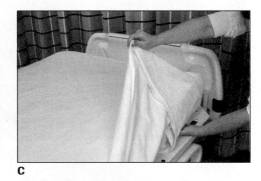

A                    B                    C

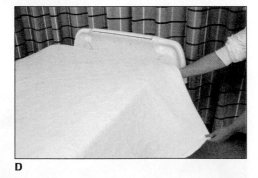
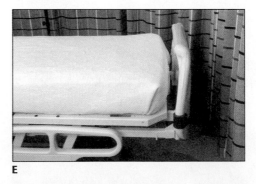

D                    E

● Mitering the corner of a bed. **A,** Tuck in the bedcover (sheet, blanket, and/or spread) firmly under the mattress at the bottom or top of the bed. **B,** Lift the bedcover so that it forms a triangle with the side edge of the bed and the edge of the bedcover is parallel to the end of the bed. **C,** Tuck the part of the cover that hangs below the mattress under the mattress while holding the triangle up or against the bed. **D,** Bring the tip of the triangle down toward the floor while the other hand holds the fold of the cover against the side of the mattress. **E,** Remove the hand and tuck the remainder of the cover under the mattress, if appropriate. The sides of the top sheet, blanket, and bedspread may be left hanging freely rather than tucked in, if desired.

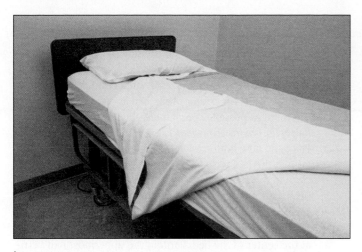

● Fold up the two outer corners of the top linens, forming a triangle.

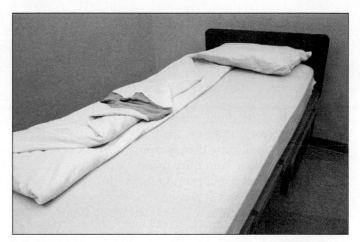

● Surgical bed. The linens are horizontally fanfolded to one side of the bed to facilitate transfer of the client into the bed.

## PRACTICE GUIDELINES

- Wash hands thoroughly after handling a client's bed linen. Clean gloves need to be used if linens and equipment have been soiled with secretions and/or excretions.

- Hold soiled linen away from uniform.

- Linen for one client is never (even momentarily) placed on another client's bed or on the floor.

- Place soiled linen directly in a portable linen hamper or tucked into a pillowcase at the end of the bed before it is gathered up for disposal.

- Do not shake soiled linen in the air because shaking can disseminate secretions and excretions and the microorganisms they contain.

- When stripping and making a bed, conserve time and energy by stripping and making up one side as much as possible before working on the other side.

- To avoid unnecessary trips to the linen supply area, gather all linen before starting to strip bed.

# Skill 12.2   Changing an Occupied Bed

## EVIDENCE-BASED NURSING PRACTICE

**Do Side Rails Prevent Falls?**

A New Zealand study of almost 2,000 clients tested a new policy of restricting side rails. The results revealed that even though the use of side rails decreased (from 29% to 7%), the mean fall rate remained the same (36.6 fall/100 admissions). However, the falls that did occur were less severe.

*Source:* Hanger, H.C., et al., (July 1999). "An analysis of falls in the hospital: Can we do without bedrails?" *Journal of American Geriatric Society*, 47(5):529; *RN*, 62(7.1).

## Delegation

Bed-making is usually delegated to UAP. Inform the UAP to what extent the client can assist or if another person will be needed to assist the UAP. Instruct the UAP about the handling of any dressings and/or tubes of the client and also the need for special equipment (e.g., footboard, heel protectors), if appropriate.

## Equipment

- Two flat sheets or one fitted and one flat sheet
- Cloth drawsheet (optional)
- One blanket
- One bedspread
- Incontinent pads (optional)
- Pillowcase(s) for the head pillow(s)
- Plastic laundry bag or portable linen hamper, if available

## Preparation

- Determine what linens the client may already have in the room. ▶*Rationale: This avoids stockpiling of unnecessary extra linens.*

## Procedure

1. Explain to the client what you are going to do, why it is necessary, and how he or she can participate. Prior to performing the procedure introduce self and verify the client's identity using agency protocol.
2. Perform hand hygiene and observe other appropriate infection control procedures. Put on disposable clean gloves if linen is soiled with body fluids.
3. Provide for client privacy.
4. Remove the top bedding.
   - Remove any equipment attached to the bed linen, such as a signal light.
   - Loosen all top linen at the foot of the bed, and remove the spread and the blanket.
   - Leave the top sheet over the client (the top sheet can remain over the client if it is being changed and if it will provide sufficient warmth), or replace it with a bath blanket as follows:
     a. Spread the bath blanket over the top sheet.
     b. Ask the client to hold the top edge of the blanket.
     c. Reaching under the blanket from the side, grasp the top edge of the sheet and draw it down to the foot of the bed, leaving the blanket in place.
     d. Remove the sheet from the bed and place it in the soiled linen hamper.
5. Change the bottom sheet and drawsheet.
   - Raise the side rail that the client will turn toward. ▶*Rationale: This protects clients from falling and allows them to support themselves in the side-lying position.* If there is no side rail, have another nurse support the client at the edge of the bed.

- Assist the client to turn on the side away from the nurse and toward the raised side rail.
- Loosen the bottom linens on the side of the bed near the nurse.
- Fanfold the dirty linen (i.e., drawsheet and the bottom sheet) toward the center of the bed as close to and under the client as possible. ▶*Rationale: Doing this leaves the near half of the bed free to be changed.*
- Place the new bottom sheet on the bed, and vertically fanfold the half to be used on the far side of the bed as close to the client as possible. Tuck the sheet under the near half of the bed and miter the corner if a contour sheet is not being used.
- Place the clean drawsheet on the bed with the center fold at the center of the bed. Fanfold the uppermost half vertically at the center of the bed and tuck the near side edge under the side of the mattress.
- Assist the client to roll over toward you, over the fanfolded bed linens at the center of the bed, onto the clean side of the bed.
- Move the pillows to the clean side for the client's use. Raise the side rail before leaving the side of the bed.
- Move to the other side of the bed and lower the side rail.
- Remove the used linen and place it in the portable hamper.
- Unfold the fanfolded bottom sheet from the center of the bed.
- Facing the side of the bed, use both hands to pull the bottom sheet so that it is smooth and tuck the excess under the side of the mattress.
- Unfold the drawsheet fanfolded at the center of the bed and pull it tightly with both hands. Pull the sheet in three divisions: (a) face the side of the bed to pull the middle division, (b) face the far top corner to pull the bottom division, and (c) face the far bottom corner to pull the top division.
- Tuck the excess drawsheet under the side of the mattress.

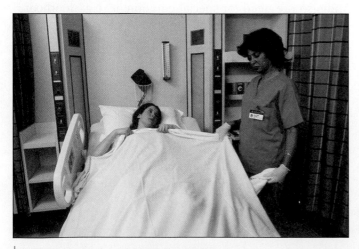

● Removing top linens under a bath blanket.

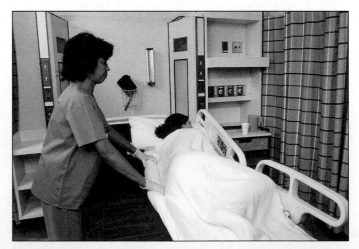

● Moving soiled linen as close to the client as possible.

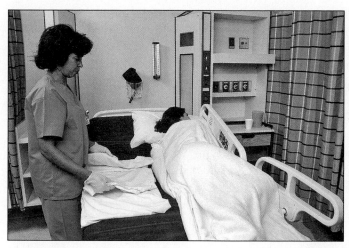

● Placing a new bottom sheet on half of the bed.

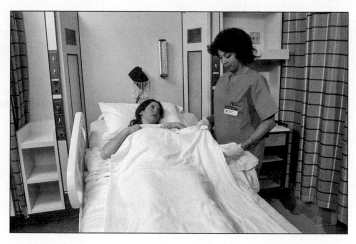

● Client holds top edge of sheet while nurse removes bath blanket.

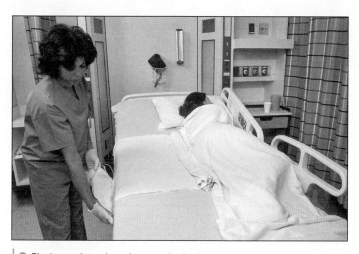

● Placing a clean drawsheet on the bed.

6. Reposition the client in the center of the bed.
   • Reposition the pillows at the center of the bed.
   • Assist the client to the center of the bed. Determine what position the client requires or prefers and assist the client to that position.

7. Apply or complete the top bedding.
   • Spread the top sheet over the client and either ask the client to hold the top edge of the sheet or tuck it under the shoulders. The sheet should remain over the client when the bath blanket or used sheet is removed.
   • Complete the top of the bed.
8. Ensure continued safety of the client.
   • Raise the side rails. Place the bed in the low position before leaving the bedside.
   • Attach the call light to the bed linen within the client's reach.
   • Put items used by the client within easy reach.
9. Bed-making is not normally recorded.

## CLINICAL ALERT

Side rail entrapment, injuries, and deaths do occur. When side rails are used, the nurse must assess the client's physical and mental status and closely monitor high-risk (frail, elderly, or confused) clients.

| UNEXPECTED OUTCOMES | CRITICAL THINKING OPTIONS |
|---|---|
| Clients refuses to have bed made. | • Assess reason for refusal. Client may be in pain or does not want to be disturbed.<br>• Offer to make the bed at a later time.<br>• Change the pillowcase and drawsheet, if client allows.<br>• Beds do not need to be changed unless soiled or damp, so allow client's independence, if possible. |
| Cross-contamination occurs from improper linen disposal. | • Provide adequate linen hampers for the nursing personnel.<br>• Attend in-service education programs on infection control. |

*(continued)*

**UNEXPECTED OUTCOMES** *(cont.)*

Client's skin becomes irritated from linen or begins to break down.

The nurse feels stress on back during bedmaking.

**CRITICAL THINKING OPTIONS** *(cont.)*

• Obtain hypoallergenic linen.
• Place special mattress under client.
• Provide skin care with lotion.

• Make sure bed is positioned for comfort of the nurse. High position is generally used.
• If client is heavy, ask for assistance with bedmaking, especially in moving side to side.
• Use full sheet or Booster Lift for turning.
• Attend in-service classes on preventing back strain.
• Use body mechanics principles during bedmaking procedure.
• Use assistive devices for large clients.

---

### DEVELOPMENTAL CONSIDERATIONS

**Child**

• Check if the child has a favorite blanket and if it was brought from home. Is so, make sure you replace it on the bed after changing the bed linens.

**Elders**

• Because of the older adult's thin, tender, and fragile skin, be sure to check that the linens are dry and free of wrinkles and be especially careful when pulling linens underneath the older client.

### SETTING OF CARE

• If the client needs to remain in bed, determine the caregiver's knowledge and experience making an occupied bed. The nurse may need to demonstrate how to change the linen. Emphasize safety for the client and use of correct body mechanics for the caregiver.

• Assess and discuss with the caregiver the following: need for linens (e.g., incontinence, drainage), available linen supply, and laundry accommodations.

---

### PRACTICE GUIDELINES

• Maintain the client in good body alignment. Never move or position a client in a manner that is contraindicated by the client's health. Obtain help if necessary to ensure safety.

• Move the client gently and smoothly. Rough handling can cause the client discomfort and abrade the skin.

• Explain what you plan to do throughout the procedure before you do it. Use terms that the client can understand.

• Use the bed-making time, like the bed bath time, to assess and meet the client's needs.

---

# Skill 12.3   Providing Morning Care

**Equipment**

Basin of warm water
Soap
Towel and washcloth
Emesis basin
Toothbrush and paste
Bedpan or urinal
Toilet tissue
Clean gloves

**Preparation**

1. Determine if client wishes morning care. ➤*Rationale: Morning care is provided to "freshen" the client in procedures occurring prior to bathing.*
2. Perform hand hygiene. ➤*Rationale: When providing morning care to several clients, it is important to perform hand hygiene between clients so that microorganisms are not transmitted from one client to another.*

3. Gather equipment and take it to client's room.
4. Explain that early morning care is available while client remains in bed. If client is able, assist him or her to the bathroom.
5. Provide privacy.

### Procedure

1. Perform hand hygiene.
2. Offer bedpan or urinal and assist client as needed. Don gloves when giving client bedpan or urinal.
3. Move bed to comfortable working height, and lower side rail.
4. Put equipment on over-bed table within reach. Place towel under client's chin. ➤*Rationale: To keep gown and linens dry.*

5. Wash client's face and hands or assist as needed. Dry face and hands.
6. Offer oral hygiene. Assist as needed. Gloves should be worn if client needs assistance with oral hygiene.
7. Hold emesis basin so client can rinse after brushing teeth.
8. Assist client to comfortable position.
9. Reposition bed, and replace side rails.
10. Remove equipment and draw curtains.
11. Remove gloves, if used.
12. Perform hand hygiene.

# Skill 12.4  Bathing an Adult or Pediatric Client

### EXPECTED OUTCOMES
- Client's skin is free of excessive perspiration, secretions, and offensive odors.
- Client feel comfortable and does not experience itching or irritation.
- Client's skin is moist and free of itching sensation.
- Client is able to take a bath or shower without excessive fatigue or anxiety.
- Client is able to bathe self using disposable cleansing system.

### Delegation

The nurse often delegates the skill of bathing to UAP. However, the nurse remains responsible *for assessment and client care.* The nurse needs to do the following:

- Inform the UAP of the type of bath appropriate for the client and precautions, if any, specific to the needs of the client.
- Remind the UAP to notify the nurse of any concerns or changes (e.g., redness, skin breakdown, rash) so the nurse can assess, intervene if needed, and document.
- Instruct the UAP to encourage the client to perform as much self-care as appropriate in order to promote independence and self-esteem.
- Obtain a complete report about the bathing experience from the UAP.

### Equipment

- Basin or sink with warm water (between 43° and 46°C or 110° and 115°F)
- Soap and soap dish

- Linens: bath blanket, two bath towels, washcloth, clean gown or pajamas or clothes as needed, additional bed linen and towels, if required
- Clean gloves, if appropriate (e.g., presence of body fluids or open lesions)
- Personal hygiene articles (e.g., deodorant, powder, lotions)
- Shaving equipment
- Table for bathing equipment
- Laundry bag

### Preparation

Before bathing a client, determine (a) the purpose and type of bath the client needs; (b) self-care ability of the client; (c) any movement or positioning precautions specific to the client; (d) other care the client may be receiving, such as physical therapy or x-rays, in order to coordinate all aspects of health care and prevent unnecessary fatigue; (e) the client's comfort level with being bathed by someone else; and (f) necessary bath equipment and linens.

Caution is needed when bathing clients who are receiving intravenous (IV) therapy. Easy-to-remove gowns that have Velcro or snap fasteners along the sleeves may be used. If a special gown is not available, the nurse needs to pay special attention when changing the client's gown after the bath (or whenever the gown becomes soiled).

In addition, special attention is needed to reassess the IV site for security of IV connections and appropriate taping around the IV site.

## Procedure

1. Prior to performing the procedure, introduce self and verify the client's identity using agency protocol. Explain to the client what you are going to do, why it is necessary, and how he or she can participate. Discuss with the client their preferences for bathing and explain any unfamiliar procedures to the client.

2. Perform hand hygiene and observe other appropriate infection control procedures.

3. Provide for client privacy by drawing the curtains around the bed or closing the door to the room. Some agencies provide signs indicating the need for privacy. ➤*Rationale: Hygiene is a personal matter.*

4. Prepare the client and the environment.
   - Invite a family member or significant other to participate if desired or requested by the client.
   - Close windows and doors to ensure the room is a comfortable temperature. ➤*Rationale: Air currents increase loss of heat from the body by convection.*
   - Offer the client a bedpan or urinal or ask whether the client wishes to use the toilet or commode. ➤*Rationale: Warm water and activity can stimulate the need to void. The*

*client will be more comfortable after voiding, and voiding before cleaning the perineum is advisable.*
   - Encourage the client to perform as much personal self-care as possible. ➤*Rationale: This promotes independence, exercise, and self-esteem.*
   - During the bath, assess each area of the skin carefully.

### For a Bed Bath

5. Prepare the bed and position the client appropriately.
   - Position the bed at a comfortable working height. Lower the side rail on the side close to you. Keep the other side rail *up*. Assist the client to move near you. ➤*Rationale: This avoids undue reaching and straining and promotes good body mechanics. It also ensures client safety.*
   - Place a bath blanket over the top sheet. Remove the top sheet from under the bath blanket by starting at the client's shoulders and moving linen down toward the client's feet. Ask the client to grasp and hold the top of the bath blanket while pulling linen to the foot of the bed. ➤*Rationale: The bath blanket provides comfort, warmth, and privacy.*

*Note:* If the bed linen is to be reused, place it over the bedside chair. If it is to be changed, place it in the linen hamper, not on the floor.

   - Remove client's gown while keeping the client covered with the bath blanket. Place gown in linen hamper.

6. Make a bath mitt with the washcloth. ➤*Rationale: A bath mitt retains water and heat better than a cloth loosely held and prevents the ends of the washcloth from dragging across the skin.*

7. Wash the face. ➤*Rationale: Begin the bath at the cleanest area and work downward toward the feet.*
   - Place towel under client's head.
   - Wash the client's eyes with water only and dry them well. Use a separate corner of the washcloth for each eye. ➤*Rationale: Using separate corners prevents transmitting microorganisms from one eye to the other.* Wipe from the inner to the outer canthus. ➤*Rationale: This prevents secretions from entering the nasolacrimal ducts.*

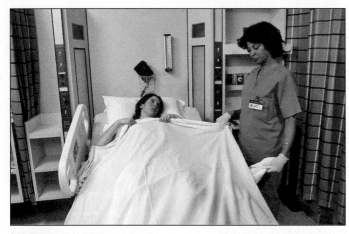

● Remove top sheet from under the bath blanket.

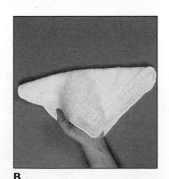
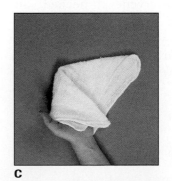
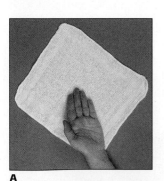
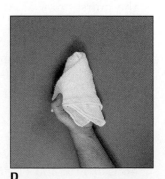

● Making a bath mitt, triangular method. **A,** Lay your hand on the washcloth; **B,** fold the top corner over your hand; **C,** fold the side corners over your hand; **D,** tuck the second corner under the cloth on the palm side to secure the mitt.

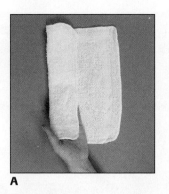
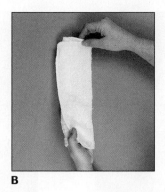
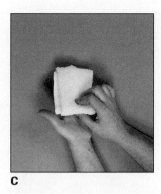

**A**        **B**        **C**

● Making a bath mitt, rectangular method. **A,** Lay your hand on the washcloth and fold one side over your hand; **B,** fold the second side over your hand; **C,** fold the top of the cloth down and tuck it under the folded side against your palm to secure the mitt.

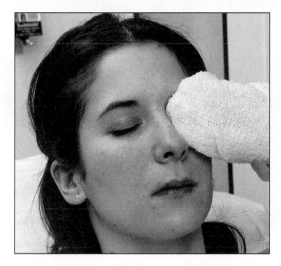

● Using a separate corner of the washcloth for each eye, wipe from the inner to the outer canthus.

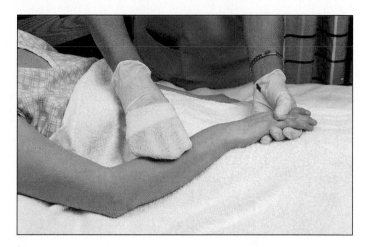

● Washing the far arm using long, firm strokes from wrist to shoulder area.

- Ask whether the client wants soap used on the face. ➤*Rationale: Soap has a drying effect, and the face, which is exposed to the air more than other body parts, tends to be drier.*
- Wash, rinse, and dry the client's face, ears, and neck.
- Remove the towel from under the client's head.

8. Wash the arms and hands. (Omit the arms for a partial bath.)
   - Place a towel lengthwise under the arm away from you. ➤*Rationale: It protects the bed from becoming wet.*
   - Wash, rinse, and dry the arm by elevating the client's arm and supporting the client's wrist and elbow. Use long, firm strokes from wrist to shoulder, including the axillary area. ➤*Rationale: Firm strokes from distal to proximal areas promote circulation by increasing venous blood return.*
   - Apply deodorant or powder if desired. Special caution is needed for clients with respiratory alterations. ➤*Rationale: Powder is not recommended due to potential adverse respiratory effects.*
   - *Optional:* Place a towel on the bed and put a washbasin on it. Place the client's hands in the basin. ➤*Rationale: Many*

*clients enjoy immersing their hands in the basin and washing themselves. Soaking loosens dirt under the nails.* Assist the client as needed to wash, rinse, and dry the hands, paying particular attention to the spaces between the fingers.
   - Repeat for hand and arm nearest you. Exercise caution if an intravenous infusion is present, and check its flow after moving the arm. Avoid submersing the IV site.

9. Wash the chest and abdomen. (Omit the chest and abdomen for a partial bath. However, the areas under a woman's breast may require bathing if this area is irritated or if the client has significant perspiration under the breasts.)
   - Place the bath towel lengthwise over the chest. Fold the bath blanket down to the client's pubic area. ➤*Rationale: This keeps the client warm while preventing unnecessary exposure of the chest.*
   - Lift the bath towel off the chest, and bathe the chest and abdomen with your mitted hand using long, firm strokes. Special attention to the skin under the breasts and any other skin folds, particularly if the client is overweight. Rinse and dry well.
   - Replace the bath blanket when the areas have been dried.

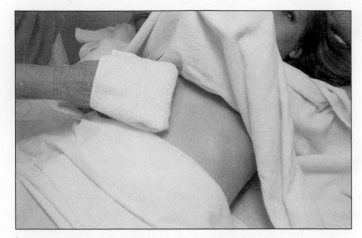

● Washing the chest and abdomen.

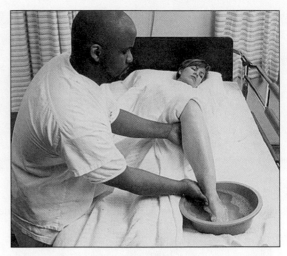

● Soaking a foot in a basin.

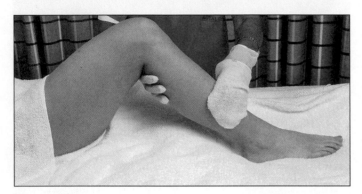

● Washing far leg.

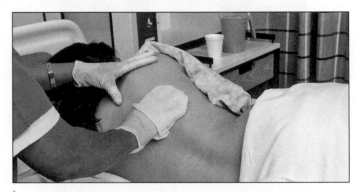

● Washing the back.

10. Wash the legs and feet. (Omit legs and feet for a partial bath.)
    • Expose the leg farthest from you by folding the bath blanket toward the other leg, being careful to keep the perineum covered. ➤*Rationale: Covering the perineum promotes privacy and maintains the client's dignity.*
    • Lift leg and place the bath towel lengthwise under the leg. Wash, rinse, and dry the leg using long, smooth, firm strokes from the ankle to the knee to the thigh. ➤*Rationale: Washing from the distal to proximal areas promotes circulation by stimulating venous blood flow.*
    • Reverse the coverings and repeat for the other leg.
    • Wash the feet by placing them in a basin of water.
    • Dry each foot. Pay particular attention to the spaces between the toes. If preferred, wash one foot after that leg before washing the other leg.
      • Obtain fresh, warm bathwater now or when necessary. ➤*Rationale: Water may become dirty or cold.* Because surface skin cells are removed with washing, the bathwater from dark-skinned clients may be dark, however, this does not mean the client is dirty. Lower the bed and raise the
      • side rails when refilling basin. ➤*Rationale: This ensures the safety of the client.*

11. Wash the back and then the perineum.
    • Assist the client into a prone or side-lying position facing away from you. Place the bath towel lengthwise alongside the back and buttocks while keeping the client covered with the bath blanket as much as possible. ➤*Rationale: This provides warmth and prevents undue exposure.*
    • Wash and dry the client's back, moving from the shoulders to the buttocks, and upper thighs, paying attention to the gluteal folds.
    • Remove and discard gloves if used.
    • Perform a back massage now or after completion of bath.
    • Assist the client to the supine position and determine whether the client can wash the perineal area independently. If the client cannot do so, drape the client and wash the area.

12. Assist the client with grooming aids such as powder, lotion, or deodorant.
    • Use powder sparingly. Release as little as possible into the atmosphere. ➤*Rationale: This will avoid irritation of the respiratory tract by powder inhalation. Excessive powder can cause caking, which leads to skin irritation.*
    • Help the client put on a clean gown or pajamas.
    • Assist the client to care for hair, mouth, and nails. Some people prefer or need mouth care prior to their bath.

### For a Tub Bath or Shower

13. Prepare the client and the tub.
    - Fill the tub about one-third to one-half full of water at 43° to 46°C (110° to 115°F). ➤*Rationale: Sufficient water is needed to cover the perineal area.*
    - Cover all intravenous catheters or wound dressings with plastic coverings, and instruct the client to prevent wetting these areas if possible.
    - Put a rubber bath mat or towel on the floor of the tub if safety strips are not on the tub floor. ➤*Rationale: These prevent slippage of the client during the bath or shower.*

14. Assist the client into the shower or tub.
    - Assist the client taking a standing shower with the initial
    - adjustment of the water temperature and water flow pressure, as needed. Some clients need a chair to sit on in the shower because of weakness. Hot water can cause elderly people to feel faint due to vasodilation and decreased blood pressure from positional changes.
    - If the client requires considerable assistance with a tub bath, a hydraulic bathtub chair may be required (see "Variation" section later in this skill).
    - Explain how the client can signal for help, leave the client for 2 to 5 minutes, and place an "Occupied" sign on the door. For safety reasons, do not leave a client with decreased cognition or clients who may be at risk (e.g., history of seizures, syncope).

15. Assist the client with washing and getting out of the tub.
    - Wash the client's back, lower legs, and feet, if necessary.
    - Assist the client out of the tub. If the client is unsteady, place a bath towel over the client's shoulders and drain the tub of water before the client attempts to get out of it. ➤*Rationale: Draining the water first lessens the likelihood of a fall. The towel prevents chilling.*

16. Dry the client, and assist with follow-up care.
    - Follow step 12.
    - Assist the client back to his or her bed.
    - Clean the tub or shower in accordance with agency practice, discard the used linen in the laundry hamper, and place the "Unoccupied" sign on the door.

17. Document the following:
    - Type of bath given (i.e., complete, partial, or self-help). This is usually recorded on a flow sheet.
    - Skin assessment, such as excoriation, erythema, exudates, rashes, drainage, or skin breakdown.
    - Nursing interventions related to skin integrity.
    - Ability of the client to assist or cooperate with bathing.
    - Client response to bathing. Also, document the need for reassessment of vital signs if appropriate.
    - Educational needs regarding hygiene.
    - Information or teaching shared with the client or the family.

### VARIATION: Bathing Using a Hydraulic Bathtub Chair

A hydraulic lift, often used in long-term care or rehabilitation settings, can facilitate the transfer of a client who is unable to ambulate to a tub. The lift also helps eliminate strain on the nurse's back.

- Bring the client to the tub room in a wheelchair or shower chair.
- Fill the tub and check the water temperature with a bath thermometer. ➤*Rationale: This avoids thermal injury to the client.*
- Lower the hydraulic chair lift to its lowest point, outside the tub.
- Transfer the client to the chair lift and secure the seat belt.
- Raise the chair lift above the tub.

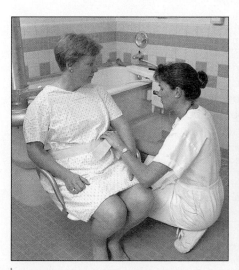

● Attach seat belt before swinging chair over the tub.

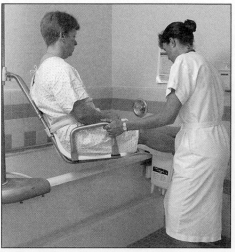

● Support client in chair as chair is swung over tub.

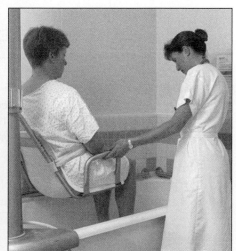

● Lower chair into tub filled with water.

- Support the client's legs as the chair is moved over the tub. ➤*Rationale: This avoids injury to the legs.*
- Position the client's legs down into the water and slowly lower the chair lift into the tub.

- Assist in bathing the client, if appropriate.
- Reverse the procedure when taking the client out of the tub.
- Dry the client and transport him or her to the room.

---

## GENERAL GUIDELINES FOR BATHING PERSONS WITH DEMENTIA

- Focus on the person rather than the task.
- Cover! Keep the person covered as much as possible to keep him or her warm.
- Time the bath to fit the person's history, preferences, and mood.
- Move slowly and let the person know when you are going to move or touch him or her.
- Evaluate to determine if the person needs pain control before the bath.
- Use a gentle touch. Use soft cloths. Pat dry rather than rubbing.
- Be flexible. Adapt your approach to meet the needs of the person.
- Consider adapting your methods (e.g., distracting the person with singing while bathing), the environment (e.g., correct size of shower chair, reducing noise, playing music), and the procedure (e.g., consistently assigning same caregiver, inviting family to help).
- Encourage flexibility in scheduling of the bath based on person's preference.
- Use persuasion, not coercion.
- Give choices and respond to individual requests.
- Help the person feel in control.

- Use a supportive, calm approach and praise the person often.
- Be prepared.
- Gather everything that you will need for the bath (e.g., towels, washcloths, clothes) before approaching the person.
- Stop when a person becomes distressed. It is not normal to have cries, screams, or protests from the person.
- Stop what you are doing and assess for causes of the distress.
- Adjust your approach.
- Shorten or stop the bath.
- Try to end on a positive note.
- Reapproach later to wash critical areas if necessary.
- Ask for help.
- Talk with others, including the family, about different ways to help make the bath more comfortable for the person.

*Note:* Adapted from *Bathing without a Battle: Personal Care of Individuals with Dementia,* by A. L. Barrick, J. Rader, B. Hoeffer, & P. D. Sloane, 2002, New York: Springer Publishing Company, Inc. Reproduced with the permission of Springer Publishing Company, CLC, New York, NY, 10036.

---

# ▌ EVIDENCE-BASED NURSING PRACTICE

### Bed Bath or Disposable Bed Bath

Very few studies have been published on the effect that bed baths or tub baths have on client comfort or healing. One study by Dunn, et al. stated that there was a high level of stress for clients receiving tub baths with the diagnosis of dementia. A study by Collins and Hampton indicated only that the bed bath was more costly than the disposable bed bath. There is a school of thought that indicates bed baths should be eliminated as part of nursing care, particularly since the average length of hospital stay is so short; however, there is insufficient evidence-based data to support this decision.

*Sources:* Dunn, J. C., B. Thiru-Chelvam, C. H. Beck. Bathing, Pleasure or pain? *Journal of Gerontologic Nursing.* 2002; 28:6. Collins, F. S. Hampton. The cost-effective use of BagBath: A new concept in Patient Hygiene. *The British Journal of Nursing.* 2003; 12:984. Moore, Katherine. Does "Arriving" Mean We Give Up the Bed Bath? *Journal of Wound, Ostomy and Continence Nursing.* September/October, 2005. Vol. 32, No. 5, pp. 285–286.

## VARIATION: Bathing Using Disposable System

### Equipment

Commercial cleansing system
Bath blanket
Clean gown
Disposable bag
Clean gloves, if appropriate.

### Preparation

1. Obtain package with cleansing cloths. Cloths are premoistened with an aloe and vitamin E formula. ➤*Rationale: The cleansing cloths are less during as they maintain the skin at pH of 4.7–4.9.*
2. Heat package in microwave for no more than 45 seconds. Check temperature before applying to skin. ➤*Rationale: Increased time could lead to excessive heat and burning of the skin. The commercial system can be used at room temperature.*
3. Explain procedure to client. ➤*Rationale: This procedure may be new to the client and an explanation is needed to ensure client understands the different between a bed bath and a bath using a cleansing system. The client may not think he has had a complete bath but only a "sponge bath."*
4. Perform hand hygiene.
5. Don gloves if there is a risk of contact with body secretions.
6. Replace top linen and gown with bath blanket or top sheet if bath blanket not available.

### Procedure

1. Open package and remove one cloth at a time.
2. Remove bath blanket at each site when cleansing with cloth.
3. Replace bath blanket when cloth removed. ➤*Rationale: To prevent client chilling.*
4. Use a new cloth for each section of the body as follows:
   a. Face, neck, and chest
   b. Right arm and axilla
   c. Left arm and axilla
   d. Perineum
   e. Right leg
   f. Left leg
   g. Back
   h. Buttocks
5. Discard cloth after cleansing each area. Do not flush down toilet. Rinsing is not required with this system. Replace bath blanket or sheet over each part of the body after it has been cleaned. ➤*Rationale: To prevent the client from becoming chilled.*
6. Place clean gown on client.
7. Place client in comfortable position.
8. Discard cloths in appropriate receptacle.
9. Perform hand hygiene.
10. Document bath on flow sheet or nurses' notes.

## DEVELOPMENTAL CONSIDERATIONS

### Factors That Can Increase Risk of Skin Breakdown and Delay Wound Healing

- Inadequate nutritional intake.
- Compromised immune system.
- Compromised circulatory and respiratory systems.
- Poor hydration.
- Decreased mobility and activity.

### Skin Changes with Age

- Delayed cellular migration and proliferation.
- Skin is less effective as barrier and slow to heal.
- There is increased vulnerability to trauma.
- There is less ability to retain water.
- Geriatric skin is dry (osteotosis) due to decreased endocrine secretion and loss of elastin. This can cause pruritus, which could lead to skin ulceration.
- Increased skin susceptibility to shearing stress leading to blister formation and skin tears.
- There is increased vascular fragility.

### The Skin of the Elderly Should Be Assessed

- Decreased temperature, degree of moisture, dryness resulting from decreased dermal vascularity.
- Skin not intact, open lesions, tears, pressure ulcers as a result of increased skin fragility.
- Decreased turgor, dehydration as a result of decreased oil and sweat glands.
- Pigmentation alterations, potential cancer.
- Pruritus—dry skin most common cause because of decreased oil and sweat glands.
- Bruises, scars from increased skin fragility.

### Bathing May Minimize Dryness

- Have client take complete bath only twice a week.
- Use superfatted or mild soap or lotions to aid in moisturizing.
- Use tepid, not hot, water.
- Apply emollient (lanolin) to skin after bathing.

## VARIATION: Bathing an Infant

### Equipment

Tub or basin filled with warm water (100°F)
Two towels
Washcloth
Suction bulb
Mild soap
Cotton balls
Blanket
Clean clothing
Clean gloves, if indicated

### Preparation

1. Provide a comfortable room environment (i.e., comfortable temperature, lighting.)
2. Check client ID.
3. Perform hand hygiene.
4. Collect necessary equipment, and place articles within reach.
5. Position the bed at a comfortable working height.
6. Place towel, laid out in diamond fashion, on bed next to basin.
7. Don gloves if there is a risk of exposure to body secretions.

### Procedure

1. Test water temperature with your wrist or elbow.
2. Lift infant using football hold.
3. Remove all clothing except shirt and diaper.
4. Cover infant with towel or blanket. Never let go of the infant during the bath. ➤*Rationale: This is a safety intervention to prevent falls or other injury.*
5. Clean infant's eyes, using a cotton ball moistened with water. Wipe from inner to outer can thus, using a new cotton ball for each eye. ➤*Rationale: This procedure prevents water and particles from entering the lacrimal duct.*
6. Make a mitt with the washcloth.
7. Wash infant's face with water.
8. Suction nose, if necessary, by compressing suction bulb prior to placing it in nostril. ➤*Rationale: This prevents aspiration of moisture.* Gently release bulb after it is placed in nostril.
9. Wash infant's ears and neck, paying attention to folds; dry all areas thoroughly. Use mild soap and rinse.
10. Remove shirt or gown.
11. Remove diaper by picking up infant's ankles in your hand.
12. Pick up infant and place feet first into basin or tub. Immerse infant in tub of water only after umbilical cord has healed. Pick up infant by placing your hand and arm around infant, cradling the infant's head and neck in your elbow. Grasp the infant's thigh with your hand. ➤*Rationale: The umbilical cord is kept dry to prevent infection and encourage it to "fall off."*
13. Wash and rinse the infant's body, especially the skin folds.

*Note:* Some facilities use disposable cleansing systems to bathe neonates and infants. There are four infant-size washcloths for infants up to 25 pounds. The bathing procedure is the same for infants and adults.

14. Wash infant's genitalia.
    a. For a female infant: Separate labia and with a cotton ball moistened with soap and water, cleanse downward once on each side. Use a new piece of cotton on each side.
    b. For an uncircumcised male infant: Do not force foreskin back. Gently cleanse the exposed surface with a cotton ball moistened with soap and water.
    c. For a circumcised male infant: Gently cleanse with plain water.
15. Wrap the infant in a towel and use a football hold when washing an infant's head. Soap your own hands and wash infant's hair and scalp paying attention to the nape of the neck and using a circular motion. Rinse hair and scalp thoroughly. ➤*Rationale: Football hold is the most secure for active infants.*
16. Place infant on a clean, dry towel with head facing the top corner and wrap infant.
17. Use the corner of the towel to dry infant's head with gentle, yet firm, circular movements.
18. Replace infant's diaper and redress in a new gown or shirt.
19. Provide comfort by holding the infant for a time following the bath procedure.
20. Perform hand hygiene.

### CLINICAL ALERT

Discharge from the eyes may be present for 2 to 3 days due to prophylactic eyedrops administered at birth.

## CLIENT TEACHING

### Dry Skin

- Use cleansing creams to clean the skin rather than soap or detergent, which cause drying and, in some cases, allergic reactions.
- Thoroughly rinse soap or detergent, if used, from the skin.
- Bathe less frequently when environmental temperature and humidity are low.
- Increase fluid intake.
- Humidify the air with a humidifier or by keeping a tub or sink full of water.
- Use moisturizing or emollient creams that contain lanolin, petroleum jelly, or cocoa butter to retain skin moisture.

### Skin Rashes

- Keep the area clean by washing it with a mild soap. Rinse the skin well, and pat it dry.
- To relieve itching, try a tepid bath or soak. Some over-the-counter preparations, such as Caladryl lotion, may help but should be used with full knowledge of the product.

- Avoid scratching the rash to prevent inflammation, infection, and further skin lesions.
- Choose clothing carefully. Too much can cause perspiration and aggravate a rash.

### Acne

- Wash the face frequently with soap or detergent and hot water to remove oil and dirt.
- Avoid using oily creams, which aggravate the condition.
- Avoid using cosmetics that block the ducts of the sebaceous glands and the hair follicles.
- Never squeeze or pick at the lesions. This increases the potential for infection and scarring.
- Condition and integrity of skin (dryness, turgor, redness, lesions, and so on).
- Client strength. Note range of motion and circulation, movement, and sensation for all extremities.
- Percentage of bath done without assistance.
- Relate to prior assessment data, if available.

---

| UNEXPECTED OUTCOMES | CRITICAL THINKING OPTIONS |
|---|---|
| Client is unwilling to accept a complete bed bath. | • Respect client's wishes and take other opportunities for assessment.<br>• Have client wash hands, face, and genitals. You should wash back and give back care. Reexplain the purpose of the bath to the client and request client participation. |
| Client is too shy to allow bath. | • Respect client's privacy and only wash areas client wishes you to do.<br>• Give assistance so client can bathe him or herself.<br>• Allow spouse or parent to give bath if this is more acceptable to client. |
| Client complains of dry, itching skin following the bath. | • Assess for cause of itching.<br>• Ask physician for an order for special lotion.<br>• Do not use soap for the bath. |

## DEVELOPMENTAL CONSIDERATIONS

### Infants

- Sponge baths are suggested for the newborn because daily tub baths are not considered necessary. After the bath, the infant should be immediately dried and wrapped. Parents need to be advised that the infant's ability to regulate body temperature has not yet fully developed and newborns' bodies lose heat readily.

### Children

- Encourage a child's participation as appropriate for developmental level.
- Closely supervise children in the bathtub. Do not leave them unattended.

### Adolescents

- Assist adolescents as needed to choose deodorants and antiperspirants. Secretions from newly active sweat glands react with bacteria on the skin, causing a pungent odor.

### Elders

- Changes of aging can decrease the protective function of the skin in elders. These changes include fragile skin, less oil and moisture, and a decrease in elasticity.
- To minimize skin dryness in elders, avoid excessive use of soap.
- The ideal time to moisturize the skin is immediately after bathing.
- Avoid powder because it causes moisture loss and is a hazardous inhalant. Cornstarch should also be avoided because in the presence of moisture it breaks down into glucose and can facilitate the growth of organisms.
- Protect elders and children from injury related to hot water burns.

## CULTURAL CONSIDERATIONS

Cultures define cleanliness in different ways. Western cultures, because of the abundance of detergents and washing machines, value clean clothes. Some underdeveloped countries have limited access to fresh water and, therefore, may not wash clothes as frequently.

Anglo-Americans are fastidious about body cleanliness and the absence of body odor. The use of perfumes, deodorants, and aftershave lotions is a major part of their hygienic care. In some cultures, natural body odor is thought to have sex appeal.

When providing hygienic care for clients, the nurse needs to assess the client's usual pattern of bathing, hygienic products usually used, and cultural rituals and beliefs.

Modesty and bathing rituals and beliefs must be considered in caring for clients. For example, some cultures and religions do not allow members of the opposite sex to see them from the waist to the knees. (Gypsy culture, Southeast Asian cultures). Hispanic women have a strong sense of modesty and do not want health care workers to see them unclothed.

## BIOCULTURAL VARIATIONS IN BODY SECRETIONS

- Most Asians and Native North Americans have a mild to absent body odor, whereas Caucasians and African Americans tend to have strong body odor.
- Eskimos have made environmental adaptation where they sweat less than Caucasians on their trunks and extremities but more on their faces. This adaptation allows for temperature regulation without the need to change clothes because of perspiration.
- The amount of chloride excreted by sweat glands varies widely. African Americans have lower salt concentrations in their sweat than Caucasians.

*Source: From Transcultural Concepts in Nursing Care*, 4th ed. (pp. 59–60), by M. M. Andrews and J. S. Boyle, 2003, Philadelphia: Lippincott, Williams & Wilkins. Adapted with permission.

# Skill 12.5  Providing Evening Care

## Equipment

Towels, washcloth
Clean linens if needed
Basin of warm water, soap
Dental items (i.e., toothbrush, dentifrice, denture cup)
Emesis basin, cup
Fresh pitcher of water if allowed
Skin care lotion and powder if desired
Personal care items (e.g., deodorant, skin moisturizers)
Bedpan, urinal, toilet paper
Miscellaneous supplies as needed (e.g., dressing, special
    equipment)
Clean gloves, if indicated

## Preparation

1. Check client's ID.
2. Explain the needs and benefits of evening care; discuss how the client can be involved.
3. Collect and arrange equipment.
4. Adjust the bed to a comfortable working height, and assist the client into a comfortable position.
5. Ensure privacy.
6. Perform hand hygiene.
7. Don gloves if indicated.

## Procedure

1. Offer bedpan or urinal if client is unable to use bathroom. Assist with handwashing.
2. If client needs or requests a bath, provide assistance as needed.
3. Assist with mouth and dental care as needed.
4. Remove equipment, extra linens, and pillows, if possible. Remove stockings, ace wraps, and binders.
5. Change dressings. Perform any required procedural techniques.
6. Wash face, hands, and back. Provide back massage.
7. Assist with combing or brushing hair if desired.
8. Replace antiembolic (elastic) stockings and binders.
9. Replace soiled linen, or straighten and tuck remaining linen. Fluff pillow and turn cool side next to client.
10. Straighten top linens. Provide additional blankets if desired.
11. Remove any additional equipment. Place cal signal and water (if allowed) within client's reach.
12. Administer sleeping medication if ordered and client requests.
13. Assess for pain.
14. Assist client into a comfortable position.
15. Ensure that the client's environment is safe and comfortable.
16. Raise side rails, place bed in LOW position, and turn lighting to low.
17. Remove gloves if used.
18. Perform hand hygiene.

*Note:* Side rails are now considered restraints by HCFA and the FDA. Check with your facility about agency policies on use of side rails.

# Skill 12.6  Providing a Back Massage

## EXPECTED OUTCOMES

- Client states he/she is comfortable and ready for sleep following evening care.
- Client states that back care has decreased muscle tension and improved comfort level.

## Delegation

The nurse can delegate this skill to UAP; however, the nurse should first assess for UAP's comfort and ability, any contraindications, and client willingness.

## Equipment

- Lotion
- Towel for excess lotion

## Preparation

Determine (a) previous assessments of the skin, (b) special lotions to be used, and (c) positions contraindicated for the client. Arrange for a quiet environment with no interruptions to promote maximum effect of the back massage.

## Procedure

1. Prior to performing the procedure, introduce self and verify the client's identity using agency protocol. Explain to the client what you are going to do, why it is necessary, and how he or she can participate. Encourage the client to give you feedback as to the amount of pressure you are using during the back rub.

2. Perform hand hygiene and observe other appropriate infection control procedures.
3. Provide for client privacy.
4. Prepare the client.
   - Assist the client to move to the near side of the bed within your reach and adjust the bed to a comfortable working height. ➤*Rationale: This prevents back strain.*
   - Establish which position the client prefers. The prone position is recommended for a back rub. The side-lying position can be used if a client cannot assume the prone position.
   - Expose the back from the shoulders to the inferior sacral area. Cover the remainder of the body. ➤*Rationale: This is to prevent chilling and minimize exposure.*
5. Massage the back.
   - Pour a small amount of lotion onto the palms of your hands and hold it for a minute. The lotion bottle can also be placed in a bath basin filled with warm water. ➤*Rationale: Back rub preparations tend to feel uncomfortably cold to people. Warming the solution facilitates client comfort.*
   - Using your palm, begin in the sacral area using smooth, circular strokes.
   - Move your hands up the center of the back and then over both scapulae.
   - Massage in a circular motion over the scapulae.
   - Move your hands down the sides of the back.
   - Massage the areas over the right and left iliac crests. Massage the back in an orderly pattern using a variety of strokes and appropriate pressure.
   - Apply firm, continuous pressure without breaking contact with the client's skin.
   - Repeat above for 3 to 5 minutes, obtaining more lotion as necessary.
   - While massaging the back, assess for skin redness and areas of decreased circulation.
   - Pat dry any excess lotion with a towel.

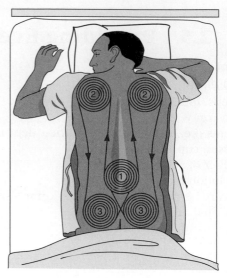

● One suggested pattern for a back massage.

6. Document that a back massage was performed and the client's response. Record any unusual findings.

**Documentation**

Sample: 6/22/2009 1400 C/o aching, intermittent back pain. Wincing and grimacing when attempting to move in bed. Rates pain at 4–5 on 0–10 scale. States uses massage to help relieve pain when at home. Back massaged. Stated the massage helped him "to relax." Lights dimmed and door to room closed.

_____ M. Black, RN

1430 Rates pain at 1–2/10. States feels "much more comfortable." Moving in bed with ease.

_____ M. Black, RN

| **UNEXPECTED OUTCOMES** | **CRITICAL THINKING OPTIONS** |
|---|---|
| Client misinterprets back care from nurse and makes sexual advances. | • Set firm limits by explaining therapeutic purpose of back care.<br>• Tell client that if he or she cannot accept back care as part of the therapeutic regimen, you will stop. |
| Client refuses back care because she or he thinks you are too busy or disinterested. | • Make sure you offer the back care in an unhurried and meaningful manner. Do not allow the client to misinterpret your offer for care.<br>• Return to client and offer back care later in the evening. |
| Client is unable to sleep even after evening care is given. | • Encourage verbalization of fears.<br>• Check to see if sleeping medication can be given.<br>• Provide additional back care. |

# Skill 12.7  Brushing and Flossing the Teeth

## EXPECTED OUTCOMES

- The oral health status of client has been assessed and documented by nurse.
- Oral hygiene care is provided without complications.
- Plaque and bacteria-producing agents are removed.

## Delegation

Oral care, brushing and flossing of teeth, and denture care can be delegated to the UAP. After performing the above assessment, the nurse should instruct the UAP as to the type of oral care and amount of assistance needed by the client. Remind the UAP to report changes in the client's oral mucosa.

## Equipment

*Brushing and Flossing*

- Towel
- Clean gloves
- Curved basin (emesis basin)
- Toothbrush (soft bristle)
- Cup of tepid water
- Dentifrice (toothpaste)
- Mouthwash
- Dental floss, at least two pieces 20 cm (8 in.) in length
- Floss holder (optional)

*For Cleaning Artificial Dentures*

- Clean gloves
- Tissue or piece of gauze
- Denture container
- Clean washcloth
- Toothbrush or stiff-bristled brush
- Dentifrice or denture cleaner
- Tepid water
- Container of mouthwash
- Curved basin (emesis basin)
- Towel

## Preparation

Assemble all necessary equipment.

## Procedure

1. Prior to performing the procedure, introduce self and verify the client's identity using agency protocol. Explain to the client what you are going to do, why it is necessary, and how he or she can participate.

2. Perform hand hygiene and observe other appropriate infection control procedures (e.g., clean gloves). ►*Rationale: Wearing gloves while providing mouth care prevents the nurse from acquiring infections. Gloves also prevent transmission of microorganisms to the client.*

3. Provide for client privacy by drawing the curtains around the bed or closing the door to the room. Some agencies provide signs indicating the need for privacy. ►*Rationale: Hygiene is a personal matter.*

4. Prepare the client.
   - Assist the client to a sitting position in bed, if health permits. If not, assist the client to a side-lying position with the head turned. ►*Rationale: This position prevents liquids from draining down the client's throat.*

5. Prepare the equipment.
   - Place the towel under the client's chin.
   - Apply clean gloves.
   - Moisten the bristles of the toothbrush with tepid water and apply the dentifrice to the toothbrush.
   - Use a soft toothbrush (a small one for a child) and the client's choice of dentifrice.
   - For the client who must remain in bed, place or hold the curved basin under the client's chin, fitting the small curve around the chin or neck.
   - Inspect the mouth and teeth.

6. Brush the teeth.
   - Hand the toothbrush to the client, or brush the client's teeth as follows:
   a. Hold the brush against the teeth with the bristles at a 45-degree angle. The tips of the outer bristles should rest against and penetrate under the gingival sulcus. The brush will clean under the sulcus of two or three

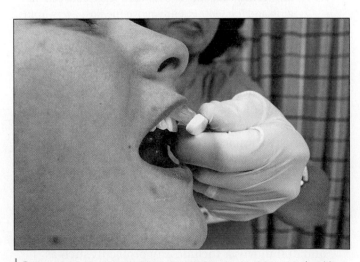

● The sulcular technique: Place the bristles at a 45-degree angle with the tops of the outer bristles under the gingival margins.

teeth at one time. ➤*Rationale: This sulcular technique removes plaque and cleans under the gingival margins.*

b. Move the bristles up and down gently in short strokes from the sulcus to the crowns of the teeth.

c. Repeat until all outer and inner surfaces of the teeth and sulci of the gums are cleaned.

d. Clean the biting surfaces by moving the brush back and forth over them in short strokes.

e. Brush the tongue gently with the toothbrush. ➤*Rationale: Brushing removes bacteria and freshens breath. A coated tongue may be caused by poor oral hygiene, low fluid intake, and side effects of medications. Brushing gently and carefully helps prevent gagging or vomiting.*

- Hand the client the water cup or mouthwash to rinse the mouth vigorously. Then ask the client to spit the water and excess dentifrice into the basin. Some agencies supply a standard mouthwash. Alternatively, a mouth rinse of normal saline can be an effective cleaner and moisturizer. ➤*Rationale: Vigorous rinsing loosens food particles and washes out already loosened particles.*

- Repeat the preceding step until the mouth is free of dentifrice and food particles.

- Remove the curved basin and help the client wipe the mouth.

7. Floss the teeth.

- Assist the client to floss independently, or floss the teeth of an alert and cooperative client as follows. Waxed floss is less likely to fray than unwaxed floss; particles between the teeth attach more readily to unwaxed floss than to waxed floss.

a. Wrap one end of the floss around the third finger of each hand.

b. To floss the upper teeth, use your thumb and index finger to stretch the floss. Move the floss up and down between the teeth. When the floss reaches the gum line, gently slide the floss into the space between the gum and the tooth. Gently move the floss away from the gum with up and down motions (American Dental Association, n.d., Cleaning your teeth). Start at the back on the right side and work around to the back of the left side, or work from the center teeth to the back of the jaw on either side.

c. To floss the lower teeth, use your index fingers to stretch the floss.

- Give the client tepid water or mouthwash to rinse the mouth and a curved basin in which to spit the water.

- Assist the client in wiping the mouth.

8. Remove and dispose of equipment appropriately.

- Remove and clean the curved basin.

- Remove and discard gloves. Perform hand hygiene.

9. Document assessment of the teeth, tongue, gums, and oral mucosa. Include any problems such as sores or inflammation, bleeding, and swelling of the gums. Brushing and flossing teeth are not usually recorded.

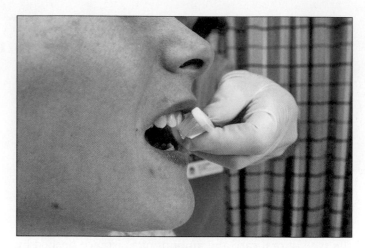

● Brushing from the sulcus to the crowns of the teeth.

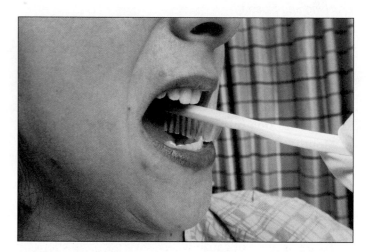

● Brushing the biting surfaces.

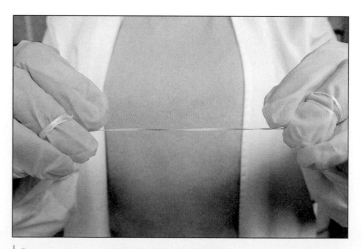

● Stretching the floss between the third finger of each hand.

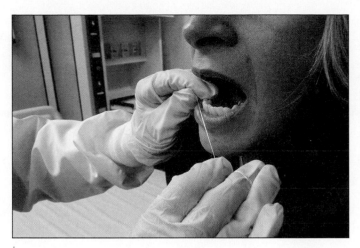

● Flossing the lower teeth by using the index fingers to stretch the floss.

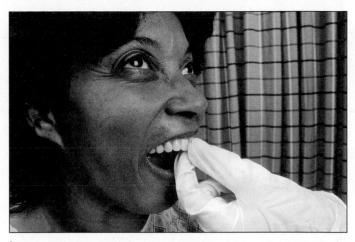

● Removing the top dentures by first breaking the suction.

## VARIATION: Artificial Dentures

1. Remove the dentures.
   * Apply gloves. ➤*Rationale: Wearing gloves decreases the likelihood of spreading infection.*
   * If the client cannot remove the dentures, using the tissue or gauze, grasp the upper plate at the front teeth with your thumb and second finger, and move the denture up and down slightly. ➤*Rationale: The slight movement breaks the suction that holds the plate on the roof of the mouth.*
   * Lower the upper plate, move it out of the mouth, and place it in the denture container.
   * Lift the lower plate, turning it so that the left side, for example, is slightly lower than the right, to remove the plate from the mouth without stretching the lips. Place the lower plate in the denture container.
   * Remove a partial denture by exerting equal pressure on the border of each side of the denture, not on the clasps, which can bend or break.

2. Clean the dentures.
   * Take the denture container to a sink. Take care not to drop the dentures. Place a washcloth in the bowl of the sink. ➤*Rationale: A washcloth prevents damage if the dentures are dropped.*
   * Using a toothbrush or special stiff-bristled brush, scrub the dentures with the cleaning agent and tepid water.
   * Rinse the dentures with tepid running water. ➤*Rationale: Rinsing removes the cleaning agent and food particles.* If the dentures are stained, soak them in a commercial cleaner. Be sure to follow the manufacturer's directions. To prevent corrosion, dentures with metal parts should not be soaked overnight.

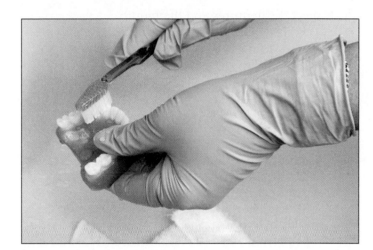

● A washcloth prevents damage if the dentures are dropped.

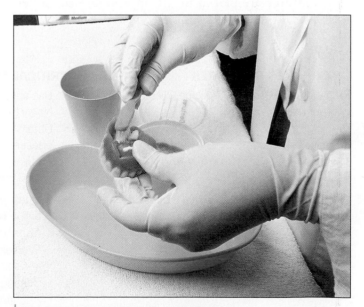

● Hold dentures securely while brushing.

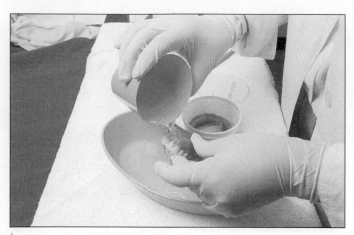

● Rinse dentures in cold water.

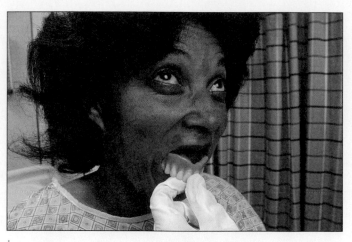

● Inserting the dentures at a slight angle.

3. Inspect the dentures and the mouth.
   • Observe the dentures for any rough, sharp, or worn areas that could irritate the tongue or mucous membranes of the mouth, lips, and gums.
   • Inspect the mouth for any redness, irritated areas, or indications of infection.
   • Assess the fit of the dentures. People who have them should see a dentist at least once a year to check the fit and the presence of any irritation to the soft tissues of the mouth. Clients who need repairs to their dentures or new dentures may need a referral for financial assistance.
4. Return the dentures to the mouth.
   • Offer some mouthwash and a curved basin to rinse the mouth. If the client cannot insert the dentures independently, insert the plates one at a time. Hold each plate at a slight angle while inserting it, to avoid injuring the lips.

*Note:* If clients perform self-cleaning of dentures, ensure that dentures are placed in the appropriate container. ➤*Rationale: Many elderly clients leave dentures on food trays and* *risk losing them when food trays are removed.* Replacement dentures may not be covered by Medicare.

5. Assist the client as needed.
   • Wipe the client's hands and mouth with the towel.
   • If the client does not want to or cannot wear the dentures, store them in a denture container with water. Label the container with the client's name and identification number. (Do not place the container on the food tray.)
6. Remove and discard gloves. Perform hand hygiene.
7. Document all assessments and include any problems such as an irritated area on the mucous membrane.

### CLINICAL ALERT

Clients in long-term care settings are at high risk for oral health problems. The nurse must assess the client's oral health and teach the UAP about the importance of and methods to promote oral hygiene.

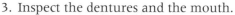

## UNEXPECTED OUTCOMES

Even with increased oral hygiene, client still has odorous breath.

## CRITICAL THINKING OPTIONS

• Use antiseptic mouthwash between oral hygiene care.
• Notify the physician, as this could be a symptom of systemic disease.
• Obtain dental consultation to check for presence of dental caries or gum disease.
• Examine client's nutritional intake. Absent nutrients or imbalanced intake of fats, protein, or carbohydrates can result in bad breath.

Client complains of extreme oral mucosal irritation or sensitivity.

• Request physician's order for one of the following solutions:
   • Saline solutions for soothing, cleansing rinses.
   • Anesthetic solutions to dull extreme pain in the oral cavity.
   • Effervescent solutions (e.g., hydrogen peroxide or ginger ale) to loosen and remove debris from the mouth.
   • Coating solutions (e.g., Maalox) to protect irritated surfaces.
   • Antibacterial—antifungal rinses (e.g., nystatin [mycostatin]) to prevent the spread of organisms that cause thrush.

| UNEXPECTED OUTCOMES *(cont.)* | CRITICAL THINKING OPTIONS *(cont.)* |
|---|---|
| Vigorous flossing results in bleeding and sore gums. | • Give client warm antiseptic mouthwash to relieve soreness.<br>• Investigate gum condition and refer for consultation. |
| Client needs care after oral surgery or oral trauma. | • Oral care following surgery or trauma is always ordered by physician. No oral hygiene care should be attempted until physician has clearly defined the specific care.<br>• Suctioning equipment should always be present.<br>• Assessment of client's head, face, neck, and general status is critical at this time. |
| Normal stimulation and cleaning is not sufficient to remove debris and plaque for the unconscious client. | • Try flossing teeth to dislodge debris.<br>• Provide mouth care with toothbrush and dentifrice at least twice daily.<br>• Check with physician and order sonic toothbrush. |
| Parotid gland inflammation can occur with improper oral hygiene. | • Rinse mouth with mouthwash.<br>• Use swab to reach back in oral cavity along mandible to temporomandibular area.<br>• Floss teeth at least daily. |

# Skill 12.8  Providing Special Oral Care for the Unconscious or Debilitated Client

## Equipment

Towel
Clean gloves
Curved basin (emesis basin)
Bite-block to hold the mouth open and teeth apart (optional)
Toothbrush
Cup of tepid water
Dentifrice or denture cleaner
Tissue or piece of gauze to remove dentures (optional)
Denture container as needed
Mouthwash
Rubber-tipped bulb syringe
Suction catheter with suction apparatus when aspiration is a concern
Foam swabs and cleaning solution for cleaning the mucous membranes
Water-soluble lip moisturizer

## Procedure

1. Prior to performing the procedure, if the client is conscious, introduce self and verify the client's identity using agency protocol. Explain to the client and the family what you are going to do and why it is necessary.
2. Perform hand hygiene and observe other appropriate infection control procedures (e.g., clean gloves).
3. Provide for client privacy by drawing the curtains around the bed or closing the door to the room. Some agencies provide signs indicating the need for privacy. ➤*Rationale: Hygiene is a personal matter.*

4. Prepare the client.
   • Position the unconscious client in a side-lying position, with the head of the bed lowered. ➤*Rationale: In this position, the saliva automatically runs out by gravity rather than being aspirated into the lung and allows for suctioning, if needed. This position is chosen for the unconscious client receiving mouth care. If the client's head cannot be lowered, turn it to one side. ➤Rationale: The fluid will readily run out of the mouth or pool in the side of the mouth, where it can be suctioned.*
   • Place the towel under the client's chin.
   • Place the curved basin against the client's chin and lower cheek to receive the fluid from the mouth.
   • Apply gloves.

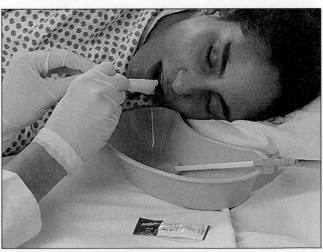

● Position of client and placement of curved basin when providing special mouth care.

5. Clean the teeth and rinse the mouth.
   - If the person has natural teeth, brush the teeth. Brush gently and carefully to avoid injuring the gums. If the client has artificial teeth, clean them.
   - Rinse the client's mouth by drawing about 10 mL of water or alcohol-free mouthwash into the syringe and injecting it gently into each side of the mouth. ➤*Rationale: If the solution is injected with force, some of it may flow down the client's throat and be aspirated into the lungs.*
   - Watch carefully to make sure that all of the rinsing solution has run out of the mouth into the basin. If not, suction the fluid from the mouth. ➤*Rationale: Fluid remaining in the mouth may be aspirated into the lungs.*
   - Repeat rinsing until the mouth is free of dentifrice, if used.
6. Inspect and clean the oral tissues.
   - If the tissues appear dry or unclean, clean them with the foam swabs or gauze and cleaning solution following agency policy.
   - Picking up a moistened foam swab, wipe the mucous membrane of one cheek. Discard the swab in a waste container; use a fresh one to clean the next area. ➤*Rationale: Using separate applicators for each area of the mouth prevents the transfer of microorganisms from one area to another.*
   - Clean all mouth tissues in an orderly progression, using separate applicators: the cheeks, roof of the mouth, base of the mouth, and tongue.
   - Observe the oral tissues closely for inflammation, dryness, or lesions.
   - Rinse the client's mouth as described in step 5.

7. Ensure client comfort.
   - Remove the basin, and dry around the client's mouth with the towel. Replace artificial dentures, if indicated.
   - Lubricate the client's lips with water-soluble moisturizer. ➤*Rationale: Lubrication prevents cracking and subsequent infection.*
   - Remove and discard gloves. Perform hand hygiene.
8. Document assessment of the teeth, tongue, gums, and oral mucosa. Include any problems such as sores or inflammation and swelling of the gums.

## CLIENT TEACHING

- Brush the teeth thoroughly after meals and at bedtime. Assist children or inspect their mouths to be sure the teeth are clean. If the teeth cannot be brushed after meals, vigorous rinsing of the mouth with water is recommended.
- Floss the teeth daily.
- Ensure an adequate intake of nutrients, particularly calcium, phosphorus, vitamins A, C, and D, and fluoride.
- Avoid sweet foods and drinks between meals. Take them in moderation at meals.
- Eat coarse, fibrous foods (cleansing foods), such as fresh fruits and raw vegetables.
- Have topical fluoride applications as prescribed by the dentist.
- Have a checkup by a dentist every 6 months.

## DEVELOPMENTAL CONSIDERATIONS

### Infants

- Most dentists recommend that dental hygiene should begin when the first tooth erupts and be practiced after each feeding. Cleaning can be accomplished by using a wet washcloth or small gauze moistened with water.

### Children

- Beginning at about 18 months of age, brush the child's teeth with a soft toothbrush. Use only a toothbrush moistened with water. Introduce toothpaste later and use one that contains fluoride.
- Frequent snacking on products containing sugar increases the child's risk for developing cavities.

### Elders

- Oral care is often difficult for certain elders to perform due to problems with dexterity or cognitive problems with dementia.

- Most long-term health care facilities have dentists that come on a regular basis to see clients with special needs.
- Dryness of the oral mucosa is a common finding in elders. Because this can lead to tooth decay, advise clients to discuss it with their dentist or primary care provider.
- Decay of the tooth root is common among elders. When the gums recede, the tooth root is more vulnerable to decay.
- Promoting good oral hygiene can have a positive effect on elders' ability to eat.

# Skill 12.9   Shaving a Male Client

### Equipment

Safety or electric razor, specific to client's needs or wishes
Shaving cream
Aftershave lotion (optional)
Two towels
Basin of warm water

### Preparation

1. Place client in sitting position.
2. Perform hand hygiene.
3. Place towel over chest and under chin.
4. Put up mirror on overbed table.
5. Determine how the client usually shaves (i.e., use of safety edge or electric razor; special products).
6. Check to see if the client has excessive bleeding tendencies due to pathologic conditions (hemophilia) or the use of specific medications (anticoagulants or large doses of aspirin). ➤*Rationale: If client is accidentally cut, it could lead to some loss of blood.*

### Procedure

1. If using a safety edge razor:
   a. Don gloves and apply a warm, moist towel to soften the hair.
   b. Apply a thick layer of soap or shaving cream to the shaving area.

c. Holding skin taut, use firm but small strokes in the direction of hair growth.
d. Gently remove soap or lather with a warm, damp towel. Inspect for areas you may have missed.
2. If using electric razor:
   a. Use rotating motion of razor and start from lateral aspect of face and move toward chin and upper lip area.
   b. Clean razor with brush or remove head and clean facial hair from head of razor.
3. Apply aftershave lotion or powder as desired.
4. Reposition client for comfort if needed.
5. Remove gloves and replace equipment.
6. Perform hand hygiene.

**CLINICAL ALERT**

According to the hospital policy, be sure to have the electric razor checked for safety aspects. Some hospitals do not allow clients to use their own electric razors.

**CLINICAL ALERT**

A beard or a mustache should not be shaved off without the client's consent.

| UNEXPECTED OUTCOMES | CRITICAL THINKING OPTIONS |
|---|---|
| Extreme matting, snarling, blood, or nonremovable substances appear in client's hair. | • Never cut a client's hair unless it is absolutely necessary. Check hospital policy regarding hair cutting.<br>• Apply alcohol to tangled hair or blood-soaked hair. Keep in place 5 minutes. Wash hair with shampoo to remove alcohol and blood.<br>• Secure permission of family or physician. |
| Client is cut during shaving procedure. | • Assess extent of cut, and place a clean towel on the area with pressure to stop bleeding.<br>• If cut appears to be more than a nick, report to physician, and fill out unusual occurrence report. |
| Shaving is difficult and painful for the client. | • Place warm towels on area to be shaved for 15 minutes.<br>• Apply more shaving cream.<br>• Ensure that razor is sharp. |

# Skill 12.10 Providing Hair Care

## EXPECTED OUTCOMES

- Hair and scalp assessment are performed without complications.
- Appropriate method of hair care was provided for client.
- Client's hair and scalp are clean, comfortable, and styled according to client's preference.
- Client is comfortable and rested following shampooing.
- Shaving is accomplished without skin nicks or discomfort.
- Lice removed following infestation.
- Client verbalizes cause of problem and preventative measures.
- Client repeats back to nurse instructions for preventing lice infestation and indicates understanding of process.
- Client and family members remain free of lice infestation.

## Delegation

Brushing and combing hair, shampooing hair, and shaving facial hair can be delegated to UAP unless the client has a condition in which the procedure would be contraindicated (e.g., cervical spinal injury or trauma). The nurse needs to assess the UAP's knowledge and experience of hair care for clients of other cultures, if appropriate.

## Equipment

- Clean brush and comb (A wide-toothed comb is usually used for many black-skinned people because finer combs pull the hair into knots and may also break the hair.)
- Towel
- Hair oil preparation, if appropriate

## Procedure

1. Prior to performing the procedure, introduce self and verify the client's identity using agency protocol. Explain to the client what you are going to do, why it is necessary, and how he or she can participate.
2. Perform hand hygiene and observe other appropriate infection control procedures.
3. Provide for client privacy by drawing the curtains around the bed or closing the door to the room. Some agencies provide signs indicating the need for privacy. ➤*Rationale: Hygiene is a personal matter.*
4. Position and prepare the client appropriately.
   - Assist the client who can sit to move to a chair. ➤*Rationale: Hair is more easily brushed and combed when the client is in a sitting position.* If health permits, assist a client confined to a bed to a sitting position by raising the head

of the bed. Otherwise, assist the client to alternate side-lying positions, and do one side of the head at a time.
   - If the client remains in bed, place a clean towel over the pillow and the client's shoulders. Place it over the sitting client's shoulders. ➤*Rationale: The towel collects any removed hair, dirt, and scaly material.*
   - Remove any pins or ribbons in the hair.
5. Remove any mats or tangles gradually.
   - Mats can usually be pulled apart with fingers or worked out with repeated brushings.
   - If the hair is very tangled, rub alcohol or an oil, such as mineral oil, on the strands to help loosen the tangles.
   - Comb out tangles in a small section of hair toward the ends. Stabilize the hair with one hand and comb toward the ends of the hair with the other hand. ➤*Rationale: This avoids scalp trauma.*
6. Brush and comb the hair.
   - For short hair, brush and comb one side at a time. Divide long hair into two sections by parting it down the middle from the front to the back. If the hair is very thick, divide each section into front and back subsections or into several layers.
7. Arrange the hair as neatly and attractively as possible, according to the individual's desires.
   - Braiding long hair helps prevent tangles.
8. Document assessments and special nursing interventions. Daily combing and brushing of the hair are not normally recorded.

## VARIATION: Hair Care for African American Clients

- Position and prepare the client.
- Separate the hair into four sections, proceeding from one section to the next.
- Untangle the hair first, if appropriate. Use fingers to reduce hair breakage and discomfort. Move fingers in a circular motion starting at the roots and gently moving up to the tip of the hair.
- Comb the hair. Dampen the hair with water or a leave-in conditioner. ➤*Rationale: This will help loosen any tangles.*
- Apply hair oil preparation as the client indicates. Using a large and open-toothed comb, grasp a small section of hair and, holding the hair at the tip, start untangling at the tip and work down toward the scalp (Jackson, 1998, p. 102).
- Ask the client if he or she would like the hair braided. ➤*Rationale: Braiding will decrease tangling; however, the choice is the client's.*

# Skill 12.11   Shampooing Hair

## Equipment

Two bath towels
Washcloth
Large container for water
Shampoo
Conditioner, if desired
Shampoo board for clients confined to bed
Hair dryer, if allowed by hospital for Disposable System
Package containing shampoo cap
Face or bath towel
Hair care products, as requested by client
Comb and/or brush

*Note:* Ensure that electrical equipment is checked by maintenance department before using. ➤*Rationale: This confirms that equipment is grounded and mechanically safe.*

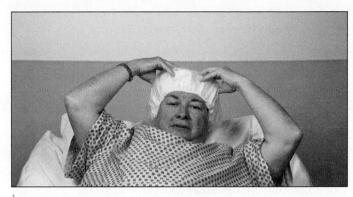

● Disposable shampoo cap can be used for clients on bed rest.

## Preparation

1. Determine client's hair care needs.
2. Perform hand hygiene.
3. Collect and assemble equipment.
4. Help client into a comfortable position to perform hair care.
5. Shampooing the hair can be accomplished in a variety of ways depending on the client's usual routine and physical condition. In many institutions, a physician's order is necessary before shampooing a client's hair.
6. If possible, the easiest way to shampoo is to assist the client while he or she is in the shower. Caution should be taken to prevent the client from becoming overly tired or weak while in the shower. (Use shower chair if necessary.)

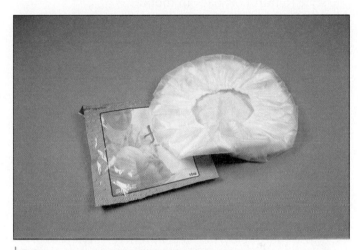

● Shampoo system activated by microwave.

## Procedure for Client in a Chair

1. Have shampoo items readily available.
2. Drape one towel over client's shoulders and around neck. Place another towel within reach.
3. Face client away from sink. Lock wheels of wheelchair.

4. Pad the edge of the sink with a towel or bath blanket.
5. Ask client to lean head and neck against sink.
6. Using a washcloth to protect client's eyes, wet hair, and gently make a lather with shampoo.
7. Rinse thoroughly, and repeat if necessary.
8. Towel dry, add conditioner if desired, and rinse again.
9. Using a dry towel, pat hair dry, and wrap turban style to transport back to bed.
10. Use hair dryer if available.
11. Style as desired.
12. Replace equipment.
13. Perform hand hygiene.

## CLINICAL ALERT

If the client is elderly, do not press the neck down on the edge of the sink—this position can diminish circulation to the brain and has been reported to be a possible cause of strokes.

**Procedure for Client on a Gurney**

1. Have shampoo items readily available.
2. Position gurney with head end at sink.
3. Lock wheels on gurney. ➤*Rationale: This prevents the gurney from moving away from the sink.*
4. Pad the edge of the sink with a towel or bath blanket.
5. Move the client's head just beyond the edge of the gurney. ➤*Rationale: To allow water to run off more easily.*
6. Put a pillow or a rolled blanket under the client's shoulders. ➤*Rationale: To help elevate and extend the head.*
7. Drape one towel over client's shoulders and around neck. Place another towel within reach.
8. Use a washcloth to protect client's eyes. Wet hair and gently make a lather with shampoo.
9. Rinse thoroughly and repeat if necessary.
10. Towel dry, add conditioner if desired, and rinse again.
11. Using a dry towel, pat hair dry, and wrap turban style to transport back to room.
12. Use hair dryer if available.
13. Style as desired.
14. Replace equipment.
15. Perform hand hygiene.

**Procedure for Client on Bed Rest**

1. Place shampoo board, if available, under the client's head. ➤*Rationale: This allows water and soap to run off into a basin at the side of the bed.*
2. Drape one towel over client's shoulders and around neck. Place another towel within reach.
3. Place client's head on shampoo board.
4. Using a washcloth to protect client's eyes, wet hair, and gently make a lather with shampoo.
5. Rinse thoroughly, and repeat if necessary.
6. Towel dry, add conditioner if desired, and rinse again.
7. Using a dry towel, pat hair dry, and wrap turban style.
8. Remove equipment from bed.

9. Change gown and linen if wet.
10. Use hair dryer if available.
11. Style as desired.
12. Replace all equipment.
13. Perform hand hygiene.

**Procedure for Client Using Disposable System**

1. Heat shampoo package in microwave for no more than 30 seconds.
2. Perform hand hygiene.
3. Open package and check temperature. ➤*Rationale: Clients react to heat at different temperatures; therefore, check the cap temperature with client before placing on client's head.*
4. Place cap on head. Ensure that all hair is contained within the cap. For longer hair, place cap on top of head and then tuck all hair up inside cap.
5. Gently massage cap with hands, 1–2 minutes for short hair and 2–3 minutes for longer hair. ➤*Rationale: This will assist in saturating the hair with the solution.*
6. Remove cap and place in appropriate receptacle.
7. Towel dry hair.
8. Complete hair care according to client's needs and desires.
9. Perform hand hygiene.

*Note:* Disposable hair care systems provide a quick and easy way to freshen client's hair with minimal client movement.

---

## CLINICAL ALERT

If hair is tangled, the cap may need to stay on for longer period of time in order to saturate hair. If blood or other secretions are present on hair, they may need to be removed using the washcloths from the disposable bath system before attempting to shampoo the hair.

---

# Skill 12.12   Identifying the Presence of Lice and Nits (Lice Eggs)

### Equipment

Bright lamp/light
Magnifying glass
Clean gloves
Isolation bag

### Procedure

*Note:* Lice become adult in 17 days. Each louse lays 4–8 eggs/day for next 18 days, then dies (each louse lays 144 eggs).

1. Perform hand hygiene. Don clean gloves.
2. Check two forms of client ID, introduce yourself, and explain procedure to client.
3. Position client so head or affected body area is well lighted by lamp.
4. Use magnifying glass to observe scalp and hair.
   a. For live lice:
      Light to dark brown in color;
      2–4 mm long; 1 mm wide;

flat body with 6 clawed legs;
live lice crawl, but do not fly, jump or hop;
feed on blood 3–4 times/day.

   b. For nits (lice eggs)
      Tiny and hard

Yellow to white in color, confused with dandruff but dandruff is flaky;
Attach to hair shaft, close to scalp;
Nits hatch after 7–10 days;
Nits are hard to remove from hair shaft.

# Skill 12.13 Removing Lice and Nits

## Equipment

Isolation bags (optional)
1% permethrin cream rinse (Nix®) or
Pyrethium® and Pyrethrins® kit(s) (RID® and R&C®)
RID®Home Lice Control Spray
Trimethoprim sulfamethoxazole (Bactrim); oral antibiotic
Clean linen
Fine-tooth "nit" comb
Disinfectant for comb
Clean gloves
Towels

## Procedure

1. Determine if client is allergic to ragweed or chrysanthemums.
2. Perform hand hygiene.
3. Don clean gloves. Gloves are used even when completing treatment at home.
4. Remove and bag client's clothing and linens. Client's clothes do not need to be bagged separately and placed in isolation bags if standard precautions are used.
5. Notify physician and other health care providers of lice infestation.
6. Begin treatment as ordered by physician.

### For Using Permethrin 1% (Nix) for Lice

   a. Shampoo hair with regular shampoo, rinse, and towel dry.
   b. Shake lotion well before applying. Nix is only used on hair, not on skin.
   c. Saturate damp hair with lotion and keep in place for 10 minutes.
   d. Rinse hair thoroughly and dry with clean towel.

> ### CLINICAL ALERT
>
> When using any of the lice treatment products, the nurse needs to check for allergies to ragweed or chrysanthemum flowers. Allergies to ragweed can cause breathing difficulties or an asthmatic attack. Allergies to chrysanthemums can cause pneumonia, muscle paralysis, or death due to respiratory failure.

   e. Inspect hair shafts daily for at least 7 days.
   f. Regular shampooing may be initiated within a day.
      ▶*Rationale: Residual deposits of the drug on the hair shaft is not reduced with regular shampooing.*
   g. Instruct client or family to monitor for side effects of drug: pruritus, transient tingling, burning, stinging, numbness, erythema, edema, rash.

7. Disinfect combs and brushes with the shampoo.
8. Remove gloves.
9. Perform hand hygiene.
10. Instruct client or parent to check hair and use "nit comb" every 2 to 3 days until lice are gone and to check skin for removal of scabies. (Pruritus may last for 2 weeks following treatment.)

> ### CLINICAL ALERT
>
> Permethrin stays on the hair shaft for up to 14 days; therefore, recurrence of lice infestations rarely happens.

> ### CLINICAL ALERT
>
> Lindane/Kwell is available only by prescription because of neurotoxicity and bone marrow suppression.

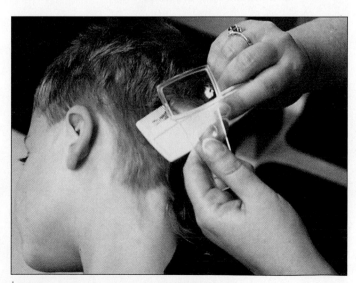

● Use magnifying glass when inspecting for head lice.

11. Wash clothes and linens in hot water (130°) or dry them using high heat.
12. Place stuffed toys in hot dryer.
13. Instruct client or family to vacuum furniture and floors to rid house of lice. ➤*Rationale: Head lice need a human host and therefore do not survive long after falling off head.*
14. Administer Bactrim if ordered. ➤*Rationale: It destroys lice.*
15. Discuss the cause, treatment, and preventive measures regarding lice infestation with client and family.

*Note:* Nix is treatment of choice and is over-the-counter. Recommended by the American Academy of Pediatrics because of its efficacy and lack of toxicity.

### For Using Pyrethium and Pyrethrins (Rid and R&C)

a. Used to treat head, pubic, and body lice (not as effective as Nix).
b. Determine if client has allergies to chrysanthemums or ragweed. ➤*Rationale: Allergic reactions may cause breathing difficulties or asthma.*
c. Assess for open lesions or sores on scalp. ➤*Rationale: Product should not be used if present as it causes burning to area.*
d. Obtain appropriate lice treatment product.
e. Place unopened tubes in a cup of warm water for 1 minute.
f. Instruct client to tightly close eyes and place towel or washcloth over eyes. ➤*Rationale: Prevents irritation to eyes.*
g. Apply product to dry hair or other affected areas. Start behind ears and back of neck. ➤*Rationale: Wetting hair dilutes treatment.* Lice can also hold their breath when immersed in water, making it difficult for active ingredients in shampoo to penetrate lice.

---

**CLINICAL ALERT**

Do not use near eyes, eyebrows, eyelids, inside nose, mouth, or vagina.

If product gets into eyes, immediately flush eyes with water. If child swallows product, immediately contact a Poison Control Center for directions on care.

---

**CLINICAL ALERT**

Stop treatment immediately if client complains of breathing difficulties, eye irritation, or skin or scalp irritation.

---

h. Leave product on hair according to manufacturer's directions, usually 10 minutes.
i. Use warm water to form lather; shampoo; and then rinse thoroughly. Towel-dry hair.
j. Comb out nits using a fine-tooth or lice/nit comb. Hair should remain slightly damp while removing nits. If hair dries during combing, dampen slightly with water. ➤*Rationale: Combing is the most important step in process of lice removal, as eggs can be left behind and hatch at a later time.*
k. Remove any remaining nits by hand (use disposable glove to remove nits).
l. Apply Rid Home Lice Control Spray to clothing, and bedding (including mattress and furniture) that cannot be dry cleaned or laundered. Do not use on sheets or pillowcase (these are to be laundered).
m. Apply second treatment in 7–10 days to kill any newly hatched lice.
n. Inspect head in 2 weeks to assess for presence of lice.
o. Inspect all members of family using magnifying glass in bright light for lice/nits (eggs). Look for tiny nits near scalp, beginning at back of neck and behind ears. Examine small section of hair at one time. Treat each member infested with lice using same treatment plan.

---

**REMOVING NITS FROM HAIR**

- Part hair into sections; start at top of head and do one section at a time.
- Lift a 1- to 2-inch-wide strand of hair. Place comb as close to scalp as possible and comb with a firm, even motion away from scalp.
- Pin back each strand of hair after combing.
- Clean comb often. Wipe nits away with tissue and discard into a plastic bag. Seal bag and discard to prevent lice from spreading.
- After combing, thoroughly recheck for lice/nits. Recomb as needed.
- Check daily for missed lice.

---

**CLINICAL ALERT**

Adverse reactions and side effects may be more frequent and severe in younger clients. Consult with physician about dose.

## EVIDENCE-BASED NURSING PRACTICE

**Head Lice Infestation**

In a randomly assigned study, 115 children, age 2–13 (mostly girls) were assigned to three groups. One group received only cream rinse (Nix), one group only the oral antibiotic (Bactrim), and one group received the combination of the oral antibiotic and the cream rinse. At both 2- and 4-week follow-up appointments, more than 90% of the children receiving the combination therapy were

lice free compared to 80% or less in the other two groups. No major side effects were noted in any of the 3 groups of children.

*Source:* Head lice infestation: single drug versus combination therapy with one percent permethrin and trimethoprim/sulfamethoxazole. *Pediatrics* 2001, March (107) E30. Authors: Hipolito, R. B., Mallorca, F. G., Zuniga-Macaraig, Z. O., et al.

# Skill 12.14   Providing Nail Care

## EXPECTED OUTCOMES

- Foot care provided without complications.
- Nail care is completed without cuts.
- Client's feet are clean and appear free of complicating conditions, such as excessive moisture, calluses, corns, blisters, abrasions, or infection.
- Client and family understand the importance and techniques for proper foot care.
- Clients with diabetes mellitus or peripheral vascular disease understand importance of appropriate foot care.

## Equipment

Basin of warm water
Towel
Scissors or nail clippers
File or emery board
Orangewood stick
Clean gloves

## Procedure

1. Check hospital policy on nail cutting. Some institutions do not allow nurses to cut client's nails if the

client has diabetes mellitus, peripheral vascular disease, or a localized condition such as a fungus infection. Thick, mycotic, or ingrown toenails should not be cut by the nurse. Request that a podiatrist see the client.
2. Perform hand hygiene and don clean gloves.
3. Position client for comfort.
4. Expose one extremity at a time.
5. Soak nails if softening is needed. Dry nails.
6. Cut toenails straight across with scissors or clippers. ▶*Rationale: Rounding off toenails may break the skin or cause ingrown toenails.*
7. Smooth cut edges with file or emery board. Be careful to not injure surrounding skin.
8. Clean under nail with orangewood stick.
9. Reposition client.
10. Remove and clean equipment.
11. Remove gloves and perform hand hygiene.

# Skill 12.15   Providing Foot Care

## Delegation

Foot care for the *nondiabetic* client can be delegated to UAP. Remind the UAP to notify the nurse of anything that looks out of the ordinary. Review with the UAP the agency policy about cutting or trimming nails.

## Equipment

Wash basin containing warm water
Pillow
Moisture-resistant disposable pad

Towels
Soap
Washcloth
Toenail cleaning and trimming equipment, if agency policy permits
Lotion or foot powder

## Preparation

Assemble all of the necessary equipment and supplies if nails need trimming and agency policy permits.

## Procedure

1. Prior to performing the procedure, introduce self and verify the client's identity using agency protocol. Explain to the client what you are going to do, why it is necessary, and how he or she can participate.
2. Perform hand hygiene and observe other appropriate infection control procedures.
3. Provide for client privacy by drawing the curtains around the bed or closing the door to the room. Some agencies provide signs indicating the need for privacy. ➤*Rationale: Hygiene is a personal matter.*
4. Prepare the equipment and the client.
   - Fill the washbasin with warm water at about 40° to 43°C (105° to 110°F). ➤*Rationale: Warm water promotes circulation, comforts, and refreshes.*
   - Assist the ambulatory client to a sitting position in a chair, or the bed client to a supine or semi-Fowler's position.
   - Place a pillow under the bed client's knees, if not contraindicated. ➤*Rationale: This provides support and prevents muscle fatigue.*
   - Place the washbasin on the moisture-resistant pad at the foot of the bed for a bed client or on the floor in front of the chair for an ambulatory client.
   - For a bed client, pad the rim of the washbasin with a towel. ➤*Rationale: The towel prevents undue pressure on the skin.*

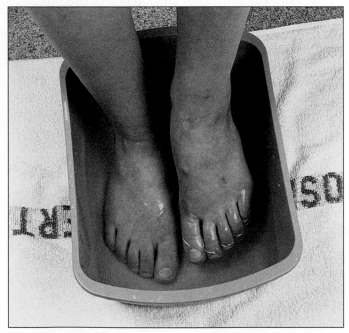

● Place towel on floor in front of client and place feet in basin for soaking.

5. Wash the foot and soak it.
   - Place one of the client's feet in the basin and wash it with soap, paying particular attention to the interdigital areas. Prolonged soaking is generally not recommended for diabetic clients or individuals with peripheral vascular disease. ➤*Rationale: Prolonged soaking may remove natural skin oils, thus drying the skin and making it more susceptible to cracking and injury.*
   - Rinse the foot well to remove soap. ➤*Rationale: Soap irritates the skin if not completely removed.*
   - Rub calloused areas of the foot with the washcloth. ➤*Rationale: This helps remove dead skin layers.*
   - If the nails are brittle or thick and require trimming, replace the water and allow the foot to soak for 10 to 20 minutes. ➤*Rationale: Soaking softens the nails and loosens debris under them.*
   - Clean the nails as required with an orange stick. ➤*Rationale: This removes excess debris that harbors microorganisms.*
   - Remove the foot from the basin and place it on the towel.
6. Dry the foot thoroughly and apply lotion or foot powder.
   - Blot the foot gently with the towel to dry it thoroughly, particularly between the toes. ➤*Rationale: Harsh rubbing can damage the skin. Thorough drying reduces the risk of infection.*
   - Apply lotion or lanolin cream to the foot but not between the toes. ➤*Rationale: This lubricates dry skin and keeps the area between the toes dry.*
     or
   - Apply a foot powder containing a nonirritating deodorant if the feet tend to perspire excessively. ➤*Rationale: Foot powders have greater absorbent properties than regular bath powders; some also contain menthol, which makes the feet feel cool.*
7. If agency policy permits, trim the nails of the first foot while the second foot is soaking.
   - See the discussion on nails in the following box for the appropriate method to trim nails. Note that in many agencies, toenail trimming requires a primary care provider's order or is contraindicated for clients with diabetes mellitus, toe infections, and peripheral vascular disease, unless performed by a podiatrist, general practice physician, or advanced practice provider such as a nurse practitioner.
8. Document any foot problems observed.
   - Foot care is not generally recorded unless problems are noted.
   - Record any signs of inflammation, infection, breaks in the skin, corns, troublesome calluses, bunions, and pressure areas. This is of particular importance for clients with peripheral vascular disease and diabetes.

## NAIL CARE

- Check the agency's policy regarding nail care. Often, podiatrists must be consulted for clients with diabetes.
- To provide nail care, the nurse needs a nail cutter or sharp scissors, a nail file, an orange stick to push back the cuticle, hand lotion or mineral oil to lubricate any dry tissue around the nails, and a basin of water to soak the nails if they are particularly thick or hard.
- One hand or foot is soaked, if needed, and dried. Then, the nail is cut or filed straight across beyond the end of the finger or toe. Avoid trimming or digging into nails at the lateral corners. ➤*Rationale: Trimming toes at the corners predisposes the client to ingrown toenails.*

- Clients who have diabetes or circulatory problems should have their nails filed rather than cut. Inadvertent injury to tissues can occur if scissors are used.
- After the initial cut or filing, the nail is filed to round the corners and the nurse cleans under the nail. Fingernails are trimmed straight across.
- Gently push back the cuticle, taking care not to injure it.
- The next finger or toe is cared for in the same manner.
- Any abnormalities, such as an infected cuticle or inflammation of the tissue around the nail, are recorded and reported.

## CLIENT TEACHING

Wash the feet daily, and dry them well, especially between the toes.

- When washing, inspect the skin of the feet for breaks or red or swollen areas. Use a mirror if needed to visualize all areas.
- To prevent burns, check the water temperature before immersing the feet.
- Cover the feet, except between the toes, with creams or lotions to moisten the skin. Lotion will also soften calluses. A lotion that reduces dryness effectively is a mixture of lanolin and mineral oil.
- To prevent or control an unpleasant odor due to excessive foot perspiration, wash the feet frequently and change socks and shoes at least daily. Special deodorant sprays or absorbent foot powders are also helpful.
- File the toenails rather than cutting them to avoid skin injury. File the nails straight across the ends of the toes. If the nails are too thick or misshapen to file, consult a podiatrist.
- Wear clean stockings or socks daily. Avoid socks with holes or darns that can cause pressure areas.
- Wear comfortable, well-fitting shoes that neither restrict the foot nor rub on any area; rubbing can cause corns and calluses. Check worn shoes for rough spots in the lining. Break in new shoes grad-

ually by increasing the wearing time 30 to 60 minutes each day.
- Avoid walking barefoot, because injury and infection may result. Wear slippers in public showers and in change areas to avoid contracting athlete's foot or other infections.
- Several times each day exercise the feet to promote circulation. Point the feet upward, point them downward, and move them in circles.
- Avoid wearing constricting garments such as knee-high elastic stockings, and avoid sitting with the legs crossed at the knees, which may decrease circulation.
- When the feet are cold, use extra blankets and wear warm socks rather than using heating pads or hot water bottles, which may cause burns. Test bathwater before stepping into it.
- Wash any cut on the foot thoroughly, apply a mild antiseptic, and notify the primary care provider.
- Avoid self-treatment for corns or calluses. Pumice stones and some callus and corn applications are injurious to the skin. Do not cut calluses or corns. Consult a podiatrist or primary care provider first.
- Notify the primary care provider if you notice abnormal sores or drainage, pain, or changes in temperature, color, and sensation of the foot.

| UNEXPECTED OUTCOMES | CRITICAL THINKING OPTIONS |
|---|---|
| Client has excessively dry, scaly skin, even after routine foot care. | • Apply alkali solutions as ordered, such as Epsom salts or bicarbonate of soda, to soften skin and remaining scales. Repeated soakings are usually necessary.<br>• Apply lanolin or shea butter moisturizer. |
| Client's feet are excessively moist. | • Give foot care twice a day.<br>• Use moisture-absorbing powder. |
| Client has large calluses on feet. | • After soaking, obtain an order to rub a pumice stone or an abrasive material on the callused skin due to possible scarring to the epidermis.<br>• For diabetic clients, obtain services of a podiatrist. |
| Client has mycotic nails. | • Report to physician so podiatrist can be consulted. |

# Skill 12.16   Providing Routine Eye Care

**Equipment**

Small basin
Water or normal saline solution
Washcloth or cotton balls
Clean gloves

**Preparation**

1. Determine client's eye care needs, and obtain physician's order if needed.
2. Explain necessity for and method of eye care to client. Discuss how client can assist you.
3. Collect necessary equipment.
4. Perform hand hygiene and don gloves.

**Procedure**

1. Use water or saline solution at room temperature.
2. Using the washcloth or cotton balls moistened in water or saline, gently wipe each eye from the inner to outer canthus. Use separate cotton ball or corner of washcloth for each eye. ➤*Rationale: To prevent cross-contamination from one eye to the other.*
3. If crusting is present, gently place a warm, wet compress over eye(s) until crusting is loosened.
4. Dispose of used supplies and return basin to appropriate area.
5. Remove and discard gloves.
6. Perform hand hygiene.

# Skill 12.17   Providing Eye Care for Comatose Client

**Equipment**

Water or normal saline solution
Washcloth, cotton balls, tissues
Sterile lubricant or eye preparations if ordered by the physician
Eye dropper or asepto bulb syringe
Eye pads or patches
Clean gloves

**Procedure**

1. Perform hand hygiene and don clean gloves.
2. Cleanse the eyes using a moistened washcloth or cotton balls moistened in water or saline. Gently wipe each eye from inner to outer canthus. Use separate cotton ball or corner of washcloth for each

eye. ➤*Rationale: Wiping from inner canthus to outer prevents particles and fluid from entering nasolacrimal duct.*
3. Use a dropper to instill a sterile ophthalmic solution (liquid tears, saline, methylcellulose) every 3 to 4 hours as ordered by physician. ➤*Rationale: To prevent corneal drying and ulceration.*
4. Keep client's eyes closed if blink reflex is absent. If eye pads or patches are used, explain their purpose to client's family. Do not tape eyes shut. ➤*Rationale: Corneal abrasions and drying occur when eyes lose blink reflex.*
5. Remove gloves and perform hand hygiene.
6. Remove patch and evaluate condition of eye every 4 hours.

# Skill 12.18 Providing Postoperative Socket Care

**Equipment**

Conformer (plastic or silicone)
Facial tissue
Washcloth
Baby shampoo
Cotton-tipped applicator sticks
Opticlude eye patch

**Procedure**

1. Explain procedure to client.
2. Provide privacy.
3. Place client in a semi to high Fowler's position
4. Instruct client to not rub his/her eyelids from nose toward side of face. This is a down and outward motion. ➤*Rationale: The conformer can become dislodged.*
5. Instruct client to close his/her eyes before wiping eye toward nose in a horizontal direction.
6. Wipe lids toward the nose with a facial tissue or warm washcloth to remove secretions and tears.

7. Clean dried secretions from lid margins with a cotton-tipped applicator soaked in baby shampoo.
8. Instruct client to take any medications that are prescribed. ➤*Rationale: Antibiotic ointment or drops can get into socket through holes in conformer.*
9. Apply Opticlude patch if desired. Usually, a few days post-op client does not need to wear a dressing, but may wish to keep socket covered.
10. Instruct client on how to replace conformer if it should fall out.
    a. Perform hand hygiene.
    b. Lift upper lid with thumb or forefinger of one hand.
    c. Slide conformer under upper lid.
    d. Hold conformer in place and pull down on lower lid. ➤*Rationale: This assists conformer to slip back into socket.*

> ## CLINICAL ALERT
>
> A conformer made of plastic or silicone is placed in socket following removal of an eye. The conformer is used to maintain orbit volume and to form lid pockets that will eventually hold artificial eye in place. The conformer is not to be removed, as it is used to maintain necessary space for artificial eye.

> ## CLINICAL ALERT
>
> Check with ophthalmologist regarding frequency of cleansing artificial eyes. Physicians are not in agreement with this procedure. Some recommend removing eye at regular intervals, while others recommend handling prosthesis only when necessary in order to prevent infection of the socket. Some clients are instructed to not remove the prosthesis between their yearly visit to the ocularist who cleans and polishes the eye. The yearly cleaning and polishing extends life of the prosthesis and returns luster to eye.

# Skill 12.19 Removing and Cleaning an Artificial Eye (Ocular Prosthesis)

**Equipment**

Suction cup (optional)
Water or hard contact lens solution
Mild soap (Ivory)
Facial tissue
Washcloth
Towel
Clean gloves
3% hydrogen peroxide, if needed
Small container
Baking soda

**Preparation**

1. If possible, encourage client or family member to care for client's artificial eye (prosthesis).
2. If assisting with artificial eye (prosthesis) care, assess client's usual method for cleansing.

3. Gather equipment.
4. Perform hand hygiene and don gloves.

**Procedure**

1. Place towel on overbed table. Remove prosthesis while working over table. ➤*Rationale: In case the prosthesis should come loose when using suction cup or you accidentally drop it.*
2. Hold the palm of your nondominant hand below prosthesis.
3. Remove prosthesis using your hand or a suction cup.
   a. When using your hands to remove prosthesis, depress lower lid and pull down and outward away from nose with index finger of dominant hand so bottom edge of prosthesis slides out of socket and into your nondominant hand.

b. When using a suction cup, lift upper eyelid with your index finger to keep eyelashes out of the way. Moisten tip of suction cup with water, squeeze suction cup and gently place tip on middle of prosthesis while releasing pressure to create suction. While pulling gently on suction cup and prosthesis, depress lower lid downward and pinch it inward slightly toward socket. Prosthesis should come out easily. Keep your nondominant hand below socket. ➤*Rationale: To prevent dropping of eye if it comes loose from suction cup.*

4. Wash prosthesis in water and a mild soap like Ivory liquid. A "hard contact" lens cleaning solution can be substituted for soap and water. ➤*Rationale: This removes most of surface accumulations and reduces irritation to eyelids.*

5. Moisten a facial tissue and rub prosthetic eye to remove surface secretions. Rinse thoroughly with water before reinserting eye.

6. Inspect tissue in and around eye for edema or drainage.

7. Wash eyelid and dry, wiping from inner to outer canthus. ➤*Rationale: Direction is more sanitary because it prevents contaminating tear duct.*

8. Moisten prosthesis, lift upper eyelid and slide into place.

9. Remove gloves and dispose of supplies.

10. Perform hand hygiene.

*for Heavy Mucus Deposit*

1. Perform hand hygiene and don gloves.

2. Explain that client will have eye removed for several hours to soak. ➤*Rationale: It takes several hours to remove heavy mucus deposits.* Instruct client on

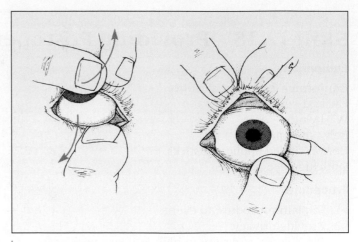

● Removal of eye prosthesis.

procedure so he/she can complete it at home if necessary.

3. Remove artificial eye using steps outlined in above skill.

4. Place artificial eye in container with 3% hydrogen peroxide. Use sufficient quantities of hydrogen peroxide to completely cover eye.

5. Soak prosthesis several hours or overnight in hydrogen peroxide solution if there is a heavy mucus deposit that is not removed with usual washing procedure.

6. Rinse prosthesis thoroughly and place in a container with ½ tsp. baking soda and cold water. Soak for 30 minutes. ➤*Rationale: This neutralizes hydrogen peroxide.*

7. Wipe surface of prosthesis with a damp facial tissue to remove any residual protein deposits.

8. Rinse well using water or soft contact lens saline solution.

9. Reinsert eye into socket.

10. Remove gloves and perform hand hygiene.

## CLINICAL ALERT

Do not clean prosthesis with abrasives or sterilizing agents, because they will attack the acrylic that encompasses artificial eye.

# Skill 12.20   Removing and Cleaning Contact Lenses

### Equipment

Towel
Contact lens container
Commercially prepared cleaning solution
Commercially prepared disinfecting solution
Commercially prepared rinsing and storing solution
Enzymatic agent (protein remover)
Clean gloves

### Procedure

1. Place client in semi-Fowler's position, and place a towel under the client's chin.

2. Perform hand hygiene and don gloves.

3. Place the tip of your thumb across the lower lid below its margin.

4. Place the tip of the forefinger of the same hand on the upper lid above its margin.

5. Spread eyelids apart as wide as possible and locate outer edges of soft lens which should appear as a rim around outer edge of iris.
6. Place thumb and forefinger directly on soft lens.
7. Gently remove soft lens from surface of eyeball by squeezing lens between thumb and fingertip. To remove rigid lens, place thumb on lower eyelid and index finger on upper lid. Press gently against eyeball to release suction; lens is released as eyelids meet lens edge. Catch lens in your hand. ➤*Rationale: Cornea is avascular and use of contact lenses interrupts flow of oxygen into cornea.* Removing lenses for a period of time allows oxygen to reach cornea and thus prevent corneal complications.
8. Release eyelids.
9. Place lens in palm of hand or place disposable lenses in trash. Disposable lenses are not to be cleaned or reused. There is not a lens cleaner available for these lenses.
10. Place 2–3 drops of cleaning solution on lens.
11. Clean lens thoroughly by rubbing between fingertip and palm of hand of 20–30 seconds.
12. Rinse lens thoroughly with sterile saline solution or rinsing solution. Use only lens cleaning system recommended by opthalmologist. Do not interchange cleaning solution systems.
13. Place lens in disinfecting solution according to physician directions. Time varies from hours to one full day. ➤*Rationale: This destroys microorganisms on lenses.*
14. Rinse lens thoroughly with rinsing solution.
15. Repeat procedure on second lens.
16. Use enzyme tablet or solution according to physician orders, usually weekly. ➤*Rationale: This removes stubborn protein and lipids.*

17. Clean lens container daily and leave open to dry. Replace as directed by physician, either weekly or monthly.
18. Remove gloves and perform hand hygiene.

*Note:* A suction sup can be placed gently against lens for easy removal of lens. Squeeze suction cup with dominant hand, place on lens, open finger slightly to create suction between lens and cup. Rock lens gently to remove it.

---

### CLIENT TEACHING

Instruct the client in the following safety issues:

- Notify physician immediately if eyes are red, not comfortable, or you can't see clearly.
- Use only rinsing solution, not saliva, to wet lenses.
- Use only commercially prepared saline solution or rinsing solution to cleanse lenses.
- Do not interchange types of lens cleaning systems.
- Maintain lens-care regimen prescribed by physician.
- Put on makeup before inserting lens.
- Use appropriate type of lenses for their intended use. Do not use daily-wear lenses at night or disposable lenses more than once.
- Do not allow soft lenses to dry out.
- Contact lens wearers should be instructed to carry appropriate identification on type and care for specific lens he/she wears.

---

# Skill 12.21   Removing, Cleaning, and Inserting a Hearing Aid

### Delegation

A nurse can delegate the task of caring for a hearing aid to the UAP. It is important, however, for the nurse to first determine that the UAP knows the correct way to care for a hearing aid. Inform the UAP to report the presence of ear inflammation, discomfort, excess wax, or drainage to the RN.

### Equipment

Client's hearing aid
Soap, water, and towels or a damp cloth
Pipe cleaner or toothpick (optional)
New battery (if needed)

### Procedure

1. Prior to performing the procedure, introduce self and verify the client's identity using agency protocol. Explain to the client what you are going to do, why it is necessary, and how he or she can participate.
2. Perform hand hygiene and observe other appropriate infection control procedures.
3. Provide for client privacy by drawing the curtains around the bed or closing the door to the room. Some agencies provide signs indicating the need for privacy. ➤*Rationale: Hygiene is a personal matter.*

4. Remove the hearing aid.
   - Turn the hearing aid off and lower the volume. The on/off switch may be labeled "O" (off), "M" (microphone), "T" (telephone), or "TM" (telephone/microphone). ➤*Rationale: The batteries continue to run if the hearing aid is not turned off.*
   - Remove the earmold by rotating it slightly forward and pulling it outward.
   - If the hearing aid is not to be used for several days, remove the battery. ➤*Rationale: Removal prevents corrosion of the hearing aid from battery leakage.*
   - Store the hearing aid in a safe place and label with client's name. Avoid exposure to heat and moisture. ➤*Rationale: Proper storage prevents loss or damage.*

5. Clean the earmold.
   - Detach the earmold if possible. Disconnect the earmold from the receiver of a body hearing aid or from the hearing aid case of behind-the-ear and eyeglass hearing aids where the tubing meets the hook of the case. Do not remove the earmold if it is glued or secured by a small metal ring. ➤*Rationale: Removal facilitates cleaning and prevents inadvertent damage to the other parts.*
   - If the earmold is detachable, soak it in a mild soapy solution. Rinse and dry it well. Do not use isopropyl alcohol. ➤*Rationale: Alcohol can damage the hearing aid.*
   - If the earmold is not detachable or is for an in-the-ear aid, wipe the earmold with a damp cloth.
   - Check that the earmold opening is patent. Blow any excess moisture through the opening or remove debris (e.g., earwax) with a pipe cleaner or toothpick.
   - Reattach the earmold if it was detached from the rest of the hearing aid.

6. Insert the hearing aid.
   - Determine from the client if the earmold is for the left or the right ear.
   - Check that the battery is inserted in the hearing aid. Turn off the hearing aid, and make sure the volume is turned all the way down. ➤*Rationale: A volume that is too loud is distressing.*
   - Inspect the earmold to identify the ear canal portion. Some earmolds are fitted for only the ear canal and concha; others are fitted for all the contours of the ear. The canal portion, common to all, can be used as a guide for correct insertion.
   - Line up the parts of the earmold with the corresponding parts of the client's ear.
   - Rotate the earmold slightly forward, and insert the ear canal portion.
   - Gently press the earmold into the ear while rotating it backward.
   - Check that the earmold fits snugly by asking the client if it feels secure and comfortable.
   - Adjust the other components of a behind-the-ear or body hearing aid.
   - Turn the hearing aid on, and adjust the volume according to the client's needs.

7. Correct problems associated with improper functioning.
   - If the sound is weak or there is no sound:
     a. Ensure that the volume is turned high enough.
     b. Ensure that the earmold opening is not clogged.
     c. Check the battery by turning the hearing aid on, turning up the volume, cupping your hand over the earmold, and listening. A constant whistling sound indicates the battery is functioning. If necessary, replace the battery. Be sure that the negative (–) and positive (+) signs on the battery match those where indicated on the hearing aid.
     d. Ensure that the ear canal is not blocked with wax, which can obstruct sound waves.
   - If the client reports a whistling sound or squeal after insertion:
     a. Turn the volume down.
     b. Ensure that the earmold is properly attached to the receiver.
     c. Reinsert the earmold.
   - Document pertinent data.
   - The removal and the insertion of a hearing aid are not normally recorded.
   - Report and record any problems the client has with the hearing aid.

---

### SETTING OF CARE

- People who need a hearing aid may not wear one because they view the hearing aid as a stigma of old age.

- It is important for the client who has just purchased a hearing aid to know that it often takes weeks or even months to adjust to the hearing aid. At first, the sounds will seem shrill as they start hearing high-frequency sounds that had been forgotten. Remind them that it is a hearing aid, not a hearing cure. Encourage them to not give up.

- The client needs to adjust to the hearing aid gradually by increasing the amount of time each day until the aid can be worn for a full day (Anderson, 1998).

- Encourage clients to purchase their hearing aids from a company that has a minimum warranty of a 30-day return policy.

- Emphasize the importance of maintaining the hearing aid, that is, having it cleaned and checked regularly.

# Skill 12.22   Providing Perineal-Genital Care

## EXPECTED OUTCOMES
- Perineal care has been comfortably and effectively provided.
- Perineal area is clean, odor-free, and without irritation or discharge.
- Skin remains intact following perineal care.

## Delegation

Perineal-genital care can be delegated to UAP; however, if the client has recently had perineal, rectal, or genital surgery, the nurse needs to assess if it is appropriate for the UAP to perform perineal-genital care.

## Equipment

*Perineal-Genital Care Provided in Conjunction with the Bed Bath*

- Bath towel
- Bath blanket
- Clean gloves
- Bath basin with warm water at 43° to 46°C (110° to 115°F)
- Soap
- Washcloth

*Special Perineal-Genital Care*

- Bath towel
- Bath blanket
- Clean gloves
- Solution bottle, pitcher, or container filled with warm water or a prescribed solution
- Bedpan to receive rinse water
- Perineal pad

## Preparation

- Determine whether the client is experiencing any discomfort in the perineal-genital area.
- Obtain and prepare the necessary equipment and supplies.

## Procedure

1. Prior to performing the procedure, introduce self and verify the client's identity using agency protocol. Explain to the client what you are going to do, why it is necessary, and how he or she can participate, being particularly sensitive to any embarrassment felt by the client.
2. Perform hand hygiene and observe other appropriate infection control procedures (e.g., clean gloves).

3. Provide for client privacy by drawing the curtains around the bed or closing the door to the room. Some agencies provide signs indicating the need for privacy. ➤*Rationale: Hygiene is a personal matter.*
4. Prepare the client:
   - Fold the top bed linen to the foot of the bed and fold the gown up to expose the genital area.
   - Place a bath towel under the client's hips. ➤*Rationale: The bath towel prevents the bed from becoming soiled.*
5. Position and drape the client and clean the upper inner thighs.

### For Female Clients

- Position the female in a back-lying position with the knees flexed and spread well apart.
- Cover her body and legs with the bath blanket positioned so a corner is at her head, the opposite corner at her feet, and the other two on the sides. Drape the legs by tucking the bottom corners of the bath blanket under and then over the inner sides of the legs. ➤*Rationale: Minimum exposure lessens embarrassment and helps to provide warmth.* Bring the middle portion of the base of the blanket up and then over the pubic area.
- Apply gloves. Wash and dry the upper inner thighs.

### For Male Clients

- Position the male client in a supine position with knees slightly flexed and hips slightly externally rotated.
- Apply gloves. Wash and dry the upper inner thighs.
6. Inspect the perineal area.
   - Note particular areas of inflammation, excoriation, or swelling, especially between the labia in females and the scrotal folds in males.
   - Also note excessive discharge or secretions from the orifices and the presence of odors.
7. Wash and dry the perineal-genital area.

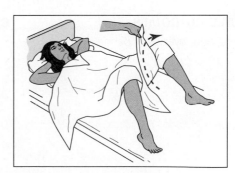

● Draping the client for perineal-genital care.

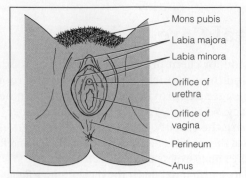

● Female genitals.

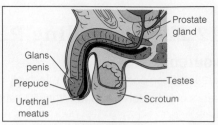

● Male genitals.

### For Female Clients

- Clean the labia majora. Then spread the labia to wash the folds between the labia majora and the labia minora. ➤*Rationale: Secretions that tend to collect around the labia minora facilitate bacterial growth.*

- Use separate quarters of the washcloth for each stroke, and wipe from the pubis to the rectum. For menstruating women and clients with indwelling catheters, use clean wipes. Use a clean wipe for each stroke. ➤*Rationale: Using separate quarters of the washcloth or new wipes prevents the transmission of microorganisms from one area to the other. Wipe from the area of least contamination (the pubis) to that of greatest (the rectum).*

- Rinse the area well. You may place the client on a bedpan and use a Peri-Wash or a solution bottle to pour warm water over the area. Dry the perineum thoroughly, paying particular attention to the folds between the labia. ➤*Rationale: Moisture supports the growth of many microorganisms.*

### For Male Clients

- Wash and dry the penis, using firm strokes.

- If the client is uncircumcised, retract the prepuce (foreskin) to expose the glans penis (the tip of the penis) for cleaning. Replace the foreskin after cleaning the glans penis. ➤*Rationale: Retracting the foreskin is neces-*

sary to remove the smegma (thick, cheesy secretion) that collects under the foreskin and facilitates bacterial growth. Replacing the foreskin prevents constriction of the penis, which may cause edema.

- Wash and dry the scrotum. The posterior folds of the scrotum may need to be cleaned when the buttocks are cleaned (see step 9). ➤*Rationale: The scrotum tends to be more soiled than the penis because of its proximity to the rectum; thus it is usually cleaned after the penis.*

8. Inspect perineal orifices for intactness.
   - Inspect particularly around the urethra in clients with indwelling catheters. ➤*Rationale: A catheter may cause excoriation around the urethra.*

9. Clean between the buttocks.
   - Assist the client to turn onto the side facing away from you.
   - Pay particular attention to the anal area and posterior folds of the scrotum in males. Clean the anus with toilet tissue before washing it, if necessary.
   - Dry the area well.
   - For post-delivery or menstruating females, apply a perineal pad as needed from front to back. ➤*Rationale: This prevents contamination of the vagina and urethra from the anal area.*

10. Remove and discard gloves. Perform hand hygiene.

11. Document any unusual findings such as redness, excoriation, skin breakdown, discharge or drainage, and any localized areas of tenderness.

---

| **UNEXPECTED OUTCOMES** | **CRITICAL THINKING OPTIONS** |
|---|---|
| Client has foul odor even after perineal care. | • Obtain order for sitz bath.<br>• Request order for medicated solution.<br>• Request culture of discharge so the appropriate treatment can be instituted. |
| Client develops urinary tract infection. | • Instruct client on proper technique for perineal care.<br>• Instruct female clients to wash from anterior to posterior aspects of perineum, using different sections of cloth for each wipe.<br>• Instruct male clients to wash from urethral opening down the shaft of the penis. |

# Skill 12.23   Assisting an Adult to Eat

## EXPECTED OUTCOMES

- Diet meets nutritional requirements and is acceptable to client's taste and cultural orientation.
- Visually impaired client is able to self-feed.
- Dysphagic client is able to eat using adaptations to prevent aspiration.

## Delegation

Assisting or feeding a client is often delegated to UAP. It is, however, the responsibility of the nurse to assess the client's ability to eat and to identify actual or potential risk factors that may impact the client's nutritional status. The nurse must instruct the UAP about strategies that promote the client's nutritional health as well as the importance of the UAP reporting any unusual or different client behaviors to the nurse.

## Equipment

Meal tray with the correct food and fluids
Extra napkin or small towel
Straw, special drinking cup, weighted glass, or other adaptive
feeding aid as required

## Preparation

Prepare the client and overbed table.

- Assist the client to the bathroom or onto a bedpan or commode if the client needs to urinate.
- Offer the client assistance in washing the hands prior to a meal. If the client has problems with oral hygiene, brushing the teeth or using a mouthwash can improve the taste in the mouth and hence the appetite.
- Clear the overbed table so that there is space for the tray. If the client must remain in a lying position in bed, arrange the overbed table close to the bedside so that the client can see the food.

## Procedure

1. Prior to performing the procedure, introduce self and verify the client's identity using agency protocol. Explain to the client what you are going to do, why it is necessary, and how he or she can participate.
2. Perform hand hygiene and observe other appropriate infection control procedures.
3. Provide for client privacy.
4. Position the client and yourself appropriately.
    - Assist the client to a comfortable position for eating. Most people sit during a meal; if it is permitted, assist the client to sit in bed or in a chair.
    - If the client is unable to sit, assist the client to a lateral position. ➤*Rationale: People will swallow more easily in these positions than in a back-lying position.*
    - If the client requires assistance with feeding, assume a sitting position, if possible, beside the client. ➤*Rationale: This conveys a more relaxed presence and encourages the client to eat an adequate meal.*

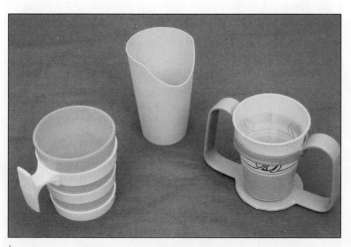

● Left to right: glass holder, cup with hole for nose, two-handled cup holder.

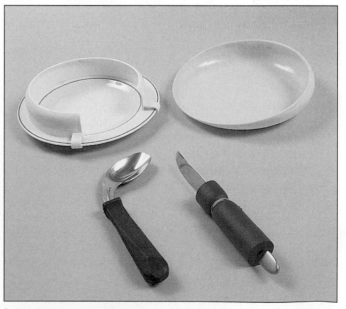

● Dinner plate with guard attached and lipped plate facilitates scooping; wide-handled spoon and knife facilitate grip.

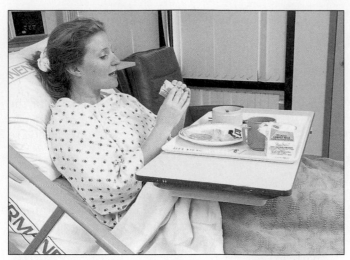

● A supported sitting position contributes to a client's comfort while eating.

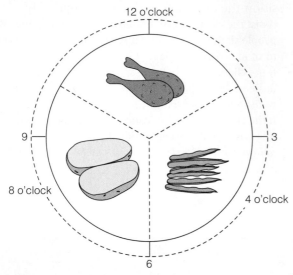

● For a client who is visually impaired, the nurse can use the clock system to describe the location of food on the plate.

5. Assist the client as required.
   • Check tray for the client's name, the type of diet, and completeness. If the diet does not seem to be correct, check it against the client's chart. Do *not* leave an incorrect diet for a client to eat.
   • Encourage the client to eat independently, assisting as needed. Do not take over the feeding process. ➤*Rationale: Participation by the client enhances feelings of independence.*
   • Remove the food covers, butter the bread, pour the drink, and cut the meat, if needed.
   • For a client with a visual impairment, identify the placement of the food as you would describe the time on a clock. For instance, say "The potatoes are at 8 o'clock, the chicken at 12 o'clock, and the green beans at 4 o'clock."

• If the client needs assistance with feeding:
   a. Ask in which order the client desires to eat the food.
   b. Use normal utensils whenever possible. ➤*Rationale: Using ordinary utensils enhances self-esteem.*
   c. If the client cannot see, tell which food you are giving.
   d. Warn the client if the food is hot or cold.
   e. Allow ample time for the client to chew and swallow the food before offering more.
   f. Provide fluids as requested or, if the client is unable to ask, offer fluids after every three or four mouthfuls of solid food.
   g. Use a straw or special drinking cup for fluids that would spill from normal containers.
   h. Make the time a pleasant one, choosing topics of conversation that are of interest to the client, if the person wants to talk.

6. After the meal, ensure client comfort.
   • Assist the client to clean the mouth and hands.
   • Reposition the client.
   • Replace the food covers and remove the food tray from the bedside.

7. Document all relevant information.
   • Note how much and what the client has eaten and the amount of fluid taken.
   • Record fluid intake and calorie count as required.
   • If the client is on a special diet or is having problems eating, record the amount of food eaten and any pain, fatigue, or nausea experienced.
   • If the client is not eating, notify the nurse in charge so that the diet can be changed or other nursing measures can be taken (e.g., rescheduling the meals, providing small, more frequent meals, or obtaining special self-feeding aids).

## DEVELOPMENTAL CONSIDERATIONS

### Elders

• Offer fluids frequently to prevent dry mouth. Initially avoid dry foods such as crackers and sticky foods such as bananas. ➤*Rationale: Saliva production decreases with age.*

• Allow the older client time to eat and offer to rewarm the food if needed. ➤*Rationale: Hand tremors and arthritic joint changes may slow the eating process for older clients.*

• Observe the dysphagia (difficulty swallowing) and adapt the older client's diet accordingly. ➤*Rationale: Esophageal nerve degeneration, which often occurs with aging, can affect the ability to swallow.*

• Older clients may need extra seasoning on food. ➤*Rationale: Aging decreases the ability to taste, especially sweet and salty foods.*

---

**SETTING OF CARE**

- Assess the home for adequate facilities to prepare and store food such as a working refrigerator and stove. Assess the client's and caregiver's ability to obtain food and prepare meals.
- Evaluate problems that can interfere with eating such as ill-fitting dentures, sore gums, constipation, diarrhea, or a special diet.

- Instruct the caregiver about the importance of regular, nutritious meals and allowing the client to remain independent when possible.
- Provide written guidelines for the client's diet and any special feeding techniques.

---

# Skill 12.24  Serving a Food Tray

## Equipment

Diet slip completed
Diet tray
Over-bed table
Utensils
Protective covering, e.g., towel

## Preparation

1. Check client's chart for physician's diet order.
2. Obtain dietary consult, if necessary, to meet client's needs.
3. Elicit food preferences of the client.
4. Check all diet trays before serving to ensure the diet provided is the one ordered.
5. Ensure that hot food is hot and cold food is cold.
6. Keep food trays attractive. Avoid spilling liquids on tray.
7. Assist client to empty bladder (if needed) and perform hand hygiene.
8. Remove unpleasant objects from area.

## Procedure

1. Identify client by checking identaband and having client state name and birth date.
2. Perform hand hygiene and assist client to do so.
3. Assist client to sit in a chair, or elevate the head of the bed to 90 degrees.
4. Place protective covering over client's chest.
5. Place food tray on over-bed table and adjust the table so client can see the food.
6. Assist client as needed (cut meat, open containers).
7. Leave call light in client's reach and check on client periodically.
8. Reposition tray table at bedside when meal is completed.
9. Assist client with hand and oral hygiene if desired.
10. Position client for comfort.
11. Note percentage and type of food eaten.
12. Remove food tray from room.
13. Document percentage and type of food eaten and, if indicated, amount of liquid intake on I&O record.
14. Perform hand hygiene.

---

**CLINICAL ALERT**

Clients sensitive to latex have potential for serious allergic reactions to some plant proteins. Cross-reactivity to latex has been shown with foods such as avocado, banana, papaya, chestnuts, kiwi, potatoes, and tomatoes. Clients with allergy to these foods may have latex allergy and vice versa.

---

# Skill 12.25  Assisting the Dysphagic Client to Eat

## Equipment

Provision for oral care and hand hygiene
Towel
Penlight to inspect oral cavity
Oral suction catheter connected to suction source

## Preparation

1. Note specific instructions for feeding technique (diet and positioning) prescribed by speech or swallowing specialist; for example, cornstarch, Thickit, or rice cereal to thicken food, as prescribed.

►*Rationale: Clients with swallowing problems find it easier to swallow thickened liquids.*

2. Check if client is receiving both oral and enteral feeding; stop the enteral solution about 1 hour before oral feeding.
3. Eliminate environmental distractors such as television, radio.
4. Ensure that temperature of food is appropriate.

**Procedure**

1. Wash your hands.
2. Check client's identaband and allergy bracelet and have client state name and birth date.
3. Provide client privacy.
4. Maintain bed in LOW position.
5. Assist client to sit upright, hips flexed slightly greater than 90 degrees with shoulders and face slightly forward, and chin parallel to the floor or slightly tucked. ►*Rationale: Gravity assists proper bolus movement to the stomach.*
6. Assist client to perform hand hygiene before eating.
7. Place towel over client's chest.
8. Place tray on over-bed table and towel under plate. ►*Rationale: This stabilizes plate while feeding.*
9. Suction oral secretions before feeding, if necessary.
10. Sit at client's side, or sit facing client.
11. Encourage self-feeding.
12. Instruct client to take (or offer) small portions of food at first (0.5 to 1 tsp at a time), bites manageable in size but large enough to require chewing.
13. Instruct client to eat food first, without accompanying liquid, reserving all liquid intake until after finishing food. ►*Rationale: Using liquids to wash down boluses of food pushes the food down too rapidly.*
14. Instruct client to perform an exaggerated sucking motion at the beginning of each swallow with chin tucked slightly. ►*Rationale: Decreases risk of aspiration.*

15. Allow client to concentrate on swallowing without distractions such as conversation or television. ►*Rationale: For the dysphagic client, swallowing takes concentration; talking increases risk for aspiration.*
16. Make sure client is swallowing every mouthful. ►*Rationale: Buildup may occur on weak side of mouth or pharynx.*
17. Observe client closely for evidence of aspiration (e.g., cough), and suction oropharynx if indicated.
18. Help with feeding only if client shows signs of weakness, fatigue.
19. Provide positive reinforcement for accomplishment.
20. Assist with oral care and hand hygiene following meal.
21. Remove food tray and raise side rails as indicated.
22. Place call bell in reach.
23. Record percentage of food eaten and amount of liquid intake (if indicated).
24. Maintain client's sitting position for 30 minutes after eating.
25. Carefully observe client with impaired communication for 30 minutes after the first few servings.

*Note:* Prescribed position is different for specific forms of dysphagia. Some types are dysphagia necessitate client positioning to one side, or with head rotated toward the stronger or weaker side, or even side-lying. Instructions should be placed in client's record, care plan, and posted at client's head of bed.

---

## CLINICAL ALERT

The use of a straw increases risk of aspiration because the dysphagic client has less control over the amount of fluid intake. Similarly, the dysphagic client should not be fed with a syringe.

---

| UNEXPECTED OUTCOMES | CRITICAL THINKING OPTIONS |
|---|---|
| Client is nauseated and vomits. | • Withhold food if client is nauseated or vomiting.<br>• Provide antiemetic or client's preferred comfort measures (cold cloth to throat, soda drink)<br>• Identify potential source for nausea: specific foods or odors, experience of pain, side effects of medication (e.g., morphine sulfate), or positional changes. |
| Visually impaired client only eats food on one half of food tray. | • Client may have homonymous hemianopia due to stroke and is unable to see the half of the tray on client's paralyzed side.<br>• Move food tray so that ignored side is within client's restricted range of vision (move tray leftward if client has had a left VCA and right side of tray has been ignored).<br>• Encourage client to turn head so that client's visual field includes the half of tray with food that has not been seen or eaten. |

**UNEXPECTED OUTCOMES (cont.)**

Client has signs of aspirating food (coughing, hoarseness, noisy breathing).

**CRITICAL THINKING OPTIONS (cont.)**

- Request speech pathologist consult for swallow evaluation.
- Ensure that assistive personnel are following individualized feeding instructions/precautions (e.g., client positioning, use of thickening agents, and avoiding use of straws).
- Remind client not to talk while eating and to concentrate on swallowing.

# Skill 12.26 Preparing for Medication Administration

## EXPECTED OUTCOMES

- Rationale for medication administration is clear.
- Client's MAR matches physician's orders.
- Dosage calculations are accurate.
- Medication sign out sheet matches remaining stock.
- Medication is administered according to the "six rights."
- Client takes medication orally without difficulty.
- Client experiences intended therapeutic drug effect.
- Topical medication has intended effect.
- Client self-administers eye medication according to instructions.
- Ear canal irrigation removes cerumen.
- Angina is relieved with ONE dose of sublingual nitroglycerin.
- Chest pain is relieved due to rapid systemic response to sublingual medication administration.
- Desired local effect of medication is achieved without undesired side effects.
- Suppository has desired effects/results.
- Injection is administered without complications.
- Injection is as painless as possible.
- Medication therapeutic effect is achieved.

## Equipment

Reference resource (e.g., PDR, pharmacology textbook, drug handbook)
Calculator (if indicated)
Medication administration record sheet (MAR)
Client's chart

## Procedure

1. Check physician's orders and client's MAR for medications client is to receive (drug, dosage, route of administration, time intervals).
2. Identify any unfamiliar drugs.
3. Research unfamiliar drugs using appropriate reference.
   a. Generic and trade name
   b. Drug classification and major uses
   c. Pharmacologic actions

d. Safe dosage, route, and time of administration
e. Side effects; adverse reactions
f. Nursing implications
g. Complete client teaching as needed

4. Review client's record for allergies, lab data, any factor (e.g., NPO status, planned procedures) that contraindicates administration of ordered medications.
5. Check client's daily MAR with previous day's MAR every 24 hours for each drug's dosage, route, and time to be given. ➤*Rationale: Pharmacy produces each daily MAR sheet.* Any new medications, discontinued medication, or altered dosage must be identified and verified with the physician's orders.
6. Validate carefully that MAR is consistent with physician's most recent order for each medication. ➤*Rationale: Some medication dosages are adjusted on a daily basis.* Errors in transmission of intentions may occur between physician, pharmacy, and client's MAR.
7. Perform hand hygiene.
8. Take medication to client's room.
9. Open medication cart; take out client's medication drawer.
10. Starting at the top of the medication record check each medication in order against the medication packages in the drawer. Ensure that all doses for your shift are there. Pharmacy restocks cart every 24 hours. ➤*Rationale: If a dose is missing, or too many doses remain, check medication record for possible error in administration.*
11. Retrieve medication to be given and compare drug label with MAR. ➤*Rationale: This is a safety check to ensure the right medication is given.*

### CLINICAL ALERT

Individual drugs are designed to be administered by specific route—be sure to check drug labels for appropriate route of administration.

12. Inspect label to ensure that medication is indicated for ordered route of administration. ➤*Rationale: Different preparations of the same medication are used for different routes of administration.*
13. Determine if any calculation is necessary to prepare the correct dosage.
14. Calculate client's dosage based on strength of medication, if indicated. Have another nurse double check your calculation.
15. Prepare medication as indicated for nonparenteral or parenteral route, checking drug label before, during, and after preparation.

## EVIDENCE-BASED NURSING PRACTICE

### Medication Administeration Errors

In a study involving 400 staff nurses, 30% of full time staff reported making at least one error in a 28-day period and another 33% reported a near error. The majority of errors or near errors involved medication administration. Of these events, 25% involved giving the wrong dose, with nurses citing interruptions and distractions during the preparation.

*Source:* Professional Update (2005). *RN, 68(3),* 20.

## LEGAL ALERT

**Transcription Error and Reconciliation Failure (*Robert Ferguson v. Baptist Health System, Inc.,* 2005)**

Robert Ferguson brought medical malpractice action against Baptist after experiencing drug toxicity due to a medication (Dilantin) transcription error on the part of the pharmacist and failure on the part of the nurse to conduct reconciliation between the MAR entry and the doctor's order. The physician's order was for Dilantin, 300 milligrams "po QHS." The MAR was generated by pharmacy for Dilantin, 300 milligrams, "t.i.d." The agency policy dictated that any time a new medication order was entered, the nurse initially undertaking to administer the medication was responsible for comparing the MAR to the actual order to "reconcile" the two. In this case, the pharmacy error was not detected by the reconciliation process. Subsequent erroneous doses were administered, but none of the nurses administering the Dilantin detected the error "due to the fact that there were no additional checks, balances, or other safeguards in place to prevent the repetition of the error." No one ever checked the original physician's order "despite the unusually large amount of Dilantin being administered." None of the nurses suspected that Ferguson's symptoms represented Dilantin toxicity. Ferguson was awarded compensatory damages and punitive damages.

---

# Skill 12.27  Converting Dosage Systems

### Procedure

1. To make conversions from the metric to apothecaries' or household systems, it is necessary to memorize or refer to equivalency tables.
2. To convert milligrams to grains, use the following formula:

$$\frac{1 \text{ gr}}{\text{milligrams per grain}} = \frac{\text{Dose desired}}{\text{Dose on hand}}$$

$$\frac{1}{60} = \frac{X}{180}$$

$$60X = 180$$

$$X = 3 \text{ gr}$$

3. You may also use ratio and proportion to calculate dosage:

$$1\text{gr}:60 \text{ mg} :: X \text{ gr}:180 \text{ mg}$$
$$60X = 180$$
$$X = 3 \text{ gr}$$

4. To convert milligrams to milliliters, you can set up a direct proportion and, following the algebraic principle, cross multiply.

# Skill 12.28  Calculating Dosages

## Equipment

Orders for dosage of medication needed
Dosage of medication on hand

## Procedure

1. To calculate oral dosages, use the following formula. (D and H must be in same unit of measure.)

$$\frac{D}{H} = X$$

   where D = dose desired; H = dose on hand; and X = dose to be administered.
   *Example:* Give 500 mg of ampicillin sodium when the dose on hand is in capsules containing 250 mg.

2. To calculate dose when in liquid form, use the following formula

$$\frac{D}{H} \times Q - X$$

   where D = dose desired; H = dose on hand; Q = quantity; and X = amount to be administered
   *Example:* Give 375 mg of ampicillin when it is supplied as 250 mg/5 mL.

$$\frac{375 \text{ mg}}{250 \text{ mg}} \times 5$$
$$1.5 \times 5 = 7.5 \text{ mL}$$

3. To calculate parenteral dosages, use the following formula:

$$\frac{D}{H} \times Q = X$$

   *Example:* Give client 40 mg gentamicin C complex sulfate. On hand is a multidose vial with a strength of 80 mg/2 mL.

$$\frac{40}{80} \times 2 = 1 \text{ mL}$$

4. To calculate dosages for infants and children using BSA (body surface area):

$$\frac{BSA}{1.7} \times \text{adult dose} = \text{pediatric dose}$$

*Note:* See *Pediatric Nursing*, 3rd ed., by Jane Ball and Ruth Bindler, 2003, Prentice Hall, for complete description of method to determine body surface area.

5. To calculate dosages for infants and children using Clark's weight rule:

$$\text{Child's dose} = \frac{\text{Child's wt. in lbs.}}{150} \times \text{Adult dose}$$

6. Check your calculations before drawing up the medications.

# Skill 12.29  Using the Narcotic Control System

## Equipment

Medication record sheet
Narcotic sign-out sheet
Medication

## Procedure

### For Client Administration

1. Check client's medication sheet for narcotic order.
2. Check dose and time last narcotic was administered.
3. Unlock and open narcotic drawer, and find appropriate narcotic container.
4. Count the number of pills, ampules, or prefilled cartridges in container.
5. Check the narcotic sign-out sheet, and check that the number of narcotics in drawer matches the number on specific narcotic sign-out sheet.
   ➤*Rationale: Laws on controlled substances require careful monitoring of narcotics.*

6. Correct any discrepancy before proceeding with narcotic administration.
7. Sign out for the narcotic on the narcotic sheet after taking narcotic out of drawer.
8. Lock drawer after dispensing medication.
9. Administer medication according to specific oral or parenteral procedure.
10. Document narcotic on client's medication record according to usual procedure. Include client's pain rating (e.g., 8/10) and sedation level before and after narcotic administration according to agency policy.

## CLINICAL ALERT

A licensed person must sign for each narcotic dispensed from the medication drawer.

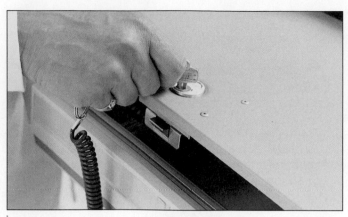

● Lock narcotic drawer after removing medication. Keep key with you at all times.

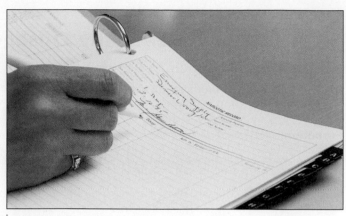

● Sign on specific narcotic sign-out sheet after taking narcotic out of drawer.

### For Unit Narcotic Stock

11. Check narcotic counts every 8 hours. One off-going and one on-coming licensed nurse must check the narcotics together. The number on each narcotic sign-out sheet must match the number of that particular narcotic remaining in the drawer.

12. Explore any discrepancy in stock and recorded dispensed narcotic numbers. ➤*Rationale: Counts must balance.* It is the nurse's responsibility to account for all controlled substances dispensed.

13. Licensed nurses cosign the narcotic record if the count is accurate.

### CLINICAL ALERT

If the narcotic depresses breathing, note client's level of sedation and respiratory rate before administering, and document assessment according to agency policy.

---

## LEGAL ALERT

### McMunn v. Mount Carmel Health et al, 1998

Plaintiff was awarded $433,415.00 for wrongful death of William Muncey, age 39, resulting from improper administration of morphine and failure to monitor and guard the client from adverse effects of the drugs he received, those known to cause respiratory depression. The client presented to Mount Carmel ED at 1635 with severe pain due to kidney stones. He received 5 mg of morphine IV at 1653, at 1700, and again at 1740. His respiratory rate was 24 and $SpO_2$ was 92%.

He then received additional 5 mg of intravenous morphine at 1805 and 1820, whereupon his $SpO_2$ dropped to 86%. The client was placed on oxygen therapy and by 1935 his $SpO_2$ had increased to 94%.

At 2015 he was admitted as an inpatient. His vital signs were taken at that time, but not again for the evening shift. The nurse had not been advised that the client's $O_2$ saturation had dropped while he was in the ED. At 2215, the nurse administered 15 mg of morphine sulfate and 50 mg Phenergan by injection. At 2300 it was documented that the client was sleeping, but no vital signs were taken.

At 0105, the nurse was notified that Mr. Muncey was unresponsive and had no pulse or respirations. A "Code Blue" was called, Narcan was given, but the client died. At autopsy, spinal fluid and blood levels of morphine were supportive of death from a respiratory depressant effect of morphine, levels unusually high explained by the combination of depressant drugs he had received.

Three areas of nursing care were found to fall below the accepted standard: coordination and communication of assessment and care, monitoring of a client receiving narcotics, and documentation of assessments for a client receiving narcotics.

# Skill 12.30   Using an Automated Dispensing System

## Equipment

Automated dispensing system (e.g., PYXIS)
Client's medication record

## Preparation

1. Touch the screen to activate the system.
2. Enter your ID code number and user password or scanned fingerprint. ➤*Rationale: This process controls access to medications.*
3. From the main menu, select command on medication management station (e.g., remove, waste, return).
4. Select client's room number, medication and name and additional identifiers (e.g., birthdate, hospital number).
5. Touch/select medication desired from client's displayed list of ordered medications.
6. Validate that client's medication record matches selected medication and dose on monitor screen.
7. Type in quantity (#) of doses desired if indicated by a range of possible doses ordered.
8. Enter a witness ID/scan (by another nurse) to validate wasted medication (if partial dose is needed).
9. Remove the medication from the automated delivery system.
10. Close drawer/storage door, and exit the system.
11. Prepare medication and administer according to route.

---

### DISPENSING MEDICATIONS—SAFE PRACTICES

- No technology system eliminates the risk for error.
- Never become complacent about what technology can do to support safe practice.
- No computer has your ability to think critically, to understand whether an ordered drug is appropriate for your client.
- Technology (e.g., bar codes) increases the amount of time spent administering medications, but does reduce time spent in documentation.

*Source:* Cohen, H., Robinson, E., & Mandrack, M. (2003). Getting to the root of medication errors. *Nursing* 2003, 33(9), 36.

---

### CLINICAL ALERT

**The usual checks** and balances between nurses and pharmacists may be bypassed with automated dispensing systems, increasing the risk for medication errors.

---

*Note:* Certain medications (e.g., cough syrup and other client-specific multiple-dose medications) may be dispensed by pharmacy and placed in the client's medication drawer rather than being accessed through the automated system.

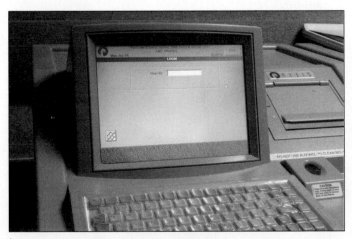

● User ID and password or scanned fingerprint control access to medications.

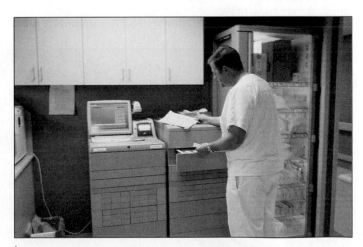

● Validate that client's MAR matches selected medications and dose on screen.

# Skill 12.31   Administering Medication Protocol

## EXPECTED OUTCOMES

- Rationale for medication administration is clear.
- Client's MAR matches physician's orders.
- Dosage calculations are accurate.
- Medication sign out sheet matches remaining stock.
- Medication is administered according to the "six rights."

## Equipment

Prepared medication
Gloves (if indicated)
Stethoscope and sphygmomanometer, if indicated

## Procedure

1. Check client's name and room number against the medication record and lock the medication cart before entering client's room, if cart is used.
   ➤*Rationale: Locking cart is a safety measure.*
2. Check client's identaband and ask client to state name and birth date.
3. Provide privacy.
4. Explain procedure and purpose of medication to client.
5. Assist client to appropriate position for medication administration.
6. Check client's vital signs if indicated before administering medication. ➤*Rationale: Medication's effects may cause hemodynamic instability if client's vital signs are at the high or low extreme of normal.*
7. Perform hand hygiene and don gloves if indicated. ➤*Rationale: Parenteral and enteral medication administration may require the use of gloves.*

> ### CLINICAL ALERT
>
> Use at least two client identifiers other than room number when administering medications or providing treatments (e.g., stated name and birth date or hospital number).

> ### CLINICAL ALERT
>
> Report any actual or potential error (e.g., sound-alike/look-alike drug names, confusion over abbreviations) to the USP Medication Errors Reporting Program: (800) 23-ERROR, or www.usp.org, or the Institute for Safe Medication Practices, www.ismp.org. A form will be sent for your completion. These agencies publicize warnings and notices in response to submitted information to help alert other professionals to potentially dangerous medication pitfalls.

8. Administer medication according to route procedure and adhering to the "Six Rights" of medication administration.
9. Dispose of equipment appropriately; then remove gloves, if used, and wash your hands.
10. Record administered medications in client's record; the time, medication given, dosage, route (including site of injection); and any relevant assessment findings.

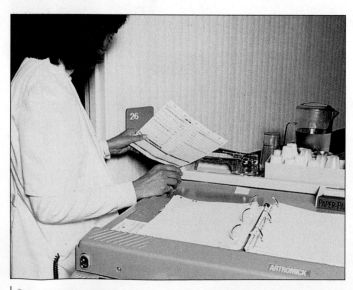

● Check client's name and room number against medication record.

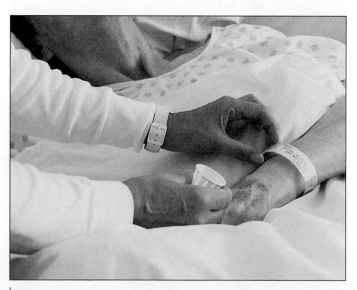

● Check client's identaband and ask client to state name and birth date.

## CLINICAL ALERT

All JCAHO-accredited agencies must have protocols developed for documenting and reconciling medications across the continuum (admission, transfer, discharge). A list of the client's home medications is compared with the admitting medication orders. Upon transfer, medications being taken are compared with orders in the new unit. Upon discharge, medications taken in the hospital are compared to the discharge medication orders. Verification, clarification, and reconciliation of discrepancies help prevent adverse drug events throughout the client's hospitalization.

## EVIDENCE-BASED NURSING PRACTICE

**Medication Errors—A Growing Problem**

One study of 5000 medication errors found that the most common errors resulting in client death were wrong dose (40.9%), wrong drug (16%), and wrong route (9.5%). In 2001, more than 100,000 medication errors were reported. Of these 2,539 resulted in injury, including 14 deaths.

*Source:* Carroll, P. (2003, January). Medication errors. *RN, 66*(1), 52–57.

## MEDICATION SAFETY MEASURES

- Keep all medicines in locked carts or cabinets.
- Do not store dangerous drugs (e.g., concentrated KCl, NaCl, magnesium sulfate) in locked carts.
- Avoid the use of stock of "borrowed" medications.
- Keep narcotics in double-locked cabinets or PYXIS. Count all narcotics with oncoming staff at the end of each shift.
- Clearly label and separate topical medicines from parenteral or oral medicines.
- Check with another nurse (1) mathematical calculations for dosages and (2) dispensed/prepared "high alert" drugs and those for high risk clients (e.g., insulins, anticoagulants, concentrated elec-

trolytes, digoxin, and hemodynamic agents if not premixed).
- Do not leave any medication at client's bedside unless there is a specific physician's order to do so.
- Report any errors in drug administration to charge nurse and client's physician immediately. Monitor the client closely for adverse effects. Document the drug given, and complete a written variance report.
- Provide complete instructions to clients regarding medication to be used at home.
- Make sure every physician involved with the client is aware of medications the client is taking at home.

## CULTURAL CONSIDERATIONS

One genetic factor noted to differ among ethnic groups is variation in metabolic pathways which may accelerate or slow drug metabolism. It is also thought that the pathophysiology of various disease states may differ among populations based on genetic determination. For example, black clients respond differently to different antihypertensives than the white population does. Blacks respond better to diuretics than they do to beta blockers and angiotensin-converting enzyme (ACE) inhibitors for hypertension.

Some agents within drug classes are more effective than others for different populations. Asians metabolize psychotropic agents more slowly then other ethnic groups, so lower does may be indicated.

The nurse should obtain a list of each client's current medications as well as any alternative therapies used so that possible untoward interactions can be prevented.

### UNEXPECTED OUTCOMES

Medication or dosage on MAR does not fit client's clinical picture.

### CRITICAL THINKING OPTIONS

- Compare new MAR with previous MAR.
- Compare new MAR with recent physician's orders.
- Discuss concerns with agency protocol.
- Contact physician for clarification.

*(continued)*

**UNEXPECTED OUTCOMES (cont.)**

Nurse is unsure of dosage calculation.

Medication sign-out sheet does not correspond to remaining stock.

Client receives wrong medication.

**CRITICAL THINKING OPTIONS (cont.)**

- Utilize helpful calculation formulas.
- Use a calculator.
- Request that another nurse check calculation or conversion.
- Seek agency pharmacist's assistance.
- Check with other nurses who may have dispensed stock medication.
- Check MARs for unclaimed stock that may have been administered.
- Complete discrepancy report if sign-out sheets and stock cannot be reconciled.
- Document the medication administered on client's MAR.
- Monitor client closely for potential undesired effects and document findings.
- Notify client's physician and document.
- Complete anonymous variance report according to agency policy.
- Always check two client identifiers before administering medication.

# Skill 12.32   Administering Oral Medications

## EXPECTED OUTCOMES
- Client takes medication orally without difficulty.
- Client experiences intended therapeutic drug effect.

## Delegation

In acute care settings, administration of oral/enteral medications is performed by the nurse and is not delegated to unlicensed assistive personnel (UAP). The nurse can inform the UAP of the intended therapeutic effects and/or specific side effects of the medication and request the UAP to report specific client observations to the nurse for follow-up. In some states, trained UAP may administer certain medications to stable clients in long-term care settings. It is important, however, for the nurse to remember that the medication knowledge of the UAP is limited and *assessment and evaluation of the effectiveness of the medication remain the responsibility of the nurse.*

## Equipment

Dispensing system
Disposable medication cups: small paper or plastic cups for tablets and capsules, waxed or plastic calibrated medication cups for liquids
MAR or computer printout
Pill crusher/cutter
Straws to administer medications that may discolor the teeth or to facilitate the ingestion of liquid medication for certain clients
Drinking glass and water or juice
Soft foods such as applesauce or pudding to use for crushed medications for clients who may choke on liquids

## Preparation

- Know the reason why the client is receiving the medication, the drug classification, contraindications, usual dosage range, side effects, and nursing considerations for administering and evaluating the intended outcomes for the medication.
- Check the medication administration record.
- Check the MAR for the drug name, dosage, frequency, route of administration, and expiration date for administering the medication, if appropriate. ➤*Rationale: Orders for certain medications (e.g., narcotics, antibiotics) expire after a specified time frame and they need to be reordered by the primary care provider.*
- If the MAR is unclear or pertinent information is missing, compare the MAR with the prescriber's most recent written order.
- Report any discrepancies to the charge nurse or the prescriber, as agency policy dictates.
- Verify the client's ability to take medication orally.
- Determine whether the client can swallow, is NPO, is nauseated or vomiting, has gastric suction, or has diminished or absent bowel sounds.
- Organize the supplies. ➤*Rationale: Organization of supplies saves time and reduces the chance of error.*

## Procedure

1. Perform hand hygiene and observe other appropriate infection control procedures.
2. Unlock the dispensing system.
3. Obtain appropriate medication.

- Read the MAR and take the appropriate medication from the shelf, drawer, or refrigerator. The medication may be dispensed in a bottle, box, or unit-dose package.
- Compare the label of the medication container or unit-dose package against the order on the MAR or computer printout. ➤*Rationale: This is a safety check to ensure that the right medication is given*. If these are not identical, recheck the prescriber's written order in the client's chart. If there is still a discrepancy, check with the nurse in charge or the pharmacist.
- Check the expiration date of the medication. Return expired medications to the pharmacy. ➤*Rationale: Outdated medications are not safe to administer.*
- Use only medications that have clear, legible labels. ➤*Rationale: This ensures accuracy.*

4. Prepare the medication.
   - Calculate the medication dosage accurately.
   - Prepare the correct amount of medication for the required dose, without contaminating the medication. ➤*Rationale: Aseptic technique maintains drug cleanliness.*
   - While preparing the medication, recheck each prepared drug and container with the MAR again. ➤*Rationale; This second safety check reduces the chance of error.*

### Tablets or Capsules

- Place packaged unit-dose capsules or tablets directly into the medicine cup. Do not remove the medication from the package until at the bedside. ➤*Rationale: The wrapper keeps the medication clean. Not removing the medication facilitates identification of the medication in the event the client refuses the drug or assessment data indicate to hold the medication. Unopened unit-dose packages can usually be returned to the medication cart.*
- If using a stock container, pour the required number into the bottle cap, and then transfer the medication to the disposable cup without touching the tablets. ➤*Rationale: This reminds the nurse to complete the needed assessment(s) in order to decide whether to give the medication or to withhold the medication if indicated.*
- Break only scored tablets if necessary to obtain the correct dosage. Use a cutting or splitting device if needed. Check agency policy as to whether unused portions of a medication can be discarded and, if so, how they are to be discarded.
- If the client has difficulty swallowing, check if the medication can be crushed. Some drug handbooks have an appendix that lists the "Do Not Crush" medications. The ISMP (2007) provides on its website an updated list of medications that should not be crushed. Some medications that should not be crushed include time-released and enteric coated medications. An example of tablets that should not be crushed is oxycodone (OxyContin), a long-acting nar-

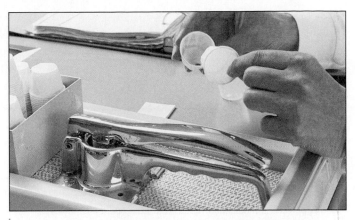

● Place med cups with tablet between to pulverize with crusher.

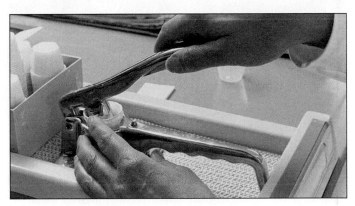

● Place pill in crusher to crush tablet, or pulverize/crush pill in unit dose container.

cotic that normally lasts 12 hours after administration. If the tablet is crushed, the client gets a surge of action in the first 2 hours, then may start having severe pain again in 4 to 6 hours, because the narcotics effect wears off too soon. The crushing of these tablets causes an uneven effect, and the long or sustained action of the medication is lost. If it is acceptable, crush the tablets to a fine powder with a pill crusher or between two medication cups. Then, mix the powder with a small amount of soft food (e.g., custard, applesauce).

## CLINICAL ALERT

Check with the pharmacy before crushing tablets. Sustainedaction, enteric-coated, buccal, or sublingual tablets should not be crushed.

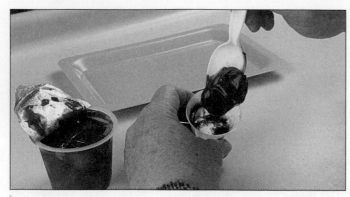

● Mix pulverized medication (for powder from opened capsule) carefully in *small* amount of soft food (pudding, jelly, applesauce).

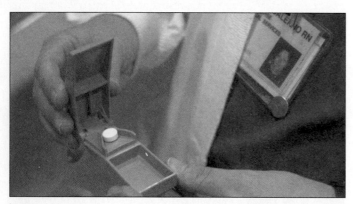

● If partial dose is ordered, place tablet in pill cutter to be cut in half.

## Liquid Medication

- Thoroughly mix the medication before pouring. Discard any medication that has changed color or turned cloudy.
- Remove the cap and place it upside down on the countertop. ➤*Rationale: This avoids contaminating the inside of the cap.*
- Hold the bottle so the label is next to the palm of the hand and pour the medication away from the label. ➤*Rationale: This prevents the label from becoming soiled and illegible as a result of spilled liquids.*
- Place the medication cup on a flat surface at eye level and fill it to the desired level, using the *bottom* of the **meniscus** (crescent-shaped upper surface of a column of liquid) to align with the container scale. ➤*Rationale: This method ensures accuracy of measurement.*
- Before capping the bottle, wipe the lip with a paper towel. ➤*Rationale: This prevents the cap from sticking.*
- When giving small amounts of liquids (e.g., <5 mL), prepare the medication in a sterile syringe without the needle or in a specially designed oral syringe. Label the syringe with the name of the medication

and the route (po) ➤*Rationale: Any oral solution removed from the original container and placed into a syringe should be labeled to avoid medications being given by the wrong route (e.g., IV). This practice facilitates client safety and avoids tragic errors.*
- Keep unit-dose liquids in their package and open them at the bedside.

**Oral Narcotics**

- If an agency uses a manual recording system for controlled substances, check the narcotic record for the previous drug count and compare it with the supply available. Some medications, including narcotics, are kept in plastic containers that are sectioned and numbered.
- Remove the next available tablet and drop it in the medicine cup.
- After removing a tablet, record the necessary information on the appropriate narcotic control record and sign it.

*Note: Computer-controlled dispensing systems allow access only to the selected drug and automatically record its use.*

*All Medications*

- Place the prepared medication and MAR together on the medication cart.
- Recheck the label on the container before returning the bottle, box, or envelope to its storage place. ➤*Rationale: This third check further reduces the risk of error.*
- Avoid leaving prepared medications unattended. ➤*Rationale: This precaution prevents potential mishandling errors.*
- Lock the medication cart before entering the client's room. ➤*Rationale: This is a safety measure because medication carts are not to be left open when unattended.*
- Check the room number against the MAR if agency policy does not allow the MAR to be removed from the medication cart. ➤*Rationale: This is another safety measure to ensure that the nurse is entering the correct client room.*

5. Provide for client privacy.
6. Prepare the client.
   - Introduce self and verify the client's identity using agency protocol. ➤*Rationale: This ensures that the right client receives the medication.*
   - Assist the client to a sitting position or, if not possible, to a side-lying position. ➤*Rationale: These positions facilitate swallowing and prevent aspiration.*
   - If not previously assessed, take the required assessment measures, such as pulse and respiratory rates or blood pressure. Take the apical pulse rate before administering digitalis preparations. Take blood pressure before giving antihypertensive drugs. Take the respiratory rate prior to

administering narcotics. ➤*Rationale: Narcotics depress the respiratory center.* If any of the findings are above or below the predetermined parameters, consult the primary care provider before administering the medication.

7. Explain the purpose of the medication and how it will help, using language that the client can understand. Include relevant information about effects; for example, tell the client receiving a diuretic to expect an increase in urine output. ➤*Rationale: Information can facilitate acceptance of and compliance with the therapy.*

8. Administer the medication at the correct time.
   * Take the medication to the client within the period of 30 minutes before or after the scheduled time.
   * Give the client sufficient water or preferred juice to swallow the medication. Before using juice, check for any food and medication incompatibilities. ➤*Rationale: Fluids ease swallowing and facilitate absorption from the gastrointestinal tract.* Liquid medications other than antacids or cough preparations may be diluted with 15 mL (1/2 oz) of water to facilitate absorption. ➤*Rationale: Putting the cup to the client's mouth maintains the cleanliness of the nurse's hands. Giving one medication at a time eases swallowing.*
   * If an older child or adult has difficulty swallowing, ask the client to place the medication on the back of the tongue before taking the water. ➤*Rationale: Stimulation of the back of the tongue produces the swallowing reflex.*
   * If the medication has an objectionable taste, ask the client to suck a few ice chips beforehand, or give the medication with juice, applesauce, or bread if there are no contraindications. ➤*Rationale: The cold temperature of the ice chips will desensitize the taste buds, and juices or bread can mask the taste of the medication.*
   * If the client says that the medication you are about to give is different from what the client has been receiving, do not give the medication without first checking the original order. ➤*Rationale: Most clients are familiar with the appearance of medications taken previously. Unfamiliar medications may signal a possible error.*
   * Stay with the client until all medications have been swallowed. ➤*Rationale: The nurse must see the client swallow the medication before the drug administration can be recorded.* The nurse may need to check the client's mouth to ensure that the medication was swallowed and not hidden inside the cheek. A primary care provider's order or agency policy is required for medications left at the bedside.

9. Document each medication given.
   * Record the medication given, dosage, time, any complaints or assessments of the client, and your signature.
   * If medication was refused or omitted, record this fact on the appropriate record; document the reason, when possible, and the nurse's actions according to agency policy.

10. Dispose of all supplies appropriately.
    * Replenish stock (e.g., medication cups) and return the cart to the appropriate place.
    * Discard used disposable supplies.

# CULTURAL CONSIDERATIONS

Cultural and genetic factors affect how a client reacts to medications. Physiologic rhythms, use of alcohol, and stress may either inhibit or accelerate drug biodynamics.

Cultural acceptance factors include values and beliefs, educational level, previous experiences, family influence, and physician/client relationship.

The concomitant use of "natural" remedies can also alter the client's response to drug therapy.

# Skill 12.33    Administering Medications by Enteral Tube

## Delegation

The administration of medications through an enteral tube is performed by the nurse and is not delegated to UAP. The nurse can inform the UAP of the intended therapeutic effects and/or specific side effects of the medication and request the UAP to report specific client observations to the nurse for follow-up.

## Equipment

Medication to be administered
Disposable medication cups: small paper or plastic calibrated medication cups for liquids
60-mL syringe with catheter tip for large-bore tube or Luer-Lok tip for small-bore tube
Pill crusher for medications that need to be crushed
Tongue blade or straw to stir dissolved medication
pH test strip
Warm water to dissolve crushed medications
Tap water (room temperature) or sterile water or normal saline for flushing tube (check agency policy)
Emesis basin
Clean gloves
MAR or computer printout

## Preparation

* Know the reason why the client is receiving the medication, the drug classification, contraindications,

usual dosage range, side effects, and nursing considerations for administering and evaluating the intended outcomes for the medication.

- Check the medication administration record.
- Check the MAR for the drug name, dosage, frequency, route of administration, and expiration date for administration of the medication, if appropriate. ➤*Rationale: Orders for certain medications (e.g., narcotics, antibiotics) expire after a specified time frame and they need to be reordered by the primary care provider.*
- If the MAR is unclear or pertinent information is missing, compare the MAR with the prescriber's most recent written order.
- Report any discrepancies to the charge nurse or the prescriber, as agency policy dictates.
- Organize the supplies.
- Gather the MAR(s) for each client so that medications can be prepared for one client at a time. ➤*Rationale: Organization of supplies saves time and reduces the chance of error.*
- Prepare the client.
- Assist the client to a Fowler's position in bed or a sitting position in a chair. If a sitting position is contraindicated, a slightly elevated right side-lying position is acceptable. ➤*Rationale: These positions enhance gravitational flow and prevent aspiration of fluid into the lungs.*

### Procedure

1. Perform hand hygiene and observe other appropriate infection control procedures.
2. Prepare medications for appropriate administration by enteral tube (e.g., use liquids or crush and dissolve tablets). Calculate medication dosage accurately.
3. Provide for client privacy.
   - Introduce self and verify the client's identity using agency protocol. ➤*Rationale: This ensures that the right client receives the medication.*
   - If not previously assessed, take the required assessment measures, such as pulse and respiratory rates or blood pressure. Take the apical pulse rate before administering digitalis preparations. Take blood pressure before giving antihypertensive drugs. Take the respiratory rate prior to administering narcotics. If any of the findings are above or below the predetermined parameters, consult the primary care provider before administering the medication.
4. Explain the purpose of the medication and how it will help, using language that the client can understand. Include relevant information about effects; for example, tell the client receiving an analgesic to expect a decrease in pain. ➤*Rationale: Information can facilitate acceptance of and compliance with the therapy.*
5. Apply clean gloves.

6. If client is receiving a continuous tube feeding, press the "Hold" button on the enteric feeding pump. ➤*Rationale: Pausing or holding the pump temporarily stops the administration of the tube feeding.*
7. Disconnect tubing that is being used for suction or feeding from gastric tube. Place cap on end of tubing. ➤*Rationale: Putting a cap on the end of the tubing prevents contamination.*
8. Assess tube placement.
9. Pinch or fold over the gastric tube. ➤*Rationale: Pinching or folding over the tubing prevents gastric contents from flowing out of the tube.*
10. Gently aspirate all the stomach contents and measure the residual volume.
11. Return residual back to stomach. ➤*Rationale: Returning the residual prevents loss of fluids and electrolytes.* Pinch or fold over the gastric tube and remove the syringe.
    - Check agency policy if residual volume greater than 100 mL.
12. Administer the medication(s).
    - Remove the plunger from the syringe and connect the syringe to a pinched or folded over tube. ➤*Rationale: Pinching or folding over the tube prevents excess air from entering the stomach and causing distention.*
    - Put 30 mL of water into the syringe barrel to flush the tube before administering the first medication. Raise or lower the barrel of the syringe to adjust the flow as needed. Pinch or clamp the tubing before all of the water is instilled. ➤*Rationale: This avoids excess air entering the stomach.*
    - Pour liquid or dissolved medication into syringe barrel and allow to flow by gravity into enteral tube.
    - If administering more than one medication, flush with 30 mL of tap water between each medication.
    - After administering the last medication, flush the tube with 30 mL of tap water. ➤*Rationale: Flushing clears the tube and prevents clogging of the tube.*
    - Pinch or fold over the gastric tube and reconnect to tubing for continuous tube feeding. If the client was previously connected to suction, keep the gastric tube clamped for 20 to 30 minutes after giving the medication. ➤*Rationale: Keeping the tube clamped for that time will help ensure that the medication is absorbed before restarting the suction.*
    - Remove and discard gloves. Perform hand hygiene.

---

### CLINICAL ALERT

Consult with pharmacist before deciding to alter the form of any medication. Have pharmacist substitute liquid form of medication if available, or substitute a short-acting formulation that can be safety crushed for administration. Contact the physician for a substitute medication if formulation alternatives are unavailable.

13. Document each medication given.
    - Record the medication given, dosage, time, any complaints or assessments of the client, and your signature.
    - If medication was refused or omitted, record this fact on the appropriate record; document the reason, when possible, and the nurse's actions according to agency policy.

- Record fluid intake accurately if client is on intake and output.
14. Dispose of all supplies appropriately.
    - Replenish stock (e.g., medication cups) and return cart to the appropriate place.
    - Discard used disposable supplies.

| UNEXPECTED OUTCOMES | CRITICAL THINKING OPTIONS |
|---|---|
| Client has an allergic or anaphylactic response to medication. | • Immediately stop or hold medication.<br>• Notify physician at once; prepare to administer epinephrine to dilate bronchi and support blood pressure.<br>• If reaction is severe:<br>  • Keep client flat in bed with head elevated.<br>  • Take vital signs every 10–15 minutes; stay with client.<br>  • Assess for hypotension or respiratory distress.<br>  • Establish airway, if necessary.<br>  • Have emergency equipment available.<br>  • Provide psychologic support to client to alleviate fears.<br>  • Record type and progression of reactions. |
| Client has difficulty swallowing medication. | • Offer water before administering oral medication.<br>• Crush medications if appropriate and administer mixed with food such as applesauce, pudding or jelly.<br>• Consult with pharmacist to dispense same medication in liquid form.<br>• If difficulty continues, consult physician for altered route of medication delivery (rectal, parenteral).<br>• Request swallow study. |
| Client is nauseated and oral medications have not been taken. | • Hold medication. Notify physician for antiemetic medication order and alternate route for administering necessary medications.<br>• Administer entiemetic if ordered, then administer medication when client's nausea is relieved. |

# Skill 12.34   Administering Sublingual Medications

### Equipment

Sublingual medication (e.g., nitroglycerin tablets in a dark bottle). Tablets lose potency when exposed to light; opened bottle should be replaced in 3 months.
*or*
Nitrolingual aerosol spray in canister

### Preparation

1. Prepare the medications.
2. Assess vital signs if administering sublingual nitroglycerin. (Systolic BP should not be lower than 90 mm Hg.)
3. Place client in a sitting position.

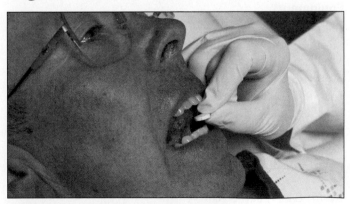

● Sublingual medication is placed under client's tongue for rapid absorption.

**Procedure**

1. Follow steps for preparing and administering oral medications, except:
   a. Explain that client must not swallow drug or eat, smoke, or drink until medication is completely absorbed.
   b. Ask client to place tablet under the tongue or to hold tongue up so tablet can be placed under tongue. ➤*Rationale: Absorption is rapid and complete due to the vast network of capillaries in this area.*
   c. Alternate: hold nitrolingual canister vertically with spray opening as close to mouth as possible. Deliver 1 or 2 metered sprays onto or under tongue, then have client close mouth immediately. Tell client not to inhale medication.
2. Evaluate client for drug action and possible side effects (e.g., headache).

> ### CLINICAL ALERT
>
> Assess client's chest discomfort: quality, location, radiation, intensity, duration and precipitating factors. When administering rapid-acting (sublingual) nitroglycerin, monitor client's response and vital signs. If chest discomfort is not relieved in 5 minutes, notify physician. Obtain order for: opiate analgesic (morphine sulfate), EKG, ST segment monitoring, and cardiac markers. No more than 3 doses of nitroglycerin should be administered in a 15-minute period because of potential hypotensive effect (BP ≤90 mm Hg) or bradycardia (HR ≤50) as this would preclude adequate dosage of morphine sulfate for pain control.

---

### EVIDENCE-BASED NURSING PRACTICE

**ACC/AHA Guidelines-Nitroglycerin**

It is recommended that clients who have been previously prescribed nitroglycerin be advised to take ONE dose sublingually promptly for chest discomfort/pain. If symptoms do not improve, or worsen in 5 minutes after ONE nitroglycerin dose, the client should call 9-1-1 immediately to access EMS. The traditional recommendation for taking up to 3 doses before calling EMS has been changed to encourage earlier EMS contact.

*Source:* Antman, E. M. et al. ACC/AHA guidelines for the management of patients with ST-elevation myocardial infarction: A report of the American College of Cardiology/American Heart Association Task Force on Practice Guidelines. *Journal of American College of Cardiology* 44(3): E1-E211, August 4, 2004 (http://www.acc.org/clinical/guidelines).

---

## Skill 12.35 Administering Ophthalmic Medications

### Delegation

Due to the need for assessment, interpretation of client status, and use of sterile technique, ophthalmic medication administration is not delegated to UAP.

### Equipment

Clean gloves
Sterile absorbent sponges soaked in sterile normal saline
Medication
Sterile eye dressing (pad) as needed and paper tape to secure it

*For irrigation, add:*
Irrigating solution (e.g., normal saline) and irrigating syringe or tubing
Dry sterile absorbent sponges
Moisture-resistant towel
Basin (e.g., emesis basin)

### Preparation

1. Check the medication administration record.
2. Check the MAR for the drug name, dose, and strength. Also confirm the prescribed frequency of the instillation and which eye is to be treated.
3. Check client allergy status.
4. If the MAR is unclear or pertinent information is missing, compare it with the most recent primary care provider's written order.
5. Report any discrepancies to the charge nurse or primary care provider, as agency policy dictates.
6. Know the reason why the client is receiving the medication, the drug classification, contraindications, usual dose range, side effects, and nursing considerations for administering and evaluating the intended outcomes of the medication.

### Procedure

1. Compare the label on the medication tube or bottle with the medication record and check the expiration date.
2. If necessary, calculate the medication dosage.
3. Introduce self and explain to the client what you are going to do, why it is necessary, and how he or she can participate. The administration of an ophthalmic medication is not usually painful. Ointments are often soothing to the eye, but some liquid prepara-

tions may sting initially. Discuss how the results will be used in planning further care or treatments.

4. Perform hand hygiene and observe other appropriate infection control procedures.

5. Provide for client privacy.

6. Prepare the client.
   - Prior to performing the procedure, verify the client's identity using agency protocol. ➤*Rationale: This ensures that the right client receives the right medication.*
   - Assist the client to a comfortable position, usually lying.

7. Clean the eyelid and the eyelashes.
   - Apply clean gloves.
   - Use sterile cotton balls moistened with sterile irrigating solution or sterile normal saline, and wipe from the inner canthus to the outer canthus. ➤*Rationale: If not removed, material on the eyelid and lashes can be washed into the eye. Cleaning toward the outer canthus prevents contamination of the other eye and the lacrimal duct.*

8. Administer the eye medication.
   - Check the ophthalmic preparation for the name, strength, and number of drops if a liquid is used. ➤*Rationale: Checking medication data is essential to prevent a medication error.* Draw the correct number of drops into the shaft of the dropper if a dropper is used. If ointment is used, discard the first bead. ➤*Rationale: The first bead of ointment from a tube is considered to be contaminated.*
   - Instruct the client to look up to the ceiling. Give the client a dry sterile absorbent sponge. ➤*Rationale: The person is less likely to blink if looking up. While the client looks up, the cornea is partially protected by the upper eyelid. A sponge is needed to press on the nasolacrimal duct after a liquid instillation to prevent systemic absorption or to wipe excess ointment from the eyelashes after an ointment is instilled.*
   - Expose the lower conjunctival sac by placing the thumb or fingers of your nondominant hand on the client's cheekbone just below the eye and gently drawing down the skin on the cheek. If the tissues are edematous, handle the tissues carefully to avoid damaging them.
     ➤*Rationale: Placing the fingers on the cheekbone minimizes the possibility of touching the cornea, avoids putting any pressure on the eyeball, and prevents the person from blinking or squinting.*
   - Holding the medication in the dominant hand, place hand on client's forehead to stabilize hand. Approach the eye from the side and instill the correct number of drops onto the outer third of the lower conjunctival sac. Hold the dropper 1 to 2 cm (0.4 to 0.8 in.) above the sac.
     ➤*Rationale: The client is less likely to blink if a side approach is used. When instilled into the conjunctival sac, drops will not harm the cornea as they might if dropped directly on it. The dropper must not touch the sac or the cornea.*
     *or*

   - Holding the tube above the lower conjunctival sac, squeeze 2 cm (0.8 in.) of ointment from the tube into the lower conjunctival sac from the inner canthus outward.
   - Instruct the client to close the eyelids but not to squeeze them shut. ➤*Rationale: Closing the eye spreads the medication over the eyeball. Squeezing can injure the eye and push out the medication.*
   - For liquid medications, press firmly or have the client press firmly on the nasolacrimal duct for at least 30 seconds. ➤*Rationale: Pressing on the nasolacrimal duct prevents the medication from running out of the eye and down the duct, preventing systemic absorption.*
   - Remove and discard gloves. Perform hand hygiene.

## VARIATION: Eye Irrigation

- Place absorbent pads under the head, neck, and shoulders. Place an emesis basin next to the eye to catch drainage. Some eye medications cause systemic reactions such as confusion or a decrease in heart rate and blood pressure if the eyedrops go down the nasolacrimal duct and get into the systemic circulation.
  ➤*Rationale: Separating the lids prevents reflex blinking. Exerting pressure on the bony prominences minimizes the possibility of pressing the eyeball and causing discomfort.*
  ➤*Rationale: At this height the pressure of the solution will not damage the eye tissue, and the irrigator will not touch the eye.*
  ➤*Rationale: Directing the solution in this way prevents possible injury to the cornea and prevents fluid and contaminants from flowing down the nasolacrimal duct.*
- Irrigate until the solution leaving the eye is clear (no discharge is present) or until all the solution has been used.
- Instruct the client to close and move the eye periodically. ➤*Rationale: Eye closure and movement help to move secretions from the upper to the lower conjunctival sac.*

9. Clean and dry the eyelids as needed. Wipe the eyelids gently from the inner to the outer canthus to collect excess medication.

10. Remove and discard gloves. Perform hand hygiene.

11. Apply an eye pad if needed, and secure it with paper eye tape.

12. Assess the client's response immediately after the instillation or irrigation and again after the medication should have acted.

13. Document all relevant assessments and interventions. Include the name of the drug or irrigating solution, the strength, the number of drops if a liquid medication, the time, and the response of the client.

# Skill 12.36 Administering Otic Medications

### Delegation

Due to the need for assessment, interpretation of client status, and use of sterile technique, otic medication administration is not delegated to UAP.

### Equipment

Clean gloves
Cotton-tipped applicator
Correct medication bottle with a dropper
Flexible rubber tip (optional) for the end of the dropper, which prevents injury from sudden motion, for example, by a disoriented client
Cotton fluff

*For irrigation, add:*
Moisture-resistant towel
Basin (e.g., emesis basin)
Irrigating solution at the appropriate temperature, about 500 mL (16 oz) or as ordered
Container for the irrigating solution
Syringe (rubber bulb or Asepto syringe is frequently used)

### Preparation

1. Check the medication administration record.
2. Check the MAR for the drug name, strength, number of drops, and prescribed frequency.
3. Check client allergy status.
4. If the MAR is unclear or pertinent information is missing, compare it with the most recent primary care provider's written order.
5. Report any discrepancies to the charge nurse or primary care provider, as agency policy dictates.
6. Know the reason why the client is receiving the medication, the drug classification, contraindications, usual dose range, side effects, and nursing considerations for administering and evaluating the intended outcomes of the medication.

### Procedure

1. Compare the label on the medication container with the medication record and check the expiration date.
2. If necessary, calculate the medication dosage.
3. Introduce self and explain to the client what you are going to do, why it is necessary, and how he or she can participate. The administration of an otic medication is not usually painful. Discuss how the results will be used in planning further care or treatments.
4. Perform hand hygiene and observe other appropriate infection control procedures.

5. Provide for client privacy.
6. Prepare the client.
   - Prior to performing the procedure, verify the client's identity using agency protocol. ➤*Rationale: This ensures that the right client receives the right medication.*
   - Assist the client to a comfortable position for eardrop administration, usually lying with the ear being treated uppermost.
7. Clean the pinna of the ear and the meatus of the ear canal.
   - Apply gloves if infection is suspected.
   - Use cotton-tipped applicators and solution to wipe the pinna and auditory meatus. ➤*Rationale: This removes any discharge present before the instillation so that it won't be washed into the ear canal.* Ensure that applicator does *not* go into the ear canal. ➤*Rationale: This avoids damage to tympanic membrane or wax becoming impacted within the canal.*
8. Administer the ear medication.
   - Warm the medication container in your hand, or place it in warm water for a short time. ➤*Rationale: This promotes client comfort and prevents nerve stimulation and pain.*
   - Partially fill the ear dropper with medication.
   - Straighten the auditory canal. Pull the pinna upward and backward for clients over 3 years of age. ➤*Rationale: The auditory canal is straightened so that the solution can flow the entire length of the canal.*
   - Instill the correct number of drops along the side of the ear canal.
   - Press gently but firmly a few times on the tragus of the ear (the cartilaginous projection in front of the exterior meatus of the ear). ➤*Rationale: Pressing on the tragus assists the flow of medication into the ear canal.*
   - Ask the client to remain in the side-lying position for about 5 minutes. ➤*Rationale: This prevents the drops from escaping and allows the medication to reach all sides of the canal cavity.*
   - Insert a small piece of cotton fluff loosely at the meatus of the auditory canal for 15 to 20 minutes. Do not press it into the canal. ➤*Rationale: The cotton helps retain the medication when the client is up. If pressed tightly into the canal, the cotton would interfere with the action of the drug and the outward movement of normal secretions.*

### VARIATION: Ear Irrigation

- Explain that the client may experience a feeling of fullness, warmth, and, occasionally, discomfort when the fluid comes in contact with the tympanic membrane.
- Assist the client to a sitting or lying position with head tilted toward the affected ear. ➤*Rationale: The solution can then flow from the ear canal to a basin.*

- Place the moisture-resistant towel around the client's shoulder under the ear to be irrigated, and place the basin under the ear to be irrigated.
- Fill the syringe with solution.
  *or*
- Hang up the irrigating container, and run solution through the tubing and the nozzle. ➤*Rationale: Solution is run through to remove air from the tubing and nozzle.*
- Straighten the ear canal.
- Insert the tip of the syringe into the auditory meatus, and direct the solution gently upward against the top of the canal. ➤*Rationale: The solution will flow around the entire canal and out at the bottom. The solution is instilled gently because strong pressure from the fluid can cause discomfort and damage the tympanic membrane.*
- Continue instilling the fluid until all the solution is used or until the canal is cleaned, depending on the

purpose of the irrigation. Take care not to block the outward flow of the solution with the syringe.
- Assist the client to a side-lying position on the affected side. ➤*Rationale: Lying with the affected side down helps drain the excess fluid by gravity.*
- Place a cotton fluff in the auditory meatus to absorb the excess fluid.
- Remove and discard gloves. Perform hand hygiene.
9. Assess the client's response and the character and amount of discharge, appearance of the canal, discomfort, and so on, immediately after the instillation and again when the medication is expected to act. Inspect the cotton ball for any drainage.
10. Document all nursing assessments and interventions relative to the procedure. Include the name of the drug or irrigating solution, the strength, the number of drops if a liquid medication, the time, and the response of the client.

# Skill 12.37   Administering Nasal Medications

## Delegation

Due to the need for assessment and interpretation of client status, nasal medication administration is not delegated to UAP.

## Equipment

Tissues
Clean gloves
Correct medication bottle with a dropper

## Preparation

- Check the medication administration record.
- Check the MAR for the drug name, strength, and number of drops. Also confirm the prescribed frequency of the instillation and which side of the nose is to be treated.
- Check client allergy status.
- If the MAR is unclear or pertinent information is missing, compare it with the most recent primary care provider's written order.
- Report any discrepancies to the charge nurse or primary care provider, as agency policy dictates.
- Know the reason why the client is receiving the medication, the drug classification, contraindications, usual dose range, side effects, and nursing considerations for administering and evaluating the intended outcomes of the medication.

## Procedure

1. Compare the label on the medication container with the medication record and check the expiration date.
2. If necessary, calculate the medication dosage.
3. Introduce self and explain to the client what you are going to do, why it is necessary, and how he or she can participate. The administration of nasal medication

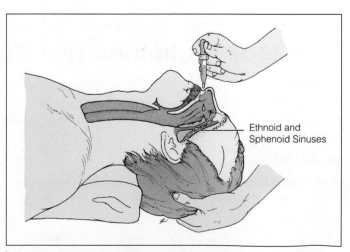

Ethnoid and Sphenoid Sinuses

● Instruct client to tilt head backwards and place dropper inside nares when instilling nose drops.

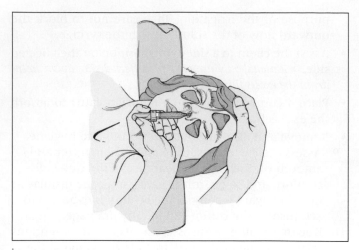

● Tilt client's head back for nose drops to reach maxillary and frontal sinuses.

is not usually painful. Discuss how the results will be used in planning further care or treatments.
4. Perform hand hygiene and observe other appropriate infection control procedures.
5. Provide for client privacy.
6. Prepare the client.
   - Prior to performing the procedure, verify the client's identity using agency protocol. ➤*Rationale: This ensures that the right client receives the right medication.*
8. Assist the client to a comfortable position.
   - To treat the opening of the eustachian tube, have the client assume a back-lying position. ➤*Rationale: The drops will flow into the nasopharynx, where the eustachian tube opens.*
   - To treat the ethmoid and sphenoid sinuses, have the client take a back-lying position with the head over the edge of

the bed or a pillow under the shoulders so that the head is tipped backward.
   - To treat the maxillary and frontal sinuses, have the client assume the same back-lying position, with the head turned toward the side to be treated. If only one side is to be treated, be sure the person is positioned so that the correct side is accessible. If the client's head is over the edge of the bed, support it with your hand so that the neck muscles are not strained.
8. Administer the medication.
   - Apply clean gloves.
   - Draw up the required amount of solution into the dropper.
   - Hold the tip of the dropper just above the nostril, and direct the solution laterally toward the midline of the superior concha of the ethmoid bone as the client breathes through the mouth. Do not touch the mucous membrane of the nares. ➤*Rationale: If the solution is directed toward the base of the nasal cavity, it will run down the eustachian tube. Touching the mucous membrane with the dropper could damage the membrane and cause the client to sneeze.*
   - Repeat for the other nostril if indicated.
   - Ask the client to remain in the position for 5 minutes. ➤*Rationale: The client remains in the same position to help the solution come in contact with all of the nasal surface or flow into the desired area.*
   - Discard any remaining solution in the dropper, and dispose of soiled supplies appropriately.
   - Remove and discard gloves. Perform hand hygiene.
9. Document all nursing assessments and interventions relative to the procedure. Include the name of the drug or irrigating solution, the strength, the number of drops if a liquid medication, the time, and the response of the client.

# Skill 12.38   Administering Metered-Dose Inhaler Medications

### Delegation

Due to the need for assessment and interpretation of client status, inhaled medication administration is not delegated to UAP.

### Equipment

- Metered-dose nebulizer with medication canister and extender if indicated

### Preparation

1. Check the medication administration record.
2. Check the MAR for the drug name, strength, and prescribed frequency.

3. Check client allergy status.
   - If the MAR is unclear or pertinent information is missing, compare it with the most recent primary care provider's written order.
   - Report any discrepancies to the charge nurse or primary care provider, as agency policy dictates.
4. Know the reason why the client is receiving the medication, the drug classification, contraindications, usual dose range, side effects, and nursing considerations for administering and evaluating the intended outcomes of the medication.

## Procedure

1. Compare the label on the medication container with the medication record and check the expiration date.
2. Introduce self and explain to the client what you are going to do, why it is necessary, and how he or she can participate. Discuss how the results will be used in planning further care or treatments.
3. Perform hand hygiene and observe other appropriate infection control procedures.
4. Provide for client privacy.
5. Prepare the client.
   - Prior to performing the procedure, verify the client's identity using agency protocol. ➤*Rationale: This ensures that the right client receives the right medication.*
   - Explain that this nebulizer delivers a measured dose of drug with each push of the medication canister, which fits into the top of the nebulizer.
6. Instruct the client to use the metered-dose nebulizer as follows:

### Metered-Dose Inhaler

1. Ensure that the canister is firmly and fully inserted into the inhaler.
2. Remove the mouthpiece cap. Holding the inhaler upright, shake the inhaler vigorously for 3 to 5 seconds to mix the medication evenly.
3. Exhale comfortably (as in a normal full breath).
4. Hold the inhaler with the canister on top and the mouthpiece at the bottom.
   a. Hold the MDI 2 to 4 cm (1 to 2 in.) from the open mouth.
   *or*
   b. Put the mouthpiece far enough into the mouth with its opening toward the throat such that the lips can tightly close around the mouthpiece. This method should not be used for steroid medications via an MDI because it is not considered as efficient in delivery of the medication (Bower, 2005).

### Metered-Dose Inhaler with Spacer

1. Insert the MDI mouthpiece into the spacer.
2. Holding the inhaler and spacer, shake vigorously for 3 to 5 seconds to mix the medication evenly.
3. An MDI with a spacer or extender is always placed in the mouth.

### Administering the Medication

1. Press down *once* on the MDI canister (which releases the dose) and inhale slowly (for 3 to 5 seconds) and deeply through the mouth.
2. Hold your breath for 10 seconds or as long as possible. ➤*Rationale: This allows the aerosol to reach deeper airways.*
3. Remove the inhaler from or away from the mouth.
4. Exhale slowly through *pursed* lips. ➤*Rationale: Controlled exhalation keeps the small airways open during exhalation.*

---

### CLINICAL ALERT

If two inhalers are to be used, the bronchodilator medication (which opens the airways) should be given prior to other medications. Bower (2005) recommends the use of the mnemonic *B before C* to remember bronchodilator before corticosteroid.

---

5. Repeat the inhalation if ordered. Wait 1 to 2 minutes between inhalations of bronchodilator medications. ➤*Rationale: The first inhalation has a chance to work and the subsequent dose reaches deeper into the lungs.*
6. Many MDIs contain steroids for an anti-inflammatory effect. Prolonged use increases the risk of fungal infections in the mouth, indicating a need for attentive mouth care.
7. Following use of the inhaler, rinse mouth with water and spit it out. ➤*Rationale: Rinsing the mouth removes any remaining medication and reduces irritation and risk of infection.* Swallowing the rinse water could increase the chance of the medication entering the bloodstream and causing adverse reactions (Bower, 2005).
8. Clean the MDI mouthpiece, and spacer if appropriate, daily. Use mild soap and water, rinse it, and let it air dry before reusing.

---

### CLINICAL ALERT

Check inhaler medication label for number of actuations (propellant-driven medication doses, e.g., 200). Have client maintain a record of actuations and discard after the number indicated. Final puffs may be nothing but propellant, which would not dilate airways in an emergency situation.

---

### CLINICAL ALERT

Inhaled steroids may not be correctly used by clients because they do not associate these medications with immediate symptom relief. The bronchodilators act to open the airways in the short term. However, it is the inhaled steroids that act as "chemical Band-Aids" to keep airway inflammation under control.

---

### WHY USE A SPACER WITH MDI?

Only 10–15% of inhaled (MDI) medications reach the small airways, but use of a spacer can increase this by about 12%.

*Source:* Togger, D., & Brenner, P. (2001). Metered dose inhalers. *American Journal of Nursing,* 101(10), 29.

9. Store the canister at room temperature. Avoid extremes of temperature.
10. Report adverse reactions such as restlessness, palpitations, nervousness, or rash to the primary care provider.

11. Document all nursing assessments and interventions relative to the procedure. Include the name of the drug, the strength, the time, and the response of the client.

---

## EVIDENCE-BASED NURSING PRACTICE

**MDI Canister Actuations—Client Monitoring**

A study evaluated how clients determined that their MDI canisters were empty. Of the clients studied, 74% did not know how many actuations were in their canisters and used their MDIs until they could no longer "hear" the medication when actuating. Additionally, while 78% knew to shake the canister before actuating, only half did so. The conclusion was that clients are likely to use the medication for up to twice the intended duration, using canisters with no active ingredients more than 50% of the time. The authors concluded that does counters appear to be the only practical solution.

*Source:* Rubin, B., & Durotoye, L. (2004). How do patients determine that their metered-dose inhaler is empty? *Chest*, 126, 1134–1137.

---

# Skill 12.39  Administering Dry Powder Inhaled (DPI) Medication

### Equipment

Dry powder capsule intended for oral inhalation
Medication package insert (instructions)
Handheld inhalation device intended for medication to be given

### Preparation

1. See Administering MDI Medications.
2. Review medication package insert instructions.
3. Perform hand hygiene.

### Procedure

1. Take dry powder capsule package and inhalation device to client's room.
2. Check client's identaband and have client state name and birth date.
3. Provide privacy.
4. Explain procedure and purpose to client.
5. Assist client to a sitting position.
6. Remove capsule from package, peeling back foil cover to expose only one capsule. ➤*Rationale: Capsules should be used immediately; unused capsules exposed to air may lose effectiveness.*
7. Open the outer cap of inhaler device (pull cap upward).
8. Open the mouthpiece.
9. Insert the capsule into center of chamber of the inhalation device.
10. Open mouthpiece and discard remaining capsule.
11. Close mouthpiece and outer cap and store at client's bedside.

12. Clean unit only as necessary, using warm water and allowing device to air dry thoroughly before next use. ➤*Rationale: No cleaning agents should be used and the device should not be wet when used.*
13. Hold the device upright, and, leaving the outer cap open, close mouthpiece/lid firmly until a click is heard and leave the outer cap open.
14. Press the side mounted piercing button in completely, then release. ➤*Rationale: The piercing button punctures the capsule, allowing medication to be released upon inhalation.*
15. Have the client breathe out completely.
16. Have the client keep his/her head in upright position and place lips tightly round the mouthpiece.

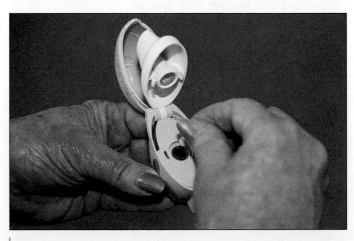

● Insert capsule into center of chamber of the inhalation device.

17. Have client breathe slowly and deeply with sufficient energy to hear the medication capsule vibrate. ➤*Rationale: As long as the capsule rattles, the client's inhalation is fast enough.*

*Note:* Some DPIs require a fast initial inhalation to activate the medication distribution.

18. Have the client hold the deep breath as long as comfortable, then return to normal breathing.
19. Have client repeat steps 12 through 15 if indicated in medication package insert. ➤*Rationale: Repeating the steps may be necessary to get the full dose of medication.*

---

# Skill 12.40 Administering Medication by Nonpressurized (Nebulized) Aerosol (NPA)

## Equipment

Nebulizer medication chamber
T-piece, mouthpiece or mask
Corrugated tubing
Air flow tubing
Prescribed medication (e.g., bronchodilator)
Prescribed diluent (normal saline)
Wall source (or other source) for compressed air, or oxygen with flowmeter

## Preparation

1. Perform hand hygiene.
2. Dilute medication as ordered and place in nebulizer chamber.
3. Attach one end of tubing to compressed air source.
4. Attach other end of tubing to nozzle at side or bottom of nebulizer.
5. Keep nebulizer chamber vertical, and connect top of chamber to mask or T-piece sidearm.
6. Hold mouthpiece in its protective cover, and attach to one end of T-piece.
7. Attach corrugated tubing to other end of T-piece.

## Procedure

1. Turn on air or oxygen (8 L/min) source, and observe for mist flow.
   a. If the client is receiving 3 L/min or less of oxygen therapy, deliver aerosolized medications with compressed air (yellow wall outlet).
   b. If the client is receiving 4 L/min or more of oxygen therapy, deliver the aerosol medication with the oxygen flowmeter (green wall outlet) set at 8 L/min.
2. Have client place mouthpiece in mouth and close lips.
3. Instruct client to breathe normally in and out of mouthpiece or mask.
4. Have client take a deep breath and hold for several seconds, then exhale slowly every 3–5 breaths. (Treatment is complete when all medication is used and no mist is seen.)
5. Turn power (air or $O_2$ flow) off, and unplug compressor (if used), or reset prescribed $O_2$ flow rate.
6. Clean mouthpiece, and place equipment in plastic bag at bedside. (Dispose of and replace components according to agency policy.)

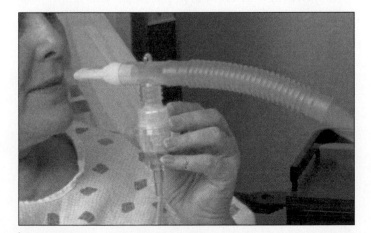

● Nonpressurized aerosol (NPA) treatment in progress.

## CLINICAL ALERT

The plastic containers with respiratory medications for nebulizers are similar to the plastic containers for single-dose eye drops. Both products have the drug name molded into the plastic, but it is difficult to see.

# Skill 12.41   Administering Vaginal Medications

## Delegation

Due to the need for assessments and interpretation of client status, vaginal medication administration is not delegated to UAP.

## Equipment

Drape
Correct vaginal suppository or cream
Applicator for vaginal cream
Clean gloves
Lubricant for a suppository
Disposable towel
Clean perineal pad

*For an irrigation, add:*
Moisture-proof pad
Vaginal irrigation set (these are often disposable) containing a nozzle, tubing and a clamp, and a container for the solution Irrigating solution

## Preparation

1. Check the medication administration record.
2. Check the MAR for the drug name, strength, and prescribed frequency.
3. Check client allergy status.
4. If the MAR is unclear or pertinent information is missing, compare it with the most recent primary care provider's written order.
5. Report any discrepancies to the charge nurse or primary care provider, as agency policy dictates.
6. Know the reason why the client is receiving the medication, the drug classification, contraindications, usual dose range, side effects, and nursing considerations for administering and evaluating the intended outcomes of the medication.

## Procedure

1. Compare the label on the medication container with the medication record and check the expiration date.
2. If necessary, calculate the medication dosage.
3. Introduce self and explain to the client what you are going to do, why it is necessary, and how she can participate. Explain to the client that a vaginal instillation is normally a painless procedure, and in fact may bring relief from itching and burning if an infection is present. Many people feel embarrassed about this procedure, and some may prefer to perform the procedure themselves if instruction is provided. Discuss how the results will be used in planning further care or treatments.

4. Perform hand hygiene and observe other appropriate infection control procedures.
5. Provide for client privacy.
6. Prepare the client.
   - Prior to performing the procedure, verify the client's identity using agency protocol. ➤*Rationale: This ensures that the right client receives the right medication.*
   - Ask the client to void. ➤*Rationale: If the bladder is empty, the client will have less discomfort during the treatment, and the possibility of injuring the vaginal lining is decreased.*
   - Assist the client to a back-lying position with the knees flexed and the hips rotated laterally.
   - Drape the client appropriately so that only the perineal area is exposed.
7. Prepare the equipment.
   - Unwrap the suppository, and put it on the opened wrapper.
   *or*
   - Fill the applicator with the prescribed cream, jelly, or foam. Directions are provided with the manufacturer's applicator.
8. Assess and clean the perineal area.
   - Apply gloves. ➤*Rationale: Gloves prevent contamination of the nurse's hands from vaginal and perineal microorganisms.*
   - Inspect the vaginal orifice, note any odor or discharge from the vagina, and ask about any vaginal discomfort.
   - Provide perineal care to remove microorganisms. ➤*Rationale: This decreases the chance of moving microorganisms into the vagina.*
9. Administer the vaginal suppository, cream, foam, jelly, or irrigation.

## Suppository

- Lubricate the rounded (smooth) end of the suppository, which is inserted first. ➤*Rationale: Lubrication facilitates insertion.*
- Lubricate your gloved index finger.
- Expose the vaginal orifice by separating the labia with your nondominant hand.
- Insert the suppository about 8 to 10 cm (3 to 4 in.) along the posterior wall of the vagina, or as far as it will go. ➤*Rationale: The posterior wall of the vagina is about 2.5 cm (1 in.) longer than the anterior wall because the cervix protrudes into the uppermost portion of the anterior wall.*
- Ask the client to remain lying in the supine position for 5 to 10 minutes following insertion. The hips may also be elevated on a pillow. ➤*Rationale: This position allows the medication to flow into the posterior fornix after it has melted.*

### Vaginal Cream, Jelly, or Foam

- Gently insert the applicator about 5 cm (2 in.).
- Slowly push the plunger until the applicator is empty.
- Remove the applicator and place it on the towel. ➤*Rationale: The applicator is put on the towel to prevent the spread of microorganisms.* Discard the applicator if disposable or clean it according to the manufacturer's directions.
- Ask the client to remain lying in the supine position for 5 to 10 minutes following the insertion.

### Irrigation

- Place the client on a bedpan.
- Clamp the tubing. Hold the irrigating container about 30 cm (12 in.) above the vagina. ➤*Rationale: At this height, the pressure of the solution should not be great enough to injure the vaginal lining.*
- Run fluid through the tubing and nozzle into the bedpan. ➤*Rationale: Fluid is run through the tubing to remove air and to moisten the nozzle.*
- Insert the nozzle carefully into the vagina. Direct the nozzle toward the sacrum, following the direction of the vagina.
- Insert the nozzle about 7 to 10 cm (3 to 4 in.), start the flow, and rotate the nozzle several times. ➤*Rationale: Rotating the nozzle irrigates all parts of the vagina.*
- Use all of the irrigating solution, permitting it to flow out freely into the bedpan.

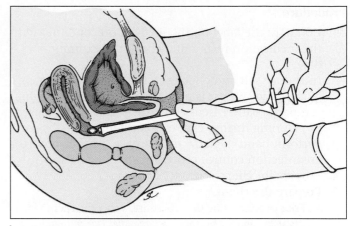

● Insert vaginal suppository at least 2 inches into vaginal canal using applicator as shown.

- Remove the nozzle from the vagina.
- Assist the client to a sitting position on the bedpan. ➤*Rationale: Sitting on the bedpan will help drain the remaining fluid by gravity.*
10. Ensure client comfort.
    - Dry the perineum with tissues as required.
    - Apply a clean perineal pad if there is excessive drainage.
    - Remove and discard gloves. Perform hand hygiene.
11. Document all nursing assessments and interventions relative to the skill. Include the name of the drug or irrigating solution, the strength, the time, and the response of the client.

# Skill 12.42  Administering Rectal Medications

### Delegation

Due to the need for assessment and interpretation of client status, rectal medication administration is not delegated to UAP.

### Equipment

Correct suppository
Clean glove
Lubricant

### Preparation

1. Check the medication administration record.
2. Check the MAR for the drug name, strength, and prescribed frequency.

3. Check client allergy status.
    - If the MAR is unclear or pertinent information is missing, compare it with the most recent primary care provider's written order.
    - Report any discrepancies to the charge nurse or primary care provider, as agency policy dictates.
    - Know the reason why the client is receiving the medication, the drug classification, contraindications, usual dose range, side effects, and nursing considerations for administering and evaluating the intended outcomes of the medication.

## Procedure

1. Compare the label on the medication container with the medication record and check the expiration date.
2. Introduce self and explain to the client what you are going to do, why it is necessary, and how he or she can participate. Discuss how the results will be used in planning further care or treatments.
3. Perform hand hygiene and observe other appropriate infection control procedures.
4. Provide for client privacy.
5. Prepare the client.
   * Prior to performing the procedure, verify the client's identity using agency protocol. ➤*Rationale: This ensures that the right client receives the right medication.*
   * Assist the client to a left lateral or left Sims' position, with the upper leg acutely flexed.
   * Fold back the top bedclothes to expose only the buttocks.
6. Prepare the equipment.
   * Unwrap the suppository, and leave it on the opened wrapper.
   * Apply glove on the hand used to insert the suppository. ➤*Rationale: The glove prevents contamination of the nurse's hand by rectal microorganisms and feces.*
   * Lubricate the smooth, rounded end of the suppository, or see the manufacturer's instructions. ➤*Rationale: The smooth, rounded end is inserted first. Lubrication prevents anal friction and tissue damage on insertion.*
   * Lubricate the gloved index finger.
7. Insert the suppository.
   * Ask the client to breathe through the mouth. ➤*Rationale: This usually relaxes the external anal sphincter.*
   * Insert the suppository gently into the anus, rounded end first (or according to the manufacturer's instructions) and along the wall of the rectum with the gloved index finger. For an adult, insert the suppository 10 cm (4 in.). ➤*Rationale: The rounded end facilitates insertion. The suppository needs to be placed along the wall of the rectum, rather than amid feces, in order to be absorbed effectively.*
   * Withdraw the finger. Press the client's buttocks together for a few minutes. ➤*Rationale: This helps minimize any urge to expel the suppository.*
   * Remove the glove by turning it inside out and discard. ➤*Rationale: Turning the glove inside out contains the rectal microorganisms and prevents their spread.*
   * Perform hand hygiene.

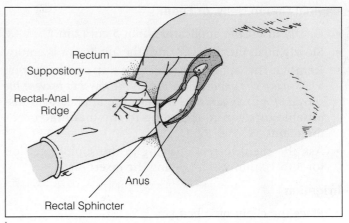

● Insert rectal suppository beyond the anal–rectal ridge to ensure it is retained.

* Ask the client to remain flat or in the left lateral position for at least 5 minutes. ➤*Rationale: This helps prevent expulsion of the suppository.* The suppository should be retained at least 30 to 40 minutes or according to manufacturer's instructions.
* If the client has been given a laxative suppository, place the call light within easy reach to summon assistance for the bedpan or toilet.
8. Document all nursing assessments and interventions relative to the procedure. Include the type of suppository given/name of the drug, the time it was given, the amount of time it was retained if it was expelled, the results or effects, and the response of the client.

---

### DEVELOPMENTAL CONSIDERATIONS

**Infants/Children**

* Obtain assistance to immobilize an infant or young child. ➤*Rationale: This prevents accidental injury due to sudden movement during the procedure.*
* For a child under 3 years, the nurse should use the gloved fifth finger for insertion. After this age, the index finger can usually be used.
* For a child or infant, insert a suppository 5 cm (2 in.) or less.

| UNEXPECTED OUTCOMES | CRITICAL THINKING OPTIONS |
|---|---|
| Client's chest discomfort is not relieved with ONE dose of sublingual nitroglycerin. | • Provide anticipatory instructions:<br>  • Check bottle for expiration date—potency is lost 3 months after opening bottle.<br>  • Recognize associated symptoms of acute MI such as dyspnea, nausea, cold sweat, lightheadedness (www.nhlbi.nih.gov/actintime).<br>  • Don't take a "wait and see" approach or deny symptoms indicative of acute MI. |
| Client's discomfort is not relieved with sublingual nitroglycerin. | • Check bottle for expiration date—potency is lost 3 months after opening bottle.<br>• Administer second tablet in 5 minutes—if discomfort continues, administer opiate analgesic, call Rapid Response Team, notify physician, and obtain stat ECG.<br>• Administer no more than three tablets/sprays in a 15-minute period.<br>• Monitor for blood pressure effect—hold medication if systolic BP is less than 90 mm Hg.<br>• Consult with physician for blood test for possible myocardial injury and need for continuous cardiac monitoring. |
| Client states that breathing has not improved after using inhaler. | • Place client in Fowler's position. Validate that MDI/spacer/NPA device is functioning properly (e.g., canister shaken before use).<br>• Check number of actuations left in MDI canister.<br>• Validate that client's lips have tight fit around MDI mouthpiece so mist is inhaled.<br>• Instruct client to hold breath 10 seconds after MDI use and to wait 2 minutes between puffs. |
| Client using MDI reports painful white patches in mouth. | • Instruct client to use spacer with MDI steroid medication.<br>• Instruct client to rinse mouth with water and expectorate after administering MDI steroid.<br>• Notify physician of findings. |
| Client fails to have BM post laxative suppository administration. | • Reassess abdomen and check client for rectal fecal impaction.<br>• Consult with physician to order oil-retention enema or cleansing enema.<br>• Teach client ways to prevent constipation. |
| Client is unable to retain vaginal suppository. | • Administer vaginal suppository at bedtime to prevent medication leakage. |

# Skill 12.43  Preparing Injections

## EXPECTED OUTCOMES

• Injection is administered without complications.
• Injection is as painless as possible.
• Medication therapeutic effect is achieved.

## Equipment

Medication in vial or ampule
Vial of compatible diluent (if necessary)
Syringe of closest capacity to hold medication
Appropriate size safety needle, filter needle for ampule medication
Antimicrobial wipes

## Procedure

1. Perform hand hygiene.
2. Obtain equipment.
3. Select the appropriate size needle, considering route, desired site, client's size, and viscosity of medication. ➤*Rationale: The larger the gauge number, the smaller the needle lumen.* Larger gauges produce less tissue trauma and are used for aqueous solutions. Smaller gauges are required for viscous solutions such as hormones.
4. Assemble the syringe and needle, maintaining sterility.
5. Fill syringe with medication or proceed to subsequent skills.

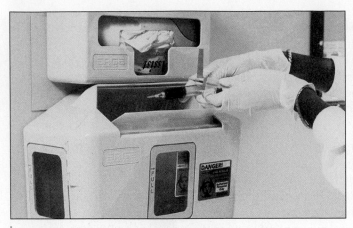

● Discard syringe in biohazard container following injection.

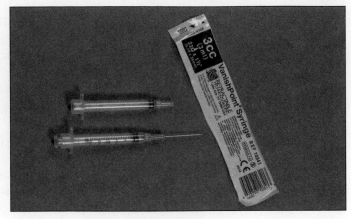

● Health care facilities must use safety needles to conform to needlestick safety legislation.

## For Withdrawing Medication from a Vial

1. Remove the vial cap.
2. Open antimicrobial wipe, and cleanse the rubber top of the vial. ➤*Rationale: Manufacturer does not guarantee sterility of rubber top.*
3. Tighten needle to syringe. Remove needle guard.

---

### CLINICAL ALERT

Federal needlestick safety legislation requires health care facilities to implement devices that protect against accidental needlesticks.

---

### SELECTING THE APPROPRIATE-SIZE NEEDLE

- Intradermal injections: 1 mL tuberculin syringe with short bevel, 25–27 gauge, 3/8–1/2 inch needle.
- Subcutaneous injections: 0.5–3 mL syringe with 25–29 gauge, 3/8–5/8 inch needle.
- Intramuscular injections: 1–5 mL syringe with needle gauge and length appropriate for muscle site and fat thickness; deltoid muscle requires 23–25 gauge, 5/8–1 inch needle; needle sizes for the vastus lateralis and gluteus muscles vary from 18 to 23 gauge, needle lengths, 1–1 1/2 inch.

---

### CLINICAL ALERT

Change needle before administering intramuscular medication that is irritating to tissue (e.g., Vistaril).

---

### EVIDENCE-BASED NURSING PRACTICE

**Needlestick Injuries**

Six percent of needlestick injuries involve safety devices with shielding, retracting, or blunting safety features. Most injuries occur after use and before disposal. In some cases, the protective features are not activated. Puncture-proof sharps disposal containers continue to play an important role in preventing injury.

*Source:* Jagger, J., & Perry, J. (2002). Realistic expectations for safety devices. *Nursing* 2002, 32(3), 72.

---

4. Pull back on plunger to fill syringe with an amount of air equal to amount of solution to be withdrawn. ➤*Rationale: The displacement of solution with air is necessary to prevent the formation of a vacuum in the sealed vial.*
5. Insert needle into upright vial. Inject air into vacant area of vial, keeping needle bevel above surface of medication. ➤*Rationale: Air creates positive pressure within vial, allowing accurate withdrawal of medication.*
6. Invert vial, and pull plunger to extract desired amount of medication. Touch only syringe barrel and plunger tip. ➤*Rationale: This prevents contamination of the plunger, inside of barrel, and medication.*
7. Expel any air bubbles from syringe at this time by tapping the side of syringe sharply with your finger or pen below the air bubble. ➤*Rationale: Air bubbles form in syringe due to dead air space in needle hub. Removing air bubbles while needle remains within the inverted vial avoids accidental contamination of needle and facilitates easy removal of air and accurate withdrawal of solution.*

8. Recheck amount of medication in syringe.
9. Turn vial to upright position and remove needle. ➤*Rationale: Removing needle from inverted vial may cause leaking of medication from needle insertion site.*
10. Replace needle guard using scoop method.
11. Recheck medication label and dosage against medication record and any dosage calculation. ➤*Rationale: This is a second safety check.*
12. Replace or dispose of medication vial, checking label once again. ➤*Rationale: This is a third safety check.*

### For Combining Medications in One Syringe Using Two Vials

1. Prepare both vials by removing caps and cleansing tops with separate antimicrobial wipes.
2. Draw air into syringe equal to amount of solution to be removed from second vial. Inject air into second vial. Do not withdraw medication at this time. ➤*Rationale: Air creates positive pressure within the vial, allowing withdrawal of solution.*
3. Draw air into syringe equal to amount of solution to be removed from first vial and inject it into first vial.
4. Invert first vial and withdraw ordered amount of medication without removing syringe.
5. Expel all air bubbles from syringe.
6. Recheck amount of solution and remove syringe from vial.
7. Insert needle into second vial, invert, and carefully withdraw exact amount of solution ordered. ➤*Rationale: Withdrawing excess solution from second vial results in an inaccurate dosage of medication. If this occurs, syringe must be discarded and procedure begun again.*

### For Withdrawing Medication from an Ampule

1. Move solution from neck to body of ampule by tapping stem sharply or holding neck of ampule between thumb and forefinger and flicking wrist.

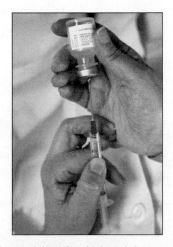

● Insert needle into upright vial and inject air into vacant area, keeping needle above surface of medication; then invert vial.

2. Using a pad, grasp neck (stem) of ampule between thumb and forefinger of one hand and grasp body of ampule with other hand. Break stem away from you. (If ampule is not scored, partially file neck of ampule.) ➤*Rationale: Gauze pad protects hands and breaking away from you prevents injury from glass fragments. Alternatively, slip a nipple from a baby bottle over the stem to prevent injury.*
3. Set the ampule upright. It is not necessary to add air prior to withdrawing the medication.
4. Use a special filter needle to withdraw solution, if indicated. ➤*Rationale: Filter needle prevents aspiration of glass when withdrawing solution from ampule.*
5. Remove needle guard and insert needle into ampule without touching sides of ampule. If needle is sufficiently long, medication may be withdrawn with ampule in upright position. When a short needle is

## TABLE 12-2 TYPES OF INJECTIONS

**Intradermal Injections**

- Injection sites: inner aspect of forearm or scapular area of back; upper chest, medial thigh.
- Purpose: to test for antigens (tubercle bacillus, allergens).
- Amount injected: ranges from 0.01 to 0.1 mL.
- Absorption rate: slow.

**Subcutaneous Injections**

- Injection sites: fatty tissue of abdomen, lateral and posterior aspects of upper arm or thigh, scapular area of back, upper ventrodorsal gluteal areas.
- Purpose: for medications that are absorbed slowly.
- Amount injected: variable—no more than 2 mL. If repeated doses are necessary, alter site accordingly.

**Intramuscular Injections**

- Purpose: to promote rapid absorption of the drug; to provide an alternate route when drug is irritating to subcutaneous tissues.
- Amount injected: variable—may be large amount of fluid. If more than 5 mL for adult or 3 mL for child and 1 mL for infant, divide dose into two syringes.
- Absorption rate: depends on circulatory state of client.
- Injection sites:

**Ventrogluteal Injection Site (preferred site for IM injection)**

Place client in side-lying position.
Use right hand for left anterior hip, or left hand for right anterior hip.
Identify greater trochanter and place palm at site.
Keep palm on greater trochanter and point index finger toward client's anterior superior iliac spine and fan out other three fingers.
Form "V" area with index finger separated from other three fingers.
Inject medication at 90° angle within "V" area.

**Dorsogluteal Injection Site (least desirable for IM injection)**

Place client in prone position.
Identify greater trochanter by placing hand on site.
Identify postero-superior spine (prominence) of iliac crest.
Draw imaginary line between greater trochanter and posterior superior iliac spine.
Locate injection site above imaginary line drawn between these two bony landmarks (this site will help to prevent injury to sciatic nerve).
Inject medication with long needle into dorsogluteal site at 90° angle.

**Vastus Lateralis Injection Site**

Place client in supine position with thigh exposed.
Identify greater trochanter and lateral femoral condyle.
Using middle third and anterior lateral aspect of thigh, select site.
Inject medication directly into muscle at 90° angle.

**Deltoid Injection Site (solution must be nonirritating)**

Expose client's upper arm.
Deltoid site is two fingerbreadths below acromion process.
Place left hand on acromion process and right index finger two fingerbreadths below.
Inject limited medication volume (0.5 to 1 mL) in deltoid IM site at 90° angle.

used, invert ampule and withdraw appropriate amount of medication. ➤*Rationale: Surface tension prevents solution from leaking out of inverted ampule.*

6. Return ampule to upright position and withdraw needle.
7. Tap syringe barrel below bubbles to dislodge air bubbles to hub of syringe.
8. Eject air with syringe in an upright position. If amount of solution is overdrawn, invert syringe and remove excess solution into a nearby receptacle.
9. Cover needle with guard, using scoop method.

### For Combining Medications Using Alternative Method

1. Draw up ordered dose from each vial or ampule into two separate syringes. First syringe must be able to hold entire volume of combined medications.
2. Remove needle from first syringe.
3. Pull back plunger of first syringe to allow space for volume of second medication to be added.
4. Insert needle of second syringe into hub of first syringe.
5. Slowly inject medication of second syringe through first syringe hub, then withdraw needle.
6. Attach new needle to first syringe.

7. Discard needles and second syringe.

### For Preparing Prefilled Medication Cartridge Syringe

1. Hold barrel of cartridge syringe (e.g., Tubex) in one hand and pull back on plunger with other hand.
2. Insert prefilled medication cartridge, needle first, into cartridge barrel.
3. Twist cartridge syringe flange clockwise until it is secure.
4. Screw plunger rod onto screw at bottom of medication cartridge until it fits firmly and tightly into rubber stopper.
5. Remove needle guard and any air bubbles.
6. Determine if dosage in cartridge is greater than required amount. If so, invert Tubex and gently expel excess medication, being careful to maintain sterility of needle. ➤*Rationale: If permanent needle is contaminated, the cartridge becomes contaminated and must be discarded.*
7. Replace needle guard, using scoop method.

## Skill 12.44   Administering Intradermal Injections

### Equipment

Medication (e.g., 0.1 mL Purified Protein Derivative Antigen for tuberculin testing)
Unit dose (1 mL) tuberculin syringe with 1/4–3/8″ 27-gauge needle
Antimicrobial wipes
Gauze pads
Clean gloves (if indicated)
Pen to mark injection site

### Procedure

1. Take prepared injection to client's room, checking room and bed number against client's medication record.
2. Check client's identaband and ask client to state name and birth date.
3. Explain procedure and purpose to client.
4. Perform hand hygiene and don gloves if exposure anticipated.

5. Select lesion-free injection site on undersurface, upper third of forearm for skin testing.
6. Cleanse area with antimicrobial wipe and allow to dry.
7. Remove needle guard.
8. Grasp the client's dorsal forearm to gently pull the skin taut on ventral forearm.
9. Holding syringe almost parallel to skin, insert needle at a 10°–15°angle with bevel facing up, about ⅛ inch. Needle point should be visible under skin. DO NOT ASPIRATE.
10. Inject medication slowly, observing for a wheal (blister) formation and blanching at the site.
    ➤*Rationale: This indicates that the medication was injected within the dermis. If no wheal develops, injection was given too deeply.*
11. Withdraw needle at same angle as inserted. Pat area gently with dry gauze pad but DO NOT MASSAGE.
    ➤*Rationale: Massaging could disperse medication.*

12. Activate needle safety feature and discard syringe unit in puncture proof container.
13. Mark injection site with pen for future assessment.
14. Return client to comfortable position.
15. Dispose of gloves and perform hand hygiene.
16. Record site and antigen in client's record.

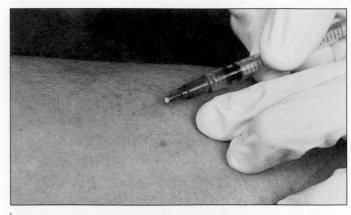

● Insert needle with bevel up for intradermal injection.

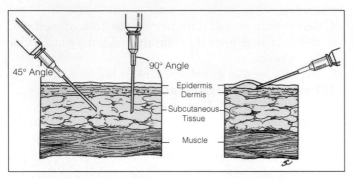

Insert needle at 45° or 90° angle into tissue for subcutaneous injection.

Insert needle at 15° angle just under the epidermis for intradermal injection.

## CLINICAL ALERT

For tuberculin testing, instruct client to return and have the site checked by the health care provider in 48 to 72 hours.

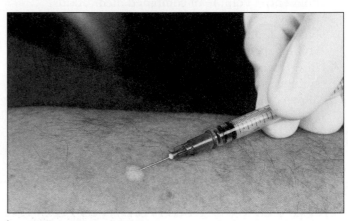

● Inject solution to form wheal on skin.

# Skill 12.45  Administering Subcutaneous Injections

## Equipment

Nonirritating medication
3-mL syringe with 5/8-inch needle (usual 25–27 gauge)
Antimicrobial wipes
Clean gloves if indicated

## Procedure

1. Take prepared injection to client's room, checking room and bed number against client's medication record.
2. Check client's identaband and ask client to state name and birth date.
3. Explain procedure and purpose to client.
4. Perform hand hygiene and don gloves.
5. Select fatty site for injection (e.g., abdomen, avoiding 2-inch radius around umbilicus), alternating sites for each injection. ➤*Rationale: This prevents repeated trauma to tissue.*

6. Cleanse area with antimicrobial wipe.
7. Remove needle guard.
8. Use thumb and forefinger and gently grasp loose area ("pinch an inch") of fatty tissue on appropriate site (e.g., posterior-lateral aspect, middle third of arm.) ➤*Rationale: This ensures insertion of medication within subcutaneous tissue, not muscle.*

*Note: Spreading the skin is acceptable when there is substantial fatty tissue.*

9. Hold syringe like a dart between the thumb and forefinger.
10. Insert needle at a 45° or 90° angle. A 90° angle is used more commonly due to short needles on prepackaged syringes. ➤*Rationale: Angle varies with the amount of subcutaneous tissue, selected site, and needle length.*

## GLOVING PROTOCOL FOR INJECTIONS

The CDC has no regulations concerning the wearing of gloves during injections. OSHA recommends that gloves are not necessary when administering IM or subcutaneous injections, as long as bleeding that could result in hand contact with blood (or other potentially infectious material) is not anticipated.

The practice of whether or not to wear gloves for subcutaneous or IM injections is in transition. Therefore, each hospital policy should dictate gloving protocol for injections.

If wearing gloves for mass inoculations, nurses must change gloves between clients and perform hand hygiene. Therefore, nurses may choose not to wear gloves in these situations (OSHA & CDC).

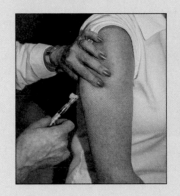
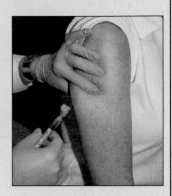

11. Continue to hold tissue and aspirate by pulling back on plunger with thumb of dominant hand. If no blood appears, administer injection. If blood appears, withdraw needle, activate safety feature and discard, then prepare a new injection. ➤*Rationale: Blood indicates needle has entered a blood vessel. Injecting the drug IV may be dangerous.*
12. Inject medication slowly.
13. Wait 10 seconds, then withdraw needle quickly and activate needle safety feature.
14. Release tissue and massage area with swab (if indicated). ➤*Rationale: Massaging area aids absorption.*

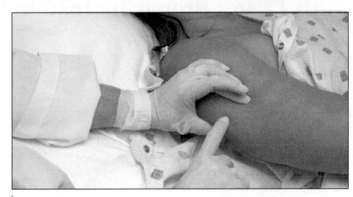

● Select site on lateral aspect of mid-upper arm for subcutaneous injection.

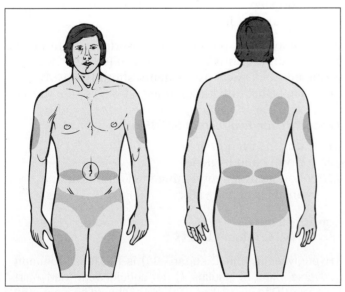

● Sites for subcutaneous injections given routinely. (Avoid umbilicus area.) Abdomen site preferred.

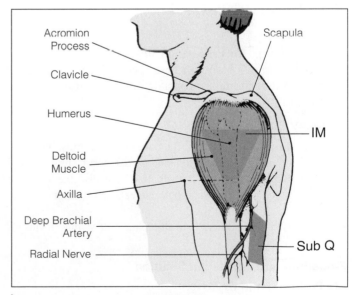

● Use upper shaded triangle for IM injection in upper arm; use lower shaded area for subcutaneous injection.

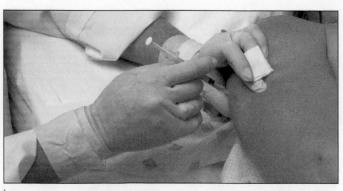

● Insert needle at 45° or 90° angle, using short needle for subcutaneous injection.

15. Discard needle/syringe unit in puncture-proof container.
16. Return client to position of comfort.
17. Discard gloves and perform hand hygiene.
18. Record medication and site used.

# Skill 12.46 Preparing Insulin Injections

## Equipment

Insulin(s) vials

Unopened vials of insulin should be stored in refrigerator

Opened vial of insulin may be refrigerated or kept at room temperature; recommend discard after 28 days

Insulin should not be exposed to light, or to temperatures over 80°F.

Do not use insulin that has clumping, frosting, or precipitation

Insulin syringe: available in 3/10 mL, 1/2mL, and 1 mL sizes (Note: syringes no longer called U40, U100, etc.)

Needles: 29–31 gauge short needles

Antimicrobial swabs

Clean gloves if indicated

## Preparation

1. Follow steps for Preparing Injections.
2. Obtain client's blood glucose level prior to preparation to determine appropriate administration of insulin.

### For Newly Diagnosed Diabetic Client

   a. Explain to client that the dose of insulin must be adjusted according to blood glucose test results.
   b. Explain that there is a variation in levels—the lowest blood glucose level is before meals and highest 1–2 hours after meals.
   c. Goal of treatment is to eliminate wide swings in glucose levels.

## Procedure for One Insulin Solution

1. Perform hand hygiene.
2. Turn intermediate or long-acting (cloudy) insulin vial top-to-bottom eight to 10 times. ➤*Rationale:* This brings cloudy insulin solution into suspension. Clear insulins do not require this.

3. Wipe top of insulin bottle with antimicrobial swab.
4. Remove needle guard and place on tray.
5. Pull plunger of syringe down to desired amount of medication (e.g., 12 units). Inject amount of air into air space, not into insulin solution. ➤*Rationale: Injecting air directly into insulin solution causes bubbles.*
6. Withdraw ordered amount of insulin into syringe.
7. Validate medication record, insulin bottle, and prepared syringe with an RN for accuracy. ➤*Rationale: Double checking insulin helps safeguard against errors.*
8. Remove needle from vial and expel air from syringe.
9. Replace needle guard.
10. Take medication to client's room.
11. Follow steps for administration of medications by subcutaneous injection.

*Note:* Some clients prefer to reuse syringes until needle becomes dull. This is practical and safe if the needle is recapped after each use. Clients should consult their physician before initiating syringe reuse.

### Procedure for Two Insulin Solutions

1. Check medication orders.
2. Perform hand hygiene.
3. Follow steps for combining medications in one syringe using two vials.

## CLINICAL ALERT

Do not shake insulin vial, as this destroys insulin potency. Rolling the vial fails to bring insulin into suspension. Turn the vial top to bottom several times instead.

4. Turn cloudy intermediate insulin Bottle (A)top to bottom 8–10 times. ➤*Rationale: This brings cloudy solution into suspension.*
5. Wipe top of both insulin bottles with alcohol.
6. Take needle guard off and place on tray.
7. Pull plunger of syringe down to desired total units of insulin.
8. Insert needle and inject prescribed amount of air into Bottle A (cloudy) insulin.
9. Inject air into insulin Bottle B and withdraw medication. ➤*Rationale: Withdrawing clear insulin first prevents inadvertent injection of intermediate-acting insulin into rapid- or short-acting insulin bottle, which would slow its rapid action.*
10. Double check your preparations with another nurse.
11. Withdraw needle from bottle and expel all air bubbles.
12. Invert Bottle A and insert needle. Take care not to inject any rapid or short-acting (clear) insulin into

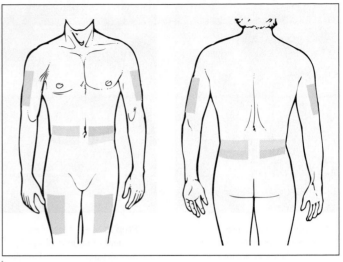

● The abdomen is the preferred site for insulin injection as absorption is more predictable. Other subcutaneous sites may be used if desired.

## CLINICAL ALERT

Do not massage site following injection of certain drugs such as insulin or heparin because this hastens absorption and drug action and may cause tissue irritation.

### TABLE 12–3  INSULIN TYPES AND THERAPEUTIC ACTION (IN MINUTES/HOURS*)

| Types | Onset | Peak | Duration |
|---|---|---|---|
| **Rapid-acting (clear solution)**<br>Humalog® (Lispro)<br>NovoLog® (Aspart) | 5–15 min | 60–90 min | 3–5 hrs |
| **Short-acting (clear solution)**<br>Novolin R<br>Humulin R | 0.5–1 hr | 2–4 hrs | 5–7 hrs |
| **Intermediate-acting (cloudy solution)**<br>Humulin N (NPH)<br>Novolin N (NPH) | 1–2 hrs<br>2 hrs | 6–12 hrs<br>6–8 hrs | 16–24 hrs<br>16–22 hrs |
| **Mixtures (cloudy solution)**<br>Humulin 70/30 (70% NPH, 30% Regular)<br>Novolin 70/30 (70% NPH, 30% Regular)<br>Humulin 50/50 (50% NPH, 50% Regular)<br>Humalog 75/25 (75% lispro protamine suspension, 25% lispro) | 30 min<br><br>15 min | 2–12 hrs<br><br>1 hr | 24 hrs<br><br>24 hrs |
| **Long-acting**<br>Lantus (glargine) (*clear solution*) | 4–6 hrs | no peak | 24 hrs |

*The time of insulin action may vary significantly in different clients, and in the same client at different times.

Insulin is biologically engineered through the process of recombinant-DNA technology. Insulin is produced by different companies who use different names for short, intermediate, or long acting forms of insulin or their mixtures.

NPH = neutral protamine Hagedorn

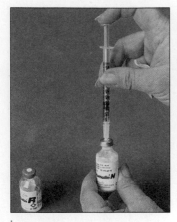

● **Step 1:** Inject prescribed amount of air into intermediate-acting (cloudy) insulin vial—withdraw needle without needle touching solution.

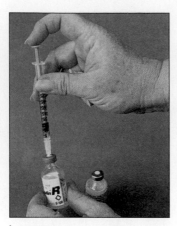

● **Step 2:** Inject prescribed amount of air into rapid- or short-acting (clear) insulin vial. Do not withdraw needle.

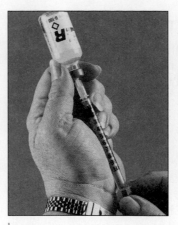

● **Step 3:** Invert vial of rapid or short-acting insulin; withdraw prescribed amount of medication and withdraw needle from vial.

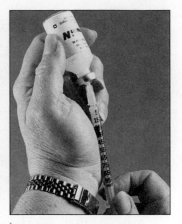

● **Step 4:** Invert intermediate-acting insulin vial and withdraw exact amount without injecting insulin into bottle.

### CLINICAL ALERT

The IV route is superior for administering sliding scale insulin to an obese client. Adipose tissue slows onset of insulin action.

### CLINICAL ALERT

Long-acting insulin, LANTUS (glargine), is a clear solution. It is not to be mixed with any other type of insulin or solution. It is given subcutaneously and is not intended for IV use.

### PREMIXING TYPES OF INSULIN

- Mixtures of rapid acting (Humalog) and intermediate or long acting insulin should be administered within 10 minutes before a meal.
- Mixtures of NPH and regular (short acting) insulin should be administered 20 to 30 minutes prior to a meal.
- Mixtures may be stored in refrigerator for up to 30 days and should be gently resuspended prior to injection.

### CLINICAL ALERT

Insulin type and brand should remain consistent for an individual client.

● Double check insulin dose with a second nurse to help prevent errors in preparation.

intermediate-acting (cloudy) insulin bottle. This can be avoided by holding steady pressure on plunger when inserting needle into bottle.

13. Pull back on plunger to obtain exact prescribed amount of intermediate or long-acting insulin. The total insulin dose now includes both the clear insulin, previously drawn up into syringe, and the intermediate cloudy insulin you have just drawn up.

14. Withdraw needle from bottle and replace needle guard.

15. Follow protocol for administration of medications by subcutaneous injections.

## EVIDENCE-BASED NURSING PRACTICE

**The Importance of Double Checking Drug Dose**

- Double checks have revealed that up to 4.2% of prescriptions are filled erroneously.
- Double checks help the nurse identify mistakes which are difficult for someone alone to recognize.

- Double checks work best when each nurse calculates desired dosages independently rather than having another nurse "verify" what has been prepared.

*Source:* Cohen, M. (2002). Double checking for errors. *Nursing 2002,* 32(3), 18.

## Skill 12.47  Teaching Client to Use Insulin Delivery System— Insulin Pen

### Equipment

Delivery device: Prefilled pen or cartridge with correct insulin type with instructions for use
Compatible needle
Antimicrobial swab

*Note:* Insulin "pens" contain a pre-filled multidose cartridge. The appropriate dose (units) is dialed before injection. Some "pens" are disposable, some are refillable for reuse. Some have a magnified dose window and some have sound clicks for each unit of insulin dialed.

### Preparation

1. Perform hand hygiene; identify client.
2. Review device instructions with the client.
3. Have client perform hand hygiene.
4. Instruct client to perform steps below.

### Procedure

1. Remove pen cap and insert insulin cartridge if indicated.
2. Turn pen up and down at least 10 times. *➤Rationale: This creates suspension of cloudy insulin.*

3. Remove needle cap and attach sterile needle immediately before injecting.
4. Prime insulin pen by pulling dose knob out in direction of arrow until a "0" appears in the dose window. *➤Rationale: A dose cannot be dialed until the dose knob is pulled out.*
5. Dial 2 units, then push plunger and repeat until drop of insulin appears at tip of needle. *➤Rationale: This removes air and ensures proper dosing.* This may require six "air shots" for the Innolet.
6. Dial required number of insulin units to be injected.
7. Swab injection site.
8. Pinch up skin, insert needle, and release skin before injection.
9. Press pen/device "push button" completely and keep depressed, counting to 6 before removing needle from skin.
10. Do not massage the area.
11. Remove needle from pen/device and dispose in sharps container.
12. Replace pen/device cap and store according to directions.

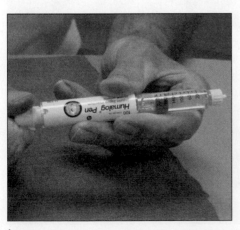

● Dial required number of insulin units to be injected.

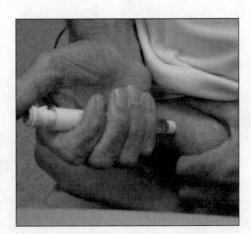

● Pinch skin, insert needle, and release skin before injecting.

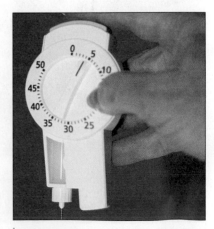

● Dial-a-dose delivery system includes a 3mL disposable prefilled syringe.

# Skill 12.48 Teaching Use of Insulin Pump

## Equipment

Insulin pump (Many types are available)

Insulin syringe

Infusion sets (e.g., Sof-Set catheter, bent and straight needles with 24–42-inch plastic tubing)

Batteries

Insertion device (e.g., Sof-Serter)

Skin prep (alcohol, Betadine, or Hibiclens)

Adhesive (Polyskin, Opsite, or Tegaderm dressing)

Humalog or NovoLog or Humulin R or Novolin Rinsulin

*Note:* There are two rapid-acting human insulin analogs: Humalog®(Lispro) and NovoLog®(Aspart). The timing of these insulins more closely resembles the way the body makes insulin when food is ingested. This type of insulin works faster and has a shorter duration of action.

## Procedure

1. Inform client of advantages of using Continuous Subcutaneous Insulin Infusion (CSII) with an insulin pump. ►*Rationale: In teaching a new method, this enhances acceptance.*

    a. CSII is a form of intensive insulin therapy used to optimize glycemic control and prevent or slow the progression of complications of diabetes.

> ## CLINICAL ALERT
>
> Insulin pump management and education should be done by a registered nurse certified in insulin pump therapy in collaboration with a physician.

> ## CLINICAL ALERT
>
> Hyperglycemia leading to diabetic ketoacidosis is the greatest risk associated with insulin pump therapy.

    b. CSII more closely mimics release of insulin by the pancreas with continuous delivery basal and bolus insulin infusion.

    - Basal: amount of insulin delivered hourly in attempt to maintain blood glucose.

    - Bolus: amount of insulin delivered immediately prior to meals or for episodes of hyperglycemia.

    c. Lifestyle advantages: flexibility; client does not have to strictly adjust meal time, exercise, or sleep schedules to coincide with peak action time of an intermediate insulin, since only rapid-acting or short-acting insulin is used.

    d. Less risk of severe hypoglycemia compared with multiple daily injections.

    e. Children as young as 2 years are now using the insulin pump.

*Note:* Continuous Subcutaneous Insulin Infusion (CSII) is a form of intensive insulin therapy utilized as an alternative to multiple daily injection for some individuals in an attempt to achieve optimal glycemic control. Insulin pumps are manufactured by a company that provides 24-hour emergency and technical information: MiniMed Technologies, Sylmar, CA (1-800-826-2099). All models are battery-powered and deliver basal and bolus doses.

2. Client selection criteria.

    a. Requires conscientious client or child committed to wear pump 24 hours per day and perform multiple daily blood glucose monitoring.

● Infusion set is primed with rapid-acting or short-acting insulin.

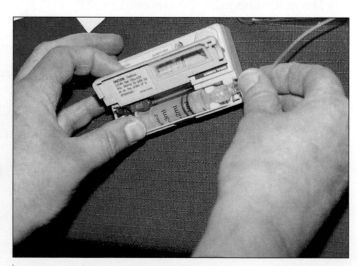

● Position syringe securely in pump.

b. Requires motivated client or child to accept greater levels of responsibility for self-care and problem-solving with CSII.

c. Availability of supportive caregiver and health care team with expertise in CSII therapy.

3. Teach client and/or caregiver how to operate insulin pump.

a. Provide instructional materials on insulin pump operation (literature and video tape tutorials available through manufacturer).

b. Instruct client on basic modalities of pump operation and programming steps (varies with model of pump).

c. Basal rate can be set in 0.1 unit increments every hour of the day and night.

d. Bolus doses can be given before meals.

e. Alarms notify client if reservoir is empty, catheter obstructed, battery "Low," or pump malfunctioning.

f. While meal timing is more flexible, review necessity of self-monitoring blood glucose before meals, bedtime, and at 0300. Additional testing is necessary for insulin dose adjustments, illness, and physical exercise. ➤*Rationale: Frequent monitoring assists proper dosage of bolus and basal rates.*

4. Instruct client on preparation of insulin infusion set.

a. Filling of reservoir/cartridge (every 72 hours or more frequently if client is on larger doses of insulin) and proper priming and placement into pump. ➤*Rationale: Changing at the same time every day establishes a routine.*

b. Selection and preparation of infusion site (abdomen is preferred site for insertion as insulin absorption is faster and more predictable due to less physical movement). Avoid areas around waistline and pantline and 1 inch from umbilicus. New insertion site should be 1–2 inches away from previous site.

c. Proper insertion of catheter-over-needle or needle.

d. Application of sterile dressing.

e. Rotation of sites and changing of catheter or needle every 72 hours. Instruct client to observe for signs of redness, tenderness, and drainage on daily basis. Reinforce to change site with new infusion set, to alternate site, and to report problems promptly to health care provider. ➤*Rationale: To prevent site problem and to ensure uniform insulin absorption.*

f. Reinforce monitoring blood glucose 3 hours after insertion and/or removal of catheter/needle. ➤*Rationale: Suspect improper insertion of catheter/needle, or accidental removal if blood glucose is 240 mg/dL with two sequential testings.*

5. Instruct client in self-management skills for episodes of acute complications of diabetes.

a. HYPOGLYCEMIA (e.g., due to physical exercise or a missed meal) = temporary stopping of insulin infusion and changes in basal/bolus rates. (See Alert.)

b. HYPERGLYCEMIA (e.g., due to sick day) = increases of basal/bolus rates.

c. Fasting states (e.g., surgery, diagnostic testing) = adjustments in basal/bolus rates as needed.

d. Instruct client to carry backup batteries, insulin, infusion sets and insulin syringes, and at least 15 g carbohydrate to be taken in event of hypoglycemic reaction.

e. Instruct client to be familiar with pump alarms and interventions for troubleshooting.

f. Instruct client to wear Med-Alert bracelet and carry medical identification, emergency phone number of health care professionals, and 24-hour emergency hotline phone number of pump manufacturer for technical support.

g. Inform client to remove pump before exposure to x-rays, MRIs, and CAT scans and have hospital personnel place pump in alternative room.

h. Advise client to avoid submersion of insulin pump in water (e.g., swimming, showering). ➤*Rationale: Not all models of insulin pumps are waterproof.*

6. Instruct client on cleaning and maintenance of pump and how to order additional supplies.

7. Provide resources for client: community insulin pump support groups, educational literature, Internet information provided online by manufacturer.

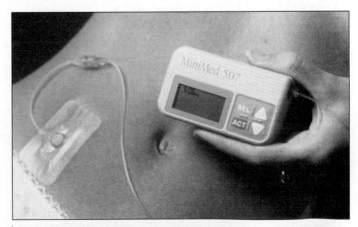

● MiniMed 507 Insulin Pump attached to fusion set. Abdominal site is preferred because insulin absorption is faster and most predictable.

# Skill 12.49 Administering Subcutaneous Anticoagulants (Heparin, LMWH, Arixtra)

## Equipment

Heparin in vial *(carefully note units per mL)*
1 mL tuberculin syringe or unit dose syringe with small (25–29) gauge needle
*or*
Low-molecular-weight heparin or Arixtra in prefilled syringe
Antimicrobial swabs
Gloves if indicated

## Preparation

1. See Preparing Injections.
2. Double check heparin calculated dose with another nurse.
3. Place client in supine position.
4. Perform hand hygiene.

*Note:* Some facilities advocate adding air to syringe to create air lock. ➤*Rationale: Prevents tracking of medication on skin and decreases bruising.* (To avoid loss of drug, do not clear prefilled syringe needle of air before injecting LMWH or Arixtra.)

## Procedure

1. Take prepared injection to client's room, check room and bed number against client's MAR.
2. Check client's identaband, and ask client to state name and birth date.
3. Provide privacy.
4. Explain procedure and purpose to client.
5. Don gloves.
6. Select site on client's lower abdomen (at least two fingerbreadths from umbilicus) or select area of fatty tissue above iliac crest. ➤*Rationale: Heparin should not be administered IM or in the extremities.*
7. Avoid ecchymotic area or lesions.
8. Cleanse site gently with antimicrobial swab, and allow to dry.
9. Gently pinch an inch of subcutaneous tissue (fat roll) between thumb and forefinger of nondominant hand and hold fat pad throughout injection.

> ### CLINICAL ALERT
>
> Heparin is available in a variety of strengths (e.g., 1000, 2500, 5000, 10,000, 25,000 units per mL vials). Carefully check vial units per mL before drawing into syringe and have another nurse double-check your calculations and prepared injection.

> ### CLINICAL ALERT
>
> Subcutaneous injection of low-molecular-weight heparin (LMWH) *or Arixtra* involves low doses that help prevent clot formation but do not alter blood coagulation studies and do not require coagulation monitoring as does unfractionated heparin. Prefilled syringe administration is less time-consuming.

10. Hold syringe between thumb and forefinger of dominant hand and insert full length of needle into skinfold at a 90° angle.
11. Inject medication slowly without aspirating first. ➤*Rationale: Aspiration can rupture small vessels and increase risk of bleeding into tissue.*

*Note:* Press prefilled syringe plunger rod firmly as far as it will go.

12. Wait 10 seconds before gently withdrawing needle at same angle in which it entered skin. ➤*Rationale: This allows heparin to absorb into tissue and minimizes bruising.*

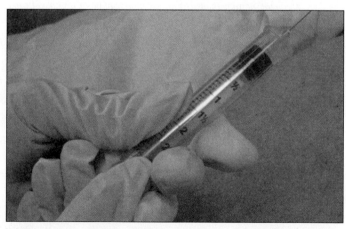

● Activate needle safety feature; then, dispose of syringe in sharps container.

> ### CLINICAL ALERT
>
> To prevent tissue damage and bruising, do not aspirate or massage anticoagulant injections.

*Note:* Release of Arixtra plunger will cause needle to retract into the security sleeve as it automatically withdraws from the skin.

13. Press and hold swab over injection site. ➤*Rationale: This prevents back-tracking of medication.*
14. Do not massage area. ➤*Rationale: This may cause bruising.*

15. Activate needle safety feature and discard syringe in puncture-proof container.
16. Return client to position of comfort.
17. Remove gloves and perform hand hygiene.
18. Document injection.

# Skill 12.50   Administering Intramuscular (IM) Injections

### Equipment

Medication vial or ampule
3-mL syringe with 1–1 1/2 inch needle (21–23 gauge)
2 antimicrobial swabs
Gloves if indicated

### Preparation

See Preparing Injections.

### Procedure

1. Check client's record for site of previous IM injections. ➤*Rationale: IM injections should be rotated to prevent local post injection complications.*
2. Take prepared injection to client's room. Check room number against client's MAR.
3. Check client's identaband, and have client state name and birth date.
4. Explain procedure to client.
5. Provide privacy for client.
6. Perform hand hygiene and don gloves if indicated.

7. Select injection site, identifying landmarks. Consider client's size, amount and viscosity of medications being injected. Alternate sites each time injections are given.

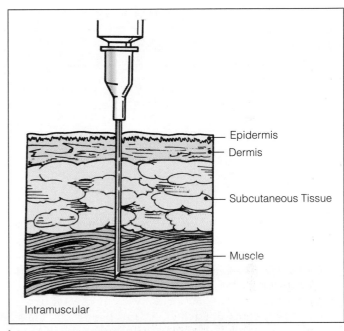

Epidermis
Dermis
Subcutaneous Tissue
Muscle
Intramuscular

● Insert needle at 90° angle for IM injections into muscle.

## CLINICAL ALERT

Ventrogluteal site is safer and preferred over dorsogluteal whenever possible, because dorsogluteal area is especially vulnerable to nerve and vascular injury.

## TECHNIQUES FOR MINIMIZING PAIN DURING IM INJECTIONS

- Encourage client to relax.
- If medication is irritating, use a new needle for injection.
- Place client on side with upper knee flexed for ventrogluteal, or flat on abdomen with toes turned inward for dorsogluteal injection.
- Avoid injecting into sensitive or hardened tissue.
- Compress tissue at injection site.
- Ensure that needle length reaches muscle for IM injection.
- Prevent antiseptic from clinging to needle during insertion by waiting until skin prep is dry.

- Reduce puncture pain by "darting" needle quickly into muscle.
- Use as small a gauge needle as possible.
- Inject medication slowly.
- Maintain grasp on syringe; do not move needle once inserted.
- Withdraw needle quickly after injection.
- Use Z-track technique.
- EMLA cream may be applied 30 to 40 minutes prior to injection.

8. Cleanse area with antimicrobial swab and allow to dry.

9. Spread skin taut between thumb and forefinger (grasping muscle is acceptable in pediatric and geriatric clients with less fatty tissue) to ensure needle placement in muscle belly.

10. Insert needle at a 90° angle to the muscle, using a quick, darting motion. ➤*Rationale: This angle facilitates medication reaching muscle.*

11. Pull back on plunger; if blood returns, discard and prepare a new injection. ➤*Rationale: The appearance of blood indicates needle has entered a blood vessel, and medication injected directly into bloodstream may be dangerous.*

12. Inject medication slowly. ➤*Rationale: This allows time for medication to disperse through tissue.*

13. Withdraw needle quickly, and massage area with antimicrobial swab.

14. Activate needle safety feature.

15. Dispose of syringe/needle unit in puncture-proof container.

16. Return client to comfortable position.

17. Discard gloves and perform hand hygiene.

18. Chart medication and site of injection.

## VARIATION: Ventrogluteal Injection Site

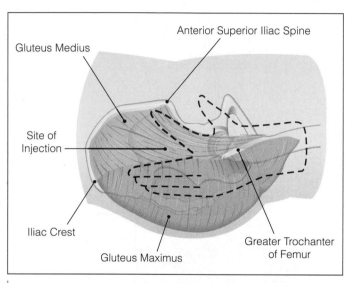

● Overlay of hand shows area of injection into ventrogluteal site for IM injections (client's right side)

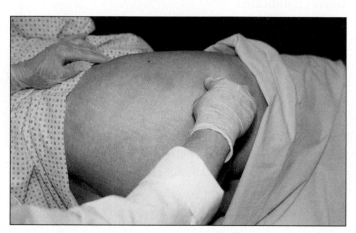

● Locate greater trochanter and anterior superior iliac spine.

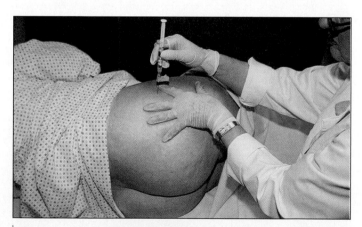

● Place palm at trochanter and index finger at anterior superior iliac spine; fan remaining fingers posteriorly.

## VARIATION: Dorsogluteal Injection Site

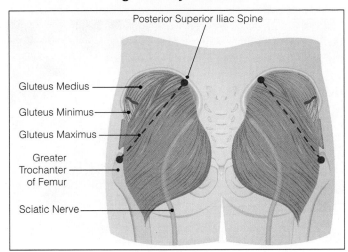

Posterior Superior Iliac Spine

Gluteus Medius

Gluteus Minimus

Gluteus Maximus

Greater Trochanter of Femur

Sciatic Nerve

- Place injection above and outside diagonal line for dorsogluteal injection.

### CLINICAL ALERT

Do not use the upper outer quadrant of the buttocks to identify the dorsogluteal injection site. The buttocks include fat tissue that extends well below the gluteal muscle and varies significantly among individuals. Intersecting vertical and horizontal lines on the buttocks can easily include the sciatic nerve and major blood vessels in the upper outer quadrant, possibly exposing them to serious and permanent injury if an injection is placed there.

### CLINICAL ALERT

Chemical injury to the sciatic nerve can occur even with injection of irritating medications near the nerve. To avoid sciatic nerve injury, locate dorsogluteal injection site above imaginary line drawn between two bony landmarks.

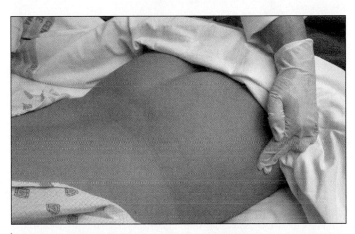

- Locate greater trochanter to identify dorsogluteal site.

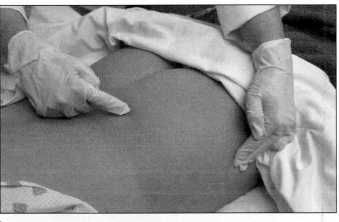

- Locate posterosuperior spine of iliac crest to identify dorsogluteal site.

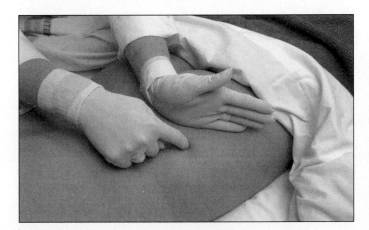

- Draw imaginary line between greater trochanter and posterior superior iliac spine.

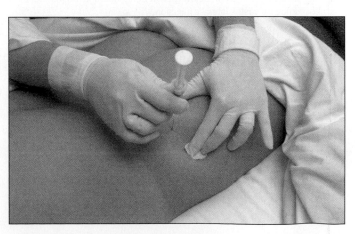

- Inject medication directly into dorsogluteal site at 90° angle.

## VARIATION: Vastus Lateralis Injection Site

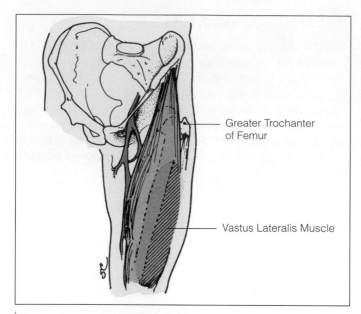

Greater Trochanter
of Femur

Vastus Lateralis Muscle

● Shaded area indicates site location for vastus lateralis injection.

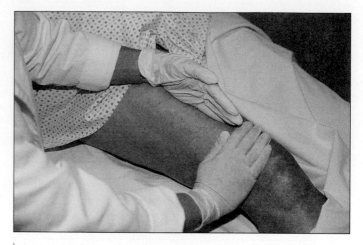

● Site is middle third and anterior lateral aspect of thigh.

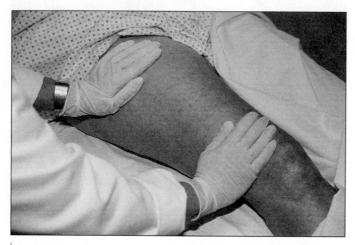

● Select site 1 hand breadth below greater trochanter and 1 hand breadth above knee for vastus lateralis injection.

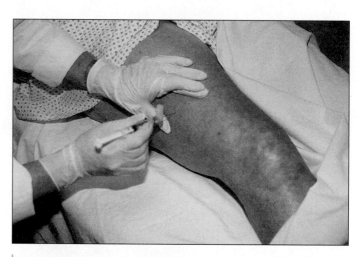

● Inject medication at 90° angle directly into muscle.

## VARIATION: Deltoid IM Injection Site

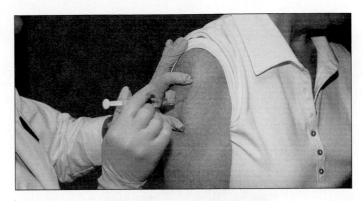

● Inject medication into deltoid area site.

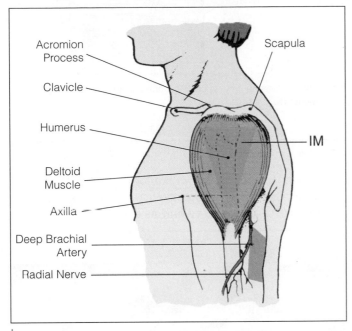

● Locate deltoid site on outer lateral aspect of upper arm.

## EVIDENCE-BASED NURSING PRACTICE

**Choose the Right Needle Size**

A 5/8-inch needle won't reach deltoid muscle in 17% of men and 50% of women. A 1-inch needle is better for men (130–260 lb) and women (132–198 lb).

*Source:* Zucherman, J. (2000, November 18). The importance of injecting vaccines into muscle. *British Medical Journal.*

# Skill 12.51 Using Z-Track Method

## Equipment

Syringe
2 needles (one 2-inch needle)
Medication
Antimicrobial swabs
Gloves

## Preparation

See Preparing Injections.

## Procedure

1. Gather equipment.
2. Draw up prescribed medication into syringe.
3. Attach new 2-inch sterile needle to syringe.
   ➤*Rationale: A new needle prevents introducing medication that could be irritating to tissue. A long needle allows medication to go deep into the muscle.*
4. Take medication to client's room; check room number against MAR.
5. Check identaband, and ask client to state name.
6. Provide privacy.
7. Explain procedure and purpose to client.
8. Perform hand hygiene and don gloves.
9. Place client in prone position, if possible. ➤*Rationale: This position provides the best perspective for identifying dorsogluteal landmarks: posterosuperior iliac crest and greater trochanter.*
10. Cleanse site with antimicrobial wipe.
11. Pull skin 1–1 1/2 inch laterally away from injection site. ➤*Rationale: This tissue displacement creates a track that keeps medication from seeping into subcutaneous tissue.*
12. Maintain displacement and insert needle at a 90° angle. Aspirate by pulling back on plunger to see if needle is in blood vessel. If so, discard and prepare new injection.
13. Inject medication and air bubble slowly and wait 10 seconds keeping skin taut. ➤*Rationale: Permits muscle relaxation and absorption of medication.*
14. Withdraw needle and release retracted skin.
   ➤*Rationale: Lateral tissue displacement interrupts needle track and seals medication in the muscle when the tissue is released.*

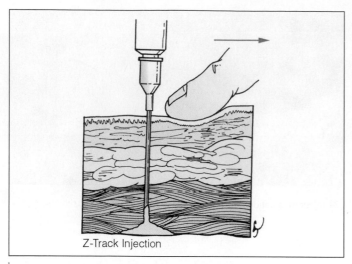

Z-Track Injection

● Z-Track Injection

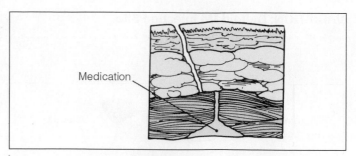

Medication

● Z-track is used to prevent backflow of medications into subcutaneous tissue.

## Z-TRACK IM SITE

Z-track technique is appropriate for any VG or DG intramuscular site. The ventrogluteal site is preferred; dorsogluteal site should be used only as a last resort.

15. Apply light pressure with swab. Do not massage. ➤*Rationale: Massage may disperse medication into subcutaneous tissue and cause tissue irritation.*
16. Activate needle safety feature.
17. Return client to a position of comfort and safety.
18. Discard gloves and equipment in appropriate area.
19. Perform hand hygiene.
20. Document administration of medications in the medication record.

## CLINICAL ALERT

The Z-track method prevents "tracking" and is used for administering medications that are especially irritating to subcutaneous and nerve tissue (e.g., imferon or Vistaril).

## CLINICAL ALERT

If client is obese, use a 2–3-inch needle so that medication is absorbed into muscle (not fat) tissue and blood level of drug is achieved.

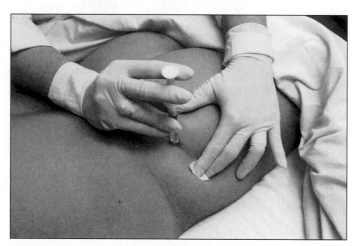

● Maintaining displacement, insert needle at 90° angle. Aspirate by pulling back on plunger, checking to see if needle is in blood vessel. If blood is aspirated, discard and prepare new injection.

## TABLE 12-4 LIST OF ABBREVIATIONS AND SYMBOLS

| | | | |
|---|---|---|---|
| aa | of each | oob | out of bed |
| a.c. | before meals | os | mouth |
| ad lib. | freely, as desired | oz | ounce |
| b.i.d. | twice each day | p.c. | after meals |
| c | with | per | by, through |
| C | carbon | PO | by mouth |
| Ca | calcium | prn, or PRN | whenever necessary |
| Cl | chlorine | q.h. | every hour |
| dr or 3 | dram | q.i.d. | four times each day |
| et | and | q.s. | as much as required, quantity sufficient |
| GI | gastrointestinal | q2h | every 2 hours |
| gt or gtt | drop(s) | q3h | every 3 hours |
| $H_2O$ | water | q4h | every 4 hours |
| $H_2O_2$ | hydrogen peroxide | RX | treatment, "take thou" |
| IM | intramuscular | S | without |
| K | potassium | STAT | immediately |
| lb or # | pound | t.i.d. | three times each day |
| m | meter | tsp | teaspoon |
| mcg | microgram | WBC | white blood count |
| mEq | milliequivalent | ° | degree |
| mg | milligram | − | minus, negative, alkaline reaction |
| mL | milliliter | + | plus, positive, acid reaction |
| mmol | millimole | % | percent |
| Na | sodium | v | Roman numeral 5 |
| NA | not applicable | vii | Roman numeral 7 |
| NG | nasogastric | ix | Roman numeral 9 |
| NPO | nothing by mouth | xiii | Roman numeral 13 |

## ABBREVIATION ALERT

**(Abbreviations to avoid: entries marked \* are prohibited by the JCAHO)**

@ (at) misinterpreted as a 2. Write out "at."

AU (each ear) misinterpreted as OU (each eye). Do not use AU. Also avoid AD (right ear) and AS (left ear).

cc (cubic centimeter) misinterpreted as units. Write "mL" for milliliters.

D/C misinterpreted as discharge or discontinue. Write out "discharge" or "discontinue."

Dram symbol (3) misinterpreted as a 3. Write out "dram."

Per os (orally) misinterpreted as OS (left eye). Use "PO."

IN (intranasal) misinterpreted as IM (intramuscular) or IV (intravenous), or as inhaled. Write out "intranasal" and "inhaled."

\*IU (international unit) misinterpreted as IV. Write "international unit."

Large doses without properly placed commas (e.g., 100000). Place commas appropriately.

\*MS, MSO4, or MgSO4 confused for one another. Write "morphine sulfate," "magnesium sulfate."

\*Q.D. (each day) misinterpreted as qid (four times a day). Write "daily."

\*Q.O.D., (every other day) misinterpreted as four times a day. Write "every other day."

qhs (at bedtime) misinterpreted as qh (every hour). Write "at bedtime."

SC or SQ, sub q (subcutaneous) misinterpreted as SL for sublingual. "sub q 2 hours before surgery" has been misinterpreted as "every 2 hours before surgery." Write "subcutaneously."

ss (one half) misinterpreted as 55. Write one half.

SSRI (sliding scale regular insulin) misinterpreted as selective-serotonin reuptake inhibitor.

\*Trailing zero after a decimal point (e.g., 5.0). Use a zero before a decimal point, never after.

\*U (unit) misinterpreted as cc, or 0. Write "unit."

μg (microgram) mistaken for milligram. Write "mcg."

x4d (for 4 days) misinterpreted as time four doses. Write out "for four days."

| UNEXPECTED OUTCOMES | CRITICAL THINKING OPTIONS |
|---|---|
| Ecchymosis occurs following heparin injection. | • Rotate injection site. Do not inject medication into ecchymotic area.<br>• Do not aspirate before injection or massage site following needle withdrawal.<br>• When forming fat pad in preparation for injection site, do not pinch tightly.<br>• Apply ice to area before injecting heparin. |
| Client complains of pain when injection is administered at dorsogluteal IM site. | • Assess site of injection, neurovascular status of extremity. Document findings.<br>• Notify physician.<br>• Obtain order for warm, moist packs.<br>• Fill out unusual occurrence form.<br>• Take greater care to identify anatomic landmarks. Place client prone (on abdomen). Use dorsogluteal site ONLY as a last resort. Administer irritating medication using Z-track technique.<br>• Locate a line from posterosuperior iliac spine to the greater trochanter of the femur; inject lateral and slightly superior to midpoint of line. Use Z-track technique. Inject into muscle at a 90° angle. |
| Medication is administered using wrong parenteral route. | • Notify physician, and complete unusual occurrence form.<br>• Medications may need to be administered to reverse the action of the medication.<br>• Monitor client's response closely and report adverse findings immediately.<br>• Medication administered IM or IV rather than sub Q leads to faster absorption rates; therefore an assessment needs to be done to determine effects. (IV administration has immediate action.) |
| Client has allergic or anaphylactic response to medication. | • Call rapid response team immediately.<br>• Maintain a patent airway and follow ABCs of emergency care.<br>• Notify client's physician.<br>• Document incident; place allergy alert bracelet on client.<br>• Complete unusual occurrence report according to agency policy. |
| Obese client fails to obtain pain relief from subcutaneous injection. | • Consult pain management team.<br>• Consider weight based dosage.<br>• Change route of analgesic administration since adipose tissue has decreased perfusion and subcutaneous medication uptake is unpredictable. |

# Skill 12.52   Adding Medications to Intravenous Fluid Containers

## EXPECTED OUTCOMES

• IV solutions from secondary IV bags infused without difficulty.
• Therapeutic blood levels of medication are maintained.
• Complications of medication administration are prevented.
• Medication is infused over appropriate time span using volume control set.
• Saline lock inserted for medication administration without compliance.

## Delegation

Adding medications to IV fluid containers involves the application of nursing knowledge and critical thinking. The nurse does not delegate this procedure to UAP. However, the nurse can inform the UAP of the intended therapeutic effects and/or specific side effects of the medication(s) in the IV and direct the UAP to report specific client observations to the nurse for follow-up.

**Equipment**

Client's MAR or computer printout
Correct sterile medication
Diluent for medication in powdered form (see manufacturer's instructions)
Correct solution container, if a new one is to be attached
Antiseptic swabs
Sterile syringe of appropriate size (e.g., 5 or 10 mL) and a 1- to 1½-inch, #20- or #21-gauge sterile safety needle if not using a needleless system
IV additive label to the drug should be available. In addition, assess the vital signs before, during, and after infusion of the drug.

**Preparation**

1. Check the medication administration record.
2. Check the label on the medication carefully against the MAR to make sure that the correct medication is being prepared.
3. Follow the three checks for administering medications. Read the label on the medication (1) when it is taken from the medication cart, (2) before withdrawing the medication, and (3) after withdrawing the medication.
5. Confirm that the dosage and route are correct.
6. Verify which infusion solution is to be used with the medication.
7. Consult a pharmacist, if required, to confirm compatibility of the drugs and solutions being mixed.
8. Organize the equipment.

**Procedure**

1. Perform hand hygiene and observe other appropriate infection control procedures.
2. Prepare the medication ampule or vial for drug withdrawal. check the agency's practice for using a filter needle to
   - withdraw premixed liquid medications from multidose vials or ampules.
3. Add the medication.

***To New IV Container***

- Locate the injection port. Clean the port with the antiseptic or alcohol swab. ➤*Rationale: This reduces the risk of introducing microorganisms into the container when the needle is inserted.*
- Remove the needle cap from the syringe, insert the needle through the center of the injection port, and inject the medication into the bag. Activate the needle safety device. Mix the medication and solution by gently rotating the bag or bottle. ➤*Rationale: This should disperse the medication throughout the solution.*
- Complete the IV additive label with name and dose of medication, date, time, and nurse's initials. Attach it on the bag or bottle. ➤*Rationale: This documents that medication has been added to the solution. The label should be easy to read when the bag is hanging.*
- Clamp the IV tubing. Spike the bag or bottle with IV tubing and hang the IV. ➤*Rationale: Clamping prevents rapid infusion of the solution.*
- Regulate infusion rate as ordered. Often a controller device such as an IV pump is used to ensure accurate rate of infusion.

***To an Existing Infusion***

- Determine that the IV solution in the container is sufficient for adding the medication. ➤*Rationale: Sufficient volume is necessary to dilute the medication adequately.*
- Confirm the desired dilution of the medication, that is, the amount of medication per milliliter of solution.
- Close the infusion clamp. ➤*Rationale: This prevents the medication from infusing directly into the client as it is injected into the bag or bottle.*
- Wipe the medication port with the alcohol or disinfectant swab. ➤*Rationale: This reduces the risk of introducing microorganisms into the container when the needle is inserted.* Remove the needle cover from the medication syringe.
- While supporting and stabilizing the bag with your thumb and forefinger, carefully insert the syringe needle through the port and inject the medication. ➤*Rationale: The bag is supported during the injection of the medication to avoid punctures.* If the bag is too high to reach easily, lower it from the IV pole. Activate the needle safety device.
- Remove the bag from the pole and gently rotate the bag. ➤*Rationale: This will mix the medication and solution.*
- Rehang the container and regulate the flow rate. ➤*Rationale: This establishes the correct flow rate.*
- Complete the medication label and apply to the IV container.

4. Dispose of the equipment and supplies according to agency practice. ➤*Rationale: This prevents inadvertent injury to others and the spread of microorganisms.*
5. Document the medication(s) on the appropriate form in the client's record.

# Skill 12.53 Administering Intermittent Intravenous Medications Using a Secondary Set

## Delegation

The administration of intermittent IV medications involves the application of nursing knowledge and critical thinking. Check the state's nurse practice act to verify the scope of practice for the licensed practical nurse/licensed vocational nurse (LPN/LVN) as it relates to IV medication administration. Agency policy also must be checked and followed. This skill is not delegated to UAP. The nurse, however, can inform the UAP of the intended therapeutic effects and/or specific side effects of the medication and direct the UAP to report specific client observations to the nurse for follow-up.

## Equipment

Client's MAR or computer printout
50- to 250-mL infusion bag with medication (most medication infusion bags are prepared by the pharmacist)
Secondary administration set
Antiseptic swabs
Sterile needle if system is not needleless
Tape
Sterile needle or needleless adapter, syringe, and saline if medication is incompatible with the primary infusion

## Preparation

1. Check the medication administration record.
2. Check the label on the medication carefully against the MAR to make sure that the correct medication is being prepared.
3. Confirm that the dosage is correct.
4. Ensure medication compatibility with primary infusion solution.
5. Consult a pharmacist, if required, to confirm compatibility of the drugs and solutions being mixed.
6. Organize the equipment.
7. Remove medication bag from the refrigerator 30 minutes before administration, if appropriate.

## Procedure

1. Perform hand hygiene and observe other appropriate infection control procedures.
2. Provide for client privacy.
3. Prepare the client.
   - Prior to performing the procedure, introduce self and verify the client's identity using agency protocol. ➤*Rationale: This ensures that the right client receives the right medication.*

   - If not previously assessed, take the appropriate assessment measures necessary for the medication.
4. Explain the purpose of the medication and how it will help, using language that the client can understand. Include relevant information about the effects of the medication. ➤*Rationale: Information can facilitate acceptance of and compliance with the therapy.*
5. Assemble the secondary infusion:
   - Close clamp on secondary infusion tubing.
   - Spike the secondary medication infusion bag.
   - Hang the secondary container at or above the level of the primary infusion. Use the extension hook to lower the primary infusion if a piggyback setup is required. Some infusion pumps do not require this.
   - Attach the needleless cannula to the tubing.
   - Attach appropriate label to the secondary tubing. *Secondary tubing is usually changed every 24 to 48 hours. Check agency policy.*
   - If the secondary tubing remains from a prior medication administration, attach a new needleless cannula. ➤*Rationale: Changing the needleless cannula will reduce the risk of transmission of microorganisms.*
6. Attach the secondary infusion to the primary infusion.
   - Clean the Y-port on the primary IV line with an antiseptic swab. Clean the **primary port** (the port furthest from the client) for a piggyback alignment and the **secondary port** (the port closest to the client) for a tandem setup.
   - If the medication is *not* compatible with the primary infusion, temporarily discontinue the primary infusion. Flush the primary line with a sterile saline solution before attaching the secondary set. To flush the line, wipe the port with an antiseptic swab, clamp the primary line, and,

---

### CLINICAL ALERT

Each IV medication bag requires its own secondary tubing. Medication from the IV infusion bag remains in the secondary tubing. It is important, therefore, when hanging subsequent IV infusion bags to hang the same medication on the same secondary tubing. This avoids the mixing of incompatible medications.

using a sterile syringe and needleless adapter, instill sufficient sterile saline solution through the port to flush any primary fluid out of the infusion tubing.

- Insert the needleless cannula of the secondary line into the primary tubing port.

7. Back prime the secondary tubing.
   - Lower the medication infusion bag below the primary IV bag.
   - Open the clamp of the medication bag.
   - Allow the solution from the primary IV bag to backfill the secondary IV tubing and one-third to one-half of the secondary tubing chamber. ➤*Rationale: This method of priming the secondary tubing allows for no loss of medication.*
   - Clamp the secondary IV tubing.
   - Hang the secondary IV bag on the IV pole.
8. Program the IV pump for the infusion rate of the IV medication bag.
9. Unclamp the secondary IV tubing and check that the secondary solution is infusing.
10. After infusion of the secondary IV medication bag, regulate the rate of the primary solution by adjusting the clamp or IV pump infusion rate. Some infusion pumps will do this automatically.
11. Leave the secondary bag and tubing in place for future administration or discard as appropriate.
12. Document relevant data.
    - Record the date, time, medication, dose, route, and solution; assessment of the IV site, if appropriate; and the client's response.
    - Record the volume of fluid of medication infusion bag on the client's intake and output record.

## VARIATION: Using a Saline Lock

Intermittent infusion devices may be attached to an intravenous catheter or needle to allow medications to be administered intravenously without requiring a continuous intravenous infusion. The device may also have a port at one end of the lock and a needleless injection cap at the other end with the extension tubing between the two ends.

---

### CLINICAL ALERT

The Joint Commission on Accreditation of Healthcare Organizations (JCAHO) 2006 National Patient Safety Goals require the labeling of all medications in syringes (including sterile saline) with the name and strength of the medication, the date, and the initials of the person preparing the label.

---

- Prepare two normal saline prefilled syringes (1 mL each).
- Spike the medication bag with minidrip (60 gtt/mL) IV tubing.
- Attach the needleless adapter to the tubing, prime the tubing, and close the clamp.
- Clean the needleless injection port of the saline lock with an antiseptic swab.
- Insert first saline syringe into the port and gently aspirate to check for patency. Flush slowly noting any resistance, swelling, pain, or burning. ➤*Rationale: This ensures placement of IV in vein.*
- Administer the medication regulating the drip rate to allow medication to infuse for appropriate time period.
- When the medication has been infused, disconnect the IV tubing maintaining sterility of the end of the IV tubing.
- Insert the second saline syringe into the port and gently flush the saline lock. ➤*Rationale: This clears the tubing and maintains patency.*
- Dispose of syringes in the appropriate container.

## VARIATION: Adding a Medication to a Volume-Control Infusion

- Withdraw the required dose of the medication into a syringe.
- Ensure that there is sufficient fluid in the volume-control fluid chamber to dilute the medication. Generally, at least 50 mL of fluid is used. Check the directions from the drug manufacturer or consult the pharmacist.
- Close the inflow to the fluid chamber by adjusting the upper roller or slide clamp above the fluid chamber; also ensure that the clamp on the air vent of the chamber is open.
- Clean the medication port on the volume-control fluid chamber with an antiseptic swab.
- Inject the medication into the port of the partially filled volume-control set.
- Gently rotate the fluid chamber until the fluid is well mixed.
- Open the line's upper clamp and regulate the flow by adjusting the lower roller or slide clamp below the fluid chamber.
- Attach a medication label to the volume-control fluid chamber.
- Document relevant data and monitor the client and the infusion.

# Skill 12.54 Administering Intravenous Medications Using IV Push

## Delegation

The administration of intravenous medication via IV push involves the application of nursing knowledge and critical thinking. This procedure is not delegated to UAP. The nurse, however, can inform the UAP of the intended therapeutic effects and/or specific side effects of the medication and direct the UAP to report specific client observations to the nurse for follow-up.

*Note:* Administration of IV push medications varies by state nurse practice acts. For example, some states may allow the RN to delegate certain medications to be given by an LPN/LVN while other states may allow only the RN to administer IV push medications. Nurses need to know their scope of practice according to their state's nurse practice act and agency policies.

## Equipment

IV push for an existing line
Client's MAR
Medication in a vial or ampule
Sterile syringe (3 to 5 mL) (to prepare the medication)
Sterile needles #21 to #25 gauge, 2.5 cm (1 in.) (needle not needed if using a needleless system)
Antiseptic swabs
Watch with a digital readout or second hand
Clean gloves

### IV Push for an IV Lock

Client's MAR
Medication in a vial or ampule
Sterile syringe (3 to 5 mL) (to prepare the medication)
Sterile syringe (3 mL) (for the saline or heparin flush)
Vial of normal saline to flush the IV catheter or vial of heparin flush solution or both depending on agency practice. ►*Rationale: These maintain the patency of the IV lock. Saline is frequently used for peripheral locks.*
Sterile needles (#21 gauge) (needle not needed if using a needleless system)
Antiseptic swabs
Watch with a digital readout or second hand
Clean gloves

## Preparation

1. Check the medication administration record.
2. Check the label on the medication carefully against the MAR to make sure that the correct medication is being prepared.
   - Follow the three checks for correct medication and dose. Read the label on the medication (1) when it is taken from the medication cart, (2) before withdrawing the medication, and (3) after withdrawing the medication.
   - Calculate medication dosage accurately.
   - Confirm that the route is correct.
   - Organize the equipment.

## Procedure

1. Perform hand hygiene and observe other appropriate infection control procedures.
2. Prepare the medication.

### For an Existing Line

- Prepare the medication according to the manufacturer's direction. ►*Rationale: It is important to have the correct dose and the correct dilution.*

### For an IV Lock

- Flushing with saline:
  a. Prepare two syringes, each with 1 mL of sterile normal saline.
- Flushing with heparin (if indicated by agency policy) and saline:
  a. Prepare one syringe with 1 mL of heparin flush solution (if indicated by agency policy).
  b. Prepare two syringes with 1 mL each of sterile, normal saline.
  c. Draw up the medication into a syringe.
3. Put a small-gauge needle on the syringe if using a needle system.
4. Perform hand hygiene and apply clean gloves. ►*Rationale: This reduces the transmission of microorganisms and reduces the likelihood of the nurse's hands contacting the client's blood.*
5. Provide for client privacy.
6. Prepare the client.
   - Prior to performing the procedure, introduce self and verify the client's identity using agency protocol. ►*Rationale: This ensures that the right client receives the right medication.*
   - If not previously assessed, take the appropriate assessment measures necessary for the medication. If any of the findings are above or below the predetermined parameters, consult the primary care provider before administering the medication.
7. Explain the purpose of the medication and how it will help, using language that the client can understand. Include relevant information about the effects of the medication. ►*Rationale: Information can facilitate acceptance of and compliance with the therapy.*

8. Administer the medication by IV push. Bunce (2003) reported that the use of the "push-stop-push-stop" technique is helpful, especially for central venous catheters. ➤*Rationale: This creates a turbulence in the flow through the catheter that reduces the residue buildup in the line and the potential for occlusion.*

## IV Lock with Needle

- Clean the injection port with the antiseptic swab. ➤*Rationale: This prevents microorganisms from entering the circulatory system during the needle insertion.*
- Insert the needle of the syringe containing normal saline through the center of the injection port and aspirate for blood. ➤*Rationale: The presence of blood confirms that the catheter or needle is in the vein. In some situations, blood will not return even though the lock is patent.*
- Flush the lock by injecting 1 mL of saline slowly. ➤*Rationale: This removes blood and heparin (if present) from the needle and the lock.*
- Remove the needle and syringe. Activate the needle safety device.
- Clean the lock's injection port with an antiseptic swab. ➤*Rationale: This prevents the transfer of microorganisms.*
- Insert the needle of the syringe containing the prepared medication through the center of the injection port.
- Inject the medication slowly at the recommended rate of infusion. Use a watch or digital readout to time the injection. Observe the client closely for adverse reactions. Remove the needle and syringe when all
- medication has been administered. ➤*Rationale: Injecting the drug too rapidly can have a serious untoward reaction.*
- Activate the needle safety device.
- Clean the injection port of the lock.
- Attach the second saline syringe, and inject 1 mL of saline. ➤*Rationale: The saline injection flushes the medication through the catheter and prepares the lock for heparin if this medication is used. Heparin is incompatible with many medications.*
- If heparin is to be used, insert the heparin syringe and inject the heparin slowly into the lock.

## IV Lock with Needleless System

- Clean the injection port of the lock.
- Insert syringe containing normal saline into the injection port.
- Flush the lock with 1 mL of sterile saline. ➤*Rationale: This clears the lock of blood.*

- Remove the syringe.
- Insert the syringe containing the medication into the port.
- Inject the medication following the precautions described previously.
- Withdraw the syringe.
- Repeat injection of 1 mL of saline.

### Existing Line

- Identify the injection port closest to the client. Some ports have a circle indicating the site for the needle insertion. ➤*Rationale: An injection port must be used because it is self-sealing. Any puncture to the plastic tubing will leak.*
- Clean the port with an antiseptic swab.
- Stop the IV flow by closing the clamp or pinching the tubing above the injection port.
- Connect the syringe to the IV system.
  a. Needle system:
- Hold the port steady.
- Insert the needle of the syringe that contains the medication through the center of the port. ➤*Rationale: This prevents damage to the IV line and to the diaphragm of the port.*
  b. Needleless system:
- Remove the cap from the needleless injection port. Connect the tip of the syringe directly to the port.
- Inject the medication at the ordered rate. Use the watch or digital readout to time the medication administration. ➤*Rationale: This ensures safe drug administration because a too rapid injection could be dangerous.*
- Release the clamp or tubing.
- After injecting the medication, withdraw the needle and activate the needle safety device. For a needleless system, detach the syringe and attach a new sterile cap to the port.

9. Dispose of equipment according to agency practice. ➤*Rationale: This reduces needlestick injuries and spread of microorganisms.*
10. Remove and dispose of gloves. Perform hand hygiene.
11. Observe the client closely for adverse reactions.
12. Determine agency policy about recommended times for changing the IV lock. Some agencies advocate a change every 48 to 72 hours for peripheral IV devices.
13. Document all relevant information.
    - Record the date, time, drug, dose, and route; client response; and assessments of infusion or heparin lock site if appropriate.

# Skill 12.55 Managing Pain with a PCA Pump

## Delegation

Initiating and maintaining a PCA pump requires application of nursing knowledge, aseptic technique, critical thinking, and administration of a controlled substance and, therefore, is not delegated to UAP. The nurse can inform UAP of the intended therapeutic effects and specific side effects of the medication and direct UAP to report specific client observations (e.g., unrelieved pain) to the nurse for follow-up. UAP must not administer a dose (push the button) for the client.

## Equipment

PCA pump and appropriate tubing
Operational manual for specific pump to be used
Alcohol swab

## Preparation

Before initiating PCA therapy, determine factors that may contraindicate use (e.g., impaired mental status, impaired respiratory status), the amount of narcotic specified by the order, bolus and continuous infusion dosage parameters, and type of primary fluid.

   Calculate:
   The initial bolus dose based on the number of milligrams of drug per milliliter of fluid.

- The dose per intermittent bolus delivery.
- The 4-hour lockout drug limit.
  1. Check the medication administration record (MAR).
     - Check the label on the medication carefully against the MAR to make sure that the correct medication is being prepared.
  2. Organize the equipment.

## Procedure

1. Prior to performing the procedure introduce self and verify the client's identity using agency protocol. Explain the purpose and operation of the PCA.
2. Perform hand hygiene and observe other appropriate infection control procedures.
3. Provide for client privacy.
4. Prepare the client.
   - If not previously assessed, take the baseline vital signs. If any of the findings are above or below the predetermined parameters, consult the primary care provider before administering the medication.
5. Set up the PCA infusion line according to the manufacturer's instructions.
   - Attach needleless adapter to end of PCA tubing.
   - Prime the PCA tubing.

- Clamp the tubing. ➤*Rationale: This prevents accidental bolusing and flushing of the primary line with the narcotic.*
- Place the medication syringe in the PCA machine according to the operational instructions.
6. Connect the PCA infusion line to the primary fluid line.
   - Cleanse injection port of primary IV with alcohol swab.
   - Connect the PCA tubing to the primary fluid line at the injection port closest to the client.
7. Deliver the loading dose, as prescribed.
   - Set the pump for a lockout time of zero minutes.
   - Set the volume to be delivered based on calculated dosage volume for the loading dose.
   - Inject the loading dose by pressing the loading dose control button.
8. Set the safety parameters for the infusion on the PCA pump according to the manufacturer's instructions. For example:
   - Dose volume limits. ➤*Rationale: This will limit the amount of drug that the client can receive when the client pushes the control button.*
   - Lockout interval between each dose. The lockout interval is generally between 5 and 15 minutes. ➤*Rationale: This sets the minimum time that must elapse before the client can receive another dose of the drug. Lockout time is based on the usual onset of the IV narcotic and the assessment of the client.*
   - Four-hour limit. Set the 4-hour dosage limit as specified on the orders. ➤*Rationale: This is an additional safety feature to limit the amount of medication delivered over 4 hours.*
9. Lock the machine. Close the door on the pump.
   - Look for any digital cues or alarms that may indicate the machine is not set, and make corrections as needed.
   - Lock the machine with the key.
10. Begin the infusion.
    - Place the client control button within reach.
11. Monitor the client.
    - Monitor the status of the client every 2 hours during the first 24 to 36 hours of infusion and regularly thereafter, depending on the client's health and agency protocol.
12. Monitor the infusion.
    - Observe the IV site for signs of infiltration and phlebitis.
    - Inspect the tubing for kinks that may occlude the line.
    - Note the total number of doses and milligrams received.
13. Document all relevant information.
    - Record the initiation of PCA, the dose setting, the doses received, pain intensity, and all assessments. See agency protocol for specific guidelines.

# Skill 12.56  Administering Blood Transfusions

## Delegation

Due to the need for sterile technique and technical complexity, blood transfusion is not delegated to UAP. The nurse must ensure that the UAP knows what complications or adverse signs can occur and should be reported to the nurse.

## Equipment

Unit of whole blood, packed RBCs, or other component
Blood administration set with 170- to 260-mL filter
IV pump, if needed
250 mL normal saline for infusion
IV pole
Venipuncture start kit containing a 20-gauge needle or catheter (if one is not already in place)
Alcohol swabs
Tape
Clean gloves

## Preparation

- Prior to performing the procedure, introduce self and verify the client's identity using agency protocol.
- Explain the procedure and its purpose to the client.
- If the client has an intravenous solution infusing, check whether the needle and solution are appropriate to administer blood. The preferred needle size is 18 to 20 gauge, and the solution *must* be normal saline. Dextrose (which causes lysis of RBCs), Ringer's solution, medications and other additives, and hyperalimentation solutions are incompatible. Refer to step 5 below if the infusing solution is not compatible.
- If the client does not have an IV solution infusing, check agency policies. In some agencies an infusion must be running before the blood is obtained from the blood bank. In this case, you will need to perform a venipuncture on a suitable vein and start an IV infusion of normal saline.

## Procedure

1. Provide for client privacy and prepare the client.
   - Assist the client to a comfortable position, either sitting or lying. Expose the IV site but provide for client privacy.
2. Perform hand hygiene and observe other appropriate infection control procedures.
3. Prepare the infusion equipment.
   - Ensure that the blood filter inside the drip chamber is suitable for the blood components to be transfused. Attach the blood tubing to the blood filter, if necessary. ➤*Rationale: Blood filters have a surface area large enough to allow the blood components through easily but are designed to trap clots.*
   - Apply gloves.
   - Close all the clamps on the Y-set: the main flow rate clamp and both Y-line clamps.
   - Insert the piercing pin (spike) into the saline solution.
   - Hang the container on the IV pole about 1 m (39 in.) above the venipuncture site.
4. Prime the tubing.
   - Open the upper clamp on the normal saline tubing, and squeeze the drip chamber until it covers the filter and one third of the drip chamber above the filter.
   - Tap the filter chamber to expel any residual air in the filter.
   - Open the main flow rate clamp, and prime the tubing with saline.
   - Close both clamps.
5. Start the saline solution.
   - If an IV solution incompatible with blood is infusing, stop the infusion and discard the solution and tubing according to agency policy.
   - Attach the blood tubing primed with normal saline to the intravenous catheter.
   - Open the saline and main flow rate clamps and adjust the flow rate. Use only the main flow rate clamp to adjust the rate.
   - Allow a small amount of solution to infuse to make sure there are no problems with the flow or with the venipuncture site. ➤*Rationale: Infusing normal saline before initiating the transfusion also clears the IV catheter of incompatible solutions or medications.*
6. Obtain the correct blood component for the client.
   - Check the order with the requisition.
   - Check the requisition form and the blood bag label with a laboratory technician or according to agency policy. Specifically, check the client's name, identification number, ABO blood type and Rh group, the blood donor number, and the expiration date of the blood. Observe the blood for abnormal color, clumping, gas bubbles, and extraneous material. Return outdated or abnormal blood to the blood bank.
   - With another nurse (most agencies require another registered nurse), compare the laboratory blood record with:
   - Two client identifiers as delineated by agency policy.
   - The number on the blood bag label.
   - The ABO blood type and Rh group on the blood bag label.
   - If any of the information does not match *exactly,* notify the charge nurse and the blood bank. Do not administer blood until discrepancies are corrected or clarified.
   - Sign the appropriate form with the other nurse according to agency policy.
   - Make sure that RBCs are left at room temperature for no more than 30 minutes before starting the transfusion.

➤*Rationale: RBCs deteriorate and lose their effectiveness after 2 hours at room temperature. Lysis of RBCs releases potassium into the bloodstream, causing hyperkalemia.*

- Agencies may designate different times at which the blood must be returned to the blood bank if it has not been started. ➤*Rationale: As blood components warm, the risk of bacterial growth also increases.* If the start of the transfusion is unexpectedly delayed, return the blood to the blood bank within 30 minutes. Do not store blood in the unit refrigerator. ➤*Rationale: The temperature of unit refrigerators is not precisely regulated and the blood may be damaged. The blood bank may not accept the returned unit if it has been out of the bank for more than 30 minutes.*

- *For platelets:* Pooled platelets usually contain 200 to 400 mL (made from 4 to 6 units). Do not refrigerate platelets, and keep them agitated at all times to prevent coagulation. Do not use microaggregate filters. Infuse at 10 mL/min or as ordered. Undulate the unit and drip chamber every 10 to 15 minutes (Weaver & McDonald, 2006).

- *For fresh frozen plasma:* 200 to 250 mL/unit. Infuse within 24 hours of thawing, at 5 to 10 mL/min or as ordered.

7. Prepare the blood bag.
   - Invert the blood bag gently several times to mix the cells with the plasma. ➤*Rationale: Rough handling can damage the cells.*
   - Expose the port on the blood bag by pulling back the tabs.
   - Insert the remaining Y-set spike into the blood bag.
   - Suspend the blood bag.

8. Establish the blood transfusion.
   - Close the upper clamp below the IV saline solution container.
   - Open the upper clamp below the blood bag. The blood will run into the saline-filled drip chamber. If necessary, squeeze the drip chamber to reestablish the liquid level with the drip chamber one-third full. (Tap the filter to expel any residual air within the filter.)
   - Readjust the flow rate with the main clamp.
   - Remove and discard gloves. Perform hand hygiene.

9. Observe the client closely for the first 15 minutes.
   - Run the blood slowly for the first 15 minutes at 20 drops/min.
   - Note adverse reactions, such as chilling, nausea, vomiting, skin rash, or tachycardia. ➤*Rationale: The earlier a transfusion reaction occurs, the more severe it tends to be. Promptly identifying such reactions helps to minimize the consequences.*
   - Remind the client to call a nurse immediately if any unusual symptoms are felt during the transfusion such as chills, nausea, itching, rash, dyspnea, or back pain.
   - If any of these reactions occur, report these to the nurse in charge, and take appropriate nursing action.

10. Document relevant data.
    - Record starting the blood, including vital signs, type of blood, blood unit number, sequence number (e.g., #1 of three ordered units), site of the venipuncture, size of the needle, and drip rate.

- Monitor the client.
- Fifteen minutes after initiating the transfusion (or according to agency policy), check the vital signs. If there are no signs of a reaction, establish the required flow rate. Most adults can tolerate receiving one unit of blood in 1½ to 2 hours. Do not transfuse a unit of blood for longer than 4 hours.
- Assess the client, including vital signs, every 30 minutes or more often, depending on the health status and agency policy. If the client has a reaction and the blood is discontinued, send the blood bag to the laboratory for investigation of the blood.

11. Terminate the transfusion.
    - Apply clean gloves.
    - If no infusion is to follow, clamp the blood tubing and remove the needle. If another transfusion is to follow, clamp the blood tubing and open the saline infusion arm. Blood administration sets are changed within 24 hours or after 4 to 6 units of blood per agency protocol.
    - If the primary IV is to be continued, flush the maintenance line with saline solution. Disconnect the blood tubing system and reestablish the intravenous infusion using new tubing. Adjust the drip to the desired rate. Measure vital signs.

12. Follow agency protocol for appropriate disposition of the used supplies.
    - Discard the administration set according to agency practice.
    - Dispose of blood bags.
      a. On the requisition attached to the blood unit, fill in the time the transfusion was completed and the amount transfused.
      b. Attach one copy of the requisition to the client's record and another to the empty blood bag.
      c. Agency policy generally involves returning the bag to the blood bank for reference in case of subsequent or delayed adverse reaction.
    - Remove and discard gloves. Perform hand hygiene.

13. Document relevant data.
    - Record completion of the transfusion, the amount of blood absorbed, the blood unit number, and the vital signs. If the primary intravenous infusion was continued, record connecting it. Also record the transfusion on the IV flow sheet and intake and output record.

### Documentation

4/21/2009 1420 c/o feeling warm, headache, & backache. Skin flushed. T 102.6°F, BP 140/90, P 112, R 28. Approximately 50 mL PRBCs infused over past 20 minutes. Infusion stopped. Tubing changed, NS infusing at 15 mL/h. Blood & admin. tubing sent to blood bank. Dr. Riley notified.

_____ C. Jones, RN

# Skill 12.57 Administering Blood Components

## Equipment

Blood component
Appropriate IV administration kit
Filter, if indicated
Clean gloves

### MODIFIED BLOOD PRODUCTS

In addition to the usual blood components such as platelets and cryoprecipitate, modified blood products are becoming more popular. Washed, irradiated, or leukocyte-removed blood is being used for clients at risk because of multiple transfusions or a weakened immune system. Testing for cytomegalovirus and matching RBC or human leukocyte antigens is also done to ensure safe transfusions.

## Procedure

1. Check physician's orders and client's signed consent for transfusion.
2. Obtain blood component from blood bank.
3. Obtain appropriate administration set.
4. Perform hand hygiene and don gloves.
5. Read directions for proper administration of the solution.
6. Identify rate at which blood component should infuse.

### CLINICAL ALERT

When infusing a blood product that has undergone leukocyte reduction it still must be filtered again through a standard blood administration set in order to trap cellular debris that may have accumulated since the original filtration.

# Skill 12.58 Managing Central Lines

## Delegation

Due to the need for sterile technique and technical complexity, the maintaining and monitoring of central venous lines are not delegated to UAP. UAP may care for clients with central lines, and the nurse must ensure that the UAP knows what complications or adverse signs should be reported to the nurse.

## Equipment

Soft-tipped clamp without teeth
Alcohol, chlorhexidine gluconate, or povidone-iodine wipes
10-mL syringe
Sterile normal saline
Heparin flush solution (e.g., 100 units heparin per milliliter of saline)

## Procedure

1. Prior to performing the procedure, introduce self and verify the client's identity using agency protocol. Explain to the client what you are going to do, why it is necessary, and how he or she can participate.
2. Perform hand hygiene and observe other appropriate infection control procedures.
3. Position the client appropriately.
   - Assist the client to a comfortable position, either sitting or lying. Expose the IV site but provide for client privacy.
4. Label each lumen of multilumen catheters.
   - Mark each lumen or port of the tubing with a description of its purpose (e.g., the distal lumen for CVP monitoring and infusing blood, the middle lumen for parenteral nutrition, and the proximal lumen for other IV solutions or for blood samples).
   *or*
   - Use a color code established by the agency to label the proximal, middle, and distal lumens. ▶*Rationale: Labeling prevents mixing of incompatible medications or infusions and reserves each lumen for specific therapies.*
5. Monitor tubing connections.
   - Ensure that all tubing connections are taped or secured according to agency protocol.
   - Check the connections every 2 hours.
   - Tape cap ends if agency protocol indicates.
6. Change tubing according to agency policy.
   - Parenteral nutrition tubing should be changed every 24 hours if the infusions contain fat emulsions and every 72 hours if no fat emulsions are used (Rosenthal, 2007).

7. Change the catheter site dressing according to agency policy.
   - Depending on the type of dressing, most agencies recommend that the dressing be changed every 2 to 7 days.
8. Administer all infusions as ordered.
   - Use a controller or pump for all fluids.
   - Maintain the fluid flow at the prescribed rate.
   - Whenever the line is interrupted for any reason, instruct the client to perform Valsalva's maneuver. If the client is unable to perform Valsalva's maneuver, place the client in a supine position, and clamp the lumen of the catheter with a soft-tipped clamp. Place a strip of tape over the catheter (about 3 in. from the end) before applying the clamp. ➤*Rationale: The clamp is placed over the taped area to prevent damage to the tubing. A clamp without teeth prevents piercing.*
9. Cap lumens without continuous infusions, and flush them regularly.
   - Close lumens not in use with an intermittent infusion cap to seal the end of a catheter.
   - Clean the adapter caps with an alcohol or povidone-iodine swab before penetration.
   - Flush lumens according to agency protocol. ➤*Rationale: Flushing prevents obstruction of the catheter by a blood clot. The exact amount and frequency of flush depends on the catheter type and agency practice.* Some agencies use normal saline solution and some use heparin solution to flush catheters. ➤*Rationale: Research indicates that heparin isn't always necessary to keep IV lines open.* A rule of thumb is to flush with heparin after infusing medications or blood, but with saline if the catheter is accessed often, for example, every 8 hours. Catheters not in active use may be flushed every 24 hours or up to once a week.
   - Always aspirate for blood before flushing (or infusing medications). ➤*Rationale: This validates that the catheter is appropriately placed in the vein and patent.*
   - Use a 10-mL or larger syringe to flush. ➤*Rationale: Smaller syringes can exert too much pressure that can damage the catheter.* Create turbulent flow with the flush by pushing, then pausing (Tilton, 2006), and then pushing again but do not use excessive force if you feel resistance. ➤*Rationale: Turbulent flow may help keep the catheter free of residue but forcing a blocked catheter can cause rupture of the catheter or push a clot free into the bloodstream.*
   - Avoid reflux of blood back into the catheter when disconnecting the syringe. Needleless systems may be negative displacement, positive displacement, or neutral displacement devices. For negative displacement devices, keep pressure on the syringe plunger as the syringe is disconnected. ➤*Rationale: Positive pressure prevents back flow of blood into the catheter.* With positive or neutral displacement devices, this technique is not used (Hadaway, 2005).

10. Administer medications as ordered.
    - If a capped lumen used for medication has been flushed with heparin solution, aspirate and discard or flush the line with 5 to 10 mL of normal saline according to agency protocol before giving the medication. ➤*Rationale: Many medications are incompatible with heparin.*
    - After the medication is instilled through the lumen, inject normal saline first and then the heparin flush solution if indicated by agency protocol. ➤*Rationale: The saline solution flushes the line of the medication. The heparin maintains the patency of the catheter by preventing blood clotting.*
11. Monitor the client for complications.
    - Assess the client's vital signs, skin color, mental alertness, appearance of the catheter site, and presence of adverse symptoms at least every 4 hours. If an air embolism is suspected, give the client 100% oxygen by mask, place the client in a left Trendelenburg position, and notify the primary care provider. ➤*Rationale: Lowering the head increases intrathoracic pressure, decreasing the flow of air into the vein during inhalation. A left side-lying position helps prevent the air from moving to the pulmonary artery.*
    - If sepsis is suspected, replace a parenteral nutrition, blood, or other infusion with 5% or 10% dextrose solution, change the IV tubing and dressing, save the remaining solution for lab analysis, record the lot number of the solution and any additives, and notify the primary care provider immediately. When changing the dressing, take a culture of the catheter site as ordered by the primary care provider or according to agency protocol.
    - If a lumen appears to be occluded, the cause could be thrombus, precipitate, or mechanical. An x-ray is done to determine if the catheter is properly located. Fluoroscopy can demonstrate the presence of a thrombus by indicating the fluid path through the catheter. If a thrombus is found, thrombolytic therapy using an enzyme such as recombinant tissue plasminogen activator (t-PA) is indicated (Hadaway, 2005). Follow agency guidelines for use of these agents. If drugs infused into the lumen may have created a precipitate, the pharmacist can assist in determining whether an acidic, alkaline, or lipid precipitate is likely and the appropriate solution to dissolve it. If the occlusion is mechanical, consult policy to determine if the nurse may reposition the catheter or if the primary care provider must be notified.
12. Document all relevant information.
    - Record the date and time of any infusion started; type of solution, drip rate, and number of milliliters infusing per hour; dressing or tubing changes; appearance of insertion site; and all other nursing assessments.

# Skill 12.59   Changing a Central Line Dressing

## EVIDENCE-BASED NURSING PRACTICE

### Antimicrobial Swabs

Studies have shown that 2% chlorhexidine gluconate solution significantly lowers catheter-related bloodstream infection rates when compared with 70% providone–iodine and 70% isopropyl alcohol.

*Sources:* LeBlanc & Cobbett. (2000). Traditional practice versus evidence-based practice for IV skin preparation. *Canadian Journal of Infection Control,* 15(1), 9–14. Maki, Ringer, & Alvarado (1991). Prospective randomized trial of providone–iodine, and chlorhexidine for prevention of infection associated with central venous and arterial catheters. *The Lancet,* 338, 339–343; Rosenthal, K. (2003). Pinpointing intravascular device infections. *Nursing Management,* 34(6), 35–43.

Another study revealed that chlorhexidine gluconate offered a broad spectrum of antimicrobial activity and long-term microbactericidal action after application.

*Source:* Hadaway, L. C. (2003a). Infusing without infecting. *Nursing,* 33(10), 58–64.

---

### PREVENTING INTRAVASCULAR CATHETER-RELATED BLOOD STREAM INFECTIONS

Catheter-related blood stream infection is 2 to 855 times higher with central vascular catheters than peripheral vascular catheters. Approximately 80,000 catheter-related infections occur in the United States each year. These infections are associated with 2,400–20,000 deaths each year. These infections can be dramatically reduced with new products that have been introduced for CVD therapy: The FDA has recently approved the use of catheters impregnated with chlorhexidine. There is still testing being done on the combination of chlorhexidine and silver sulfadiazine because of some anaphylactoid reactions in Japan. Use of minocycline–rifampin impregnated catheters show promise of even lower infection rates.

- Catheters impregnated with chlorhexidine–silver sulfadiazine or catheters impregnated with minocycline–rifampin
- Catheter hubs containing iodinated alcohol
- Chlorhexidine-impregnated sponge dressings placed at the catheter insertion site: Infection rate decreased from 5.2% to 3% for catheters in place less than 10 days.

*Source:* Mermel, L. A. (2001, March–April). New technologies to prevent intravascular catheter-related bloodstream infections. *Emerging Infectious Diseases,* CDC, 7(2).

---

### Delegation

Due to the need for sterile technique and technical complexity, changing a central line dressing is not delegated to UAP. UAP may care for clients with central lines, and the nurse must ensure that the UAP knows what complications or adverse signs should be reported to the nurse.

### Equipment

Central line dressing set
*or*
Two face masks (one for the nurse and one for the client)
Three 70% isopropyl alcohol swabs
Three antiseptic swabs (e.g., 2% chlorhexidine gluconate, 1% iodine tincture, or povidone-iodine solutions)
Tincture of benzoin or other skin protection swabs
Clean gloves
Sterile gloves

4 × 4 gauze sponges
Catheter securement device (according to agency policy)
Precut sterile drain gauze or 2 × 2 gauze and sterile scissors
Transparent semipermeable polyurethane dressing such as Op-Site or Tegaderm
Nonallergenic 2.5-cm (1-in.) tape
Dressing label
Sterile drape

### Procedure

1. Prior to performing the procedure, introduce self and verify the client's identity using agency protocol. Explain to the client what you are going to do, why it is necessary, and how he or she can participate.
2. Provide for client privacy and position the client.
   - Assist the client to a comfortable position, either sitting or lying. The client should be supine if the tubing or

injection cap is also being changed. ➤*Rationale: An upright position during these techniques increases the chances of an air embolism forming.* Expose the central line site but provide for client privacy.

3. Perform hand hygiene and observe other appropriate infection control procedures.
4. Prepare the client.
   - Apply a mask, and have the client apply a mask (if tolerated or as agency protocol indicates), and/or ask the client to turn the head away from the insertion site. ➤*Rationale: This helps protect the insertion site from the nurse's and client's nasal and oral microorganisms. Turning the client's head also makes the site more accessible.*
5. Prepare the equipment.
   - Establish a sterile field and place the sterile supplies.
6. Remove the old dressing.
   - Apply clean gloves.
   - For a transparent dressing, pull both sides away from the insertion site, stretching it to lift it off the skin (Hadaway, 2005). For taped dressings, hold the catheter with one hand and gently pull the tape in the direction of the catheter. ➤*Rationale: This prevents catheter displacement and skin irritation.*
   - Inspect the skin for signs of irritation or infection. Inspect the catheter for signs of leakage or other problems. If infection is suspected, take a swab of the drainage for culture, label it, send it to the laboratory, and notify the primary care provider. Measure the length of the external portion of the catheter extending from the skin exit site to the injection cap or infusion tubing. ➤*Rationale: This measurement allows comparison with previous measurements to determine if the catheter is migrating in or out.*
   - Remove and discard gloves. Perform hand hygiene.
7. Cleanse the site.
   - Apply sterile gloves.
   - Clean the catheter insertion site with three alcohol swabs in a circular motion, moving from the insertion site outward and let the skin dry. Extend the cleansed area about 2 inches in diameter from the insertion site. ➤*Rationale: Cleaning from the insertion site outward and discarding the sponges after each wipe avoids introducing contaminants from the uncleaned area to the site.*
   - Repeat the procedure with the antiseptic swabs and let the skin dry. If using povidone-iodine, cleanse in a circular motion. If using chlorhexidine gluconate, scrub in a back-and-forth motion for 30 seconds (Tilton, 2006).
   - If possible, use one hand to lift the catheter so you can clean under it.
8. Apply the new dressing.
   - Apply benzoin or other skin protectant to the dressing area, and allow it to air dry about 1 minute. ➤*Rationale: This protects the skin when adhesive is applied and promotes adhesion of the cover dressing. Appropriate drying time is essential to prevent skin breakdown when the dressing is removed.*
   - Secure the catheter to the skin with a catheter securement device following the manufacturer's instructions, tape, or Steri-Strips.
   - Cover with one or two 4 × 4 gauze dressings. ➤*Rationale: This protects the catheter and skin surrounding the insertion site from airborne contaminants. Gauze is recommended for the first 24 hours after initial central line insertion to absorb exudate.* or
   - Apply a transparent semipermeable polyurethane dressing. Be sure to pinch the dressing around the catheter so no air gaps exist. ➤*Rationale: This type of dressing allows gas exchange but is impermeable to liquids and microorganisms. It also allows visualization of the site.*
   - Label the dressing with catheter information, date and time of the dressing change, and your initials.
   - Remove and discard gloves. Perform hand hygiene.
9. Document all relevant information.
   - Record the appearance of catheter insertion site: presence of drainage, the type of dressing applied, client complaints or concerns, and patency of tubing (if evaluated).

### Documentation

4/13/2009 2030 Dressing changed on Broviac catheter. External portion 12.7 cm unchanged from previous. Skin redness, drainage, or swelling. IV infusing freely. No c/o discomfort. Transparent dressing reapplied c̄ sterile technique.

———————————————— J. Valenzuela, RN

## EVIDENCE-BASED NURSING PRACTICE

**Evaluation of BIOPATCH Antimicrobial Dressing**

A controlled, randomized study of 687 clients with 1,699 central venous or arterial catheter insertion sites was conducted in two centers. Results indicated as 44% reduction in local infections and a 60% reduction in catheter-related blood stream infections. There were no serious device-related adverse events during the study. Data regarding use of patch on children under 16 is limited. Patch should not be used on premature infants as hypersensitivity reactions and necrosis of the skin have occurred.

*Source:* Maki, D. G., et al. (2000). An evaluation of Biopatch Antimicrobial Dressing compared to routine standard of care in the prevention of catheter-related bloodstream infection. Johnson & Johnson Medical Division of ETHICON, Inc.

# Skill 12.60   Working with Implanted Vascular Access Devices

## Delegation

Due to the need for sterile technique and technical complexity, accessing an IVAD is not delegated to UAP. UAP may care for clients with such devices, and the nurse must ensure that the UAP knows what complications or adverse signs should be reported to the nurse.

## Equipment

IV solution container and administration set
*or*
Blood or blood product with transfusion set and priming saline
*or*
Blood specimen tubes and syringe and needle
Sterile gloves
10-mL syringes of normal saline flush and 5-mL syringes of heparinized saline (100 units/mL of heparin) according to agency policy
2% lidocaine with subcutaneous syringe and needle (optional)
Povidone-iodine or chlorhexidine gluconate and alcohol swabs
Straight or right-angled Huber needle, (with extension tubing if indicated)
Adhesive or nonallergenic tape
Dressing materials (e.g., 2 × 2 gauze, semipermeable transparent dressing)

## Preparation

1. Assemble the equipment.
2. Attach the IV tubing to the infusion or transfusion container.
3. Prime the infusion tubing with fluid.
4. Prepare and label syringes of normal saline and heparinized saline. Connect the first of these to be used to the Huber needle. Saline followed by heparinized saline is used to flush the device before and after medications or periodically if not in use (check agency policy). ▶*Rationale: Heparinized saline may help prevent clotting. There is also some risk of heparininduced thrombocytopenia so that heparin is not used without clear policy.*

## Procedure

1. Prior to performing the procedure, introduce self and verify the client's identity using agency protocol. Explain to the client what you are going to do, why it is necessary, and how he or she can participate.
2. Provide for client privacy and prepare the client.
   - Assist the client to a comfortable position, either sitting or lying. Expose the IVAD site but provide for client privacy.

3. Perform hand hygiene and observe other appropriate infection control procedures.
4. Prepare the site.
   - Locate the IVAD device and its septum, the disk at the center of the port where the needle will be inserted.
   - Prepare the skin in accordance with agency policy and let the area dry after applying such solutions as povidone iodine, chlorhexidine gluconate, and alcohol.
   - Apply sterile gloves.
   - *Optional:* Inject 2% lidocaine subcutaneously over the needle insertion site. ▶*Rationale: This anesthetizes the area for injection.* It may be ordered during the first few weeks after the implant surgery, when the area is tender and swollen and more pain from the needle puncture is felt. Other topical anesthetics may be used.
   - An ice pack may be placed over the site for several minutes to reduce discomfort from the needle puncture.
5. Insert the Huber needle.
   - Grasp the base of the IVAD device between two fingers of your nondominant hand to stabilize it. IVADs may have top entry or side entry ports, depending on the design.
   - Insert the needle at a 90-degree angle to the septum, and push it firmly through the skin and septum until it contacts the base of the IVAD chamber.
   - Avoid tilting or moving the needle when the septum is punctured. ▶*Rationale: Needle movement can damage the septum and cause fluid leakage.*
   - When the needle contacts the base of the septum, aspirate for blood to determine correct placement. If no blood is obtained, remove the needle and repeat the procedure after having the client move the arms and change position. ▶*Rationale: Movement can free the catheter tip from the vessel wall, where it may be lodged.*
   - Infuse the saline flush. There should be no discomfort or sign of subcutaneous infiltration with infusion of the flush.
6. Prevent manipulation or dislodgement of the needle.
   - If the needle will remain in place for longer than needed to withdraw a blood sample or flush an unused port, secure the needle.
   - Support the Huber needle with 2 × 2 dressings and apply an occlusive transparent dressing to the needle site. Some manufacturer's devices include a safety lock to decrease accidental needlesticks and a patient comfort pad that sits between the needle hub and the skin.
   - Loop and tape the tubing. ▶*Rationale: Looping prevents tension on the needle.*
7. Attach infusion tubing or an intermittent infusion access cap to the Huber needle.
   - A Huber needle can remain in place for 1 week before it needs to be changed.

8. After use, perform a final flush with heparinized saline.
   - When flushing, maintain positive pressure, and clamp the tubing immediately before the flush is finished.
   ➤*Rationale: These actions avoid reflux of the heparinized saline.*

### VARIATION: Obtaining a Blood Specimen

- Withdraw 10 mL of blood (or an amount according to agency policy) and discard it. ➤*Rationale: This initial specimen may be diluted with saline and heparin from previous flushes.*
- Draw up the required amount of blood and transfer it to the appropriate containers.
- Slowly instill 10 mL of normal saline, according to agency policy. ➤*Rationale: This thoroughly flushes the catheter of blood.*
- Inject 5 mL of heparin flush solution to prevent clotting.

9. Remove and discard gloves. Perform hand hygiene.

10. Document all relevant information.
    - Record the appearance of the IVAD site; any difficulty accessing the port and interventions used; presence of drainage; the type of dressing applied; infusions given; and client complaints or concerns. Note any clinical signs indicating venous thrombosis (pain in the neck, arm, and/or shoulder on the side of the insertion site; neck and/or supraclavicular swelling); infection (redness and swelling at the site); and dislodgement of the needle or catheter (shortness of breath, chest pain, coolness in the chest).

### Documentation

4/14/09 0900 Implanted port r chest c̄ skin intact and no swelling. Accessed c̄ 20G 1″ Huber needle. Prompt blood return, flushed s̄ difficulty. IV infusion begun. No c/o of discomfort.

_____ G. Young, RN

| UNEXPECTED OUTCOMES | CRITICAL THINKING OPTIONS |
|---|---|
| Secondary bag solution does not infuse adequately. | • Check that primary IV bag is lower than secondary bag (if infusion device requires).<br>• Ensure that cannula is positioned properly in the primary injection port and second bag is sufficiently spiked.<br>• Check that the roller clamp of the secondary tubing is open fully. |
| Solution in primary IV tubing is incompatible with medication to be administered via secondary "piggyback." | • Prior to administering medication, flush primary tubing with solution compatible with medication (e.g., normal saline, 5% D/W0.<br>• Hang a separate solution compatible with medication and run through line to flush during drug administration. |
| Solution does not infuse through peripheral lock. | • Gently turn lock to establish flow.<br>• Reposition client's extremity.<br>• Initiate a new IV site. |
| Transfusion reaction occurs. | • Stop blood administration and begin infusion of normal saline or ordered solution, to keep IV open.<br>• Check transfusion reaction form for appropriate nursing intervention.<br>• Complete all relevant nursing actions. |
| Blood does not flow through tubing. | • Check client's IV site and gauge of needle (at least 18 or 20 gauge).<br>• Gently agitate blood bag to mix blood cells with the anticoagulant.<br>• Raise blood bag higher on IV pole. Squeeze flexible tubing to promote blood flow.<br>• Adjust clamp on tubing. As the blood passes over the filter, more blood microaggregates clog the filter and slow drip rate.<br>• Replace tubing.<br>• Utilize an infusion pump, especially if administering blood through a small catheter or lock.<br>• Consider using blood warmer. |

| UNEXPECTED OUTCOMES (cont.) | CRITICAL THINKING OPTIONS (cont.) |
|---|---|
| Blood has been hanging for more than 4 hours. | • Take down blood bag and send to laboratory.<br>• Document amount of blood administered.<br>• Maintain IV with normal saline or ordered IV solution.<br>• Monitor vital signs for complications.<br>• Notify physician. |
| Potential circulatory overload occurs. | • Monitor symptoms: sudden dyspnea, tachypnea, tachycardia, chest discomfort, distended neck veins, moist crackle and rales, restlessness, sudden increase in blood pressure.<br>• Stop transfusion and place client in Fowler's position.<br>• Start oxygen at 2 L/min per nasal cannula.<br>• Be prepared for ECG and chest x-ray.<br>• Be prepared to administer lasix and morphine sulfate. |
| Air enters central vein, producing air embolism from system being open at atmosphere. | • Immediately clamp catheter and place client in Trendelenburg position (turned to the left so right ventricle is uppermost).<br>• Immediately inform physician and monitor until physician arrives. Assess vital signs and breath sounds.<br>• Administer high-flow $O_2$ as necessary.<br>• Prevent air embolism by having client perform Valsalva's maneuver any time catheter is open to air, or use in-line catheter clamp.<br>• Ensure client has a patent peripheral IV line. |
| Infection at insertion site. | • Prepare for catheter removal and possible reinsertion at another site.<br>• If catheter is removed, cut off catheter tip with sterile scissors and place in sterile container, send tip to laboratory for culture.<br>• Administer antibiotics as ordered.<br>• Observe client carefully for signs of systemic infection. |
| Dysrhythmia detected. | • Change client's position.<br>• Notify physician.<br>• Verify catheter position on chest x-ray (right atrium placement causes dysrhythmias.<br>• Prepare for catheter repositioning or removal of catheter by physician. |
| Catheter becomes dislodged. | • Check the exact length of catheter to determine extent of problem.<br>• Secure catheter and extension tubing with tape to prevent further migration of tube.<br>• Notify physician immediately. |
| Catheter appears to be or becomes occluded. | • Reposition client.<br>• Ask client to raise arms overhead.<br>• Follow facility policy and procedure.<br>• Assess mechanical problem: tubing, pumps, catheter, clamps, insertion site, or sutures.<br>• Assess nonthrombotic problem: medications infused, fluids or withdrawal of blood. Use of precipitate clearance agent is established by individual facility policies and procedures.<br>• Assess thrombotic problem: use of thrombolytic clearance agents is established by individual facility policy and procedures.<br>• Perform Valsalva's maneuver. Turn head to one side.<br>• Attempt to flush catheter with normal saline, using gentle pressure.<br>• Notify physician for order to administer fibrinolytic agent or other agents. |

*(continued)*

**UNEXPECTED OUTCOMES (cont.)**

CVP system does not infuse.

CVP readings vary greatly.

**CRITICAL THINKING OPTIONS (cont.)**

- Check lines for kinks. Change client's position. Check to make sure the manometer stopcock is in the IV—>client position.
- Obtain order for placing heparin in IV bottle to maintain patency.
- Notify physician and prepare for possible reinsertion.

- Assess patency of setup.
- Assess client's level of pain; pain increases the CVP reading.
- Assess if position of client has been changed; raising the head of the bed alters the reading unless setup is adjusted.
- Check that the marked area at midaxillary level is at the level of the client's right atrium (4th ICS).
- If client has COPD, heart failure, or hypovolemia, expect readings to differ from normal range. However, once baseline is established for individual client, trends should be watched and evaluated against goals of therapy.

# Skill 12.61  Home Setting: Bathing Client in the Home

## Equipment

Personal care items (i.e., soap, deodorant, toothbrush)
Tray for personal items
Beach towel
Large piece of plastic
Call bell, dinner bell, or smoke alarm
Nonskid strips for tub
Shower chair or suction tips for chair legs

## Procedure

1. Keep all personal care items (soap, deodorant, lotion, powder, cosmetics, cologne, hair products, oral hygiene supplies, and other personal items) on a tray or in a handy carry tote (e.g., the type of rubber or plastic tote that can be purchased to carry household cleaning supplies).
2. Use beach towel for bath blanket.

3. Place plastic under towel to protect mattress prior to beginning the bath.
4. Ensure that nonskid strips or mats are on the floor of tub or shower.
   a. Ask family to purchase strips.
   b. Place wet terrycloth towel on floor of tub or shower if strips or mat not available. ➤*Rationale: A wet towel provides a temporary nonskid surface during bath or shower.*
5. Provide tub or shower stool or chair.
   a. Order from supply company, if family desires and can afford.
   b. Improvise shower chair by using straight-backed chair and attaching suction cups to legs to prevent sliding. (Suction cups are available at hardware stores.)
6. Simulate a client call bell by placing dinner bell or battery-powered smoke detector that emits a loud alarm within easy reach of client.

# Skill 12.62  Home Setting: Transferring Client to Tub or Shower

## Equipment

Towels
Shower or tub chair
Grips in bathtub or bath mat
Safety bars on tub or wall
Assistive devices (e.g., walker, wheelchair, cane) to assist to shower or tub if needed
Mechanical lift device, if needed

## Procedure

1. Gather equipment.
2. Place wet bath towel on the floor of tub or shower if safety grips or mats are not available.

3. Position chair or shower stool securely in the tub or shower. Place second chair or wheelchair outside tub.
4. Assist client to bathroom.
5. Transfer client to tub or shower chair before putting water in tub. Use mechanical lift device, or:
   a. Stand in front of client.
   b. Lower client into chair, bending your knees and keeping your back straight. ➤*Rationale: This provides most secure balance and aids in preventing back injuries.*
   c. Flex your knees, move to kneeling position, and keep your back straight while assisting client to swing legs over side of tub.

# Skill 12.63   Home Setting: Adapting Bedmaking to the Home

## Equipment

Sheets
Pillowcases
Plastic trash bag
Cotton flannel
Plastic shower curtain

## Procedure

1. Follow directions for making an occupied or unoccupied bed outlined in Skills 12.1 and 12.2.
2. Turn pillowcase inside out and use as laundry bag, or use plastic trash bag.
3. Place one knee on bed if bed cannot be moved away from wall. This is especially useful when making water beds.
4. Make incontinent pads with cotton flannel if commercial pads are not available. ➤*Rationale: This material is soft and easily laundered.*
5. Make bed protectors by cutting a piece of plastic shower curtain or heavy trash bag. Cover with drawsheet or cotton flannel. ➤*Rationale: This protects skin from direct contact with plastic.*

# Skill 12.64   Home Setting: Providing Wound Care

## Equipment

Normal saline solution
Medicated ointment (if prescribed)
Irrigation set (if needed)
Asepto syringe
Dressings—hydrocolloid or transparent adhesive film
Nonallergic tape
Clean gloves
Plastic bags

## Procedure

1. Perform hand hygiene.
2. Don clean gloves.
3. Remove dressings. Discard in plastic bag.
4. Cleanse with normal saline solution, or irrigate the wound with warm, soapy water, rinsing thoroughly, according to physician orders.
5. Allow to dry or apply medicated ointment, as ordered.
6. Apply dressing as ordered.
7. Dispose of waste according to protocol.
8. Remove gloves and perform hand hygiene.

*Note:* For pressure ulcer care, follow specific directions for pressure ulcer care in Chapter 10, "Tissue Integrity."

# Skill 12.65   Home Setting: Removing Lice

## Equipment

Isolation bag or plastic bag
Treatment solution as ordered
Clean linen
Fine-tooth comb
Disinfectant for comb
Clean towel
Spray for fomites

## Procedure

1. Obtain order for treatment and notify family members and health care givers. ➤*Rationale: All household members and caregivers must be treated to prevent the spread of lice to others.*
2. Remove and bag client's clothing and linens, and place in plastic bag. Launder these articles separately. Use hot water at 130°F and detergent. ➤*Rationale: This prevents cross-contamination of lice to other family members.*
3. Items that cannot be washed should be dry cleaned. Place in plastic bag, seal, and take to dry cleaner.
4. Begin treatment as ordered by physician. Common treatments include cream, lotion, or shampoo. ➤*Rationale: Head lice infestation requires shampoo.* Body and pubic lice require shower with soap followed by lotion application. Common treatments include:
    Permethrin (Elimit Nix)
    Pyrethrum extract (Rid)
    Any OTC pediculicide product that contains permethrin or pyrethrum

5. Shake lotion well, and apply thin film of lotion over entire body (excluding face, urethral meatus, and soles of feet). Rub in, allow skin to dry and cool. Leave in place 8–12 hours. Remove by washing.
6. Apply shampoo, and leave in place 4 minutes.
   ▶*Rationale: Prolonged use of shampoo can burn scalp.*
7. Rinse thoroughly.
8. Comb through hair with fine-tooth comb.
9. Disinfect comb and brushes in rubbing alcohol or Lysol for 1 hour; rinse in hot water.
10. Perform hand hygiene.
11. Instruct client to vacuum rugs, upholstery, and furniture. Then, spray with a commercial spray. Empty vacuum cleaner bag into trash bag, and seal.
12. Discuss with client and family the cause, treatment, and preventive measures regarding lice infestation.
13. Instruct client or family to repeat treatment in 7–10 days only if living lice are present.

# Skill 12.66  Home Setting: Administering Medications

## Procedure

1. Examine all medications taken by the client during the admission visit and subsequent visits. Include all over-the-counter (OTC) as well as prescription drugs. Document on assessment sheet.
2. Discuss lifestyle with client and family as it relates to medication schedule and their beliefs about medications.
3. Establish the medication regimen based on physician's orders or prescribed drugs and client's schedule.
4. Teach client and family the medication regimen.
5. Teach client and family how to monitor for effects and side effects of drugs.
6. Design medication aids, such as a calendar of drugs or daily/weekly pill reminder boxes, to help client and family remember to take medications.
   a. Investigate and share with the client and family those aids that are commercially available.
   b. Improvise using household items, such as egg cartons, tiny paper cups attached together or stacked, or empty match boxes glued together to make a row of pill containers that can be labeled with time and day.
7. Design creative methods to assist client and family to administer medication.
   a. If client has trouble seeing the markings on a syringe or on medication bottles, the nurse may recommend a magnifying glass, magnifying syringe, or marking the bottles or syringes with tape at the appropriate dosage.
   b. If a client lives alone, needs daily insulin, and knows the procedures but cannot see well enough to fill the syringes accurately, the nurse may prefill the syringes and leave them in the refrigerator for use between visits. Check if mixed insulin can be prefilled and is allowed to be refrigerated before using. ▶*Rationale: NPH or lente insulin mixed with regular must be administered immediately, otherwise it loses its potency.*
   c. Take syringe out of refrigerator 1 hour before administration.
   d. If other medications are prefilled in a syringe, determine if any qualifiers exist, such as how long before medication must be administered.
8. Discard uncapped needles and syringes in sharps container.
9. Document all teaching and learning outcomes, administration of medication, and client response to medications.

---

### CLINICAL ALERT

Home health aides and homemakers are not allowed to administer medications to clients in the home setting. Families should be instructed not to ask home health aides or homemakers to give medication.

### CLINICAL ALERT

New insulin pens have a magnified dose window for easier viewing of dosage. These dose pens are safer to use for clients with impaired vision.

# Skill 12.67 Home Setting: Sterilizing Nondisposable Medication Equipment

## Equipment

Large pan or kettle
Jar or container with lid for storage
Equipment to be sterilized
Tongs or forceps for handling sterile equipment

## Procedure

1. Place jar, lid, tongs, and equipment in large clean pan.
2. Fill pan with cold water until all equipment is covered.
3. Place pan on stove.
4. Boil water for 20 minutes.
5. Pour off water.
6. Lift equipment out of pan, using tongs. Remove jar from pan by touching only the outside.
7. Position jar so sterile equipment can easily be inserted without touching edges of the jar.
8. Place lid on jar by grasping outside edge and twisting tightly.

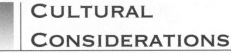

## CULTURAL CONSIDERATIONS

Home health care nurses are being asked to decrease the amount of time spent with home care clients. They are also being asked to provide high-quality and culturally competent care and be cost effective. In some areas of the United States, folk remedies are common to the clients but unknown to the nurses. Some clients do not trust nurses who are not of their culture and who do not seem to understand their need for folk remedies. To provide the necessary care and be cost effective, it is imperative that the nurse assess each client's cultural norms and mores, determine their experience with Western medicine, and ask about the folk remedies they are currently using. It is very important to identify any herbs or other remedies the client is taking, as they could affect medications being prescribed by the physician. Completing a cultural assessment will provide necessary information for the nurse to develop an effective treatment plan for the client to follow.

# 13

# Safety

**Skill 13.1**    Providing Safety for Clients during a Fire    675

**Skill 13.2**    Preventing Thermal/Electrical Injuries    676

**Skill 13.3**    Managing Clients in Restraints    677

     VARIATION: Applying Torso/Belt Restraints    678

**Skill 13.4**    Using a Bed or Chair Exit Safety Monitoring Device    678

**Skill 13.5**    Applying Wrist or Ankle Restraint    680

**Skill 13.6**    Applying a Papoose Board Immobilizer    681

**Skill 13.7**    Applying a Mummy Immobilizer    682

**Skill 13.8**    Implementing Seizure Precautions    683

**Skill 13.9**    Identifying Eligibility for Medicare Reimbursement    685

**Skill 13.10**    Completing Admission Documentation    687

**Skill 13.11**    Maintaining Nurse's Safety    687

**Skill 13.12**    Assessing Home for Safe Environment    688

**Skill 13.13**    Evaluating Client's Safety    689

**Skill 13.14**    Assessing Caregiver's Safety    690

**Skill 13.15**    Assessing for Elder Abuse    690

A safe physical environment is one in which people can function without injury and feel a sense of security. The skills in this chapter focus on those measures the nurse can take to reduce the risk of client injury as a result of unsafe movement within and out of a bed or chair. These include measures that are taken in anticipation of and in the event of a seizure during which the client cannot control physical movement and is at risk of sustaining an injury. Attention to the dignity and well being of clients must be maintained at all times. Many clients will have strong emotional responses around issues of falling, being restrained, and having a seizure. Embarrassment, fear, and a decreased sense of autonomy and control can all compromise a client's healing potential. The holistic nurse will demonstrate therapeutic presence while providing the skills presented in this chapter.

# Skill 13.1   Providing Safety for Clients during a Fire

## Equipment

Appropriate extinguisher for fire:
Water type
Soda-acid type
Foam type
Dry chemical type
Carbon dioxide type
ABC extinguisher

## Procedure

1. Follow hospital policy and procedure for type of fire safety program and for ringing the fire alarm to summon help.
2. Remove all clients from the immediate area to a safe place. Be familiar with fire exits and agency evacuation plan.
3. To remove a client safely from the fire, use carrying method that is most comfortable for you and safe for client.
   a. Place blanket (or bedspread) on floor. Lower client onto blanket. Lift up head end of blanket and drag client out of danger.
   b. Use two-person swing method. Place client in sitting position. Form a seat by having two people clasp forearms or shoulders. Lift client into "seat" and carry out of danger.
   c. Carry client using "back-strap" carry method. Step in front of client. Place client's arms around your neck. Grasp client's wrists and hold tight against your chest. Pull client onto your back and carry to safety.

4. Activate fire alarm.
5. Secure the burning area by closing all doors and windows.
6. Shut off all possible oxygen sources and electrical appliances in the fire area.
7. If possible, employ the appropriate extinguishing method without endangering yourself. Fire extinguishers should not be used directly on a person.
8. Be familiar with the different types of fire extinguishers and their location.

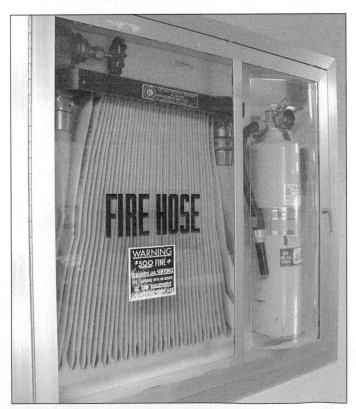

● Become familiar with the location and use of fire extinguishers in the hospital.

---

### PRIORITIES FOR FIRE SAFETY

R   rescue and remove all clients in immediate danger

A   activate fire alarm

C   confine the fire; close doors, window, turn off oxygen supplies and electrical equipment

E   Extinguish fire when possible

### Class A

a. Water-under-pressure type or soda-acid type.
b. Use on cloth, wood, paper, plastic, rubber, or leather.
c. Never use on electrical or chemical fires due to danger of shock.

### Class B

a. Foam, dry chemical, carbon dioxide types.
b. Use on fires such as gasoline, alcohol, acetone, oil, grease, or paint thinner and remover.
c. Class A extinguisher is never used on class B fires.

### Class C

a. Dry chemical or carbon dioxide types.
b. Use on electrical wiring, electrical equipment, or motors.
c. Class A or class B extinguishers are never used on class C fires.

### Class ABC combination

a. Contains graphite.
b. Use on any type of fire.
c. Most common extinguisher in use.

9. Keep fire exits clear at all times.

# Skill 13.2   Preventing Thermal/Electrical Injuries

## Equipment

Fire extinguishers
Covers for heat and cold application devices

## Procedure

1. Make sure that all electrical apparatuses are routinely checked and maintained. Look for safety inspection expiration dates on biomedical equipment.
2. Have all electrical appliances brought to the hospital by client (radios, electric razors, hair dryers, etc.) inspected by hospital maintenance staff. It is best to discourage use of nonhospital equipment.
3. Make sure water in the tub or shower is not more than 110°F (95°F for those with circulatory insufficiency).
4. When heating pads, sitz bath, or hot compresses are used, check the client frequently for redness. Maximum temperature should not exceed 105°F (95°F for those with circulatory insufficiency).
5. Hospitals do not allow smoking in the facility. There may be designated smoking areas outside the building. Inform clients and visitors about the hospital's smoking regulations. Do not allow confused, sedated, or severely incapacitated clients to smoke without direct supervision.
6. Store all combustible materials securely to prevent spontaneous combustion.
7. Make sure that all staff and employees participate in and understand fire safety measures, such as extinguishing fires and plan for evacuating clients.
8. Report and do not use any apparatus that produces a shock, has a broken plug or ground pin, or has a frayed cord.
9. Never apply direct heat (e.g., heating pad) to ischemic tissue—doing so increases the tissue's need for oxygen.
10. Turn equipment off before unplugging it. ➤*Rationale: This prevents sparks that can cause a fire.*
11. Plug devices that require a high current (i.e., ventilators or radiant warmers) into separate outlets. ➤*Rationale: This prevents overloading the circuit that could lead to a fire.*
12. Use only three-pronged grounded plugs.

---

### CLINICAL ALERT

The elderly, diabetic, or comatose client is especially vulnerable to thermal injuries.

# Skill 13.3   Managing Clients in Restraints

## Equipment

Appropriate restraint, limb, torso, and vest

## Preparation

1. Identify and evaluate if less restrictive measures have been explored before the client is placed in restraints.
2. Call physician or LIP for restraint order before applying restraints. If restraints must be placed before the order is obtained, ensure the order is obtained within 1 hour for either a nonbehavioral health client or a behavioral health client. ➤*Rationale: Physician's order is required to apply restraints.*

*Note:* Follow guidelines for obtaining restraint orders and updating orders according to hospital policy.

3. Ensure that a face-to-face assessment is completed on the client within 8 hours for a nonbehavioral health client, and 1 hour for a behavioral (psychiatric) health client. ➤*Rationale: Frequent assessments prevent complications.*
4. Ensure that restraint orders are renewed every 24 hours or sooner according to facility policy for nonbehavioral health clients, or every 2 to 4 hours for behavioral health clients. Children from 12 to 17 must have orders renewed every 2 hours, for a maximum of 24 hours. ➤*Rationale: Restraints should be discontinued as soon as possible.*
5. Establish and implement a plan of care for the client to eliminate the need for restraints.
6. Discuss the use of restraints with the client and family members. If possible, elicit the support of the family or use sitters to stay with the client rather than place the client in restraints.

## Procedure

1. Gather appropriate restraint and perform hand hygiene.
2. Seek the client's cooperation with restraint procedure, if possible.
3. Apply restraint according to manufacturer's specific directions.
4. Monitor and assess the client every 15 minutes.

---

**CLINICAL ALERT**

Restraints are indicated only if there is no other viable option available to protect the client; and then they are implemented only when the client is assessed and evaluated by an appropriate licensed independent practitioner.

---

**CLINICAL ALERT**

There are three types of restraints used in clinical practice:

1. *Chemical:* Sedating psychotropic drugs to manage or control behavior. Psychoactive medication used in this manner is an inappropriate use of medication.
2. *Physical:* Direct application of physical force to a client, without the client's permission, to restrict his or her freedom of movement.
3. *Seclusion:* Involuntary confinement of a client in a locked room.

Physical force may be applied by individuals, mechanical devices, or a combination of any of them.

---

5. Release restraint at least every 2 hours or sooner (JCAHO, 2004). ➤*Rationale: Releasing restraints allows the client to be provided with the following:*
   a. Toileting.
   b. Fluids and food.
   c. Hygiene care such as brushing teeth or washing face and hands.
   d. Circulation checked; skin care provided.
   e. Body alignment checked.
   f. Range of motion to all joints, particularly those in restraints.
6. Avoid application of force on long bone joints and pad bony prominences beneath restraint. ➤*Rationale: Reduces pressure on skin.*
7. Take vital signs every 8 hours unless indicated more frequently.

---

**CLINICAL ALERT**

In acute medical and post-surgical care, a restraint may be necessary to ensure that an IV or tube feeding is not removed, or the client cannot be allowed out of bed following surgery. This type of medical restraint may be used temporarily to limit mobility or prevent injury to the client.

Additional types of activities that may constitute a restraint include:

- Tucking a client's sheet so tight that he/she cannot move.
- Using a side rail to prevent a client from voluntarily getting out of bed.
- Placing the client in a geri-chair with a table.
- Placing a wheelchair-bound client so close to the wall that it prevents them from moving.

8. Bathe client every 24 hours or more often as needed.
9. Do not interrupt the client's sleep unless indicated by his/her medical condition.
10. Ensure that a new order and the physician or LIP completes a medical assessment every 24 hours.
11. Obtain a physician's order and discontinue restraints as soon as it is clinically indicated.
12. Document all assessments and findings on appropriate forms.

### VARIATION: Applying Torso/Belt Restraints

#### Equipment

Safety belt restraint (usually 2 inch soft webbing material) with waist and side belts (for bed)

#### Procedure

1. Check physician's order and client care plan for torso/belt restraint. Perform hand hygiene.
2. Obtain belt. Belts usually have a key-locked buckle. ➤*Rationale: To prevent slipping and to provide a snug fit.*
3. Explain necessity for safety belt to client and family.
4. Apply torso restraint as follows:
   a. Slip waist belt through flat buckle, adjusting to client's size.
   b. Snap hinged plate shut by hooking plain end of key over cross bar and lifting upward.
   c. Attach side belts to bed frame in similar manner.
   d. Release restraint by hooking green end of key over cross bar from below and pulling downward.

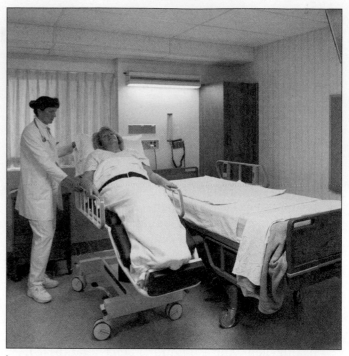

● Some belts have a key-locked buckle to prevent slipping and to provide a snug fit.

5. Document time, rationale, and type of safety belt used in nurses' notes, along with client monitoring, client response, frequency of care measures, and time and rationale for discontinuing restraint. Documentation must be done every 15 minutes.

# Skill 13.4   Using a Bed or Chair Exit Safety Monitoring Device

### Delegation

Risk factors for falls may be observed and recorded by persons other than the nurse. The nurse is responsible for assessing the client and confirming that there is a risk of the client falling when getting out of a chair or bed unassisted. The nurse develops a plan of care that includes a variety of interventions that will protect the client. If indicated, use of a safety monitoring device may be delegated to unlicensed assistive personnel (UAP) who have been trained in its application and monitoring.

### Equipment

• Alarm and control device
• Sensor
• Connection to nurse call system

### Procedure

1. Prior to performing the procedure, introduce self and verify the client's identity using agency protocol. Explain to client and family the purpose and procedure of using a safety monitoring device. Explain that the device does not limit mobility in any manner; rather, it alerts the staff when the client is about to get out of bed or a chair. Explain that the nurse must be called when the client needs to get out of bed or a chair.
2. Perform hand hygiene and observe appropriate infection control procedures.
3. Provide for client privacy.
4. Test the battery device and alarm sound. ➤*Rationale: Testing ensures that the device is functioning properly prior to use.*

5. Apply the leg band or sensor pad.
   - Place the leg band according to the manufacturer's recommendation. Place the client's leg in a straight horizontal position. ➤*Rationale: The alarm device is position sensitive; that is, when it approaches a near-vertical position (such as in walking, crawling, or kneeling as the client attempts to get out of bed), the audio alarm will be triggered.*
   - For the bed or chair device, the sensor is usually placed under the buttocks area.
   - For a bed or chair device, set the time delay to 1 to 12 seconds for determining the client's movement patterns.
   - Connect the sensor pad to the control unit and the nurse call system.
6. Instruct the client to call the nurse when the client wants or needs to get up, and assist as required.
   - When assisting the client up, deactivate the alarm.
   - Assist the client back to bed or chair, and reattach the alarm device.
7. Ensure client safety with additional safety precautions.
   - Place call light within client reach, lift side rails per agency policy, and lower the bed to its lowest position.

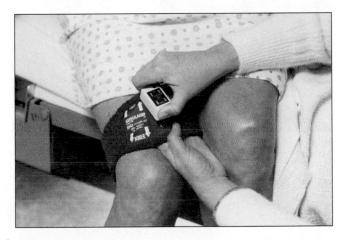

● Placing the leg band alarm.
(Courtesy of Alert Care, Mill Valley, CA)

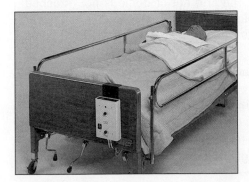

   ➤*Rationale: The alarm device is not a substitute for other precautionary measures.*
   - Place ambulation monitoring stickers on the client's door, chart, and other relevant locations.
8. Document the type of alarm used, where it was placed, and its effectiveness in the client record using forms or checklists supplemented by narrative notes when appropriate. Record all additional safety precautions and interventions discussed and employed.

### Documentation

Sample: 7/2/09 1130 Found out of bed despite frequent verbal reminders to use call light for assistance. Explained about using a magnetic box mobility alarm to ensure own safety from possible fall. Verbalized agreement. Alarm device applied. Reminded again of importance to call the nurse for assistance. Call light placed within client's reach.
—————————————————— J. Wallace, RN

### SETTING OF CARE

If a monitoring device is used in the home, instruct caregivers to do the following:
- Test the monitoring device every 12 to 24 hours to ensure that it is working.
- Check the volume of the alarm to ascertain they can hear it.
- Although these devices are sensitive and alarms can be triggered by normal movement, instruct family to investigate all alarms, and not to assume a false alarm. They may, however, adjust the alarm controls.

Use of the device does not take the place of proper supervision of clients at risk for falling. Assessment of the reasons for falling, especially among elders, can lead to effective prevention.

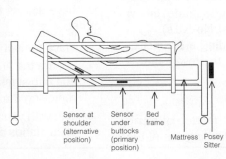

● Placement of a bed exit monitoring device.
(Courtesy of J. T. Posey, Co.)

Sensor at shoulder (alternative position) | Sensor under buttocks (primary position) | Bed frame | Mattress Posey Sitter

# Skill 13.5   Applying Wrist or Ankle Restraint

## Delegation

The nurse must make the determination that restraints are appropriate in specific situations, select the proper type of restraints, evaluate the effectiveness of the restraints, and assess for potential complications from their use. Application of ordered restraints and their temporary removal for skin monitoring and care may be delegated to UAP who have been trained in their use.

## Equipment

Appropriate type and size of restraint.

## Procedure

1. Prior to performing the procedure, introduce self and verify the client's identity using agency protocol. Explain to the client and family what you are going to do, why it is necessary, and how they can participate. Allow time for the client to express feelings about being restrained. Provide needed emotional reassurance that the restraints will be used only when absolutely necessary and that there will be close contact with the client in case assistance is needed.
2. Perform hand hygiene and observe appropriate infection control procedures.
3. Provide for client privacy if indicated.
4. Apply the selected restraint.

### Wrist or Ankle Restraint

- Pad bony prominences on the wrist or ankle if needed to prevent skin breakdown.
- Apply the padded portion of the restraint around the ankle or wrist.

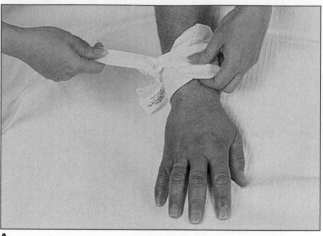

**A**

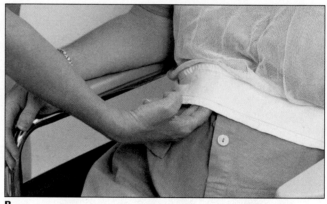

**B**

 Ensure that a finger can be inserted between the restraint and **A,** the wrist; and **B,** the chest.

---

## DEVELOPMENTAL CONSIDERATIONS

### Infants

Elbow restraints are used to prevent infants or small children from flexing their elbows to touch or reach their face or head, especially after surgery. Ready-made elbow restraints are available commercially (e.g., No-No's).

A mummy restraint is made by folding a blanket or sheet around the infant, in a certain way to prevent movement during a blood specimen.

### Children

A crib net is simply a device placed over the top of a crib to prevent active young children from climbing out of the crib. At the same time, it allows them freedom to move about in the crib. The crib net or dome is not attached to the movable parts of the crib so that the caregiver can have access to the child without removing the dome or net.

- Place the net over the sides and ends of the crib.
- Secure the ties to the springs or frame of the crib. The crib sides can then be freely lowered without removing the net.
- Test with your hand that the net will stretch if the child stands against it in the crib.

- Pull the tie of the restraint through the slit in the wrist portion or through the buckle and ensure the restraint is not too tight.
- Using a half-bow knot, attach the other end of the restraint to the movable portion of the bed frame. ➤*Rationale: If the ties are attached to the movable portion, the wrist or ankle will not be pulled when the bed position is changed.*

5. Adjust the plan of care as required, for example, to include releasing the restraint, all other interventions implemented in an attempt to avoid the use of restraints and their outcomes, and the time the primary care provider was notified of the need for restraint. Also record:
   - The type of restraint applied, the time it was applied, and the goal for its application.
   - The client's response to the restraint, including a rationale for its continued use (Anstine, 2007).
   - The times that the restraints were removed and skin care given.
   - Any other assessments and interventions.
   - Explanations given the client and significant others.

### Documentation

Sample: 7/10/2009 1200 Confused. Disoriented to time and place. Reoriented frequently. Pulling at central IV line, NG tube and chest tube. Medicated for pain relief. Lights dimmed.

_____ M. Murray, RN

1245 Continues to pull at IV and tubes. Dr. Jones notified. Received an order to apply mitt restraints. Family notified and situation explained. Family member to come and sit with client. Mitt restraints applied, relaxation music initiated. _____ M. Murray, RN

1330 Son arrived and sitting with client. Calm though still disoriented. Mitts removed, skin intact, hands warm with good color and mobility. Vital signs stable.

_____ M. Murray, RN

---

### SETTING OF CARE

While other measures should always be tried first, restraints may be necessary for clients in wheelchairs or in the home. Safety guidelines apply in all cases. Assess the knowledge and skill of all caregivers in the use of restraints and educate as indicated.

- Use means other than restraints as much as possible, and stay with the client. Remember that the goal is a restraint-free environment.
- Pad bony prominences, such as wrists and ankles, if needed before applying a restraint over them.
- Tie restraints with half-bow (quick release) knots that will not tighten when pulled, and to parts of the wheelchair that do not move and release quickly in case of emergency.
- Assess restrained limbs for signs of impaired blood circulation.
- Always stay with a client whose restraint is temporarily removed.

---

# Skill 13.6   Applying a Papoose Board Immobilizer

### Preparation

1. Gather equipment and supplies for the procedure. ➤*Rationale: Having supplies prepared reduces the time the child spends in temporary restrain devices and reduces the anxiety felt by the child.*
2. Explain the reason for immobilization to the child and parent and how long it will be needed. ➤*Rationale: Young children will be less anxious if the explanation about what they will feel is placed in nonthreatening, developmentally appropriate terms.*
3. Have an assistant (or the parent) available to help position and hold a body part if needed. ➤*Rationale: The papoose is most often used when the nurse does not have an assistant available or a parent willing to restrain the child for a procedure.*

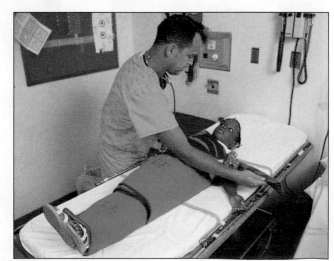

● Child on a papoose board.

**Equipment**

- Immobilization board (papoose) to fit the child's size
- Sheet
- Infection control supplies as needed.

**Procedure**

1. Place a towel or sheet over the board.
2. Have the child lie supine on the board, with the head at the top.

3. Place the fabric wrappings around the child, and secure the Velcro fasteners. To be most effective, the fabric wrappings should be secure over the elbows, hips, and knees to prevent flexion. ➤*Rationale: This action prevents the child from pulling apart the wrappings or from kicking.*
4. After the procedure, release the child and allow the parents to provide comfort.

# Skill 13.7   Applying a Mummy Immobilizer

**Preparation**

1. Have supplies and materials for the procedure collected and ready for use.
2. Explain the procedure to the child and parent.

**Equipment**

- Soft blanket or sheet two to three times larger than the child.

**Procedure**

*Infant*

1. Put the blanket (or sheet) on the bed or examination table. Fold down one corner until it reaches the middle of the blanket.

2. Place the infant in a diagonal position with his or her neck on the folded edge.
3. Bring one side of the blanket over the infant's arm and then under the back. Tuck that edge under and over the other arm and around the back. It may be helpful to roll the infant on the side to smooth the blanket behind the back, and then roll the infant onto the back over the smoothed section of blanket.
4. Bring the other side of the blanket around the body and tuck underneath the body.
5. Bring the bottom corner of the blanket up and over the abdomen.

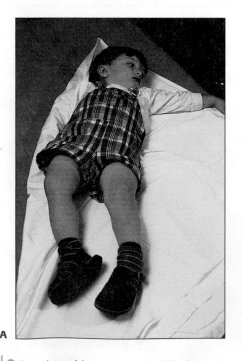

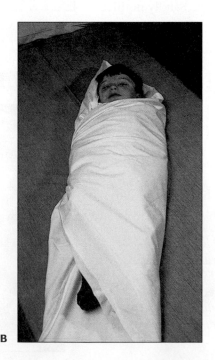

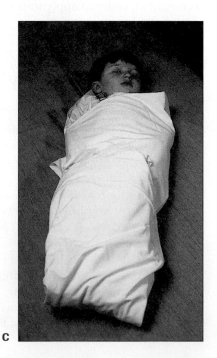

A          B          C

● Steps in applying mummy immobilization.

### Toddler and Older Child

1. Put the blanket (or sheet) on the bed or examination table. Fold down one corner until it reaches the middle of the blanket.
2. Place the child on the blanket, positioning so that there is sufficient material to wrap the knees and lower legs. If necessary, fold down the top edges of the blanket to the shoulders.

3. Bring one side of the blanket over the arm, body, and legs, and tuck it under the other arm and around the back and legs.
4. Bring the other side of the blanket up and around the body, and tuck underneath the back and legs. ➤*Rationale: The child should not be able to flex the knees and kick or it may be impossible to perform the procedure.*

# Skill 13.8  Implementing Seizure Precautions

### Delegation

UAP should be familiar with establishing and implementing seizure precautions and methods of obtaining assistance during a client's seizure. Care of the client during a seizure, however, is the responsibility of the nurse due to the importance of careful assessment of respiratory status and the potential need for intervention.

### Equipment

- Blankets or other linens to pad side rails
- Oral suction equipment and clean gloves
- Oxygen equipment

### Procedure

1. Prior to performing the procedure, introduce self and verify the client's identity using agency protocol. Explain to the client what you are going to do, why it is necessary, and how he or she can participate.

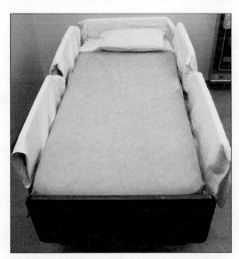

● Padding a bed for seizure precautions.

2. Perform hand hygiene and observe appropriate infection control procedures. If the client is actively seizing, apply clean gloves in preparation for performing respiratory care measures.
3. Provide for client privacy.
4. Pad the bed of any client who might have a seizure. Secure blankets or other linens around the head, foot, and side rails of the bed.
5. Put oral suction equipment in place and test to ensure that it is functional. ➤*Rationale: Suctioning may be needed to prevent aspiration of oral secretions.*
6. If a seizure occurs:
   - Remain with the client and call for assistance. Do not restrain the client.
   - If the client is not in bed, assist client to the floor and protect the client's head by holding it in your lap or on a pillow. Loosen any clothing around the neck and chest.
   - Turn the client to a lateral position if possible. ➤*Rationale: Turning to the side allows secretions to drain out of the mouth, decreasing the risk of aspiration, and helps keep the tongue from occluding the airway.*
   - Move items in the environment to ensure the client does not experience an injury.
   - Do not insert anything into the client's mouth.
   - Time the seizure duration.
   - Observe the progression of the seizure, noting the sequence and type of limb involvement. Observe skin color. When the seizure allows, check pulse and respirations.
   - Apply oxygen via mask or nasal cannula.
   - Use equipment to suction the mouth if the client vomits or has excessive oral secretions.
   - Administer anticonvulsant medications, as ordered.
   - When the seizure has subsided, assist client to a comfortable position. Reorient. Explain what happened. Reassure the client. Provide hygiene as necessary. Allow the client to verbalize feelings about the seizure.

## DEVELOPMENTAL CONSIDERATIONS

### Infants

- The most common cause of seizures in young infants is birth injury (e.g., intracranial trauma, hemorrhage, anoxia) or congenital brain defects. Onset of epilepsy is highest in the first few months of life (Hockenberry & Wilson, 2007).

### Children

- In children over 3 years of age, the most common cause of seizures is idiopathic epilepsy.
- Febrile seizures associated with acute infections occur more commonly in children than in adults and are usually preventable through the use of antipyretics and tepid baths.

- Determine oxygenation. Apply oxygen if pulse oximetry reading is less than 95%. Oxygen can be applied via head hood, tent, nasal cannula, or mask, depending on the age and response of the child. Oxygen is drying and must be humidified. Tents are cooling, and the child's thermal balance must be monitored. The concentration of oxygen in tents is more difficult to regulate.
- Children who have frequent seizures may need to wear helmets for protection.
- Children on anticonvulsant medications should wear a medical identification tag (bracelet or necklace).

## SETTING OF CARE

- If clients have frequent or recurrent seizures or take anticonvulsant medications, they should wear a medical identification tag (bracelet or necklace) and carry a card delineating any medications they take.
- When making home visits, inspect anticonvulsant medications and confirm that clients are taking them correctly. Blood level measurements may be required periodically.
- Assist clients in determining which persons in the community should or must be informed of their

seizure disorder (e.g., employers, health care providers such as dentists, motor vehicle department if driving, and companions).
- Discuss safety precautions for inside and out of the home. If seizures are not well controlled, activities that may require restriction or direct supervision by others include tub bathing, swimming, cooking, using electric equipment or machinery, and driving.
- Discuss with the client and family factors that may precipitate a seizure.

---

- If applied, remove and discard gloves. Perform hand hygiene.
7. Document the event in the client record using forms or checklists supplemented by narrative notes when appropriate.

### Documentation

Sample: 7/8/09 1815 Upon entering room, observed generalized muscle spasms/contractions of arms and legs lasting 25 seconds. Seizure padding previously placed on bed. Incontinent of urine. Cyanotic. Placed on left side.

Suctioned. Airway clear. Respirations 14/min with irregular pattern. Oxygen applied at 4 L/min via mask. Oxygen sat 90% on O2. Not currently responding to verbal stimuli. Dr. Smith notified.

_____ M. Faustino, RN

1835 Respirations 15/min, regular. Responding to verbal stimuli, oriented to person, place and time. Oxygen sat 95% on $O_2$. $O_2$ discontinued per doctor's order. VS taken every 15 min. See neuro flow sheet.

_____ M. Faustino, RN

## HOME SETTING

# Skill 13.9   Identifying Eligibility for Medicare Reimbursement

**Procedure**

1. Complete OASIS forms.
   a. Integrate information with H485 data.
   b. Complete all sections of document. ➤*Rationale: Denial of service can result if documentation incomplete.*
   c. Complete forms within 7 days.
   d. Ensure information from forms is transcribed accurately onto H485 forms. ➤*Rationale: To prevent denial of service.*
2. Check required criteria for Medicare coverage eligibility. ➤*Rationale: This prevents administering care for which reimbursement will not be received.*
3. Identify client as homebound.
   a. Client's condition severely restricts leaving the home.
   b. Leaving the home requires considerable effort and assistance of another person.
   c. Special transportation is necessary.
   d. Absences from the home are infrequent and short.
4. Check that home service is considered skilled. To be skilled, service must be under the supervision of a registered nurse or a physical therapist.
   a. Registered nurse performs specific functions:
   Client teaching
   Dressings or irrigations
   Catheterization
   Parenteral therapies
   Medication administration and teaching
   b. Physical therapist performs certain functions:
   Gait training
   Therapeutic exercises
   Ultrasound, diathermy, TENS
   Restorative therapy
   c. Speech therapist performs certain functions:
   Therapy for clients with certain diagnoses (e.g., CVA, laryngectomies)
   Selected diagnostic and evaluative services
5. Provide supplemental services from home health aide, social worker, or occupational therapist; care is reimbursed by Medicare only when one of the three skilled services is required.
   a. Supplemental services may be obtained even if one of the skilled services is not needed; however, Medicare does not reimburse, and client is responsible for payment.
   b. Home health aide services are reimbursable only if plan of care is established and supervised by registered nurse. Personal care (ADL) Light housekeeping (e.g., food preparation, client's laundry) Selected semiskilled care (e.g., PROM exercises).

   c. Social worker.
   Interventions must contribute significantly to the improvement of the client's medical condition. Indication that social, environmental, or family conditions inhibit progress of recovery from medical condition
   d. Occupational therapy.
   Design maintenance program
   Teach compensatory techniques and activities of daily living (ADL)
   Design self-help devices to assist ADL
   Provide restorative therapy
6. Provide care that is part-time and intermittent.
   a. Care must be episodic or acute and not chronic.
   b. Medically predictable recurring need for care must be present.
   c. Knowledge that condition will improve in a limited time frame.
   d. Frequency of service ranges from daily to every 90 days, depending on individual client's need.
7. Check that plan of treatment is authorized by physician and recertified every 60 days.
   a. Health Care Financing Administration form (H485) is standardized for plan of treatment. This form is used by all home health agencies for Medicare clients.
   b. Form must include:
   Identifying data
   Diagnosis (ICD-9CM)
   Start of care
   Types of services required and frequency
   Functional limitations
   Activities permitted
   Safety measures
   Treatments
   Medications
   Mental status
   Nutritional status and diet orders
   Medical supplies and DME
      Goals and discharge plans
      Significant clinical findings
      Prognosis
      Physician's name, address, signature
      Certification of homebound status
8. Assess that care is medically reasonable and necessary.
   a. Entire plan of care must correlate with client's medical problems and client's clinical status.
   b. Each service's goals (client outcomes) must be clearly stated and realistic for the client.

**Outcome and Assessment Information Set (OASIS-B1)**

**START OF CARE VERSION**
(also used for Resumption of Care Following Inpatient Stay)

Items to be Used at this Time Point------------------------------------------ M0080–M0825

## CLINICAL RECORD ITEMS

**(M0080) Discipline of Person Completing Assessment:**
☐ 1-RN  ☐ 2-PT  ☐ 3-SLP/ST  ☐ 4-OT

**(M0090) Date Assessment Completed:** ___/___/___
month  day  year

**(M0100) This Assessment is Currently Being Completed for the Following Reason:**
**Start/Resumption of Care**
☐ 1 – Start of care—futher visits planned
☐ 3 – Resumption of care (after inpatient stay)

## DEMOGRAPHICS AND PATIENT HISTORY

**(M0175)** From which of the following **Inpatient Facilities** was the patient discharged during the past 14 days?
(**Mark all that apply.**)
☐ 1 – Hospital
☐ 2 – Rehabilitation facility
☐ 3 – Skilled nursing facility
☐ 4 – Other nursing home
☐ 5 – Other (specify)
☐ NA – Patient was not discharged from an inpatient facility [ If NA, go to *M0200* ]

**(M0180) Inpatient Discharge Date** (most recent):
___/___/___
month  day  year
☐ UK – Unknown

**(M0190) Inpatient Diagnoses** and ICD-9-CM code categories (three digits required; five digits optional) for only those conditions treated during an inpatient facility stay within the last 14 days (no surgical or V-codes):

| Inpatient Facility Diagnosis | ICD-9-CM |
|---|---|
| a. _____ | (___ ___ ___ . ___ ___) |
| b. _____ | (___ ___ ___ . ___ ___) |

**Effective 10/1/2003**
List each Inpatient Diagnosis and ICD-9-CM code at the level of highest specificity for only those conditions treated during an inpatient stay within the last 14 days (no surgical, E-codes, or V-codes):

| Inpatient Facility Diagnosis | ICD-9-CM |
|---|---|
| a. _____ | (___ ___ ___ . ___ ___) |
| b. _____ | (___ ___ ___ . ___ ___) |

● Sample of first page of discharge documentation form (OASIS-B1—required by HCFA).

---

**(M0790) Management of Inhalant/Mist Medications:** Patient's ability to prepare and take all prescribed inhalant/mist medications (nebulizers, metered dose devices) reliably and safely, including administration of the correct dosage at the appropriate times/intervals. **Excludes all other forms of medications (oral tabets, injectable and IV medications).**

Prior Current
☐ ☐ 0 – Able to independently take the correct medication and proper dosage at the correct times.
☐ ☐ 1 – Able to take medication at correct times if:
 (a) individual dosages are prepared in advance by another person, OR
 (b) given daily reminders.
☐ ☐ 2 – Unable to take medication unless administered by someone else.
☐ ☐ NA – No inhalant/mist medications prescribed.
☐ ☐ UK – Unknown

**(M0800) Management of Injectable Medications:** Patient's ability to prepare and take all prescribed injectable medications reliably and safely, including administration of the correct dosage at the appropriate times/intervals. **Excludes IV medications.**

Prior Current
☐ ☐ 0 – Able to independently take the correct medication and proper dosage at the correct times.
☐ ☐ 1 – Able to take injectable medication at correct times if:
 (a) individual syringes are prepared in advance by another person, OR
 (b) given daily reminders
☐ ☐ 2 – Unable to take injectable medications unless administered by someone else.
☐ ☐ NA – No injectable medications prescribed.
☐ ☐ UK – Unknown

## EQUIPMENT MANAGEMENT

**(M0810) Patient Management of Equipment (includes ONLY oxygen, IV/infusion therapy, enteral/parenteral nutrition equipment or supplies):** Patient's ability to set up, monitor and change equipment reliably and safely, add appropriate fluids or medication, clean/store/dispose of equipment or supplies using proper technique. (**NOTE: This refers to ability, not compliance or willingness.**)

☐ 0 – Patient manages all tasks related to equipment completely independently.
☐ 1 – If someone else sets up equipment (i.e., fills portable oxygen tank, provides patient with prepared solutions), patient is able to manage all other aspects of equipment.
☐ 2 – Patient requires considerable assistance from another person to manage equipment, but independently completes portions of the task.
☐ 3 – Patient is only able to monitor equipment (e.g., liter flow, fluid in bag) and must call someone else to manage the equipment.
☐ 4 – Patient is completely dependent on someone else to manage all equipment.
☐ NA – No equipment of this type used in care [ If NA, go to *M0825* ]

**(M0820) Caregiver Management of Equipment (includes ONLY oxygen, IV/infusion equipment, enteral/parenteral nutrition, ventilator therapy equipment or supplies):** Caregiver's ability to set up monitor, and change equipment reliably and safely, add appropriate fluids or medication, clean/store/dispose of equipment or supplies using proper technique. (**NOTE: This refers to ability, not compliance or willingness.**)

☐ 0 – Caregiver manages all tasks related to equipment completely independently.
☐ 1 – If someone else sets up equipment, caregiver is able to manage all other aspects.
☐ 2 – Caregiver requires considerable assistance from another person to manage equipment, but independently completes significant portions of task.
☐ 3 – Caregiver is only able to complete small portions of tasks (e.g., administer nebulizer treatment, clean/store/dispose of equipment or supplies).
☐ 4 – Caregiver is completely dependent on someone else to manage all equipment.
☐ NA – No caregiver
☐ UK – Unknown

● Sample of equipment management form (OASIS-HCFA).

---

**Outcome and Assessment Information Set (OASIS-B1)**

**DISCHARGE VERSION**
(also used for Transfer to an Inpatient Facility or Patient Death at Home)

**Items to be Used at Specific Time Points**

**Transfer to an Inpatient Facility** ---------------- M0080–M0100, M0830–M0855, M0890–M0906
Transferred to an inpatient facility—patient not discharged from an agency
Transferred to an inpatient facility—patient discharged from agency

**Discharge from Agency — Not to an Inpatient Facility**
Death at home ---------------------------------------- M0080–M0100, M0906
Discharge from agency ----------------------------- M0080–M0100, M0200–M220, M250, M0280–M0380, M0410–M0820, M0830–M0880, M0903–M0906

## CLINICAL RECORD ITEMS

**(M0080)** Discipline of Person Completing Assessment:
☐ 1-RN  ☐ 2-PT  ☐ 3-SLP/ST  ☐ 4-OT

**(M0090)** Date Assessment Completed: ___/___/___
month  day  year

**(M0100)** This Assessment is Currently Being Completed for the Following Reason:
**Transfer to an inpatient facility**
☐ 6 – Transferred to an inpatient facility—patient not discharged from agency [ Go to *M0830* ]
☐ 7 – Transferred to an inpatient facility—patient discharged from agency [ Go to *M0830* ]
**Discharge from Agency — Not to an Inpatient Facility**
☐ 8 – Death at home [ Go to *M0906* ]
☐ 9 – Discharge from agency [ Go to *M0200* ]

## DEMOGRAPHICS AND PATIENT HISTORY

**(M0200) Medical or Treatment Regimen Change Within Past 14 days:** Has this patient experienced a change in medical or treatment regimen (e.g., medication, treatment, or service change due to new or additional diagnosis, etc.) within the last 14 days?
☐ 0 – No [ If, No go to *M0250* ]
☐ 1 – Yes

**(M0210)** List the patient's **Medical Diagnoses** and ICD-9-CM code categories (three digits required; five digits optional) for those conditions requiring changed medical or treatment regimen (no surgical or V-codes):

| Changed Medical Regimen Diagnosis | ICD-9-CM |
|---|---|
| a. _____ | (___ ___ ___ . ___ ___) |
| b. _____ | (___ ___ ___ . ___ ___) |
| c. _____ | (___ ___ ___ . ___ ___) |
| d. _____ | (___ ___ ___ . ___ ___) |

● Sample of outcome and assessment form (OASIS-HCFA).

---

**(M0420) Frequency of Pain** interfering with patient's activity or movement:
☐ 0 – Patient has no pain or pain does not interfere with activity or movement
☐ 1 – Less often than daily
☐ 2 – Daily, but not constantly
☐ 3 – All of the time

**(M0430) Intractable Pain:** Is the patient experiencing pain that is not easily relieved, occurs at least daily, and affects the patient's sleep, appetite, physical or emotional energy, concentration, personal relationships, emotions, or ability or desire to perform physical activity?
☐ 0 – No
☐ 1 – Yes

## INTEGUMENTARY STATUS

**(M0440)** Does this patient have a **Skin Lesion** or an **Open Wound**? This excludes "OSTOMIES."
☐ 0 – No [ If No, go to *M0490* ]
☐ 1 – Yes

**(M0445)** Does this patient have a **Pressure Ulcer**?
☐ 0 – No [ If No, go to *M0468* ]
☐ 1 – Yes

**(M0450) Current Number of Pressure Ulcers at Each Stage:** (Circle one response for each stage.)

| | Pressure Ulcers Stages | Number of Pressure Ulcers | | | | |
|---|---|---|---|---|---|---|
| a) | Stage 1: Nonblanchable erythema of intact skin; the heralding of skin ulceration. In darker-pigmented skin, warmth, edema, hardness, or discolored skin may be indicators. | 0 | 1 | 2 | 3 | 4 or more |
| b) | Stage 2: Partial thickness skin loss involving epidermis and/or dermis. The ulcer is superficial and presents clinically as an abrasion, blister, or shallow crater. | 0 | 1 | 2 | 3 | 4 or more |
| c) | Stage 3: Full-thickness skin loss involving damage or necrosis of subcutaneous tissue which may extend down to, but not through, underlying fascia. The ulcer presents clinically as a deep crater with or without undermining of adjacent tissue. | 0 | 1 | 2 | 3 | 4 or more |
| d) | Stage 4: Full-thickness skin loss with extensive destruction, tissue necrosis, or damage to muscle, bone, or supporting structures (e.g., tendon, joint capsule, etc.). | 0 | 1 | 2 | 3 | 4 or more |
| e) | In addition to the above, is there at least one pressure ulcer that cannot be observed due to the presence of eschar or a nonremovable dressing, including casts? ☐ 0 – No ☐ 1 – Yes | | | | | |

**(M0460) Stage of Most Problematic (Observable) Pressure Ulcer:**
☐ 0 – Stage 1
☐ 1 – Stage 2
☐ 2 – Stage 3
☐ 3 – Stage 4
☐ NA – No observable pressure ulcer

**(M0464) Status of Most Problematic (Observable) Pressure Ulcer:**
☐ 1 – Fully granulating
☐ 2 – Early/partial granulation
☐ 3 – Not healing
☐ NA – No observable pressure ulcer

● Sample of assessment tool (OASIS-HCFA).

# Skill 13.10 Completing Admission Documentation

**Procedure**

1. Complete all sections of the OASIS document.
   a. Demographic data: address, referring physician, payment source, etc.
   b. Present history.
   c. Present illness.
   d. Living arrangements.
   e. Supportive assistance.
   f. Physical assessment/Review of systems.
   g. ADLs.
   h. Medications.
   i. Equipment management.
   j. Homebound status.
   k. Therapy modalities required.
   l. Unmet needs.
   m. Lack of Knowledge section.
   n. Treatment/Procedures Performed.
   o. Response to Teaching/Training Performed.
   p. Patient Rights and Responsibilities.
   q. Coordination of Patient Services.
   r. Discharge Planning.

2. Signed consent forms.
   a. IV therapy.
   b. Consent for treatment.
   c. Consent for service.
3. Signed HIPAA form.
4. Signed Advanced-Directive document.
5. Signed Patient's Bill of Rights document.
6. Billing Data Base.
7. Discipline Specific Evaluation, if therapy was instituted.
8. Plan of Care.
9. H485 Worksheet.
10. Aide Assignment and Duties, if appropriate.
11. Physician Plan of Care.
12. Home Health Plan of Care.
13. Nurses' Notes as necessary.
14. Identify if prehospital "Do Not Resuscitate" form has been signed.

# Skill 13.11 Maintaining Nurse's Safety

**Procedure**

1. Evaluate safety of nurse prior to the visit.
   a. Call the client before the visit to determine convenient time.
   b. Confirm directions to home.
   c. Determine if household pets are present; if so, ask that they be secured during visit.
   d. Check neighborhood to determine need for assistance from police to make home visit.
2. Wear identifying name badge. Most agencies request that the nurse wear a lab coat.
3. Wear flat shoes to allow you to walk quickly or to run if necessary.
4. Maintain personal safety while traveling in the car.
   a. Keep car in good working order and stocked with necessary equipment.
   b. Keep gas tank at least half full at all times.
   c. Obtain automobile club membership for emergency use. ►*Rationale: To call for assistance with car problems.*
   d. Keep a windshield cover with CALL POLICE sign available. ►*Rationale: To alert neighbors you need immediate assistance.*

**CLINICAL ALERT**

If your safety is in jeopardy, use one of the following defensive strategies: Scream or yell FIRE or STRANGER. Kick the person in the shin or groin. Bite or scratch the person. Use chemical spray or blow a whistle. If you feel your personal safety is in question, do not make a visit or stay in the residence.

e. Have car phone available and charged at all times.

f. Keep blanket in car. ➤*Rationale: To keep warm in the winter if you need to wait for assistance.*

g. Keep thermos of water in car at all times. ➤*Rationale: In case you need to wait for assistance in hot weather.*

h. Keep doors locked and windows up at all times.

i. Park in full view of neighbors, preferably directly in front of home.

j. Lock all personal items in trunk of the car before leaving home or office.

k. Keep all equipment in the trunk of the car. Restock the nurses' bag before the visits for the day.

l. Keep nurses' bag on front seat.

m. Keep change in car for phone calls if necessary.

n. Place all valuable objects out of direct sight in car, i.e., laptop computers, phone. Place these under the seat if possible. ➤*Rationale: To prevent car break-in and theft.*

5. Maintain personal safety while walking on the street.

a. Keep one arm and hand free when walking from car to house.

b. Walk directly to client's residence.

c. When approaching a group of strangers, cross the street or walkway, if appropriate.

d. When leaving a residence, keep keys in your hand with the pointed end of the key facing outward. ➤*Rationale: The keys can act as a weapon if necessary.*

e. Carry a chemical spray and whistle within easy reach.

*Note:* Attendance at a class is necessary before it is legal to carry a chemical spray such as Mace.

6. Maintain personal safety when making home visit.

a. Use common walkways or hallways. Do not park behind a building or in a dark area.

b. Knock on the door and wait for permission to enter.

c. Keep a clear pathway to the door if the situation is potentially unsafe.

d. Observe home environment for safety hazards, i.e., weapons.

e. Make a joint visit with another agency staff member or ask for an escort if there is a potentially unsafe situation.

f. Call for police support if the visit is essential and the situation is unsafe. ➤*Rationale: There may be times when a visit is essential, but it is unsafe for one individual to make a visit.*

g. Make visit in the morning when good visual support exists if neighborhood is unsafe.

h. Close the case if the nurse feels the situation is unsafe and there are no alternative actions that can guarantee the nurse's safety.

# Skill 13.12    Assessing Home for Safe Environment

### Equipment

Home Assessment Checklist
Outcome and Assessment Information Act (OASIS-B1)

### Procedure

1. Identify type of dwelling, i.e., client-owned, boarding home, rental, mobile home.

2. Identify water source.

3. Identify sewer source.

4. Identify type of plumbing available.

5. Determine if any pollutants are present in the environment.

6. Assess exterior of the home for
   a. Condition of sidewalks and steps.
   b. Presence of railings on steps.
   c. Barriers that prevent easy access to the home.
   d. Adequacy of lighting.
   e. Adequacy of roof and windows.

7. Assess interior of the home for
   a. Presence of scatter rugs or worn carpeting.
   b. Uncluttered pathways throughout the house.
   c. Adequacy of lighting.
   d. Doorways wide enough to permit assistive devices.
   e. Cleanliness of house.
   f. Presence of insects, rodents, or infective agents.
   g. Presence of functioning smoke detectors.
   h. Adequate heating and cooling systems.
   i. Presence of running water.

8. Determine if hazardous materials are safely stored.

9. Assess for presence of lead-based paint.

10. Determine if medications can be adequately stored out of reach of children and impaired individuals.

11. Assess stairway and halls for
    a. Adequacy of light.
    b. Handrails that are securely fastened to wall.
    c. Flooring in good repair.
    d. Rugs or carpeting in good repair.
    e. Light switches in easy reach and accessible at both ends of stairs or hallway.
12. Assess kitchen for
    a. Properly functioning stove.
    b. Adequacy of light surrounding stove and sink.
    c. Condition of small appliances.
    d. Accessibility of appliances to clients in wheelchairs.
    e. Adequacy of sewage disposal.

13. Assess bathroom for
    a. Skidproof strips or mat in tub or shower.
    b. Handrails around toilet and tub or shower.
    c. Accessibility of medicine cabinet.
    d. Adequate space if wheelchairs or walkers are used.
    e. Temperature of hot water from faucets in sink, tub, or shower.
14. Assess bedroom for
    a. Accessibility of closets and cabinets.
    b. Ease in getting into and out of bed.
    c. Adequate space, if commode or wheelchair is required.
    d. Night light availability.
    e. Accessibility of medications, water on a nightstand.
    f. Calling system to alert health care provider.
    g. Flooring in good repair and nonslippery surface.

# Skill 13.13    Evaluating Client's Safety

## Procedure

1. Evaluate client's cognitive abilities: level of consciousness, orientation, ability to make appropriate judgments, ability to follow commands and directions.
    a. Knowledge of how to operate appliances, e.g., stoves and heaters.
    b. History of alcohol or drug abuse.
    c. Knowledge of medication times and doses to be taken.
    d. Knowledge of how to call for help: physician, nurse, fire, police.
2. Evaluate client's sensory and motor function.
    a. Hearing and vision acuity.
    b. Ability to ambulate with assistance.
    c. Need for assistive devices or support in ambulation.
3. Assess if client needs alternatives to physical restraints.
    a. Determine if environment needs to be modified by removing unsafe objects or barriers.
    b. Remove wheels from chairs or bed.
    c. Install bed check system or alarm device.
    d. Decrease auditory and visual stimuli.
    e. Place supplies close to bed or chair (e.g., tissues, water).
    f. Develop routine for client.

4. Evaluate most effective type of restraint, if absolutely necessary.
    a. Determine that less restrictive methods have been attempted.
    b. Assess purpose of restraint to determine most appropriate type.
    c. Obtain physician's order for restraint. Order must include reason, type, and time of restraints.
    d. Obtain informed consent from client or guardian before applying.
    e. Explain purpose of restraints to client and family members.
    f. Ensure caregiver is instructed on use of restraints.
    g. Evaluate effectiveness and continued need for restraints. The safety issues are the same as for clients in the hospital.
5. Determine client's ability to manage self-care.
    a. Bathing, grooming, and dressing.
    b. Preparing food and feeding.
    c. Toileting.
    d. Housekeeping, shopping, transportation to physician and pharmacy.
6. Determine client's financial support.
    a. Determine health care insurance plan, workers' compensation, Medicare, Medicaid.
    b. Determine need for social service intervention.

# Skill 13.14   Assessing Caregiver's Safety

**Procedure**

1. Determine caregiver's cognitive function.
   a. Ability to understand and carry out interventions.
   b. Ability to make safe decisions and judgments.
   c. Willingness to care for client.
2. Determine caregiver's sensory and motor function.
   a. Ability to hear client's needs.
   b. Visual acuity to read directions, medication labels.
   c. Ability to feel temperature changes, e.g., water for bathing.

3. Determine caregiver's motor function and strength.
   a. Ability to assist client in transfer, moving, turning, and ADLs.
   b. Ability to provide treatments and care for client.
   c. Ability to prepare food and do housekeeping chores.
   d. Ability to do shopping and provide transportation for physician visits.

# Skill 13.15   Assessing for Elder Abuse

**Procedure**

1. Assess client for indications of neglect: failure to provide adequate food, clothing, medical assistance, or assistance with ADLs. Check body for signs of cleanliness. Determine if emotional abuse is present. Ask about threats, intimidation, or isolation.
2. Identify if financial abuse has occurred, such as misuse of finances or property.
3. Assess for signs of physical abuse: signs of restraining; hitting, biting, burning; black and blue marks on trunk, abdomen, buttocks, upper thighs; scars, and abrasions. Bilateral bruises or parallel injuries may indicate forceful restraining; shaking may cause parallel injuries of upper arms. Accidental injuries affect knees, back of hands, forehead, and elbows.
4. Assess for signs of malnourishment or dehydration.
5. Check skin for pressure ulcers.
6. Assess for signs of sprains or dislocations from pulling or pushing the client.
7. Ask about visits to the hospital ER. Ask why client sought medical care, how much time elapsed between injury and visit to ER.
8. Assess for signs of emotional abuse. Observe if client is fearful of strangers, becomes quiet when caregiver enters room, craves attention and socialization.

**QUESTIONS TO ASK IF SUSPICION OF ABUSE**

- Who cares for you at home?
- Did someone hurt you?
- Are you happy with where you live?
- Tell me about your daily routine.
- Who assists you with ADLs?
- Do you feel safe living here?
- Who manages your money?
- How did the injury (or bruises) occur?
- Did you receive medical attention?
- Has this type of injury happened before?

# 14

# Assisting with Medical Procedures

**Skill 14.1**  Assisting with Invasive Procedures    692

**Skill 14.2**  Assisting with Thoracentesis    693

**Skill 14.3**  Assisting with Paracentesis    694

**Skill 14.4**  Assisting with Lumbar Puncture    695

**Skill 14.5**  Assisting with Bone Marrow Aspiration    697

**Skill 14.6**  Assisting with Chest Tube Insertion    700

**Skill 14.7**  Assisting with Chest Tube Removal    703

**Skill 14.8**  Assisting with Percutaneous Central Vascular Catheterization    706

When procedures are performed by the physician or other health care provider, the nurse may be asked to participate in a number of different ways: preparing the client and/or the support persons, monitoring and assisting the client during the procedure, caring for the client after the procedure, and documenting the client's response to the procedure. The procedure may be performed at the bedside, in an examining room, or sometimes in the emergency or special procedures department of a hospital. Many proce-

dures are invasive, involving insertion of an instrument, often a needle, through the skin and withdrawing some fluid or tissue. The fluid or tissue is usually placed in a special container and sent to the hospital laboratory for examination. Although the techniques for taking specimens are considered safe, complications can occur with each of them. The knowledge and skill of the assisting nurse can help minimize complications and maximize the therapeutic value of the procedure.

# Skill 14.1    Assisting with Invasive Procedures

## Delegation

Unlicensed personnel may be delegated the task of assisting the nurse or other health care provider with some skills. However, if these activities require the assistant to perform skills not generally expected of unlicensed personnel, such as sterile technique, they may not be delegated to the UAP. As always, the nurse must verify the individual UAP's abilities and experience, the individual client's needs, and be knowledgeable about agency and individual state regulatory policies and procedures.

## Equipment

- Varies according to the procedure.
- Always have extra sterile gloves and other common supplies available.

## Preparation

- Ensure that the results of relevant laboratory tests are available.
- Determine if a consent form has been signed. Some agencies require a signed consent from the client for special procedures.
- Coordinate the services of personnel from other departments who are involved in the procedure.

## Procedure

1. Prior to performing the procedure, introduce self and verify the client's identity using agency protocol. Explain to the client what you and any other health care providers are going to do, why it is necessary, and how he or she can participate. Discuss how the results will be used in planning further care or treatments.
2. Observe appropriate infection control procedures.
3. Provide for client privacy and safety.

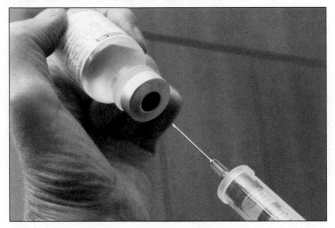

● Holding a vial.

4. Prepare the client.
   - Have the client empty the bladder and bowels prior to the procedure. ➤*Rationale: This prevents discomfort resulting from a need to use the bathroom during the procedure.*
   - Position the client as required for the procedure.
   - Drape the client to expose only the necessary area.
5. Open any sterile trays or equipment that is needed. Fill in labels and laboratory slips with the client's identification data.
   - Check with the person performing the procedure to determine the best time for opening supplies.
6. Prepare and provide equipment and medications needed during the procedure.
   - Maintain sterility of dressings, needles, syringes, specimen containers, and other equipment.
   - Draw up or pour medications or solutions as needed. If another practitioner is wearing sterile gloves and will be drawing the medication from a vial that you are holding (nonsterile outside), show the practitioner the label and

say the name and concentration of the fluid before it is aspirated. For example, show the label while you say "epinephrine one to ten thousand" or "Xylocaine one percent without epinephrine" and then tilt the vial top so the practitioner can access it.

7. Support the client during the procedure.
   • If you are not needed to handle equipment or supplies for the practitioner, position yourself where you can observe and reassure the client.
   • Observe the client closely for signs of distress, for example, abnormal pulse, respirations, or blood pressure; altered level of consciousness; or change in skin color.

8. Label any specimens and arrange for them to be sent immediately to the laboratory. ➤*Rationale: Incorrect identification of specimens can lead to subsequent error of diagnosis or therapy for the client.*

9. Provide required nursing care after the procedure.
   • Assist the client to a comfortable position.
   • Measure vital signs.
   • Wash off any antiseptic or other product applied to the skin.
   • Observe the insertion site for swelling or bleeding.

10. Document the procedure and findings in the client record using forms or checklists supplemented by narrative notes when appropriate.

# Skill 14.2 Assisting with Thoracentesis

Normally, only sufficient fluid to lubricate the pleura is present in the pleural cavity. However, excessive fluid can accumulate as a result of injury, infection, or other pathology. In such a case or in the case of pneumothorax, a primary care provider may perform a thoracentesis to remove the excess fluid or air to ease breathing. Thoracentesis is also performed to introduce chemotherapeutic drugs intrapleurally.

The nurse assists the client to assume a position that allows easy access to the intercostal spaces. This is usually a sitting position with the arms above the head, which spreads the ribs and enlarges the intercostal space. Two positions commonly used are one in which the arm is elevated and stretched forward and one in which the client leans forward over a pillow. To make sure that the needle is inserted below the fluid level when fluid is to be removed (or above any fluid if air is to be removed), the primary care provider will palpate and percuss the chest and select the exact site for insertion of the needle. A site

on the lower posterior chest is often used to remove fluid, and a site on the upper anterior chest is used to remove air. A chest x-ray prior to the procedure will help pinpoint the best insertion site.

The primary care provider and the assisting nurse follow strict sterile technique. The primary care provider attaches a syringe and/or stopcock to the aspirating needle. The stopcock must be in the closed position so that no air will enter the pleural space. The primary care provider inserts the needle through the intercostal space to the pleural cavity. In some instances, the primary care provider threads a small plastic tube through the needle and then withdraws the needle. (The tubing is less likely to puncture the pleura.)

If a syringe is used to collect the fluid, the plunger is pulled out to withdraw the pleural fluid as the stopcock is opened. If a large container is used to receive the fluid, the tubing is attached from the stopcock to the adapter on the receiving bottle. When the adapter and stopcock are

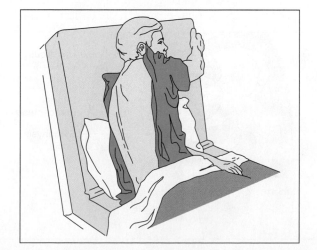

**A**

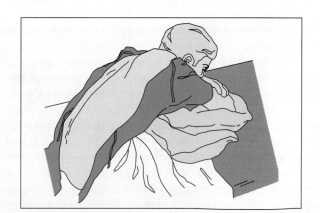

**B**

● Two positions commonly used for a thoracentesis: **A,** sitting on one side with arm held to the front and up; **B,** sitting and leaning forward over a pillow.

## DEVELOPMENTAL CONSIDERATIONS

**Elders**

- Some elders will need help maintaining the proper position due to arthritis, tremors, or weakness.
- Provide support with pillows during the procedure.
- Absence of body fat in elders can help the primary care provider locate the intercostal spaces.
- Provide an extra blanket to keep your client warm during the procedure. Elders have a decreased metabolism and less subcutaneous fat.

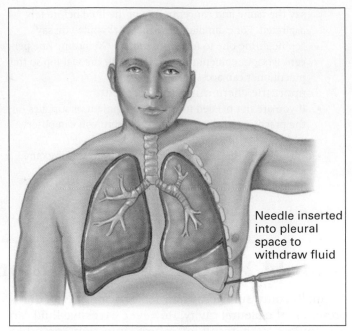

Needle inserted into pleural space to withdraw fluid

● Needle is inserted into the pleural space on the lower posterior chest to withdraw fluid. Note: From *Medical Terminology: A Living Language*, 3rd ed. (p. 219, Fig 7.15), by B. Fremgen, and S. Frucht, 2005. Upper Saddle River, NJ: Pearson Education, Inc.

opened, gravity allows fluid to drain from the pleural cavity into the container, which should be kept below the level of the client's lungs. After the fluid has been withdrawn, the primary care provider removes the needle or plastic tubing. A small sterile dressing is applied over the puncture site.

## Skill 14.3 Assisting with Paracentesis

Normally the body creates just enough peritoneal fluid for lubrication. The fluid is continuously formed and absorbed into the lymphatic system. However, in some disease processes, a large amount of fluid accumulates in the abdominal cavity; this condition is called ascites. Normal ascitic fluid is serous, clear, and light yellow in color. An abdominal paracentesis is carried out to obtain a fluid specimen for laboratory study and to relieve pressure on the abdominal organs due to the presence of excess fluid.

A primary care provider performs the procedure with the assistance of a nurse. Strict sterile technique is followed. A common site for abdominal paracentesis is midway between the umbilicus and the symphysis pubis on the midline. The primary care provider makes a small incision with a scalpel, inserts the trocar (a sharp, pointed instrument) and cannula (tube), and then withdraws the trocar, which is inside the cannula. Tubing is attached to the cannula and the fluid flows through the tubing into a receptacle. If the purpose of the paracentesis is to obtain a specimen, the primary care provider may use a long aspirating needle attached to a syringe rather than making an incision and using a trocar and cannula. Normally about

1500 mL is the maximum amount of fluid drained at one time to avoid hypovolemic shock. The fluid is drained very slowly for the same reason. Some fluid is placed in the specimen container before the cannula is withdrawn. The small incision may or may not be sutured; in either case, it is covered with a small sterile bandage.

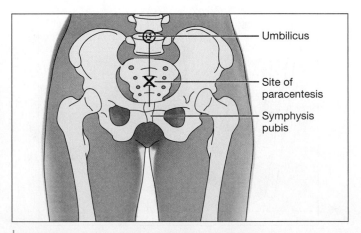

Umbilicus

Site of paracentesis

Symphysis pubis

● A common site for an abdominal paracentesis.

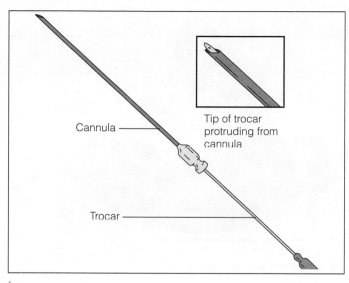

A trocar and cannula may be used for an abdominal paracentesis.

**DEVELOPMENTAL CONSIDERATIONS**

**Elders**

- Provide pillows and blankets to help elders remain comfortable during the procedure.
- Ask the client to empty the bladder just before the procedure. Elders may need to void more frequently and in smaller amounts.
- Remove ascitic fluid slowly and monitor the client for signs of hypovolemia. Elders have less tolerance for fluid loss and may develop hypovolemia if a large volume of fluid is drained rapidly.

# Skill 14.4 Assisting with Lumbar Puncture

In a lumbar puncture (LP, or spinal tap), cerebrospinal fluid (CSF) is withdrawn through a needle inserted into the subarachnoid space of the spinal canal between the third and fourth lumbar vertebrae or between the fourth and fifth lumbar vertebrae. At this level the needle avoids damaging the spinal cord and major nerve roots. The client is positioned laterally with the head bent toward the chest, the knees flexed onto the abdomen, and the back at the edge of the bed or examining table. In this position the back is arched, increasing the spaces between the vertebrae so that the spinal needle can be inserted readily. The nurse helps the client maintain this position to help prevent accidental needle displacement (Dulak, 2005). During a lumbar puncture, the primary care provider frequently takes CSF pressure readings using a manometer, a glass or plastic tube calibrated in millimeters. The primary care provider collects samples of CSF. After the procedure, apply a small sterile dressing over the puncture site.

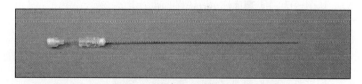

A spinal needle with the stylet protruding from the hub.

**DEVELOPMENTAL CONSIDERATIONS**

**Children**

- Briefly demonstrate the procedure on a doll or stuffed animal. Allow time to answer questions.
- One member of the health care team should stay in close physical contact with the child, maintain eye contact, and talk to and reassure the child during the process.

**Elders**

- Some clients need help maintaining the flexed position due to arthritis, weakness, or tremors.
- Provide an extra blanket to keep the client warm during the procedure. Elders have a decreased metabolism and less subcutaneous fat.
- If the client has a hearing loss, speak slowly, distinctly, and loud enough, especially when unable to make eye contact.

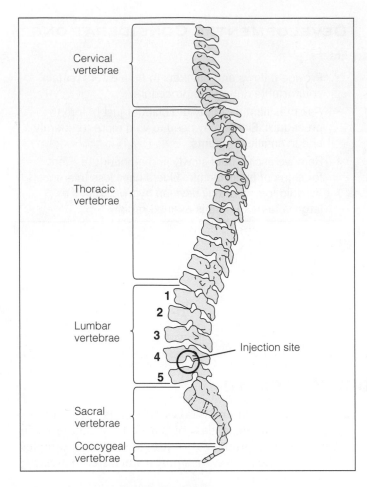

Cervical vertebrae

Thoracic vertebrae

Lumbar vertebrae

1
2
3
4
5

Injection site

Sacral vertebrae

Coccygeal vertebrae

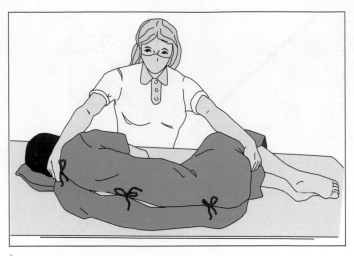

● Supporting the client for a lumbar puncture.

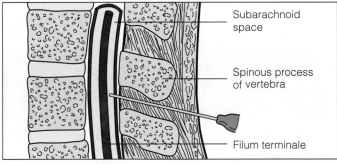

Subarachnoid space

Spinous process of vertebra

Filum terminale

● A diagram of the vertebral column, indicating a site for insertion of the lumbar puncture needle into the subarachnoid space of the spinal canal.

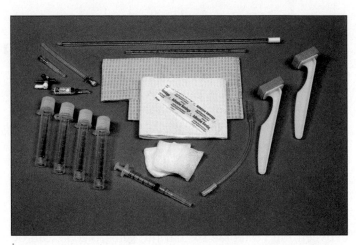

● A preassembled lumbar puncture set. Note the manometer at the top of the set.

# Skill 14.5  Assisting with Bone Marrow Aspiration

Another type of diagnostic study is the *biopsy*. A biopsy is a procedure whereby tissue is obtained for examination. Biopsies are performed on many different types of tissues, for example, bone marrow, liver, breast, lymph nodes, and lung.

A bone marrow biopsy is the removal of a specimen of bone marrow for laboratory study. The biopsy is used to detect specific diseases of the blood, such as pernicious anemia and leukemia. The bones of the body commonly used for a bone marrow biopsy are the sternum, iliac crests, anterior or posterior iliac spines, and proximal tibia in children. The *posterior superior iliac crest* is the preferred site with the client placed prone or on the side.

After injecting a local anesthetic, a small incision may be made with a scalpel to avoid tearing the skin or pushing skin into the bone marrow with a needle. The primary care provider then introduces a bone marrow needle with stylet into the red marrow of the spongy bone.

Once the needle is in the marrow space, the stylet is removed and a 10-mL syringe is attached to the needle. The plunger is withdrawn until 1 to 2 mL of marrow has been obtained. The primary care provider replaces the stylet in the needle, withdraws the needle, and places the specimen in test tubes and/or on glass slides. The nurse places a small sterile dressing over the puncture site.

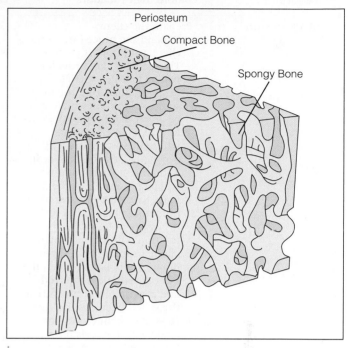

● A cross section of a bone.

## DEVELOPMENTAL CONSIDERATIONS

### Children

- Young clients need emotional support due to the pain and pressure associated with this procedure.
- Young clients may require gentle restraint to prevent movement during the procedure.

### Elders

- Elders with osteoporosis will experience less needle pressure.
- Ask the client to empty the bladder for comfort before the procedure.
- Provide pillows and blankets to help elders remain comfortable during the procedure.

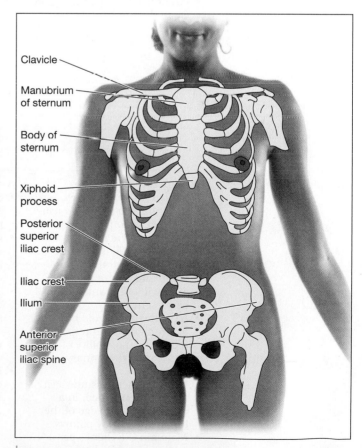

● The sternum and the iliac crests are common sites for a bone marrow biopsy.

## TABLE 14–1 ASSISTING WITH ASPIRATION AND BIOPSY PROCEDURES

| Procedure | Before the Procedure | During the Procedure | After the Procedure |
|---|---|---|---|
| Lumbar puncture | Prepare the client:<br>• Explain the procedure to the client and support persons. The primary care provider will be taking a small sample of spinal fluid from the lower spine. A local anesthetic will be given to minimize discomfort. Explain when and where the procedure will occur (e.g., the bedside or in a treatment room) and who will be present (e.g., the primary care provider and the nurse). Explain that it will be necessary to lie in a certain position without moving for about 15 minutes. A slight pinprick will be felt when the local anesthetic is injected and a sensation of pressure as the spinal needle is inserted.<br>• Have the client empty the bladder and bowels prior to the procedure to prevent unnecessary discomfort.<br>• Position and drape the client.<br>• Open the lumbar puncture set. | Support and monitor the client throughout:<br>• Stand in front of the client and support the back of the neck and knees if the client needs help remaining still.<br>• Reassure the client throughout the procedure by explaining what is happening. Encourage normal breathing and relaxation.<br>• Observe the client's color, respirations, and pulse during the procedure. Ask the client to report headache or persistent pain at the insertion site.<br><br>Handle specimen tubes appropriately:<br>• Wear gloves when handling test tubes.<br>• Label the specimen tubes in sequence.<br>• Send the CSF specimens to the lab immediately.<br><br>Place a small sterile dressing over the puncture site. | Ensure the client's comfort and safety:<br>• Assist the client to a dorsal recumbent position with only one head pillow. The client may remain in this position for a prescribed time period. It has been thought that lying flat prevents a post–lumbar puncture headache but this has not been supported by research.<br>• Determine whether analgesics are ordered and can be given for headaches.<br>• Offer oral fluids frequently, unless contraindicated, to help restore the volume of CSF.<br><br>Monitor the client:<br>• Observe for swelling or bleeding at the puncture site.<br>• Monitor changes in neurologic status.<br>• Determine whether the client is experiencing any numbness, tingling, or pain radiating down the legs.<br><br>Document the procedure on the client's chart:<br>• Include date and time performed; the primary care provider's name; the color, character (e.g., clear, cloudy, bloody), and amount of CSF; and the number of specimens obtained. Also document nursing assessments and interventions. |
| Abdominal paracentesis | Prepare the client:<br>• Explain the procedure: obtaining the specimen usually takes about 15 minutes. Emphasize the importance of remaining still during the procedure. Tell the client when and where the procedure will occur and who will be present.<br>• Have the client void just before the paracentesis to reduce the possibility of puncturing the urinary bladder.<br>• Help the client assume a sitting position in bed, in a chair, or on the edge of the bed supported by pillows.<br>• Maintain the client's privacy and provide blankets for warmth. | Assist and monitor the client:<br>• Support the client verbally and describe the steps of the procedure as needed.<br>• Observe the client closely for signs of distress (e.g., abnormal pulse rate, skin color, and blood pressure).<br>• Observe for signs of hypovolemic shock induced by the loss of fluid: pallor, dyspnea, diaphoresis, drop in BP, and restlessness or increased anxiety.<br>• Place a small sterile dressing over the site of the incision after the cannula or aspirating needle is withdrawn. | Monitor the client closely:<br>• Observe for hypovolemic shock.<br>• Observe for scrotal edema with male clients.<br>• Monitor vital signs, urine output, and drainage from the puncture site every 15 minutes for at least 2 hours and every hour for 4 hours or as the client's condition indicates.<br>• Measure the abdominal girth at the level of the umbilicus.<br><br>Document all relevant information:<br>• Include date and time performed; the primary care provider's name; abdominal girth before and after; the color, clarity, and amount of drained fluid; and the nurse's assessments and interventions.<br><br>Transport the correctly labeled specimens to the laboratory. |

| Procedure | Before the Procedure | During the Procedure | After the Procedure |
|---|---|---|---|
| Thoracentesis | Prepare the client:<br>• Explain the procedure to the client. Normally, the client may experience some discomfort and a feeling of pressure when the needle is inserted. The procedure may bring considerable relief if breathing has been difficult. The procedure takes only a few minutes, depending primarily on the time it takes for the fluid to drain from the pleural cavity. To avoid puncturing the lungs, it is important for the client not to cough while the needle is inserted. Explain when and where the procedure will occur and who will be present.<br>• Help position the client and cover the client as needed with a bath blanket. | Support and monitor the client throughout:<br>• Support the client verbally and describe the steps of the procedure as needed.<br>• Observe the client for signs of distress, such as dyspnea, pallor, and coughing.<br>Collect drainage and laboratory specimens.<br>Place a small sterile dressing over the site of the puncture. | Monitor the client:<br>• Assess pulse rate and respiratory rate and skin color.<br>• Don't remove more than 1000 mL of fluid from the pleural cavity within the first 30 minutes.<br>• Observe changes in the client's cough, sputum, respiratory depth, and breath sounds; note complaints of chest pain.<br>Position the client appropriately:<br>• Some agency protocols recommend that the client lie on the unaffected side with the head of the bed elevated 30 degrees for at least 30 minutes because this position facilitates expansion of the affected lung and eases respirations.<br>Document all relevant information:<br>• Include date and time performed; the primary care provider's name; the amount, color, and clarity of fluid drained; if any specimens were obtained; and nursing assessments and interventions provided.<br>Transport the specimens to the laboratory. |
| Bone marrow biopsy | Prepare the client:<br>• Explain the procedure. The client may experience pain when the marrow is aspirated and hear a crunching sound as the needle is pushed through the cortex of the bone. The procedure usually takes 15 to 30 minutes. Explain when and where the procedure will occur, who will be present, and which site will be used.<br>• Help the client assume a supine position (with one pillow if desired) for a biopsy of the sternum (sternal puncture) or a prone position for a biopsy of either iliac crest. Fold the bedclothes back or drape the client to expose the area.<br>• Administer a sedative as ordered. | Monitor and support the client throughout:<br>• Describe the steps of the procedure as needed and provide verbal support.<br>• Observe the client for pallor, diaphoresis, and faintness due to bleeding or pain.<br>Place a small sterile dressing over the site of the puncture after the needle is withdrawn.<br>• Some agency protocols recommend direct pressure over the site for 5 to 10 minutes to prevent bleeding.<br>Assist with preparing specimens as needed. | Monitor the client:<br>• Assess for discomfort and bleeding from the site. The client may experience some tenderness in the area. Bleeding and hematoma formation need to be assessed for several days. Report bleeding or pain to the nurse in charge.<br>• Provide an analgesic as needed and ordered.<br>Document all relevant information:<br>• Include date and time of the procedure; the primary care provider's name; and any nursing assessments and interventions. Document any specimens obtained.<br>Transport the specimens to the laboratory. |

*(continued)*

TABLE 14–1 **ASSISTING WITH ASPIRATION AND BIOPSY PROCEDURES** (CONTINUED)

| Procedure | Before the Procedure | During the Procedure | After the Procedure |
|---|---|---|---|
| Liver biopsy | Prepare the client:<br>• Give preprocedural medications as ordered. Vitamin K may be given for several days before the biopsy to reduce the risk of hemorrhage.<br>• Explain the procedure and tell the client that the primary care provider will take a small sample of liver tissue by putting a needle into the client's side or abdomen. Explain that a sedative and local anesthetic will be given, so the client will feel no pain. Explain when and where the procedure will occur, who will be present, the time required, and what to expect as the procedure is being performed (e.g., the client may experience mild discomfort when the local anesthetic is injected and slight pressure when the biopsy needle is inserted).<br>• Ensure that the client fasts for at least 2 hours before the procedure.<br>• Administer the appropriate sedative about 30 minutes beforehand or at the specified time.<br>• Help the client assume a supine position with the upper right quadrant of the abdomen exposed. Cover the client with the bedclothes so that only the abdominal area is exposed. | Monitor and support the client throughout:<br>• Support the client in a supine position.<br>• Instruct the client to take a few deep inhalations and exhalations and to hold the breath after the final exhalation for up to 10 seconds as the needle is inserted, the biopsy obtained, and the needle withdrawn. Holding the breath after exhalation immobilizes the chest wall and liver and keeps the diaphragm in its highest position, avoiding injury to the lung and laceration of the liver.<br>• Instruct the client to resume breathing when the needle is withdrawn.<br>• Apply pressure to the site of the puncture to help stop any bleeding.<br><br>Apply a small dressing to the site of the puncture. | Position the client appropriately:<br>• Assist the client to a right side-lying position with a small pillow or folded towel under the biopsy site. Instruct the client to remain in this position for several hours.<br><br>Monitor the client:<br>• Assess the client's vital signs every 15 minutes for the first hour following the test or until the signs are stable. Then monitor vital signs every hour for 24 hours or as needed.<br>• Determine whether the client is experiencing abdominal pain. Severe abdominal pain may indicate bile peritonitis.<br>• Check the biopsy site for localized bleeding. Pressure dressings may be required if bleeding does occur.<br><br>Document all relevant information:<br>• Include date and time performed; the primary care provider's name; and all nursing assessments and interventions.<br><br>Transport the specimens to the laboratory. |

# Skill 14.6 Assisting with Chest Tube Insertion

## Delegation

Assisting the primary care provider with insertion of a chest tube is not delegated to unlicensed assistive personnel (UAP).

## Equipment

- Sterile chest tube tray that includes:
  - Drapes
  - 10-mL syringe
  - Gauze sponges
  - 22-gauge needle
- 25-gauge needle
- #11 blade scalpel
- Forceps
- Two rubber-tipped tube clamps
- Extra 4 × 4 gauze sponges or other occlusive bandage material
- Split drain sponges
- Chest tube and trocar or hemostat
- Suture materials
- Drainage system (water or dry seal)

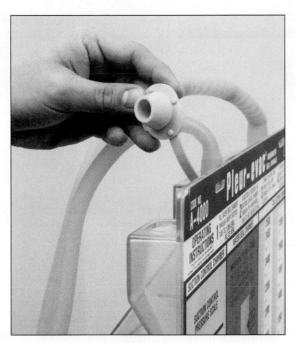

● Opening the water-seal filling port.

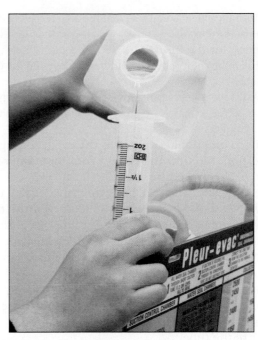

● Filling the water-seal chamber with sterile water.

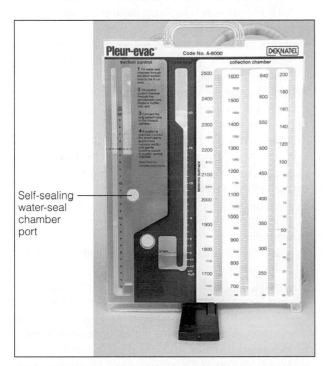

Self-sealing water-seal chamber port

● A three-chamber wet-suction/wet-seal disposable chest drainage system.

- Suction source, if indicated
- Sterile gloves (for primary care provider and nurse)
- Local anesthetic vial
- Skin cleansing solution (e.g., povidone-iodine)
- Adhesive or foam tape
- Petrolatum gauze (optional)

## Preparation

- Although the primary care provider will have already done initial client and family teaching, the nurse reinforces key elements. Review the technique of chest tube insertion and its purpose with the client and family.
- Confirm with the primary care provider the desired types and numbers of equipment needed. Primary care providers have personal preferences for styles and sizes of chest tubes, and needs vary with the purpose of the tube.
- Premedicate the client for pain. Incorporate nonpharmacologic pain and stress-reducing strategies as much as possible.

## Procedure

1. Prior to performing the procedure, introduce self and verify the client's identity using agency protocol. Explain to the client what your role will be, why it is necessary, and how he or she can participate. Discuss how the results will be used in planning further care or treatments.
2. Perform hand hygiene and observe appropriate infection control procedures.
3. Provide for client privacy.
4. Position the client as directed by the primary care provider.
   - The client may be placed flat or in semi-Fowler's position. ➤*Rationale: The flat position is preferred for best access to the second or third intercostal space; a semi-Fowler's position is preferred for access into the sixth to eighth intercostal space.*

- Turn the client laterally so that the area receiving the tube is facing upward.
5. Prepare for the insertion.
   - Open the chest tube tray and sterile gloves on the overbed table.
   - Assist the primary care provider to clean the insertion site.
   - Assist the primary care provider to draw up the local anesthetic.
6. Provide emotional support to the client during insertion. Monitor the client's condition and reaction to the procedure.
7. Dress the site. The primary care provider will usually place a purse-string suture to anchor the tube.
   - Apply sterile gloves and wrap the petrolatum gauze (if desired) around the chest tube at the insertion site.
   - Place drain gauze around the chest tube, one from the top and one from the bottom.
   - Place several additional gauze squares and tape or occlusive bandage materials over the drain gauze. These form an airtight seal at the insertion site.
8. Secure the tube.
   - Assist with connecting the chest tube to the valve or drainage system.
   - Attach the longer tube from the collection chamber to the client's chest tube.
   - Remove and discard gloves. Perform hand hygiene.
   - Tape the chest tube to the client's skin.
   - Tape all connections using spiral turns, but do not completely cover the collection tubing with tape. ➤*Rationale: Taping prevents inadvertent separation. Not covering all the collection tubing allows drainage to be seen.*

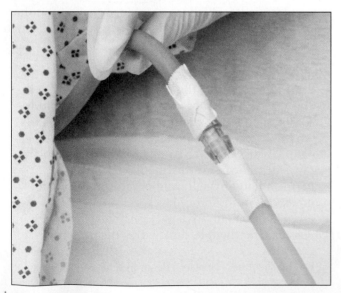

● Taped tubing connection with the connector exposed for observation of drainage.

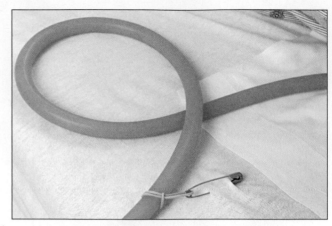

● Coiled drainage tubing secured on bed linen.

- Coil the drainage tubing and secure it to the linen, ensuring slack for the client to turn and move. ➤*Rationale: This prevents kinking of the tubing and impairment of drainage.*
- If suction is ordered, attach the remaining shorter tube from the suction chamber to the suction source, and turn it on. If wet suction is used, inspect the suction chamber for bubbling. Gentle bubbling indicates an appropriate suction level.
- If suction has not been ordered, keep the shorter rubber tube unclamped. This maintains negative or equal pressure in the system.
9. When all drainage connections are complete, ask the client to take a deep breath and hold it for a few seconds, then slowly exhale. These actions facilitate drainage from the pleural space and lung reexpansion.
10. Prepare the client for a chest x-ray to check for placement of the tube and lung expansion.
11. Ensure client safety.
    - Keep rubber-tipped chest tube clamps at the bedside..
    - Assess the client for signs of a new or worsening pneumothorax.
    - Assess the client for signs of subcutaneous emphysema (collection of gas under the skin). Palpate around the dressing site for crackling indicative of subcutaneous emphysema. ➤*Rationale: Subcutaneous emphysema can result from a poor seal at the chest tube insertion site.* This is not an emergency but should be reported, documented, and monitored. It should reabsorb in a few days.
    - Assess drainage and vital signs every 15 minutes for the first hour and then as ordered. Mark the collection chamber with a line and the date and time. Report bleeding or drainage greater than 100 mL/h.
12. Document the insertion in the client record using forms or checklists supplemented by narrative notes when appropriate. Include the name of the primary care provider, site of placement, type of tube, type of drainage system, characteristics of the immediate drainage, and other assessment findings.

## MANAGING VENTILATOR-RELATED EVENTS

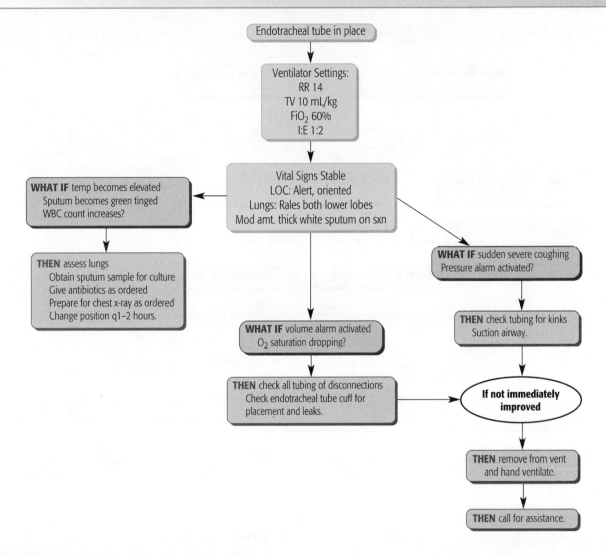

### Documentation

5/12/09 0130 32-Fr chest tube inserted into l chest by Dr. Novarty & connected to water-seal drainage unit. Suction at 20 cm $H_2O$. Immediately drained 120 mL straw-colored fluid. Moderate coughing after insertion, eased in 10 minutes. All connections taped, tubing taped to chest wall & attached to draw sheet. Tidaling c̄ respirations. Client instructed re: positioning & care of tube & collection device. Expresses understanding. VS 101 F, 100, 26, 170/94. _____ J. Lygas, RN

# Skill 14.7   Assisting with Chest Tube Removal

### Delegation

Assisting with the removal of a chest tube is not delegated to UAP. However, many effects of the removal may be observed during usual care and may be recorded by persons other than the nurse. Abnormal findings must be validated and interpreted by the nurse.

### Equipment

- Clean gloves
- Sterile gloves
- Suture removal set with forceps and scissors
- Sterile petrolatum gauze

## ASSESSING CHEST TUBE FUNCTIONING

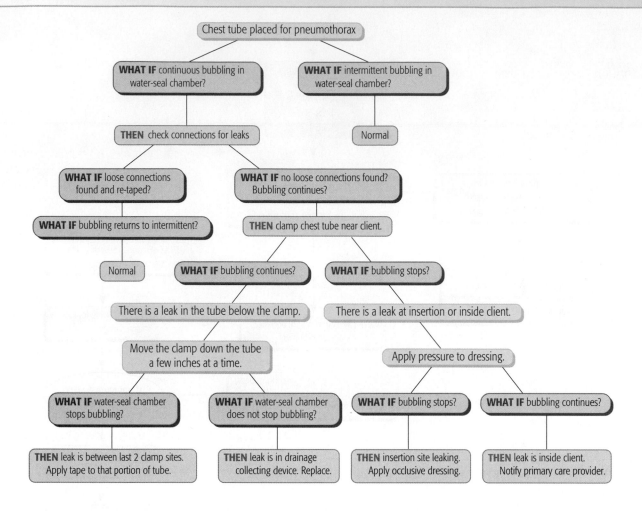

- 4 × 4 gauze sponges
- Adhesive tape
- Moisture-proof bag
- Linen-saver pad

### Preparation

- Ensure that the client has been informed that the chest tube will be removed and when. Clamp the tube, if ordered. Administer analgesics as ordered.

### Procedure

1. Prior to performing the procedure, introduce self and verify the client's identity using agency protocol. Explain to the client what you are going to do, why it is necessary, and how he or she can participate. Discuss how the results will be used in planning further care or treatments.
2. Perform hand hygiene and observe other appropriate infection control procedures.
3. Provide for client privacy.

4. Prepare the client:
   - Assist the client to a side-lying or semi-Fowler's position with the chest tube site exposed.
   - Place the linen-saver pad under the client, beneath the chest tube. ➤*Rationale: This protects the bed linens and provides a place for the chest tube after removal.*
   - Instruct the client on how to hold the breath during removal. Some experts recommend holding a full inhalation, others recommend holding a full exhalation (Coughlin & Parchinsky, 2006), and still others recommend the Valsalva maneuver—exhaling against the closed glottis (Roman & Mercado, 2006).
5. Prepare the sterile field and supplies. Have the petrolatum gauze opened and ready for quick application.
6. Remove the dressing around the chest tube.
   - Apply clean gloves and dispose of the dressing in the moisture-proof bag.
   - Remove and discard gloves. Perform hand hygiene.
7. Assist with removal of the tube.
   - Apply sterile gloves.

- Assist the client with the breathing technique and provide emotional support during the primary care provider's removal of the sutures and tube.
- Immediately apply the petrolatum gauze, and cover it with dry gauze and adhesive tape. ➤*Rationale: This forms an airtight bandage.*
- Remove and discard gloves. Perform hand hygiene.

8. Assess and monitor the client's response to tube removal.
   - Obtain vital signs every 15 minutes for the first hour and, if stable, then as indicated.
   - Auscultate lung sounds every hour for the first 4 hours to determine that the lung is remaining inflated.
   - Observe for signs of pneumothorax.

---

## CLINICAL ALERT

The chest tube can be removed when drainage is less than 50–100 mL in 24 hours, or, if inserted for blood removal, drainage has become serous or sero serosanguineous and less than 100 mL in the past 8 hours.

---

9. Document the date and time of removal, any drainage noted, and the client's response to the procedure in the client record using forms or checklists supplemented by narrative notes when appropriate.
10. Prepare the client for a chest x-ray 1 to 2 hours after chest tube removal and possibly again in 12 to 24 hours.

---

| UNEXPECTED OUTCOMES | CRITICAL THINKING OPTIONS |
|---|---|
| Air leak is present. | • Check for specific leak area by briefly clamping chest drainage tube between client and bottle closest to client.<br>    a) If water-seal bottle continues to bubble, the leak is in the tubing<br>    b) If water-seal bottle stops bubbling, the leak is in the client's chest tube at insertion site.<br>• Secure all connections with tape.<br>• Change tubing if necessary (obtain physician's order).<br>• Apply sterile petrolatum gauze around chest tube insertion site if leak is at that site. |
| Drainage system is obstructed. | • Assess tubing for kinks or clots.<br>• Loop tubing on bed to allow straight drainage to collection system.<br>• Obtain physician's order to milk or strip tubing. |
| Client develops signs of mediastinal shift (trachea deviated to unaffected side, paradoxical pulse develops, jugular veins distend, cardiac output decreases). | • Note signs of respiratory distress and call a "CODE" or rapid response team immediately. Check drainage tube for patency. Prepare to assist with thoracentesis. |
| Chest tube becomes disconnected from drainage system. | • Clamp chest tube near chest insertion site.<br>    a) Replace extension tubing leading from chest tube and submerge into open bottle of sterile water to create underwater seal.<br>    b) Unclamp chest tube as soon as extension tubing is placed under water or connected to new system.<br>• Secure connecting sites with tape to prevent disconnection.<br>• Assess client for signs of respiratory distress due to pneumothorax and report. |
| Chest tube becomes dislodged. | Notify physician.<br>Instruct client with external chest disruption to exhale and apply sterile non-porous 4 × 4 gauze dressing with tape on three sides to allow air to escape on exhalation but inhibit air intake on inspiration. |

# Skill 14.8 Assisting with Percutaneous Central Vascular Catheterization

## Equipment

Specific nontunneled catheter
Routine IV setup (tubing and solution)
Through-the-needle radiopaque central catheter
Local anesthetic, syringes, and needles
Sterile gloves, sterile gown, masks, drapes, and sutures
Antimicrobial swabs 2% chlorhexidine
Intermittent infusion caps or positive pressure device
Flush solution and syringes
Transparent semipermeable dressing
Securement device

## Procedure

1. Identify client using two descriptors and validate signed consent for catheter insertion.
2. Perform hand hygiene and explain procedure to client, including rationale for mask, positioning and Valsalva's maneuver.
3. Place client in Trendelenburg's position. ➤*Rationale: This position prevents air embolism and helps distend subclavian and jugular veins.*
4. According to physician's preference, extend client's neck and upper chest by placing a rolled pillow or blanket between shoulder blades. ➤*Rationale: Usual insertion sites are either subclavian or right jugular vein.*
5. Place mask on client, and turn client's head away from side of venipuncture. ➤*Rationale: This facilitates filling the vessel with blood and prevents contamination.*
6. Maintain sterility while opening glove packet and sterile drape pack.
7. Open antimicrobial prep pads.

*Note:* New guidelines to prevent catheter-related blood stream infection recommend physicians don cap and ster-

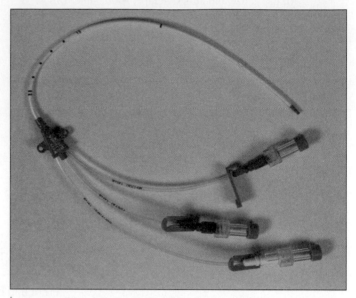

● Triple-lumen central venous catheter.

ile gown in addition to mask and sterile gloves (Institute for Healthcare Improvement).

8. Don mask and gloves and assist with central catheter insertion.
   a. Physician dons mask, gown, and sterile gloves for this procedure.
   b. Physician prepares the client's skin, drapes area, and, using a sterile syringe and needle, draws up anesthetic to infiltrate the site.

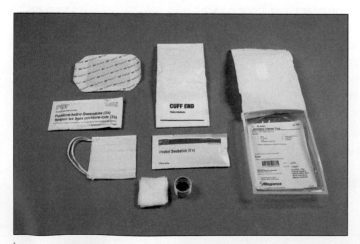

● Equipment for changing a central line dressing: gauze and paper tape are used 24 hours and then removed.

### CLINICAL ALERT

Required drying time needed in order to prevent skin breakdown as a result of chemical reaction between solutions and dressings.

| Solutions | Required Drying Time |
|---|---|
| Chlorhexidine gluconate 2% with alcohol | 30 seconds |
| Chlorhexidine gluconate without alcohol | 2 minutes |
| Povidone–iodine | 2 minutes |
| 70% isopropyl alcohol | Dries quickly, kills bacteria only when first applied. No lasting bactericidal effect; can excessively dry the skin. |

*Source*: Hadaway L. C. *Nursing*, 32(9), 36–48. Hadaway, L. C. *Journal of Infusion Nursing*, 26(1), 44–48.

# GUIDELINES TO PREVENT CATHETER-RELATED BLOOD STREAM INFECTIONS

**Hand Hygiene**

- Decontaminate hands with alcohol-based hand cleaner; if hands are visibly contaminated with blood or body fluids, use antimicrobial soap and water.
- Use hospital-provided hand lotions compatible with antiseptic agents to maintain integrity of skin. Home lotions may neutralize antibacterial agents in antiseptic agents used in hospitals.
- Decontaminate hands before and after putting on or removing gloves, providing direct client care, assisting with insertion of central venous catheter, inserting peripheral catheter, changing central venous dressing, or accessing catheter to administer medication or flush.
- Do not use artificial nails when working in the health care facility.

**Barrier Precautions**

- Use maximum barrier precautions when inserting or assisting with insertion of central venous catheters, including PICC lines. Include: cap that covers all hair, mask covering mouth and nose, sterile gown, and sterile gloves.
- Cover client from head to toe with large sterile drape leaving small opening for insertion of catheter.
- Place mask on client when PICC insertion is done, and cover face if subclavian or jugular vein placement site for central venous catheters.
- Keep all supplies together to prevent need to look for additional supplies as CVC insertion is begun.

**Site Preparation Using Chlorhexidine Gluconate**

- Prepare site using 2% chlorhexidine gluconate.
- Pinch wings on chlorhexidine applicator to break open ampule. Hold applicator down to allow solution to saturate pad.
- Press sponge against skin.
- Swab with applicator using a gentle back-and-forth motion. This motion creates friction and lets solution more effectively penetrate epidermal layers.
- Swab site for 30 seconds and then allow to dry thoroughly, approximately 2 minutes. Do not wipe or blot area.

**Catheter Site Selection**

- Use central venous catheters (CVCs) impregnated with antimicrobial agents.
- Nontunneled percutaneously inserted CVCs are available with three different agents: chorhexidine/silver sulfadiazine; rifampin/minocycline; and silver/platinum ionic metals. PICC brand uses rifampin/minocycline agents.
- These catheters should be used for clients with dwell time of more than 5 days and in health care facilities where the catheter-resistance blood stream infection rates are high.
- There is inconclusive evidence that multiple-lumen catheters should not be used; even though they have higher infection rates, they also have fewer mechanical complications than single lumen catheters.

*Source:* Institute for Healthcare Improvement, http://www.ihi.org/IHI.

# ▌ EVIDENCE-BASED NURSING PRACTICE

**Antimicrobial Swabs**

Studies have shown that 2% chlorhexidine gluconate solution significantly lowers catheter-related bloodstream infection rates when compared with 70% providone–iodine and 70% isopropyl alcohol.

*Sources:* LeBlanc & Cobbett. (2000). Traditional practice versus evidence-based practice for IV skin preparation. *Canadian Journal of Infection Control,* 15(1), 9–14. Maki, Ringer, & Alvarado (1991). Prospective randomized trial of providone–iodine, and chlorhexidine for prevention of infection associated with central venous and arterial catheters. *The Lancet,* 338, 339–343; Rosenthal, K. (2003). Pinpointing intravascular device infections. *Nursing Management,* 34(6), 35–43.

Another study revealed that chlorhexidine gluconate offered a broad spectrum of antimicrobial activity and long-term microbactericidal action after application.

*Source:* Hadaway, L. C. (2003a). Infusing without infecting. *Nursing,* 33(10), 58–64.

## CLINICAL ALERT

To decrease pressure in the catheter, use a 10-mL syringe.

## CLINICAL ALERT

All continuous IV infusions administered via a central line must have an electric infusion controller device in place.

c. As physician inserts catheter, client is instructed to perform Valsalva's maneuver to prevent air embolism.
   (1) Instruct client to exhale against a closed glottis or to hum.
   (2) If client is unable to do this, compress client's abdomen. ➤*Rationale: Both these procedures help to decrease chances of air embolism.*

*Note:* A 14-gauge needle is inserted into the subclavian vein, using the clavicle as a guide. When blood returns in the syringe, the syringe is removed from the needle and a wire is threaded through the needle into the subclavian vein. The needle is removed and the catheter is fed over the wire into the subclavian and brachio-cephalic vein. The wire is removed when the tip of the catheter rests in superior vena cava.

9. When physician has completed catheterization, insert injection cap, flush with 5 mL NS, then heparinize with 3 mL dilute heparin (according to agency policy).
10. Apply securement device to skin and place catheter in clamp.
11. Cover securement device and catheter with sterile transparent dressing (according to hospital policy).
12. Label insertion site dressing with date, nurse's initials, and time of insertion.
13. Obtain x-ray for validation of placement into superior vena cava before initiating infusion (unless emergency placement performed).
14. Monitor client's vital signs. ➤*Rationale: Bleeding or pneumothorax may occur.*

## EVIDENCE-BASED NURSING PRACTICE

**Preventing Intravascular Catheter-Related Blood Stream Infections**

Catheter-related blood stream infection is 2 to 855 times higher with central vascular catheters than peripheral vascular catheters. Approximately 80,000 catheter-related infections occur in the United States each year. These infections are associated with 2,400–20,000 deaths each year. These infections can be dramatically reduced with new products that have been introduced for CVD therapy: The FDA has recently approved the use of catheters impregnated with chlorhexidine. There is still testing being done on the combination of chlorhexidine and silver sulfadiazine because of some anaphylactoid reactions in Japan. Use of minocycline–rifampin impregnated catheters show promise of even lower infection rates.

- Catheters impregnated with chlorhexidine–silver sulfadiazine or catheters impregnated with minocyclinerifampin
- Catheter hubs containing iodinated alcohol
- Chlorhexidine-impregnated sponge dressings placed at the catheter insertion site: Infection rate decreased from 5.2% to 3% for catheters in place less than 10 days.

*Source:* Mermel, L. A. (2001, March–April). New technologies to prevent intravascular catheter-related bloodstream infections. *Emerging Infectious Diseases,* CDC, 7(2).

# INDEX

12-lead ECG recording, 350–352

## A

Abdomen, assessing, 494–498
  auscultation, 495
  bladder palpation, 497
  bowel sounds, 495
  care setting, 497
  developmental considerations, 497–498
  palpation, 496
  percussion, 496
  peritoneal friction rubs, 495
  vascular sounds, 495
Abdominal binder, 413
Acid-base imbalance, arterial blood gas
    values in, 112
Acid-base imbalance, causes of, 110
African Americans, 31
  hypertension in, 100
  pain, expression of, 4
AIDS client, 185
Airway obstruction, clearing, 320–323. *See also*
    Obstructed airway
Alginate, 414–415
Allen test, 108
Ambulation, 249–251
  care setting, 251
  developmental considerations, 251
  variation, 250
American Heart Association (AHA), 538
Amniocentesis, 375–376
Amniotomy, 381
Amputee, 443
Ankle-brachial index (ABI), 422
Antepartal assessment, 359–363
Antiemboli stockings, 337–338
  care setting, 338
  developmental considerations, 338
  measuring for graduated compression
    stockings, 337
  safe practice issues, 337
Anus, assessing, 515
  developmental considerations, 515
APGAR scores, assessing, 396
Apical pulse, assessing, 531–533
Apical-radial pulse, assessing, 529–531
  care setting, 530
  developmental considerations, 530
  one-nurse technique, 529
  two-nurse technique, 529
Arab Americans, 31
  pain, expression of, 4
Arterial blood pressure, 109–110
Arterial blood samples, 111–112
Arterial catheter, 112–114
Arterial line insertion, 108–109
Arterial ulcer, 423. *See also* Ulcer
Asepsis, 157

Asian Americans
  pain, expression of, 4
Assessments, 445–558
  abdomen, 494–498
  abdominal girth, measuring, 548
  anus, 515
  apical pulse, 531–533
  apical-radial pulse, 529–530
  appearance and mental status, 448–451
  blood pressure, 537–542, 549–550
  body language, 447
  body mass index, measuring, 546
  body temperature, 522–529
  breasts and axillae, 489–493
  chest circumference, measuring, 547
  cultural considerations and, 447–448
  ears and hearing, 466–469
  eye contact, 447
  eyes and vision, 460–465
  female genitals, 510–512
  Glasgow coma scale, 553
  hair, 456–457
  head circumference, measuring, 547
  head-to-toe framework, 447
  hearing acuity, 557–558
  heart and central vessels, 484–487
  heart rate, 548
  height, measuring, 545
  intracranial pressure monitoring, 554–555
  length, measuring, 544–545
  male genitalia, 512–514
  measurements, 544–548
  mouth and oropharynx, 471–474
  musculoskeletal system, 498–501
  nails, 457–459
  neck, 475–476
  neurologic system, 501–510
  neurovascular, 554
  nose and sinuses, 469–471
  pain, client in, 516–522
  peripheral pulses, 533–535
  peripheral vascular system, 487–489
  pulse oximeter, 543–544
  respiration, 535–537
  respiratory rate, 549
  skin, 451–456
  skull and face, 459–460
  temperature, child's body, 551–552
  thorax and lungs, 477–484
  touch and personal space, 447
  visual acuity, 555–557
  vital signs, 446
  weight, measuring, 546
Association of PeriOperative Registered Nurses
    (AORN), 176
Automated external defibrillation (AED), 332–333
  care setting, 333
  developmental considerations, 332, 333

## B

Bandages, 416–419
Bar code medication administration (BCMA)
    system, 140
Bathing
  bed bath, 572–574, 576
  biocultural variations in body secretions, 580
  cultural considerations and, 580
  dementia clients, 576
  developmental considerations, 577, 580
  disposal system use, 577
  home setting care, 670
  hydraulic bathtub chair, 575–576
  infant, 578
  skin problems, 579
  transferring client to tub or shower in home
    setting, 670
  tub or shower, 575
Bath, newborn, 400
Bath, sitz, 17
Bed, air-fluidized, 427
Bed, changing, 562–570
  care setting, 570
  developmental considerations, 570
  guidelines, 567, 570
  in home setting, 671
  occupied, 567–570
  side rails and falls, 567
  surgical, 565–567
  unoccupied, 562–567
Bed, low-air-loss, 427
Bed, nonhospital, 271
  developmental considerations, 271–273
Bedpan, 33–34
Bed, positioning in, 221–225, 227–234
  care setting, 234
  cultural considerations and, 229
  dangle, 232–233
  developmental considerations, 228–229,
    233–234
  dorsal recumbent, 223
  draw sheet use, 227
  Fowler's position, 221
  lateral, 224
  logrolling technique, 231–232
  moving client up, 227–228
  positions, 222
  prone, 223
  Sims', 224–225
  turning patient, 229–230
Benson, Herbert, 4
Biopatch antimicrobial dressing, 666
Blackhall, I. J., 27
Bladder
  irrigation of, 55–58
Bladder irrigation
  open irrigation, 56

Blood components, 663–664
  modified blood products, 663
Blood glucose, measuring, 212–215
Blood pressure, 109–110
  mean arterial, 112
  monitoring arterial, 110
Blood pressure, assessing, 537–542, 549–550
  body position factor, 538
  care setting, 542
  cultural considerations and, 542
  developmental considerations, 541
  electronic monitoring device, 541
  forearm, 537
  manual sphygmomanometer, 550
  music, effect on vital signs, 537
  oscillometry, 550
  palpation method, 540, 550
  sources of error in, 542
  sphygmomanometer, 539
  stethoscope accuracy in measuring, 537
  thigh blood pressure, 540–541
Blood transfusions, 661–663
Body language, in assessment, 447
Body mass index (BMI), 546
Body mechanics, 219–220
  back brace, 220
  gait belt, 219
Body temperature assessment. *See*
    Temperature, assessing body
Bone marrow aspiration, 697–700
  aspiration and biopsy procedures, 698–700
  developmental considerations, 697
Bowel diversion ostomy appliance, 89–94
  care setting, 94
  irrigating a colostomy, 92
  one-piece pouching system, 91
  two-piece pouching system, 93
Bowel management, Zassi system, 74–78
Bowel movement
  terminology, 34
Bowel routine, 66–67
  constipation management, 66
  developmental considerations, 67
  training, 67
Breastfeeding, 392–394
Breasts and axillae, assessing, 489–493
  developmental considerations, 493
  self-exam, 492–493
Breathing. *See* Oxygenation
Breathing, controlled, 2–4
  CAM techniques, 2
  nonpharmacological approaches to pain, 3
Breathing, deep, 275–276
Bronchial hygiene therapy, 287
Bulb syringe, 395–396
Butterfly needle, 128, 132

### C

Calorie, calculation for IV, 135
Cane, using, 251–252
Cannula, in oxygenation, 282–283
Capillary blood specimen, obtaining, 212–215
  care setting, 214
  developmental considerations, 214
  home setting care, 214–215
Cardiac pacing, 352

Cardiopulminary resuscitation (CPR), 328–332. *See
    also* External cardiac compressions
Caring interventions, 559–673, 592
  back massage, 581–582
  bathing, 571–580
  bed, changing, 562–570
  blood components, 663–664
  blood transfusions, 661–663
  brushing and flossing teeth, 583–587
  central lines, managing, 663–665
  eating assistance, 605–609
  evening care, 581
  eye care, 598–601
  foot care, 595–596, 597
  hair care, 590
  hair problems, 562
  hearing aid, 601–602
  implanted vascular access devices, 667–670
  injections, 633–643
  massage, 561–562
  medicine administration, 609–660
  morning care, 570–571
  nail care, 595
  oral hygiene, 587–589
  perineal-genital care, 603–604
  personal hygiene, 560–561
  shaving male client, 589
Cast care, 260–266
  care setting, 262
  child with cast, 265–266
  developmental considerations, 261–262
  initial, 260–263
  ongoing, 263–265
  plaster, 264
  synthetic, 264–265
Catheter, catheterization, 46–55
  arterial catheter, removing, 112–114
  care and removal, 53–55
  care setting, 52
  catheter sizes, 50, 51
  central venous dual-lumen dialysis catheter
      (DLC), 102–104
  developmental considerations, 51
  Foley, 46, 47
  Foley catheter cautions, 46
  irritation/inflammation with, 49
  peritoneal dialysis catheter, 94–96
  risks for urinary retention, 46
  self-cathertization, 104
  suprapubic catheter care, 58–60, 105
  voiding ability, 46
*C. difficile*, 160
Center for Disease Control (CDC), 117, 133, 157,
    159, 211, 292
Central line
  changing dressing, 665–667
  in infusions, 124, 153–155
  managing, 663–665
  preventing intravascular catheter-related blood
      stream infections, 665
Central venous dual-lumen dialysis catheter (DLC),
    102–104
  care setting, 103
Chest percussion, 288
Chest physiotherapy (CPT), 287
  bronchial hygiene therapy, 287

Chest tube, 312–320
  assessing functioning of, 320, 704
  chest tube functioning assessment, 704
  developmental considerations, 318
  drainage, 315–318
  insertion, 312–314, 700–703
  managing ventilator-related events, 703
  removal, 319, 703–705
Chest vibration, 288–289
Childbirth. *See* Reproduction
Chinese-Americans, 31
Circumcision, 399
Client care preparation, 183–184
Colostomy irrigation, 107–108
Comfort, 1–31
  compresses and moist packs, 15–16
  controlled breathing, 2–4
  cooling blankets, 21–24
  cultural considerations and, 2
  dry cold measures, 20–21
  dry heat measures, 13–15
  dying patient needs, 25–28
  guided imagery, 6–7
  infant radiant warmer, 18–20
  muscle relaxation, 4–6
  postmortem care, 28–31
  sitz bath, 17
  TENS unit, 8–12
  tepid sponges, 17–18
Commode, 36–37
  cultural considerations, 37
Compresses and moist packs, 15–16
Computerized prescriber order entry (CPOE), 140
Constipation, 66
Contaminated equipment, disposal of, 170
Continuous ambulatory peritoneal dialysis (CAPD),
    105–106, 107
  transfer sets, 106
Cooling blanket, 21–24
  hypothermia and, 21
COPD, 283
Cough/coughing, 275–276
Crutches, using, 253–257
  chair, 255
  gaits, 253–255
  measuring clients for, 257
  stairs, 255–256
Cultural diversity, at end of life, 28

### D

Dehydration, 120
Dentures, 585–586
Digital pressure, 335
  pulse sites, 335
Discharge, client teaching, 182
Diversity, cultural
  at end of life, 28
Dressing(s)
  Biopatch antimicrobial, 666
  changing, 179–181
  dry, 405–407
  hydrocolloid, 431–432
  hydrogel, 430
  moisture-retentive, comparing, 433
  moist wound, 432

transparent film, 429–430
transparent wound barrier, 440–441
venous ulcer, 422–426
wet-to-moist, 410–412
wound with drain, 408–410
Drug(s). *See* Medication
Dry cold measures, 20–21
postoperative cold therapy, 20
Dry heat measures, 13–15
Aquathermia (or K-pad), 14
disposable cold pack, 20–21
disposable hot pack, 14
heating pad, 14
hot water bottle, 13
ice bag, 21
Dying patient, 24, 25–31
care setting, 27
children, 30
client teaching considerations of, 27
clinical manifestations of, 27
cultural considerations of, 27
cultural diversity and, 28
cultural rituals, 31
elderly, 30
physiological needs of, 25–28
three dimensions with cultural variations
in, 28

**E**

Ears and hearing, assessing, 466–469
auricles, 467
care setting, 469
developmental considerations, 469
external ear canal, 467
hearing acuity tests, 467–468
Eating assistance, 190–191, 605–608
care setting, 191, 607
developmental considerations, 191, 606
dysphagic client, 607–609
food trays, 607
ECG, recording 12-lead, 350–352
ECG strip interpretation, 345–349
atrial fibrillation, 348
atrial flutter, 348
hemodynamic instability signs, 349
multifocal premature ventricular contraction
(PVCs), 347
normal sinus rhythm, 346
oscilloscope, 346
selected cardiac rhythms and dysrhythmias,
347–349
sinus bradycardia, 347
sinus tachycardia, 347
third-degree heart block, 349
ventricular fibrillation, 349
ventricular tachycardia, 347
Elder abuse, assessing, 690
Electrical stimulation (in tissue therapy), 435–436
candidates for, 435
Electrolytes (and fluids), 115–155
Elimination, 32–114
Allen test, 108
arterial blood pressure, monitoring, 109–110
arterial blood samples, withdrawing, 111–112
arterial catheter, removing, 112–114

arterial line insertion, 108–109
bacterial culture, collecting stool for, 72
bedpan, 33–34
bladder irrigation, 55–57
bladder irrigation, maintaining, 57–58
bowel diversion ostomy appliance, 89–94
bowel routine, developing regular, 66–67
care setting, 103–104
catheter care and removal, 53–55
central venous dual-lumen dialysis catheter
(DLC), 102–104
changing dressing for CAPD client, 107
colostomy irrigation, 107–108
commode, 36–37
continuous ambulatory peritoneal dialysis
(CAPD), 105–106
enema, 78–80
external urinary device, 37–39
fecal impaction, 65
fecal ostomy pouch, applying, 82–88
hemodialysis, providing, 98–101
hemodialysis, terminating, 101–102
home setting care, 104–108
ova and parasites, collecting stool for, 73
peritoneal dialysis catheter, 94–95
peritoneal dialysis procedures, 96–98
pinworm testing, 73
rectal tube insertion, 67–69
retention enema, 80–82
self-cathertization, 104
stool specimen, collecting from infant, 72
stool specimen testing, 69–71
suprapubic catheter care, 58–60, 105
urinal, 34–36
urinary, 32–64
urinary catheterization, 46–53
urinary diversion pouch, 62–63
urinary ostomy care, 60–62
urine specimen, 24-hour collecting, 41–42
urine specimen, clean-catch method, 42–45
urine specimen, collecting, 39–40
urine specimen, collecting from infant, 41
urine specimen from ileal conduit, 64
urine tests, 45–46
of waste products, 64–94
Zassi bowel management system, 74–78
Endotracheal intubation, 291–292
Endotracheal tube, 294
Enema, 73, 78–82
administering, 78–80
care setting, 81
developmental considerations, 82
retention enema, 80–82
Enteral nutrition (EN), or total enteral nutrition
(TEN), 190
Epidural, during labor, 386–387
Ethnicity, 28
Exercises
passive range of motion, 240–246
Expiratory flow, peak, 286–287
External cardiac compressions, 328–332
care setting, 331
developmental considerations, 330–331
new resuscitation guidelines, 328
External urinary device, 37–39
Extravasation, 147

Eye care, 598–601
Eye contact, in assessment, 447
Eyes and vision, assessing, 460–465
care setting, 465
developmental considerations, 465
external eye structures, 460–462
extraocular muscle tests, 463
visual acuity, 463–464
visual fields, 462

**F**

Face mask, for oxygenation, 282
Face mask, in oxygenation, 283
Face tent, in oxygenation, 282, 283–284
Fecal impaction, 65
Fecal ostomy pouch, 82–88
applying two-piece, 86–87
changing one-piece, 84–85
client teaching, 87
developmental considerations, 88
loop colostomy, 87
Feeding tubes, 190. *See also* Tube feeding
Fetal heart rate, 381–382
Fetal monitoring, external electronic, 382–383
Fetal monitoring, internal electronic, 384–385
Fetal well-being biophysical profile (BPP), 378
criteria for scoring, 378
Fetal well-being contraction stress test (CST),
377–378
test interpretation, 378
Fetal well-being nonstress test (NST), 376–377
Fever, 4
reducing, 17–18
Flow rate, infusion, 134–137
factors influencing, 135
Fluids, 115–155
care setting, 120
dehydration and, 120
developmental considerations, 119
homeostasis, 116
increasing intake of, 119
infusing through central line, 153–155
infusion devices, discontinuing, 150–152
infusion flow rate, 134
infusion pump, 138–139
infusions, maintaining, 144–147
intake, adult daily average, 116
intake and output, 116–121
intake and output, monitoring, 118
intake, maintaining, 118–119
intermittent infusion devices, 147–149
intravenous infusions, 122–125
output, adult daily average, 116
restricting intake of, 119–120
"smart" pump, 140–142
syringe pump, 142–144
venipuncture, 126
Food and Drug Administration (FDA), 198
Food/eating. *See also* Nutrition
eating assistance, 190–191
enteral nutrition, 190
gastrostomy or jejunostomy feeding, 202–204
IV lipids, 209–212
nasogastric tube, 192–198
parental nutrition, 208–209

small-bore nasointestinal/jejunostomy tube, 204–207
total nutrient admixture (TNA), 215–217
tube feeding, 198–202
Foot care, 595–596, 597

**G**

Gastric lavage, 196
Gastric (Salem) sump tube, 193
Gastrostomy feeding, open system, 203
Gastrostomy tube, 190, 192–197, 202–204
Genitalia, male, assessing, 512–515
    developmental considerations, 514
    Tanner stages of pubic hair development, 514
Genitals, female, assessing, 510–512
    developmental considerations, 511–512
    stages of pubic hair development, 512
GI motility, postoperative, 198
Glasgow coma scale, 553
    infants and children, 553
Gloves, in preventing contamination, 161–163
Glucose, 46, 212–215
Glue, for wound closure, 182
Gown, changing for client with IV, 150
Guided imagery, 6–7

**H**

Hair, assessing, 456–457
    care setting, 457
    developmental considerations, 457
Hair care, 590
    lice, 592–595
Hand hygiene (medical asepsis), 157–160
    compliance, 158
    cultural considerations and, 160
    nail polish and, 160
    waterless antiseptic agents, 159
Hand washing, 157
Hearing acuity, assessing, 557, 557–558
    care setting, 558
    developmental considerations, 558
    passing standards with pure tone audiometer, 558
    pure tone audiometry, 557, 558
    tympanogram, 558
    tympanometry, 558
Hearing aid, 601–602
Heart and central vessels, assessing, 484–487
    carotid arteries, 485–486
    developmental considerations, 487
    jugular veins, 486
Heart rate, assessing, 548
    normal rates for children, 548
Heat and cold measures
    applying, 10
    contraindications to use of, 12
    developmental considerations, 12
    indications for use of, 11
    physiological effects of, 10
    temperatures for, 11
    tolerance variables for, 11
Hemodialysis, 98–102
    arteriorvenous fistula, assessing, 100
    blood flow and, 100

fistula or graft, 99, 100
    ongoing patient care, 100–102
    process, 99
    providing, 98–100
    survival rate, 102
Heparin, in IV flushing, 148
HIV client, 185
*Holistic Nursing: A Handbook for Clinical Practice*, 160
Home care, guidelines for, 687
Homeostasis, 116
Home setting care, 104–108, 184–185
Home-setting safety, 685–690
Hydraulic lift, 238–239
Hydrocolloid dressing, 431–432
Hydrogel dressing, 430
Hygiene, 560–561
    factors influencing, 562
Hyperventilation, 300
Hypothermia, 21
    classifications of, 22
    stroke outcome and, 21
Hypoxia, 285

**I**

Ileal conduit, 64
Implanted vascular access devices, 667–670
Incentive spirometer, 280–281
    care setting, 281
    developmental considerations, 281
Incranial pressure monitoring, 554–555
    IPC waveforms and implications, 554
    signs of increased pressure, 555
Inducing labor, 385–386
Infant radiant warmer
    legalities and, 19
Infant radiant warmer, monitoring, 18–20
Infection, 156–188
    AIDS or HIV client, 185
    ambulatory and community settings, 188
    client care preparation, 183–184
    client preparion for surgery, 175–178
    client teaching considerations, 187–188
    disposing of waste material in home, 184–185
    double-bagging, 167–168
    dressing changes, 179–181
    gloves, 161–163
    hand hygiene (medical asepsis), 157–160
    hand washing in reducing, 157
    isolation attire, 163–165
    isolation room, removing equipment from, 169–170
    isolation room, removing items from, 166–167
    isolation room, removing specimen from, 168
    latex precautions, 161
    lifespan considerations, 187
    mask usage, 165–166
    preventative measures, 185–186
    safer IV drug user practices, 186–187
    staple removal, 182–183
    sterile container, 178
    sterile field preparation, 179
    sterile gown and gloves, 173
    surgical hand antisepsis/scrubs, performing, 170–173

surgical site preparation, 174–175
    surgical technique, 170–173
    suture removal, 181–182
    transporting client from isolation room, 169
    vital signs, assessing, 166
Infection control, 187–188
Infusing IV fluids, through central line, 153–155
Infusion devices, discontinuing, 150–152
    developmental considerations, 151
Infusion devices, maintaining intermittent, 147–149
    client teaching considerations, 149
    low-dose heparin, flushing with, 148
Infusion pump, 138–139
    developmental considerations, 139
Infusions, maintaining, 144–147
    care setting, 146
    client teaching considerations, 146
    therapy record, 145
Injections, 225, 633–643
    combining in one syringe, 635
    deltoid injection site, 651
    dorsogluteal injection site, 649
    gloving protocol, 639
    insulin, 640–643
    insulin pen, 643
    insulin pump, 644–645
    insulin types and therapeutic action, 641
    intradermal, 637–638
    intramuscular (IM) injections, 647–651
    minimizing pain during, 647
    needle size, 634, 651
    needlestick injuries, 634
    premixing types of insulin, 642
    preparing, 633–637
    reconstituting powdered medication, 635
    sites for, 639
    subcutaneous, 638–640
    subcutaneous anticoagulants, 646–647
    types of, 636
    vastus lateralis injection site, 650
    ventrogluteal injection site, 648
    withdrawing medication from ampule, 635, 637
    withdrawing medication from vial, 634
    Z-track method, 651–652
Insulin, 640–645
Intake (of fluids), monitoring, 116–121
    care setting, 120
    dehydration and, 120
    developmental considerations, 119
Intrapartal assessment, 363–365
Intravenous, 122
Intravenous infusion, 122–125
    *Dial-A-Flo* in-line device, 136
    IV calorie calculation, 135
    IV flow rates factors, 135
    pump, 136
    regulating flow rate, 134–137
    therapy record, 125
Invasive medical procedure assistance, 692–693
Irrigation, wound, 412–413
Isolation attire, 163–165
Isolation room, protocol, 169
Isolation room, removal procedures, 166–169
IV. *See* Intravenous
IV drug user, 186–187

IV lipids
  administration sets, 210
  guidelines for infusion, 211
  infusing, 209–212
  side effects of, 211

**J**

Jejunostomy tube, 190, 202–207

**K**

Kagawa-Singer, M., 27
Ketone bodies, 46

**L**

Labor, induction of, 385–386
  Pitocin and cervical ripening agents, 385
Latex, 161
Lice, 592–595, 671–672
Lipids, IV infusion of, 209–212. *See also*
  IV lipids
Lochia, 389–390
Logrolling technique, 231–232
Lumbar puncture, 225–226, 695–696
  developmental considerations, 695
  lumbar puncture set, 696
  needle insertion site, 696
  spinal needle, 695

**M**

Mask, in preventing contamination, 165–166
Massachusetts General Hospital, 142
Massage, 581–582
Maternal
  assessment, 359–367
Maternity. *See* Reproduction
Mayo Clinic, 148
Measurement assessment, 544–548
  abdominal girth, 548
  body mass index, 546
  chest circumference, 547
  head circumference, 547
  height, 545
  length, 544–545
  weight, 546
Mechanical ventilator, 307–311
  care setting, 310
  cultural considerations and, 310
  developmental considerations, 310
  enteral nutrition, 307
  kinetic rotation, 307
  patient delirium, 307
  pneumonia prevention, 311
Mechanics. *See* Body mechanics
Medical asepsis. *See* Hand hygiene
Medical procedures assistance, 691–708
  bone marrow aspiration, 697–700
  chest tube insertion, 700–703
  chest tube removal, 703–705
  invasive procedures, 692–693
  lumbar puncture, 695–696
  paracentesis, 694–695
  percutaneous central vascular
    catheterization, 706–708
  thoracentesis, 693–694

Medicare reimbursement eligibility, home care,
    685–687
Medication. *See also* Injections
  abbreviations and symbols, 653
  automated dispensing system, 613
  calculating dosages, 611
  converting dosage systems, 610
  cultural considerations and, 615, 617
  developmental considerations, 632
  double checking dosage, 643
  dry powder inhaled (DPI), 628–629
  enteral tube administration, 619–621
  errors in administration, 610, 615
  home administration, 672
  injections, 633–643
  intermittent intravenous using secondary set,
    656–657
  intravenous fluid containers, 654–655
  intravenous using IV push, 658–659
  legalities and, 610, 612
  MDI canister actuations, 627, 628
  medication protocol, 614–616
  metered-dose inhaler, 626–628
  narcotic control system, 611–612
  nasal, 625–626
  nitroglycerin, ACC/AHA guidelines, 622
  nonpressurized (nebulized) aerosol (NPA), 629
  ophthalmic, 622–623
  oral, 616–617
  otic, 624–625
  PCA pump for pain management, 660
  preparing for administration, 609–610
  rectal, 631–633
  safe practices for dispensing, 613
  safety measures, 615
  sterilizing nondisposable medication equipment
    in home setting, 673
  sublingual, 621–622
  vaginal, 630–631
Medication equipment, sterilizing in home
    setting, 673
Mental status, assessing, 448–451
  developmental considerations, 451
Metabolic complications (associated with
    TNA), 217
Metabolism, 189–217
Mexican Americans
  pain, expression of, 4
Mobility, 218–273, 227–229
  ambulatory assistance, 249–251
  bed and chair transfer, 234–237
  bed and stretcher transfer, 237–238
  bed, nonhospital, positioning of, 271
  bed, supporting client position in, 221–224,
    227–234
  body mechanics, 219–220
  cane, assistance with using, 251–252
  cast care, 260–266
  child, positioning for injections, 225
  child, positioning for lumbar puncture, 225–226
  child, positioning for otoscopic exam, 226–227
  crutches, assistance with using, 253–257
  hydraulic lift use, 238–239
  passive motion device, 247–248
  passive range of motion exercises, 240–246

  skin traction, child, 270–271
  traction, 266–270
  transporting an infant, 258
  transporting a toddler, 259
  walker, assistance with using, 257–258
Mouth and oropharynx, assessing, 471–474
  developmental considerations, 474
  lips and buccal mucosa, 472
  oropharynx and tonsils, 473–474
  palates and uvula, 473
  teeth and gums, 472–473
  tongue, 473
Movement. *See* Mobility
Muscle
  relaxation of, 4–6
Musculoskeletal system, assessing, 498–501
  bones, 500
  care setting, 498
  developmental considerations, 500–501
  joints, 500

**N**

Nail care, 595
Nails, assessing, 457–459
  care setting, 459
  developmental considerations, 458
Nasal cannula, 284
Nasal pharyngeal suctioning, 394–395
Nasal trumpet, 290
Nasogastric tube, 192–195
  auscultation to determine placement, 194
  developmental considerations, 195
  flushing/maintaining, 195
  gastric (Salem) sump tube, 193
  measuring, 192, 193
  removing, 197–198
Nasopharyngeal airway (nasal trumpet), 290
National Institute of Occupational Safety and Health
    (NIOSH), 220
Native Americans, 31
  pain, expression of, 4
Neck, assessing, 475–477
  lymph nodes, 476
  muscles, 475–476
  tracheal tube cuff inflation, 477
Negative pressure wound therapy, 437–439
  VAC® Unit, 438, 439
  vacuum-assisted closure, 327
"Negotiating Cross-Cultural Issues at the End of
    Life" (Kagawa-Singer and Blackhall), 27
Neurologic system, assessing, 501–510
  attention span, 502
  Babinski reflex, 504
  consciousness level, 502
  cranial nerve functions, 503
  cranial nerves, 502–504
  developmental considerations, 509–510
  Glasgow coma scale, 502, 553
  language, 501
  memory, 502
  motor function, 504–509
  orientation, 501–502
  reflexes, 504
  Romberg test, motor function, 505
Neurovascular assessment, 554

Newborn
  APGAR scoring, 372
  assessment, 359, 367–372
Newborn assessment, 367–372
Noncontact normothermis wound therapy,
    435–436
  legalities and, 436
*Norovirus,* 160
Nose and sinuses, assessing, 469–471
  developmental considerations, 471
  facial sinuses, 471
  nose, 470
Nose and throat specimens, 277–279
Nutrients, 190
Nutrition, 190
  eating assistance, 190–191
  enteral nutrition (EN), 190
  feeding tubes, 190
  total enteral nutrition (TEN), 190
Nutritional variations (with TNA
    complications), 217

## O

Obesity, metabolism and, 205
Obstructed airway, 320–323
  care setting, 323
  clearing, 320–322
  developmental considerations, 322–323
Oral hygiene, 587–589
Oropharyngeal airway, 289
Oropharyngeal, nasopharyngeal, and
    nasotracheal suctioning
  attaching catheter to suction unit, 296
  care setting, 298
  closed airway suction system, 295
  developmental considerations, 298
  oral suction tube, 296
  wall suction unit, 297
OSHA, 160
Otoscopic exam, 226–227
Outake (of fluids), monitoring, 116–121
  care setting, 120
  developmental considerations, 119
Ova and parasites, 73
Oxygen, administering, 282–286
Oxygenation, 274–333
  automated external defibrillation, 332–333
  cannula, 282–283
  capping tracheostomy tube, 306–307
  chest percussion, 288
  chest physiotherapy (CPT), 287
  chest tube drainage, 315–318
  chest tube insertion, 312–315
  chest tube removal, 319
  chest vibration, 288–289
  clearing obstructed airway, 320–323
  deep breathing and coughing, 275–276
  endotracheal intubation, 291–292
  endotracheal tube care, 294
  endotracheal tube, extubating, 294
  external cardiac compressions, 328–332
  face mask, 282, 283
  face tent, 282, 283–284
  incentive spirometer, 280–281
  measuring peak respiratory flow, 286–287

  mechanical ventilator, 307–312
  nasopharyngeal airway insertion, 290
  nose and throat specimens, 277–279
  oropharyngeal airway insertion, 289
  oropharyngeal, nasopharyngeal, and
      nasotracheal suctioning, 295–298
  oxygen cylinder, 284–285
  pediatric tent, 285–286
  rescue breathing, performing, 324–328
  saturation (using pulse oximeter), 279–280
  sputum specimen, 276–277
  tracheal tube cuff inflation, 293
  tracheostomy care, 302–306
  tracheostomy or endotracheal tube suctioning,
      298–301
Oxygen cylinder, 284–285
  hypoxia symptoms, 285
Oxygen saturation, 279–280
  care setting, 280
  developmental considerations, 279
  oximeter sensors, 280

## P

Pacemaker function, 355
  pacemaker failure alert, 355
Pacemaker insertion, 353–354
  electrical safety, 353
  revised NASPE/BPEG generic code for
      antibradycardia pacing, 354
Pacemaker, permanent, 356
  pacemaker clinics, 356
Pain, 3–4
  cultural expression of, 4
  nonpharmacological approaches to, 3
Pain, assessing, 516–522
  care setting, 519
  child pain, 519
  daily pain diary, 519
  FLACC behavioral pain assessment scale,
      519, 521
  neonatal infant pain scale (NIPS), 519, 520
  Oucher scale, 519, 522
  pain management flow sheet, 517
Paracentesis, 694–695
  developmental considerations, 695
Parasites, 73
Passive motion device, continuous, 247–248
  care setting, 248
  developmental considerations, 248
Passive range of motion exercises, 240–246
  care setting, 247
  developmental considerations, 246
Pediatric tent, in oxygenation, 285–286
Pelvic exam, 372–373
Percutaneous central vascular catheterization,
      706–708
  antimicrobial swabs, 707
  guidelines to prevent catheter-related blood
      stream infections, 707, 708
Perfusion, 334–357
  12-lead ECG recording, 350–352
  antiemboli stockings, 337–338
  cardiac pacing, monitoring, 352
  digital pressure, 335
  ECG strip interpretation, 345–349

  pacemaker function, 355
  pacemaker insertion, 353–355
  permanent pacemaker, 356–357
  pneumatic compression devices, 339
  pressure dressing, 336
  sequential compression devices (SCDs), 340
  telemetry, 343–345
Perineal-genital care, 603–604
Peripheral pulses, assessing, 533–535
  pulse rate measurement, 535
  using a DUS, 535
Peripheral vascular system, assessing, 487–489
  capillary refill test, 488
  developmental considerations, 489
  other assessments, 488
  peripheral perfusion, 488
  peripheral pulses, 487
  peripheral veins, 488
Peritoneal dialysis catheter, 94–95
Peritoneal dialysis procedures, 96–98
  care setting, 98
Personal hygiene, 560–561
Personal space, 447
Phlebitis, 147
Phototherapy, 400–402
Pinworms, 73
Pneumatic compression devices, 339
Poison control agents, 197
  activated charcoal, 197
Postmortem care, 28–31
  cultural considerations and, 31
  developmental considerations and, 30
  family needs inventory, 28
  shroud kit, 29
Postpartal (PP) maternal assessment, 366–367
Postpartum perineal, 391–392
  REEDA scale, 392
Preanesthesia evaluation form, 177
Pressure dressing, 336
Pressure ulcer, 426–429. *See also* Ulcer
Prolapsed cord, during labor, 388
Puerto Ricans
  pain, expression of, 4
Pulse, 529–535, 543
Pulse oximeter, 279–280
Pulse oximeter, assessing, 543–544
  care setting, 544
  developmental considerations, 544
  fingertip oximeter sensor, 543
Pump, infusion, 138–139
  controller, 138
  developmental considerations, 139

## R

Rectal tube, 67–69
REEDA scale, 392
Refeeding syndrome, 205
Reflexes, assessment of, 373–374
Reiki, 2
Relaxation, muscle, 4–6
*Relaxation Response, The* (Benson), 4
Reproduction, 358–402
  amniocentesis, 375–376
  amniotomy, 381
  APGAR scores assessment, 396

bath, newborn, 400
breastfeeding, 392–394
bulb syringe, suctioning with, 395–396
circumcision, 399
deep tendon reflexes and clonus, 373–374
epidural, 386–388
external electronic fetal monitoring, 382–383
fetal heart rate, 381–382
fetal well-being assessments, 376–378
inducing labor, 385–386
internal electronic fetal monitoring, 384–385
intrapartal vaginal exam, 379–380
lochia evaluation, 389–390
maternal assessment, 359–367
nasal pharyngeal suctioning, 394–395
newborn assessment, 359, 367–372
pelvic exam, 372–373
phototherapy, 400–402
postpartum perineal assessment, 391–392
prolapsed cord, 388
Rh immune globulin, 374  375
thermoregulation of newborn, 397–398
umbilical cord clamp, 398
uterine fundus assessment, 388–389
Rescue breathing, 324–328
care setting, 328
developmental considerations, 327
Respiration, assessing, 535–537
altered breathing patterns and sounds, 536
care setting, 537
counting accuracy, 535
developmental considerations, 537
Respiratory function. *See* Oxygenation
Respiratory rate, assessing, 549
normal changes per age group, 549
Restraints, 677–684
care setting, 681
developmental considerations, 680
managing clients in, 677–678
mummy immobilizer, 682–683
papoose board immobilizer, 681–682
torso/belt, 678
wrist or ankle, 680–681
Retention enema, 80–82
Rh immune globulin (RhoGAM, HypRho-D),
374–375
Romberg test, motor function, 509

**S**

Safety, 674–690
bed or chair exit safety device, 678–680
caregiver's, in home setting, 690
client's, in home setting, 689
clients in restraints, 677–678
elder abuse assessment, 690
fire, during, 675–676
home environment assessment, 688–689
in home setting, 685–690
mummy immobilizer, 682–683
nurse's, in home setting, 687
papoose board immobilizer, 681–682
priorities for fire safety, 675
seizure precautions, 683–684
thermal/electrical injury prevention, 676
wrist or ankle restraints, 680–681

Saline, in IV flushing, 148
*Scope and Standards of Pain: Pain Management
Nursing,* 4
Seizures, 683–684
care setting, 684
developmental considerations, 684
Sequential compression devices (SCDs), 340–342
care setting, 341
contraindications to use of, 341
developmental considerations, 340
DVT and, 341
pneumatic compression devices, 340
Sitz bath, 17
Skin, 404. *See also* Tissue
Skin, assessing, 451–456
care setting, 456
developmental considerations, 455
edema grading scale, 453
primary skin lesions, 454
secondary skin lesions, 453
skin lesions, charting, 453
Skin traction, child, 270–271
Skull and face, assessing, 459–460
developmental considerations, 460
"Smart" pump, for infusions, 140–142
bar code medication administration system
(BCMA), 140
computerized prescriber order entry
(CPOE), 140
error reduction and, 142
legalities and, 142
Sponges, tepid, 17–18
Sputum specimen, 276–277
Staple removal, 182–183
Stent, 63
Sterile container, pouring from, 178
Sterile field preparation, 179
care setting, 179
Sterile gown and gloves (closed method), 173
Stockings, compression, 337–338. *See also*
Antiemboli stockings
Stool specimen, 69–73
bacterial culture, collecting stool for, 72
care setting, 71
collecting infant, 72
developmental considerations, 71
obtaining and testing, 69–71
ova and parasites, collecting stool for, 73
pinworm testing, 73
Stress
cognitive-behavioral approach to managing, 4
managing, 4–5
opposite of stress response, 4
relaxation approach to managing, 4
Stroke
hypothermia and, 21
Stump, 442–444
positioning and exercising, 442
postoperative care, 442
preoperative care, 442
shrinking/molding, 443–444
Suctioning
oropharyngeal, nasopharyngeal, and
nasotracheal, 295–298
tracheostomy or endotracheal tube, 298–301

Supplies, 179–180
Surgery, preparing client, 175–178
Surgical consent form, 177
Surgical hand antisepsis/scrubs, performing,
170–173
alcohol-based surgical hand rub, 172–173
Surgical preoperative checklist, 176
Surgical site infection (SSI), 174
Surgical site preparation, 174–175
Suture removal, 181–182
Syringe pump, 142–144

**T**

Teeth
brushing and flossing, 583–587
care setting, 589
dentures, 585–586
developmental considerations, 588
special oral care, 587–589
Telemetry, 343–345
electrode placement, 343, 344–345
electrode system for monitoring, 344
Temperature, assessing body, 522–533
care setting, 529
developmental considerations, 528
electronic thermometer, 526
Glasgow coma scale, 553
head-to-toe framework, 527
infant or child, 523–524, 551–552
legalities and, 525
mercury, 524
sites for temperature measurement, 525
temperature-sensitive skin tape, 526
temporal artery thermometer, 526
tympanic, correct technique, 524
tympanic thermometer, 526
TENS unit, managing, 8–12
care setting, 9
developmental considerations, 9–10
heat and cold, effects of, 10
Tepid sponges, 17–18
Thermoregulation, of newborn, 397–398
actions to help maintain stable temperature, 397
Thoracentesis, 693–694
developmental considerations, 694
Thorax and lungs, assessing, 477–483
adventitious breath sounds, 483
developmental considerations, 481–482
normal breath sounds, 483
posterior thorax, 478–481
Tissue, 403–444, 404
ankle-brachial index (ABI), 422
dressings, 404–411, 422–426, 429–433
electrical stimulation, 434–435
Medieval remedies, 405
negative pressure wound therapy, 437–440
noncontact normothermic wound therapy,
435–436
pressure ulcer formation, 405
pressure ulcers, 426–429
stump positioning, 442
stump shrinking, 443–444
venous ulcer, 422–426
wounds, 404, 408–421, 432, 435–441, 440–441
Total enteral nutrition (TEN), 190

Total nutrient admixture (TNA), 215–217
  complications with, 217
  discontinuing infusion, 216–217
  monitoring client on TNA, 216
  nutritional assessment, 215
Tracheal tube cuff, inflating, 293
Tracheostomy care, 302–306
  capping tube, 306–307
  care setting, 305
  developmental considerations, 305
  disposal inner cannula, 305
  one-way speaking valve, 306
Tracheostomy tube suctioning, 298–301
  care setting, 301
  closed-suction system (in-line catheter), 301
  developmental considerations, 301
  hyperventilation, 300
Traction, 266–270
  Buck's, 267
  care setting, 270
  developmental considerations, 269
  lifting extremity with external fixator, 267
  pin site care, 267
  skin traction care, 266–267
  traction *vs.* no traction in hip fracture, 266
Transferring client, 234–239
  bed and chair, between, 234–237
  bed and stretcher, between, 237–238
Transfer sets, for CAPD, 106
Transporting infant, 258
Transporting toddler, 259
Tube feeding, 198–207, 198–212
  administering, 198–207
  care setting, 202
  client teaching considerations, 201
  continuous-drip feeding, 200–201
  developmental considerations, 201
  documentation for enteral, 206
  feeding bag (open system), 199
  gastrostomy feeding, open system, 203
  gastrostomy or jejunostomy, 202–204
  IV lipids, 209–212
  obese clients, 205
  pH method for placement, 206
  prefilled bottle (closed system), 200
  refeeding syndrome, 205
  small-bore nasointestinal/jejunostomy tube, 204–207
  syringe (open system), 199–200
  total parental, 208–209

**U**

Ulcer, 422–429
  arterial, 423
  moist wound dressings, 432
  nutritional assessment, 431
  pressure, 426–429
  pressure relief, 427
  pressure ulcer assessment guide, 430
  pressure ulcer formation, 427
  venous, 422–426
  warming therapy, 426
Umbilical cord clamp, 398
Universal protocol for wrong site, wrong procedure,
  and wrong person surgery, 177
Unlicensed assistive personnel (UAP), 33
Urinal, 34–36
Urinary tract
  bladder irrigation, maintaining, 57–58
  bladder irrigation, performing, 55–57
  catheter care and removal, 53–55
  catheterization, 46–53
  diversion pouch, applying, 62–64
  elimination, 32–64
  infection, 54
  ostomy care, 60–62
  suprapubic catheter care, 58–60
Urine specimen
  care setting, 40
  clean-catch method, 42–45
  closed drainage system, 44
  collecting, 39–40
  collecting 24-hour, 41–42
  collecting from infant, 41
  developmental considerations, 40
  from ileal conduit, 64
Urine tests, 45–46
Uterine fundus, 388–389

**V**

VAC® unit, 438, 439
Vaginal exam, 379–380
Vascular system, 122
Vein, selecting for IV, 126
Venipuncture, 126–133
  butterfly needle, 128, 132–133
  developmental considerations, 133
  IV administration set, 127
  IV catheter/needle, 127
  peripheral IV, 128
  vein selection, 126
Venous ulcer, 422–426. *See also* Ulcer
Ventilator, 307–312
Ventilator-related events, managing, 315
Vesicant, 147
Visual acuity, assessing, 555–557
  HOTV, Snellen E., or picture chart, 555–556
  passing standards based on age, 557
  Snellen letter chart, 555
Vital signs, assessing, 166, 446, 447

**W**

Walker, using, 257–258
  care setting, 258
  developmental considerations, 258
Waste, elimination of, 64–94
  fecal impaction, 65
Waste, elimination of
  Allen test, 108
  arterial blood pressure, monitoring, 109–110
  arterial blood samples, withdrawing, 111–112
  arterial catheter, removing, 112–114
  arterial line insertion, 108
  bacterial culture, collecting stool for, 72
  bowel diversion ostomy appliance, 89–94
  central venous dual-lumen dialysis catheter
    (DLC), 102–104
  enema, 78–80
  fecal ostomy pouch, applying, 82–88
  hemodialysis, 98–102
  hemodialysis, providing ongoing care, 100–101
  hemodialysis, terminating, 101–102
  home setting care, 104–108
  ova and parasites, collecting stool for, 73
  peritoneal dialysis catheter, 94–95
  peritoneal dialysis procedures, 96–98
  pinworm testing, 73
  rectal tube insertion, 67–69
  regular bowel routine, 66–67
  retention enema, 80–82
  stool specimen, collecting from infant, 72
  stool specimen, testing, 69–71
  Zassi bowel management system, 74–78
Waste material, disposal of, 184–185
Wound(s)
  abdominal binder application, 413
  alginate dressings, 414–415
  bandages and binders, 416–419
  care, client, 415
  cleaning, 408–410
  developmental considerations, 415
  with drain, 408–410
  drainage maintenance, 419–420
  drainage specimen, 420–422
  dressing, 410–412, 432–433
  in-home care of, 671
  irrigating, 412–413
  moist environment, 404
  negative pressure therapy, 437–439
  noncontact normothermic therapy, 435–436
  pressure relief, 404
  transparent barrier application, 440–441
  types of, 404

**Z**

Zassi bowel management system, 74–78
Zborowski, M., 2